Mosby's

2002-2003 Medical Drug Reference

Allan J. Ellsworth, Pharm.D.

Professor of Pharmacy and Family Medicine,
University of Washington Schools of Pharmacy and Medicine,
Seattle, Washington

Daniel M. Witt, Pharm.D.

Chief,
Clinical Pharmacy Anticoagulation Cardiac Risk Services,
Kaiser Permanente, Colorado Region,
Westminster, Colorado

David C. Dugdale, M.D.

Associate Professor of Medicine,
University of Washington School of Medicine,
Seattle, Washington

Lynn M. Oliver, M.D.

Assistant Professor of Family Medicine,
University of Washington School of Medicine,
Seattle, Washington

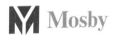 Mosby

An Affiliate of Elsevier Science

St. Louis   London   Philadelphia   Sydney   Toronto

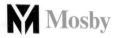
Mosby

An Affiliate of Elsevier Science

Editor: Steven Merahn
Publishing Services Manager: Linda McKinley
Senior Designer: Julia Dummitt
Cover Art: Adam Cohen

NOTICE

Pharmacology is an ever-changing field. Standard safety precautions must be followed, but as new research and clinical experience broaden our knowledge, changes in treatment and drug therapy may become necessary or appropriate. Readers are advised to check the most current product information provided by the manufacturer of each drug to be administered to verify the recommended dose, the method and duration of administration, and contraindications. It is the responsibility of the licensed prescriber, relying on experience and knowledge of the patient, to determine dosages and the best treatment for each individual patient. Neither the publisher nor the editor assumes any liability for any injury and/or damage to persons or property arising from this publication.

Mosby, Inc.
An Affiliate of Elsevier Science
11830 Westline Industrial Drive
St. Louis, Missouri 63146

Printed in the United States of America

ISBN 0-323-02219-7

00 01 02 03 04 GW/FF 9 8 7 6 5 4 3 2 1

Instructions for Use

Mosby's Medical Drug Reference was conceived in response to the demands of physicians and other healthcare providers who require an up-to-date, authoritative, comprehensive, portable drug prescribing reference for use at the point of care. This compact, easily accessible manual has been created in part from the renowned and objective drug database, *Mosby's GenRx*, which is updated quarterly to provide timely drug information for accurate and efficient prescribing. As a standard reference, *Mosby's GenRx* is indispensable in its print and CD-ROM formats; for those situations when the demands of patient care require a more portable drug prescribing guide, we proudly present *Mosby's 2002-2003 Medical Drug Reference*.

Mosby's 2002-2003 Medical Drug Reference is organized into several highly functional parts. The body of the book is a listing, by generic name, of nearly 900 drugs in common clinical use, representing over 2600 products. An appendix of the book contains tables of comparative drug data and other information useful for choosing drug therapy. The comprehensive index provides rapid reference by listing all generic and trade names; index searches are further aided by the colored index paper. The inside front and back covers contain formulas for calculating drug dosages and useful conversion information. The comprehensive Therapeutic Index, which allows prescribers to locate drugs appropriate for a broad range of clinical indications, has been updated for this edition.

Drug monographs in *Mosby's 2002-2003 Medical Drug Reference* are organized in a uniform fashion as follows (when there is no information in a category applicable to a given drug, the category has been deleted entirely):

Drug Name (generic)
Pronunciation (phonetic)
Trade Names
Chemical Class
Therapeutic Class
DEA Schedule (if applicable, see p. ix)
Clinical Pharmacology (including information about the mechanism of
    action and pharmacokinetics of the drug)
Indications and Uses (non–FDA-approved uses marked with *
    if applicable)
Dosage
Available Forms and Cost of Therapy (the range of average wholesale
    prices [AWPs] of generic brands are given)

Contraindications (if the only contraindication is hypersensitivity, this category has been deleted)

Precautions

Pregnancy and Lactation (see p. x)

Side Effects/Adverse Reactions (listed by organ system; *common side effects* [greater than 5% incidence] italicized, ***potentially life-threatening side effects*** bold and italicized)

Drug Interactions, if applicable. The clinical significance of each drug interaction is derived from data presented in Hansten PD, Horn JR: Drug interactions analysis and management. Interactions are classified by potential severity as: **A**—Avoid combination, risk always outweighs benefit; **❷**—Usually avoid combination, use combination only under special circumstances; or **❸**—Minimize risk, take action as necessary to reduce risk of adverse outcome as a result of drug interaction. Interactions of lesser significance, either because they are minor or poorly documented, are not included. If no drug interactions are known, or if the interactions are of minimal risk, this category has been deleted.

Lab Test Interactions (if applicable). Only laboratory interactions that are well documented and are analytical in nature are included. Changes in lab results that reflect the physiologic action of the drug or an adverse metabolic effect of the drug are not included. If no lab interactions are known, this category has been deleted.

Special Considerations (if applicable) such as patient education or monitoring or information about the place of the drug in therapy.

Every possible effort has been made to ensure the accuracy and currency of the information contained within *Mosby's 2002-2003 Medical Drug Reference*. However, drug information is constantly changing and is subject to interpretation. The authors, editors, or publishers cannot be responsible for information that has either changed or been erroneously published or for the consequences of such errors. Decisions regarding drug therapy for a specific patient must be based on the independent judgment of the clinician.

Allan J. Ellsworth
Daniel M. Witt
David C. Dugdale
Lynn M. Oliver

ACKNOWLEDGMENTS

We are grateful for the support, stimulus, and suggestions of our colleagues in the Departments of Family Medicine, Medicine, and Pharmacy, University of Washington, Seattle, Washington, and the Medical and Pharmacy Staff of Kaiser Permanente of Colorado, Denver, Colorado. As usual, to our families and friends, whose support, patience, love, and understanding allow many things to go undone during the completion of the project, we thank you all.

Abbreviations

ABG arterial blood gas
ac before meals
ACE angiotensin-converting enzyme
ACTH adrenocorticotropic hormone
AD right ear
ADH antidiuretic hormone
aer aerosol
AIDS acquired immunodeficiency syndrome
ALT alanine aminotransferase, serum
ANA antinuclear antibody
aPTT activated partial thromboplastin time
AS left ear
AST aspartate aminotransferase, serum
AU each ear
AUC area under curve
AV atrioventricular
bid twice a day
BP blood pressure
BUN blood urea nitrogen
c-AMP cyclic adenosine monophosphate
cap capsule
°C degrees Celsius (centigrade)
Ca calcium
CAD coronary artery disease
cath catheterize
cc cubic centimeter
CBC complete blood count
chew tab tablet, chewable
CHF congestive heart failure
Cl chloride
cm centimeter
CMV cytomegalovirus
CNS central nervous system
CO₂ carbon dioxide
COPD chronic obstructive pulmonary disease
CPAP continuous positive airway pressure

CPK creatine phosphokinase
CrCl creatinine clearance
cre cream
Creat creatinine
CSF cerebrospinal fluid
CV cardiovascular
CVA cerebrovascular accident
CVP central venous pressure
CXR chest x-ray
D5W 5% dextrose in water
DIC disseminated intravascular coagulation
dL deciliter
D_LCO diffusing capacity of carbon monoxide
DNA deoxyribonucleic acid
DUB dysfunctional uterine bleeding
ECG electrocardiogram
EDTA ethylenediaminetetraacetic acid
EEG electroencephalogram
EENT eye, ear, nose, throat
elix elixir
ESR erythrocyte sedimentation rate
ET via endotracheal tube
EXT REL extended release
°F degrees Fahrenheit
FEV₁ forced expiratory volume in 1 second
FSH follicle stimulating hormone
g gram
G6PD glucose-6-phosphate dehydrogenase
GGTP gamma glutamyl transpeptidase
GI gastrointestinal
gtt drop
GU genitourinary
H₂ histamine₂
Hct hematocrit

HCG	human chorionic gonadotropin	**Na**	sodium
HEME	hematologic	**neb**	nebulizer
Hgb	hemoglobin	**NPO**	nothing by mouth
5-HIAA	5-hydroxyindoleacetic acid	**NS**	normal saline
HIV	human immunodeficiency virus	**NSAID**	nonsteroidal antiinflammatory drug
H_2O	water	**O_2**	oxygen
HMG CoA	3-hydroxy-3-methylglutaryl coenzyme A	**OD**	right eye
		oint	ointment
HPA	hypothalamic-pituitary-adrenal	**OS**	left eye
hr	hour	**OTC**	over the counter
hs	at bedtime	**OU**	each eye
HSV	herpes simplex virus	**oz**	ounce
IgG	immunoglobulin G	**$PaCO_2$**	arterial partial pressure of carbon dioxide
IM	intramuscular	**PaO_2**	arterial partial pressure of oxygen
in	inch		
INF	infusion	**pc**	after meals
INH	inhalation	**PCWP**	pulmonary capillary wedge pressure
inj	injection		
INR	international normalized ratio	**P_i**	inorganic phosphorus
IO	intraosseous	**po**	by mouth
IPPB	intermittent positive pressure breathing	**PO_4**	phosphate
		pr	per rectum
IU	international units	**prn**	as needed
IV	intravenous	**PT**	prothrombin time
K	potassium	**PTH**	parathyroid hormone
kg	kilogram	**PTT**	partial thromboplastin time
L	liter	**PVC**	premature ventricular contraction
L-A	long acting		
lb	pound	**q**	every
LDH	lactate dehydrogenase	**qAM**	every morning
LDL	low density lipoprotein	**qd**	every day
LFTs	liver function tests	**qh**	every hour
LH	luteinizing hormone	**qid**	four times a day
liq	liquid	**qod**	every other day
LMP	last menstrual period	**qPM**	every night
loz	lozenge	**q2h**	every 2 hours
lyphl	lyophilized	**q3h**	every 3 hours
m	meter	**q4h**	every 4 hours
m^2	square meter	**q6h**	every 6 hours
MAOI	monoamine oxidase inhibitor	**q8h**	every 8 hours
μg	microgram	**q12h**	every 12 hours
MDI	metered dose inhaler	**RAIU**	radioactive iodine uptake
mEq	milliequivalent	**RBC**	red blood cell or count
mg	milligram	**RESP**	respiratory
Mg	magnesium	**RNA**	ribonucleic acid
MI	myocardial infarction	**sc**	subcutaneous
min	minute	**sl**	sublingual
ml (mL)	milliliter	**sol**	solution
mm	millimeter	**SO_4**	sulfate
mmol	millimole	**ss**	one half
mo	month	**supp**	suppository
MS	musculoskeletal		

sus rel	sustained release
susp	suspension
sust	sustained
syr	syrup
T$_3$	triiodothyronine
T$_4$	thyroxine
tab	tablet
tid	three times a day
tinc	tincture
top	topical
trans	transdermal
TSH	thyroid stimulating hormone
TT	thrombin time

U	unit
UA	urinalysis
URI	upper respiratory infection
UTI	urinary tract infection
UV	ultraviolet
vag	vaginal
VMA	vanillylmandelic acid
vol	volume
VS	vital signs
WBC	white blood cell or count
wk	week
yr	year

Federal Controlled Substances Act Schedules

SCHEDULE I: No accepted medical use in the United States and a high abuse potential. Examples include heroin, marijuana, LSD, peyote, mescaline, psilocybin, and methaqualone.

SCHEDULE II: High abuse potential with severe dependence liability. Examples include opium, morphine, codeine, fentanyl, hydromorphone, methadone, meperidine, oxycodone, oxymorphone, cocaine, amphetamine, methamphetamine, phenmetrazine, methylphenidate, phencyclidine, amobarbital, pentobarbital, and secobarbital.

SCHEDULE III: Lesser abuse potential with moderate dependence liability. Examples include compounds containing limited quantities of certain narcotic or nonnarcotic drugs, such as barbiturates, glutethimide, methyprylon, nalorphine, benzphetamine, chlorphentermine, clortermine, phendimetrazine, and paregoric; suppository dosage form containing amobarbital, secobarbital, or pentobarbital.

SCHEDULE IV: Low abuse potential. Examples include barbital, phenobarbital, mephobarbital, chloral hydrate, ethchlorvynol, ethinamate, meprobamate, paraldehyde, methohexital, fenfluramine, diethylpropion, phentermine, chlordiazepoxide, diazepam, oxazepam, clorazepate, flurazepam, clonazepam, prazepam, lorazepam, alprazolam, halazepam, temazepam, triazolam, mebutamate, dextropropoxyphene, and pentazocine.

SCHEDULE V: Low abuse potential. These products contain limited quantities of certain narcotic drugs generally for antitussive or antidiarrheal purposes.

FDA Pregnancy Categories

A: Adequate studies in pregnant women have not demonstrated a risk to the fetus in the first trimester of pregnancy, and there is no evidence of risk in later trimesters.

B: Animal studies have not demonstrated a risk to the fetus, but there are no adequate studies in pregnant women; OR animal studies have shown an adverse effect, but adequate studies in pregnant women have not demonstrated a risk to the fetus during the first trimester of pregnancy, and there is no evidence of risk in later trimesters.

C: Animal studies have shown an adverse effect on the fetus, but there are no adequate studies in humans; OR there are no animal reproduction studies and no adequate studies in humans.

D: There is evidence of human fetal risk, but the potential benefits from the use of the drug in pregnant women may be acceptable despite its potential risks.

X: Studies in animals or humans demonstrate fetal abnormalities or adverse reaction; reports indicate evidence of fetal risk. The risk of use in a pregnant woman clearly outweighs any possible benefit.

Contents

abacavir

(ah-bah´cah-veer)

Rx: Ziagen

Chemical Class: Nucleoside analog

Therapeutic Class: Antiretroviral

CLINICAL PHARMACOLOGY

Mechanism of Action: Converted intracellularly to carbovir then phosphorylated to carbovir triphosphate; carbovir triphosphate interferes with HIV reverse transcriptase thus inhibiting viral replication

Pharmacokinetics

PO: Peak 1 hr; oral bioavailability 83%; 50% protein bound; extensively metabolized by liver (primary routes are alcohol dehydrogenase and glucuronyl transferase; metabolism by cytochrome P450 enzymes is insignificant), inactive metabolites excreted in urine (1% excreted unchanged); $t_{1/2}$ 1.5 hr; crosses placenta, excreted in breast milk, CSF level 18-33% of plasma level

INDICATIONS AND USES: HIV infection

DOSAGE

Adult and Child >16 yr

• PO 300 mg bid

• For latest treatment guidelines, see www.hivatis.org

Child 3 months-16 yr

• PO 8 mg/kg (max 300 mg) bid

• For latest treatment guidelines, see www.hivatis.org

$ AVAILABLE FORMS/COST OF THERAPY

• Liq—Oral: 20 mg/ml, 240 ml: **$111.64**

• Tab—Oral: 300 mg, 60's: **$336.31**

CONTRAINDICATIONS: Hypersensitivity to carbovir

PRECAUTIONS: Use as monotherapy (rapid resistance develops), prior resistance to antiretroviral agents, pregnancy, hepatic insufficiency

PREGNANCY AND LACTATION: Pregnancy category C; breast feeding not recommended due to drug secretion and potential for HIV transmission

SIDE EFFECTS/ADVERSE REACTIONS

CNS: Dizziness (16%), headache (41%), insomnia (18%)

GI: Hepatic steatosis, *nausea (57%)*

METAB: **Lactic acidosis**

SKIN: Rash

MISC: **Hypersensitivity (fever, rash in 2-5%; rechallenge may be fatal)**

INTERACTIONS

Drugs

3 *Amprenavir:* Mild increase in amprenavir plasma level with co-administration

SPECIAL CONSIDERATIONS

PATIENT/FAMILY EDUCATION

• May administer without regard for food

• If you miss a dose: take the missed dose as soon as you remember, then go back to your normal dosing schedule; skip the missed dose if it is time for your next dose; do not take 2 doses at the same time

MONITORING PARAMETERS

• CBC, metabolic panel, CD4 lymphocyte count, HIV RNA level

---

italic = common side effects   ***bold italic*** = life-threatening reactions

abciximab

(ab-six′ih-mab)

Rx: ReoPro
Chemical Class: Glycoprotein (GP) IIb/IIIa inhibitor
Therapeutic Class: Antiplatelet agent

CLINICAL PHARMACOLOGY

Mechanism of Action: Reversibly prevents fibrinogen, von Willebrand's factor, and other adhesion ligands from binding to platelet GP IIb/IIIa receptors, thereby inhibiting platelet aggregation

Pharmacokinetics

Duration of action on platelets approximately 48 hr although abciximab remains in the circulation for up to 10 days in a platelet-bound state; initial $t_{1/2}$ <10 min, second phase $t_{1/2}$ 30 min

INDICATIONS AND USES: Adjunct to percutaneous transluminal coronary angioplasty (PCTA) for the prevention of acute cardiac ischemic complications in patients at high risk for abrupt closure of the treated coronary vessel; myocardial infarction in combination with fibrinolytic therapy*; unstable angina refractory*; acute ischemic stroke*

DOSAGE

Adult

• *Adjunct to PCTA:* IV 0.25 mg/kg bolus 10-60 min prior to start of PCTA, followed by a continuous INF of 10 µg/min for 12 hr

• *Refractory unstable angina:* IV 0.25 mg/kg bolus followed by 10 µg/min IV infusion × 18-24 hr (w/heparin and ASA if tolerated)

$ **AVAILABLE FORMS/COST OF THERAPY**

• Inj, Sol—IV: 2 mg/ml, 4 ml: **$562.50**

CONTRAINDICATIONS: Active internal bleeding; recent (within 6 wk) GI or GU bleeding of clinical significance; history of CVA within 2 yr or CVA with a significant residual neurological deficit; bleeding diathesis; administration of oral anticoagulants within 7 days unless prothrombin time is <1.2 × control; thrombocytopenia (<100,000 cells/µl); recent (within 6 wk) major surgery or trauma; intracranial neoplasm, arteriovenous malformation or aneurysm; severe uncontrolled hypertension; presumed or documented history of vasculitis; use of IV dextran before PCTA or intent to use it during PCTA; hypersensitivity to murine proteins

PRECAUTIONS: Elderly, children, weight <75 kg, prior thrombolytic therapy, history of GI disease; IM injections, urinary catheters, nasotracheal intubation, nasogastric tubes

PREGNANCY AND LACTATION: Pregnancy category C; excretion into breast milk unknown, use caution in nursing mothers

SIDE EFFECTS/ADVERSE REACTIONS

CNS: Hypesthesia, confusion
CV: Hypotension, bradycardia, ***bleeding*** (major bleeding 11.1%-14%)
EENT: Abnormal vision
GI: Nausea, vomiting
HEME: Anemia, leukocytosis, ***thrombocytopenia***
RESP: Pleural effusion, pneumonia
MISC: Pain, peripheral edema, human anti-chimeric antibody development, ***anaphylaxis***

INTERACTIONS

Drugs

3 *Antithrombotics (aspirin, heparin, warfarin, ticlopidine, clopidogrel):* Increased risk of bleeding

---

* = non-FDA-approved use

SPECIAL CONSIDERATIONS
PATIENT/FAMILY EDUCATION

• Fab fragment of the chimeric human-murine monoclonal antibody 7E3

• Intended to be used with aspirin and heparin

• In the event of serious bleeding that cannot be controlled by compression, discontinue abciximab and heparin

• In patients with failed PCTAs, stop INF

• Eptifibitide, tirofiban, and abciximab can all decrease the incidence of cardiac events associated with acute coronary syndromes; direct comparisons are needed to establish which, if any, is superior; for angioplasty, until more data become available, abciximab appears to be the drug of choice

MONITORING PARAMETERS

• Baseline platelet count, prothrombin time, aPTT; during INF closely monitor platelet count and aPTT (heparin therapy)

---

acarbose

(a-car'bose)

Rx: Precose

Chemical Class: α-amylase/α-glucosidase inhibitor

Therapeutic Class: Antidiabetic

CLINICAL PHARMACOLOGY

Mechanism of Action: Inhibits intestinal α-glucosidase, the enzyme responsible for digesting complex starches to oligosaccharides; delays postprandial absorption of glucose; attenuates postprandial plasma glucose peaks; does not increase insulin secretion

Pharmacokinetics

PO: Minimally absorbed in unchanged form; 35% of dose is absorbed as metabolites; biotransformation by intestinal microorganisms; metabolites excreted by urinary and fecal routes; $t_{1/2}$ 2.7-9 hr

INDICATIONS AND USES: Diabetes mellitus, type 1 and 2: adjunctive therapy in those insufficiently managed with other antidiabetic agents

DOSAGE

Adult

• PO 25 mg tid, taken at beginning of each meal; increase after 6-8 wk to 50-100 mg tid

$ AVAILABLE FORMS/COST OF THERAPY

• Tab—Oral: 25 mg, 100's: **$59.94**; 50 mg, 100's: **$59.94**; 100 mg, 100's: **$70.02**

CONTRAINDICATIONS: Inflammatory bowel disease, colonic ulceration, partial intestinal obstruction, chronic intestinal disease associated with marked disorders of absorption or digestion, cirrhosis

PREGNANCY AND LACTATION: Pregnancy category B; excreted into breast milk in rats; no human data available

SIDE EFFECTS/ADVERSE REACTIONS

GI: Abdominal distension, borborygmus, diarrhea, elevated transaminases (15%), flatulence (70%)

METAB: Potential for hypoglycemia only with insulin or sulfonylureas

INTERACTIONS

Drugs

3 *Charcoal, digestive enzyme preparations:* Reduced effects of acarbose

3 *Cholestyramine:* Enhanced side effects of acarbose

3 *Neomycin:* Enhanced reduction of postprandial blood glucose and exacerbation of adverse effects

---

italic = common side effects　　　　**bold italic** = life-threatening reactions

3 *Metformin:* Decreased metformin peak serum and AUC concentrations

SPECIAL CONSIDERATIONS
• Does not cause hypoglycemia
• Reduces HbA1c 0.5-1%

MONITORING PARAMETERS
• Self-monitored blood glucose; glucose, HbA1c 3-6 mo
• Consider ALT/AST during first yr

PATIENT/FAMILY EDUCATION
• Take glucose rather than complex carbohydrates to abort hypoglycemic episodes
• Decrease adverse GI effects by reducing dietary starch content

---

acebutolol
(a-se-byoo'-toe-lole)
Rx: Sectral
Chemical Class: β_1-selective (cardioselective) adrenoreceptor blocker
Therapeutic Class: Antihypertensive; antianginal

CLINICAL PHARMACOLOGY
Mechanism of Action: Competitive beta-adrenergic antagonist at β_1-receptor sites (cardioselective at usual doses; β_2-receptor blockade noted at higher doses); produces negative inotropic and chronotropic responses; slows AV nodal conduction; decreases heart rate; decreases myocardial oxygen consumption; antiarrhythmic effects (class II); reduction in platelet aggregation and blood viscosity; suppression of renin release; inhibition of central sympathetic outflow; decreases presynaptic receptor neurotransmitter release; no intrinsic sympathomimetic or membrane stabilizing activity; low lipid solubility

*= non-FDA-approved use

Pharmacokinetics
PO: Incomplete GI absorption (40%-60% bioavailable); peak serum concentrations, 2-4 hr; not metabolized by liver; excreted unchanged in urine and feces; $t_{1/2}$ 6-7 hr; crosses placenta in measurable, but not significant concentrations

INDICATIONS AND USES: Angina pectoris,* anxiety,* performance anxiety,* arrhythmia (class II), congestive heart failure,* hypertension, migraine headache,* post myocardial infarction,* alcohol withdrawal syndrome,* esophageal varices with cirrhosis*

DOSAGE
Adult
• *Hypertension:* PO 400 mg qd or in 2 divided doses; increase to desired response; usual range 400-800 mg/day
• *Ventricular premature beats:* PO 200 mg bid, may increase gradually; usual range 600-1200 mg daily

$ AVAILABLE FORMS/COST OF THERAPY
• Cap, Gel—Oral: 200 mg, 100's: **$74.88-$134.60**; 400 mg, 100's: **$99.56-$178.96**

CONTRAINDICATIONS: Cardiogenic shock, heart block (2nd, 3rd degree), sinus bradycardia

PRECAUTIONS: Anesthesia/surgery (myocardial depression), avoid abrupt withdrawal, bronchospastic airways, congestive heart failure, diabetes mellitus, hyperthyroidism/thyrotoxicosis (acebutolol, unlike propranolol does not decrease T_3 levels), concurrent clonidine (discontinue acebutolol several days prior to withdrawal of clonidine), peripheral vascular disease, renal disease

PREGNANCY AND LACTATION: Pregnancy category D; frequently used in the third trimester for treatment of hypertension (many studies of efficacy and safety of atenolol in pregnancy induced hypertension); long-term use has been associated with intrauterine growth retardation; excreted into breast milk; observe for signs of beta-blockade

SIDE EFFECTS/ADVERSE REACTIONS

CNS: Catatonia, depression, *dizziness,* drowsiness, *fatigue,* hallucinations, *headache,* insomnia, lethargy, memory loss, strange dreams

CV: Bradycardia, **CHF,** cold extremities, postural hypotension, **2nd or 3rd degree heart block, shock**

EENT: Dry burning eyes, sore throat

GI: Diarrhea, elevated transaminases, **ischemic colitis, mesenteric arterial thrombosis,** nausea, vomiting

GU: Impotence

HEME: **Agranulocytosis,** positive ANA, **purpura, thrombocytopenia**

METAB: Hyperglycemia, decreased hypoglycemic response to insulin

RESP: **Bronchospasm,** dyspnea, wheezing

SKIN: Alopecia, fever, rash

INTERACTIONS

Drugs

3 *Alpha-1 adrenergic blockers:* Potential enhanced first dose response (marked initial drop in blood pressure, particularly on standing [especially prazocin])

3 *Amiodarone:* Bradycardia/ventricular dysrhythmia

3 *Anesthetics, local:* Enhanced sympathomimetic effects, hypertension due to unopposed α-receptor stimulation

3 *Antacids:* May reduce β-blocker absorption

3 *Antidiabetics:* Delayed recovery from hypoglycemia, hyperglycemia, attenuated tachycardia during hypoglycemia, hypertension during hypoglycemia

3 *Digoxin:* Additive prolongation of atrioventricular (AV) conduction time

3 *Dihydropyridine calcium channel blockers:* Severe hypotension or impaired cardiac performance; most prevalent with impaired left ventricular function, cardiac arrhythmias, or aortic stenosis

3 *Diltiazem:* Severe hypotension or impaired cardiac performance; most prevalent with impaired left ventricular function, cardiac arrhythmias, or aortic stenosis

3 *Dipyridamole:* Bradycardia

3 *Disopyramide:* Additive decreases in cardiac output

3 *Epinephrine:* Enhanced pressor response resulting in hypertension

3 *Neostigmine:* Bradycardia

3 *Neuroleptics:* Increased serum levels of both resulting in accentuated pharmacologic response to both drugs

3 *NSAIDs:* Reduced hypotensive effects

3 *Phenylephrine:* Acute hypertensive episodes

3 *Prazosin:* First-dose hypotensive response enhanced

3 *Tacrine:* Additive bradycardia

2 *Theophylline:* Antagonist pharmacodynamics

3 *Verapamil:* Severe hypotension or impaired cardiac performance; most prevalent with impaired left ventricular function, cardiac arrhythmias, or aortic stenosis

SPECIAL CONSIDERATIONS

• Properties of low lipid solubility and competitive cardioselectivity yields less CNS and bronchospastic adverse effects

MONITORING PARAMETERS

• Angina: Reduction in nitroglycerin usage; frequency, severity, onset, and duration of angina pain; heart rate

• Arrhythmias: Heart rate

• Congestive heart failure: Functional status, cough, dyspnea on exertion, paroxysmal nocturnal dyspnea, exercise tolerance, and ventricular function
• Hypertension: Blood pressure
• Migraine headache: Reduction in the frequency, severity, and duration of attacks
• Postmyocardial infarction: Left ventricular function, lower resting heart rate
• Toxicity: Blood glucose, bronchospasm, hypotension, bradycardia, depression, confusion, hallucination, sexual dysfunction

PATIENT/FAMILY EDUCATION
• Do not discontinue abruptly; may require taper; rapid withdrawal may produce rebound hypertension or angina

---

acetaminophen
(ah-seet′ah-min-oh-fen)
OTC: Acephen, Apacet, Arthritis Pain Formula, Aspirin Free Pain Relief, Feverall, Genapap, Liquiprin, Neopap, Panadol, Tapanol Tempra, Tylenol

Combinations

Rx: with butalbital (Phrenilin); with butalbital and caffeine (Fioricet, Esgic, Isocet); with butalbital, caffeine and codeine (Amaphen, Fioricet w/codeine); with codeine (Tylenol, Phenaphen No. 2,3,4); with dichloralphenazone and isometheptene (Midrin, Midchlor); with hydrocodone (Vicodin, Lorcet, Lortab); with oxycodone (Percocet, Roxicet, Tylox); with pentazocine (Talacen); with propoxyphene (Wygesic, Darvocet-N)

OTC: with pamabrom + pyrilamine (Midol PMS, Pamprin); with antihistamine and decongestant (Actifed Plus, Drixoral Cold & Flu, Benadryl Sinus, Sine-Off, Sinarest); with decongestant, antihistamine, dextromethorphan (Nyquil)

Chemical Class: Nonsalicylate, para-aminophenol derivative
Therapeutic Class: Nonnarcotic analgesic; antipyretic

CLINICAL PHARMACOLOGY
Mechanism of Action: Potent inhibitor of cyclo-oxygenase in the CNS; analgesic and antipyretic

properties; no antiinflammatory properties

Pharmacokinetics

PO: Onset 10-30 min, peak ½-2 hr, duration 3-4 hr; 60%-70% bioavailable

PR: Onset slow, peak 1-2 hr, duration 3-4 hr; 30%-40% bioavailable; widely distributed; $t_{\frac{1}{2}}$ 3-4 hr; 85%-90% metabolized by liver, excreted by kidneys

INDICATIONS AND USES: Analgesia, antipyresis; arthritic and rheumatic conditions involving musculoskeletal pain; diseases accompanied by discomfort and fever (i.e., common cold, flu, and other bacterial and viral infections); headache, dysmenorrhea, toothaches, vaccine reaction prophylaxis

DOSAGE

Adult and Child >14 yr

• PO 325-1000 mg q4h prn, not to exceed 4 g/day; PR 325-1000 mg q4h prn, not to exceed 4 g/day

Child

• 10-15 mg/kg q4h, not to exceed 5 doses/24h

$ AVAILABLE FORMS/COST OF THERAPY

• Cap—Oral: 500 mg, 100's: **$1.50-$6.99**; 650 mg, 24's: **$3.12**
• Drops—Oral: 80 mg/0.8 ml, 15 ml: **$1.25-$5.99**
• Elixir—Oral: 160 mg/5 ml, 120 ml: **$1.21-$5.79**; 500 mg/15 ml, 240 ml: **$2.42-$13.44**
• Supp—Rect: 80 mg, 6's: **$4.56**; 120 mg, 12's: **$3.20-$9.30**; 325 mg, 12's: **$5.06-$9.48**; 650 mg, 12's: **$4.29-$11.60**
• Tab—Oral: 325 mg, 100's: **$0.70-$10.88**; 500 mg, 100's: **$1.05-$22.44**; 650 mg, 100's: **$7.12**
• Tab, Chewable—Oral: 80 mg, 30's: **$0.84-$3.69**; 160 mg, 24's: **$1.12-$4.10**

PRECAUTIONS: Hepatic disease, renal disease, chronic alcoholism (≥ 3 drinks/day), elderly

PREGNANCY AND LACTATION: Pregnancy category B; low concentrations in breast milk (1%-2% of maternal dose); compatible with breast feeding

SIDE EFFECTS/ADVERSE REACTIONS

HEME: Hemolytic anemia (long-term use), leukopenia, neutropenia, pancytopenia, thrombocytopenia

MISC: Overdosage: ***acute hepatic and renal failure,*** confusion, ***delirium followed by vascular collapse, convulsions, coma, death,*** drowsiness, jaundice, nausea, vomiting

SKIN: ***Angioedema,*** rash, urticaria

INTERACTIONS

Drugs

❸ *Anticoagulants:* Enhanced hypoprothrombinemic response
❸ *Anticonvulsants, Barbiturates, Rifabutin, Rifampin:* Enhanced hepatoxic potential in overdose
❸ *Cholestyramine/Colestipol:* Reduced acetaminophen levels and response
❸ *Ethanol:* Increased hepatoxicity in chronic, excessive alcohol ingestion
❸ *Isoniazid:* Increased acetaminophen levels & hepatoxicity

Overdosage

• Specific antidote is acetylcysteine; administer as serum level of acetaminophen indicates high risk of hepatotoxicity. Minimal toxic dose 10g (140 mg/kg), can occur with less, ≥ 20-25g potentially fatal

Labs

• *False decrease:* Amylase
• *False increase:* Urine 5-HIAA
• *Interference:* Cannot assay ticarillin levels

---

italic = common side effects　　　**bold italic** = life-threatening reactions

SPECIAL CONSIDERATIONS
PATIENT/FAMILY EDUCATION
• Many OTC drugs contain acetaminophen; additive dosage may exceed 4 g/day maximum and increase risk of hepatotoxicity

---

acetazolamide
(a-set-a-zole′a-mide)
Rx: AK-Zol, Diamox, Storzolamide
Chemical Class: Sulfonamide derivative; carbonic anhydrase inhibitor
Therapeutic Class: Diuretic, anticonvulsant; antiglaucoma agent; acute mountain sickness

---

CLINICAL PHARMACOLOGY
Mechanism of Action: Kidney: increased excretion of sodium, potassium, bicarbonate, and water—alkaline diuresis; *CNS:* reduction in rate of aqueous humor formation—decreased intraocular pressure (IOP); *Resp:* resultant metabolic acidosis yields compensatory enhanced ventilatory oxygenation at high altitude
Pharmacokinetics
PO: Onset 1-1½ hr, peak 2-4 hr, duration 6-12 hr
PO-SUS REL: Onset 2 hr, peak 8-12 hr, duration 18-24 hr
IV: Onset 2 min, peak 15 min, duration 4-5 hr
65% absorbed if fasting (oral), 75% absorbed if given with food; $t_{1/2}$ 2½-5½ hr; excreted unchanged by kidneys (80% within 24 hr); crosses placenta
INDICATIONS AND USES: Open-angle glaucoma, narrow-angle glaucoma (preoperatively, if surgery delayed), epilepsy (petit mal, grand mal, mixed), edema in CHF, drug-induced edema, acute mountain sickness (prevention and treatment)
DOSAGE
Adult
• *Narrow-angle glaucoma:* PO/IV 250 mg q4h or 250 mg bid, to be used for short-term therapy
• *Open-angle glaucoma:* PO/IV 250-1000 mg/day in divided doses for amounts over 250 mg
• *Seizures:* PO/IV 8-30 mg/kg/day, usual range 375-1000 mg/day
• *Mountain sickness:* Treatment: PO 250 mg q8-12h; Prophylaxis: PO 125 mg bid; Periodic breathing at altitude: PO 62.5-125 mg with dinner or hs
Child
• *Seizures:* PO/IV 8-30 mg/kg/day in divided doses tid or qid, or 300-900 mg/m^2/day, not to exceed 1.5 g/day
Ⓢ AVAILABLE FORMS/COST OF THERAPY
• Cap, Gel, Sus Action—Oral: 500 mg, 100's: **$120.36**
• Inj, Powder—IV: 500 mg, 1 vial: **$19.86-$41.63**
• Tab, Uncoated—Oral: 125 mg, 100's: **$9.05-$39.21**; 250 mg, 100's: **$4.00-$51.48**
CONTRAINDICATIONS: Hypersensitivity to sulfonamides, severe renal disease, severe hepatic disease, electrolyte imbalances (hyponatremia, hypokalemia), hyperchloremic acidosis, Addison's disease, long-term use in narrow-angle glaucoma
PRECAUTIONS: Hypercalciuria
PREGNANCY AND LACTATION: Pregnancy category C; premature delivery and congenital anomalies in humans; teratogenic (defects of the limbs) in mice, rats, hamsters, and rabbits; not recommended for nursing mothers

---

* = non-FDA-approved use

SIDE EFFECTS/ADVERSE REACTIONS

CNS: Anxiety, confusion, depression, dizziness, drowsiness, fatigue, headache, nervousness, paresthesia, sedation, **seizures,** stimulation
EENT: Myopia, tinnitus
GI: Anorexia, constipation, diarrhea, **hepatic insufficiency,** melena, *nausea,* taste alterations, *vomiting,* weight loss
GU: Crystalluria, glucosuria, *hypokalemia,* polyuria, renal calculi, **uremia**
HEME: **Agranulocytosis, aplastic anemia, hemolytic anemia, leukopenia, pancytopenia, purpura, thrombocytopenia**
METAB: Hyperglycemia
SKIN: Fever, photosensitivity, pruritus, *rash,* **Stevens-Johnson syndrome,** urticaria
MISC: Loss of taste of carbonated beverages

INTERACTIONS

Drugs
3 *Cyclosporine:* Increased trough cyclosporine levels with potential for neurotoxicity and nephropathy
3 *Flecainide, quinidine:* Alkalinization of urine increases quinidine serum levels
3 *Methenamine compounds:* Alkalinization of urine decreases antibacterial effects
3 *Phenytoin:* Increased risk of osteomalacia
3 *Primidone:* Decreased primidone levels
2 *Salicylates:* Increased serum levels of acetazolamide—CNS toxicity
Labs
• *False increase:* 17 hydroxysteroid

SPECIAL CONSIDERATIONS
PATIENT/FAMILY EDUCATION

• Carbonated beverages taste flat
• If GI symptoms occur, take with food

MONITORING PARAMETERS

• Intraocular pressure, reduction in AMS symptoms, serum electrolytes, creatinine, CO_2

acetic acid

(a-cee´tic)
Rx: Acetasol, Burow's Otic, VoSol
Combinations
  Rx: with hydrocortisone (VoSol HC Otic, AA HC Otic, Acetasol HC) with oxyquinolone (Aci-Jel)
Chemical Class: Organic acid
Therapeutic Class: Antibacterial, antifungal

CLINICAL PHARMACOLOGY

Mechanism of Action: Bacteriostatic, fungistatic; penetrates bacterial cells, disrupts cell membrane; restores normal vaginal acidity
INDICATIONS AND USES: Prophylactically in surgical dressings, burns; bladder/urinary catheter irrigant; therapeutically for otitis externa (particularly *Pseudomonas* sp., *Candida* sp., and *Aspergillus* sp.) and to maintain vaginal acidity in vaginitis

DOSAGE

Adult
• *Otitis externa:* Instill 4-5 drops to affected ear tid
• *Urinary bladder catheter irrigant:* 30-50 ml flush
• *Vaginitis:* 1 applicatorful intravaginally bid
Child
• *Otitis externa:* Instill 3-4 drops to affected ear tid

$ AVAILABLE FORMS/COST OF THERAPY

• Gel—Vaginal: 0.92%, 85 g: **$28.20**

• Otic drops: 2%, 15 ml: **$2.10-$31.00**
• Sol, Bladder Irrigation: 0.25%, 1000 ml: **$2.61-$2.90**

PREGNANCY AND LACTATION: Pregnancy category C when combined with oxyquinoline

SIDE EFFECTS/ADVERSE REACTIONS

EENT: Burning on instillation, irritation

GU: Irritation, local burning and stinging

---

acetohydroxamic acid

(a-set'oh-hye-drox-am'ic)

Rx: Lithostat

Chemical Class: Hydroxylamine, ethyl acetate compound
Therapeutic Class: Urinary tract product

CLINICAL PHARMACOLOGY

Mechanism of Action: Inhibits bacterial enzyme urease, which decreases conversion of urea to ammonia; the reduced ammonia levels and decreased pH increase the effectiveness of concurrent urinary antimicrobial agents

Pharmacokinetics

PO: Peak 15-60 min, $t_{1/2}$ 3½-10 hr; hepatic metabolism, excreted in urine as unchanged drug (15%-60%)

INDICATIONS AND USES: Adjunctive treatment in chronic urinary tract infections due to urea-splitting organisms

DOSAGE

Adult

• PO 250 mg q6-8h when stomach is empty, not to exceed 1.5 g/day

Child

• PO 10 mg/kg/day in 2-3 divided doses

⬛ AVAILABLE FORMS/COST OF THERAPY

• Tab—Oral: 250 mg, 100's: **$103.13**

CONTRAINDICATIONS: Severe renal disease, infection by nonurease-producing organisms

PRECAUTIONS: Deep vein thrombosis, hepatic disease, renal disease, lactation

PREGNANCY AND LACTATION: Pregnancy category X; teratogenic (retarded and clubbed rear leg at 750 mg/kg and above and exencephaly and encephalocele at 1500 mg/kg) when given intraperitoneally to rats

SIDE EFFECTS/ADVERSE REACTIONS

CNS: Anxiety, depression, headache, malaise, nervousness, restlessness

CV: Deep vein thrombosis, palpitations, phlebitis, pulmonary embolism

GI: Anorexia, nausea, vomiting

HEME: **Hemolytic anemia (Coombs' negative; 15%)**

SKIN: Alopecia, rash on face, arms

SPECIAL CONSIDERATIONS
PATIENT/FAMILY EDUCATION

• Avoid alcohol: Promotes skin rash
• Concurrent contraception recommended during treatment

---

acetylcysteine

(a-see-til-sis´tay-een)
Rx: Mucomyst, Mucosil
Chemical Class: Amino acid,
L-cysteine
Therapeutic Class: Mucolytic;
acetaminophen antidote

CLINICAL PHARMACOLOGY
Mechanism of Action: Decreases
viscosity of secretions by breaking
disulfide links of mucoproteins; increases hepatic glutathione, which
is necessary to inactivate toxic metabolites in acetaminophen overdose
Pharmacokinetics
NEB/INSTILL: Onset 1 min, duration
5-10 min
PO: Peak levels within 1-2 hr (0.35-4
mg/L); 50% protein binding; terminal t$_{1/2}$ 6.25 hr; metabolized by liver,
excreted in urine
INDICATIONS AND USES: Antidote
for acetaminophen overdose; mucolytic: adjuvant therapy for abnormal, viscid, or inspissated mucus secretions in chronic bronchopulmo-
nary disease; diagnostic bronchial
scans (bronchograms, bronchos-
pirometry, bronchial wedge catheterization); keratoconjunctivitis
sicca* (as ophthalmic solution);
bowel obstruction due to meconium
ileus* (as an enema)
DOSAGE
Adult and Child
• *Mucolytic:* Instill 1-2 ml
(10%-20% sol) q1-4h prn; neb 3-5
ml (20% sol) or 6-10 ml (10% sol)
tid
• *Acetaminophen toxicity:* PO 140
mg/kg, then 70 mg/kg q4h × 17
doses to total of 1330 mg/kg; (dilute
20% solution to concentration of
5%; dilutions should be freshly prepared and utilized within 1 hr)

💲 AVAILABLE FORMS/COST OF THERAPY
• Sol, INH—Oral: 10%, 4 ml, 10 ml,
30 ml: **$1.68-$5.31**/4 ml
• Sol, INH—Oral: 20%, 4 ml, 10 ml,
30 ml: **$2.25-$6.56**/4 ml
PRECAUTIONS: Asthma, hepatic
disease, renal disease, COPD, alco-
holism
PREGNANCY AND LACTATION:
Pregnancy category B
SIDE EFFECTS/ADVERSE REAC-TIONS
CNS: Chills, dizziness, drowsiness,
fever, headache
EENT: Rhinorrhea
GI: Anorexia, nausea, stomatitis,
vomiting
RESP: Bronchospasm, chest tight-
ness
SKIN: Clamminess, fever, rash, urti-
caria
INTERACTIONS
• Avoid contact with iron, copper,
rubber
SPECIAL CONSIDERATIONS
• Disagreeable odor may be noted
• Solution in opened bottle may
change color; of no significance

acitretin

(a-si-tre´tin)
Rx: Soriatane
Chemical Class: Retinoid
Therapeutic Class: Antipsori-
atic agent

CLINICAL PHARMACOLOGY
Mechanism of Action: Unknown;
accelerated reappearance of stratum
corneum and inhibition of neutrophil migration from dermal capillar-
ies are among proposed mechanisms

Pharmacokinetics
PO: Peak serum level 3-4 hr; bioavailability enhanced by food; 99% protein bound, not stored in adipose tissue; metabolized by liver to active metabolites, excreted equally in bile and urine; $t_{1/2}$ 50-100 hr

INDICATIONS AND USES: Psoriasis, cutaneous lupus erythematosus*; Darier's disease*; lichen planus*; lichen sclerosis et atrophicus*; X-linked ichthyosis*

DOSAGE
Adult
• *Psoriasis:* PO 25-50 mg qd with food
• *Nonpsoriatic dermatoses:* PO 25-50 mg qd with food
Child
• *Psoriasis:* PO 1 mg/kg qd with food
• *Nonpsoriatic dermatoses:* PO 1 mg/kg qd with food

💲 **AVAILABLE FORMS/COST OF THERAPY**
• Cap—Oral: 10 mg, 30's: **$266.98**; 25 mg, 30's: **$351.24**

CONTRAINDICATIONS: Pregnancy, alcohol, concurrent use of vitamin A preparations

PRECAUTIONS: Women of childbearing age should use contraception during therapy and for 3 yr after therapy; renal insufficiency, liver disease, hyperlipidemia, pancreatitis, excessive exposure to sun or sun lamps

PREGNANCY AND LACTATION: Pregnancy category X; breast milk excretion unknown

SIDE EFFECTS/ADVERSE REACTIONS
CNS: Dizziness, dysesthesia, fatigue, headache, pseudotumor cerebri
EENT: Cheilitis (80%), conjunctivitis (40%), decreased night vision, dry eyes (40%), dry nose (50%), epistaxis, stomatitis (6%), xerostomia (50%)

GI: Increased transaminase levels (16%), nausea
HEME: Thrombocytosis
METAB: Hypertriglyceridemia, hyperglycemia
MS: Arthralgia, hyperostosis, *myalgia*
SKIN: Alopecia, dry skin (70%), nail fragility, pruritus, rash
MISC: Chills, diaphoresis (25%)

INTERACTIONS
Drugs
❷ *Methotrexate:* Increased potential for hepatotoxicity
❷ *Ethanol:* Drastically increases the $t_{1/2}$ of acitretin metabolite, etretinate
❷ *Progestin only contraceptives:* Decreased contraceptive effects

SPECIAL CONSIDERATIONS
PATIENT/FAMILY EDUCATION
• Avoid progestin only contraceptives
MONITORING PARAMETERS
• Transaminase levels monthly for first 6 mo then every 3 mo
• Lipid levels monthly for first 4 mo then every 2-3 mo
• Yearly radiographs to monitor for drug-induced vertebral abnormalities
• In children, measure PO_4, Ca levels in blood and urine and vitamin D and PTH levels every 6 mo

---

acyclovir
(ay-sye'kloe-ver)
Rx: Zovirax
Chemical Class: Acyclic purine nucleoside analog
Therapeutic Class: Antiviral

CLINICAL PHARMACOLOGY
Mechanism of Action: Interferes with DNA synthesis by conversion to acyclovir triphosphate, causing decreased viral DNA replication
Pharmacokinetics
IV: Onset unknown, peak 1 hr

---

* = non-FDA-approved use

PO: Onset unknown, peak 1½-2 hr, bioavailability 10%-20%; $t_{1/2}$ 3½ hr; distributed widely, CSF concentrations are 50% of plasma, crosses placenta; metabolized by liver, excreted by kidneys as unchanged drug (95%)

INDICATIONS AND USES: *PARENTERAL:* Initial and recurrent mucosal and cutaneous HSV-1, HSV-2, herpes zoster in immunocompromised patients; HSV encephalitis in patients >6 months; severe initial clinical episodes of genital herpes in patients who are not immunocompromised

Oral: Initial and recurrent genital herpes, acute treatment of herpes zoster and chicken pox; CMV and HSV following bone marrow or renal transplant*; disseminated primary eczema herpeticum*; herpes simplex—associated with erythema multiforme*; herpes simplex—labialis, ocular infections, proctitis, whitlow*; herpes zoster encephalitis*; infectious mononucleosis*; varicella*; pneumonia*

Top: Initial herpes genitalis and limited non-life-threatening mucocutaneous herpes simplex in immunocompromised patients

DOSAGE

Adult

• *Herpes simplex:* IV 500 mg/m² over 1 hr q8h × 5 days

• *Genital herpes:* PO 200 mg q4h 5 × /day while awake for 10 days

• *Genital herpes, intermittent therapy:* 200 mg q4h 5x/day while awake for 5 days

• *Genital herpes, suppressive therapy:* 400 mg bid × 12 mos, then reevaluate need off drug; alternate regimens: 200 mg tid to 200 mg 5 × /day

• *Herpes simplex encephalitis:* IV 10 mg/kg over 1 hr q8h × 10 days

• *Herpes zoster:* PO 800 mg q4h 5 × /day × 7-10 days; IV 500 mg/m² over 1 hr q8h

• *Chicken pox:* PO adults and children >40 kg: 800 mg qid for 5 days at the earliest sign or symptom. With immunosuppression IV 10 mg/kg over 1 h q8h × 10 days

• *Renal failure:* IV CrCl 25-50 ml/min/1.73 m²: give dose q12h; CrCl 10-25: give dose q24h; CrCl 0-10: reduce dose 50%, give q24h

• *Renal failure:* PO CrCl <10 ml/min/1.73 m²: give dose q12h

Child

• *Herpes simplex:* IV 250 mg/m² over 1 hr q8h × 5 days

• *Herpes simplex encephalitis:* Child >6 mo: IV 500 mg/m² q8h × 10 days; child >2 yr with immunosuppression: 20 mg/kg qid × 5 days

• *Chicken pox:* 2 yr and older: 20 mg/kg per dose qid (80 mg/kg/day), 5 days

$ AVAILABLE FORMS/COST OF THERAPY

• Cap, Gel—Oral: 200 mg, 100's: **$92.25-$145.78**

• Inj, Powder—IV: 500 mg: **$10.00-$65.00**

• Oint—Top: 5%, 3 g, 15 g: **$20.69-$25.62**/3 g

• Susp—Oral: 200 mg/5 ml, 480 ml: **$100.19-$126.81**

• Tab, Uncoated—Oral: 400 mg, 100's: **$179.05**; 800 mg, 100's: **$348.20-$550.05**

PRECAUTIONS: Hepatic disease, renal disease, electrolyte imbalance, dehydration

PREGNANCY AND LACTATION: Pregnancy category B; excreted into breast milk; compatible with breast feeding

SIDE EFFECTS/ADVERSE REACTIONS

CNS: Confusion, dizziness, hallucinations, headache, lethargy, ***seizures,*** tremors

---

italic = common side effects   ***bold italic*** = life-threatening reactions

EENT: Gingival hyperplasia

GI: Abdominal pain, diarrhea, nausea, transaminase elevation, vomiting

GU: **Acute renal failure,** *elevated* **BUN/Creat (5-10%), glomerulonephritis,** hematuria, oliguria, proteinuria

HEME: Anemia, leukocytoclastic vasculitis, leukopenia, lymphadenopathy, thrombocytopenia

MS: Joint pain, leg pain, muscle cramps

SKIN: Pain or phlebitis at IV site

SPECIAL CONSIDERATIONS

• In recurrent herpes genitalis and herpes labialis in non-immunocompromised patients, no evidence of clinical benefit from topical acyclovir

---

adapalene

(a-dap´pa-leen)

Rx: Differin

Chemical Class: Naphthoic acid derivative (retinoid-like)

Therapeutic Class: Antiacne agent

CLINICAL PHARMACOLOGY

Mechanism of Action: Modulates DNA transcription and thereby cell differentiation; causes comedolysis and reduces inflammation

Pharmacokinetics

TOP: Minimal absorption; primarily biliary excretion

INDICATIONS AND USES: Acne vulgaris

DOSAGE

Adult

• Apply thin film to affected area after washing in the evening at bedtime

---

$ **AVAILABLE FORMS/COST OF THERAPY**

• Cre—Top: 0.1%, 15, 45 g: **$37.19**/15 g
• Gel—Top: 0.1%, 15, 45 g: **$27.31**/15 g
• Sol—Top: 0.1%, 30 ml: **$72.56**

PRECAUTIONS: May aggravate acne early in treatment; do not use if sunburned or if using topical preparations containing sulfur, resorcinol, or salicylic acid

PREGNANCY AND LACTATION: Pregnancy category C; excretion in breast milk unknown

SIDE EFFECTS/ADVERSE REACTIONS

SKIN: Burning, dryness, erythema, pruritus, scaling (most common during first month of therapy; one or more adverse effects in 30-60% with solution, 10-40% with gel)

SPECIAL CONSIDERATIONS

• Avoid excessive exposure to sunlight
• Do not apply to lips or mucous membranes, or to cut, abraded, or sunburned skin
• May aggravate acne early in course of therapy
• Therapeutic results noticed in 8-12 wks

---

adenosine

(ah-den´oh-seen)

Rx: Adenocard

Chemical Class: Endogenous nucleoside

Therapeutic Class: Antidysrhythmic

CLINICAL PHARMACOLOGY

Mechanism of Action: Slows conduction through AV node; interrupts reentry pathways through AV node

Pharmacokinetics

IV: Cleared from plasma in <30 sec, $t_{1/2}$ 10 sec

INDICATIONS AND USES: PSVT, including PSVT associated with Wolff-Parkinson-White syndrome; does *not* convert atrial flutter, atrial fibrillation, or ventricular tachycardia to normal sinus rhythm; symptomatic relief of varicose vein complications with stasis dermatitis

DOSAGE

Adult

• *PSVT:* IV bolus 6 mg; if conversion to normal sinus rhythm does not occur within 1-2 min, give 12 mg by rapid IV bolus; may repeat 12 mg dose again in 1-2 min

• *Varicose veins:* IM 25 mg once or twice daily until relief is obtained and then 25 mg 2 or 3 times weekly for maintenance

Child

• *PSVT:* IV bolus 0.05 mg/kg; if not effective within 2 min, increase dose in 0.05 mg/kg increments every 2 min to a maximum of 0.25 mg/kg or until termination of PSVT; median dose, 0.15 mg/kg; do not exceed 12 mg/dose

🖫 AVAILABLE FORMS/COST OF THERAPY

• Inj, Sol—IM: 25 mg/ml, 10 ml: **$3.29-$15.95**

• Inj, Sol—IV: 3 mg/ml, 2 ml: **$26.97**

CONTRAINDICATIONS: Second or third degree AV block, sick sinus syndrome, bradycardia, bronchoconstrictive lung disease

PRECAUTIONS: Cardiac arrest, hypertension, hypotension, proarrhythmic events, unstable angina

PREGNANCY AND LACTATION: Pregnancy category C; fetal effects unlikely

SIDE EFFECTS/ADVERSE REACTIONS

CNS: Apprehension, arm tingling, blurred vision, dizziness, headache, lightheadedness, numbness

CV: **Atrial tachydysrhythmia,** atrioventricular and ventricular proarrhythmic events, bradycardia, chest pain, *facial flushing (18%),* hypotension, hypertension, palpitations, sweating, negative inotropic events

GI: Groin pressure, metallic taste, nausea, throat tightness

RESP: *Chest pressure, dyspnea,* hyperventilation

INTERACTIONS

Drugs

🔳 *β-blockers:* Bradycardia

🔳 *Dipyridamole:* Increased serum adenosine levels, potentiates pharmacologic effects of adenosine

🔳 *Nicotine:* Greater hemodynamic response to adenosine (hypotension, chest pain)

🔳 *Theophylline/caffeine:* Inhibits hemodynamic effects of adenosine

---

albendazole

(al-ben´da-zole)
Rx: Albenza
Chemical Class: Benzimidazole derivative
Therapeutic Class: Anthelminthic

CLINICAL PHARMACOLOGY

Mechanism of Action: Causes selective degeneration of cytoplasmic microtubules in cells of intestinal helminths and their tissue-dwelling larvae

Pharmacokinetics

PO: Onset 30 min, peak 2 hr, elimination $t_{1/2}$ 8 hr; absorption less than 5% of oral dose (serum level increased 4-fold with fatty meal); rapidly metabolized by liver, excreted in urine; active metabolite, albendazole sulfoxide, penetrates hydatid cyst fluid and CSF and is 70% protein bound

INDICATIONS AND USES: Hydatid disease, neurocysticercosis, infestations by susceptible protozoa* and helminths*

DOSAGE

Adult

• *Capillariasis:* PO 200 mg bid × 10 days

• *Clonorchiasis:* PO 400 mg qd × 7 days

• *Cysticercosis, neurocysticercosis (echinococciasis):* PO 7.5 mg/kg bid with food × 8-30 days, maximum dose 400 mg bid

• *Filariasis (loiasis):* PO 400 mg bid × 21 days

• *Giardiasis, Hymenolepsis nana, cutaneous larva migrans (toxocariasis):* PO 400 mg qd × 3 days

• *Hookworm (ancylostomiasis), pinworm (enterobiasis), roundworm (ascariasis), whipworm (trichuriasis):* PO 400 mg, may repeat dose in 3 wk

• *Hydatid cyst disease (echinococciasis):* PO 7.5 mg/kg bid with food × 28 days, maximum dose 400 mg bid; repeat after 14 drug-free days for total of 3 cycles

• *Microsporidiosis:* PO 400 mg qd × 30 days, maintenance therapy may be required in HIV-infected persons

• *Opisthorchiasis:* PO 400 mg bid × 3 days

• *Strongyloidiasis, tapeworm (taeniasis):* PO 400 mg qd × 3 days, may repeat treatment in 3 wk

• *Trichinosis:* PO 400 mg bid × 15 days

• *Trichostrongyliasis:* PO 400 mg

• *Visceral larva migrans (toxocariasis):* PO 10 mg/kg/day in 2-3 divided doses × 5 days

Child

• *Capillariasis:* Age 1-12 yr: PO 200 mg bid × 10 days

• *Clonorchiasis:* Age 2-12 yr: PO 400 mg qd × 7 days

• *Giardiasis, Hymenolepsis nana, cutaneous larva migrans (toxocariasis):* Age 2-12 yr: PO 400 mg qd × 3 days

• *Hookworm (ancylostomiasis), pinworm (enterobiasis), roundworm (ascariasis), whipworm (trichuriasis):* Age 2-12 yr: PO 400 mg, repeat dose in 3 wk; Age 0-2 yr: PO 200 mg, may repeat dose in 3 wk

• *Hydatid cyst disease (echinococciasis):* Age 2-12 yr: PO 7.5 mg/kg bid with food × 28 days, maximum dose 400 mg bid; repeat after 14 drug-free days for total of 3 cycles

• *Neurocysticercosis (echinococciasis):* Age 1-12 yr: PO 7.5 mg/kg bid with food × 8-30 days, maximum dose 400 mg bid

• *Opisthorchiasis:* Age 2-12 yr: PO 400 mg bid × 3 days

• *Strongyloidiasis, tapeworm (taeniasis):* Age 2-12 yr: PO 400 mg qd × 3 days, may repeat treatment in 3 wk; Age 0-2 yr: PO 200 mg qd × 3 days, may repeat treatment in 3 wk

• *Trichinosis:* Age 2-12 yr: PO 400 mg bid × 15 days

• *Trichostrongyliasis:* Age 1-12 yr: PO 400 mg

• *Visceral larva migrans (toxocariasis):* Age 0-12 yr: PO 10 mg/kg/day in 2-3 divided doses × 5 days

$ **AVAILABLE FORMS/COST OF THERAPY**

• Tab, Uncoated—Oral: 200 mg, 112's: **$154.55**

PRECAUTIONS: Administer with corticosteroids in patients with neurocysticercosis, avoid during pregnancy

PREGNANCY AND LACTATION: Pregnancy category C, excreted in breast milk

---

* = non-FDA-approved use

SIDE EFFECTS/ADVERSE REACTIONS

CNS: Dizziness, headache

GI: Abdominal pain, *abnormal LFTs* anorexia, constipation, diarrhea, dry mouth, hepatotoxicity (5%, high dose only), nausea, vomiting

HEME: Eosinophilia, neutropenia (5%, high dose only)

SKIN: Alopecia, pruritus, rash

MISC: Fever

INTERACTIONS

Drugs

3 *Dexamethasone:* 56% increase in serum level of albendazole

3 *Praziquantel:* 50% increase in serum level of albendazole

SPECIAL CONSIDERATIONS

• For appropriate infections, retest stool 3 wk after treatment to detect residual ova

• Patients treated for neurocystircercosis should receive steroid and anticonvulsant therapy

---

albuterol

(al-byoo´ter-ole)

Rx: Airet, Proventil, Proventil-HFA, Proventil Repetabs, Respirol, Ventolin, Ventolin Rotacaps, Volmax Combinations

   Rx: with ipratropium (Combivent)

Chemical Class: Sympathomimetic amine; β_2- adrenergic agonist

Therapeutic Class: Antiasthmatic, bronchodilator

CLINICAL PHARMACOLOGY

Mechanism of Action: Bronchodilation by β_2-stimulation, resulting in relaxation of bronchial smooth muscle; inhibits mast cell degranulation; stimulates cilia to remove secretions

Pharmacokinetics

PO: Onset ½ hr, peak 2½ hr, duration 4-6 hr

PO SUS ACTION: Onset ½ hr, peak 2-3 hr, duration 12 hr

INH: Onset 5-15 min, peak 1-1½ hr, duration 4-6 hr

Metabolized in liver to inactive sulfate; 28% appears unchanged in urine; $t_{1/2}$ 2½-4 hr

INDICATIONS AND USES: Relief and prevention of bronchospasm in reversible airway disease; exercise-induced bronchospasm

DOSAGE

Adult

• *Prevention of exercise-induced bronchospasm:* MDI 2 puffs, 15 min before exercising

• *Bronchospasm:* MDI (Rotohaler) 1-2 puffs (capsules for inhalation) q4-6h; NEB 2.5 mg (3 ml of 0.083% soln) tid-qid; PO 2-4 mg tid-qid, max 8 mg qid; Sus Action PO 4-8 mg q12h, max 16 mg q12h

Child (6-12 yr)

• *Bronchospasm:* PO 2 mg tid-qid, max 24 mg/day; Sus Action PO 4 mg q12h, max 12 mg q12h

Child (≥4 yr)

• *Bronchospasm:* MDI (Rotahaler) 1-2 puffs (capsules for inhalation) q4-6h

• *Prevention of exercise-induced bronchospasm:* MDI 2 puffs 15-30 min before exercise; Rotahaler 1 capsule for inhalation 15 min before exercise

Child (≥2 yr)

• *Bronchospasm:* PO (syrup) 0.1 mg/kg tid, may increase stepwise to 0.2 mg/kg tid, max 4 mg tid; NEB 0.1-0.15 mg/kg (0.12-0.18 ml/kg of 0.083% soln) q1h initially then q4-6h, max 2.5 mg tid-qid

---

italic = common side effects   ***bold italic*** = life-threatening reactions

💲 AVAILABLE FORMS/COST OF THERAPY

• Cap, Gel—INH: 200 µg/puff, 100's: **$32.15**
• MDI—INH: 0.09 mg/puff, 17 g (200 puffs): **$9.24-$38.39**
• Sol—INH: 0.083%, 3 ml: **$1.10-$2.13**; 0.5%, 20 ml: **$8.99-$28.98**
• Syr—Oral: 2 mg/5 ml, 480 ml: **$8.24-$44.72**
• Tab, Coated, Sus Action—Oral: 4 mg, 100's: **$85.24-$109.21**; 8 mg, 100's: **$218.42**
• Tab, Uncoated—Oral: 2 mg, 100's: **$3.89-$48.92**; 4 mg, 100's: **$5.34-$86.77**

CONTRAINDICATIONS: Tachydysrhythmias, severe cardiac disease

PRECAUTIONS: Ischemic heart disease, cardiac dysrhythmias, hyperthyroidism, diabetes mellitus, hypertension, prostatic hypertrophy, convulsive disorders, use in labor and delivery

PREGNANCY AND LACTATION: Pregnancy category C; excretion into breast milk unkown

SIDE EFFECTS/ADVERSE REACTIONS

CNS: Anxiety, *dizziness,* flushing, hallucinations, *headache,* insomnia, irritability, restlessness, *stimulation, tremors*
CV: Angina, dysrhythmias, hypertension, hypotension, *palpitations, tachycardia*
EENT: Dry nose, irritation of nose and throat, angle-closure glaucoma
GI: Heartburn, *nausea,* vomiting
METAB: Hypokalemia
MS: Inhibition of uterine contractions, muscle cramps
RESP: Cough

INTERACTIONS
Drugs

🔳 β-*blockers:* Decreased action of albuterol, cardioselective beta-blockers preferable if concurrent use necessary
🔳 *Furosemide:* Potential for additive hypokalemia
🔳 *MAOIs:* Action of albuterol on the vascular system may be potentiated, caution if administered concomitantly or within 2 weeks of discontiuation of MAOIs
🔳 *Tricyclic antidepressants:* Action of albuterol on the vascular system may be potentiated, caution if administered concomitantly or within 2 weeks of discontinuation of Tricyclics

SPECIAL CONSIDERATIONS
• Inhalation technique critical
• Consider spacer devices

PATIENT/FAMILY EDUCATION
• See clinician if using ≥4 inhalations/day on regular basis or >1 canister (200 inhalations) in 8 wks

---

alclometasone
(al-clo-met´a-sone)
Rx: Aclovate
Chemical Class: Glucocorticoid
Therapeutic Class: Topical corticosteroid, low potency

CLINICAL PHARMACOLOGY
Mechanism of Action: Depresses formation, release, and activity of endogenous mediators of inflammation such as prostaglandins, kinins, histamine, liposomal enzymes, and the complement system resulting in decreased edema, erythema, and pruritus

Pharmacokinetics

TOP: Approximately 3% absorbed during 8 hr of contact with intact, normal skin; metabolized primarily in liver and then excreted by kidneys and into bile

INDICATIONS AND USES: Psoriasis, eczema, contact dermatitis, pruritus of corticosteroid responsive dermatoses

DOSAGE

Adult and Child

• TOP: Apply to affected area bid, rub completely into skin

$ AVAILABLE FORMS/COST OF THERAPY

• Cre/Oint—Top: 0.05%, 15, 45, 60 g: **$11.20-$18.08**/15 g

PRECAUTIONS: Viral infections, bacterial infections, children

PREGNANCY AND LACTATION: Pregnancy category C; unknown whether topical application could result in sufficient systemic absorption to produce detectable amounts in breast milk (systemic corticosteroids are secreted into breast milk in quantities not likely to have detrimental effects on infant)

SIDE EFFECTS/ADVERSE REACTIONS

SKIN: Acne, allergic contact dermatitis, atrophy, burning, dryness, folliculitis, hypertrichosis, hypopigmentation, irritation, itching, miliaria, perioral dermatitis, secondary infection, striae

MISC: Systemic absorption of topical corticosteroids has produced reversible HPA axis suppression (more likely with occlusive dressings, prolonged administration, application to large surface areas, liver failure, and in children)

SPECIAL CONSIDERATIONS

PATIENT/FAMILY EDUCATION

• Apply sparingly only to affected area

• Avoid contact with the eyes

• Do not put bandages or dressings over treated area unless directed by clinician

• Discontinue drug, notify clinician if local irritation or fever develops

• Do not use on weeping, denuded, or infected areas

---

alendronate

(a-len´dro-nate)

Rx: Fosamax

Chemical Class: Synthetic analog of pyrophosphate

Therapeutic Class: Bisphosphonate

CLINICAL PHARMACOLOGY

Mechanism of Action: Highly selective binding to hydroxyapatite at sites of bone resorption, inhibits normal and abnormal bone resorption ("crystal poison"); minimal secondary reduction in bone formation (resorption coupled to formation); bone formation exceeds bone resorption at these remodeling sites, leading to progressive gains in bone mass

Pharmacokinetics

PO: Onset 3-4 wk; bioavailability <1%, food decreases bioavailability by 40%; protein binding 78%; $t_{1/2}$ *(in bone)* up to 10 yr

INDICATIONS AND USES: Treatment and prophylaxis of osteoporosis in postmenopausal women; Paget's disease of bone; prevention of glucocorticoid-induced osteoporosis, hyperparathyroidism,* bone pain in prostatic carcinoma and metastatic breast cancer,* hypercalcemia of malignancy*

DOSAGE

Adult

• *Osteoporosis (prophylaxis):* PO 5 mg qd (Treatment): PO 10 mg qd

---

• *Paget's disease:* PO 40 mg qd for 6 mo

Child

• Safety and efficacy not established

$ **AVAILABLE FORMS/COST OF THERAPY**

• Tab—Oral: 5 mg, 100's: **$231.29**; 10 mg, 100's: **$231.29**; 35 mg, 20's: **$323.83**; 40 mg, 30's: **$165.64**

CONTRAINDICATIONS: Hypocalcemia, esophageal abnormalities, delayed esophageal emptying, patient unable to stand or sit upright for at least 30 min after administration

PRECAUTIONS: CrCl <35 ml/min; uncorrected mineral deficiencies (i.e., calcium, vitamin D)

PREGNANCY AND LACTATION: Pregnancy category C; contraindicated in nursing mothers

SIDE EFFECTS/ADVERSE REACTIONS

CNS: Headache

GI: Abdominal distention, *abdominal pain,* acid regurgitation, dysphagia, esophageal ulcer, flatulence, gastritis

METAB: Hypocalcemia, hypophosphatemia

MS: Musculoskeletal pain

SKIN: Erythema, rash

MISC: Drug fever

INTERACTIONS

Drugs

3 *Antacids:* Calcium, magnesium and aluminum bind alendronate and reduce absorption

3 *Food (including coffee and orange juice):* Decreases bioavailability of alendronate by 40%-60%

3 *Aspirin:* Increased risk of upper GI adverse effects

SPECIAL CONSIDERATIONS

PATIENT/FAMILY EDUCATION

• Patients should receive supplemental calcium and vitamin D if dietary intake is inadequate

• Administer 30 min before the first food/beverage/medication of the day with 6-8 oz plain water; avoid lying down for at least 30 min

---

allopurinol

(al-oh-pure'i-nole)

Rx: Aloprim, Lopurin, Zurinol, Zyloprim

Chemical Class: Enzyme (xanthine oxidase) inhibitor

Therapeutic Class: Antigout agent

CLINICAL PHARMACOLOGY

Mechanism of Action: Xanthine oxidase inhibitor; reduces uric acid synthesis

Pharmacokinetics

PO: Peak 2-4 hr; excreted in feces and urine; $t_{1/2}$ 2-3 hr, active metabolite $t_{1/2}$ 18-30 hr

INDICATIONS AND USES: Chronic primary or secondary gout (prevention of acute attacks, tophi, joint destruction, uric acid lithiasis or nephropathy), hyperuricemia associated with malignancies, recurrent calcium oxalate calculi, prevention of fluorouracil-induced stomatitis (as mouthwash 1 mg/ml in methylcellulose)*

DOSAGE

Adult

• *Gout/hyperuricemia:* PO 200-600 mg qd depending on severity, not to exceed 800 mg/day

• *Impaired renal function:* PO 200 mg qd when CrCl is 10-20 ml/min; 100 mg qd when CrCl 3-10 ml/min; 100 mg qod when CrCl <3 ml/min

• *Recurrent urinary calculi:* PO 200-300 mg qd

• *Uric acid nephropathy prevention:* PO 600-800 mg qd × 2-3 days

Child (6-10 yr)

• PO 300 mg qd

---

* = non-FDA-approved use

Child (<6 yr)
• PO 150 mg qd

§ AVAILABLE FORMS/COST OF THERAPY
• Inj, Sol—IV: 500 mg/vial: **$500.00**
• Tab, Uncoated—Oral: 100 mg, 100's: **$3.94-$29.30**; 300 mg, 100's: **$9.38-$76.15**

PRECAUTIONS: Renal disease, hepatic disease, children

PREGNANCY AND LACTATION: Pregnancy category C; allopurinol and oxypurinol have been found in the milk of a mother who was receiving allopurinol

SIDE EFFECTS/ADVERSE REACTIONS
CNS: Drowsiness, headache, neuritis, paresthesia
EENT: Cataracts, epistaxis, retinopathy
GI: Anorexia, cholestatic jaundice, cramps, diarrhea, hepatomegaly, hepatotoxicity, malaise, metallic taste, nausea, peptic ulcer, stomatitis, vomiting
*GU: **Renal failure***
*HEME: **Bone marrow suppression***
MS: Arthralgia, myopathy
SKIN: Alopecia, ecchymosis, erythema, dermatitis, pruritus, purpura, ***Stevens-Johnson syndrome***
MISC: Chills, fever

INTERACTIONS
Drugs
❷ *Angiotensin-converting enzyme inhibitors:* Predisposed to hypersensitivity reactions including Stevens-Johnson syndrome, skin eruptions, fever, and arthralgias
❸ *Antacids:* Aluminum hydroxide inhibits the response to allopurinol
❷ *Azathioprine:* Increased toxicity of azathioprine; requires dose adjustment
❸ *Cyclophosphamide:* May increase cyclophosphamide toxicity
❸ *Cyclosporine/tacrolimus:* Increased toxicity of immunosuppressive drug
❷ *Mercaptopurine:* Increased effect of mercaptopurine with increased risk of toxicity
❸ *Oral anticoagulants:* Enhanced hypoprothrombinemic response
❸ *Theophylline:* Large doses may increase serum theophylline levels

SPECIAL CONSIDERATIONS
• Increased acute attacks of gout during early stages of allopurinol administration—cover with colchicine (see next bullet)
• Maintenance doses of colchicine (0.6 mg qd-bid) should be given prophylactically along with starting with low doses of allopurinol
• Parenteral formulation available as orphan drug and in Canada
• Gel formulation FDA-approved, not yet marketed

---

almotriptan
(al-moe-trip'tan)
Rx: Axert
Chemical Class: Serotonin derivative
Therapeutic Class: Antimigraine agent

CLINICAL PHARMACOLOGY
Mechanism of Action: Selectively activates vascular 5-HT$_1$-receptors in cranial arteries causing vasoconstriction and inhibition of proinflammatory neuropeptide release, actions correlating with the relief of migraine in humans
Pharmacokinetics
PO: Peak 1-3 hr; well absorbed (PO bioavailability 70%); 35% bound to plasma proteins; metabolized mainly by MAO-mediated oxidation (27% of dose), and cytochrome P450-mediated oxidation (12% of

---

italic = common side effects   ***bold italic*** = life-threatening reactions

dose); eliminated primarily by renal excretion (40% unchanged); $t_{1/2}$ 3-4 hr

INDICATIONS AND USES: Acute migraine headache with or without aura

DOSAGE

Adult and Child >16 yr

• PO 6.25-12.5 mg at first sign of headache: may repeat after 2 hr if the headache returns (no more than 2 doses should be given within a 24 hr period); the maximum dose should not exceed 12.5 mg/24 hr in patients with hepatic or renal function impairment

$ AVAILABLE FORMS/COST OF THERAPY

• Tab—Oral: 6.25 mg, 6's: **$65.93**; 12.5 mg, 6's: **$65.93**

CONTRAINDICATIONS: Ischemic heart disease; hemiplegic or basilar migraine; Prinzmetal's angina; uncontrolled hypertension; within 24 hr of ergotamine-containing product or other 5-HT$_1$-receptor agonist

PRECAUTIONS: Children <18 yr; hypertension; impaired hepatic or renal function

PREGNANCY AND LACTATION: Pregnancy category C; excretion in human breast milk unknown (lactating rats had milk concentrations 7 times higher than maternal plasma concentrations 6 hr after almotriptan dosing), use caution in nursing mothers

SIDE EFFECTS/ADVERSE REACTIONS

CNS: Somnolence, dizziness, headache, paresthesia, tremor, vertigo, anxiety, hypesthesia, restlessness, stimulation, insomnia, shakiness

CV: Vasodilation, palpitation, tachycardia, hypertension, syncope

EENT: Ear pain, conjunctivitis, eye irritation, hyperacusis

GI: Nausea, dry mouth, abdominal cramps, diarrhea, vomiting, dyspepsia, taste alteration

GU: Dysmenorrhea

MS: Myalgia, muscular weakness

METAB: Hyperglycemia, increased serum creatine phosphokinase

RESP: Pharyngitis, rhinitis, dyspnea, laryngismus, sinusitis, bronchitis, epistaxis

SKIN: Diaphoresis, dermatitis, erythema, pruritus, rash

MISC: Chest pain, back pain, neck pain, fatigue, rigid neck

INTERACTIONS

Drugs

⚠ *Egotomine-containing drugs:* Increased vasoconstriction

⚠ *Other 5-HT$_1$-agonists:* Increased vasoconstriction

🅱 *MAO inhibitors:* Decreased almotriptan clearance

🅱 *Ketoconazole, itraconazole, ritonavir, erythromycin:* Increased plasma concentrations of almotriptan

❷ *Sibutramine:* Theoretical increase in the risk of serotonin syndrome

SPECIAL CONSIDERATIONS

• Safety of treating, on average, more than 4 headaches in a 30-day period has not been established

• Controlled trials have not adequately established the effectiveness of a second dose if the initial dose is ineffective

• Superiority over other triptan migraine headache agents has not been demonstrated

PATIENT/FAMILY EDUCATION

• Use only to treat migraine headache, not for prevention

alprazolam

(al-pray'zoe-lam)
Rx: Xanax
Chemical Class: Benzodiaz-
epine
Therapeutic Class: Anxiolytic

CLINICAL PHARMACOLOGY
Mechanism of Action: CNS depressant via facilitation of inhibitory
GABA at benzodiazepine receptor
sites (BZ_1—associated with sleep;
BZ_2—associated with memory, motor, sensory, and cognitive function); effects include muscle relaxation (spinal cord), anticonvulsant
activity (brain stem), ataxia (cerebellum), emotional behavior (limbic and cortical areas), and anxiolytic effects (separate from general
CNS depression); other effects include sedative, appetite-stimulating, and weak analgesic actions
Pharmacokinetics
PO: Onset 30 min, peak serum conc
1-2 hr, duration 4-6 hr, therapeutic
response 2-3 days, metabolized by
liver, excreted by kidneys; crosses
placenta; $t_{1/2}$ 12-15 hr
INDICATIONS AND USES: Anxiety,
panic disorder, anxiety with depressive symptoms, agoraphobia with
social phobia (2-8 mg/day),* depression,* premenstrual syndrome*
DOSAGE
Adult
• *Anxiety:* PO 0.25-0.5 mg tid, up to
4 mg/day in divided doses
• *Panic disorder:* PO 0.5 mg tid; increase dose q3-4 days in 1 mg/day
increments to 10 mg/day
• *Geriatric:* PO 0.25 mg bid-tid
**$ AVAILABLE FORMS/COST
    OF THERAPY**
• Sol—Oral: 0.5 mg/5ml, 500 ml:
$51.75; 1 mg/ml w/dropper, 30 ml:
$37.50

• Tab, Plain Coated—Oral: 0.25 mg,
100's: **$46.40-$98.21**; 0.5 mg,
100's: **$57.75-$122.35**; 1 mg,
100's: **$77.05-$163.25**; 2 mg,
100's: **$136.28-$277.56**
CONTRAINDICATIONS: Untreated
narrow-angle glaucoma, psychosis,
concurrent treatment with itraconazole, ketaconazole, nefazadone
PRECAUTIONS: Elderly, debilitated, hepatic disease, renal disease,
suicidal patients, addictive patients
PREGNANCY AND LACTATION:
Pregnancy category D; children
born of a mother receiving benzodiazepines may be at risk for withdrawal symptoms; neonatal flaccid-
ity and respiratory problems have
been reported; chronic administration of diazepam to nursing mothers
has been reported to cause infants to
become lethargic and lose weight
SIDE EFFECTS/ADVERSE REAC-
    TIONS
CNS: Anxiety, ataxia, confusion, depression, *dizziness, drowsiness,* fatigue, hallucinations, headache, insomnia, stimulation, tremors
CV: Bradycardia, hypertension,
orthostatic hypotension, tachycardia
EENT: Blurred vision, mydriasis, tinnitus
GI: Anorexia, constipation, diarrhea, dry mouth, hepatic dysfunction, nausea, vomiting
SKIN: Dermatitis, itching, rash
INTERACTIONS
Drugs
3 *Cimetidine:* Cimetidine inhibits
metabolism, increases plasma levels
3 *Digoxin:* Inconsistently raises
digoxin levels
3 *Erythromycin, clarithromycin,
troleandomycin:* Possible increased
sedation

---

italic = common side effects   ***bold italic*** = life-threatening reactions

3 *Ethanol:* Enhanced adverse psychomotor effects; difficulty performing tasks that require alertness

3 *Fluoxetine, fluvoxamine, ketoconazole, itraconazole, nefazadone (see contraindications):* Increases alprazolam plasma concentrations; increases in psychomotor impairment

3 *Grapefruit juice:* Increased alprazolam levels due to inhibition of presystemic (intestinal) enzyme CYP34A

3 *Phenytoin, carbamazepine:* Decreased benzodiazepine effect

SPECIAL CONSIDERATIONS

PATIENT/FAMILY EDUCATION

• Not for "everyday" stress or longer than 3 mo; avoid driving, activities that require alertness

• Caution when medication discontinued abruptly after long-term (>4 wks) use—may precipitate withdrawal syndrome

---

alprostadil
(al-pros'ta-dil)

Rx: Caverject, Edex, MUSE, Prostin VR Pediatric
Chemical Class: Prostaglandin E$_1$ (PGE$_1$)
Therapeutic Class: Anti-impotence agent; patent ductus arteriosus

---

CLINICAL PHARMACOLOGY

Mechanism of Action: Relaxes vascular smooth muscle, especially of ductus arteriosus and corpus cavernosum

Pharmacokinetics

INTRACAVERNOSAL (CAVERJECT): Peak 5-20 min; INTRAURETHRAL (MUSE): onset 5-10 min, duration 30-60 min: 80% metabolized in lungs, excreted in urine (metabolites)

INDICATIONS AND USES: Temporary maintenance of patency of the ductus arteriosus until definitive surgery can be performed, erectile dysfunction, primary pulmonary hypertension,* severe peripheral arterial occlusive disease*

DOSAGE

Adult

• *Erectile dysfunction:* Intracavernosal 2.5 µg prior to intercourse, increase by 2.5-5 µg depending on response. Mean dose 20 µg; Intraurethral-administer pellet via applicator (supplied) with at least 24 hr between uses

Infants

• IV INF 0.1 µg/kg/min, until desired response, then reduce to lowest effective amount; 0.4 µg/kg/min not likely to produce greater beneficial effects

S **AVAILABLE FORMS/COST OF THERAPY**

• Inj, Sol—IV: 500 µg/ml, 1 ml: **$216.00**

• Kit-IV: 10 µg: **$15.34-$40.16**; 20 µg: **$20.54-$54.28**; 40 µg: **$32.80-$35.70**

• Pellet, urethral: 125 µg, 6's: **$118.50**; 250 µg, 6's: **$124.13**; 500 µg, 6's: **$132.75**; 1000 µg, 6's: **$143.25**

CONTRAINDICATIONS: Conditions that might predispose to priapism (e.g., sickle-cell anemia/trait, multiple myeloma, leukemia), patients with anatomical deformation of penis (e.g., Peyronie's disease), penile implants, for sexual intercourse with a pregnant woman (unless a condom is used)

PRECAUTIONS: Bleeding disorders; men for whom sexual activity is inadvisable

---

SIDE EFFECTS/ADVERSE REACTIONS

CNS: **Cerebral bleeding,** *fever,* hyperextension of the neck, hyperirritability, hypothermia, jitteriness, lethargy, **seizures,** stiffness

CV: *Bradycardia,* **CHF,** edema, *flushing,***hypotension (4%),** tachycardia, **ventricular fibrillation**

GI: Diarrhea, hyperbilirubinemia, regurgitation

GU (PENILE ADMINISTRATION): Injection site hematoma, *penile fibrosis,* (3-8%), *penile pain,* (36%), prolonged erection

HEME: **Bleeding, DIC, thrombocytopenia**

METAB: Hyperkalemia, hypoglycemia, hypokalemia

MS: Cortical proliferation of the long bones

RESP: **Apnea** (10% of neonates), **bradypnea,** hypercapnia, tachypnea, wheezing

SPECIAL CONSIDERATIONS

• For intracavernosal use administer 1st dose under medical supervision. Use ½-inch 27-30 gauge needle along dorso-lateral aspect of proximal third of penis. Alternate sides

• Urinate prior to intraurethral use to disperse pellet

• Use lowest dose allowing satisfactory erection lasting ≥1 h

MONITORING PARAMETERS

• Infant ABG's, arterial pH, arterial pressure, continuous ECG

alteplase

(al-teep′lase)
Rx: Activase
Chemical Class: Tissue plasminogen activator (tPA)
Therapeutic Class: Thrombolytic

CLINICAL PHARMACOLOGY

Mechanism of Action: Promotes thrombolysis by promoting conversion of plasminogen to plasmin

Pharmacokinetics

IV: Cleared by liver, 80% cleared within 10 min after infusion is terminated

INDICATIONS AND USES: Acute myocardial infarction; pulmonary embolism; acute ischemic stroke within 3h of onset; unstable angina pectoris*; peripheral arterial thromboembolism*

DOSAGE

Adult

• *Acute MI:* IV 15 mg bolus, then 0.75 mg/kg over 30 min (max 50 mg), then 0.5 mg/kg over 60 min (max 35 mg)

• *Pulmonary embolism:* IV 100 mg over 2 hr

• *Acute ischemic stroke:* IV 0.9 mg/kg (max 90 mg) over 60 min with 10% of total dose administered as an initial IV bolus over 1 min; initiate treatment within 3 hr after onset of stroke symptoms after exclusion of intracranial hemorrhage by CT scan

⑤ AVAILABLE FORMS/COST OF THERAPY

• Inj, Lyphl-Sol—IV: 1 mg/ml, 50 mg: **$1,375.00**; 1 mg/ml, 100 mg: **$2,750.00**

CONTRAINDICATIONS: Active bleeding, recent GI/GU bleed, hemorrhagic stroke, severe uncontrolled hypertension, recent surgery/trauma, aneurysm, arterio-venous malformation, brain tumor, prolonged or traumatic CPR, bleeding disorder, diabetic hemorrhagic retinopathy, suspected aortic dissection, pregnancy, liver or kidney dysfunction

PRECAUTIONS: Recent (within 10 days) major surgery (e.g., coronary artery bypass graft, obstetrical delivery, organ biopsy); previous puncture of noncompressible vessels; cerebrovascular disease; recent trauma (within 10 days); hypertension (systolic BP ≥ 180 mm Hg and/or diastolic BP ≥ 110 mm Hg); high likelihood of left heart thrombus (e.g., mitral stenosis with atrial fibrillation); acute pericarditis; bacterial endocarditis; hemostatic defects including those secondary to severe hepatic or renal disease; significant liver dysfunction; septic thrombophlebitis or occluded arteriovenous cannula at seriously infected site; advanced age (>75 yr); patients currently receiving oral anticoagulants (e.g., warfarin); any other condition in which bleeding constitutes a significant hazard or would be particularly difficult to manage because of its location; readministration

PREGNANCY AND LACTATION: Pregnancy category C. Unknown if excreted in breast milk

SIDE EFFECTS/ADVERSE REACTIONS

CV: Accelerated idioventricular rhythm, sinus bradycardia, ventricular tachycardia

HEME: Intracranial, retroperitoneal, surface, GI, GU bleeding; increased PT, aPTT, TT

SKIN: Rash, urticaria

INTERACTIONS

Drugs

3 *Heparin, oral anticoagulants, drugs that alter platelet function (i.e., aspirin, dipyridamole, abciximab, eptifibitide, tirofiban):* May increase the risk of bleeding

Labs

• *Decrease:* Fibrinogen (mitigated by collecting blood in presence of aprotinin)

SPECIAL CONSIDERATIONS

• Heparin (in doses sufficient to prolong the aPTT to 1.5-2 times control value) is usually administered in conjunction with thrombolytic therapy; aspirin may also be administered to inhibit platelet aggregation during and/or following post-thrombolytic therapy

• Compress arterial puncture sites at least 30 min

MONITORING PARAMETERS

• Prior to initiation of therapy: coagulation tests, hematocrit, platelet count

• During therapy: ECG, mental status, neurological status, vital signs

---

aluminum chloride hexahydrate

Rx: Drysol (20%), Xerac AC (6.25%)

Chemical Class: Aluminum salt
Therapeutic Class: Antihidrotic

CLINICAL PHARMACOLOGY

Mechanism of Action: Astringent or increased permeability of the sweat duct causing reabsorption of sweat

INDICATIONS AND USES: Hyperhidrosis

DOSAGE
Adult
• TOP: Apply to affected area at bedtime; to help prevent irritation, area should be completely dry prior to application; wash treated area the following morning; excessive sweating may be stopped after 2 or more treatments; thereafter, apply once or twice weekly or as needed

💲 AVAILABLE FORMS/COST OF THERAPY
• Sol—Top: 6.25%, 35, 60 ml: **$6.28**/35 ml; 20%, 35, 60 ml: **$6.44**/35 ml

PRECAUTIONS: Broken, irritated, or recently shaved skin

SIDE EFFECTS/ADVERSE REACTIONS
SKIN: Burning or prickling sensation, transient stinging or itching

SPECIAL CONSIDERATIONS
PATIENT/FAMILY EDUCATION
• Do not apply to broken or irritated skin
• For maximum effect, cover treated area with saran wrap held in place by snug-fitting shirt, mitten or sock (never hold saran wrap in place with tape)
• Avoid contact with eyes

---

aluminum salts
OTC: *Aluminum hydroxide:* AlternaGEL, Alu-Cap, Alu-Tab, Amphojel
OTC: *Aluminum carbonate:* Basaljel
Combinations
　OTC: with magnesium hydroxide (Maalox, Rulox, Mylanta, Gelusil, Aludrox)
Chemical Class: Aluminum salt
Therapeutic Class: Antacid; phosphate adsorbent

CLINICAL PHARMACOLOGY
Mechanism of Action: Neutralizes gastric acidity; binds phosphates in GI tract; enhances phosphate excretion
Pharmacokinetics
PO: Onset 20-40 min; non-absorbable; excreted in feces

INDICATIONS AND USES: Antacid (symptomatic relief of hyperacidity, GERD, peptic ulcer disease); phosphate renal stones (prevention); phosphate binder, reduction of hyperphosphatemia in chronic renal failure

DOSAGE
ALUMINUM CARBONATE GEL
Adult
• *Urinary phosphate stones:* Susp 5-10 ml 1 hr pc, hs; extra str susp 2.5-5 ml 1 hr pc, hs; PO 2-6 tabs 1 hr pc, hs
• *Antacid:* Susp 15-45 ml 1 hr pc, hs; extra str susp 5-15 ml 1 hr pc, hs; PO chew 1-2 tabs or caps as needed
ALUMINUM HYDROXIDE
Adult
• *Antacid:* PO susp 5-15 ml 1 hr pc, hs; PO tab 600 mg 1 hr pc, hs, chewed with milk or water

---

• *Hyperphosphatemia in renal failure:* PO susp 5-30 ml bid-qid; PO tab 600-1800 mg bid-qid; titrate to normal serum phosphorus

Child

• *Hyperphosphatemia in renal failure:* PO susp 50-150 mg/kg/24 hr in divided doses q4-6 hr; titrate to normal serum phosphorus

$ AVAILABLE FORMS/COST OF THERAPY

Aluminum Carbonate Gel

• Cap—Oral: 500 mg, 100's: **$20.66**
• Tab—Oral: 500 mg, 100's: **$20.44**

Aluminum Hydroxide

• Susp—Oral: 320 mg/5 ml, 480 ml: **$4.75-$9.80**; 600 mg/5 ml, 480 ml: **$4.08-$8.00**
• Tab—Oral: 300 mg, 100's: **$4.29**; 600 mg, 100's: **$11.48**

CONTRAINDICATIONS: Appendicitis

PRECAUTIONS: Elderly, fluid restriction, decreased GI motility, GI obstruction, dehydration, sodium-restricted diets

PREGNANCY AND LACTATION: Pregnancy category C

SIDE EFFECTS/ADVERSE REACTIONS

GI: Anorexia, **bowel obstruction, constipation,** fecal impaction

METAB: Hypophosphatemia, hypercalciuria

MISC: Aluminum intoxication, osteomalacia

INTERACTIONS

Drugs

3 *Allopurinol, atenolol, ketoconazole, itraconazole (not fluconazole):* Aluminum hydroxide inhibits GI absorption

3 *Cefpodoxime, cefuroxime:* Reduced bioavailability and serum concentration of cefpodoxime

3 *Cyclosporine:* Reduced cyclosporine blood concentrations possible

3 *Glipizide, glyburide:* Enhanced absorption of hypoglycemic agent

3 *Iron:* Reduced GI absorption of iron; separate doses by 1-2 hr

3 *Isoniazid:* Some antacids reduce plasma concentration of isoniazid

3 *Penicillamine:* Reduced penicillamine bioavailability

3 *Quinolones:* Antacids reduce the serum concentration of all the quinolone antibiotics and may inhibit their efficacy

3 *Salicylates:* Decreased serum salicylate concentrations

3 *Sodium polystyrene sulfonate resin:* Combined use may result in systemic alkalosis

3 *Tetracycline:* Reduced serum concentration and efficacy of tetracycline

3 *Vitamin C:* Increases aluminum absorption

SPECIAL CONSIDERATIONS

PATIENT/FAMILY EDUCATION

• Thoroughly chew chewable tablets before swallowing, follow with a glass of water
• May impair absorption of many drugs; do not take other drugs within 1-4 hr of aluminum hydroxide administration
• Stools may appear white or speckled

MONITORING PARAMETERS

• Monitor for hypophosphatemia: anorexia, weakness, fatigue, bone pain, hyporeflexia; urinary pH, Ca^{++}, electrolytes

---

* = non-FDA-approved use

amantadine

(a-man'ta-deen)

Rx: Symmetrel

Chemical Class: Tricyclic amine

Therapeutic Class: Antiviral; antiParkinson's agent

CLINICAL PHARMACOLOGY

Mechanism of Action: Prevents uncoating of nucleic acid in viral cell, preventing penetration of virus to host; causes release of dopamine from dopaminergic terminals in the substantia nigra

Pharmacokinetics

PO: Onset 48 hr (Parkinson's disease), $t_{1/2}$ 15-17 hr; 67% protein bound, 90% excreted unchanged in urine; excretion increased with acidic urine

INDICATIONS AND USES: Influenza A prophylaxis or treatment, Parkinson's disease, drug-induced extrapyramidal reactions

DOSAGE

Adult

• *Influenza type A:* PO 200 mg/day in single dose or divided bid; start treatment as soon as possible after onset of symptoms and continue for 24-48 hr after symptoms disappear; start prophylaxis in anticipation of contact or as soon as possible after exposure, continue at least 10 days following a known exposure

• *Parkinson's disease:* PO 100 mg qd for 1 wk then increase gradually to 400 mg/day in divided doses if needed

• *Drug-induced extrapyramidal reactions:* PO 100 mg bid, increase to 300 mg/day in divided doses if needed

• *Dosage with renal impairment* (based on CrCl in ml/min/1.73 m^2): CrCl 30-50: PO 200 mg 1st day followed by 100 mg qd thereafter; CrCl 15-29: PO 200 mg 1st day followed by 100 mg qod thereafter; CrCl <15: PO 200 mg every 7 days

Elderly

• *Influenza type A:* 100-200 mg/day

Child

• *Influenza type A:* (1-9 yr) PO 4.4-8.8 mg/kg/day divided bid, do not exceed 150 mg/day; (9-12 yr) PO 100 mg bid

$ AVAILABLE FORMS/COST OF THERAPY

• Cap—Oral: 100 mg, 100's: **$23.24-$90.94**

• Syr—Oral: 50 mg/5 ml, 480 ml: **$34.35-$90.56**

CONTRAINDICATIONS: Child <1 yr

PRECAUTIONS: Seizure disorder, CHF, orthostatic hypotension, psychiatric disorders, hepatic disease, renal disease, peripheral edema, eczematoid rash, abrupt discontinuation

PREGNANCY AND LACTATION: Pregnancy category C; excreted in human milk, exercise caution when administering to nursing mothers because of potential for urinary retention, vomiting, and skin rash

SIDE EFFECTS/ADVERSE REACTIONS

CNS: Anorexia, anxiety, ataxia, confusion, depression, fatigue, hallucinations, headache, *insomnia, lightheadedness,* psychosis, **seizures**

CV: **CHF,** orthostatic hypotension, peripheral edema

EENT: Blurred vision

GI: Constipation, dry mouth, *nausea,* vomiting

GU: Increased BUN, urinary retention

HEME: **Leukopenia**

SKIN: Eczematoid dermatitis, livedo reticularis, photosensitivity, rash

---

italic = common side effects   ***bold italic*** = life-threatening reactions

INTERACTIONS
Drugs
3 *Benztropine:* Potentiation of amantadine's CNS side effects

3 *Triamterene:* Increased amantadine toxicity

3 *Trihexyphenidyl:* Potentiation of amantadine's CNS side effects

SPECIAL CONSIDERATIONS
PATIENT/FAMILY EDUCATION
• Administer at least 4 hr before bedtime to prevent insomnia

• Take with meals for better absorption and to decrease GI symptoms

• Arise slowly from a reclining position; avoid hazardous activities if dizziness or blurred vision occurs

• Do not discontinue abruptly in Parkinson's disease

---

ambenonium
(am-be-noe′nee-um)
Rx: Mytelase
Chemical Class: Synthetic quaternary ammonium derivative
Therapeutic Class: Cholinergic

CLINICAL PHARMACOLOGY
Mechanism of Action: An acetylcholinesterase inhibitor, inhibits destruction of acetylcholine, facilitating transmission of impulses across myoneural junction

Pharmacokinetics
PO: Onset 20-30 min, duration 3-8 hr

INDICATIONS AND USES: Myasthenia gravis (particularly useful in patients sensitive to bromides)

DOSAGE
Adult
• PO 5 mg q3-4h while awake, gradually increased q1-2 days to optimal muscle strength and no GI disturbances (range 5-75 mg per dose), doses above 200 mg/day require close supervision to avoid overdosage

S **AVAILABLE FORMS/COST OF THERAPY**
• Tab, Scored—Oral: 10 mg, 100's: **$111.52**

CONTRAINDICATIONS: Urinary or intestinal obstruction

PRECAUTIONS: Seizure disorder, asthma, coronary occlusion, hyperthyroidism, dysrhythmias, peptic ulcer, bradycardia, hypotension, children, presence of other cholinergics (atropine sulfate should be available for cholinergic crisis)

PREGNANCY AND LACTATION: Pregnancy category C; would not be expected to cross placenta or be excreted into breast milk because it is ionized at physiologic pH; although apparently safe for the fetus, may cause transient muscle weakness in the newborn

SIDE EFFECTS/ADVERSE REACTIONS
CNS: Dizziness, drowsiness, headache, incoordination, *loss of consciousness, paralysis, seizures*

CV: **AV block,** bradycardia, *cardiac arrest, dysrhythmias, hypotension,* non-specific ECG changes, tachycardia

EENT: Blurred vision, conjunctival hyperemia, diplopia, lacrimation, miosis, spasm of accommodation, visual changes

GI: Cramps, diarrhea, dysphagia, flatulence, *increased gastric secretions,* increased peristalsis, *increased salivation,* nausea, vomiting

GU: Frequency, incontinence, urgency

MS: Arthralgia, fasciculation, muscle cramps and spasms, weakness

---

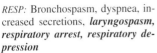

RESP: Bronchospasm, dyspnea, increased secretions, ***laryngospasm, respiratory arrest, respiratory depression***

SKIN: Rash, sweating, urticaria

INTERACTIONS

Drugs

3 *Tacrine:* Increased cholinergic effects

SPECIAL CONSIDERATIONS

PATIENT/FAMILY EDUCATION

• Notify clinician of nausea, vomiting, diarrhea, sweating, increased salivation, irregular heartbeat, muscle weakness, severe abdominal pain or difficulty in breathing

• Administer on an empty stomach

MONITORING PARAMETERS

• Therapeutic response: Increased muscle strength, improved gait, absence of labored breathing (if severe)

• Appearance of side effects: Narrow margin between 1st appearance of side effects and serious toxicity

• Symptoms of increasing muscle weakness may be due to cholinergic crisis (overdosage) or myasthenic crisis (increased disease severity); if crisis is myasthenia, patient will improve after 1-2 mg edrophonium; if cholinergic, withdraw ambinonium and administer atropine

---

amcinonide

(am-sin′oh-nide)

Rx: Cyclocort

Chemical Class: Synthetic fluorinated glucocorticoid

Therapeutic Class: Topical corticosteroid, high potency

CLINICAL PHARMACOLOGY

Mechanism of Action: Depresses formation, release, and activity of endogenous mediators of inflammation such as prostaglandins, kinins,

histamine, liposomal enzymes, and the complement system resulting in decreased edema, erythema, and pruritus

Pharmacokinetics

Absorbed through skin (increased by inflammation and occlusive dressings); metabolized primarily in the liver

INDICATIONS AND USES: Psoriasis, eczema, contact dermatitis, pruritus

DOSAGE

Adult and Child

• Apply to affected area bid; rub completely into skin

$ **AVAILABLE FORMS/COST OF THERAPY**

• Cre—Top: 0.1%, 15, 30 and 60 g: **$15.34**/15 g

• Oint—Top: 0.1%, 15, 30 and 60 g: **$19.60**/15 g

CONTRAINDICATIONS: Fungal infections, use on face, groin, or axilla

PRECAUTIONS: Viral infections, bacterial infections, children

PREGNANCY AND LACTATION: Pregnancy category C; unknown whether topical application could result in sufficient systemic absorption to produce detectable amounts in breast milk (systemic corticosteroids are secreted into breast milk in quantities unlikely to have detrimental effects on breast feeding infant)

SIDE EFFECTS/ADVERSE REACTIONS

SKIN: Acne, allergic contact dermatitis, atrophy, burning, dryness, folliculitis, hypertrichosis, hypopigmentation, irritation, itching, miliaria, perioral dermatitis, secondary infection, striae

MISC: Systemic absorption of topical corticosteroids has produced reversible HPA axis suppression (more likely with occlusive dressings, prolonged administration, application to large surface areas, liver failure, and in children)

SPECIAL CONSIDERATIONS
PATIENT/FAMILY EDUCATION
• Apply sparingly only to affected area
• Avoid contact with eyes
• Do not put bandages or dressings over treated area unless directed by clinician
• Do not use on weeping, denuded, or infected areas
• Discontinue drug, notify clinician if local irritation or fever develops

---

amikacin
(am-i-kay´sin)
Rx: Amikin
Chemical Class: Aminoglycoside
Therapeutic Class: Antibiotic

CLINICAL PHARMACOLOGY
Mechanism of Action: Interferes with protein synthesis in bacterial cell by binding to ribosomal subunit, which causes misreading of genetic code; inaccurate peptide sequence forms in protein chain, causing bacterial death

Pharmacokinetics
IM: Onset rapid, peak 1-2 hr
IV: Onset immediate
Plasma $t_{1/2}$ 2-3 hr; not metabolized, excreted unchanged in urine

INDICATIONS AND USES: Severe systemic infections of CNS, respiratory, GI, urinary tract, bone, skin, soft tissues caused by susceptible organisms

Antibacterial spectrum usually includes:
• Gram-positive organisms: *Staphylococcus* sp. including methicillin-resistant strains (in general has a low order of activity against other Gram-positive organisms)
• Gram-negative organisms: *Pseudomonas* sp.; *E. coli, Proteus* sp. (indole-positive and indole-negative); *Providencia* sp.; *Klebsiella, Enterobacter,* and *Serratia* sp.; *Acinetobacter* sp.; *Citrobacter freundii*

DOSAGE
Adult
• *Severe systemic infections:* IV INF 15 mg/kg/day (use ideal body weight) in 2-3 divided doses q8-12h in 100-200 ml diluent over 30-60 min, not to exceed 1.5 g/day; decreased doses are needed in poor renal function as determined by blood levels and renal function studies; IM 15 mg/kg/day in divided doses q8-12h
• *Uncomplicated urinary tract infections:* IM 250 mg bid
• *Decreased renal function:* 7.5 mg/kg initially, then adjusted as determined by blood levels and renal function studies

Child
• *Severe systemic infections:* Same as adult

Neonate
• IV INF 10 mg/kg initially, then 7.5 mg/kg q12h in diluent over 1-2 hr

§ AVAILABLE FORMS/COST OF THERAPY
• Inj, Sol—IM, IV: 50 mg/ml, 2 ml: **$32.50-$317.12**; 250 mg/ml, 2 ml: **$4.37-$99.30**

CONTRAINDICATIONS: Long-term therapy (ototoxic and nephrotoxic)

PRECAUTIONS: Neonates, renal disease, myasthenia gravis, hearing deficits, Parkinson's disease, elderly, sulfite sensitivity (contains sodium bisulfite), dehydration

---

PREGNANCY AND LACTATION: Pregnancy category C; although fetal ototoxicity has occurred after *in utero* exposure to other aminoglycosides, 8th cranial nerve toxicity has not been reported with amikacin; excreted into breast milk in low concentrations; poor oral bioavailability reduces potential for ototoxicity for the infant

SIDE EFFECTS/ADVERSE REACTIONS

CNS: Confusion, depression, dizziness, muscle twitching, neurotoxicity, numbness, *seizures,* tremors, vertigo

CV: Hypotension or hypertension, palpitations

EENT: Ototoxicity: hearing loss, deafness; tinnitus, visual disturbances

GI: Nausea, vomiting

GU: Azotemia, hematuria, ***nephrotoxicity,*** oliguria, ***renal failure***

HEME: ***Agranulocytosis,*** anemia, eosinophilia, ***leukopenia, thrombocytopenia***

SKIN: Alopecia, dermatitis, *rash,* urticaria

INTERACTIONS

Drugs

3 *Amphotericin B:* Synergistic nephrotoxicity

2 *Atracurium:* Amikacin potentiates respiratory depression by atracurium

3 *Carbenicillin:* Potential for inactivation of amikacin in patients with renal failure

3 *Carboplatin:* Additive nephrotoxicity or ototoxicity

3 *Cephalosporins:* Increased potential for nephrotoxicity in patients with preexisting renal disease

3 *Cisplatin:* Additive nephrotoxicity or ototoxicity

3 *Cyclosporine:* Additive nephrotoxicity

2 *Ethacrynic acid:* Additive ototoxicity

3 *Indomethacin:* Reduced renal clearance of amikacin in premature infants

3 *Methoxyflurane:* Additive nephrotoxicity

3 *Neuromuscular blocking agents:* Amikacin potentiates respiratory depression by neuromuscular blocking agents

3 *NSAIDs:* May reduce renal clearance of amikacin

3 *Pencillins (extended spectrum):* Potential for inactivation of amikacin in patients with renal failure

3 *Piperacillin:* Potential for inactivation of amikacin in patients with renal failure

2 *Succinylcholine:* Amikacin potentiates respiratory depression by succinylcholine

3 *Ticarcillin:* Potential for inactivation of amikacin in patients with renal failure

3 *Vancomycin:* Additive nephrotoxicity or ototoxicity

2 *Vecuronium:* Amikacin potentiates respiratory depression by vecuronium

Labs

• *False increase:* Urine amino acids

• *False decrease:* Bilirubin, cholesterol, serum creatine kinase, serum glucose, LDH, BUN

• *False positive:* Urine oligosaccharides

• *Interference:* Serum tobramycin, kanamycin

SPECIAL CONSIDERATIONS

PATIENT/FAMILY EDUCATION

• Report headache, dizziness, loss of hearing, ringing, roaring in ears, or feeling of fullness in head

MONITORING PARAMETERS

• Urine output, serum creat

• Serum peak, drawn 30-60 min after IV INF or 60 min after IM inj; trough level drawn just before next dose; adjust dosage per levels (usual therapeutic plasma levels; peak 20-35 mg/L, trough ≤10 mg/L)

---

amiloride
(a-mill'oh-ride)
Rx: Midamor
Combinations
  Rx: with hydrochlorothiazide (Moduretic)
Chemical Class: Pyrazine
Therapeutic Class: Potassium-sparing diuretic, antihypertensive

---

CLINICAL PHARMACOLOGY
Mechanism of Action: Inhibits renal sodium reabsorption in exchange for potassium and hydrogen ions directly in the distal renal tubule; weak diuretic and antihypertensive effects when used alone
Pharmacokinetics
PO: Onset 2 hr, peak 6-10 hr, duration 24 hr; excreted unchanged in urine (60%), feces (40%); $t_{1/2}$ 6-9 hr
INDICATIONS AND USES: Adjunctive treatment with thiazide or loop diuretics in congestive heart failure or hypertension to help restore potassium balance; lithium-induced polyuria*; aerosolized administration (drug dissolved in 0.3% saline delivered by nebulizer) in cystic fibrosis*
DOSAGE
Adult
• PO 5 mg qd, may be increased to 10-20 mg qd if needed
$ AVAILABLE FORMS/COST OF THERAPY
• Tab, Uncoated—Oral: 5 mg, 100's: **$28.00-$57.65**
CONTRAINDICATIONS: Hyperkalemia (serum potassium >5.5 mEq/L), impaired renal function, anuria, severe renal disease, antika-liuretic therapy (including angiotensin converting enzyme inhibitors, angiotensin II receptor blockers, and potassium supplements)
PRECAUTIONS: Dehydration, diabetes, acidosis, hepatic function impairment, children
PREGNANCY AND LACTATION: Pregnancy category B; therapy for preexisting hypertension can be continued throughout pregnancy with minimal risk; initiating for simple edema not recommended; few unequivocal indications for diuretic therapy in pregnancy except for pulmonary edema or congestive heart failure; excretion into breast milk unknown; use caution in nursing mothers
SIDE EFFECTS/ADVERSE REACTIONS
CNS: Anxiety, decreased libido, depression, dizziness, encephalopathy, fatigue, *headache,* insomnia, mental confusion, nervousness, paresthesias, tremor, vertigo, weakness
CV: Angina, **dysrhythmias,** orthostatic hypotension
EENT: Blurred vision, increased intraocular pressure, loss of hearing, nasal congestion, tinnitus
GI: Abdominal pain, anorexia, constipation, cramps, *diarrhea,* dry mouth, dyspepsia, flatulence, GI bleeding, jaundice, *nausea, vomiting*
GU: Dysuria, frequency, impotence, polyuria
*HEME: **Agranulocytopenia, leukopenia, thrombocytopenia** (rare)*
METAB: Acidosis, hyperkalemia, hypochloremia, hyponatremia
MS: Cramps, joint pain
SKIN: Alopecia, pruritus, rash, urticaria
INTERACTIONS
Drugs
3 *ACE inhibitors:* Hyperkalemia in predisposed patients

---

* = non-FDA-approved use

3 *Angiotensin II receptor antagonists:* Concurrent mechanisms to decrease potassium excretion; increased risk of hyperkalemia

2 *Potassium preparations:* Hyperkalemia in predisposed patients

3 *Quinidine:* Increased ventricular arrhythmias

SPECIAL CONSIDERATIONS
PATIENT/FAMILY EDUCATION
• Notify clinician of muscle weakness, fatigue, flaccid paralysis
• Take with food or milk for GI symptoms
• Take early in day to prevent nocturia
• Avoid large quantities of potassium-rich foods: oranges, bananas, salt substitutes

MONITORING PARAMETERS
• Blood pressure, edema, urine output, ECG (if hyperkalemia exists), urine electrolytes, BUN, creatinine, gynecomastia, impotence

---

aminocaproic acid
(a-mee-noe-ka-proe´ik)
Rx: Amicar
Chemical Class: Synthetic monoaminocarboxylic acid
Therapeutic Class: Hemostatic

CLINICAL PHARMACOLOGY
Mechanism of Action: Inhibits fibrinolysis by inhibiting plasminogen activators and, to a lesser degree, by antiplasmin activity

Pharmacokinetics
PO: Rapidly absorbed, peak 2 hr; excreted by kidneys as unmetabolized drug; $t_{1/2}$ 2 hr

INDICATIONS AND USES: Hemorrhage from systemic hyperfibrinolysis and urinary fibrinolysis; adjunctive therapy in hemophilia*; recurrent subarachnoid hemorrhage*; amegakaryocytic thrombocytopenia,* proposed for topical treatment of traumatic hyphema of the eye*; TOPICAL: Hemostatic mouthwash — prevents bleeding during dental procedures in anticoagulated patients

DOSAGE
Adult
• IV 4-5 g in 250 ml NS, D_5W, or LR, infused over 1 hr, followed by continuous infusion at the rate of 1-1.25 g/hr diluted in 50-100 ml of compatible solution, not to exceed 30 g/day; use infusion pump; do not give by direct IV; PO 5 g loading dose during first hour, then 1-1.25 g qh if needed, not to exceed 30 g/day; TOP 5 g vial for injection qs to 100 mL, hold in area of procedure for 2 min starting 30 minutes before procedure and ql-2 hr after procedure until gone

Child
• IV 100 mg/kg or 3 g/m² loading dose followed by continuous infusion at the rate of 33.3 mg/kg/hr or 1 g/m²/hr; do not exceed 18 g/m²/day; PO 100-200 mg/kg loading dose followed by 100 mg/kg/dose q6h, not to exceed 30 g/day

$ AVAILABLE FORMS/COST OF THERAPY
• Inj, Sol—IV: 250 mg/ml, 20 ml: **$16.24**
• Syr—Oral: 1.25 g/5 ml, 480 ml: **$458.25**
• Tab, Uncoated—Oral: 500 mg, 100's: **$172.43**

CONTRAINDICATIONS: DIC, upper urinary tract bleeding, neonates (injectable contains benzyl alcohol)
PRECAUTIONS: Renal disease, hepatic disease, thrombosis, cardiac disease
PREGNANCY AND LACTATION: Pregnancy category C; excretion in milk unknown; use caution in nursing mothers

---

SIDE EFFECTS/ADVERSE REACTIONS

*CNS: **Cerebral ischemia**, delirium, dizziness,*hallucinations, *headache,* psychosis, ***seizures*** (in treatment of subarachnoid hemorrhage)

CV: Bradycardia, ***dysrhythmias***, hypotension

EENT: Conjunctival suffusion, nasal congestion, tinnitus

GI: Abdominal cramps, diarrhea, nausea, vomiting

GU: Dysuria, ejaculatory failure, frequency, menstrual irregularities, myoglobinuria, oliguria, ***renal failure***

HEME: Thrombosis

MS: Fatigue, malaise, myopathy, rhabdomyolysis, weakness

SKIN: Rash

INTERACTIONS

Labs

• *False increase:* Urine amino acids

SPECIAL CONSIDERATIONS

PATIENT/FAMILY EDUCATION

• Report any signs of bleeding or myopathy

• Change position slowly to decrease orthostatic hypotension

• No need to adjust INR in warfarin anticoagulated patients with topical hemostatic mouthwash use

MONITORING PARAMETERS

• Do **not** administer without a definite diagnosis and laboratory findings indicative of hyperfibrinolysis

• Blood studies including coagulation factors, platelets, fibrinolysin; CPK, urinalysis

---

aminophylline (theophylline ethylenediamine)

(am-in-off'i-lin)

Rx: Truphylline

Chemical Class: Xanthine derivative; ethylenediamine

Therapeutic Class: Antiasthmatic bronchodilator; COPD agent

CLINICAL PHARMACOLOGY

Mechanism of Action: Activity due to theophylline; directly relaxes bronchial and pulmonary smooth muscle; stimulates CNS; induces diuresis; increases gastric acid secretion, decreases lower esophageal sphincter pressure; central respiratory stimulant

Pharmacokinetics

PO: Well absorbed, onset ¼ hr, peak 1-2 hr, duration 6-8 hr

PO SUS ACTION: Peak 4-7 hr, duration 8-12 hr

IV: Onset rapid, duration 6-8 hr

PR: Absorption slow and erratic, onset erratic, peak 3-5 hr, duration 6-8 hr

Metabolized by liver; excreted in urine; $t_{1/2}$ 3-12 hr, $t_{1/2}$ increased in geriatric patients, hepatic disease, cor pulmonale, and CHF, $t_{1/2}$ decreased in children and smoking

INDICATIONS AND USES: Asthma, reversible bronchospasm associated with chronic bronchitis and emphysema; apnea and bradycardia of prematurity*

DOSAGE

Adult and Child

• *PO acute therapy (patients not currently receiving theophylline products):* Following a 6.3 mg/kg loading dose, maintenance dose as follows: children age 1-9 yr, 5.1 mg/kg q6h; children age 9-16 yr and

---

smokers, 3.8 mg/kg q6h; otherwise healthy non-smoking adults, 3.8 mg/kg q8h; older patients/patients with CHF, cor pulmonale, 2.5 mg/kg q8h

• *PO acute therapy (patients currently receiving theophylline products):* Defer loading dose if serum theophylline concentration can be rapidly obtained; base loading dose on the principle that each 0.63 mg/kg of aminophylline will increase serum theophylline concentration by 1 µg/ml; if this is not possible and sufficient respiratory distress is present (without signs of theophylline toxicity), use 3.1 mg/kg of a rapidly available form of aminophylline; will likely increase serum theophylline concentration 5 µg/ml; maintenance dosage as described above

• *PO chronic therapy:* Initial dose 20.3 mg/kg/24 hr or 500 mg/24 hr (whichever is less) divided q6-8h; increase q 3 days by 25% as tolerated until clinical response or maximum dose is reached (below); monitor serum theophylline concentrations; do not exceed the following (or 1140 mg, whichever is less without serum level monitoring): Age 1-9 yr, 30.4 mg/kg/day; age 9-12 yr, 25.3 mg/kg/day; age 12-16 yr, 22.8 mg/kg/day; age 16 yr and older, 16.5 mg/kg/day

• *IV (patients not currently receiving theophylline products):* Following a 6.3 mg/kg IV loading dose, maintenance dose follows: Children age 1-9 yr, 1 mg/kg/hr; children age 9-16 yr and smokers, 0.8 mg/kg/hr; otherwise healthy non-smoking adults, 0.5 mg/kg/hr; older patients/patients with cor pulmonale, 0.3 mg/kg/hr; patients with CHF, 0.1-0.2 mg/kg/hr

• *IV (patients currently receiving theophylline products):* Defer loading dose if serum theophylline concentration can be rapidly obtained. Base loading dose on the principle that each 0.63 mg/kg of aminophylline will increase serum theophylline concentration by 1 µg/ml; if this is not possible and sufficient respiratory distress is present, use 3.1 mg/kg of aminophylline; will likely increase serum theophylline concentration 5 µg/ml (administer only if theophylline toxicity is not present); maintenance dosage as described above

§ AVAILABLE FORMS/COST OF THERAPY

• Inj, Sol—IV: 25 mg/ml, 10 ml: **$1.12**
• Sol—Oral: 105 mg/5 ml, 240 ml: **$11.16-$14.00**
• Supp—Rect: 250mg, 10's: **$13.12-$17.33**; 500 mg, 10's: **$16.47-$19.25**
• Tab, Uncoated—Oral: 100 mg, 100's: **$0.74-$6.05**; 200 mg, 100's: **$1.00-$7.55**

CONTRAINDICATIONS: Hypersensitivity to xanthines or ethylenediamine; underlying seizure disorder (not on anticonvulsant therapy); suppositories are contraindicated in the presence of irritation or infection of the rectum or lower colon

PRECAUTIONS: Elderly, CHF, cor-pulmonale, hepatic disease, pre-existing dysrhythmias, hypertension, infants <1 yr, hypoxemia, sustained high fever, history of peptic ulcer, alcoholism

PREGNANCY AND LACTATION: Pregnancy category C; pharmacokinetics of theophylline may be altered during pregnancy, monitor serum concentrations carefully; excreted into breast milk; may cause irritability in the nursing infant, otherwise compatible with breast feeding

SIDE EFFECTS/ADVERSE REACTIONS

CNS: Anxiety, *dizziness,* headache, insomnia, lightheadedness, muscle twitching, reflex hyperexcitability, restlessness, seizures

CV: **Circulatory failure,** flushing, hypotension, *palpitations, sinus tachycardia,* **ventricular dysrhythmias**

GI: Anal irritation (suppositories), anorexia, bitter taste, black stools, diarrhea, dyspepsia, epigastric pain, esophageal reflux, hematemesis, *nausea, vomiting*

GU: Proteinuria, urinary frequency

METAB: Hyperglycemia, SIADH

RESP: Tachypnea

SKIN: Urticaria, alopecia

INTERACTIONS

Drugs

3 *Adenosine:* Decreased hemodynamic effects of adenosine

3 *Allopurinol, Amiodarone, Cimetidine, Ciprofloxacin, Disulfiram, Erythromycin, Interferon alfa, Isoniazid, Methimazole, Metoprolol, Norfloxacin, Pefloxacin, Pentoxifylline, Propafenone, Propylthiouracil, Radioactive iodine, Tacrine, Thiabendazole, Ticlopidine, Verapamil:* Increased theophylline concentrations

3 *Aminoglutethamide, Barbiturates, Carbamazepine, Moricizine, Phenytoin, Rifampin, Ritonavir, Thyroid hormone:* Reduced theophylline concentrations; decreased serum phenytoin levels

3 *Beta-blockers:* Reduced bronchodilating response to theophylline

❷ *Enoxacin, Fluvoxamine, Mexiletine, Propranolol, Troleandomycin:* Markedly increased theophylline concentrations

3 *Imipenem:* Some patients on theophylline have developed seizures following addition of imipenem

3 *Lithium:* Reduced lithium concentrations

3 *Smoking:* Increased aminophylline dosing requirements

SPECIAL CONSIDERATIONS
PATIENT/FAMILY EDUCATION

• Avoid large amounts of caffeine-containing products

• If GI upset occurs, take with 8 oz water

• Notify clinician if nausea, vomiting, insomnia, jitteriness, headache, rash, palpitations occur

MONITORING PARAMETERS

• Serum theophylline concentrations every 6-12 mo or with status changes (therapeutic level is 10-20 µg/ml); toxicity may occur with small increase above 20 µg/ml, especially in the elderly

• Serious side effects (ventricular dysrhythmias, seizures, death) may occur without preceding signs of less serious toxicity (nausea, restlessness)

---

aminosalicylate
(a-mee-noe-sal-i'si-late)
Rx: P.A.S. Sodium
Chemical Class: Salicylate derivative
Therapeutic Class: Antituberculosis agent

CLINICAL PHARMACOLOGY

Mechanism of Action: Prevents synthesis of folic acid by competitively blocking the conversion of aminobenzoic acid to dihydrofolic acid; bacteriostatic against *Mycobacterium tuberculosis;* inhibits onset of bacterial resistance to isoniazid and streptomycin

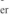

Pharmacokinetics

PO: Peak 0.5-1 hr; concentrates in pleural and caseous tissue; metabolized by liver, excreted in urine; $t_{1/2}$ 1 hr

INDICATIONS AND USES: Alternative treatment of tuberculosis (always in combination with streptomycin, isoniazid, or both), Crohn's disease*

DOSAGE

Adult

• PO 14-16 g/day in 2-3 divided doses

Child

• PO 275-420 mg/kg/day in 3-4 divided doses

💲 AVAILABLE FORMS/COST OF THERAPY

• Tab, Coated—Oral: 500 mg, 100's: **$30.00**

CONTRAINDICATIONS: Severe renal disease; G-6-PD deficiency

PRECAUTIONS: Impaired renal or hepatic function, acidic urine, gastric ulcer, CHF, and other situations in which excess sodium is potentially harmful

PREGNANCY AND LACTATION: Pregnancy category C; excreted into breast milk; use caution in nursing mothers

SIDE EFFECTS/ADVERSE REACTIONS

GI: Abdominal pain, diarrhea, hepatitis, jaundice, *nausea, vomiting*

GU: Crystalluria

HEME: **Agranulocytosis, hemolytic anemia,** increased PT, **leukopenia, thrombocytopenia**

METAB: Goiter with or without myxedema

SKIN: Skin eruptions

MISC: Encephalopathy, fever, infection, Loeffler's syndrome, mononucleosis-like syndrome, vasculitis

INTERACTIONS

Drugs

❸ *Rifampin:* Reduced serum rifampin concentrations

Labs

• *False increase:* BUN, CSF protein serum bilirubin, serum glucose, serum phosphate, urine bile, urine phenylketones, urine porphobilinogen, urine protein, urine vanillylmandelic acid

SPECIAL CONSIDERATIONS

PATIENT/FAMILY EDUCATION

• Administer with food to decrease stomach upset

• Protect from moisture, light, and extremes of temperature

• Notify clinician if fever, sore throat, unusual bleeding, bruising, or skin rashes occur

• 500-mg tablet contains 54.5 mg sodium

---

amiodarone

(a-mee′oh-da-rone)

Rx: Cordarone

Chemical Class: Iodinated benzofuran derivative

Therapeutic Class: Antidysrhythmic (class III)

CLINICAL PHARMACOLOGY

Mechanism of Action: Prolongs action potential duration and effective refractory period; noncompetitive α- and β-adrenergic inhibition

Pharmacokinetics

PO: Slowly and variably absorbed, peak 3-7 hr, onset 1-3 wk; extensive distribution; $t_{1/2}$ 26-107 days; eliminated via hepatic metabolism (CYP3A4) and excretion into bile

INDICATIONS AND USES: Life-threatening recurrent ventricular fibrillation and hemodynamically unstable ventricular tachycardia unresponsive to adequate doses of other

---

antiarrhythmics; refractory-sustained or paroxysmal atrial fibrillation and paroxysmal supraventricular tachycardia,* symptomatic atrial flutter,* CHF (low dose), hypertrophic cardiomyopathy*

DOSAGE

Adult

• IV Loading dose 1000 mg over first 24 hr; 150 mg (15 mg/min) for first 10 min, 360 mg (1 mg/min) over next 6 hr, 540 mg (0.5 mg/min) over remaining 18 hr; maintenance 0.5 mg/min (720 mg/24 hr) up to 3 wk

• PO loading dose 800-1600 mg/day for 1-3 wk; then 600-800 mg/day for 1 mo; maintenance 200-600 mg/day (lower doses effective for supraventricular arrhythmias)

Child

• (The safety and effectiveness of of amiodarone in pediatric patients have not been established)

• PO loading dose 10-15 mg/kg/day or 600-800 mg/1.73 m^2/day for 4-14 days or until adequate control of dysrhythmia or prominent adverse effects occur; maintenance 5 mg/kg/day or 200-400 mg/1.73 m^2/day qd for several weeks; reduce to lowest effective dosage possible

• IV 5 mg/kg over 30 min followed by PO 800 mg qd × 7 days, then 600 mg qd × 3 days, then 200-400 mg qd maintenance; IV load allows shorter time to arrhythmic control than PO load; *or* IV 5 mg/kg bolus followed 15 min later by continuous IV infusion of 20 mg/kg/day for 3-5 days

$ **AVAILABLE FORMS/COST OF THERAPY**

• Inj, Sol—IV: 50 mg/ml, 3 ml: **$98.87**

• Tab, Uncoated—Oral: 200 mg, 100's: **$197.93-$375.78**

CONTRAINDICATIONS: Severe sinus-node dysfunction, with resultant marked sinus bradycardia; 2nd and 3rd degree AV block; syncope caused by episodes of bradycardia (except when used in conjunction with a pacemaker); hypersensitivity

PRECAUTIONS: Thyroid disease, 2nd or 3rd degree AV block, electrolyte imbalances, bradycardia, pulmonary disease (poorer prognosis should pulmonary toxicity develop)

PREGNANCY AND LACTATION: Pregnancy category D; due to a very long t$_{1/2}$, amiodarone should be discontinued several months prior to conception to avoid early gestational exposure, reserve for refractory dysrhythmias; newborns exposed to amiodarone should have TFTs; excreted into breast milk; contains high proportions of iodine; breast feeding not recommended

SIDE EFFECTS/ADVERSE REACTIONS

Adverse reactions occur in about 75% of patients receiving doses ≥400 mg/day and cause discontinuation of drug in 7%-18% of patients

CNS: Ataxia, *dizziness,* fatigue, *headache,* insomnia, involuntary movements, lack of coordination, malaise, paresthesias, peripheral neuropathy, tremors

CV: Bradycardia, **cardiac conduction abnormalities,** CHF, *dysrhythmias,* hypotension, *sinoatrial node dysfunction, sinus arrest*

EENT: Blurred vision, corneal microdeposits, dry eyes, halos, loss of vision, optic neuritis, optic neuropathy, photophobia

GI: Abdominal pain, anorexia, constipation, diarrhea, hepatotoxicity, nausea, vomiting

METAB: Hyperthyroidism or hypothyroidism

MS: Pain in extremities, weakness

RESP: Cough, dyspnea, ***pulmonary fibrosis(^{1}/$_{1000}$),*** pulmonary inflammation

---

* = non-FDA-approved use

SKIN: Alopecia, angioedema, blue-gray skin discoloration, photosensitivity, rash, spontaneous ecchymosis

MISC: Abnormal salivation, abnormal taste or smell, coagulation abnormalities, edema, flushing

INTERACTIONS

Drugs

3 *Aprinidine:* Increased aprinidine concentrations

3 β-*adrenergic blockers:* Bradycardia, cardiac arrest, or ventricular arrhythmia shortly after initiation of β-adrenergic blockers that undergo extensive hepatic metabolism (propranolol, sotalol, metoprolol)

3 *Calcium channel blockers:* Cardiotoxicity with bradycardia and decreased cardiac output with diltiazem and, potentially, verapamil

3 *Cholestyramine, Colestipol:* Decreased amiodarone plasma concentrations

3 *Cimetidine:* Increased amiodarone plasma concentrations (other H$_2$ blockers likely have no effect)

3 *Cyclosporine, Tacrolimus:* Increased cyclosporine, tacrolimus concentrations

3 *Digitalis glycosides:* Accumulation of digoxin

3 *Fentanyl:* In combination with amiodarone may cause hypotension, bradycardia, and decreased cardiac output

3 *Flecainide, Ecainide:* Increased flecainide, ecainide serum concentrations

3 *Methotrexate:* Impaired methotrexate metabolism with >2 weeks oral amiodarone administration

3 *Oral anticoagulants:* Enhanced hypoprothrombinemic response to warfarin (prothrombin time increased 100%), reduce warfarin dose 1/3-1/2

3 *Phenytoin:* Increased serum phenytoin concentrations, decreased amiodarone concentrations

3 *Procainamide:* Increased procainamide concentrations

3 *Protease inhibitors (Indinavir):* Inceased amiodarone plasma concentrations

3 *Quinidine:* Increased quinidine plasma concentrations, reduce quinidine dose by 1/3

3 *Rifampin:* Decreased amiodarone plasma concentrations

3 *St. John's Wort (Hypericum perforatum):* Potential for decreased amiodarone plasma concentrations

3 *Theophylline:* Increased theophylline levels

3 *Volatile anesthetic agents:* Increased sensitivity to myocardial depressant and conduction effects of halogenated inhalational anesthetics

Labs

• *Increase:* Serum T4 and serum reverse T3

• *Decrease:* Serum T3

SPECIAL CONSIDERATIONS

• **Should be administered only by clinicians experienced in treatment of life-threatening dysrhythmias who are thoroughly familiar with the risks and benefits of amiodarone therapy**

• IV amiodarone contains the preservative benzyl alcohol which has been associated with fatal gasping syndrome in neonates

PATIENT/FAMILY EDUCATION

• Take with food and/or divide doses if GI intolerance occurs, do not take oral form with grapefruit juice

• Use sunscreen or stay out of sun to prevent burns

• Report side effects immediately

• Skin discoloration is usually reversible

MONITORING PARAMETERS
• Chest x-ray, ophth referral, and PFTs (baseline and q3 mo)
• Electrolytes
• LFTs
• ECG (measure PR, QRS, QT intervals; check for PVCs, other dysrhythmias); QT interval prolongation of 10%-15% suggests therapeutic effect
• TFTs
• CNS symptoms

---

amitriptyline
(a-mee-trip'ti-leen)
Rx: Elavil
Combinations
  Rx: with chlordiazepoxide (Limbitrol); with perphenazine (Triavil)
Chemical Class: Tertiary amine Dibenzocycloheptadiene derivative
Therapeutic Class: Antidepressant; anxiolytic; antineurolgic

CLINICAL PHARMACOLOGY
Mechanism of Action: Inhibits reuptake of norepinephrine and serotonin (blocking activity moderate and very high, respectively) at the presynaptic neuron, prolonging neuronal activity; inhibits histamine and acetylcholine activity; mild peripheral vasodilator effects and possible "quinidine-like" actions on cardiac conduction; high anticholinergic and sedative, moderate orthostatic hypotensive side effects
Pharmacokinetics
PO/IM: Onset 45 min, peak 2-4 hr, therapeutic response 2-4 wk once adequate dosage achieved; metabolized by liver (active metabolite, nortriptyline), excreted in urine/feces; crosses placenta; $t_{1/2}$ 10-50 hr
INDICATIONS AND USES: Depression, chronic pain (chronic tension headache, migraine, diabetic neuropathy, cancer pain, postherpetic neuralgia),* panic disorder,* eating disorders,* myofacial pain syndromes*
DOSAGE
Adult
• PO 50-100 mg hs, may increase to 200 mg/day, not to exceed 300 mg/day (chronic pain doses usually at lower end of range)
• IM (do not administer IV) 20-30 mg qid, or 80-120 mg hs
Adolescent/Geriatric
• PO 30 mg/day in divided doses, may be increased to 150 mg/day
Child
• *Chronic pain management:* PO 0.1 mg/kg/day in 3 divided doses initially, advance as tolerated over 2-3 weeks to 0.5-2 mg/kg qhs
• *Depression:* PO 1 mg/kg/day in 3 divided doses initially with increases to 1.5 mg/kg/day
$ AVAILABLE FORMS/COST OF THERAPY
• Inj, Sol—IM: 10 mg/ml, 10 ml: **$0.33-$12.16**
• Tab, Coated—Oral: 10 mg, 100's: **$2.25-$25.39**; 25 mg, 100's: **$1.96-$69.95**; 50 mg, 100's: **$3.25-$116.45**; 75 mg, 100's: **$2.45-$124.04**; 100 mg, 100's: **$6.00-$2,156.88**; 150 mg, 100's: **$7.75-$223.19**
CONTRAINDICATIONS: Acute recovery phase of MI, concurrent use of MAOIs
PRECAUTIONS: Suicidal patients, convulsive disorders, prostatic hypertrophy, psychiatric disease, severe depression, increased intraocular pressure, narrow-angle glaucoma, urinary retention, cardiac disease (2nd or 3rd degree heart block or sick sinus syndrome), hepatic disease/renal disease, hyperthyroidism, electroshock therapy, elective surgery, elderly, abrupt discontinuation

---

* = non-FDA-approved use

PREGNANCY AND LACTATION:
Pregnancy category D; excreted into breast milk; effect on nursing infant unknown but may be of concern

SIDE EFFECTS/ADVERSE REACTIONS

CNS: Anxiety, confusion (especially in elderly), *dizziness, drowsiness,* extra-pyramidal symptoms (elderly), fatigue, headache, increased psychiatric symptoms, insomnia, memory impairment, nervousness, nightmares, panic, stimulation, tremors, weakness

CV: **Dysrhythmias,** hypertension, *orthostatic hypotension,* palpitations, syncope, tachycardia

EENT: Blurred vision, mydriasis, nasal congestion, ophthalmoplegia, tinnitus

GI: Constipation, cramps, diarrhea, *dry mouth,* epigastric distress, hepatitis, increased appetite, jaundice, nausea, paralytic ileus, stomatitis, vomiting, weight gain

GU: Urinary retention

HEME: **Agranulocytosis, eosinophilia, leukopenia, thrombocytopenia**

SKIN: Photosensitivity, pruritus, rash, sweating, urticaria

INTERACTIONS

Drugs

3 *Altretamine:* Orthostatic hypotension

3 *Amphetamines:* Theoretical increase in effect of amphetamines, clinical evidence lacking

3 *Anticholinergics:* Excessive anticholinergic effects

3 *Barbiturates:* Reduced serum concentrations of cyclic antidepressants

2 *Bethanidine:* Reduced antihypertensive effect of bethanidine

3 *Carbamazepine:* Reduced antidepressant serum concentrations

3 *Cimetidine (other H$_2$ blockers less likely to have effect):* Inhibition of TCA metabolism

2 *Clonidine:* Reduced antihypertensive response to clonidine; enhanced hypertensive response with abrupt clonidine withdrawal

2 *Epinephrine, norepinephrine:* Enhanced pressor response

3 *Ethanol:* Additive impairment of motor skills; abstinent alcoholics may eliminate cyclic antidepressants more rapidly than non-alcoholics

3 *Fluoxetine, paroxetine:* Marked increases in cyclic antidepressant plasma concentrations

3 *Guanabenz, guanfacine, debrisoquin:* Inhibition of antihypertensive effect

2 *Guanethidine, guanadrel:* Inhibited antihypertensive response to guanethidine

3 *Hypoglycemics:* Enhanced hypoglemic effects

3 *Isoproterenol:* Increased cardiac arrhythmias

3 *Lithium:* Increased risk of neurotoxicity

2 *MAOIs:* Excessive sympathetic response, mania, or hyperpyrexia possible

2 *Moclobemide:* Potential association with fatal or non-fatal serotonin syndrome

3 *Neuroleptics:* Increased therapeutic and toxic effects of both drugs

2 *Norepinephrine:* Markedly enhanced pressor response to norepinephrine

3 *Phenylephrine:* Enhanced pressor response

3 *Propoxyphene:* Enhanced effect of cyclic antidepressants

3 *Quinidine:* Increased cyclic antidepressant serum concentrations

3 *Rifampin:* Possible decreased TCA levels

3 *Ritonavir, indinavir:* Increased TCA levels

Labs

• *False increase:* Carbamazepine levels

SPECIAL CONSIDERATIONS
PATIENT/FAMILY EDUCATION
• Therapeutic effects may take 2-3 wk
• Use caution in driving or other activities requiring alertness
• Avoid rising quickly from sitting to standing, especially elderly
• Avoid alcohol ingestion, other CNS depressants
• Do not discontinue abruptly after long-term use
• Wear sunscreen or large hat to prevent photosensitivity
• Increase fluids, bulk in diet if constipation occurs
• Gum, hard sugarless candy, or frequent sips of water for dry mouth
MONITORING PARAMETERS
• Mental status: mood, sensorium, affect, suicidal tendencies
• Determination of amitriptyline plasma concentrations is not routinely recommended but may be useful in identifying toxicity, drug interactions, or noncompliance (adjustments in dosage should be made according to clinical response not plasma concentrations)
• Therapeutic plasma levels 125-250 µg/L (including active metabolites)

amlexanox
(am-lex′a-nox)
Rx: Aphthasol
Chemical Class: Benzopyranobipyridine carboxylic acid derivative
Therapeutic Class: Antiallergic, antiinflammatory

CLINICAL PHARMACOLOGY
Mechanism of Action: Accelerates healing probably via inhibition of formation or release of inflammatory mediators

INDICATIONS AND USES: To reduce the duration, pain, size and erythema of aphthous ulcers
DOSAGE
Adult
• *Aphthous ulcers:* TOP apply qid after oral hygiene until ulcer heals
$ AVAILABLE FORMS/COST OF THERAPY
• Top—5% paste: 5 g: **$20.88**
PRECAUTIONS: History of contact dermatitis
SIDE EFFECTS/ADVERSE REACTIONS
SKIN: Contact mucositis; transient pain, stinging, or burning at the site of application

amlodipine
(am-low′di-peen)
Rx: Norvasc
Combinations
Rx: with benazepril (Lotrel)
Chemical Class: Dihydropyridine
Therapeutic Class: Calcium channel blocker: antihypertensive; antianginal

CLINICAL PHARMACOLOGY
Mechanism of Action: Inhibits calcium ion influx across cell membrane in vascular smooth muscle and cardiac muscle; produces relaxation of coronary and peripheral vascular smooth muscle; hemodynamics: increases myocardial contractility and cardiac output; significantly decreases peripheral vascular resistance
Pharmacokinetics
PO: Peak serum conc 6-9 hr, bioavailability 60%-65% $t_{1/2}$ 30-50 hr, metabolized by liver, excreted in urine (5%-10% unchanged)

INDICATIONS AND USES: Chronic stable angina pectoris,* hypertension, vasospastic (Prinzmetal's or variant) angina,* CHF*, Raynaud's phenomenon*

DOSAGE

Adult

• *Angina:* PO 5-10 mg qd

• *Hypertension:* PO 5 mg qd initially, may increase up to 10 mg/day (small, fragile, or elderly patients or patients with hepatic insufficiency may be started on 2.5 mg qd)

§ AVAILABLE FORMS/COST OF THERAPY

• Tab, Uncoated—Oral: 2.5 mg, 90's: **$130.60**; 5 mg, 90's: **$113.10**; 10 mg, 90's: **$195.70**

PRECAUTIONS: CHF, hypotension, hepatic insufficiency, aortic stenosis, elderly

PREGNANCY AND LACTATION: Pregnancy category C; unknown if excreted into milk; use caution in nursing mothers

SIDE EFFECTS/ADVERSE REACTIONS

CNS: Anxiety, asthenia, depression, dizziness, lightheadedness, fatigue, headache (7.5%), insomnia, malaise, nervousness, paresthesia, somnolence, tremor

CV: Bradycardia, **dysrhythmia,** hypotension, palpitations, *peripheral edema,* syncope, tachycardia

GI: Abdominal cramps, constipation, diarrhea, dry mouth, flatulence, gastric upset, nausea (3%), vomiting

GU: Nocturia, polyuria

SKIN: Hair loss, pruritus, rash, urticarial

MISC: Cough, epistaxis, flushing, muscle cramps, nasal congestion, sexual dysfunction, shortness of breath, sweating, tinnitus, weight gain

INTERACTIONS

Drugs

❸ *Barbiturates:* Reduced plasma concentrations of amlodipine

❸ *Diltiazem:* Reduced clearance of amlodipine

❸ *Erythromycin:* Reduced clearance of amlodipine

❸ *Fentanyl:* Severe hypotension or increased fluid volume requirements

❸ *Grapefruit juice:* Reduced clearance of amlodipine

❸ *H₂ blockers:* Increased plasma concentration of amlodipine possible

❸ *Proton pump inhibitors:* Increased plasma concentration of amlodipine possible

❸ *Quinidine:* Increased plasma concentration of amlodipine; reduced plasma quinidine level

❸ *Rifampin:* Reduced plasma concentration of amlodipine

❸ *Vincristine:* Reduced vincristine clearance

SPECIAL CONSIDERATIONS

PATIENT/FAMILY EDUCATION

• Notify clinician of irregular heart beat, shortness of breath, swelling of feet and hands, pronounced dizziness, hypotension

---

ammonium lactate
Rx: Lac-Hydrin
Chemical Class: Alpha hydroxy acid
Therapeutic Class: Emollient

CLINICAL PHARMACOLOGY

Mechanism of Action: Natural skin humectant; reduces excessive epidermal keratinization (e.g., ichthyosis)

INDICATIONS AND USES: Dry, scaly skin (xerosis); ichthyosis vulgaris; itching associated with these conditions

---

italic = common side effects   ***bold italic*** = life-threatening reactions

DOSAGE
Adult and Child
• TOP rub in thoroughly to affected areas bid

💲 AVAILABLE FORMS/COST OF THERAPY
• Cre, Top—12%: 140, 280, 385 g: **$58.06**/385 g
• Lotion, Top—12%: 225, 240, 400, 420 g: **$12.95-$42.36**/225 g **$21.50-$66.67**/400 g
• Lotion, Top—5%: 120, 240 ml: **$10.54**/120 ml
• Sol: 500, 2500 ml: **$27.85**/500 ml

PREGNANCY AND LACTATION: Pregnancy category C; unknown if excreted in breast milk; lactic acid is a normal constituent of blood and tissues

SIDE EFFECTS/ADVERSE REACTIONS
SKIN: Burning, erythema, hyperpigmentation, irritation, peeling, stinging

SPECIAL CONSIDERATIONS
• Side effects greater in fair-skinned individuals, if applied to abraded or inflamed areas, and in ichthyosis (where incidence of burning, stinging, and erythema is 10%)

---

amobarbital
(am-oh-bar'bi-tal)
Rx: Amytal
Combinations
  Rx: with secobarbital (Tuinal)
Chemical Class: Barbituric acid derivative
Therapeutic Class: Sedative/hypnotic
DEA Class: Schedule II

CLINICAL PHARMACOLOGY
Mechanism of Action: CNS depressant: depresses the sensory cortex, decreases motor activity, alters cerebellar function, produces drowsiness, sedation, and hypnosis; little analgesic action at subanesthetic doses (may increase reaction to painful stimuli); anticonvulsant activity in anesthetic doses; dose-dependent respiratory depression (hypnotic doses produce respiratory depression similar to physiologic sleep)

Pharmacokinetics
PO: Onset 45-60 min, duration 6-8 hr
IV: Onset 5 min, duration 3-6 hr
Metabolized by liver, excreted by kidneys (inactive metabolites), highly protein bound; $t_{1/2}$ 16-40 hr

INDICATIONS AND USES: Sedation, preanesthetic sedation, short-term (up to 2 wk) treatment of insomnia, anticonvulsant (status epilepticus),* adjunct in psychiatry*

DOSAGE
Adult
• *Preanesthetic sedation:* PO/IM 200 mg 1-2 hr preoperatively
• *Anticonvulsant/psychiatry:* IV 65-500 mg given over several min, not to exceed 100 mg/min; not to exceed 1 g
• *Insomnia:* PO/IM 65-200 mg hs

Child >6 yr
• *Sedation:* PO 2 mg/kg/day in 4 divided doses
• *Anticonvulsant/psychiatry:* IV 65-500 mg given over several min, not to exceed 100 mg/min; not to exceed 1 g
• *Insomnia:* IM 2-3 mg/kg hs

💲 AVAILABLE FORMS/COST OF THERAPY
• Inj, Lyphl-Sol—IM, IV: 0.5 g/vial: **$8.94**
• Cap—Oral (combined with secobarbital): 100 mg/100 mg, 100's: **$25.78**; 200 mg/200 mg, 100's: **$33.08**

CONTRAINDICATIONS: Hypersensitivity to barbiturates, respiratory depression, severe liver impairment, porphyria

---

* = non-FDA-approved use

PRECAUTIONS: Anemia, addiction to barbiturates, hepatic disease, COPD/emphysema, renal disease, hypertension, elderly, acute/chronic pain, mental depression, history of drug abuse, abrupt discontinuation

PREGNANCY AND LACTATION: Pregnancy category D; small amount excreted in breast milk, use caution in nursing mothers

SIDE EFFECTS/ADVERSE REACTIONS

CNS: CNS depression, dizziness, *drowsiness, hangover,* headache, *lethargy,* lightheadedness, mental depression, physical dependence, slurred speech, stimulation in the elderly and children, vertigo

CV: Bradycardia, hypotension

GI: Constipation, diarrhea, nausea, vomiting

HEME: **Agranulocytosis, megaloblastic anemia** (long-term treatment), **thrombocytopenia**

RESP: **Apnea, bronchospasm, depression, laryngospasm**

SKIN: Abscesses at injection site, angioedema, erythema multiforme, pain, *rash,* **Stevens-Johnson syndrome,** thrombophlebitis, urticaria

MISC: Osteomalacia (prolonged use), rickets

INTERACTIONS

Drugs

3 *Acetaminophen:* Enhanced hepatotoxic potential of acetaminophen overdoses

3 *Antidepressants:* Reduced serum concentration of cyclic antidepressants

3 *β-adrenergic blockers:* Reduced serum concentrations of β-blockers which are extensively metabolized

3 *Calcium channel blockers:* Reduced serum concentrations of verapamil and dihydropyridines

3 *Chloramphenicol:* Increased barbiturate concentrations; reduced serum chloramphenicol concentrations

3 *Corticosteroids:* Reduced serum concentrations of corticosteroids; may impair therapeutic effect

3 *Cyclosporine:* Reduced serum concentration of cyclosporine

3 *Digitoxin:* Reduced serum concentration of digitoxin

3 *Disopyramide:* Reduced serum concentrations of disopyramide

3 *Doxycycline:* Reduced serum doxycycline concentrations

3 *Estrogen:* Reduced serum concentration of estrogen

3 *Ethanol:* Excessive CNS depression

3 *Griseofulvin:* Reduced griseofulvin absorption

3 *Methoxyflurane:* Enhanced nephrotoxic effect

3 *MAOIs:* Prolonged effect of barbiturates

3 *Narcotic analgesics:* Increased toxicity of meperidine; reduced effect of methadone; additive CNS depression

3 *Neuroleptics:* Reduced effect of either drug

❷ *Oral anticoagulants:* Decreased hypoprothrombinemic response to oral anticoagulants

3 *Oral contraceptives:* Reduced efficacy of oral contraceptives

3 *Phenytoin:* Unpredictable effect on serum phenytoin levels

3 *Propafenone:* Reduced serum concentration of propafenone

3 *Quinidine:* Reduced quinidine plasma concentrations

3 *Tacrolimus:* Reduced serum concentration of tacrolimus

3 *Theophylline:* Reduced serum theophylline concentrations

3 *Valproic acid:* Increased serum concentration of amobarbital

---

italic = common side effects   ***bold italic*** = life-threatening reactions

❷ *Warfarin:* See oral anticoagulants

SPECIAL CONSIDERATIONS
PATIENT/FAMILY EDUCATION
• Indicated only for short-term treatment of insomnia; probably ineffective after 2 wk; physical dependency may result when used for extended time (45-90 days depending on dose)
• Avoid driving or other activities requiring alertness
• Avoid alcohol ingestion or CNS depressants
• Do not discontinue medication abruptly after long-term use
MONITORING PARAMETERS
• Serum folate, vitamin D (if on long-term therapy)
• PT in patients receiving anticoagulants

---

amoxapine
(a-mox´a-peen)
Rx: Asendin
Chemical Class: Dibenzoxazepine derivative: secondary amine
Therapeutic Class: Tricyclic antidepressant

CLINICAL PHARMACOLOGY
Mechanism of Action: Inhibits reuptake of norepinephrine and serotonin (blocking activity high and moderate, respectively); blocks postsynaptic dopamine receptors; inhibits activity of histamine and acetylcholine; mild peripheral vasodilator effects and possible "quinidine-like" actions; high anticholinergic, moderate sedative, and slight orthostatic hypotension side effects

Pharmacokinetics
PO: Steady state 7 days; metabolized by liver, excreted by kidneys; $t_{1/2}$ 8 hr

INDICATIONS AND USES: Depression in patients with neurotic or reactive depressive disorders; endogenous and psychotic depressions; depression accompanied by anxiety or agitation

DOSAGE
Adult
• PO 50 mg bid-tid, may increase to 100 mg bid-tid by the end of the 1st wk, not to exceed 300 mg/day unless lower doses have been given for at least 2 wk; may be given daily dose hs; not to exceed 600 mg/day in hospitalized patients
Adolescents
• PO 25-50 mg/day, increase gradually to 100 mg/day (divided or as single hs dose)
Child
• Not recommended for patients <16 yr

§ AVAILABLE FORMS/COST OF THERAPY
• Tab, Uncoated—Oral: 25 mg, 100's: **$46.70-$83.24**; 50 mg, 100's: **$76.48-$135.38**; 100 mg, 100's: **$128.99-$225.00**; 150 mg, 30's: **$60.73-$102.30**

CONTRAINDICATIONS: Acute recovery phase of MI, concurrent use of MAOIs

PRECAUTIONS: Suicidal patients, severe depression, increased intraocular pressure, narrow-angle glaucoma, urinary retention, cardiac disease, hepatic disease, hyperthyroidism, electroshock therapy, elective surgery, elderly, convulsive disorders, prostatic hypertrophy

PREGNANCY AND LACTATION: Pregnancy category C; excreted into breast milk; effect on nursing infant unknown but may be of concern

SIDE EFFECTS/ADVERSE REACTIONS
CNS: Anxiety, ataxia, confusion, *dizziness, drowsiness,* EPS, headache, impairment of sexual functioning,

increased psychiatric symptoms, insomnia, **neuroleptic malignant syndrome,** nightmares, paresthesia, **seizures,** stimulation, syncope, tardive dyskinesia, tremor, weakness

CV: Hypertension, *orthostatic hypotension,* palpitations, *tachycardia*

EENT: *Blurred vision,* mydriasis, ophthalmoplegia, tinnitus

GI: Constipation, cramps, diarrhea, *dry mouth,* epigastric distress, hepatitis, increased appetite, jaundice, nausea, paralytic ileus, peculiar taste, stomatitis, vomiting

GU: Urinary retention

HEME: **Agranulocytosis, eosinophilia, leukopenia, thrombocytopenia**

METAB: Breast enlargement, galactorrhea, menstrual irregularity, SIADH

SKIN: Photosensitivity, pruritus, rash, sweating, urticaria

INTERACTIONS

Drugs

3 *Barbiturates:* Reduced serum concentrations of cyclic antidepressants

2 *Bethanidine:* Reduced antihypertensive effect of bethanidine

3 *Carbamazepine:* Reduced serum concentrations of cyclic antidepressants

3 *Cimetidine:* Increased serum concentrations of cyclic antidepressants

3 *Clonidine:* Reduced antihypertensive effect of clonidine; enhanced hypertensive response with abrupt clonidine withdrawal

3 *Debrisoquin:* Reduced antihypertensive effect of debrisoquin

3 *Dilitiazem:* Increased serum concentrations of cyclic antidepressants

2 *Epinephrine:* Markedly enhanced pressor response to IV epinephrine

3 *Ethanol:* Additive impairment of motor skills; abstinent alcoholics may eliminate cyclic antidepressants more rapidly than non-alcoholics

3 *Fluoxetine:* Marked increases in serum concentrations of cyclic antidepressants

3 *Fluvoxamine:* Marked increases in serum concentrations of cyclic antidepressants

3 *Guanabenz, guanadrel, guanethidine, guanfacine:* Reduced antihypertensive effect

3 *Lithium:* Increased risk of neurotoxicity

2 *Moclobemide:* Potential association with fatal or non-fatal serotonin syndrome

⚠ *MAOIs:* Excessive sympathetic response, mania, or hyperpyrexia possible

3 *Neuroleptics:* Increased therapeutic and toxic effects of both drugs

2 *Norepinephrine:* Markedly enhanced pressor response to IV norepinephrine

3 *Paroxetine:* Marked increases in serum concentrations of cyclic antidepressants

3 *Propoxyphene:* Increased serum concentrations of cyclic antidepressants

3 *Quinidine:* Increased serum concentrations of cyclic antidepressants

3 *Rifampin:* Reduced serum concentrations of cyclic antidepressants

3 *Ritonavir:* Marked increases in serum concentrations of cyclic antidepressants

3 *Sulfonylureas:* Cyclic antidepressants may increase hypoglycemic effect

SPECIAL CONSIDERATIONS

PATIENT/FAMILY EDUCATION

• Therapeutic effects may take 2-3 wk

• Use caution in driving or other activities requiring alertness

---

italic = common side effects   ***bold italic*** = life-threatening reactions

• Avoid rising quickly from sitting to standing, especially elderly
• Avoid alcohol ingestion, other CNS depressants
• Do not discontinue abruptly after long-term use
• Wear sunscreen or large hat to prevent photosensitivity
• Increase fluids, bulk in diet if constipation occurs
• Use gum, hard sugarless candy, or frequent sips of water for dry mouth
• Potential for tardive dyskinesia

MONITORING PARAMETERS
• Mental status: mood, sensorium, affect, suicidal tendencies

---

amoxicillin
(a-mox´i-sill-in)

Rx: Amoxil, Moxilin, Senox, Trimox, Wymox
Chemical Class: Aminopenicillin
Therapeutic Class: Antibiotic

CLINICAL PHARMACOLOGY
Mechanism of Action: Inhibits bacterial wall synthesis, bactericidal
Pharmacokinetics
PO: Peak 1 hr, duration 6-8 hr, $t_{1/2}$ 1-1.3 hr; excreted largely unchanged in urine by glomerular filtration and active tubular secretion (can be delayed by concomitant administration of probenecid)
INDICATIONS AND USES: Infections of the ear, nose, throat, GU tract, skin and soft tissues, lower respiratory tract caused by susceptible organisms; gonococcal infections; prevention of bacterial endocarditis Antibacterial spectrum usually includes:

• Gram-positive organisms: Streptococci (including *S. faecalis, S. pyogenes, S. pneumoniae*) and non-penicillinase-producing staphylococci
• Gram-negative organisms: *Haemophilus influenzae, E. coli, Proteus mirabilis,* and *Neisseria gonorrhoeae*

DOSAGE
Adult
• *Systemic infections:* PO 250-500 mg q8h or PO 875 mg q12h
• *Gonorrhea:* PO 3 g given with 1 g probenecid as a single dose (not first line); follow with doxycycline
• *Bacterial endocarditis prophylaxis:* PO 3 g 1 hr before procedure, then 1.5 g 6 hr after initial dose
Child
• *Otitis media:* PO 80-90 mg/kg/day divided q8-12
• *Systemic infections:* PO 20-40 mg/kg/day in divided doses q8h or 25-45 mg/kg/day in divided doses q12h
• *Bacterial endocarditis prophylaxis:* PO 50 mg/kg × 1 (max 2 g dose)

§ AVAILABLE FORMS/COST OF THERAPY
• Cap, Gel—Oral: 250 mg, 100's: **$8.73-$29.59**; 500 mg, 100's: **$16.80-$58.69**; 875 mg, 100's: **$87.21-$96.90**
• Powder, Reconst—Oral: 50 mg/ml, 15 ml: **$1.78-$2.65**; 125 mg/5 ml, 150 ml: **$2.49-$9.55**; 200 mg/5 ml, 100 ml: **$10.15**; 250 mg/5 ml, 150 ml: **$2.19-$10.43**; 400 mg/5 ml; 100 ml: **$10.90**
• Tab, Chewable—Oral: 125 mg, 100's: **$10.90-$23.10**; 200 mg, 100's: **$50.75**; 250 mg, 100's: **$20.58-$33.25**; 400 mg, 100's: **$62.00**

---

* = non-FDA-approved use

PRECAUTIONS: Hypersensitivity to cephalosporins, renal insufficiency, prolonged or repeated therapy, mononucleosis

PREGNANCY AND LACTATION: Pregnancy category B; excreted into breast milk in low concentrations; no adverse effects have been observed, but potential exists for modification of bowel flora and allergy/sensitization in nursing infant

SIDE EFFECTS/ADVERSE REACTIONS

CNS: Fever, headache

GI: Abdominal pain, colitis, *diarrhea,* glossitis, increased AST, ALT, *nausea,* pseudomembranous colitis, *vomiting*

HEME: **Bone marrow depression,** eosinophilia, increased bleeding time

RESP: **Anaphylaxis,** respiratory distress

MISC: Hypersensitivity reactions (rashes, urticaria, erythema multiforme, **exfoliative dermatitis, anaphylaxis**)

INTERACTIONS

Drugs

🔳 *Atenolol:* Reduced serum concentration of atenolol

🔳 *Chloramphenicol:* Inhibited antibacterial activity of amoxicillin; administer amoxicillin 3 hours before chloramphenicol

🔳 *Macrolide antibiotics:* Inhibited antibacterial activity of amoxicillin; administer amoxicillin 3 hours before macrolides

🔳 *Methotrexate:* Increased serum methotrexate concentrations

🔳 *Oral contraceptives:* Occasional impairment of oral contraceptive efficacy; consider use of supplementary contraception during cycles in which amoxicillin is used

🔳 *Tetracyclines:* Inhibited antibacterial activity of amoxicillin; administer amoxicillin 3 hours before tetracycline

SPECIAL CONSIDERATIONS

PATIENT/FAMILY EDUCATION

• May administer on a full or empty stomach

• Administer at even intervals

• Shake oral suspensions well before administering; discard after 14 days

• High rates of rash in patients on allopurinol, with mononucleosis, lymphocytic leukemia

---

amoxicillin/clavulanate

(a-mox′i-sill-in clav-u-lan′ate)

Rx: Augmentin

Chemical Class: Aminopenicillin; β-lactamase inhibitor

Therapeutic Class: Antibiotic

CLINICAL PHARMACOLOGY

Mechanism of Action: Inhibits bacterial wall synthesis; bactericidal; clavulanate protects amoxicillin from degradation by β-lactamase enzymes, extending the spectrum of activity

Pharmacokinetics

PO: Peak 2 hr, duration 6-8 hr, $t_{1/2}$ 1-1.3 hr; excreted largely unchanged in urine

INDICATIONS AND USES: Infections of the lower respiratory tract, ear, sinuses, skin and soft tissues, urinary tract caused by susceptible organisms

Antibacterial spectrum usually includes:

• Gram-positive organisms: *Staphylococcus aureus, S. epidermidis, S. saprophyticus, Enterococcus, S. pneumoniae, S. pyogenes, S. viridans*

• Gram-negative organisms: *Hemophilus influenzae, Moraxella catarrhalis, Escherichia coli, Klebsiella* sp., *Enterobacter* sp., *Proteus mirabilis, P. vulgaris, Neisseria gonorrhoeae, Legionella* sp.

• Anaerobes: *Clostridium* sp., *Peptococcus* sp., *Peptostreptococcus* sp., *Bacteroides* sp., including *B. fragilis*

DOSAGE

Adult

• PO 250-500 mg (amoxicillin) q8h depending on severity of infection or 875 mg bid

Child

• PO 20-40 mg/kg/day (amoxicillin) in divided doses q8h; use chewable tablets under 40 kg for correct clavulanate dose

§ AVAILABLE FORMS/COST OF THERAPY

• Powder, Reconst—Oral: 125 mg/31.25 mg/5 ml, 150 ml: **$27.00-$41.54**; 200 mg/28.5 mg/5 ml 100 ml: **$30.95-$44.46**; 250 mg/62.5 mg/5 ml, 150 ml: **$51.40-$80.88**; 400 mg/57 mg/5 ml, 100 ml: **$56.15-$77.50**; 600 mg/42.9 mg/5 ml, 100 ml: **$52.03**

• Tab, Chewable—Oral: 125 mg/31.25 mg, 30's: **$27.40-$41.54**; 200 mg/28.5 mg, 20's: **$30.95**; 250 mg/62.5 mg, 30's: **$51.70-$79.22**; 400 mg/57 mg, 20's: **$58.95**

• Tab, Uncoated—Oral: 250 mg/125 mg, 30's: **$56.00-$91.00**; 500 mg/125 mg, 20's: **$62.65-$84.10**; 875 mg/125 mg, 20's: **$88.60-$117.97**

NOTE: Due to clavulanate strength, 2 × 250 mg tabs do not equal a 500 mg tab

CONTRAINDICATIONS: Hypersensitivity to penicillins

PRECAUTIONS: Hypersensitivity to cephalosporins, renal insufficiency, prolonged or repeated therapy, mononucleosis

PREGNANCY AND LACTATION: Pregnancy category B; excreted into breast milk in low concentrations; no adverse effects have been observed

SIDE EFFECTS/ADVERSE REACTIONS

CNS: Fever, headache

GI: Abdominal pain, black tongue, colitis, *diarrhea,* (9%) glossitis, increased AST, ALT, nausea, pseudomembranous colitis, vomiting

GU: Moniliasis, vaginitis

HEME: **Bone marrow depression,** eosinophilia, increased bleeding time

METAB: Alkalosis, hyperkalemia, hypernatremia, hypokalemia

MISC: Hypersensitivity reactions (rash, urticaria, erythema multiforme, *exfoliative dermatitis, anaphylaxis*)

INTERACTIONS

Drugs

§ *Atenolol:* Reduced serum concentration of atenolol

§ *Chloramphenicol:* Inhibited antibacterial activity of amoxicillin; administer amoxicillin 3 hours before chloramphenicol

§ *Macrolide antibiotics:* Inhibited antibacterial activity of amoxicillin; administer amoxicillin 3 hours before macrolides

§ *Methotrexate:* Increased serum methotrexate concentrations

§ *Oral contraceptives:* Occasional impairment of oral contraceptive efficacy; consider use of supplementary contraception during cycles in which amoxicillin is used

§ *Tetracyclines:* Inhibited antibacterial activity of amoxicillin; administer amoxicillin 3 hours before tetracycline

SPECIAL CONSIDERATIONS

PATIENT/FAMILY EDUCATION

• Administer with food to decrease GI side effects

---

* = non-FDA-approved use

• Administer at even intervals
• Shake oral suspensions well before administering; discard after 14 days; must be refrigerated

---

amphetamine

(am-fet´a-meen)
Combinations
  Rx: with dextroamphetamine: (Adderall, Adderall XR)
Chemical Class: β-phenylisopropylamine (racemic)
Therapeutic Class: CNS stimulant
DEA Class: Schedule II

CLINICAL PHARMACOLOGY

Mechanism of Action: Sympathomimetic amines with CNS stimulant activity; increases release of norepinephrine from central noradrenergic neurons; at higher doses dopamine may be released in the mesolimbic system; peripheral alpha and beta activity includes elevation of systolic and diastolic blood pressures and weak bronchodilator and respiratory stimulation action; heart rate reflexly slowed at standard doses, arrhythmias with overdose

Pharmacokinetics

PO: Immed Rel: Onset 30 min, peak 1-3 hr, duration 4-20 hr; metabolized by liver, excreted by kidneys, crosses placenta; $t_{1/2}$ dependent on urinary pH; at urinary pH <5.6, $t_{1/2}$ is 7-8 hr (increases with alkalinization of urine)

INDICATIONS AND USES: Attention Deficit Hyperactivity Disorder; narcolepsy; short-term adjunct to caloric restriction in exogenous obesity* **(high potential for abuse, use only when alternative therapies have failed)**

DOSAGE

Adult

• *Narcolepsy:* Immed Rel PO 5-60 mg qd in divided doses
• *Obesity:* Immed Rel PO 5-30 mg in divided doses 30-60 min before meals

Child

• *Attention Deficit Hyperactivity Disorder:* >6 yr: Immed Rel PO 5 mg qd-bid increasing by 5 mg/day at weekly intervals (will rarely exceed 40 mg/day); Sus Action PO 10 mg qd increasing by 10 mg/day at weekly intervals (max recommended dose is 30 mg/day); 3-5 yr: Immed Rel PO 2.5 mg qd increasing by 2.5 mg/day at weekly intervals (usual range 0.1-0.5 mg/kg/dose)
• *Narcolepsy:* >12 yr: Immed Rel PO 10 mg qd increasing by 10 mg/day at weekly intervals; 6-12 yr: Immed Rel PO 5 mg qd increasing by 5 mg/wk (max 60 mg/day)

⑤ AVAILABLE FORMS/COST OF THERAPY

• Tab, Combination—Oral: 5, 7.5, 10, 12.5, 15, 20, 30 mg, 100's: all: **$128.17**
• Tab, Combination, Sus Action—Oral: 10, 20, 30 mg, 100's: all: **$234.00**

CONTRAINDICATIONS: Hyperthyroidism, moderate to severe hypertension, glaucoma, severe arteriosclerosis, history of drug abuse, cardiovascular disease, agitated states, within 14 days of MAOI administration

PRECAUTIONS: Mild hypertension, child <3 yr, Tourette's syndrome, motor and phonic tics

PREGNANCY AND LACTATION: Pregnancy category C; use of amphetamine for medical indications not a significant risk to the fetus for congenital anomalies, mild withdrawal symptoms may be observed

---

italic = common side effects   ***bold italic*** = life-threatening reactions

in the newborn; illicit maternal use presents significant risks to the fetus and newborn, including intrauterine growth retardation, premature delivery, and the potential for increased maternal, fetal, and neonatal morbidity; concentrated in breast milk; contraindicated during breast feeding

SIDE EFFECTS/ADVERSE REACTIONS

CNS: Addiction, aggressiveness, changes in libido, chills, dependence, dizziness, dyskinesia, dysphoria, euphoria, headache, *hyperactivity, insomnia,* irritability, overstimulation, psychotic episodes, *restlessness, talkativeness,* tremor

CV: **Dysrhythmias** (at larger doses), hypertension, *palpitations,* reflex decrease in heart rate, *tachycardia*

GI: Anorexia, constipation, cramps, diarrhea, dry mouth, metallic taste, nausea, vomiting, weight loss

GU: Impotence

METAB: Reversible elevations in serum thyroxine (T_4) with heavy use

SKIN: Urticaria

INTERACTIONS

Drugs

🔳 *Antacids:* May inhibit amphetamine excretion

🔳 *Ethosuximide:* Intestinal absorption of ethosuximide may be delayed

🔳 *Furazolidone:* Hypertensive reactions

🔳 *Guanadrel:* Inhibits antihypertensive response to guanadrel

🔳 *Guanethidine:* Inhibits antihypertensive response to guanethidine

🔳 *Lithium:* May inhibit effects of amphetamines

⚠️ *MAOIs:* Severe hypertensive reactions possible

🔳 *Methenamine:* Urinary excretion of amphetamine is increased by acidifying agents

❷ *Norepinephrine:* Adrenergic effect of norepinephrine enhanced

🔳 *Phenobarbital:* Intestinal absorption of phenobarbital may be delayed; synergistic anticonvulsant effect possible

🔳 *Phenytoin:* Intestinal absorption of phenytoin may be delayed; synergistic anticonvulsant effect possible

⚠️ *Propoxyphene:* In cases of propoxyphene overdosage, amphetamine CNS stimulation is potentiated, fatal convulsions can occur

❷ *Selegiline:* Severe hypertensive reactions possible

🔳 *Sodium bicarbonate:* May inhibit amphetamine excretion

❷ *Tricyclic antidepressants:* May enhance activity of tricyclics; increased amphetamine levels in the brain; CV effects potentiated

Labs

• *False positive:* Urine amino acids

• May interfere with urinary steroid determinations

SPECIAL CONSIDERATIONS

PATIENT/FAMILY EDUCATION

• Take early in the day

• Do not discontinue abruptly

• Avoid hazardous activities until stabilized on medication

---

amphotericin B, amphotericin B cholesteryl, amphotericin B lipid complex, liposomal amphotericin B

(am-foe-ter'i-sin)

Rx: Abelcet (ABLC); AmBisome, Amphotec, Fungizone (IV and topical)
Chemical Class: Amphoteric polyene; lipid complex (ABLC)
Therapeutic Class: Antifungal

CLINICAL PHARMACOLOGY

Mechanism of Action: Binds to sterols in the cell membrane of susceptible fungi with a resultant change in cell permeability allowing leakage of intracellular components; fungistatic or fungicidal depending on concentration obtained in body fluids and the susceptibility of the fungus

Pharmacokinetics

IV: Peak 1-2 hr, initial plasma $t_{1/2}$ 24 hr, elimination $t_{1/2}$ 15 days; metabolic pathways are not known, very slowly excreted by the kidneys (metabolites), highly bound to plasma proteins; poorly penetrates CSF, bronchial secretions, aqueous humor, muscle, bone, brain, pancreas; not removed by hemodialysis

ABLC: Metabolic pathways unknown, pharmacokinetics not linear; clearance from blood increases with increasing doses; terminal elimination $t_{1/2}$ approx 173 hr; effect of hepatic and renal impairment on disposition unknown

INDICATIONS AND USES: TOP: Cutaneous and mucocutaneous mycotic infections caused by *Candida* sp. IV: Potentially life-threatening fungal infections: aspergillosis *(A. fumigatus),* cryptococcosis (torulo-sis), North American blastomycosis, systemic candidiasis, coccidioidomycosis and histoplasmosis, mucormycosis due to susceptible species of the genera *Absidia* sp., *Mucor* sp., *Rhizopus* sp., *Entomophthora* sp., and *Basidiobolus* sp., sporotrichosis *(S. schenckii);* American mucocutaneous leishmaniasis (not drug of choice as primary therapy); empirical therapy for presumed fungal infection in febrile neutropenic patients

ABLC: Treatment of aspergillosis in patients refractory to or intolerant of conventional amphotericin B therapy (may have less nephrotoxicity)

Do not use IV form of amphotericin B to treat noninvasive fungal infections, such as oral thrush, vaginal candidiasis and esophageal candidiasis in patients with normal neutrophil counts

DOSAGE

Adult and Child

• TOP bid-qid for 7-21 days or longer if needed

• IV INF (minimum dilution 0.1 mg/ml) infuse 1 mg test dose slowly over 20-30 min to determine patient tolerance; initial therapeutic dose (if test dose tolerated) 0.25 mg/kg/day over 4-6 hr; individualize subsequent doses by increasing in 0.25 mg/kg/day increments (usual range 0.25-1 mg/kg/day); do not exceed 1.5 mg/kg/day; amphotericin cholesteryl IV INF 3-4 mg/kg/day at a rate of 1 mg/kg/hr; ABLC IV INF 5.0 mg/kg/day at a rate of 2.5 mg/kg/hr; liposomal amphotericin B IV INF 3-5 mg/kg/day over 2 hr; INTRATHECAL 25-100 µg q48-72 hr; increase to 500 µg as tolerated; BLADDER IRRIGATION 5-15 mg/100 ml of sterile water irrigation solution at 100-300 ml/day; instill into bladder, clamp catheter for 60-120 minutes then drain; repeat 3-4 times/day for 2-5 days

§ AVAILABLE FORMS/COST OF THERAPY

ABLC
• Inj, Sol—IV: 5 mg/ml, 10 ml: **$134.66**

Amphotericin B
• Cre—Top: 3%, 20 g: **$32.71**
• Inj, Lyphl, Sol—IV: 50 mg vial, 1's: **$10.00-$45.48**
• Lotion—Top: 3%, 30 ml: **$44.86**
• Susp—Oral: 100 mg/ml, 24 ml, 1's: **$27.21**

Amphotericin B Cholesteryl Sulfate
• Inj, Lyphl, Sol—IV: 50 mg vial, 1's: **$84.00**; 100 mg vial, 1's: **$160.00**

Amphotericin B Liposomal
• Inj, Lyphl—IV: 50 mg vial, 1's: **$196.25**

PRECAUTIONS: Renal disease, rapid IV infusion, prior total body irradiation, leukocyte infusions, avoid eye contact

PREGNANCY AND LACTATION: Pregnancy category B; excretion in human milk unknown: due to the potential toxicity, consider discontinuing nursing

SIDE EFFECTS/ADVERSE REACTIONS

Severe reactions may be lessened by giving acetaminophen, antihistamines, and antiemetics before infusion and by maintaining sodium balance; meperidine or hydrocortisone may also help

CNS: Chills, dizziness, *fever, headache,* paresthesias, peripheral nerve pain, peripheral neuropathy, *seizures*

CV: Cardiac arrest, dysrhythmias, hypertension, hypotension, *ventricular fibrillation*

EENT: Blurred vision, deafness, diplopia, tinnitus

GI: Acute liver failure, anorexia, cramps, diarrhea, epigastric pain, hemorrhagic gastroenteritis, *nausea, vomiting*

GU: Anuria, azotemia, *hypokalemia,* hyposthenuria, nephrocalcinosis, oliguria, *permanent renal impairment (especially with doses >5 g),* renal tubular acidosis

HEME: Agranulocytosis, eosinophilia, hypomagnesemia, hyponatremia, *leukopenia,* normochromic, normocytic anemia, *thrombocytopenia*

MS: Arthralgia, generalized pain, myalgia, weakness, weight loss

SKIN: Burning, irritation, pain, necrosis at injection site with extravasation; contact dermatitis, dry skin, erythema, flushing, pruritus, staining of nail lesions, stinging, urticaria

INTERACTIONS

Drugs

3 *Aminoglycosides:* Synergistic nephrotoxicity

3 *Cyclosporine:* Increased nephrotoxicity of both drugs

3 *Neuromuscular blocking agents:* Prolonged muscle relaxation due to hypokalemia

Labs

• *Increase:* Serum bilirubin, serum conjugated bilirubin, serum cholesterol

• *Decrease:* Serum unconjugated bilirubin

SPECIAL CONSIDERATIONS

PATIENT/FAMILY EDUCATION

• Long-term therapy may be needed to clear infection (2 wk-3 mo depending on type of infection)

MONITORING PARAMETERS

• BUN, serum creatinine; if BUN exceeds 40 mg/dl or serum creatinine exceeds 3 mg/dl, discontinue the drug or reduce dosage until renal function improves

A

• Regular monitoring of CBC, K, Na, Mg, LFTs
• Total dosage

---

ampicillin

(am'pi-sill-in)

Rx: Marcillin, Principen, Totacillin

Combinations

Rx: with probenecid (Polycillin PRB, Probampicin)

Chemical Class: Aminopenicillin

Therapeutic Class: Antibiotic

CLINICAL PHARMACOLOGY

Mechanism of Action: Inhibits bacterial wall synthesis; bactericidal

Pharmacokinetics

PO: Peak 2 hr

IV: Peak 5 min

IM: Peak 1 hr

$t_{1/2}$ 50-110 min, excreted largely unchanged in urine by glomerular filtration and active tubular secretion (can be delayed by concomitant administration of probenecid)

INDICATIONS AND USES: Infections of the respiratory tract and soft tissues caused by susceptible organisms; bacterial meningitis caused by susceptible organisms; septicemia; gonococcal infections; prevention of bacterial endocarditis; prophylaxis in cesarean section*

Antibacterial spectrum usually includes:

• Gram-positive organisms: α- and β-hemolytic streptococci, *Streptococcus pneumoniae,* nonpenicillinase-producing staphylococci, *Bacillus anthracis,* and most strains of enterococci and clostridia

• Gram-negative organisms: *Haemophilus influenzae, Neisseria gonorrhoeae, N. meningitidis, N. ca-* tarrhalis, *Escherichia coli, Proteus mirabilis, Bacteroides funduliformis, Salmonella* sp. and *Shigella* sp.

DOSAGE

Adult

• *Systemic infections:* PO 250-500 mg q6h; IV/IM 500 mg-3 g q4-6h

• *Meningitis:* IV 8-14 g/day in divided doses q3-4h

• *Gonorrhea:* PO 3.5 g given with 1 g probenecid as a single dose

• *Renal impairment:* CrCl 10-30 ml/min: administer q6-12h; CrCl <10 ml/min: administer q12h

Child

• *Systemic infections:* PO 50-100 mg/kg/day in divided doses q6h; IV/IM 100-200 mg/kg/day in divided doses q4-6h; max 2-3 g/day

• *Meningitis:* IV 200-400 mg/kg/day in divided doses q4-6h; max 12 g/day

⑤ AVAILABLE FORMS/COST OF THERAPY

• Cap, Gel—Oral: 250 mg, 100's: **$7.43-$18.56**; 500 mg, 100's: **$15.85-$33.12**

• Inj, Dry-Sol—IM, IV: 125 mg/vial, 1's: **$0.98-$2.47**; 250 mg/vial, 1's: **$0.62-$9.50**; 500 mg/vial, 1's: **$1.04-$10.50**; 1 g/vial, 1's: **$1.30-$18.75**; 2 g/vial, 1's: **$2.30-$29.50**

• Powder, Reconst—Oral: 125 mg/5 ml, 200 ml: **$2.95-$9.69**; 250 mg/5 ml, 200 ml: **$2.10-$3.43**

PRECAUTIONS: Hypersensitivity to cephalosporins, renal insufficiency, prolonged or repeated therapy, mononucleosis, neonates

PREGNANCY AND LACTATION: Pregnancy category B; excreted into breast milk in low concentrations; no adverse effects have been observed

---

SIDE EFFECTS/ADVERSE REACTIONS

CNS: Anxiety, *coma,* depression, hallucinations, lethargy, *seizures* twitching

GI: Black "hairy" tongue, *diarrhea,* glossitis, *nausea,* pseudomembranous colitis, stomatitis, *vomiting,* increased AST/ALT

GU: Glomerulonephritis, hematuria, *moniliasis,* oliguria, proteinuria, *vaginitis*

HEME: **Bone marrow depression,** increased bleeding time, eosinophilia

MISC: Hypersensitivity reactions (rashes, urticaria, erythema multiforme, **exfoliative dermatitis anaphylaxis**)

INTERACTIONS

Drugs

3 *Atenolol:* Reduced serum concentration of atenolol

3 *Chloramphenicol:* Inhibited antibacterial activity of ampicillin; administer ampicillin 3 hr before chloramphenicol

3 *Macrolide antibiotics:* Inhibited antibacterial activity of ampicillin; administer amoxicillin 3 hr before macrolides

3 *Methotrexate:* Increased serum methotrexate concentrations

3 *Oral contraceptives:* Occasional impairment of oral contraceptive efficacy; consider use of supplemental contraception during cycles in which ampicillin is used

3 *Tetracyclines:* Inhibited antibacterial activity of ampicillin; administer ampicillin 3 hr before tetracycline

Labs

• *False positive:* Urine amino acids

• *Increase:* Urine glucose (Clinitest method), plasma phenyldanine (dried blood spot method), CSF protein (Ektachem method), serum protein (Biuret method), serum theophylline (3M Diagnostics TheoFast method), serum uric acid

• *Decrease:* Serum cholesterol (CHOD-iodide method only), serum folate (bioassay method only), urine glucose (Clinistix and Diastix methods)

SPECIAL CONSIDERATIONS
PATIENT/FAMILY EDUCATION

• Administer on an empty stomach

• Administer at even intervals

• Shake oral suspensions well before administering, discard after 14 days

• High rates of rash in patients on allopurinol, with mononucleosis, lymphatic leukemia

• Amoxicillin is better oral choice given greater ease of dosing and lower incidence of diarrhea

---

ampicillin/sulbactam

(am'pi-sill-in/sul-bac'tam)
Rx: Unasyn
Chemical Class: Aminopenicillin (ampicillin); penicillinate (sulbactam)
Therapeutic Class: Antibiotic

CLINICAL PHARMACOLOGY

Mechanism of Action: Inhibits bacterial cell wall synthesis; sulbactam inhibits β-lactamase; bactericidal

Pharmacokinetics

IV: Immediate peak, serum $t_{1/2}$ 1 hr; 75%-85% excreted unchanged in urine

IM: Peak levels lower than for IV administration

INDICATIONS AND USES: Infections of skin and skin structures; gynecological infections; intraabdominal infections caused by susceptible organisms

---

* = non-FDA-approved use

Antibacterial spectrum usually includes:
• Gram-positive organisms: *Staphylococcus aureus, S. epidermidis, S. saprophyticus, Enterococcus, Streptococcus pneumoniae, S. pyogenes, S. viridans*
• Gram-negative organisms: *Hemophilus influenzae, Moraxella catarrhalis, Escherichia coli, Klebsiella* sp., *Proteus mirabilis, P. vulgaris, Providencia* sp., *Morganella morganii, Neisseria gonorrhoeae*
• Anaerobes: *Clostridium* sp., *Peptococcus* sp., *Peptostreptoccoccus* sp., *Bacteroides* sp. including *B. fragilis*

DOSAGE
Adult and Child ≥40 kg
• IV/IM 1.5-3.0 g (ampicillin + sulbactam) q6h
• Child <40 kg, ≥1 yr old, IV 300 mg/kg/day (200 mg ampicillin/100 mg sulbactam) in divided doses q6h
• *Impaired renal function:*

CREATININE CLEARANCE (ML/MIN/1.73 M²)	T½ (HR)	DOSAGE
≥30	1	1.5-3.0 g q6-8h
15-29	5	1.5-3.0 g q12h
5-14	9	1.5-3.0 g q24h

💲 AVAILABLE FORMS/COST OF THERAPY
• Inj, Dry-Sol—IM, IV: 1.5 g, (1 g ampicillin + 0.5 g sulbactam) 1's: **$8.13-$9.15**; 3.0 g, (2 g ampicillin + 1 g sulbactam) 1's: **$15.35-$16.23**
CONTRAINDICATIONS: Hypersensitivity to penicillins
PRECAUTIONS: Mononucleosis (incidence of rash 43%-100%); safety not established in children
PREGNANCY AND LACTATION: Pregnancy category B; animal studies at doses 10× the human dose reveal no evidence of harm; low concentrations excreted in breast milk

SIDE EFFECTS/ADVERSE REACTIONS
CNS: Fatigue, headache, malaise, *seizures* (overdosage)
EENT: Epitaxis, glossitis, stomatitis
GI: Abdominal distension, diarrhea (3%), elevated LFTs, flatulence, gastritis, nausea, *pseudomembranous colitis,* vomiting
GU: Dysuria, increased BUN/creatinine, urinary retention
HEME: **Bone marrow depression**
SKIN: Erythema multiforme, *exfoliative dermatitis,* pain at injection site (16% for IM, 3% for IV), rash (2%), thrombophlebitis (3%), urticaria
MISC: **Anaphylaxis**
INTERACTIONS
Drugs
🩸 *Chloramphenicol:* Inhibited antibacterial activity of ampicillin/sulbactam; administer ampicillin/sulbactam 3 hr before chloramphenicol
🩸 *Macrolide antibiotics:* Inhibited antibacterial activity of ampicillin/sulbactam; administer ampicillin/sulbactam 3 hr before macrolides
🩸 *Methotrexate:* Increased serum methotrexate concentrations
🩸 *Oral contraceptives:* Occasional impairment of oral contraceptive efficacy; consider use of supplemental contraception during cycles in which ampicillin/sulbactam is used
🩸 *Tetracyclines:* Inhibited antibacterial activity of ampicillin/sulbactam; administer ampicillin/sulbactam 3 hr before tetracyclines
Labs
• *False positive:* Urine amino acids
• *Increase:* Urine glucose (Clinitest method), plasma phenyldanine (dried blood spot method), CSF protein (Ektachem method), serum protein (biuret method), serum theophylline (3M Diagnostics TheoFast method), serum uric acid, serum creatinine

---

• *Decrease:* Serum cholesterol (CHOD-iodide method only), serum folate (bioassay method only)

SPECIAL CONSIDERATIONS

• Do not reconstitute or administer with aminoglycosides (ampicillin inactivates aminoglycosides, may be administered separately)

• Safety and efficacy established for pediatric skin and soft tissue infections only

---

amprenavir

(am-prehn´-eh-veer)

Rx: Agenerase
Chemical Class: HIV protease inhibitor
Therapeutic Class: HIV infection

CLINICAL PHARMACOLOGY
Mechanism of Action: Inhibits HIV protease preventing cleavage of viral polypeptides resulting in the formation of immature noninfectious viral particles

Pharmacokinetics
PO: Peak 1-2 hr; bioavailability 70% with capsule, 60% with liquid; 90% protein bound; metabolized by CYP 3A4 isoenzyme with metabolites found in stool and urine; 3% excreted unchanged in urine; inhibits CYP 3A4 to a degree similar to nelfinavir; $t_{1/2}$ 7-10 hr

INDICATIONS AND USES: HIV infection treatment

DOSAGE
Adult and Child >16 yr
• PO 1200 mg bid
• For hepatic insufficiency, reduce dose: Child-Pugh score 5-8: 450 mg bid; Child-Pugh score 9-12: 300 mg bid
• For latest treatment guidelines, see www.hivatis.org

Child 4-16 yr
• PO CAP 20 mg/kg bid (max 2400 mg per day); LIQ 22.5 mg/kg bid (max 2800 mg per day)
• For latest treatment guidelines, see www.hivatis.org

💲 AVAILABLE FORMS/COST OF THERAPY
• Cap—Oral: 50 mg, 480's: **$211.48**; 150 mg, 240's: **$317.22**
• Liq—Oral: 15 mg/ml, 240 ml: **$36.77**

NOTE: Capsules of amprenavir contain 109 IU of vitamin E; liquid contains 46 IU per ml

PRECAUTIONS: Blood coagulation defects related to vitamin K deficiency, child under 4 yr old, diabetes mellitus, hemophilia A or B, hepatic insufficiency (adjust dose), hypersensitivity to other protease inhibitors, oral contraceptive use, sulfonamide allergy

PREGNANCY AND LACTATION: Pregnancy category C; excreted in breast milk of animals

SIDE EFFECTS/ADVERSE REACTIONS

CNS: Depression or mood disorder (15%), headache (10%), paresthesia (8%), perioral paresthesia (26%)
GI: Abdominal pain, *diarrhea (10%), nausea, vomiting*
METAB: Hyperglycemia, hypertriglyceridemia
SKIN: Rash (10%)

INTERACTIONS
Drugs
3 *Abacavir:* Mild increase in amprenavir plasma level when given with abacavir
⚠ *Astemizole:* Increased plasma levels of astemizole
3 *Barbiturates:* Increased clearance of amprenavir; reduced clearance of barbiturates

---

❷ *Carbamazepine:* Increased clearance of amprenavir; reduced clearance of carbamazepine

▲ *Cisapride:* Increased plasma levels of cisapride

▲ *Ergot alkaloids:* Increased plasma levels of ergot alkaloids

❸ *Erythromycin:* Reduced clearance of amprenavir; amprenavir reduces clearance of erythromycin

▲ *Lovastatin:* Amprenavir reduces clearance of lovastatin

▲ *Midazolam:* Increased plasma levels of midazolam and prolonged effect

❸ *Nevirapine:* Reduces plasma amprenavir levels

❸ *Oral contraceptives:* Amprenavir may reduce efficacy

❸ *Phenytoin:* Increased clearance of amprenavir; reduced clearance of phenytoin

❷ *Rifabutin:* Increased clearance of amprenavir; reduced clearance of rifabutin

▲ *Rifampin:* Increased clearance of amprenavir

❸ *Ritonavir:* Decreased clearance of amprenavir

❸ *Saquinavir:* Decreased clearance of saquinavir; reduce dose of Fortovase (saquinavir soft gel capsule) to 800 mg tid

❸ *Sildenafil:* Decreased clearance of sildenafil

▲ *Simvastatin:* Amprenavir reduces clearance of simvastatin

▲ *Terfenadine:* Increased plasma levels of terfenadine

▲ *Triazolam:* Increased plasma levels of triazolam and prolonged effect

SPECIAL CONSIDERATIONS
PATIENT/FAMILY EDUCATION
• May take with or without food, but do not take with a high-fat meal
• Do not take supplemental vitamin E; capsule and liquid forms have vitamin E in them

MONITORING PARAMETERS
• CBC, metabolic panel, hepatic function panel, CD4 lymphocyte count, HIV RNA level

---

amrinone

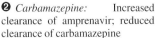

(am´ri-none)
Rx: Inocor
Chemical Class: Bipyrimidine derivative
Therapeutic Class: Cardiac inotropic agent

CLINICAL PHARMACOLOGY
Mechanism of Action: Cardiac inotrope distinct from digitalis glycosides or catecholamines; direct vasodilator, which reduces preload and afterload; not a β-adrenergic agonist; dose-related increases in cardiac output occur (28% at 0.75 mg/kg to about 61% at 3 mg/kg IV bolus); pulmonary capillary wedge pressure, total peripheral resistance, and diastolic and mean arterial pressures show dose-related decreases; heart rate generally unchanged

Pharmacokinetics

Onset of action 2-5 min, peak 10 min, duration variable, $t_{1/2}$ 4-6 hr; metabolized in liver, 60%-90% excreted in urine as drug and metabolites; in patients with compromised renal and hepatic perfusion, plasma levels of amrinone may rise during the infusion period

INDICATIONS AND USES: Short-term management of congestive heart failure unresponsive to other medication

DOSAGE
Adult

• IV bolus 0.75 mg/kg over 2-3 min; start infusion of 5-10 µg/kg/min; may give another 0.75 mg/kg bolus 30 min after start of therapy; daily dose should not exceed 10 mg/kg;

the above dosing regimen will yield a plasma concentration of amrinone of 3 μg/ml; increases in cardiac index show a linear relationship to plasma concentration in a range of 0.5 μg/ml to 7 μg/ml

💲 AVAILABLE FORMS/COST OF THERAPY

• Inj, Sol—IV: 5 mg/ml, 20 ml vial: **$61.90-$85.20**

CONTRAINDICATIONS: Hypersensitivity to bisulfites, severe aortic or pulmonic obstructive valvular disease, acute MI

PRECAUTIONS: Diuretic therapy (decreased cardiac filling pressure may cause decreased response to amrinone), arrhythmias, aortic or pulmonic valvular disease

PREGNANCY AND LACTATION: Pregnancy category C

SIDE EFFECTS/ADVERSE REACTIONS

CV: Chest pain, *dysrhythmias (3%),* headache, hypotension (1.3%)

GI: Abdominal pain, anorexia, hepatotoxicity, hiccups, nausea, vomiting

HEME: Thrombocytopenia (2.4%); dose dependent

RESP: Pleuritis

SKIN: Allergic reactions, burning at injection site

MISC: Fever, hypersensitivity reaction manifested by pleuritis, pericarditis, myositis, or interstitial pulmonary infiltrates

INTERACTIONS

Drugs

• *Furosemide:* Precipitates when furosemide is injected into an IV line infusing amrinone

Labs

• *Increase:* Serum digoxin (Abbott TdX method)

SPECIAL CONSIDERATIONS
MONITORING PARAMETERS

• BP and pulse q5 min during infusion; if BP drops 30 mm Hg, stop infusion

• Cardiac output and pulmonary capillary wedge pressure

• Monitor platelet count and serum K, Na, Cl, Ca, BUN, creatinine, ALT, AST, and bilirubin daily

---

amyl nitrite
(am´il)
Rx: Amyl nitrite
Chemical Class: Organic nitrate
Therapeutic Class: Vasodilator: Anti-anginal; cyanide antidote

---

CLINICAL PHARMACOLOGY

Mechanism of Action: Stimulation of c-GMP production yields vascular smooth muscle relaxation; venous dilation predominates but dose-dependent dilation of arterial beds occurs; dilation of postcapillary vessels promotes venous pooling, decreases venous return to the heart, reducing left ventricular end-diastolic pressure (preload); arteriolar relaxation reduces systemic vascular resistance and arterial pressure (afterload); myocardial oxygen consumption/demand is decreased; blood pressure decreases with reflex tachycardia; converts hemoglobin to methemoglobin, which binds to cyanide

Pharmacokinetics

INH: Onset 30 sec, duration 3-5 min; metabolized by liver, ⅓ excreted in urine

INDICATIONS AND USES: Acute angina pectoris, cyanide poisoning, diagnostic aid in cardiac auscultation*

---

* = non-FDA-approved use

DOSAGE

With the patient seated or recumbent, a capsule of amyl nitrite is crushed with the fingers and held to the nostrils for inhalation of the vapors

Adult

• *Angina pectoris, cardiac diagnostic aid:* INH 0.18-0.3 ml cap as needed, 1-6 INH from 1 cap, may repeat in 3-5 min

• *Cyanide poisoning:* INH 0.3 ml cap inhaled for 15 sec until sodium nitrite infusion is ready

$ AVAILABLE FORMS/COST OF THERAPY

• Sol—INH: 0.3 ml: **$2.99-$7.44**

CONTRAINDICATIONS: Severe anemia, increased intracranial pressure, hypertension, cerebral hemorrhage

PRECAUTIONS: Volatile nitrites abused for sexual stimulation; transient dizziness, weakness, or other signs of cerebral hypoperfusion may develop following inhalation; glaucoma

PREGNANCY AND LACTATION: Pregnancy category: markedly reduces systemic blood pressure and blood flow on maternal side of the placenta

SIDE EFFECTS/ADVERSE REACTIONS

CNS: Dizziness, headache, syncope, weakness

*CV: **Cardiovascular collapse,*** palpitations, *postural hypotension,* tachycardia

GI: Abdominal pain, nausea, vomiting

GU: Urinary incontinence

HEME: Hemolytic anemia, methemoglobinemia

MS: Muscle twitching

SKIN: Flushing, pallor, sweating

INTERACTIONS

Drugs

3 *Alcohol:* Exaggerated hypotension and cardiac collapse

3 *Calcium channel blockers:* Exaggerated symptomatic orthostatic hypotension

3 *Dihydroergotamine:* Increases the bioavailability of dihydroergotamine with resultant increase in mean standing systolic blood pressure; functional antagonism, decreasing effects

3 *Sildenafil:* Excessive hypotensive effects

Labs

• False decrease in cholesterol via Zlatkis-Zak color reaction

SPECIAL CONSIDERATIONS
PATIENT/FAMILY EDUCATION

• Drug should be inhaled while the patient is seated or lying down

• Taking after drinking alcohol may worsen side effects

• Alert to probable headache, dizziness, or flushing side effects

• Amyl nitrite is very flammable

• Tolerance may develop with repeated use

---

anagrelide

(ah-na′ greh-lide)
Rx: Agrylin
Chemical Class: Quinazoline derivative
Therapeutic Class: Anti-platelet agent

CLINICAL PHARMACOLOGY

Mechanism of Action: Reduces blood platelet count, perhaps via a dose-related reduction in platelet production resulting from a decrease in megakaryocyte hypermaturation

---

Pharmacokinetics
PO: Peak 1 hr, bioavailability reduced by food; extensively metabolized; metabolites eliminated in urine (>70%) and feces (10%); $t_{1/2}$ 1.3 hr, terminal elimination $t_{1/2}$ approximately 3 days

INDICATIONS AND USES: Essential thrombocythemia—secondary to myeloproliferative disorders

DOSAGE

Adult

• PO 0.5 mg qid or 1 mg bid; dose may be adjusted after at least 1 wk to the lowest amount required to maintain platelet count <600,000; do not increase dose by >0.5 mg/day in any 1 wk period; do not exceed 10 mg/day or 2.5 in a single dose

$ **AVAILABLE FORMS/COST OF THERAPY**

• Cap, opaque—Oral: 0.5 mg, 100's: **$590.90**; 1 mg, 100's: **$1,181.78**

PRECAUTIONS: Known or suspected heart disease; renal or hepatic function impairment

PREGNANCY AND LACTATION: Pregnancy category C; not recommended in women who are or may become pregnant; excretion into breast milk unknown

SIDE EFFECTS/ADVERSE REACTIONS

CNS: Dizziness, headache (44.5%)
*CV: **Arrhythmia, cerebrovascular accident,** chest pain, **CHF,** edema,* hemorrhage, *palpitations,* postural hypotension, syncope, *tachycardia,* vasodilation
EENT: Abnormal vision, amblyopia, diplopia, epistaxis, rhinitis, sinusitis, tinnitus
GI: Abdominal pain, anorexia, aphthous stomatitis, constipation, *diarrhea* (24.3%), *dyspepsia,* elevated liver enzymes, *flatulence,* gastritis, **GI hemorrhage,** melena, *nausea, vomiting*

GU: Dysuria, hematuria
HEME: Anemia, ecchymosis, lymphadenoma, ***thrombocytopenia***
MS: Arthralgia, *back pain,* leg cramps, myalgia
RESP: Asthma, *dyspnea*
SKIN: Alopecia, photosensitivity, pruritus, rash
MISC: Asthenia, chills, fever, flu symptoms, *malaise,* neck pain, *pain, paresthesia*

SPECIAL CONSIDERATIONS
MONITORING PARAMETERS

• Platelet count q2 days during first wk, then weekly thereafter until maintenance dose reached

---

anistreplase

(an-ih-strep´layz)
Rx: Eminase
Chemical Class: Anisoylated plasminogen streptokinase activator complex
Therapeutic Class: Thrombolytic

CLINICAL PHARMACOLOGY
Mechanism of Action: Promotes thrombolysis by promoting conversion of plasminogen to plasmin; made *in vitro* from lys-plasminogen and streptokinase

Pharmacokinetics
IV: Onset immediate, $t_{1/2}$ of fibrinolytic activity of circulating anistreplase 70-120 min

INDICATIONS AND USES: Acute myocardial infarction

DOSAGE

Adult

• IV 30 U over 4-5 min as soon as possible after onset of symptoms

$ **AVAILABLE FORMS/COST OF THERAPY**

• Powder—Inj: 30 U/vial, 1 vial: **$2,511.93**

CONTRAINDICATIONS: History of severe allergic reactions to anistreplase or streptokinase, active internal bleeding, intraspinal or intracranial surgery within 2 mo, neoplasms of CNS, severe hypertension, cerebral embolism/thrombosis/hemorrhage, known bleeding diathesis

PRECAUTIONS: Recent major surgery, previous puncture of noncompressible vessels, cerebrovascular disease, recent gastrointestinal or genitourinary bleeding, recent trauma; hypertension: systolic BP ≥180 mm Hg and/or diastolic BP ≥110 mm Hg; high likelihood of left heart thrombosis; acute pericarditis, subacute bacterial endocarditis, hemostatic defects, including those secondary to severe hepatic or renal disease; severe hepatic or renal dysfunction; pregnancy; diabetic hemorrhagic retinopathy or other hemorrhagic ophthalmic conditions; septic thrombophlebitis; advanced age; patients currently receiving oral anticoagulants; any other condition in which bleeding constitutes a significant hazard

Readministration
Because of the increased likelihood of resistance due to antistreptokinase antibody, anistreplase may not be effective if administered between 5 days and 12 mo after prior anistreplase or streptokinase therapy; risk of allergic reactions also increased following readministration

PREGNANCY AND LACTATION: Pregnancy category C

SIDE EFFECTS/ADVERSE REACTIONS
CNS: Agitation, dizziness, fever, headache, paresthesia, sweating, tremor, vertigo
*CV: **Dysrhythmias and conduction disorders (38%)**, hypotension (10%)*
EENT: Epistaxis

GI: Elevated transaminase levels, nausea, vomiting
GU: Hematuria
*HEME: GI (2%), GU (2%), **intracranial (1%), retroperitoneal**, or surface bleeding (total incidence 15%), **thrombocytopenia***
MS: Arthralgia, low back pain
*RESP: **Bronchospasm**, dyspnea, hemoptysis*
SKIN: Flushing, itching, phlebitis at infusion site, rash, urticaria
*MISC: **Anaphylaxis (0.2%)***
INTERACTIONS
Drugs
3 *Heparin, oral anticoagulants, drugs that alter platelet function (i.e., aspirin, dipyridamole, abciximab, eptifibitide, tirofiban):* May increase the risk of bleeding

---

anthralin
(anth-rah'lin)
Rx: Dritho-Scalp, Drithocreme, Micanol
Chemical Class: Anthratriol derivative
Therapeutic Class: Anti-psoriatic; keratolytic

CLINICAL PHARMACOLOGY
Mechanism of Action: Reduces the mitotic rate and proliferation of epidermal cells in psoriasis by inhibiting the synthesis of nucleic protein
Pharmacokinetics
Absorption in humans has not been determined; appears to be low
INDICATIONS AND USES: Psoriasis
DOSAGE
Adult
• Begin with the lowest concentration (0.1%) and gradually increase until desired effect is obtained

• *Skin:* TOP apply at bedtime to plaque sites; wash off remaining drug in the morning
• *Scalp:* TOP massage into affected areas; shampoo in the morning

§ AVAILABLE FORMS/COST OF THERAPY

• Cre—Top: 0.1%, 50 g: **$38.35-$65.49**; 0.25%, 50 g: **$30.24-$36.29**; 0.5%, 50 g: **$46.15-$54.50**; 1%, 50 g: **$47.23-$65.44**

CONTRAINDICATIONS: Acute psoriasis (where inflammation is present)

PRECAUTIONS: Excessive irritation, renal and hepatic impairment, inflammation, application to face, genitalia, or intertriginous skin

PREGNANCY AND LACTATION: Pregnancy category C; excretion into human milk unknown; because of the potential for tumorigenicity shown in animal studies, use with caution in nursing mothers

SIDE EFFECTS/ADVERSE REACTIONS

SKIN: Discoloration of fingernails, *irritation of normal skin,* sensitivity reaction, staining of hair

SPECIAL CONSIDERATIONS
PATIENT/FAMILY EDUCATION

• Use plastic gloves for application and wear a plastic cap over treated scalp at bedtime to avoid staining
• Apply a protective film of petrolatum to areas surrounding plaque
• May stain fabrics

---

argatroban
(ar-gat′tro-ban)
Rx: Acova
Chemical Class: Peptide
Therapeutic Class: Anticoagulant; direct thrombin inhibitor

CLINICAL PHARMACOLOGY
Mechanism of Action: Direct thrombin inhibitor that reversibly binds to the thrombin active site; does not require the co-factor antithrombin for antithrombotic activity; exerts anticoagulant effects by inhibiting thrombin-catalyzed or induced reactions, including fibrin formation, activation of coagulation factors V, VIII, and XIII, protein C and platelet aggregation; capable of inhibiting the action of both free and clot-associated thrombin

Pharmacokinetics
IV: Onset immediate, steady-state concentrations of drug and anticoagulant effect within 1-3 hr and maintained until infusion is discontinued; 54% bound to plasma proteins; metabolized by liver, excreted primarily in the feces, presumably through biliary secretion; $t_{1/2}$ 39-51 min

INDICATIONS AND USES: Anticoagulant for prophylaxis or treatment of thrombosis in patients with heparin-induced thrombocytopenia (HIT)

DOSAGE
Adult
• IV (dilute with 0.9% NS, D_5W or LR to a final concentration of 1 mg/ml prior to administration) 2 µg/kg/min administered as a continuous infusion; check aPTT 2 hr after initiation and adjust infusion rate to achieve aPTT of 1.5-3 times

the initial baseline value (infusion rate adjustment should not exceed 10 µg/kg/min)

• For patients with moderate hepatic impairment, an initial dose of 0.5 µg/kg/min is recommended

$ AVAILABLE FORMS/COST OF THERAPY

• Inj, Sol—IV: 100 mg/ml, 2.5 ml: **$780.00**

CONTRAINDICATIONS: Overt major bleeding

PRECAUTIONS: All parenteral anticoagulants should be discontinued prior to argatroban administration; disease states and other circumstances in which there is an increased danger of bleeding (severe hypertension, recent lumbar puncture, spinal anesthesia, major surgery, gastrointestinal lesions, congenital or acquired bleeding disorders); hepatic impairment; children <18 yr

PREGNANCY AND LACTATION: Pregnancy category B; excretion into human milk unknown, use caution in nursing mothers

SIDE EFFECTS/ADVERSE REACTIONS

CNS: **Intracranial hemorrhage,** cerebrovascular disorder

CV: Hypotension, **cardiac arrest, ventricular tachycardia**

GI: **Gastrointestinal hemorrhage,** diarrhea, nausea, vomiting, abdominal pain

GU: Hematuria, abnormal renal function

HEME: Decreased hemoglobin/hematocrit

RESP: Hemoptysis, dyspnea, coughing

MISC: **Multisystem hemorrhage,** allergic reactions, pain

INTERACTIONS

Drugs

3 *Antiplatelet agents:* Increased bleeding risk

3 *Heparin:* Allow heparin's effect on the aPTT to decrease prior to initiation of argatroban; co-administration is unlikely since heparin is contraindicated in patients with HIT

3 *Warfarin:* Increased prolongation of prothrombin time and INR (see SPECIAL CONSIDERATIONS)

Labs

• *Increased:* aPTT, PT, INR, activated clotting time, thrombin time

SPECIAL CONSIDERATIONS

• Recognize the potential for combined effects on INR with co-administration of argatroban and warfarin; an INR should be measured daily while argatroban and warfarin are co-administered; in general, with doses of argatroban up to 2 µg/kg/min, argatroban can be discontinued when the INR is >4 on combined therapy; after argatroban is discontinued, repeat the INR measurement in 4-6 hr; resume the argatroban infusion if the repeat INR is below the desired therapeutic range; repeat this procedure daily until the desired therapeutic range on warfarin alone is reached; for argatroban doses greater than 2 µg/kg/min, temporarily reduce the dose of argatroban to a dose of 2 µg/kg/min; repeat the INR on argatroban and warfarin 4-6 hr after reduction of the argatroban dose and follow the process outlined above for administering argatroban at doses up to 2 µg/kg/min

MONITORING PARAMETERS

• aPTT, hemoglobin, hematocrit, platelet count

---

italic = common side effects   **bold italic** = life-threatening reactions

ascorbic acid (vitamin C)
(a-skor'bic)

Rx: injection: Cenolate, CEE-500, Mega-C/A Plus, Ortho/CS

OTC: Ascorbicap, Cecon, Cevi-Bid, Ce-Vi-Sol, C-Crystals, Cebid Timecelles, Dull-C, Flavorcee, N'ice Vitamin C Drops

Chemical Class: Water soluble vitamin

Therapeutic Class: Urinary acidifier; vitamin

CLINICAL PHARMACOLOGY
Mechanism of Action: Needed for wound healing, collagen synthesis, carbohydrate metabolism; antioxidant

Pharmacokinetics

PO: Readily absorbed; metabolized in liver by oxidation and sulfation, unused amounts excreted in urine (unchanged) and as metabolites

INDICATIONS AND USES: Prevention and treatment of scurvy; urinary acidifying agent; dietary supplementation

DOSAGE
Adult

• *Scurvy:* PO/SC/IM/IV 100 mg-500 mg qd for at least 2 wk, then 50 mg or more qd

• *Urinary acidification:* PO/SC/IM/IV 4-12 g qd in divided doses

• *Dietary supplementation:* PO/SC/IM/IV 50-200 mg qd

Child

• *Scurvy:* PO/SC/IM/IV 100-300 mg qd for at least 2 wk, then 35 mg or more qd

• *Urinary acidification:* PO/SC/IM/IV 500 mg q6-8h

• *Dietary supplementation:* PO/SC/IM/IV 35-100 mg qd

$ AVAILABLE FORMS/COST OF THERAPY

• Inj, Sol—IM, IV, SC: 250 mg/ml, 2 ml: **$3.68**; 500 mg/ml, 2 ml: **$3.79-$7.50**

• Sol—Oral: 100 mg/ml, 50 ml: **$18.68**; 250 mg/ml, 500 ml: **$33.20**

• Syr—Oral: 500 mg/ml, 480 ml: **$14.00**

• Tab—Oral: 100 mg, 100's: **$1.03-$5.65**; 250 mg, 100's: **$1.30-$5.32**; 500 mg, 100's: **$1.54-$7.26**; 1000 mg, 100's: **$3.25-$9.25**

• Tab, Chewable—Oral: 250 mg, 100's: **$1.80-$4.60**; 500 mg, 100's: **$2.70-$9.69**

PRECAUTIONS: Gout, excessive doses for prolonged periods of time (diabetics, patients with recurrent renal calculi, patients undergoing anticoagulant therapy), tartrazine sensitivity, sulfite sensitivity, G-6-PD deficiency

PREGNANCY AND LACTATION: Pregnancy category A if doses do not exceed the RDA, otherwise pregnancy category C; excreted into breast milk via a saturable process; the RDA during lactation is 90-100 mg; maternal supplementation up to the RDA is needed only in those women with poor nutritional status

SIDE EFFECTS/ADVERSE REACTIONS

CNS: Dizziness, fatigue, flushing, headache, insomnia

GI: Anorexia, cramps, diarrhea, heartburn, nausea, vomiting

GU: Crystalluria, oxalate or urate renal stones, polyuria, urine acidification

HEME: Hemolysis (after large doses in patients with G-6-PD deficiency), *sickle-cell crisis*

INTERACTIONS
Drugs
3 *Antacids:* Vitamin C increases the amount of aluminum absorbed from aluminum-containing antacids

Labs
• *False negative:* Amine-dependent stool occult blood, urine bilirubin, blood, leukocyte determinations
• *False positive:* Urine glucose
• *Decrease:* Urine amphetamine, serum AST (Ames Seralyzer method), urine barbiturate (Abbott TDx method) serum bicarbonate (Kodak Ektachem 700 method), serum bilirubin (Jendrassik method), serum cholesterol (Olympus, Abbott TDx, CHOD-PAP methods), serum CK (Kodak Ektachem Systems), serum creatinine (Merck, Wako, Boehringer Mannheim methods), urine glucose (glucose oxidase methods), serum HDL-cholesterol (Kodak Ektachem Systems), urine oxalate (oxalate decarboxylase methods), urine porphobilinogen, serum triglycerides (GPO-PAP, Boehringer Mannheim methods), serum urea nitrogen (Ames Seralyzer), serum uric acid (Ames Seralyzer), urine uric acid (Kodak Ektachem Systems)
• *Increase:* Serum amylase (only at toxic ascorbic acid levels), serum AST (SMA 12/60 method), serum bilirubin (SMA 12/60 method), serum glucose (SMA 12/60 and O-toluidine methods), serum HbAlc (electrophoretic method), urine β-hydroxybutyrate, urine 17-hydroxy corticosteroids, urine iodide, urine 17-ketosteroids, urine oxalate (chromatographic methods), serum phosphate (Boehringer-Mannheim method), CSF and urine protein (Kodak Ektachem Systems), serum uric acid (Klein and phosphotungstate methods)

aspirin

A

(as′pir-in)
Rx: Aspirin CR, Aspirin Delayed Release, Easprin, ZORprin
OTC: Ascriptin, Aspergum, Bayer, Bayer Children's Aspirin, Ecotrin, Ecotrin Maximum Strength, 8-Hour Bayer Extended Release, Empirin, Maximum Bayer, Norwich
Combinations
 Rx: with butalbital (Fiorinal); with codeine (Empirin); with dihydrocodeine and caffeine (Synalgos DC); with dipyridamole (Aggrenox); with oxycodone (Percodan); with propoxyphene (Darvon)
 OTC: with antacids (Ascriptin, Bufferin, Magnaprin)
Chemical Class: Salicylate derivative
Therapeutic Class: Nonnarcotic analgesic; antiinflammatory; antiplatelet agent; antipyretic

CLINICAL PHARMACOLOGY
Mechanism of Action: Inhibits prostaglandin synthesis and release; acts on the hypothalamus heat-regulating center to reduce fever; blocks prostaglandin synthetase action, which prevents formation of the platelet-aggregating substance thromboxane A_2

Pharmacokinetics
PO: Well-absorbed; enteric coated product may exhibit erratic absorption; onset 15-30 min (delayed with enteric coated), peak 1-2 hr, duration 4-6 hr
PR: Absorption erratic, onset slow, duration 4-6 hr

---

italic = common side effects   ***bold italic*** = life-threatening reactions

Metabolized by liver, metabolites excreted by kidneys; $t_{1/2}$ 3 hr at lower doses (300-600 mg), 5-6 hr (1000 mg) up to 30 hrs in larger doses (due to saturable metabolic pathways)

INDICATIONS AND USES: Mild to moderate pain and fever; inflammatory conditions such as rheumatic fever, rheumatoid arthritis; osteoarthritis; thromboembolic disorders; reducing risk of recurrent transient ischemic attacks; reducing the risk of death or nonfatal MI in patients with previous MI or unstable angina; prevention of systemic embolism in patients with atrial fibrillation or prosthetic heart valves*; low doses may be useful in preventing toxemia of pregnancy*; to reduce the risk of stroke in patients who have had transient ischemia of the brain or completed ischemic stroke due to thrombosis (Aggrenox)

DOSAGE

Adult

• *Arthritis:* PO 2.6-5.2 g/day in divided doses q4-6h

• *Pain/fever:* PO/PR 325-650 mg q4h prn, not to exceed 4 g/day

• *Acute ischemic stroke:* PO (within 48 hours) 160-325 mg qd

• *Transient ischemic attacks:* PO 50-325 mg qd

• Heart disease (stable angina, unstable angina, acute MI, clinical or laboratory evidence of CAD): PO 160-325 mg qd

• *Atrial fibrillation* (<65 yr and no risk factors or unable to take warfarin): PO 75-325 mg qd

• Following CABG with no risk factors: PO 325 mg qd for 1 yr

• *Mechanical caged ball heart valve:* PO 80-100 mg (given with warfarin)

• *Any mechanical heart valve and additional clot risk factors:* PO 80 mg qd (given with warfarin)

• *Mechanical heart valve patients who develop systemic embolism:* PO 80 mg qd (given with warfarin)

• *Bioprosthetic heart valve and sinus rhythm after warfarin for 3 mo:* PO 160 mg qd

Child

• *Arthritis:* PO 60-90 mg/kg/day in divided doses; usual maintenance dose 80-100 mg/kg/day divided q6-8h; maintain serum salicylate level of 150-300 µg/ml

• *Pain/fever:* PO/PR 10-15 mg/kg/dose q4-6h prn

§ AVAILABLE FORMS/COST OF THERAPY

• Gum Tab, Chewable—Oral: 227.5 mg, 16's: **$2.18**

• Supp—Rect: 60 mg, 12's: **$2.19-$3.25**; 125 mg, 12's: **$1.88-$4.95**; 300 mg, 12's: **$1.47-$3.56**; 600 mg, 12's: **$1.61-$3.75**; 1200 mg, 12's: **$2.13**

• Tab, Chewable—Oral: 81 mg, 100's: **$6.89**

• Tab, Enteric Coated—Oral: 81 mg, 60's: **$4.86**; 162 mg, 60's: **$3.08-$4.20**; 300 mg, 100's: **$3.70**; 325 mg, 100's: **$0.94-$22.30**; 500 mg, 60's: **$2.50-$6.48**; 650 mg, 100's: **$3.95**; 975 mg, 100's: **$8.19-$59.15**

• Tab, Film Coated—Oral: 325 mg, 100's: **$0.56-$14.04**; 500 mg, 100's: **$1.10-$7.44**; 650 mg, 100's: **$2.79-$13.55**

• Tab, Sus Action—Oral: 800 mg, 100's: **$7.66-$90.61**; 975 mg, 100's: **$11.48-$14.50**

CONTRAINDICATIONS: Hypersensitivity to salicylates, NSAIDs, or tartrazine (FDC yellow dye #5); GI bleeding; hemophilia; hemorrhagic states

PRECAUTIONS: Anemia, asthma, nasal polyps, nasal allergies, hepatic disease, renal disease, Hodgkin's disease, pre/postoperatively, children or teenagers with flu-like symptoms (may be associated with the development of Reye's syndrome), gout, history of coagulation defects, bleeding disorders

PREGNANCY AND LACTATION: Pregnancy category C (category D if full doses used in 3rd trimester); use in pregnancy should generally be avoided; in pregnancies at risk for the development of pregnancy-induced hypertension and preeclampsia, and in fetuses with intrauterine growth retardation, low-dose aspirin (40-150 mg/day) may be beneficial; excreted into breast milk in low concentrations

SIDE EFFECTS/ADVERSE REACTIONS

CNS: Confusion, dizziness, drowsiness, headache

EENT: Dimness of vision, reversible hearing loss, tinnitus

GI: Acute reversible hepatotoxicity, anorexia, cholestasis, diarrhea, *dyspepsia,* epigastric discomfort, **GI bleeding,** heartburn, increased transaminase levels, *nausea*

HEME: Decreased plasma iron concentration, hyperuricemia (low dose), hyperuricosuria (high dose), *leukopenia,* prolonged bleeding time, shortened erythrocyte survival time, ***thrombocytopenia***

METAB: Hypoglycemia, hypokalemia, hyponatremia

RESP: Hyperpnea, wheezing

SKIN: Angioedema, bruising, hives, rash, urticaria

MISC: Fever, thirst

INTERACTIONS

Drugs

3 *ACE inhibitors:* Reduced antihypertensive effect

2 *Acetazolamide:* Increased concentrations of acetazolamide, possibly leading to CNS toxicity

3 *Antacids:* Decreased serum salicylate concentrations; high dose salicylates only

3 *Corticosteroids:* Increased incidence and/or severity of GI ulceration; enhanced salicylate excretion

3 *Diltiazem:* Enhanced antiplatelet effect of aspirin

3 *Ethanol:* Enhanced aspirin-induced GI mucosal damage and aspirin-induced prolongation of bleeding time

3 *Griseofulvin:* Reduced serum salicylate level

3 *Intrauterine contraceptive device:* May reduce contraceptive effectiveness

2 *Methotrexate:* Increased serum methotrexate concentrations and enhanced methotrexate toxicity

2 *Oral anticoagulants:* Increased risk of bleeding by inhibiting platelet function and possibly by producing gastric erosions

3 *Probenecid:* Salicylates inhibit the uricosuric activity of probenecid

3 *Sulfinpyrazone:* Salicylates inhibit the uricosuric activity of sulfinpyrazone

3 *Sulfonylureas:* Enhanced hypoglycemic response to sulfonylureas

2 *Warfarin:* Enhanced hypoprothrombinemic effect of warfarin

3 *Zafirlukast:* Increased plasma concentrations of zafirlukast

Labs

• *Increase:* Serum acetaminophen (Glynn-Kendal method), urine acetoacetate (Gerhardt ferric chloride procedure), urine glucose (Ames Clinitest method), serum HbAlc (chromatographic and electrophoretic, but not colorimetric methods), urine hippuric acid, urine homogentisic acid, urine homovanillic acid, urine ketones (Gerhardt's test), urine phenyl ketones, CSF and urine protein (Folm-Ciocalteu method), serum and urine uric acid (non-specific methods only)

• *Decrease:* Serum albumin, urine glucose (glucose oxidase methods), total serum phenytoin (but not free serum phenytoin)

SPECIAL CONSIDERATIONS
PATIENT/FAMILY EDUCATION
• Administer with food
• Do not exceed recommended doses
• Read label on other OTC drugs, many contain aspirin
• Therapeutic response may take 2 wk (arthritis)
• Avoid alcohol ingestion, GI bleeding may occur
• **Not to be given to children with flu-like symptoms, Reye's syndrome may develop**

MONITORING PARAMETERS
• AST, ALT, bilirubin, creatinine, CBC, hematocrit if patient is on long-term therapy

---

atenolol
(a-ten´oh-lol)
Rx: Tenormin
Combinations
  Rx: with chlorthalidone
    (Tenoretic)
Chemical Class: β_1-selective (cardioselective) adrenoreceptor blocker
Therapeutic Class: Antihypertensive; antianginal

CLINICAL PHARMACOLOGY
Mechanism of Action: Competitive beta-adrenergic agonist inhibition at β_1 receptor sites (cardioselective at usual doses; β_2-blockade noted at higher doses); produces negative inotropic and chronotropic responses; slows AV nodal conduction; decreases heart rate; decreases myocardial oxygen consumption; antiarrhythmic effects (class II); reduction in platelet aggregation and blood viscosity; suppression of renin release; inhibition of central sympathetic outflow; decreases presynaptic receptor neurotransmitter release; no intrinsic sympathomimetic, membrane stabilizing activity; low lipid solubility

Pharmacokinetics
PO: Incomplete GI absorption (40%-60% bioavailable); peak serum concentrations, 2-4 hr; not metabolized by liver; excreted unchanged in urine and feces; $t_{1/2}$ 6-7 hr; crosses placenta in measurable, but not significant concentrations

INDICATIONS AND USES: Angina pectoris, anxiety,* performance anxiety,* arrhythmia (class II),* congestive heart failure,* migraine headache,* post myocardial infarction,* alcohol withdrawal syndrome,* esophageal varices with cirrhosis*

DOSAGE
Adult and Child >16 yr
• *Post myocardial infarction:* IV 5 mg over 5 min; repeat in 10 min if initial dose tolerated; start PO 50 mg q12h × 2 doses immediately after last IV dose; then 100 mg qd × 10 days
• *Hypertension:* PO 50-100 mg qd
• *Angina pectoris:* PO 50-200 mg qd
Child
• PO initial 1-1.2 mg/kg/dose qd; maximum 2 mg/kg/day qd
• *Renal impairment:*

CREATININE CLEARANCE	MAXIMUM DOSE	DOSING INTERVAL
15-35 ml/min	50 mg or 1 mg/kg/dose	Daily
<15 ml/min	50 mg or 1 mg/kg/dose	Every other day

$ AVAILABLE FORMS/COST OF THERAPY
• Inj, Sol—IV, Buffered: 5 mg/10 ml, 10 ml: **$40.25**

---

* = non-FDA-approved use

• Tab, Uncoated—Oral: 25 mg, 100's: **$6.23-$120.84**; 50 mg, 100's: **$5.31-$129.46**; 100 mg, 100's: **$5.31-$129.46**

CONTRAINDICATIONS: Cardiogenic shock, 2nd or 3rd degree heart block, sinus bradycardia, overt cardiac failure

PRECAUTIONS: Anesthesia/surgery (myocardial depression), avoid abrupt withdrawal, bronchospastic airways, congestive heart failure, diabetes mellitus, hyperthyroidism/thyrotoxicosis (atenolol, unlike propranolol does not decrease T_3 levels), concurrent clonidine (discontinue atenolol several days prior to withdrawal of clonidine), peripheral vascular disease, renal disease

PREGNANCY AND LACTATION: Pregnancy category D; frequently used in the third trimester for treatment of hypertension (many studies of efficacy and safety of atenolol in pregnancy-induced hypertension); long-term use has been associated with intrauterine growth retardation; excreted into breast milk; observe for signs of beta-blockade

SIDE EFFECTS/ADVERSE REACTIONS

CNS: Ataxia, depression, *dizziness,* drowsiness, *fatigue,* hallucinations, insomnia, *lethargy,* memory loss, mental changes, strange dreams

CV: Bradycardia, CHF, cold extremities, postural hypotension, profound hypotension, **2nd or 3rd degree heart block, withdrawal angina, rebound hypertension**

EENT: Dry burning eyes, sore throat, visual disturbances

GI: Diarrhea, dry mouth, **ischemic colitis, mesenteric arterial thrombosis,** nausea, vomiting

GU: Impotence, sexual dysfunction

METAB: Hyperglycemia, hyperlipidemia (increase TG, total cholesterol, LDL; decrease HDL), **masked hypoglycemic response** (sweating excepted)

RESP: **Bronchospasm,** dyspnea, wheezing

SKIN: Alopecia, pruritis, rash

INTERACTIONS

Drugs

3 *Adenosine:* Bradycardia aggravated

3 *Alpha-1 adrenergic blockers:* Potential enhanced first dose response (marked initial drop in blood pressure, particularly on standing [especially prazocin])

3 *Amoxicillin, Ampicillin:* Reduced atenolol bioavailability

3 *Antacids:* Reduced atenolol absorption

3 *Calcium channel blockers:* See dihydropyridine and verapamil

3 *Clonidine:* Exacerbation of rebound hypertension upon discontinuation of clonidine

3 *Digoxin:* Additive prolongation of atrioventricular (AV) conduction time

3 *Dihydropyridines:* Additive hemodynamic effects; increased serum concentration of atenolol

3 *Dipyridamole:* Bradycardia aggravated

3 *Disopyramide:* Additive decreases in cardiac output

3 *Lidocaine:* Increased serum lidocaine concentrations possible

3 *Neostigmine:* Bradycardia aggravated

3 *NSAIDs:* Reduced antihypertensive effects of atenolol

3 *Physostigmine:* Bradycardia aggravated

3 *Prazosin:* First-dose response to prazosin may be enhanced by β-blockade

3 *Tacrine:* Bradycardia aggravated

❷ *Theophylline:* Antagonistic pharmacodynamic effects

❸ *Verapamil:* Enhanced effects of both drugs, particularly AV node conduction slowing; reduced atenolol clearance

SPECIAL CONSIDERATIONS
• Properties of low lipid solubility and competitive cardioselectivity yield less CNS and bronchospastic adverse effects

PATIENT/FAMILY EDUCATION
• Do not discontinue drug abruptly, may precipitate angina
• Report bradycardia, dizziness, confusion, depression, fever, shortness of breath, swelling of the extremities
• Take pulse at home, notify clinician if <50 beats/min
• Avoid hazardous activities if dizziness, drowsiness, lightheadedness are present
• May mask the symptoms of hypoglycemia, except for sweating, in diabetic patients

MONITORING PARAMETERS
• Angina: Reduction in nitroglycerin usage; frequency, severity, onset, and duration of angina pain; heart rate
• Arrhythmias: Heart rate
• Congestive heart failure: Functional status, cough, dyspnea on exertion, paroxysmal nocturnal dyspnea, exercise tolerance, and ventricular function
• Hypertension: Blood pressure
• Migraine headache: Reduction in the frequency, severity, and duration of attacks
• Postmyocardial infarction: Left ventricular function, lower resting heart rate
• Toxicity: Blood glucose, bronchospasm, hypotension, bradycardia, depression, confusion, hallucination, sexual dysfunction

---

atorvastatin
(a-tor′va-sta-tin)
Rx: Lipitor
Chemical Class: Substituted hexahydronaphthalene
Therapeutic Class: Antilipemic (HMG-CoA reductase inhibitor); "statin"

CLINICAL PHARMACOLOGY
Mechanism of Action: Competitively inhibits 3-hydroxy-3-methylglutaryl-coenzyme A (HMG-CoA) reductase, an early rate-limiting step in cholesterol biosynthesis; increases HDL-cholesterol mildly [5%-14%], decreases total and LDL cholesterol [28%-45%, 27%-60% respectively], and lowering effect on triglycerides [20%-50%]

Pharmacokinetics
PO: Peak 1-2 hours; 12% bioavailability; food decreases absorption 30% (not clinically significant); >98% protein bound; metabolized via CYP-3A4; $t_{1/2}$ 14 hours

INDICATIONS AND USES: Primary hypercholesterolemia (heterozygous familial and nonfamilial hypercholesterolemia), mixed dyslipidemia (Fredrickson types IIa and IIb), hypertriglyceridemia (includes Fredrickson type IV), primary dysbetalipoproteinemia (Fredrickson type III), and homozygous familial hyperlipidemia

DOSAGE
Adult
• PO: 10-80 mg qd; dose can be administered without regard to meals

🄢 AVAILABLE FORMS/COST OF THERAPY
• Tab, Film-Coated—Oral: 10 mg, 90's: **$207.84**; 20 mg, 90's: **$303.60**; 40 mg, 90's: **$327.92**; 80 mg, 90's: **$327.92**

---

* = non-FDA-approved use

CONTRAINDICATIONS: Active liver disease; unexplained persistent elevations of serum transaminases; pregnancy and lactation

PRECAUTIONS: Liver dysfunction

PREGNANCY AND LACTATION: Pregnancy category X; not recommended for nursing mothers

SIDE EFFECTS/ADVERSE REACTIONS

CNS: Headache

CV: Migraine, palpitation, postural hypotension, syncope, vasodilation

EENT: Amblyopia, dry eyes, taste disturbances, tinnitus

GI: Abdominal pain, constipation, diarrhea, dyspepsia, flatulence, gastroenteritis, LFT abnormalities

HEME: Anemia, ecchymosis, petechia, thrombocytopenia

METAB: Hyperglycemia, increased creatinine phosphokinase

MS: Arthralgia, leg cramps, *myalgia*

SKIN: Pruritus, rash

MISC: Face edema, fever, flu-like syndrome, malaise, photosensitivity

INTERACTIONS

Drugs

3 *Azole antifungals (fluconazole, itraconazole, ketoconazole, miconazole):* Increased atorvastatin levels; increased risk of rhabdomyolysis

3 *Bile acid sequestrants (cholestyramine, colestipol):* 25% reduction in atorvastatin plasma levels if coadministered

3 *Cyclosporine:* Concomitant administration increases risk of severe myopathy or rhabdomyolysis

3 *Digoxin:* Elevation of digoxin level (approximately 20%)

3 *Erythromycin:* Increased atorvastatin concentrations (approximately 40%); increased risk of rhabdomyolysis

3 *Fibric acid:* Increased risk of severe myopathy, especially with high statin doses

3 *Nefazodone:* Increased atorvastatin levels; increased risk of rhabdomyolyisis

3 *Niacin:* Concomitant administration increases risk of severe myopathy or rhabdomyolysis

3 *Oral contraceptives:* Coadministration increases AUC for norethindrone and ethinyl estradiol by approximately 30% and 20%, respectively

SPECIAL CONSIDERATIONS

• Statin selection based on lipid-lowering prowess, cost, and availability

• Potency and ability to lower serum triglycerides is unique among the HMG-CoA reductase inhibitors. However, no outcome data available

PATIENT/FAMILY EDUCATION

• Report symptoms of myalgia, muscle tenderness, or weakness

• Take daily doses in the evening for increased effect

MONITORING PARAMETERS

• Cholesterol (max therapeutic response 4-6 wk)

• LFT's (AST, ALT) at baseline and at 12 wk of therapy: if no change, no further monitoring necessary (discontinue if elevations persist at $>3 \times$ upper limit of normal)

• CPK in patients complaining of diffuse myalgia, muscle tenderness, or weakness

---

atovaquone
(a-toe′va-kwone)
Rx: Mepron
Chemical Class: Hydroxy-napthoquinone derivative
Therapeutic Class: Antiprotozoal

CLINICAL PHARMACOLOGY
Mechanism of Action: Inhibits synthesis of nucleic acid and ATP
Pharmacokinetics
PO: Peak 1-8 hr; bioavailability 23% fasting, 47% with food; highly lipophilic, with low aqueous solubility (CSF:plasma ratio <1%); 99.9% protein bound; $t_{1/2}$, 2.2-2.9 days, fecal elimination with enterohepatic circulation

INDICATIONS AND USES: Acute oral treatment of mild to moderate *Pneumocystis carinii* pneumonia (PCP) in patients who are intolerant to co-trimoxazole
DOSAGE
Adult
• PO 750 mg bid with food for 21 days

$ **AVAILABLE FORMS/COST OF THERAPY**
• Susp—Oral: 750 mg/5 ml, 210 ml: **$599.14-$738.64**

CONTRAINDICATIONS: GI disorders that inhibit absorption
PREGNANCY AND LACTATION: Pregnancy category C; human breast milk studies not available; in rats, concentrations in milk 30% of maternal serum

SIDE EFFECTS/ADVERSE REACTIONS
CNS: Headache, insomnia
GI: Diarrhea, nausea, vomiting
METAB: Fever
RESP: Cough
SKIN: Skin rash

SPECIAL CONSIDERATIONS
• Plasma concentrations have been shown to correlate with the likelihood of successful treatment and survival

atropine
(a′troe-peen)
Rx: Atropine Care, Atropisol, Atrosulf-1, Isopto Atropine, Ocu-Tropine, Sal-Tropine
Chemical Class: Belladonna alkaloid
Therapeutic Class: Anticholinergic; ophthalmic anticholinergic; gastrointestinal antispasmodic; antiasthmatic, bronchodilator; mydriatic

CLINICAL PHARMACOLOGY
Mechanism of Action: Blocks acetylcholine at parasympathetic neuroeffector sites; increases cardiac output and heart rate by blocking vagal stimulation in heart; dries secretions by blocking vagus; blocks response of iris sphincter muscle, muscle of accommodation of ciliary body to cholinergic stimulation, resulting in dilation, paralysis of accommodation
Pharmacokinetics
PO/IM/SC: Well absorbed
PO: Onset ½ hr, peak ½-1 hr, duration 4-6 hr
IM/SC: Onset 15-50 min, peak 30 min, duration 4-6 hr
IV: Peak 2-4 min, duration 4-6 hr
OPHTH: Peak 30-40 min (mydriasis), 60-180 min (cycloplegia), duration 6-12 days, $t_{1/2}$ 13-40 hr; excreted by kidneys unchanged (70%-90% in 24 hr); metabolized in liver, 40%-50% crosses placenta, excreted in breast milk

INDICATIONS AND USES: Bradycardia, bradydysrhythmia; anticholinesterase insecticide poisoning; blockade of cardiac vagal reflexes; antisialagogue (preanesthetic to prevent or reduce secretions of the respiratory tract and end of life comfort measure); rigidity and tremor of parkinsonism; antispasmodic with GU, biliary surgery; bronchodilator; mydriasis/cycloplegia for iritis, cycloplegic refraction; INH via neb for bronchospasm with COPD* (replaced with ipratropium bromide)

DOSAGE

Adult

• *Bradycardia/bradydysrhythmias:* IV BOL 0.5-1 mg given q3-5 min, not to exceed 2 mg

• *Insecticide poisoning:* IM/IV 2 mg qh until muscarinic symptoms disappear; may need 6 mg qh

• *Pre-surgery:* SC/IM/IV 0.4-0.6 mg before anesthesia

• *Iritis/cycloplegic refraction:* Instill sol 1-2 gtt of a 1% sol qd-tid for iritis or 1 hr before refracting

• *Parkinsonism:* PO 0.4 mg

Child

• *Bradycardia/bradydysrhythmias:* IV BOL 0.01-0.03 mg/kg up to 0.4 mg or 0.3 mg/m²; may repeat q4-6h

• *Insecticide poisoning:* IM/IV 2 mg qh until muscarinic symptoms disappear; may need 6 mg qh

• *Pre-surgery:* SC 0.1-0.4 mg 30 min before surgery

• *Iritis/cycloplegic refraction:* Instill sol 1-2 gtt of a 0.5% sol qd-tid for iritis or bid × 1-3 days before exam (cycloplegic refraction); instill oint qd-bid 2-3 days before exam

§ AVAILABLE FORMS/COST OF THERAPY

• Inj, Sol—IM, IV, SC: 0.05 mg/ml, 5 ml: **$11.19**; 0.1 mg/ml, 5 ml: **$3.24-$12.35**; 0.4 mg/ml, 1 ml: **$0.43-$1.12**; 0.5 mg/ml, 1 ml: **$0.98-$1.33**; 1 mg/ml, 1 ml: **$0.44-$1.12**

• Oint—Ophth: 1%, 3.5 g: **$1.35-$3.80**

• Sol—Ophth: 0.5%, 5 ml: **$10.94**; 1%, 5 ml: **$1.40-$16.94**; 2%, 2 ml: **$4.76**

• Tab—Oral: 0.4 mg, 100's: **$28.95**

CONTRAINDICATIONS: Hypersensitivity to belladonna alkaloids, angle-closure glaucoma, GI obstructions, myasthenia gravis, thyrotoxicosis, ulcerative colitis, prostatic hypertrophy, tachycardia/tachydysrhythmias, asthma, acute hemorrhage, myocardial ischemia

PRECAUTIONS: Renal disease, lactation, CHF, hyperthyroidism, COPD, hepatic disease, child <6 yr, hypertension, elderly, intraabdominal infections, Down's syndrome, spastic paralysis, gastric ulcer

PREGNANCY AND LACTATION: Pregnancy category C; passage into breast milk still controversial; neonates particularly sensitive to anticholinergic agents; compatible with breast feeding

SIDE EFFECTS/ADVERSE REACTIONS

CNS: Anxiety, coma, confusion, dizziness, drowsiness, flushing, headache, insomnia, involuntary movement, psychosis, weakness

CV: Angina, ectopic ventricular beats, hypertension, hypotension, *paradoxical bradycardia*, PVCs, tachycardia

EENT: Blurred vision, eye pain, glaucoma, nasal congestion, photophobia, pupil dilation

GI: Abdominal distension, abdominal pain, altered taste, anorexia, constipation, dry mouth, nausea, *paralytic ileus*, vomiting

GU: Dysuria, hesitancy, impotence, retention

---

italic = common side effects   ***bold italic*** = life-threatening reactions

SKIN: Contact dermatitis, dry skin, flushing, rash, urticaria

MISC: Decreased sweating, suppression of lactation

INTERACTIONS

Drugs

3 *Amantadine:* Enhanced anticholinergic effect of atropine; enhanced CNS effect of amantadine

3 *Neuroleptics:* Reduced neuroleptic effect

3 *Rimantadine:* Enhanced anticholinergic effect of atropine; enhanced CNS effect of rimantadine

3 *Tacrine:* May reduce anticholinergic effect of atropine; atropine may reduce CNS effect of tacrine

---

auranofin

(ah-ran´-oh-fin)

Rx: Ridaura

Chemical Class: Gold compound

Therapeutic Class: Disease-modifying arthritis drug (DMARD)

CLINICAL PHARMACOLOGY

Mechanism of Action: Unknown; best hypothesis relates to uptake of gold by macrophages with resultant inhibition of phagocytosis and activities of lysosomal enzymes; decreases both polymorphonuclear and monocyte function; decreased concentration of rheumatoid factor and immunoglobulins; impairs mitogen-induced proliferation of lymphocytes

Pharmacokinetics

PO: 25% of the gold absorbed by GI tract, peak 2 hr, steady state 8-16 wk; excreted in urine (60% of the absorbed gold) and feces; terminal plasma $t_{1/2}$ (steady state) 26 days; terminal body $t_{1/2}$ 80 days

INDICATIONS AND USES: Asthma,* rheumatoid arthritis; psoriatic arthritis*

DOSAGE

Adult

• PO 6 mg qd or 3 mg bid, may increase to 9 mg/day after 3 mo

Child

• PO (initial) 0.1 mg/kg/day, (maintenance) 0.15 mg/kg/day, (max) 0.2 mg/kg/day

$ **AVAILABLE FORMS/COST OF THERAPY**

• Cap, Gel—Oral: 3 mg, 60's: **$78.75-$170.26**

CONTRAINDICATIONS: Necrotizing enterocolitis, bone marrow aplasia, child <6 yr, lactation, pulmonary fibrosis, exfoliative dermatitis, blood dyscrasias, recent radiation therapy, renal/hepatic disease, marked hypertension, uncontrolled CHF

PRECAUTIONS: Skin rash, renal disease, liver disease

PREGNANCY AND LACTATION: Pregnancy category C; nursing not recommended; gold appears in breast milk

SIDE EFFECTS/ADVERSE REACTIONS

CNS: Confusion, dizziness, EEG abnormalities, hallucinations, *seizures*

EENT: Corneal ulcers, gold deposits in ocular tissues, iritis

GI: Abdominal cramping, anorexia, constipation, *diarrhea,* dyspepsia, *enterocolitis,* flatulence, gingivitis, glossitis, increased AST/ALT, jaundice, melena, metallic taste, *nausea, stomatitis, vomiting*

GU: **Hematuria,** increased BUN/creatinine, proteinuria, vaginitis

HEME: **Agranulocytosis, aplastic anemia,** eosinophilia, **leukopenia, neutropenia, thrombocytopenia**

RESP: Cough, dyspnea, **fibrosis, interstitial pneumonitis**

SKIN: Alopecia, *dermatitis,* ***exfoliative dermatitis,*** photosensitivity, *pruritus, rash,* urticaria

MISC: Gold toxicity: decreased Hgb, WBC $<4000/mm^3$, granulocytes $<1500/mm^3$, platelets $<150,000/mm^3$, hematuria, itching, proteinuria, rash, severe diarrhea, stomatitis

SPECIAL CONSIDERATIONS
MONITORING PARAMETERS

• Rheumatoid arthritis: tender, swollen joints, visual analogue scale for pain; acute phase reactants (ESR, C-reactive protein), duration of early morning stiffness, preservation of function; persistence of loose stools and/or severe diarrhea may be a drug effect; pruritus is a warning sign for development of cutaneous reactions, metallic taste may be a warning sign of stomatitis development; CBC with differential, platelet count, urinalysis, renal function, and hepatic function tests should be done prior to treatment; CBC with differential, platelet count, and urinalysis should be done every month during therapy

---

aurothioglucose/gold sodium thiomalate
(aur-oh-thye-oh-gloo′kose/gold sodium thye-oh-maa′late)
Rx: Solganol (aurothioglucose); Aurolate, Myochrysine (gold sodium thiomalate)
Chemical Class: Heavy metal, active gold compound (50%)
Therapeutic Class: Gold salt, slowly-acting antiarthritic drug, disease-modifying arthritis drug (DMARD)

CLINICAL PHARMACOLOGY
Mechanism of Action: Unknown; best hypothesis relates to uptake of gold by macrophages with resultant inhibition of phagocytosis and activities of lysosomal enzymes; decreases both polymorphonuclear and monocyte function; decreased concentration of rheumatoid factor and immunoglobulins; impairs mitogen-induced proliferation of lymphocytes

Pharmacokinetics
IM: Peak 4-6 hr; excreted in urine, feces; $t_{1/2}$ 3-27 days, increases up to 168 days with 11th dose

INDICATIONS AND USES: Asthma,* Felty's syndrome, rheumatoid arthritis; Sjögren's syndrome; pemphigus*; psoriatic arthritis

DOSAGE
Adult

• *Aurothioglucose:* IM administer weekly; 1st dose 10 mg; 2nd, 3rd doses 25 mg; then 50 mg q wk up to 0.8-1.0 g; continue 25-50 mg q3-4 wk if improvement without toxicity

• *Gold sodium thiomalate:* IM 10 mg, then 25 mg after 1 wk, then 50 mg q wk for total of 14-20 doses,

---

then 50 mg q2 wk × 4, then 50 mg q3 wk × 4, then 50 mg qmo for maintenance

Child 6-12 yr
• *Aurothioglucose:* IM 1 mg/kg/wk × 20 wk, or ¼ of adult dose
• *Gold sodium thiomalate:* IM 1 mg/kg/wk × 20 wk, then q3-4wk if improvement without toxicity; not to exceed 50 mg/dose

$ **AVAILABLE FORMS/COST OF THERAPY**
Aurothioglucose
• Inj, Susp in Oil—IM: 50 mg/ml, 10 ml: **$153.42-$167.70**
Gold Sodium Thiomalate
• Inj, Sol—IM: 50 mg/ml, 1 ml: **$8.30-$15.68**

CONTRAINDICATIONS: Systemic lupus erythematosus, uncontrolled diabetes mellitus, marked hypertension, recent radiation therapy, CHF, renal disease, liver disease, agranulocytosis, blood dyscrasias, hemorrhagic diathesis, history of hepatitis, colitis, urticaria, eczema

PREGNANCY AND LACTATION: Pregnancy category C; gold has been demonstrated in breast milk and in the serum and red blood cells of a nursing infant; the slow excretion and persistence of gold in the mother, even after discontinuing therapy, must also be considered

SIDE EFFECTS/ADVERSE REACTIONS
CNS: Confusion, *dizziness,* EEG abnormalities, *encephalitis,* hallucinations
CV: Bradycardia, rapid pulse
EENT: Corneal ulcers, iritis
GI: Cramping, diarrhea, flatulence, hepatitis, jaundice, metallic taste, nausea, stomatitis, vomiting
GU: Hematuria, *nephrosis,* proteinuria, *tubular necrosis*
HEME: **Agranulocytosis, aplastic anemia,** eosinophilia, *leukopenia, neutropenia,* thrombocytopenia

RESP: Interstitial pneumonitis, pharyngitis, ***pulmonary fibrosis***
SKIN: Alopecia, ***angioedema,*** dermatitis, ***exfoliative dermatitis,*** photosensitivity, *pruritus, rash,* urticaria
MISC: **Anaphylaxis:** "nitritoid" reaction (vasomotor reaction manifests as nausea, weakness, flushing, tachycardia, and/or syncope in 5% of patients receiving gold sodium thiomalate; not reported with aurothioglucose, hence probably related to vehicle or preservative in alternative product); gold toxicity (decreased Hgb, WBC <4000/mm^3, granulocytes <1500/mm^3, platelets <150,000/mm^3, severe diarrhea, stomatitis, hematuria, rash, itching, proteinuria)

SPECIAL CONSIDERATIONS
• Administer in gluteal muscle with patient recumbent for 10 min after injection

MONITORING PARAMETERS
• Rheumatoid arthritis: tender, swollen joints, visual analogue scale for pain; acute phase reactants (ESR, C-reactive protein), duration of early morning stiffness, preservation of function; persistence of loose stools and/or severe diarrhea may be a drug effect; pruritus is a warning sign for development of cutaneous reactions, metallic taste may be a warning sign of stomatitis development; CBC with differential, platelet count, urinalysis, renal function, and hepatic function tests should be done prior to treatment; CBC with differential, platelet count, and urinalysis should be done every month during therapy

azatadine

(a-za'ta-deen)

Rx: Optimine

Chemical Class: Piperidine derivative

Therapeutic Class: Antihistamine

CLINICAL PHARMACOLOGY

Mechanism of Action: Decreases allergic response by blocking histamine at H_1-receptors

Pharmacokinetics

PO: Peak 4 hr; metabolized in liver, excreted by kidneys; crosses placenta, crosses blood-brain barrier; minimally bound to plasma proteins; $t_{1/2}$ 9-12 hr

INDICATIONS AND USES: Perennial and seasonal allergic rhinitis; chronic urticaria

DOSAGE

Adult

• PO 1-2 mg bid, not to exceed 4 mg/day

Child >12 yr

• PO 1-2 mg bid

$ **AVAILABLE FORMS/COST OF THERAPY**

• Tab, Uncoated—Oral: 1 mg, 100's: **$131.25**

CONTRAINDICATIONS: Concurrent acute asthma attack, lower respiratory tract disease, child <12 yr

PRECAUTIONS: Increased intraocular pressure, renal disease, cardiac disease, asthma, seizure disorder, stenosed peptic ulcers, hyperthyroidism, prostatic hypertrophy, bladder neck obstruction, elderly

PREGNANCY AND LACTATION: Pregnancy category B; excretion into breast milk unknown

SIDE EFFECTS/ADVERSE REACTIONS

CNS: Anxiety, chills, confusion, *dizziness, drowsiness,* euphoria, fatigue, neuritis, paresthesia, poor coordination, sweating

CV: Hypotension, palpitations, tachycardia

EENT: Blurred vision; dilated pupils; dry nose, throat; tinnitus

GI: Anorexia, constipation, dry mouth, nausea, vomiting

GU: Dysuria, frequency, impotence, retention

*HEME: **Agranulocytosis, hemolytic anemia, thrombocytopenia***

RESP: Chest tightness, increased thick secretions, wheezing

SKIN: Photosensitivity, rash, urticaria

azathioprine

(ay-za-thye'oh-preen)

Rx: Imuran

Chemical Class: Purine analog; derivative of 6-mercaptopurine

Therapeutic Class: Immunosuppressant

CLINICAL PHARMACOLOGY

Mechanism of Action: Immunosuppressive by inhibiting purine synthesis in cells

Pharmacokinetics

PO: Peak 1-2 hr; metabolized in liver (cleaved to mercaptopurine then inactivated by xanthine oxidase); 30% bound to serum proteins; excreted in urine (both parent and metabolite) rapidly; crosses placenta

INDICATIONS AND USES: Renal homotransplantation to prevent graft rejection; refractory rheumatoid arthritis, refractory ITP*; glomerulonephritis*; nephrotic syndrome*; bone marrow transplant*;

---

ulcerative colitis*; myasthenia gravis* (2-3 mg/kg/day); Behçet's syndrome*; Crohn's disease*

DOSAGE

Adult

• *Prevention of rejection:* PO/IV 3-5 mg/kg/day, then maintenance (PO) of at least 1-2 mg/kg/day

• *Refractory rheumatoid arthritis:* PO 1 mg/kg/day; may increase dose after 2 mo by 0.5 mg/kg/day; not to exceed 2.5 mg/kg/day

Child

• *Prevention of rejection:* PO/IV 3-5mg/kg/day, then maintenance (PO) of at least 1-2 mg/kg/day

$ AVAILABLE FORMS/COST OF THERAPY

• Inj, Lyphl-Sol—IV: 100 mg/vial: **$85.00-$137.10**

• Tab, Uncoated—Oral: 50 mg, 100's: **$131.05-$187.63**

PRECAUTIONS: Severe leukopenia and/or thrombocytopenia may occur as well as macrocytic anemia and bone marrow depression; fungal, viral, bacterial, and protozoal infections may be fatal; may increase the patient's risk of neoplasia via mutagenic and carcinogenic properties (skin cancer and reticulum cell or lymphomatous tumors); temporary depression in spermatogenesis

PREGNANCY AND LACTATION: Pregnancy category D

SIDE EFFECTS/ADVERSE REACTIONS

GI: Esophagitis, hepatotoxicity, jaundice, nausea, *pancreatitis,* stomatitis, vomiting

HEME: Anemia (macrocytic), *leukopenia, pancytopenia, thrombocytopenia*

MS: Arthralgia, muscle wasting

SKIN: Rash

MISC: Fungal, viral, bacterial, and protozoal infections

INTERACTIONS

Drugs

❷ *Allopurinol:* Allopurinol may increase toxicity of azathioprine; dosage adjustment is necessary

❸ *Warfarin:* Reduced warfarin effect

SPECIAL CONSIDERATIONS

MONITORING PARAMETERS

• Hgb, WBC, platelets monthly

• D/C if leukocytes are $<3000/mm^3$

• Therapeutic response may take 3-4 mo in rheumatoid arthritis

---

azelaic acid

(a-zuh-lay′ick)

Rx: Azelex

Chemical Class: Dicarboxylic acid

Therapeutic Class: Antiacne agent

CLINICAL PHARMACOLOGY

Mechanism of Action: Normalizes keratinization, resulting in decreased microcomedo formation; antimicrobial activity against *S. epidermidis* and *P. acnes*

Pharmacokinetics

TOP: 4% absorbed systemically; elimination $t_{1/2}$ 12 hr, onset of action within 4 wk; renal excretion, primarily as unchanged azelaic acid

INDICATIONS AND USES: Acne

DOSAGE

Adult and Child >12 yr

• Apply thin film to affected area bid

$ AVAILABLE FORMS/COST OF THERAPY

• Cre—Top: 20%, 30, 50 g: **$36.95-$48.53**/30 g

PREGNANCY AND LACTATION: Pregnancy category B; distributed in breast milk but little absorbed systemically and unlikely that concen-

---

* = non-FDA-approved use

trations of this normal dietary constituent would exceed baseline endogenous concentrations

SIDE EFFECTS/ADVERSE REACTIONS

SKIN: Burning and itching (1%-5%), contact dermatitis, dryness and redness (<1%), hypopigmentation (especially in darker-skinned individuals), keratosis pilaris

SPECIAL CONSIDERATIONS

• Wash hands after application; avoid contact with mucous membranes; if drug gets into eyes, wash with large quantities of water

• If skin irritation occurs, decrease frequency of application or temporarily discontinue treatment

• Azelaic acid is a naturally occurring substance found in the human diet

---

azelastine

(a'zel-ah-steen)

Rx: Astelin (nasal), Optivar (ophthalmic)

Chemical Class: Phthalazinone derivative

Therapeutic Class: Antihistamine

CLINICAL PHARMACOLOGY

Mechanism of Action: Decreases allergic response by blocking histamine at H_1-receptors

Pharmacokinetics

NASAL: Onset within 3 hr, duration 12 hr; systemic absorption occurs despite inhaled route; metabolized by hepatic cytochrome P-450 system, metabolites excreted in feces

OPHTH: Onset within 3 min, duration 8 hr, minimal systemic absorption

INDICATIONS AND USES: *Nasal:* Seasonal allergic rhinitis; vasomotor rhinitis, perennial rhinitis*

Ophthalmic: Itching of the eye associated with allergic conjunctivitis

DOSAGE

Adult

• INH 2 sprays in each nostril bid

• OPHTH 1 gtt in each affected eye bid

Child ≥12 yr

• INH ≥12 yr: 2 sprays in each nostril bid; 5-11 yr: 1 spray in each nostril bid (allergic rhinitis)

• OPHTH 3 yr: 1 gtt in each affected eye bid

💲 AVAILABLE FORMS/COST OF THERAPY

• Spray, Nasal—INH: 17 ml (twin pack), 1 mg/spray (200 sprays/twin pack): **$47.00**

• Sol—Ophth: 0.05%, 3, 6 ml: **$46.51**/3 ml

PREGNANCY AND LACTATION: Pregnancy category C, excretion into breast milk unknown

SIDE EFFECTS/ADVERSE REACTIONS

CNS: Headache, *somnolence*

EENT: Bitter taste, transient eye burning/stinging

METAB: Weight gain

SPECIAL CONSIDERATIONS

• Low sedating antihistamine nasal spray with first-dose activity; note: onset of action not as fast as decongestant nasal sprays, but appropriate for prn use

PATIENT/FAMILY EDUCATION

• Advise caution with use concomitant with activities that require concentration or while operating machinery; may cause drowsiness

• Preservative in ophth sol, benzlkonium chloride, may be absorbed by soft contact lenses, wait at least 10 min after instilling ophth sol before inserting soft contacts

---

---

azithromycin

(ay-zi-thro-mye'sin)
Rx: Zithromax
Chemical Class: Macrolide
(azalide) derivative
Therapeutic Class: Antibiotic

CLINICAL PHARMACOLOGY
Mechanism of Action: Binds to 50S
ribosomal subunits of susceptible
bacteria and suppresses protein synthesis
Pharmacokinetics
PO: Peak 2.2 hr, duration 24 hr, rapidly absorbed and widely distributed
into tissues (higher concentrations
in tissues than in plasma), protein
binding 51%, bioavailability 40%,
$t_{1/2}$ 68 hr; excreted in bile, feces, urine
primarily as unchanged drug
INDICATIONS AND USES: Mild to
moderate infections of the upper and
lower respiratory tract; uncomplicated skin and skin structure infections; nongonococcal urethritis or
cervicitis caused by susceptible organisms; gonococcal urethritis*;
chancroid; otitis media; prevention
of *Mycobacterium avium* complex
infection in AIDS patients*
Antibacterial spectrum usually includes:
• Gram-positive organisms: *Staphylococcus aureus, Streptococcus
pneumoniae, S. pyogenes, S. agalactiae,* streptococci (Groups
C,F,G), *S. viridans* group streptococci
• Gram-negative organisms: *Moraxella catarrhalis, Haemophilus
influenzae, Bordetella pertussi,
Campylobacter jejuni, H. ducreyi,
Legionella pneumophilia*
• Anaerobes: *Bacteroides bivivu,
Clostridium perfringens,* other *Clostridium* sp., *Peptostreptococcus* sp.

• Misc: *Chlamydia trachomatis,
Borrelia burgdorferi, Mycoplasma
pneumoniae, Treponema pallidum,
Ureaplasma urealyticum*
DOSAGE
Adult
• *Pneumonia:* PO 500 mg on day 1,
then 250 mg qd on days 2-5 for a total dose of 1.5 g; IV 500 mg qd for 2
days followed by 5-8 days by PO
500 mg qd
• *Nongonococcal urethritis or cervicitis:* 1 g single PO dose for
chlamydial infections
• *Chancroid:* 1 g as a single dose
• *Gonococcal urethritis or cervici-
tis:* 2 g PO as single dose
• *Pelvic inflammatory disease:* 500
mg IV then 250 mg PO qd for 6 days
• *Prevention of Mycobacterium
avium complex infection in AIDS
patients:* PO 1200 mg once per week
Child
• *Acute otitis media:* PO 10 mg/kg ×
1, then 5 mg/kg qd for next 4 days;
alternate: 30 mg/kg single dose
• *Pharyngitis/tonsillitis:* PO 12
mg/kg qd × 5 days
• *Community-acquired pneumonia:*
PO 10 mg/kg × 1, then 5 mg/kg qd
for next 4 days
**⑤ AVAILABLE FORMS/COST
OF THERAPY**
• Cap—Oral: 250 mg, 6's: **$40.05-
$63.78**
• Inj, Dry-Sol—IV: 500 mg/vial:
$24.44-$25.98
• Sachet—Oral: 1 g: **$20.98**
• Susp—Oral: 100 mg/5 ml, 15 ml:
$28.60-$38.26; 200 mg/5 ml, 15 ml:
$28.60-$38.26
• Tab—Oral: 600 mg, 30's: **$516.95**
CONTRAINDICATIONS: Hyper-
sensitivity to erythromycin
PRECAUTIONS: Hepatic, renal,
cardiac disease
PREGNANCY AND LACTATION:
Pregnancy category B; excretion
into breast milk unknown

---

* = non-FDA-approved use

SIDE EFFECTS/ADVERSE REACTIONS

CV: Chest pain, palpitations

CNS: Dizziness, headache, somnolence, vertigo

GI: Abdominal pain, cholestatic jaundice, diarrhea, dyspepsia, flatulence, heartburn, hepatotoxicity, melena, nausea, stomatitis, vomiting

GU: Moniliasis, nephritis, vaginitis

SKIN: Photosensitivity, pruritus, rash, urticaria

INTERACTIONS

Drugs

3 *Penicillins:* Azithromycin may inhibit antibacterial activity of penicillins

Labs

• *Increase:* Serum 17 Hydroxycorticosteroids, 17 ketosteroids

• *Decrease:* Serum folate (bioassay only)

SPECIAL CONSIDERATIONS
PATIENT/FAMILY EDUCATION

• New formulation can be taken without regard to food

• Tablet and capsule may be taken without regard to food. Suspension should be taken on an empty stomach

---

aztreonam

(az-tree'oo-nam)

Rx: Azactam

Chemical Class: Monobactam

Therapeutic Class: Antibiotic

CLINICAL PHARMACOLOGY

Mechanism of Action: Inhibits bacterial wall synthesis; bactericidal

Pharmacokinetics

IV: Peak, following single 1 g dose 204 µg/ml; trough, at 8 hr 3 µg/ml; $t_{1/2}$ 1.7 hr, $t_{1/2}$ prolonged in renal disease; protein binding 56%; metabolized by liver, excreted in urine; small amounts appear in breast milk, placenta

INDICATIONS AND USES: Infections of the respiratory, urinary, and gynecologic tracts, skin, muscle, and bone; intra-abdominal septicemia caused by susceptible organisms.

Antibacterial spectrum usually includes:

• Gram-negative organisms: *E. coli, Klebsiella pneumoniae, Proteus mirabilis, P. aeruginosa, Enterobacter* sp., *K. oxytoca, Citrobacter* and *S. marcescens, Haemophilus influenzae*

DOSAGE
Adult

• *Urinary tract infections:* IV/IM 500 mg-1 g q8-12h

• *Systemic infections:* IV/IM 1-2 g q8-12h

• *Severe systemic infections:* IV/IM 2 g q6-8h; do not exceed 8 g/day; continue treatment for 48 hr after negative culture or until patient is asymptomatic

Child

• Postnatal age <7 days, <2000 g: IM/IV 30 mg/kg q12h; >2000 g 30 mg/kg q8h

• Postnatal age >7 days, <2000 g:

• 30 mg/kg q8h; >2000 g: 30 mg/kg q6h

• Children >1 mo: 90-120 mg/kg/day divided q6-8h

• *Cystic Fibrosis:* 50 mg/kg/dose q6-8h (max 6-8 g/day)

§ AVAILABLE FORMS/COST OF THERAPY

• Inj, Lyphl-Sol—IM, IV: 500 mg/vial: **$84.50**; 1 g/vial: **$16.15-$18.89**; 2 g/vial: **$34.00-$37.69**

PRECAUTIONS: Children; impaired renal, hepatic function; elderly; hypersensitivity to penicillins, cephalosporins

PREGNANCY AND LACTATION: Pregnancy category B; excreted in breast milk in concentrations <1% of maternal serum concentrations

SIDE EFFECTS/ADVERSE REACTIONS

CNS: Anxiety, **coma,** depression, hallucinations, lethargy, malaise, **seizures,** twitching

EENT: Diplopia, nasal congestion, tinnitus

GI: Abdominal pain, colitis, *diarrhea,* glossitis, increased AST/ALT, *nausea, vomiting*

GU: Breast tenderness, vaginal candidiasis, vaginitis

HEME: **Bone marrow depression,** increased bleeding time

INTERACTIONS

Drugs

3 *Aminoglycosides:* Potential increased nephrotoxicity, ototoxicity

3 *Cephalosporins, imipenem:* Antagonism secondary to antibiotic-induced high levels of β-lactamase

SPECIAL CONSIDERATIONS

• Minimal cross-reactivity between aztreonam and penicillins and cephalosporins; aztreonam and aminoglycosides have been shown to be synergistic *in vitro* against most strains of *P. aeruginosa,* many strains of *Enterobacteriaceae,* and other gram-negative aerobic bacilli

---

bacitracin

(bass-i-tray´sin)

Rx: Ak-Tracin, Baci-Rx, Bacticin, Ocu-Tracin, Spectro-Bacitracin

Combinations

  Rx: with neomycin, polymixin, and hydrocortisone (Cortisporin)

  OTC: with neomycin and polymixin (Neosporin); with polymixin (Polysporin)

Chemical Class: Bacillus subtilis derivative

Therapeutic Class: Antibacterial; ophthalmic antibacterial

CLINICAL PHARMACOLOGY

Mechanism of Action: Inhibits bacterial cell wall synthesis (bactericidal)

Pharmacokinetics

IM: Peak 1-2 hr, duration >12 hr; widely distributed (demonstrable in ascitic and pleural fluids after IM injection); metabolized in liver, excreted in urine

INDICATIONS AND USES: Ophth for superficial ocular infections involving the conjunctiva and/or cornea caused by susceptible organisms; IM for infants with pneumonia and empyema caused by susceptible staphylococci; PO for antibiotic-associated colitis (Orphan Drug status); top treatment of impetigo due to *Staphylococcus aureus*

DOSAGE

Adult

• OPHTH: Apply to conjunctival sac bid-qid

• IM: 20,000-25,000 U q6h × 7-10 days

• PO: 25,000 U qid × 10 days

Child

• OPHTH: Apply to conjunctival sac bid-qid; IM: infants <2.5 kg 900 U/kg/day in divided doses q8-12h; infants >2.5 kg 1000 U/kg/day in divided doses q8-12h

💲 AVAILABLE FORMS/COST OF THERAPY

• Inj, Lyphl-Sol—IM: 50,000 U/vial: **$4.20-$11.88**

• Oint—Ophth: 500 unit/g, 3.5 g: **$1.30-$11.96**

• Oint—Top: 500 unit/g, 15, 30, 60, 120, 144, 454, 480 g: **$0.80-$9.01**/30 g

CONTRAINDICATIONS: Severe renal disease

PRECAUTIONS: Overgrowth of non-susceptible organisms; skin sensitivity due to neomycin in combination products

PREGNANCY AND LACTATION: Pregnancy category C

SIDE EFFECTS/ADVERSE REACTIONS

EENT: Poor corneal wound healing, visual haze (temporary)

GI: Diarrhea, nausea, vomiting

GU: Albuminuria, casts, cylindruria, proteinuria, ***renal failure due to tubular and glomerular necrosis***

SKIN: Rash

MISC: Pain at injection site

SPECIAL CONSIDERATIONS

• Administer IM in deep muscle mass; rotate injection site; do *not* give IV/SC

---

baclofen

(bak'loe-fen)

Rx: Lioresal, Lioresal Intrathecal

Chemical Class: GABA chlorophenyl derivative

Therapeutic Class: Skeletal muscle relaxant

CLINICAL PHARMACOLOGY

Mechanism of Action: Inhibits synaptic responses at the spinal level by decreasing excitatory neurotransmitter release; decreases frequency, severity of muscle spasms; structural analog of the inhibitory neurotransmitter gamma-aminobutyric acid (GABA); general CNS depressant properties

Pharmacokinetics

PO: Peak 2-3 hr, duration >8 hr

INTRATHECAL: (CSF/plasma levels 100 times oral route); bolus: onset ½-1 hr, peak 4 hr, duration 4-8 hr; continuous INF: peak 24-48 hr, $t_{1/2}$ 2½-4 hr; partially metabolized in liver, excreted in urine (unchanged)

INDICATIONS AND USES: Spasticity with spinal cord injury; spasticity in multiple sclerosis; intractable spasticity in children with cerebral palsy* (intrathecal); trigeminal neuralgia*; tardive dyskinesia in combination with neuroleptics*

DOSAGE

Adult

• PO 5 mg tid × 3 days, then 10 mg tid × 3 days, then 15 mg tid × 3 days, then 20 mg tid × 3 days, then titrated to response, not to exceed 80 mg/day

• INTRATHECAL use implantable intrathecal INF pump; use screening trial of 3 separate bolus doses if needed (50 µg/ml, 75 µg/1.5 ml, 100 µg/2 ml); initial: double screening

---

italic = common side effects   ***bold italic*** = life-threatening reactions

dose that produced result and give over 24 hr, increase by 10%-30% q24h only; maintenance: 12-1500 µg/day (limited experience with doses >1000 µg/day)

Child

• 2-7 yr: initial: PO 10-15 mg/24 hr divided q8h; titrate dose every 3 days in increments of 5-15 mg/day to a max of 40 mg/day

• ≥8 yr: PO max 60 mg/day in 3 divided doses

$ AVAILABLE FORMS/COST OF THERAPY

• Kit—Intrathecal: 500 µg/ml, 20 ml: **$208.00**; 2000 µg/ml, 5 ml: **$213.50**

• Tab, Uncoated—Oral: 10 mg, 100's: **$31.75-$72.88**; 20 mg, 100's: **$51.11-$124.80**

PRECAUTIONS: Peptic ulcer disease, renal disease, hepatic disease, stroke, seizure disorder, diabetes mellitus, elderly

PREGNANCY AND LACTATION: Pregnancy category C; present in breast milk, 0.1% of mother's dose; compatible with breast feeding

SIDE EFFECTS/ADVERSE REACTIONS

CNS: Disorientation, *dizziness, drowsiness, fatigue,* headache, insomnia, paresthesias, *seizures* (decreased seizure threshold); tremors; *weakness*

CV: Chest pain, edema, hypotension, palpitations

EENT: Blurred vision, mydriasis, nasal congestion, tinnitus

GI: Abdominal pain, anorexia, constipation, dry mouth, increased AST, alk phosphatase, *nausea,* vomiting

GU: Urinary frequency

METAB: Hyperglycemia

SKIN: Pruritus, rash

SPECIAL CONSIDERATIONS

• Abrupt discontinuation may lead to hallucinations, spasticity, tachycardia; drug should be tapered off over 1-2 wk

---

balsalazide

(ball-sal´a-zide)

Rx: Colazal

Chemical Class: 5-amino derivative of salicylic acid

Therapeutic Class: GI antiinflammatory

CLINICAL PHARMACOLOGY

Mechanism of Action: A prodrug that is enzymatically cleaved in the colon to produce mesalamine (5-aminosalicylic acid) which may act by blocking cyclooxygenase and inhibiting prostaglandin production in the colon

Pharmacokinetics

PO: Peak 1-2 hr; systemic absorption very low and variable (greater in patients with ulcerative colitis compared to healthy subjects); 99% bound to plasma proteins; unabsorbed drug eliminated in feces; absorbed drug metabolized and eliminated in urine (mainly as N-acetyl metabolite)

INDICATIONS AND USES: Mildly to moderately active ulcerative colitis (safety and effectiveness beyond 12 wk has not been established)

DOSAGE

Adult

• PO: 2250 mg (three 750 mg capsules) tid (total daily dose 6.75 g) for a total duration of 8 wk (some patients in clinical trials required treatment for up to 12 wk)

$ AVAILABLE FORMS/COST OF THERAPY

• Cap—Oral: 750 mg, 280's: **$280.00**

CONTRAINDICATIONS: Hypersensitivity to salicylates

PRECAUTIONS: Children; pyloric stenosis (may have prolonged gastric retention of capsules); renal dysfunction

PREGNANCY AND LACTATION: Pregnancy category B; excretion into breast milk unknown, mesalamine has produced adverse effects in a nursing infant and should be used with caution during breast feeding; observe nursing infant closely for changes in stool consistency

SIDE EFFECTS/ADVERSE REACTIONS

CNS: Headache, dizziness
EENT: Rhinitis, pharyngitis
GI: Abdominal pain, diarrhea, nausea, vomiting, rectal bleeding, flatulence, dyspepsia, frequent stools, dry mouth, cramps, constipation, *hepatotoxicity*
MS: Arthralgia, back pain, myalgia
RESP: Coughing
MISC: Insomnia, fatigue, fever, pain, anorexia

INTERACTIONS
Drugs

3 *Orally administered antibiotics:* Theoretical interference with the release of mesalamine in the colon

SPECIAL CONSIDERATIONS
• The recommended dose of 6.75 g/day provides approximately 2.4 g of free mesalamine to the colon

MONITORING PARAMETERS
• Amount of rectal bleeding, stool frequency, abdominal pain

---

becaplermin
(beck-a-pler′min)
Rx: Regranex
Chemical Class: Recombinant human platelet-derived growth factor (rhPDGF-BB)
Therapeutic Class: Diabetic neuropathic ulcer agent

CLINICAL PHARMACOLOGY
Mechanism of Action: Has biological activity similar to that of endogenous platelet-derived growth factor, which includes promoting the chemotactic recruitment and proliferation of cells involved in wound repair and enhancing the formation of granulation tissue

Pharmacokinetics
TOP: Systemic bioavailability <3%

INDICATIONS AND USES: Adjunctive treatment of lower extremity diabetic neuropathic ulcers that extend into the subcutaneous tissue or beyond and have an adequate blood supply

DOSAGE
Adult
• TOP Apply a 2/3-inch length of gel squeezed from a 15 g or 7.5 g tube or a 1 1/3-inch length of gel squeezed from a 2 g tube for each square inch of ulcer surface qd until complete ulcer healing has occurred; recalculate the amount of gel to be applied at weekly or biweekly intervals depending on the rate of change in ulcer area; the calculated length of gel should be squeezed onto a clean measuring surface, e.g., wax paper; the measured gel is transferred from the clean measuring surface using an application aid and then spread over the entire ulcer area to yield a thin continuous layer of approximately 1/16 of an inch thickness; the site(s) of application should then be cov-

---

ered by a saline moistened dressing and left in place for approximately 12 hours; the dressing should then be removed and the ulcer rinsed with saline or water to remove residual gel and covered again with a second moist dressing (without gel) for the remainder of the day

$ **AVAILABLE FORMS/COST OF THERAPY**
• Gel—Top: 100 µg/g, 15 g: **$477.23**
CONTRAINDICATIONS: Known neoplasm(s) at the site(s) of application; wounds that close by primary intention (non-sterile product)
PRECAUTIONS: Exposed joints, tendons, ligaments and bone; children <16 yr
PREGNANCY AND LACTATION: Pregnancy category C; excretion into breast milk is unknown but would be expected to be low given the systemic bioavailability of the drug
SIDE EFFECTS/ADVERSE REACTIONS
SKIN: Erythematous rash
SPECIAL CONSIDERATIONS
PATIENT/FAMILY EDUCATION
• Store refrigerated
• Wash hands before applying
MONITORING PARAMETERS
• If the ulcer does not decrease in size by approximately 30% after 10 wk of treatment or complete healing has not occurred in 20 wk, continued treatment should be reassessed

beclomethasone
(be-kloe-meth´a-sone)
Rx: INH: Beclovent, Vanceril; NASAL: Beconase AQ, Beconase, Vancenase, Vancenase AQ, Vancenase AQ Double Strength
Chemical Class: Halogenated synthetic glucocorticoid
Therapeutic Class: Anti-inflammatory corticosteroid, synthetic

CLINICAL PHARMACOLOGY
Mechanism of Action: Anti-inflammatory via inhibition of migration of polymorphonuclear leukocytes, fibroblasts, reversal of increased capillary permeability and lysosomal stabilization
Pharmacokinetics
INH: Despite inhaled routes, systemic absorption occurs; absorption occurs rapidly from all respiratory and gastrointestinal tissues; metabolized in lungs, liver, GI system; excreted in feces (with metabolites), less than 10% excreted in urine; $t_{1/2}$ 3-15 hr, crosses placenta
INDICATIONS AND USES: INH for chronic asthma; nasal for seasonal or perennial rhinitis; prevention of recurrence of nasal polyps; non-allergic (vasomotor) rhinitis
DOSAGE
Adult
• INH 2-4 puffs tid-qid, not to exceed 20 INH/day; NASAL 1-2 sprays in each nostril bid-qid; double strength NASAL 1-2 sprays each nostril qd
Child (6-12 yr)
• INH 1-2 puffs tid-qid, not to exceed 10 INH/day
Child (>12 yr)
• NASAL 1-2 sprays in each nostril bid-qid

AVAILABLE FORMS/COST OF THERAPY

• MDI Aer—INH: 42 µg/INH, 6.7 g: **$17.23-$49.11**; 42 µg/INH, 16.8 g: **$32.78-$49.71**
• MDI Aer—Nasal INH: 42 µg/INH, 6.7-7 g: **$17.23-$49.11**; 42 µg/INH, 16.8 g: **$32.78-$57.10**
• MDI Double Strength Aer—INH: 84 µg/INH; 12.2 g: **$53.33**
• Spray—Nasal: 42 µg/spray, 25 g: **$32.75-$58.56**; 84 µg/INH, 19 g: **$55.78**

CONTRAINDICATIONS: Primary treatment for status asthmaticus; nonasthmatic bronchial disease; bacterial, fungal, or viral infections of mouth, throat, or lungs; children <3 yr

PRECAUTIONS: Nasal disease/surgery, children <12 yr (potential reduction in bone growth velocity), nasal ulcers, recurrent epistaxis; suppression of HPA-axis observed when administered at doses of 2000 µg/day by oral aerosol; not a bronchodilator; not indicated for rapid relief of bronchospasm; systemic effects such as mental disturbances, increased bruising, weight gain, cushingoid features, and cataracts

PREGNANCY AND LACTATION: Pregnancy category C; breast milk excretion unknown; other corticosteroids excreted in low concentrations with systemic administration; compatible with breast feeding

SIDE EFFECTS/ADVERSE REACTIONS

CNS: Headache, paresthesia
EENT: Burning, candidal infection, *dryness,* earache, *nasal irritation,* nasal ulcerations, perforation of nasal septum, secretions with blood, *sneezing,* sore throat
GI: Dry mouth, dysphonia
METAB: Adrenal suppression
*RESP: **Bronchospasm***
SKIN: Pruritus, urticaria

SPECIAL CONSIDERATIONS
PATIENT/FAMILY EDUCATION

• Rinse mouth with water following INH to decrease possibility of fungal infections, dysphonia
• Review proper MDI administration technique regularly
• Systemic corticosteroid effects from inhaled and nasal steroids inadequate to prevent adrenal insufficiency in patients withdrawn from corticosteroids abruptly
• Response to nasal steroids seen in 3 days-2 wk; D/C if no improvement in 3 wk
• For prophylactic use, no role in acute treatment of asthma/allergy

---

belladonna alkaloids
(bell-a-don'a)
Rx: Belladonna Tincture
Combinations
   Rx: with butalbital (Butibel); with ergotamine and phenobarbital (Bellergal-S, Phenerbel-S); with phenobarbital (Donnatal, Donnatal Extentabs)
Chemical Class: Belladonna alkaloid
Therapeutic Class: Anticholinergic; gastrointestinal antispasmodic

---

CLINICAL PHARMACOLOGY
Mechanism of Action: Belladonna inhibits muscarinic actions of acetylcholine at postganglionic parasympathetic neuroeffector sites including smooth muscle, secretory glands, and CNS sites
Pharmacokinetics
PO: Duration 4-6 hr: metabolized by liver, excreted in urine

INDICATIONS AND USES: Adjunctive therapy in treatment of peptic ulcer, functional digestive disorders, diarrhea, diverticulitis, pancreatitis; dysmenorrhea; nocturnal enuresis; Parkinsonism; motion sickness; nausea and vomiting

DOSAGE
Adult
• PO 0.6-1 ml of tincture tid-qid
Child
• PO 0.03 ml/kg of tincture tid

$ AVAILABLE FORMS/COST OF THERAPY
• Tincture—Oral: 27-33 mg/100 ml, 120 ml: **$8.52**

CONTRAINDICATIONS: Hypersensitivity to anticholinergics, narrow-angle glaucoma, GI obstruction, myasthenia gravis, paralytic ileus, GI atony, toxic megacolon, obstructive uropathy

PRECAUTIONS: Hyperthyroidism, coronary artery disease, dysrhythmias, CHF, ulcerative colitis, hypertension, hiatal hernia, hepatic disease, renal disease, elderly, children, prostatic hypertrophy, chronic lung disease, high environmental temperatures

PREGNANCY AND LACTATION: Pregnancy category C; excretion into breast milk is controversial; neonates may be particularly sensitive to anticholinergic agents; use caution in nursing mothers

SIDE EFFECTS/ADVERSE REACTIONS
CNS: Anxiety, confusion, dizziness, drowsiness, hallucinations, headache, insomnia, nervousness, stimulation in elderly, weakness
CV: Palpitations, tachycardia
EENT: Blurred vision, cycloplegia, increased ocular pressure, mydriasis, photophobia
GI: Altered taste, *constipation, dry mouth,* dysphagia, heartburn, nausea, *paralytic ileus,* vomiting
GU: Hesitancy, impotence, *retention*
SKIN: Allergic reactions, anhidrosis, flushing, pruritus, rash, urticaria

INTERACTIONS
Drugs
3 *Amantadine:* Enhanced anticholinergic effect; enhanced CNS effect of amantadine
3 *Neuroleptics:* Reduced neuroleptic effect
3 *Rimantadine:* Enhanced anticholinergic effect; enhanced CNS effect of rimantadine
3 *Tacrine:* May reduce anticholinergic effect of atropine; belladonna may reduce CNS effect of tacrine

SPECIAL CONSIDERATIONS
• Product contains hyoscyamine, atropine, and scopolamine

PATIENT/FAMILY EDUCATION
• Avoid hot environments, heat stroke may occur
• Use sunglasses when outside to prevent photophobia

---

belladonna and opium

(bell-a-don'a)
Rx: B & O Supprettes
Chemical Class: Belladonna alkaloid/opiate
Therapeutic Class: Antispasmodic; narcotic analgesic
DEA Class: Schedule II

CLINICAL PHARMACOLOGY
Mechanism of Action: Belladonna inhibits muscarinic actions of acetylcholine at postganglionic parasympathetic neuroeffector sites including smooth muscle, secretory glands, and CNS sites; opium contains many narcotic alkaloids including morphine, which inhibit gastric motility and provide sedation and analgesic properties
Pharmacokinetics
PR: Onset 30 min (opium), 1-2 hr (belladonna); opium metabolized in the liver

INDICATIONS AND USES: Ureteral spasm not responsive to non-narcotic analgesics; rectal or bladder tenesmus occurring in postoperative states and neoplastic situations

DOSAGE

Adult

• PR 1 supp 1-2 times daily, up to 4 doses/day

Child

• Not recommended for children <12

$ **AVAILABLE FORMS/COST OF THERAPY**

• Supp—Rect: 16.2 mg/30 mg, 12's: **$31.30-$35.44**; 16.2 mg/60 mg, 12's: **$25.30-$38.06**

CONTRAINDICATIONS: Hypersensitivity to anticholinergics or opium, narrow-angle glaucoma, severe hepatic or renal disease, bronchial asthma, respiratory depression, seizure disorders, acute alcoholism, delirium tremens, premature labor

PRECAUTIONS: Elderly, debilitated patients, increased intracranial pressure, toxic psychosis, myxedema

PREGNANCY AND LACTATION: Pregnancy category C; excretion of belladonna into breast milk is controversial; neonates may be particularly sensitive to anticholinergic agents, therefore use caution in nursing mothers

SIDE EFFECTS/ADVERSE REACTIONS

CNS: CNS depression, confusion, *drowsiness,* headache, memory loss, sedation, tiredness, weakness

CV: **Dysrhythmias,** bradycardia, flushing, hypotension, increased intracranial pressure, orthostatic hypotension, palpitations, peripheral vasodilation, tachycardia

EENT: Blurred vision, dry mouth, intraocular pain, mydriasis, photophobia

GI: Bloated feeling, *constipation,* nausea, vomiting

GU: Hesitancy, retention

RESP: **Respiratory depression**

SKIN: Decreased sweating, rash

MISC: Physical and psychological dependence

INTERACTIONS

Drugs

❸ *Amantadine:* Enhanced anticholinergic effect; enhanced CNS effect of amantadine

❸ *Neuroleptics:* Reduced neuroleptic effect

❸ *Rimantadine:* Enhanced anticholinergic effect; enhanced CNS effect of rimantadine

❸ *Tacrine:* May reduce anticholinergic effect; belladonna may reduce CNS effect of tacrine

SPECIAL CONSIDERATIONS
PATIENT/FAMILY EDUCATION

• Moisten finger and suppository with water before inserting

• May cause drowsiness, dry mouth, and blurred vision

• Store at room temperature; DO NOT refrigerate

---

benazepril

(be-naze′a-pril)

Rx: Lotensin

Combinations

   Rx: with hydrochlorothiazide (Lotensin HCT)

   Rx: with amlodipine (Lotrel)

Chemical Class: Nonsulfhydryl, angiotensin-converting enzyme (ACE) inhibitor

Therapeutic Class: Antihypertensive

CLINICAL PHARMACOLOGY

Mechanism of Action: Antihypertensive, hypoproliferative, and cardioprotective effects attributable to competitive inhibition of angiotensin-converting enzyme (ACE) yielding decreased plasma concentrations of angiotensin II, plasma aldosterone concentrations, systemic vascular resistance, blood pressure, preload and afterload, not accompanied by changes in heart rate, pressor sensitivity to exogenous norepinephrine, or baroreceptor sensitivity

Pharmacokinetics

PO: Peak ½-1 hr, serum protein binding 97%, $t_{1/2}$ 10-11 hr; metabolized by liver to active metabolite (benazeprilat), which is excreted by the kidneys

INDICATIONS AND USES: Hypertension, CHF, MI, erythrocytosis,* nephropathy,* retinopathy*

DOSAGE

Adult

• PO 10 mg qd initially, increase as needed to 20-40 mg/day divided bid or qd
• *Renal impairment:* PO 5 mg qd with CrCl <30 ml/min/1.73 m²; increase as needed to maximum of 40 mg/day

$ AVAILABLE FORMS/COST OF THERAPY

• Tab, Uncoated—Oral: 5 mg, 100's: **$97.43**; 10 mg, 100's: **$86.64-$98.69**; 20 mg, 100's: **$86.64-$97.43**; 40 mg, 100's: **$88.95-$97.43**

PRECAUTIONS: History of anaphylaxis, renal insufficiency (<30 ml/min), hypotension (CHF, elderly, volume depletion—diuretics, dialysis, cirrhosis), aortic stenosis, hyperkalemia (potassium supplements, potassium-sparing diuretics, renal disease, diabetes), neutropenia (autoimmune diseases, collagenvascular, febrile illness, immunosuppressant drug therapy), proteinuria, renal artery stenosis, surgery/anesthesia (excessive hypotension, correctable with fluids)

PREGNANCY AND LACTATION: Pregnancy category C (1st trimester), category D (2nd and 3rd trimesters); ACE inhibitors can cause fetal and neonatal morbidity and death when administered to pregnant women; detectable in breast milk in trace amounts, a newborn would receive <0.1% of the mg/kg maternal dose; effect on nursing infant has not been determined

SIDE EFFECTS/ADVERSE REACTIONS

CNS: Anxiety, *dizziness, fatigue, headache,* insomnia, paresthesia
CV: Angina, hypotension, palpitations, postural hypotension, syncope (especially with first dose)
GI: Abdominal pain, constipation, melena, nausea, vomiting
GU: Decreased libido, impotence, increased BUN/creatinine, urinary tract infection
HEME: **Agranulocytosis, neutropenia**
METAB: Hyperkalemia, hyponatremia
MS: Arthralgia, arthritis, myalgia
RESP: Asthma, bronchitis, *cough,* dyspnea, sinusitis
SKIN: Angioedema, flushing, rash, sweating

INTERACTIONS

Drugs

❷ *Allopurinol:* Combination may predispose to hypersensitivity reactions
❸ *Alpha adrenergic blockers:* Exaggerated first dose hypotensive response when added to benazepril
❸ *Aspirin:* May reduce hemodynamic effects of benazepril; less likely at doses under 236 mg; less likely with nonacetylated salicylates
❸ *Azathioprine:* Increased myelosuppression
❸ *Cyclosporine:* Combination may cause renal insufficiency

---

* = non-FDA-approved use

3 *Insulin:* Benazepril may enhance insulin sensitivity

3 *Iron:* Benazepril may increase chance of systemic reaction to IV iron

3 *Lithium:* Reduced lithium clearance

3 *Loop diuretics:* Initiation of benazepril may cause hypotension and renal insufficiency in patients taking loop diuretics

3 *NSAIDs:* May reduce hemodynamic effects of benazepril

3 *Potassium-sparing diuretics:* Increased risk of hyperkalemia

3 *Trimethoprim:* Additive risk of hyperkalemia, especially in patient predisposed to renal insufficiency

Labs
• ACE inhibition can account for approximately 0.5 mEq/L rise in serum potassium

SPECIAL CONSIDERATIONS
PATIENT/FAMILY EDUCATION
• Caution with salt substitutes containing potassium chloride
• Rise slowly to sitting/standing position to minimize orthostatic hypotension
• Dizziness, fainting, lightheadedness may occur during 1st few days of therapy
• May cause altered taste perception or cough; persistent dry cough usually does not subside unless medication is stopped; notify clinician if these symptoms persist

MONITORING PARAMETERS
• BUN, creatinine, potassium within 2 wk after initiation of therapy (increased levels may indicate acute renal failure)

bentoquatum
(ben'toe-kwa-tum)
OTC: Ivy Block
Chemical Class: Organoclay compound
Therapeutic Class: Rhus dermatitis protectant

CLINICAL PHARMACOLOGY
Mechanism of Action: May interfere with allergen absorption by physical blocking
INDICATIONS AND USES: Prevention of poison ivy, oak, and sumac
DOSAGE
Adult and Child
• TOP apply 15 min prior to potential exposure; wash with soap and water after exposure
$ **AVAILABLE FORMS/COST OF THERAPY**
• Lotion—Top: 5%, 120 ml: **$11.95**
CONTRAINDICATIONS: Preexisting rash
PRECAUTIONS: Children <6 yr
SPECIAL CONSIDERATIONS
PATIENT/FAMILY EDUCATION
• To be used prior to exposure only

benzocaine

(ben'zoe-kane)

Rx: Americaine;

OTC: Anbesol, Bicozene, Boil-ease, Chigger-tox, Dermoplast, Foille, Hurricaine, Orajel, Orabase, Solarcaine

Combinations

> **Rx:** with antipyrine (Allergen, Auralgan, Auroto); with benzethonium chloride (Americaine, Otocain); with phenylephrine (Tympagesic)

Chemical Class: Aminobenzoate derivative; ester
Therapeutic Class: Topical local anesthetic

CLINICAL PHARMACOLOGY

Mechanism of Action: Benzocaine reversibly stabilizes the neuronal membrane, which decreases its permeability to sodium ions; depolarization of the neuronal membrane is inhibited thereby blocking the initiation and conduction of nerve impulses, topical anesthetic

Pharmacokinetics
TOP: Peak 1 min, duration 0.5-1 hr

INDICATIONS AND USES: Lubricant and topical anesthetic on intratracheal catheters, nasogastric and endoscopic tubes, urinary catheters, laryngoscopes, proctoscopes, sigmoidoscopes, vaginal specula; topical anesthetic for pharyngeal and nasal airways to obtund the pharyngeal and tracheal reflexes; relief of pain and pruritis in acute congestive and serous otitis media, acute swimmer's ear, and other forms of otitis externa

DOSAGE

Adult and Child >1 yr
• *Anesthetic lubricant:* TOP apply evenly to exterior of tube or instrument prior to use
• *Cerumen removal:* Instill tid for 2-3 days to help cerumen detach and facilitate removal
• *Otic drops:* Instill 4-5 gtts in the external auditory canal, then insert a cotton pledget into the external ear; repeat every 1-2 hr if necessary to relieve pain

§ AVAILABLE FORMS/COST OF THERAPY

• Cre—Top: 5%, 10, 30 g: **$1.00**/30 g
• Gel—Top: 10%, 5, 10, 30 g: **$2.03-$4.33**/10 g; 20%, 2, 5, 20, 30, 120 g: **$5.67**/30 g; 6.3%, 7.5 g: **$4.18**; 7.5%, 10, 15 g: **$3.32**/15 g
• Liq—Top: 20%, 30 ml: **$5.67**
• Oint—Rect: 20%, 30 g: **$3.85**
• Oint—Top: 10%, 30 g: **$11.25**
• Paste—Top: 20%, 5, 15 g: **$6.38**/15 g
• Sol—Otic: (with antipyrine) 10 ml-15 ml: **$1.73-$12.27**/15 ml
• Spray/Aerosol—Top: 20%, 60, 120 ml: **$3.85-$23.85**/60 ml

CONTRAINDICATIONS: Perforated tympanic membrane or ear discharge (otic drops)

PREGNANCY AND LACTATION: Pregnancy category C; excretion in breast milk unknown; use caution in nursing mothers

SIDE EFFECTS/ADVERSE REACTIONS

EENT: Irritation in ear, itching
HEME: Methemoglobinemia in infants
SKIN: Burning, edema, erythema, pruritis, rash, stinging, tenderness, urticaria

SPECIAL CONSIDERATIONS
PATIENT/FAMILY EDUCATION

• Protect the solution from light and heat, do not use if it is brown or contains a precipitate

• Discard this product 6 mo after dropper is first placed in the drug solution

---

benzonatate

(ben-zoe'na-tate)

Rx: Tessalon Perles
Chemical Class: Tetracaine derivative
Therapeutic Class: Antitussive

CLINICAL PHARMACOLOGY

Mechanism of Action: Acts peripherally by anesthetizing the stretch receptors located in the respiratory passages, lungs, and pleura; reduces cough reflex at its source; has no inhibitory effect on the respiratory center in recommended dosage

Pharmacokinetics

PO: Onset 15-20 min, duration 3-8 hr

INDICATIONS AND USES: Symptomatic relief of cough

DOSAGE

Adult and Child >10 yr

• PO 100 mg tid, not to exceed 600 mg/day

S AVAILABLE FORMS/COST OF THERAPY

• Cap, Elastic—Oral: 100 mg, 100's: **$54.12-$117.94**

CONTRAINDICATIONS: Hypersensitivity to ester-type local anesthetics

PREGNANCY AND LACTATION: Pregnancy category C; excretion into breast milk unknown; use with caution in nursing mothers

SIDE EFFECTS/ADVERSE REACTIONS

CNS: Dizziness, drowsiness, headache
CV: Chest numbness
EENT: Burning eyes, nasal congestion
GI: Constipation, *nausea,* upset stomach
SKIN: Pruritus, rash, urticaria

SPECIAL CONSIDERATIONS
PATIENT/FAMILY EDUCATION

• Avoid driving, other hazardous activities until stabilized on this medication

• Do not chew or break capsules, will anesthetize mouth

---

benzoyl peroxide

(ben'zoe-ill per-ox'ide)

Rx: Benzac, Benzagel, Benzashave, Benzox, Brevoxyl, Delaqua, Desquam-E, Desquam-X, Pan-Oxyl, Persa-Gel;
OTC: Acetoxyl, Acne-10, Acnomel, Advanced Formula Oxy Sensitive, Ambi-10, Benoxyl, Clearasil, Clear by Design, Dermoxyl, Dryox, Exact, Fostex, Loroxide, Neutrogena, Oxyderm, Oxy-10, Perfectoderm, Solugel
Chemical Class: Benzoic acid derivative
Therapeutic Class: Antiacne agent

CLINICAL PHARMACOLOGY

Mechanism of Action: Antibacterial activity against *Propionibacterium acnes,* the predominant organism in sebaceous follicles and comedones; aided by mild drying action, removal of excess sebum; mild desquamation and sebostatic effects

---

italic = common side effects   ***bold italic*** = life-threatening reactions

Pharmacokinetics
TOP: 50% absorbed through skin; metabolized to benzoic acid, excreted in urine as benzoate
INDICATIONS AND USES: Mild to moderate acne
DOSAGE
Adult and Child
• TOP apply to affected area qd or bid
$ AVAILABLE FORMS/COST OF THERAPY
• Bar—Top: 5%, 10%, 4 oz: **$4.76-$9.34**
• Cre—Top: 5%, 45, 60, 120 g: **$1.70-$15.89**/45 g; 10%, 30, 45, 120, 450 g: **$1.98-$4.91**/30 g
• Gel—Top: 2.5%, 45, 60, 90 g: **$5.89-$30.75**/45 g; 4%, 42, 90 g: **$67.71**/90 g; 5%, 30, 45, 60, 90 g: **$5.68-$25.51**/45 g; 10%, 45, 60, 90 g: **$5.89-$30.75**/45 g
• Liq—Top: 2.5%, 240 ml: **$22.54**; 5%, 30, 90, 120, 150, 240 ml: **$25.36-$30.19**/240 ml; 10%, 30, 60, 90, 120, 150, 240 ml: **$14.59-$33.00**/240 ml
• Lotion—Top: 5%, 30, 60 ml: **$1.61-$5.61**/30 ml; 10%, 30, 60, 90, 360 ml: **$8.71-$19.44**/60 ml
PRECAUTIONS: Concurrent use with tretinoin may cause excess skin irritation
PREGNANCY AND LACTATION: Pregnancy category C; excretion into milk unknown
SIDE EFFECTS/ADVERSE REACTIONS
SKIN: Allergic and contact dermatitis, dryness, edema, erythema, local skin irritation, scaling, stinging
SPECIAL CONSIDERATIONS
PATIENT/FAMILY EDUCATION
• Keep away from eyes, mouth, inside of nose and other mucous membranes
• May cause transitory feeling of warmth or slight stinging

• Expect dryness and peeling, discontinue use if rash or irritation develops
• Water-based cosmetics may be used over drug; don't counter-treat dryness with emollients

---

benztropine

(benz'troe-peen)
Rx: Cogentin
Chemical Class: Tertiary amine
Therapeutic Class: Anticholinergic, anti-Parkinson's agent

CLINICAL PHARMACOLOGY
Mechanism of Action: Blocks striatal cholinergic receptors, which helps balance cholinergic and dopaminergic activity
Pharmacokinetics
IM/IV: Onset 15 min, duration 6-10 hr
PO: Onset 1 hr, duration 6-10 hr
INDICATIONS AND USES: Adjunctive treatment of all forms of Parkinson's disease; drug-induced extrapyramidal symptoms
DOSAGE
Adult
• *Parkinsonism:* PO 0.5-6 mg/day in 1-2 divided doses, begin with 0.5 mg/day and increase in 0.5 mg increments at 5-6 day intervals to achieve desired effect
• *Drug-induced extrapyramidal symptoms:* PO/IM/IV 1-4 mg/dose 1-2 times/day; switch to PO as soon as possible
Child >3 yr
• *Drug-induced extrapyramidal symptoms:* PO/IM/IV 0.02-0.05 mg/kg/dose 1-2 times/day
$ AVAILABLE FORMS/COST OF THERAPY
• Inj, Sol—IM, IV: 1 mg/ml, 2 ml: **$8.22**

---

* = non-FDA-approved use

• Tab, Uncoated—Oral: 0.5 mg, 100's: **$3.13-$22.06**; 1 mg, 100's: **$5.40-$24.06**; 2 mg, 100's: **$6.93-$30.34**

CONTRAINDICATIONS: Narrow-angle glaucoma, myasthenia gravis, GI/GU obstruction, child <3 yr, peptic ulcer, megacolon, prostatic hypertrophy

PRECAUTIONS: Elderly, tachycardia, liver/kidney disease, drug abuse history, dysrhythmias, hypotension, hypertension, psychiatric patients, children, tardive dyskinesia

PREGNANCY AND LACTATION: Pregnancy category C; an inhibitory effect on lactation may occur; infants may be particularly sensitive to anticholinergic effects

SIDE EFFECTS/ADVERSE REACTIONS

CNS: Anxiety, confusion, delusions, depression, dizziness, hallucinations, headache, incoherence, irritability, memory loss, restlessness, sedation

CV: Hypotension, mild bradycardia, palpitations, postural hypotension, tachycardia

EENT: Angle-closure glaucoma, blurred vision, difficulty swallowing, dilated pupils, dry eyes, increased intraocular tension, mydriasis, photophobia

GI: Abdominal distress, *constipation, dry mouth,* epigastric distress, nausea, ***paralytic ileus,*** vomiting

GU: Dysuria, hesitancy, retention

MS: Cramping, muscular weakness

SKIN: Dermatoses, rash, urticaria

MISC: Decreased sweating, erectile dysfunction, flushing, heat stroke, hyperthermia, increased temperature, numbness of fingers

INTERACTIONS

Drugs

3 *Anticholinergics:* Excess anticholinergic side effects

3 *Amantadine:* Potentiates CNS side effects of amantadine

3 *Neuroleptics:* Inhibition of therapeutic response to neuroleptics; excessive anticholinergic effects

3 *Tacrine:* Reduced therapeutic effects of both drugs

SPECIAL CONSIDERATIONS

PATIENT/FAMILY EDUCATION

• Do not discontinue abruptly

• Administer with or after meals to prevent GI upset

• Drug may increase susceptibility to heat stroke

---

benzylpenicilloyl-polylysine

(ben'zill-pen-i-cill'oyl-poly-ly-'seen)

Rx: Pre-Pen
Chemical Class: Penicillin derivative
Therapeutic Class: Penicillin allergy skin test

CLINICAL PHARMACOLOGY

Mechanism of Action: Elicits IgE antibodies that produce type I accelerated urticarial reactions to penicillins

INDICATIONS AND USES: Adjunct in assessing the risk of administering penicillin (benzylpenicillin or penicillin G) when it is the preferred drug of choice in patients who have a history of clinical penicillin hypersensitivity

DOSAGE

Adult and Child

• *Scratch Test* (always perform first): A sterile 20 gauge needle should be used to make a 3-5 mm scratch of the epidermis; apply a small drop of Pre-Pen solution to the scratch and rub gently with an applicator, toothpick, or the side of the needle; a positive reaction consists of the development within 10 min of a pale wheal, usually with pseudopods, surrounding the scratch site and varying in diameter from 5 to 15 mm (or more)

• *Intradermal Test* (use only if scratch test completely negative): Use a tuberculin syringe with a 26 to 30 gauge, short, bevel needle to inject a volume of 0.01-0.02 ml; use a separate syringe and needle to inject a like amount of saline as a control at least 1.5 in removed from the test site; most skin reactions will develop within 5-15 min; a positive reaction consists of itching and marked increase in size of original bleb; wheal may exceed 20 mm in diameter and exhibit pseudopods; the control site should be completely reactionless

§ AVAILABLE FORMS/COST OF THERAPY

• Inj, Sol—Intradermal: 0.25 ml: **$19.42-$20.77**

CONTRAINDICATIONS: Extreme hypersensitivity

PRECAUTIONS: Repeated skin testing

PREGNANCY AND LACTATION: Pregnancy category C

SIDE EFFECTS/ADVERSE REACTIONS

SKIN: Edema, erythema, pruritus, urticaria, wheal

MISC: Systemic allergic reactions occur rarely

SPECIAL CONSIDERATIONS

• Does not identify those patients who react to a minor antigenic determinant (i.e., anaphylaxis); does not reliably predict the occurrence of late reactions; patients with a negative skin test may still have allergic reactions to therapeutic penicillin

---

bepridil
(beh´prih-dill)
Rx: Vascor
Chemical Class: Diarylaminopropylamine ether
Therapeutic Class: Calcium-channel blocker; Antianginal

CLINICAL PHARMACOLOGY
Mechanism of Action: Inhibits both calcium and sodium ion flux across cell membrane during cardiac depolarization; produces relaxation of coronary vascular smooth muscle; dilates coronary arteries; slows SA/AV node conduction times; dilates peripheral arteries; hemodynamics: decreases myocardial contractility, no effect on cardiac output, decreases peripheral vascular resistance

Pharmacokinetics
PO: Peak serum concentration 2-3 hr, 99% bound to plasma proteins, $t_{1/2}$ 24 hr; completely metabolized in the liver, excreted in urine and feces

INDICATIONS AND USES: Chronic stable angina; because of potential side effects (ventricular arrhythmias, agranulocytosis), should be reserved for patients who are unresponsive to, or intolerant of, other antianginal medication; may be used alone or in combination with β-blockers and/or nitrates

DOSAGE
Adult
• PO 200 mg qd initially, increase after 10 days depending on response, max 400 mg/day; most patients maintained on 300 mg/day

§ AVAILABLE FORMS/COST OF THERAPY

• Tab, Plain Coated—Oral: 200 mg, 90's: **$323.34**; 300 mg, 90's: **$361.01**; 400 mg, 90's: **$327.68**

CONTRAINDICATIONS: Sick sinus syndrome, 2nd or 3rd degree heart block, Wolff-Parkinson-White syndrome, hypotension <90 mm Hg systolic, uncompensated cardiac insufficiency, history of serious ventricular dysrhythmias, congenital QT interval prolongation or taking other drugs that prolong QT interval

PRECAUTIONS: CHF, renal disease, hepatic disease, children, hypokalemia, left bundle branch block, sinus bradycardia, recent MI

PREGNANCY AND LACTATION: Pregnancy category C; excreted in breast milk; use caution in nursing mothers

SIDE EFFECTS/ADVERSE REACTIONS

CNS: Anxiety, *asthenia,* confusion, depression, *dizziness,* drowsiness, fatigue, *headache,* insomnia, lightheadedness, nervousness, tremor, weakness

*CV: **AV block,** bradycardia, CHF, **dysrhythmia (torsades de pointes, ventricular tachycardia),*** edema, hypotension, palpitations

EENT: Blurred vision, tinnitus

GI: Constipation, *diarrhea,* dry mouth, *gastric upset,* increased liver function studies, *nausea,* vomiting

GU: Nocturia, polyuria

*HEME: **Agranulocytosis** (rare)*

RESP: Shortness of breath

SKIN: Rash

INTERACTIONS

Drugs

3 *Beta-blockers:* Additive depressant effects on myocardial contractility or AV conduction

3 *Digitalis glycosides:* Reduced clearance; increased digitalis levels; potential toxicity

SPECIAL CONSIDERATIONS

PATIENT/FAMILY EDUCATION

• ECGs will be necessary during initiation of therapy and after dosage changes

• Notify provider immediately for irregular heartbeat, shortness of breath, pronounced dizziness, constipation, or hypotension

• May be taken with food or meals

MONITORING PARAMETERS

• Blood pressure, pulse, respiration, ECG intervals (PR, QRS, QT) at initiation of therapy and again after dosage increases prologation of QT interval by >0.52 sec predisposes to proarrythmia

• Serum potassium (normalize before initiation)

---

betamethasone

(bay-ta-meth′a-sone)

Rx: Systemic: Celestone, Celstone Soluspan

Rx: Topical: Alphatrex, Betatrex, Diprolene, Diprosone, Luxiq Qualisone, Maxivate, Valisone Combinations

   Rx: with clotrimazole (Lotrisone)

Chemical Class: Synthetic glucocorticoid

Therapeutic Class: Topical corticosteroid, intermediate potency (benzoate [cream, gel, lotion, ointment], valerate [cream, lotion, ointment, powder]), high potency (dipropionate [cream, lotion, ointment, spray]); systemic corticosteroid

---

CLINICAL PHARMACOLOGY

Mechanism of Action: Decreases inflammation by depressing migration of polymorphonuclear leukocytes and activity of endogenous mediators of inflammation; has many profound metabolic effects; does not possess mineralocorticoid activity

---

italic = common side effects   ***bold italic*** = life-threatening reactions

Pharmacokinetics

Extensive metabolism in liver; t½ 300+ min, duration 36-54 hr

INDICATIONS AND USES: *Systemic:* Antiinflammatory or immunosuppressant agent in the treatment of a variety of diseases of hematologic, allergic, inflammatory, neoplastic, and autoimmune origin; Addison's disease, congenital adrenal hyperplasia, thyroiditis, hypercalcemia, serum sickness; prevention of neonatal respiratory distress syndrome (by administration to mother)*

Topical: Psoriasis, eczema, contact dermatitis, pruritus, and other corticosteroid responsive dermatoses

DOSAGE

Adult

• PO 0.6-7.2 mg/day; IM 0.5-9 mg/day divided q12h (usually ⅓-½ the oral dose); IM (to mother for prophylaxis of infant lung prematurity) 12.5 mg q24h × 2 doses; IV (sodium phosphate salt only) up to 9 mg; Intra-articular and soft tissue (sodium phosphate/acetate salt): large joints 6-12 mg (1-2 ml), smaller joints 1.5-3 mg (0.25-1 ml), bursitis 6 mg, ganglia 3 mg, tendonitis 1.5-3 mg; TOP apply to affected area bid-tid

Child

• PO 0.0175-0.25 mg/kg/day divided q6-8h or 0.5-7.5 mg/m²/day divided q6-8h; IM 0.0175-0.125 mg base/kg/day divided q6-12h or 0.5-7.5 mg/m²/day divided q6-12h; TOP apply to affected area bid-tid

$ AVAILABLE FORMS/COST OF THERAPY

• Aer, Spray (dipropionate)—Top: 0.1%, 85 g: **$25.97**

• Cre (dipropionate)—Top: 0.05%, 15, 45, 60 g: **$7.50-$52.31**/45 g

• Cre (valerate)—Top: 0.1%, 15, 45 g: **$4.67-$29.63**/45 g

• Cre, Augmented (dipropionate)—Top: 0.05%, 15, 45 g, 50 g: **$9.07-$62.19**/45 g

• Gel, Augmented (dipropionate)—Top: 0.05%, 15, 45, 50 g: **$51.30**/45 g

• Inj, Susp (sodium phosphate)—Intra-articular, Intradermal, IM: 3 mg/ml, 5 ml: **$14.60-$31.53**

• Lotion (dipropionate)—Top: 0.05%, 20, 60 ml: **$10.30-$74.11**/60 ml

• Lotion (valerate)—Top: 0.1%, 20, 60 ml: **$7.80-$39.62**/60 ml

• Lotion, Augmented (dipropionate)—Top: 0.05%, 30, 60 ml: **$41.83**/30 ml

• Oint (dipropionate)—Top: 0.05%, 15, 45 g: **$7.50-$52.31**/45 g

• Oint (valerate)—Top: 0.1%, 15, 45 g: **$4.67-$29.63**/45 g

• Oint, Augmented (dipropionate)—Top: 0.05%, 15, 45, 50 g: **$41.42-$51.30**/45 g

• Syr—Oral: 0.6 mg/5 ml, 120 ml: **$41.22**

• Tab—Oral: 0.6 mg, 100's: **$186.54**

CONTRAINDICATIONS: Systemic fungal infection; use on face, groin, or axilla (topical)

PRECAUTIONS: Psychosis, diabetes mellitus, glaucoma, osteoporosis, seizure disorders, ulcerative colitis (intestinal perforation), CHF, hypertension, myesthenia gravis (if used with anticholinesterase agents), renal disease, esophagitis, peptic ulcer, latent tuberculosis or amebiasis (reactivation of disease)

PREGNANCY AND LACTATION: Pregnancy category C; used in patients with premature labor at about 24-36 wk gestation to stimulate fetal lung maturation (see dosage); excreted in breast milk, could suppress infant's growth and interfere with endogenous corticosteroid production

SIDE EFFECTS/ADVERSE REACTIONS

CNS: Depression, headache, *mood changes,* **seizures,** vertigo

CV: **CHF,** hypertension, tachycardia, thromboembolism, thrombophlebitis

EENT: Blurred vision, cataracts, increased intraocular pressure

GI: Abdominal distention, diarrhea, **hemorrhage,** increased appetite, *nausea, **pancreatitis***

METAB: Cushingoid state, decreased glucose tolerance, growth suppression in children, **HPA suppression**

MS: Aseptic necrosis of femoral and humeral heads, fractures, muscle mass loss, osteoporosis, weakness

SKIN: Acne, allergic contact dermatitis, atrophy, bruising, burning, dryness, ecchymosis, folliculitis, hypertrichosis, hypopigmentation, irritation, itching, miliaria, perioral dermatitis, petechiae, poor wound healing, secondary infection, striae, suppression of skin test reactions

INTERACTIONS

Drugs

⊠ *Aminoglutethamide:* Enhanced elimination of corticosteroids; marked reduction in corticosteroid response; increased clearance of prednisone; doubling of dose may be necessary

⊠ *Antidiabetics:* Increased blood glucose

⊠ *Barbiturates, carbamazepine:* Reduced serum concentrations of corticosteroids; increased clearance of prednisone

⊠ *Cholestyramine, colestipol:* Possible reduced absorption of corticosteroids

⊠ *Cyclosporine:* Possible increased concentration of both drugs, seizures

⊠ *Erythromycin, troleandomycin, clarithromycin, ketoconazole:* Possible enhanced steroid effect

⊠ *Estrogens, oral contraceptives:* Enhanced effects of corticosteroids

⊠ *Isoniazid:* Reduced plasma concentrations of isoniazid

⊠ *IUDs:* Inhibition of inflammation may decrease contraceptive effect

⊠ *NSAIDs:* Increased risk GI ulceration

⊠ *Rifampin:* Reduced therapeutic effect of corticosteroids; may reduce hepatic clearance of prednisone

⊠ *Salicylates:* Subtherapeutic salicylate concentrations possible

Labs

• *False negative:* Skin allergy tests

SPECIAL CONSIDERATIONS

• Recommend single daily doses in AM

• Signs of adrenal insufficiency include fatigue, anorexia, nausea, vomiting, diarrhea, weight loss, weakness, dizziness and low blood sugar; drug-induced secondary adrenocorticoid insufficiency may be minimized by gradual systemic dosage reduction; relative insufficiency may exist for up to 1 yr after discontinuation of therapy; be prepared to supplement in situations of stress

• May mask infections

• Do not give live virus vaccines to patients on prolonged therapy

• Patients on chronic steroid therapy should wear medic alert bracelet

• Do not use topical products on weeping, denuded, or infected areas

MONITORING PARAMETERS

• Serum K and glucose

• Growth of children on prolonged therapy

betaxolol

(bay-tax′oh-lol)
Rx: Betoptic, Betoptic S,
Kerlone
Chemical Class: β_1-selective
(cardioselective) adrenorecep-
tor blocker
Therapeutic Class: Antihyper-
tensive; antiglaucoma agent

CLINICAL PHARMACOLOGY
Mechanism of Action: Preferentially competes with β-adrenergic
agonists for available β_1-receptor
sites inhibiting the chronotropic and
inotropic responses to β_1-adrener-
gic stimulation (cardioselective);
blocks β_2 receptors in bronchial system at higher doses; weak mem-
brane stabilizing activity; lacks intrinsic sympathomimetic (partial
agonist) activity; reduces aqueous
humor production; slight increase in
outflow may be an additional mechanism; little or no effect on pupil size
or accommodation
Pharmacokinetics
PO: Peak 1.5-6 hr
OPHTH: Onset 30 min, duration 12
hr
50% protein bound; metabolized by
liver, excreted in urine as metabolites and unchanged drug; $t_{1/2}$ 14-22
hr
INDICATIONS AND USES: Hypertension; chronic open-angle glaucoma
DOSAGE
Adult
• PO 10 mg qd, increased to 20 mg
qd after 7-14 days if desired response is not achieved; doses >20
mg/day have not produced additional antihypertensive effect
• OPHTH 1 gtt bid
Elderly
• PO reduce initial dose to 5 mg qd

$ **AVAILABLE FORMS/COST
OF THERAPY**
• Sol—Ophth: 0.5%, 2.5, 5, 10, 15
ml: **$26.17-$28.11**/5 ml
• Susp—Ophth: 0.25%, 2.5, 5, 10,
15 ml: **$26.94-$32.44**/5 ml
• Tab, Plain Coated—Oral: 10 mg,
100's: **$95.35**; 20 mg, 100's:
$142.85
CONTRAINDICATIONS: Cardiogenic shock, 2nd or 3rd degree heart
block, sinus bradycardia, CHF unless secondary to a tachydysrhythmia treatable with β-blockers
PRECAUTIONS: Major surgery, diabetes mellitus, renal disease, thyroid disease, COPD, asthma, well-
compensated heart failure, abrupt
withdrawal, peripheral vascular disease; ophthalmic preparations can
be absorbed systemically
PREGNANCY AND LACTATION:
Pregnancy category C; excretion
into breast milk unknown; use caution in nursing mothers
**SIDE EFFECTS/ADVERSE REAC-
TIONS**
CNS: Depression, *dizziness,* drowsiness, *fatigue,* hallucinations, insomnia, *lethargy,* memory loss, mental
changes, strange dreams
CV: Bradycardia, **CHF,** cold extremities, profound hypotension,
2nd or 3rd degree heart block
EENT: Blepharoptosis, diplopia, dry
burning eyes, keratitis, ptosis, sore
throat, visual disturbances
GI: Diarrhea, dry mouth, ***ischemic
colitis, mesenteric arterial thrombosis,*** *nausea,* vomiting
GU: Impotence, sexual dysfunction
HEME: ***Agranulocytosis, thrombocytopenia***
METAB: Hyperlipidemia (increase
TG, total cholesterol, LDL; decrease HDL), masked hypoglycemic response to insulin (sweating
excepted)
RESP: ***Bronchospasm,*** dyspnea

SKIN: Alopecia, pruritis, rash
INTERACTIONS
Drugs

3 *Adenosine:* Increased risk of bradycardic response

3 *Antacids:* Decreased absorption of oral betaxolol

3 *Antidiabetics:* Altered response to hypoglycemia, prolonged recovery of normoglycemia, hypertension, blockade of tachycardia; may increase blood glucose and impair peripheral circulation

3 *Dipyridamole:* Bradycardia

3 *Neostigmine:* Additive risk of bradycardia

3 *NSAIDs:* Reduced hypotensive effects of β-blockers

3 *Tacrine:* Additive bradycardia

3 *Theophylline:* Antagonistic pharmacodynamic effects

3 *Verapamil:* Enhanced effects of both drugs, particularly atrioventricular conduction slowings

SPECIAL CONSIDERATIONS

• Do not discontinue oral drug abruptly, may precipitate angina or MI

• Anaphylactic reactions may be more severe and not be as responsive to usual doses of epinephrine

• Transient stinging/discomfort is relatively common with ophthalmic preparations, notify clinician if severe

MONITORING PARAMETERS

• Blood pressure, pulse, intraocular pressure (ophth)

---

bethanechol
(be-than´e-kole)
Rx: Duvoid, Urecholine
Chemical Class: Synthetic choline ester
Therapeutic Class: Cholinergic stimulant

CLINICAL PHARMACOLOGY
Mechanism of Action: Stimulates muscarinic acetylcholine receptors directly mimicking the effects of parasympathetic nervous system stimulation; stimulates gastric motility and micturition

Pharmacokinetics
PO: Onset 30-90 min, duration 1-6 hr

SC: Onset 5-15 min, duration 1 hr

INDICATIONS AND USES: Acute postoperative and postpartum nonobstructive (functional) urinary retention; neurogenic atony of the urinary bladder with retention; gastric atony or stasis*; congenital megacolon*; gastroesophageal reflux*

DOSAGE
Adult
• PO 10-50 mg bid-qid; SC 2.5-5 mg tid-qid, up to 7.5-10 mg q4h for neurogenic bladder

Child
• *Abdominal distention or urinary retention:* PO 0.6 mg/kg/day divided tid-qid

• *Gastroesophageal reflux:* PO 0.1-0.2 mg/kg/dose given 30 min to 1 hr before each meal, max qid; SC 0.12-0.2 mg/kg/day divided tid-qid

$ AVAILABLE FORMS/COST OF THERAPY

• Inj, Sol—SC: 5 mg/ml, 1 ml: **$5.62**
• Tab, Uncoated—Oral: 5 mg, 100's: **$2.75-$40.74**; 10 mg, 100's: **$2.95-$123.83**; 25 mg, 100's: **$3.95-$165.09**; 50 mg, 100's: **$7.25-$194.18**

---

italic = common side effects   ***bold italic*** = life-threatening reactions

CONTRAINDICATIONS: Severe bradycardia, asthma, severe hypotension, hypertension, hyperthyroidism, peptic ulcer, parkinsonism, seizure disorders, coronary artery disease, coronary occlusion, mechanical bladder neck obstruction, possible GI obstruction, peritonitis, recent urinary or GI surgery, atrioventricular conduction defects, vasomotor instability, IM/IV inj

PRECAUTIONS: Child <8 yr, urinary retention due to obstruction; not for IM or IV administrations (severe cholinergic overstimulation)

PREGNANCY AND LACTATION: Pregnancy category C; abdominal pain and diarrhea have been reported in a nursing infant exposed to bethanechol in milk; use caution in nursing mothers

SIDE EFFECTS/ADVERSE REACTIONS

More common after SC injection

CNS: Dizziness, headache, lightheadedness or fainting

CV: Fall in blood pressure with reflex tachycardia, vasomotor response

EENT: Lacrimation, miosis

GI: Abdominal cramps, *belching,* borborygmi, colicky pain, *diarrhea, nausea,* salivation

GU: Urinary urgency

RESP: **Bronchospasm, may precipitate asthmatic attack**

SKIN: Flushing, sweating

MISC: Malaise

INTERACTIONS

Drugs

3 *β-blockers:* Additive bradycardia

3 *Tacrine:* Increased cholinergic effects

SPECIAL CONSIDERATIONS

• Recommend taking on an empty stomach to avoid nausea and vomiting

biperiden
(bye-per'i-den)
Rx: Akineton
Chemical Class: Tertiary amine
Therapeutic Class: Anticholinergic; anti-Parkinson's agent

CLINICAL PHARMACOLOGY

Mechanism of Action: Blocks striated cholinergic receptors, which helps balance cholinergic and dopaminergic activity

Pharmacokinetics

PO: Onset 1 hr, duration 6-10 hr

INDICATIONS AND USES: Adjunctive treatment of all forms of Parkinson's syndrome; drug-induced extrapyramidal symptoms

DOSAGE

Adult

• *Parkinson symptoms:* PO 2 mg tid-qid; max 16 mg/24 hr

• *Extrapyramidal symptoms:* PO 2 mg qd-tid

$ AVAILABLE FORMS/COST OF THERAPY

• Tab, Uncoated—Oral: 2 mg, 100's: **$29.76-$43.15**

CONTRAINDICATIONS: Narrow-angle glaucoma, myasthenia gravis, GI/GU obstruction, megacolon, stenosing peptic ulcers, prostatic hypertrophy

PRECAUTIONS: Elderly, tachycardia, dysrhythmias, liver or kidney disease, drug abuse, hypotension, hypertension, psychiatric patients; give parenteral dose with patient recumbent to prevent postural hypotension; isolated instances of mental confusion, euphoria, agitation, and disturbed behavior have been reported in susceptible patients

PREGNANCY AND LACTATION:
Pregnancy category C; breast milk excretion not known, nursing infants particularly sensitive to anticholinergic effects

SIDE EFFECTS/ADVERSE REACTIONS

CNS: Anxiety, confusion, delusions, depression, dizziness, euphoria, hallucinations, headache, incoherence, irritability, memory loss, restlessness, sedation, tremor

CV: Bradycardia, palpitations, postural hypotension, tachycardia

EENT: Angle-closure glaucoma, blurred vision, difficulty swallowing, dilated pupils, increased intraocular tension, mydriasis, photophobia

GI: Abdominal distress, *constipation, dry mouth,* nausea, **paralytic ileus,** vomiting

GU: Dysuria, hesitancy, retention

MS: Cramping, weakness

SKIN: Dermatoses, rash, urticaria

MISC: Decreased sweating, flushing, heat stroke, hyperthermia, increased temperature, numbness of fingers

INTERACTIONS

Drugs

3 *Amantadine:* Potentiates CNS side effect of amantadine

3 *Anticholinergics:* Increased anticholinergic effects

3 *Neuroleptics:* Inhibition of therapeutic response to neuroleptics; excessive anticholinergic effects

3 *Tacrine:* Reduced therapeutic effects of both drugs

SPECIAL CONSIDERATIONS

PATIENT/FAMILY EDUCATION

• May increase susceptibility to heatstroke

• Do not discontinue drug abruptly; taper off over 1 wk

---

bisacodyl

(bis-a-koe′dill)

OTC: Bisac-Evac, Bisco-Lax, Dulagen, Dulcolax, Fleet Bisacodyl

Chemical Class: Diphenylmethane derivative

Therapeutic Class: Stimulant laxative

CLINICAL PHARMACOLOGY

Mechanism of Action: Acts directly on intestine by increasing motor activity; irritates colonic intramural plexus

Pharmacokinetics

PO: Onset 6-8 hr

PR: Onset 15-60 min

Absorption is minimal; absorbed drug metabolized by liver; excreted in urine, bile, feces, breast milk

INDICATIONS AND USES: Short-term treatment of constipation; bowel or rectal preparation for surgery, examination

DOSAGE

Adult

• PO 5-15 mg; up to 30 mg for bowel or rect preparation; PR 10 mg, 37.5 ml enema

Child

• PO 5-10 mg (or 0.3 mg/kg) for age >3 yr; PR 5-10 mg for age 2-11 yr; 5 mg for age <2 yr

\$ AVAILABLE FORMS/COST OF THERAPY

• Liq—Rect: 10 mg/37.5 ml: **$1.43**

• Supp—Rect: 10 mg, 12's: **$1.19-$8.37**

• Tab, Enteric Coated—Oral: 5 mg, 100's: **$1.28-$32.61**

CONTRAINDICATIONS: Rectal fissures, abdominal pain, nausea, vomiting, appendicitis, acute surgical abdomen, ulcerated hemor-

---

rhoids, acute hepatitis, fecal impaction, intestinal/biliary tract obstruction

PREGNANCY AND LACTATION: Pregnancy category B; excreted in breast milk

SIDE EFFECTS/ADVERSE REACTIONS

GI: Anorexia, cramps, diarrhea, *nausea,* rectal burning (suppositories), *vomiting*

METAB: Alkalosis, hypokalemia, protein-losing enteropathy, *tetany*

MS: Muscle weakness

INTERACTIONS

Labs

• Glucose: Falsely low with Clinistix, Diastix; no effect with Tes-tape

SPECIAL CONSIDERATIONS

PATIENT/FAMILY EDUCATION

• Do not take within 1 hr of antacids or milk

---

bismuth subsalicylate

(bis′meth)

OTC: Pepto-Bismol, Pink Bismuth

Combinations

  Rx: with metronidazole, tetracycline (Helidac)

Chemical Class: Salicylate derivative

Therapeutic Class: Antidiarrheal; gastrointestinal antiulcer agent

---

CLINICAL PHARMACOLOGY

Mechanism of Action: Inhibits prostaglandin synthesis responsible for GI hypermotility (salicylate moiety); bismuth moiety may have direct antimicrobial effect

Pharmacokinetics

PO: Onset 1 hr, peak 2 hr, duration 4 hr; salicylate moiety absorbed (262 mg bismuth subsalicylate yields 102 mg salicylate)

INDICATIONS AND USES: Diarrhea; indigestion; nausea, abdominal cramps, prevention of travelers' diarrhea; as part of combination therapy for *Helicobacter pylori;* infantile diarrhea*

DOSAGE

Adult

• *Diarrhea:* PO 30 ml or 2 tabs q30-60 min; not to exceed 8 doses for >2 days

• *Prevention of travelers' diarrhea:* PO 30 ml or 2 tabs qid

• *Helicobacter pylori:* PO 2 tabs qid (in combination with other agents)

Child

• *Diarrhea:* Age 9-12 yr PO 15 ml or 1 tab q30-60 min, not to exceed 8 doses for >2 days; Age 6-9 yr PO 10 ml or ⅔ tab q30-60 min, not to exceed 8 doses for >2 days; Age 3-6 yr PO 5 ml or ⅓ tab q30-60 min, not to exceed 8 doses for >2 days

$ **AVAILABLE FORMS/COST OF THERAPY**

• Susp—Oral: 262 mg/15 ml, 30, 120, 240, 360, 480 ml: **$1.66-$4.21**/240 ml; 524 mg/15 ml, 120, 240, 360 ml: **$1.65-$4.03**; 690 mg/30 ml, 240, 480 ml: **$1.51-$4.08**/240 ml

• Tab, Chewable—Oral: 262 mg, 30's: **$1.85-$3.75**; 300 mg, 30's: **$1.23-$2.93**

CONTRAINDICATIONS: Child <3 yr

PRECAUTIONS: Anticoagulant therapy; stop use if symptoms do not improve within 2 days or become worse, or if diarrhea is accompanied by high fever or severe abdominal pain

PREGNANCY AND LACTATION: Pregnancy category C; salicylate excreted in breast milk

SIDE EFFECTS/ADVERSE REACTIONS

CNS: Confusion, twitching

EENT: Blue gums, hearing loss, metallic taste, tinnitus

GI: Black tongue, *dark stools,* fecal impaction (high doses)
HEME: Increased bleeding time
INTERACTIONS
Drugs
❷ *Tetracyclines:* Decreased absorption of tetracyclines
Labs
• *Color:* Blackens or discolors stool
• *Glucose (urine):* Interferes with Benedict's reaction
SPECIAL CONSIDERATIONS
PATIENT/FAMILY EDUCATION
• Chew or dissolve in mouth; do not swallow whole
• Shake suspension before using

---

bisoprolol
(bis-ope′pro-lal)
Rx: Zebeta
Combinations
  Rx: with hydrochlorothiazide: (Ziac)
Chemical Class: β₁-selective (cardioselective) adrenoreceptor blocker
Therapeutic Class: Antihypertensive

CLINICAL PHARMACOLOGY
Mechanism of Action: Competitive β-adrenergic antagonist at $β_1$-receptor sites (cardioselective at usual doses; $β_2$-blockade noted at doses >20 mg); produces negative inotropic and chronotropic responses; slow AV nodal conduction; decreases heart rate; decreases myocardial oxygen consumption; antiarrhythmic effects (class II); reduction in platelet aggregation and blood viscosity; suppression of renin release; inhibition of central sympathetic outflow; decreases presynaptic receptor neurotransmitter release; no

intrinsic sympathomimetic, or membrane stabilizing activity; low to moderate lipid solubility
Pharmacokinetics
PO: Peak plasma level 2-4 hr, plasma $t_{1/2}$ 9-12 hr; 50% excreted unchanged in urine; protein binding 30%; metabolized in liver to inactive metabolites; full antihypertensive effect after 1 wk of therapy; if creatinine clearance <40 ml/min, plasma $t_{1/2}$ tripled; in cirrhotics, plasma $t_{1/2}$ is 8.3 to 21.7 hours

INDICATIONS AND USES: Angina pectoris,* postmyocardial infarction,* hypertension, migraine headache,* psychiatric disorders* (anxiety,* performance anxiety,* panic attacks,* neuroleptic induced akathisia*)
DOSAGE
Adult and Child >16 yr
• *Hypertension:* PO 5-20 mg qd; reduce dose in renal or hepatic impairment
🖫 AVAILABLE FORMS/COST OF THERAPY
• Tab, Plain Coated—Oral: 5 mg, 30's: **$34.24-$39.32**; 10 mg, 30's: **$34.24-$39.32**
• Tab, Plain Coated—Oral: with hydrochlorothiazide: 2.5 mg/6.25 mg, 100's: **$113.50-$131.14**; 5 mg/6.25 mg, 100's: **$113.50-$131.14**; 10 mg/6.25 mg, 30's: **$114.00**
CONTRAINDICATIONS: Cardiogenic shock, heart block (2nd, 3rd degree), sinus bradycardia, overt cardiac failure
PRECAUTIONS: Anesthesia/surgery (myocardial depression), avoid abrupt withdrawal; bronchospastic airways, congestive heart failure, diabetes mellitus, hyperthyroidism/thyrotoxicosis (bisoprolol, unlike propranolol, does not decrease T_3 levels), concurrent clonidine (discontinue bisoprolol several days

prior to withdrawal of clonidine), peripheral vascular disease, renal disease

PREGNANCY AND LACTATION: Pregnancy category C; similar drug, atenolol frequently used in the third trimester for treatment of hypertension (many studies of efficacy and safety of atenolol in pregnancy-induced hypertension); long-term use has been associated with intrauterine growth retardation; excreted into breast milk; observe for signs of beta-blockade

SIDE EFFECTS/ADVERSE REACTIONS

CNS: Catatonia, depression, dizziness, drowsiness, *fatigue,* hallucinations, headache, insomnia, lethargy, memory loss, mental changes, peripheral neuropathy, strange dreams, vertigo

CV: Bradycardia, **CHF,** cold extremities, postural hypotension, ***profound hypotension, 2nd or 3rd degree heart block, ventricular dysrhythmias***

EENT: Dry burning eyes, rhinitis, sinusitis, sore throat

GI: Diarrhea, flatulence, gastric pain, gastritis, increased AST/ALT (1-2 times normal in 4%), ischemic colitis, mesenteric arterial thrombosis, nausea, vomiting

GU: Decreased libido, impotence

HEME: Purpura

METAB: Azotemia, hyperglycemia, hyperkalemia, hypertriglyceridemia, hyperuricemia, increased hypoglycemic response to insulin

MS: Arthralgia, joint pain

RESP: **Bronchospasm,** cough, dyspnea, wheezing

SKIN: Alopecia, fever, pruritus, rash, sweating

MISC: Decreased exercise tolerance, edema, facial swelling, weight gain

INTERACTIONS
Drugs

🔳 *Adenosine:* Additive bradycardia

🔳 *Alpha-1 adrenergic blockers:* Potential enhanced first dose response [marked initial drop in blood pressure, particularly on standing (especially prazocin)]

🔳 *Amiodarone:* Increased bradycardic effect of bisoprolol

🔳 *Antidiabetics:* Reduced response to hypoglycemia (sweating persists)

🔳 *Barbiturates:* Enhanced bisoprolol metabolism

🔳 *Cimetidine:* Plasma levels of β-blocker may be elevated

🔳 *Cocaine:* Bisoprolol potentiates cocaine-induced coronary vasoconstriction

🔳 *Contrast media:* Increased risk for anaphylaxis

🔳 *Digoxin, digitoxin:* Potentiation of bradycardia; additive prolongation of atrioventricular (AV) conduction time

🔳 *Dipyridamole:* Additive bradycardia

🔳 *Disopyramide:* Additive decreases in cardiac output

🔳 *Fluoxetine:* Fluoxetine inhibits CYPD26, partially responsible for bisoprolol metabolism; increased β-blocker effects

🔳 *Lidocaine:* β-blocker-induced reductions in cardiac output and hepatic blood flow may yield increased lidocaine concentrations

🔳 *Neostigmine:* Additive bradycardia

🔳 *Neuroleptics:* Decreased bisoprolol metabolism; decreased neuroleptic metabolism

🔳 *NSAIDs:* Reduced antihypertensive effect

🔳 *Physostigmine:* Additive bradycardia

🔳 *Prazosin:* Enhanced 1st-dose response to prazosin

3 *Rifampin:* Increases clearance by 51%, reduced β-blocker effects

3 *Tacrine:* Additive bradycardia

2 *Theophylline:* Bisoprolol reduces clearance of theophylline; antagonistic pharmacodynamics

SPECIAL CONSIDERATIONS

• Property of competitive cardioselectivity yields less bronchospastic adverse effects

MONITORING PARAMETERS

• Arrhythmias: Heart rate
• Hypertension: Blood pressure
• Migraine headache: Reduction in the frequency, severity, and duration of attacks
• Postmyocardial infarction: Left ventricular function, lower resting heart rate
• Toxicity: Blood glucose, bronchospasm, hypotension, bradycardia, depression, confusion, hallucination, sexual dysfunction

---

bitolterol

(bye-tole´ter-ol)

Rx: Tornalate

Chemical Class: Sympathomimetic amine; β₂-adrenergic agonist

Therapeutic Class: Antiasthmatic, bronchodilator

CLINICAL PHARMACOLOGY

Mechanism of Action: Causes bronchodilation by β_2-stimulation, resulting in relaxation of bronchial smooth muscle; inhibits mast cell degranulation; stimulates cilia to remove secretions

Pharmacokinetics

INH: Onset 3 min, peak 30-60 min, duration 5-8 hr; bitolterol is a prodrug that is hydrolyzed by esterases in tissue and blood to the active moiety colterol

INDICATIONS AND USES: Prophylaxis and treatment of bronchial asthma and reversible bronchospasm

DOSAGE

Adult and Child >12 yr

• *Bronchospasm:* MDI 1-3 puffs at intervals of 1-3 min, not to exceed 3 puffs q6h or 2 puffs q4h; via neb 1.5-3.5 mg (continuous flow) or 0.5-1.5 mg (intermittent flow) tid-qid, interval between treatments should not be <4 hr

• *Prophylaxis of bronchospasm:* MDI 2 puffs at intervals of 1-3 min q8h

AVAILABLE FORMS/COST OF THERAPY

• MDI—INH: 0.37 mg/puff, 15 ml in metered dose inhaler: **$35.23**
• Sol—INH: 0.2%, 30 ml: **$16.54**; 0.2%, 60 ml: **$31.34**

PRECAUTIONS: Ischemic heart disease, cardiac dysrhythmias, hyperthyroidism, diabetes mellitus, hypertension

PREGNANCY AND LACTATION: Pregnancy category C; excretion into breast milk unknown

SIDE EFFECTS/ADVERSE REACTIONS

CNS: Dizziness, hallucinations, headache, hyperkinesia, insomnia, lightheadedness, nervousness, *tremors*

CV: Chest discomfort, palpitations, tachycardia

EENT: Throat irritation

GI: Heartburn, nausea

MS: Muscle cramps

RESP: **Bronchospasm,** coughing, dyspnea

INTERACTIONS

Drugs

2 *β-blockers:* Decreased action of bitolterol, cardioselective beta-blockers preferable if concurrent use necessary

---

italic = common side effects   ***bold italic*** = life-threatening reactions

3 *Furosemide:* Potential for additive hypokalemia

SPECIAL CONSIDERATIONS
• No real clinical advantage over less expensive agents (e.g., albuterol, metaproterenol)

PATIENT/FAMILY EDUCATION
• Wash inhaler in warm water and dry qd
• If previously effective dosage regimen fails to provide usual relief, seek medical advice immediately

---

bivalirudin

(bye-va-leer´u-din)

Rx: Angiomax
Chemical Class: Peptide
Therapeutic Class: Anticoagulant; direct thrombin inhibitor

CLINICAL PHARMACOLOGY
Mechanism of Action: Directly inhibits thrombin by specifically binding both to the catalytic site and to the anion-binding exosite of circulating and clot-bound thrombin

Pharmacokinetics
IV: Onset immediate, coagulation times return to baseline approximately 1 hr following cessation of infusion; cleared from plasma by combination of renal mechanisms and proteolytic cleavage (clearance reduced 20% with moderate and severe renal impairment, 80% in dialysis-dependent patients); $t_{1/2}$ 25 min (normal renal function)

INDICATIONS AND USES: Anticoagulant in patients with unstable angina undergoing percutaneous transluminal coronary angioplasty (PTCA); intended for use with aspirin and has been studied only in patients receiving concomitant aspirin

DOSAGE
Adult
• IV 1 mg/kg bolus followed by a 4 hr infusion at a rate of 2.5 mg/kg/hr; an additional infusion of 0.2 mg/kg/hr for up to 20 hr can be initiated following completion of the initial 4 hr infusion if necessary; initiate treatment just prior to PTCA; use in conjunction with aspirin (300-325 mg daily); dilute in D_5W or 0.9% NS to yield a final concentration of 5 mg/ml prior to administration
• Dose reductions and anticoagulation status monitoring may be necessary in patients with renal impairment

$ **AVAILABLE FORMS/COST OF THERAPY**
• Inj, Lyophilized—IV: 250 mg/vial: **$418.75**

CONTRAINDICATIONS: Active major bleeding; IM administration

PRECAUTIONS: Children; renal impairment; disease states associated with an increased risk of bleeding

PREGNANCY AND LACTATION: Pregnancy category B; because of possible adverse effects on the neonate and the potential for increased maternal bleeding, particularly during the third trimester, should be used during pregnancy only if clearly needed; excretion into breast milk unknown, use caution in nursing mothers

SIDE EFFECTS/ADVERSE REACTIONS
*CNS: Headache, **cerebral ischemia,** facial paralysis*
*CV: **Hemorrhage,** hypotension, hypertension, bradycardia, syncope, **ventricular fibrillation***
GI: Nausea, vomiting, dyspepsia, abdominal pain
*GU: Urinary retention, **kidney failure,** oliguria*

RESP: Lung edema

MISC: Back pain, pain, injection site pain, insomnia, pelvic pain, insomnia, fever, anxiety, nervousness

INTERACTIONS

Drugs

3 *Heparin, thrombolytics, warfarin:* Increased risk of major bleeding

SPECIAL CONSIDERATIONS

• Safety and effectiveness have not been established in patients with unstable angina who are not undergoing PTCA or in patients with other acute coronary syndromes

MONITORING PARAMETERS

• In clinical trials, the dose of bivalirudin was not titrated according to the activated clotting time (ACT)

---

bosentan
(bo'sen-tan)

Rx: Tracleer

Chemical Class: Substituted pyrimidine derivative

Therapeutic Class: Endothelin-1 receptor antagonist - antihypertensive

---

CLINICAL PHARMACOLOGY

Mechanism of Action: Endothelin-1 antagonist; endothelin-1 is an endogenous peptide (neurohormone) with potent vasoconstrictor activity that is implicated in the pathogenesis of hypertension, congestive heart failure, myocardial infarction, and renal failure

Pharmacokinetics

PO: Peak response 4-8 hr after dose; duration 24 hours

50% bioavailablity without food effect (PO); >98% bound to albumin; extensively metabolized by liver CYP2C9 and CYP3A4 (3 metabolites - 1 active; contributes 10-20% of activity), excreted minimally by kidneys (3%), but extensively in bile
$t_{1/2}$ 5-8 hr

INDICATIONS AND USES: Pulmonary hypertension (WHO Class III, IV), systemic hypertension,* congestive heart failure*

DOSAGE

Adult and Child >16 yr

• PO initially 62.5 mg bid for 4 weeks; maintenance dose may increased to 125 mg bid; no adjustments for decreased renal function

$ **AVAILABLE FORMS/COST OF THERAPY**

• Tab, Film-Coated—Oral: 62.5, 125 mg, 100's: *cost not available*

CONTRAINDICATIONS: Pregnancy

PRECAUTIONS: Potential liver injury

PREGNANCY AND LACTATION: Pregnancy category X; expected to cause fetal harm if administered to pregnant women

SIDE EFFECTS/ADVERSE REACTIONS

CNS: Headache, fatigue

CV: Flushing, edema, hypotension, palpitations

EENT: Nasopharyngitis

GI: Nausea, vomiting, **hepatotoxicity**, dyspepsia

INTERACTIONS

Drugs

3 *Hormonal contraceptives:* Induction of CYP3A4 by bosentan may increase metabolism of contraceptive with possible failure

2 *Cyclosporine A:* Increased bosentan trough concentrations of 3-30 fold and decreased cyclosporine A levels by 50% with concomitant administration

2 *Ketoconazole:* Ketoconazole is a potent CYP3A4 inhibitor; concurrent administration increases bosentan levels 2 fold

---

3 *Simvastatin and other statins:* Concurrent administration decreased simvastatin and metabolites by 50%

3 *Warfarin:* Concurrent administration reduces both S-warfarin (CYP2C9 substrate) and R-warfarin (CYP3A4 substrate) by 29% and 38% respectively, but without clinical changes in INR

SPECIAL CONSIDERATIONS

• Because of potential liver injury and in an effort to make the chance of fetal exposure to bosentan as small as possible, the drug may only be prescribed through the TRACLEER Access Program by calling 1-866-228-3546

MONITORING PARAMETERS

• Blood pressure, blood chemistries to include transaminases, monthly pregnancy test, hemoglobin levels at 1 and 3 months

---

bretylium

(bre-til'ee-um)

Chemical Class: Bromobenzyl quaternary ammonium compound

Therapeutic Class: Antidysrhythmic (class III)

CLINICAL PHARMACOLOGY

Mechanism of Action: Causes an early release of norepinephrine from postganglionic nerve terminals, then selectively accumulates in sympathetic ganglia and their postganglionic adrenergic neurons where it inhibits norepinephrine release; suppresses ventricular fibrillation and ventricular dysrhythmias; increases action potential duration and effective refractory period without changes in heart rate

Pharmacokinetics

IV: Onset 5 min for suppression of ventricular fibrillation, onset 20-120 min for suppression of ventricular tachycardia

IM: Onset 20-120 min for suppression of ventricular tachycardia, duration 6-24 hr; 80% excreted unchanged by kidneys in 24 hr

INDICATIONS AND USES: Ventricular tachycardia and other life threatening ventricular dysrhythmias that have failed to respond to 1st-line agents; ventricular fibrillation

DOSAGE

Adult

• *Ventricular fibrillation:* IV bolus 5 mg/kg, then 10 mg/kg repeated q15 min, up to total 30-35 mg/kg; maintenance therapy is IV INF 1-2 mg/min or 5-10 mg/kg over 10 min q6h

• *Ventricular dysrhythmias:* IV INF 500 mg diluted in 50 ml D_5W or NS, infuse over 10-30 min, may repeat in 1 hr, maintain with 1-2 mg/min or 5-10 mg/kg over 10-30 min q6h; IM 5-10 mg/kg undiluted, repeat in 1-2 hr if needed, maintain with same dose q6-8h

Child

• *Ventricular fibrillation:* IV bolus 5 mg/kg, then 10 mg/kg if ventricular fibrillation persists

$ **AVAILABLE FORMS/COST OF THERAPY**

• Inj, Sol—IM, IV: 50 mg/ml, 10 ml: **$2.31-$41.08**

CONTRAINDICATIONS: Digitalis toxicity (initial release of norepinephrine caused by bretylium may aggravate digitalis toxicity)

PRECAUTIONS: Renal disease; postural hypotension, hypertension or increased frequency of PVCs and other dysrhythmias may occur transiently in some patients; aortic stenosis, pulmonary hypertension

---

PREGNANCY AND LACTATION:
Pregnancy category C
SIDE EFFECTS/ADVERSE REACTIONS
CNS: Anxiety, confusion, dizziness, psychosis, syncope
CV: Angina, bradycardia, *hypotension, postural hypotension (50%),* PVCs, transient hypertension
GI: Nausea, vomiting
RESP: **Respiratory depression**
INTERACTIONS
Drugs
❸ *Catecholamines:* Enhanced pressor effects
❸ *Digoxin:* Digitalis toxicity may be aggravated by the initial norepinephrine release
SPECIAL CONSIDERATIONS
MONITORING PARAMETERS
• ECG, electrolytes, BP

---

bromocriptine
(broe-moe-krip′teen)
Rx: Parlodel
Chemical Class: Ergot alkaloid derivative
Therapeutic Class: Anti-Parkinson's agent; ovulation stimulant; dopaminergic

---

CLINICAL PHARMACOLOGY
Mechanism of Action: Inhibits prolactin release by activating postsynaptic dopamine receptors; activation of striatal dopamine receptors may be reason for improvement in Parkinson's disease
Pharmacokinetics
PO: Peak 1-3 hr, duration 4-8 hr; 90%-96% protein bound; $t_{1/2}$ 3 hr; metabolized by liver (inactive metabolites), 85%-98% of dose excreted in feces
INDICATIONS AND USES: Hyperprolactinemia-associated dysfunctions (including amenorrhea with or without galactorrhea, infertility, or hypogonadism); prolactin-secreting adenomas (may be used to reduce the tumor mass prior to surgery); female infertility associated with hyperprolactinemia; acromegaly; Parkinson's disease; prevention of physiological lactation* (after parturition when the mother elects not to breast-feed the infant, when breast feeding is contraindicated, after stillbirth or abortion); neuroleptic malignant syndrome,* cocaine addiction*; cyclic mastalgia*

DOSAGE
Adult
• *Hyperprolactinemic indications:* PO 1.25-2.5 mg with meals; may increase by 2.5 mg q3-7 days; usual 5-7.5 mg/day with range from 2.5-15 mg/day
• *Acromegaly:* PO 1.25-2.5 mg qPM with food × 3 days; may increase by 1.25-2.5 mg q3-7 days until optimal therapeutic benefit; usual range 20-30 mg/day; max 100 mg/day (monitor growth hormone levels)
• *Parkinson's disease:* PO 1.25 mg bid with meals; may increase q2-4 wk by 2.5 mg/day; not to exceed 100 mg qd
• *Postpartum lactation:* (After vital signs have stabilized and no sooner than 4 hr after delivery) PO 2.5 mg bid with meals × 14 days; an additional 7 days may be necessary
(NOTE: this indication has been withdrawn by the manufacturer)
$ **AVAILABLE FORMS/COST OF THERAPY**
• Cap, Gel—Oral: 5 mg, 100's: **$268.21-$389.81**
• Tab, Uncoated—Oral: 2.5 mg, 100's: **$156.05-$255.45**

---

italic = common side effects   ***bold italic*** = life-threatening reactions

CONTRAINDICATIONS: Severe ischemic disease, uncontrolled hypertension, toxemia of pregnancy, sensitivity to any ergot alkaloids, severe peripheral vascular disease

PRECAUTIONS: Hepatic disease, renal disease, children, pituitary tumors, hypotension, concurrent BP-lowering medications

PREGNANCY AND LACTATION: Pregnancy category D; since it prevents lactation, should not be administered to mothers who elect to breast-feed infants

SIDE EFFECTS/ADVERSE REACTIONS

CNS: Abnormal involuntary movements, anxiety, ataxia, cerebrospinal fluid rhinorrhea (treatment of prolactinomas), confusion, depression, *dizziness,* drowsiness, fatigue, hallucinations, *headache,* insomnia, nervousness, "on-off" phenomenon, psychosis, restlessness, *seizures,* visual disturbance

CV: Bradycardia, decreased BP, *dysrhythmias,* extrasystole, orthostatic hypotension, palpitation, *shock, stroke*

EENT: Blurred vision, burning eyes, diplopia, nasal congestion

GI: Anorexia, constipation, cramps, diarrhea, dry mouth, *GI hemorrhage, nausea (49%), vomiting*

GU: Diuresis, frequency, incontinence, retention

SKIN: Alopecia, rash on face, arms

INTERACTIONS

Drugs

3 *Erythromycin:* Marked elevations in bromocriptine levels

⚠ *Isometheptene:* Case report of hypertension and ventricular tachycardia with combination

3 *Neuroleptics:* Neuroleptic drugs probably inhibit the ability of bromocriptine to lower serum prolactin concentrations in patients with pituitary adenomas; theoretically, bromocriptine should inhibit the antipsychotic effects of neuroleptic agents, but clinical evidence suggests that this may be uncommon

⚠ *Phenylpropanolamine:* Increased risk of hypertension and seizures

SPECIAL CONSIDERATIONS

• Routine use for suppression of lactation not recommended

PATIENT/FAMILY EDUCATION

• Use measures to prevent orthostatic hypotension

brompheniramine

(brome-fen-ir′a-meen)
Rx: Colhist, ND Stat, Nasahist-B
OTC: Dimetane Extentabs
Combinations
  Rx: with phenylpropanolamine, codeine (Bromanate DC, Bromphen DC with Codeine, Dimetane-DC Cough, Myphetane DC Cough, Polyhistine CS); with pseudoephedrine, dextromethorphan (Bromadine-DM, Bromarest DX, Bromatane DX, Bromfed DM, Bromphen DX, Dimetane DX, Myphetane DX)
  OTC: with phenylpropanolamine (Bromaline, Bromanate, Dimaphen, Dimetane Decongestant, Dimetapp, Vicks DayQuil Allergy); with pseudo-ephedrine (Bromfed, Drixoral)
Chemical Class: Alkylamine derivative
Therapeutic Class: Antihistamine

CLINICAL PHARMACOLOGY
Mechanism of Action: Decreases allergic response by blocking histamine at H_1-receptors
Pharmacokinetics
PO: Peak 2-5 hr; metabolized in liver, excreted in urine as inactive metabolites; $t_{1/2}$ 12-34 hr
INDICATIONS AND USES: Perennial and seasonal allergic rhinitis (PO); allergic reactions to blood and plasma, adjunctive anaphylactic therapy (parenteral)

DOSAGE
Adult
• PO 4-8 mg tid-qid, not to exceed 24 mg/day; PO TIME REL 8-12 mg bid-tid or 12 mg q12h, not to exceed 24 mg/day; IM/IV/SC 5-20 mg q6-12h, not to exceed 40 mg/day
Child 6-12 yr
• PO 2-4 mg q4-6h, not to exceed 16 mg/day; IM/IV/SC 0.5 mg/kg/day divided q6-8h
Child <6 yr
• PO 0.125 mg/kg/dose q6h, not to exceed 8 mg/day

$ **AVAILABLE FORMS/COST OF THERAPY**
• Elixir—Oral: 2 mg/5 ml, 120, 480 ml: **$4.32-$4.85**/480 ml
• Inj, Sol—IM, IV, SC: 10 mg/ml, 10 ml: **$4.00-$20.30**
• Tab, Sus Action—Oral: 12 mg, 100's: **$24.38**
• Tab, Uncoated—Oral: 4 mg, 100's: **$2.93-$2.95**
CONTRAINDICATIONS: Narrow-angle glaucoma, bladder neck obstruction
PRECAUTIONS: Liver disease, elderly, increased intraocular pressure, hyperthyroidism, cardiovascular disease, hypertension, urinary retention, newborn or premature infants, renal disease, stenosed peptic ulcers
PREGNANCY AND LACTATION: Pregnancy category C; an association between 1st trimester exposure and congenital defects has been found in humans; excreted into breast milk, compatible with breast feeding
SIDE EFFECTS/ADVERSE REACTIONS
CNS: Anxiety, confusion, *dizziness, drowsiness,* euphoria, fatigue, neuritis, paresthesia, poor coordination
CV: Hypotension, palpitations, tachycardia

---

italic = common side effects   ***bold italic*** = life-threatening reactions

EENT: Blurred vision, dry nose, throat; mydriasis, nasal stuffiness, tinnitus

GI: Anorexia, *constipation,* diarrhea, *dry mouth,* nausea, vomiting

GU: Dysuria, frequency, impotence, retention

HEME: **Agranulocytosis, hemolytic anemia, thrombocytopenia**

RESP: Chest tightness, increased thick secretions, wheezing

SKIN: Photosensitivity

INTERACTIONS

Labs

• *Aminoacids:* Urine, increase; on thin-layer chromatography

• *Amphetamine:* Urine, increase; false positives

• *False negative:* Skin allergy tests

SPECIAL CONSIDERATIONS

PATIENT/FAMILY EDUCATION

• Do not crush or chew sustained release forms

• Use hard candy, gum, frequent rinsing of mouth for dryness

---

budesonide

(bu-dess´ah-nide)

Rx: Powder INH: Pulmicort Turbuhaler; Suspension INH: Pulmicort Respules; Nasal: Rhinocort Aqua

Chemical Class: Glucocorticoid

Therapeutic Class: Antiasthmatic, antiinflammatory corticosteroid

---

CLINICAL PHARMACOLOGY

Mechanism of Action: Decreases inflammation by suppression of migration of polymorphonuclear leukocytes, fibroblasts, reversal of increased capillary permeability, and lysosomal stabilization

Pharmacokinetics

INH: 20% of dose reaches systemic circulation; extensive first-pass metabolism, no unchanged drug excreted in urine; peak effect 3-7 days

INDICATIONS AND USES: Management of symptoms of seasonal or perennial rhinitis in adults and children and nonallergic perennial rhinitis in adults (nasal); chronic asthma (oral inhaler)

DOSAGE

Adult

• *Allergic rhinitis:* NASAL INH 2 inh each nostril bid or 4 inh each nostril q AM; when response achieved taper dose q2-4 wks to minimum effective dose

• *Asthma:* ORAL INH 1-4 inh bid

Child ≥6 yr

• Allergic rhinitis: NASAL INH same as adult

• Asthma: Powder INH 1-2 inh bid; Solution INH (child 12 mo - 8 yr) 0.25-1 mg total daily dose administered qd or bid

$ **AVAILABLE FORMS/COST OF THERAPY**

• MDIAer—INH: 200 μg/inh, 200 doses: **$123.86**

• MDIAer—Nasal INH: 32 μg/inh, 200 doses: **$39.50**

• Sol—INH: 0.125 mg/2 ml: **$4.20**; 0.25 mg/2 ml: **$4.20**

• Spray—Nasal INH: 32 μg/inh, 120 doses: **$50.40**

CONTRAINDICATIONS: Treatment of acute asthma

SIDE EFFECTS/ADVERSE REACTIONS

EENT: Dry mouth (nasal use), epistaxis, nasal irritation, pharyngitis

GI: Difficulty swallowing (oral use), dyspepsia, hoarseness, oral thrush

RESP: Cough

SPECIAL CONSIDERATIONS
• May allow discontinuation of chronic systemic corticosteroids in many patients with asthma
• 3-7 days required for maximum benefit (nasal)

PATIENT/FAMILY EDUCATION
• To be used on regular basis, not for acute symptoms
• Use bronchodilators before oral inhaler (for patients using both)
• Nasal vehicle may cause rhinitis

MONITORING PARAMETERS
• Monitor children for growth as well as for effects on the HPA axis during chronic therapy
• Monitor patients switched from chronic systemic corticosteroids to avoid acute adrenal insufficiency in response to stress

---

bumetanide
(byoo-met'a-nide)
Rx: Bumex
Chemical Class: Sulfonamide derivative
Therapeutic Class: Loop diuretic

CLINICAL PHARMACOLOGY
Mechanism of Action: Inhibits sodium and chloride reabsorption in the ascending limb of the loop of Henle; potassium excretion is increased in a dose-related fashion; more chloruretic than natriuretic; may have an additional action in the proximal tubule

Pharmacokinetics
PO: Onset 0.5-1 hr, duration 4 hr
IM: Onset 40 min, duration 4 hr
IV: Onset 5 min, duration 0.5-1 hr
94-96% bound to plasma proteins; excreted by kidneys; $t_{1/2}$ 1-1.5 hr

INDICATIONS AND USES: Edema (congestive heart failure, hepatic cirrhosis, nephrotic syndrome); hypertension; adult nocturia*

DOSAGE
Adult
• PO 0.5-2.0 mg qd, may give 2nd or 3rd dose at 4-5 hr intervals up to max of 20 mg/day, may be given on alternate days or intermittently; IV/IM 0.5-1.0 mg/day, may give 2nd or 3rd dose at 2-3 hr intervals up to max of 10 mg/day

Child >6 months
• PO/IM/IV 0.015 mg/kg/dose qd or qod, maximum 0.1 mg/kg/day or 10 mg

$ AVAILABLE FORMS/COST OF THERAPY
• Inj, Sol—IM, IV: 0.25 mg/ml, 2 ml: **$1.34-$2.15**
• Tab, Uncoated—Oral: 0.5 mg, 100's: **$27.18-$41.48**; 1 mg, 100's: **$38.15-$58.24**; 2 mg, 100's: **$64.53-$98.45**

CONTRAINDICATIONS: Anuria, hepatic coma, severe electrolyte depletion

PRECAUTIONS: Fluid and electrolyte imbalance (including sodium, chloride, potassium, magnesium, calcium), renal disease, hepatic disease (may precipitate hepatic encephalopathy), gout, COPD, lupus erythematosus, diabetes mellitus, hyperparathyroidism, vomiting, diarrhea, elevated cholesterol/triglycerides

PREGNANCY AND LACTATION: Pregnancy category C; cardiovascular disorders such as pulmonary edema, severe hypertension, or CHF are probably the only valid indications for loop diuretics during pregnancy; excretion into breast milk unknown

---

italic = common side effects   ***bold italic*** = life-threatening reactions

SIDE EFFECTS/ADVERSE REACTIONS

CNS: Dizziness, fatigue, headache, vertigo, weakness

CV: ECG changes, *hypotension*

EENT: Blurred vision, ear pain, ototoxicity, tinnitus

GI: Abdominal pain, anorexia, cramps, diarrhea, dry mouth, *nausea,* upset stomach, vomiting

GU: Glycosuria, *polyuria,* **renal failure,** sexual dysfunction

HEME: **Thrombocytopenia**

METAB: Hyperglycemia, hyperuricemia, hypocalcemia, hypochloremic alkalosis, *hypokalemia,* hypomagnesemia, hyponatremia

MS: Arthritis, hyperuricemia, *muscular cramps,* stiffness, tenderness

SKIN: Photosensitivity, pruritus, purpura, rash, **Stevens-Johnson syndrome,** sweating

INTERACTIONS

Drugs

🖪 *Aminoglycosides (gentamicin, kanamycin, neomycin, streptomycin):* Additive ototoxicity (ethacrynic acid > furosemide, torsemide, bumetanide)

🖪 *Angiotensin converting enzyme inhibitors:* Initiation of ACEI with intensive diuretic therapy may result in precipitous fall in blood pressure; ACEIs may induce renal insufficiency in the presence of diuretic-induced sodium depletion

🖪 *Barbiturates (phenobarbital):* Reduced diuretic response

🖪 *Bile acid-binding resins (cholestyramine, colestipol):* Resins markedly reduce the bioavailability and diuretic response of furosemide

🖪 *Carbenoxolone:* Severe hypokalemia from coadministration

🖪 *Cephalosporins (cephaloridine, cephalothin):* Enhanced nephrotoxicity with coadministration

❷ *Cisplatin:* Additive ototoxicity (ethacrynic acid > furosemide, torsemide, bumetanide)

🖪 *Clofibrate:* Enhanced effects of both drugs, especially in hypoalbuminemic patients

🖪 *Corticosteroids:* Concomitant loop diuretic and corticosteroid therapy can result in excessive potassium loss

🖪 *Digitalis glycosides (digoxin, digitoxin):* Diuretic-induced hypokalemia may increase risk of digitalis toxicity

🖪 *Nonsteroidal antiinflammatory drugs (flurbiprofen, ibuprofen, indomethacin, naproxen, piroxicam, sulindac):* Reduced diuretic and antihypertensive effects

🖪 *Phenytoin:* Reduced diuretic response

🖪 *Serotonin-reuptake inhibitors (fluoxetine, paroxetine, sertraline):* Case reports of sudden death; enhanced hyponatremia proposed; causal relationships not established

🖪 *Terbutaline:* Additive hypokalemia

🖪 *Tubocurarine:* Prolonged neuromuscular blockade

Labs

• *Cortisol:* False increases

• *Glucose:* Falsely low urine tests with Clinistix and Diastix

• *Thyroxine:* Increased serum concentration

• *T_3 uptake:* Interference causes increased serum values

SPECIAL CONSIDERATIONS

• Cross-sensitivity with furosemide rare; may substitute bumetanide at a 1:40 ratio with furosemide in patients allergic to furosemide; may show cross-hypersensitivity to sulfonamides

PATIENT/FAMILY EDUCATION

• Take early in the day

MONITORING PARAMETERS
• Urine volume, creatinine clearance, BUN, electrolytes, reduction in edema, increased diuresis, decrease in body weight, reduction in blood pressure, glucose, uric acid, serum calcium (tetany), tinnitus, vertigo, hearing loss (especially in those at risk for ototoxicity—IV doses >120 mg; concomitant ototoxic drugs; renal disease)

---

bupivacaine
(byoo-piv´a-caine)
Rx: Marcaine, Marcaine Spinal, Sensorcaine, Sensorcaine-MPF
Combinations
   Rx: with epinephrine (Marcaine with Epinephrine, Sensorcaine with Epinephrine, Sensorcaine-MPF with Epinephrine)
Chemical Class: Amide; aminoacyl derivative
Therapeutic Class: Local anesthetic

CLINICAL PHARMACOLOGY
Mechanism of Action: Blocks the generation and conduction of nerve impulses; the order of loss of nerve function is: (1) pain, (2) temperature, (3) touch, (4) proprioception, and (5) skeletal muscle tone
Pharmacokinetics
INJ: Peak 30-45 min, duration 3-6 hr; 96% bound to plasma proteins; metabolized in liver, excreted in urine; $t_{1/2}$ 3.5 hr
INDICATIONS AND USES: Local or regional anesthesia; analgesia for surgery, oral surgical procedures, diagnostic and therapeutic procedures, obstetrical procedures

DOSAGE
Dose varies with procedure, depth of anesthesia, vascularity of tissues, duration of anesthesia, and condition of patient
Adult
• *Caudal block:* Inj 15-30 ml of 0.25% or 0.5%
• *Epidural block:* Inj 10-20 ml of 0.25% or 0.5%
• *Peripheral nerve block:* Inj 5 ml of 0.25% or 0.5% (12.5-25 mg), max 2.5 mg/kg or 400 mg/day
• *Sympathetic nerve block:* Inj 20-50 ml of 0.25%
Child
• *Caudal block:* Inj 1-3.7 mg/kg
• *Epidural block:* Inj 1.25 mg/kg/dose
💲 **AVAILABLE FORMS/COST OF THERAPY**
• Inj, Sol—Caudal Block, Epidural: 0.25%, 10 ml: **$3.07-$4.45**; 0.5%, 10 ml: **$3.36-$4.81**; 0.75%, 10 ml: **$3.70-$5.30**
CONTRAINDICATIONS: Obstetrical paracervical block anesthesia
PRECAUTIONS: Obstetrical anesthesia (0.75% concentration), intravenous regional anesthesia, hypotension, heart block, hepatic disease, impaired cardiovascular function, use in head and neck area, retrobulbar blocks, elderly, anaphylaxis
PREGNANCY AND LACTATION: Pregnancy category C; excretion into breast milk unknown; regional use may prolong labor and delivery
SIDE EFFECTS/ADVERSE REACTIONS
CNS: Anxiety, disorientation, drowsiness, *loss of consciousness,* restlessness, *seizures,* shivering, tremors
CV: Bradycardia, *cardiac arrest, dysrhythmias,* fetal bradycardia, hypertension, hypotension, *myocardial depression*

---

italic = common side effects   ***bold italic*** = life-threatening reactions

EENT: Blurred vision, miosis, tinnitus

GI: Nausea, vomiting

RESP: Respiratory arrest

SKIN: Allergic reactions, burning, edema, rash, skin discoloration at injection site, tissue necrosis, urticaria

INTERACTIONS

Drugs

3 β-*blockers:* Hypertensive reactions possible, especially with local anesthetics containing epinephrine; acute discontinuation of β-blockers before local anesthesia may increase the risk of side effects due to anesthetic

SPECIAL CONSIDERATIONS

• Amide-type local anesthetic

MONITORING PARAMETERS

• Blood pressure, pulse, respiration during treatment, ECG

• Fetal heart tones if drug is used during labor

---

buprenorphine

(byoo-pre-nor′feen)

Rx: Buprenex

Chemical Class: Semisynthetic opiate (thebaine) derivative

Therapeutic Class: Narcotic agonist-antagonist analgesic

DEA Class: Schedule V

CLINICAL PHARMACOLOGY

Mechanism of Action: Analgesia via binding to μ subclass opiate receptors in the CNS; μ receptors mediate morphinelike supraspinal analgesia, euphoria, and respiratory and physical depression; narcotic antagonist activity is approximately equipotent to naloxone

Pharmacokinetics

IM: Onset 15 min, peak 1 hr, duration 6 hr

IV: Onset 1 min, peak 5 min, duration 2-5 hr

Metabolized by liver, excreted predominantly in feces; 96% bound to plasma proteins; $t_{1/2}$ 2-3 hr

INDICATIONS AND USES: Moderate to severe pain

DOSAGE

NOTE: Parenteral dose of 0.3 mg equivalent to 10 mg morphine

Adult

• IM/IV 0.3 mg q6h prn (reduce dosage by half in the elderly, debilitated patients, or in the presence of respiratory disease); repeat once (up to 0.3 mg) prn 30-60 min after initial dose

Child >2 yr

• IM/IV 2 μg/kg/dose q6-8h prn

$ **AVAILABLE FORMS/COST OF THERAPY**

• Inj, Sol—IM, IV: 0.3 mg/ml:1 ml: **$2.55-$3.06**

PRECAUTIONS: Addictive personality, narcotic-dependent patients (may cause withdrawal), increased intracranial pressure, respiratory depression, hepatic disease, renal disease, hypothyroidism, biliary tract dysfunction, prostatic hypertrophy

PREGNANCY AND LACTATION: Pregnancy category C; safe use in labor and delivery has not been established; excretion into breast milk unknown

SIDE EFFECTS/ADVERSE REACTIONS

CNS: Coma, confusion, depression, *dizziness,* euphoria, hallucinations, headache, nervousness, paresthesia, psychosis, *sedation,* slurred speech, tremor, weakness

CV: Bradycardia, hypertension, hypotension, tachycardia

EENT: Blurred vision, conjunctivitis, diplopia, miosis, tinnitus

GI: Constipation, dry mouth, dyspepsia, flatulence, loss of appetite, nausea

GU: Urinary retention

RESP: Apnea, cyanosis, dyspnea, *respiratory depression*

SKIN: Injection site reactions, pallor, pruritus, rash, sweating, urticaria

SPECIAL CONSIDERATIONS
• Effective long-acting opioid agonist-antagonist; unconfirmed reported lower physical dependence; no significant advantages

MONITORING PARAMETERS
• Respiration rate

---

bupropion

(byoo-proe′pee-on)
Rx: Wellbutrin, Wellbutrin SR, Zyban
Chemical Class: Aminoketone derivative
Therapeutic Class: Antidepressant

CLINICAL PHARMACOLOGY
Mechanism of Action: Inhibits neuronal reuptake of dopamine and norepinephrine (slight) at the presynaptic neuron; moderate anticholinergic, sedation; slight orthostatic hypotensive activity

Pharmacokinetics
PO: Peak 2 hr, onset 2-4 wk, $t_{1/2}$ 12-14 hr; metabolized by liver

INDICATIONS AND USES: Depression; smoking cessation, bipolar disorder

DOSAGE
Adult
• *Depression:* PO 100 mg bid initially, increase based on clinical response to 100 mg tid no sooner than 3 days after initiating therapy, may increase after 1 month to 150 mg tid; **no single dose should exceed 150 mg; at least 6 hr should elapse between doses;** or PO Sus Action 150 mg bid

• Smoking cessation:150 mg Sus Action qd × 3 days; then 150 mg Sus Action bid × 7-12 weeks (target quit date to follow 1 week of therapy)

AVAILABLE FORMS/COST OF THERAPY
• Tab, Coated—Oral: 75 mg, 100's: **$72.00-$93.74**; 100 mg, 100's: **$96.06-$125.04**
• Tab, Sus Action—Oral: 100 mg, 60's: **$74.41-$102.62**; 150 mg, 60's: **$79.75-$109.99**
• Advantage pack—tab, Sus Action—Oral: 150 mg, 60's: **$83.74** plus behavioral modification program

CONTRAINDICATIONS: Seizure disorder, prior or current diagnosis of bulimia or anorexia nervosa (increased risk of seizure), concurrent use of MAOI

PRECAUTIONS: Renal and hepatic disease, recent MI, unstable heart disease, history of drug abuse or dependence, bipolar affective disorder

PREGNANCY AND LACTATION: Pregnancy category B; excretion into breast milk unknown

SIDE EFFECTS/ADVERSE REACTIONS
CNS: Agitation, anxiety, confusion, decreased libido, dizziness, dry mouth, *headache/migraine, insomnia,seizures,* sweating, tremor
CV: Arrhythmias, edema, hypertension, hypotension, palpitations, syncope, tachycardia
EENT: Auditory disturbance, blurred vision
GI: Appetite increase, constipation, dyspepsia, *nausea, vomiting*
GU: Impotence, menstrual complaints, urinary frequency
METAB: Glycosuria, gynecomastia
MS: Arthritis
SKIN: Pruritus, rash

italic = common side effects   ***bold italic*** = life-threatening reactions

SPECIAL CONSIDERATIONS

• Equal efficacy as tricyclic antidepressants; advantages include minimal anticholinergic effects, lack of orthostatic hypotension, no cardiac conduction problems, absence of weight gain, no sedation

• Prescribe in equally divided doses of 3 or 4 times daily to minimize risk of seizures

PATIENT/FAMILY EDUCATION

• Ability to perform tasks requiring judgment or motor and cognitive skills may be impaired

• Therapeutic effects may take 2-4 wk

• Do not discontinue medication quickly after long-term use

---

buspirone

(byoo-spir'own)
Rx: BuSpar
Chemical Class: Azaspirodecanedione
Therapeutic Class: Anxiolytic

CLINICAL PHARMACOLOGY

Mechanism of Action: Anxiolytic activity presumed secondary to high affinity for serotonin (5-HT$_{1A}$) receptors; there is also moderate affinity for brain D$_2$-dopamine receptors and increases norepinepherine metabolism in the locus ceruleus; the drug has no affinity for benzodiazepine receptors; there are no anticonvulsant, muscle relaxant, or sedative effects

Pharmacokinetics

PO: Peak 40-90 min; 95% bound to plasma proteins; metabolized by liver (CYP3A4), excreted in urine and feces; t$_{1/2}$ 2-3 hr

INDICATIONS AND USES: Anxiety disorders, premenstrual syndrome*

DOSAGE

Adult

• PO 5 mg tid, may increase by 5 mg/day q2-3 days, not to exceed 60 mg/day

Ⓢ AVAILABLE FORMS/COST OF THERAPY

• Tab, Uncoated—Oral: 5 mg, 100's: **$68.94-$94.10**; 10 mg, 100's: **$134.50-$164.10**; 15 mg, 60's: **$121.15-$147.11**; 30 mg, 60's: **$218.10-$264.83**

PRECAUTIONS: Liver disease, renal disease, elderly, children <18 yr

PREGNANCY AND LACTATION: Pregnancy category B; excretion into breast milk unknown; use caution in nursing mothers

SIDE EFFECTS/ADVERSE REACTIONS

CNS: Akathisia, confusion, depression, *dizziness, drowsiness,* excitement, headache, incoordination, insomnia, involuntary movements, lightheadedness, nervousness, paresthesia, stimulation, tremor

CV: Bradycardia, hypertension, hypotension, non-specific chest pain, palpitations

EENT: Altered taste, smell; blurred vision; nasal congestion; red, itchy eyes; sore throat; tinnitus

GI: Constipation, diarrhea, dry mouth, dyspepsia, flatulence, increased appetite, *nausea,* rectal bleeding

GU: Change in libido, frequency, hesitancy, menstrual irregularity

MS: Muscle cramps, pain, spasms, weakness

RESP: Chest congestion, hyperventilation, shortness of breath

SKIN: Alopecia, dry skin, edema, pruritus, rash

MISC: Fatigue, fever, sweating, weight gain

---

* = non-FDA-approved use

INTERACTIONS
Drugs
3 *Fluoxetine:* Reduced therapeutic response to both drugs

A *MAOIs:* Elevated blood pressure, don't give concomitantly

3 *Haloperidol:* Increased serum conc. of haloperidol

3 *CYP3A4 inhibitors:* Diltiazem, verapamil, erythromycin, itraconazole, nefazodone, ketoconazole, ritonavir, grapefruit juice; plasma buspirone concentration increased, adverse events likely, may need to adjust dose

3 *CYP3A4 inducers:* Rifampin, dexamethasone, phenytoin, phenobarbital, carbamazepine; plasma buspirone concentration decreased, may need to adjust dose to maintain anxiolytic effect

SPECIAL CONSIDERATIONS
• Advantages include less sedation (preferable in elderly), less effect on psychomotor and psychologic function, minimal propensity to interact with ethanol and other CNS depressants
• Will not prevent benzodiazepine withdrawal

PATIENT/FAMILY EDUCATION
• Optimal results may take 3-4 wk of treatment, some improvement may be seen after 7-10 days

---

butabarbital
(byoo-tah-bar´bi-tal)
Rx: Butisol
Chemical Class: Barbituric acid derivative
Therapeutic Class: Sedative/hypnotic
DEA Class: Schedule III

CLINICAL PHARMACOLOGY
Mechanism of Action: Non-selective CNS depressant: depresses the sensory cortex, decreases motor activity, alters cerebellar function, produce drowsiness, sedation, and hypnosis; little analgesic action at subanesthetic doses (may increase reaction to painful stimuli); anticonvulsant activity in anesthetic doses; dose-dependent respiratory depression (hypnotic doses produce respiratory depression similar to physiologic sleep)

Pharmacokinetics
PO: Onset 0.5-1 hr, $t_{1/2}$ 66-140 hr; metabolized by liver, excreted in urine as metabolites

INDICATIONS AND USES: Hypnotic in the short-term treatment of insomnia for periods up to 2 wk in duration (may lose efficacy for sleep induction and maintenance after this period of time)

DOSAGE
Adult
• *Daytime sedation:* PO 15-30 mg tid-qid
• *Bedtime hypnotic:* PO 50-100 mg
• *Preoperative sedation:* PO 50-100 mg 60-90 min before surgery

Child
• *Preoperative sedation:* PO 2-6 mg/kg; max 100 mg
• *Daytime sedation:* PO 7.5-30 mg; depending on age, weight, and sedation desired

---

💲 AVAILABLE FORMS/COST OF THERAPY

• Elixir—Oral: 30 mg/5 ml, 480 ml: **$5.95-$149.03**
• Tab, Uncoated—Oral: 15 mg, 100's: **$59.40**; 30 mg, 100's: **$105.68**; 50 mg, 100's: **$137.47**; 100 mg, 100's: **$109.42**

CONTRAINDICATIONS: Respiratory depression, addiction to barbiturates, severe liver impairment, porphyria

PRECAUTIONS: Anemia, hepatic disease, renal disease, hypertension, elderly, acute/chronic pain, mental depression, history of drug abuse, abrupt discontinuation

PREGNANCY AND LACTATION: Pregnancy category D; small amounts excreted in breast milk; use caution in nursing mothers

SIDE EFFECTS/ADVERSE REACTIONS

CNS: CNS depression, dizziness, *drowsiness,* headache, *lethargy,* light-headedness, mental depression, physical dependence, slurred speech, stimulation in the elderly and children, vertigo
CV: Bradycardia, hypotension
EENT: **Laryngospasm**
GI: Constipation, diarrhea, nausea, vomiting
HEME: **Agranulocytosis,** megaloblastic anemia, (long-term treatment), **thrombocytopenia**
MS: Osteomalacia (prolonged use), rickets
RESP: **Apnea, bronchospasm, respiratory depression**
SKIN: Abscesses at injection site, angioedema, erythema multiforme, pain, *rash,* **Stevens-Johnson syndrome,** thrombophlebitis, urticaria

INTERACTIONS
Drugs

🔳 *Acetaminophen:* Enhanced hepatotoxic potential of acetaminophen; reduced therapeutic response to acetaminophen
🔳 *Antidepressants:* Reduced serum concentrations and therapeutic response of cyclic antidepressants
🔳 *β-adrenergic blockers:* Reduced serum concentrations of β-blockers that are extensively metabolized
🔳 *Calcium channel blockers:* Reduced plasma concentrations of verapamil and nifedipine
🔳 *Chloramphenicol:* Increased serum barbiturate concentrations; reduced serum chloramphenicol concentrations
🔳 *Corticosteroids:* Induced metabolism leads to decreases in steroid levels and therapeutic effect
🔳 *Cyclosporine A:* Barbiturates, as inducers of metabolism, reduce cyclosporine levels
🔳 *Digitoxin:* Induced hepatic metabolism leads to reduced serum levels of digitoxin
🔳 *Disopyramide:* Reduced serum concentrations of disopyramide
🔳 *Doxycycline:* Reduced serum doxycycline concentrations
🔳 *Ethanol:* Excessive CNS depression
🔳 *Furosemide:* Reduced diuretic effect
🔳 *Lamotrigine:* Induced metabolism leads to decreased lamotrigine levels and therapeutic effect
🔳 *MAOIs:* Prolonged effect of barbiturates
🔳 *Methoxyflurane:* Enhanced nephrotoxicity of methoxyflurane
🔳 *Narcotic analgesics:* Increased toxicity of meperidine; reduced effect of methadone; excessive CNS depression
🔳 *Neuroleptics:* Possible reduction in neuroleptic effect

---

❷ *Oral anticoagulants:* Inhibited hypoprothrombinemic response to oral anticoagulants; fatal bleeding episodes have occurred when barbiturates were discontinued in patients stabilized on an anticoagulant

❸ *Oral contraceptives:* Reduced efficacy of oral contraceptives; menstrual irregularities and unintended pregnancies may occur

❸ *Phenytoin:* Barbiturates usually decrease phenytoin levels; monitor closely when concurrent therapy is stopped, started, or changed

❸ *Quinidine:* Reduced serum quinidine plasma concentrations

❸ *Theophylline:* Reduced serum theophylline concentrations; potential of reduced therapeutic response to theophylline

❸ *Valproic acid:* Increases barbiturate concentrations

Labs

• *Barbiturates:* Positive urine

• *Phenobarbital:* Increased serum levels; significant interference

SPECIAL CONSIDERATIONS
PATIENT/FAMILY EDUCATION

• Not chronic medication; indicated only for short-term treatment of insomnia and is probably ineffective after 2 wk

• Physical dependency may result when used for extended time (45-90 days depending on dose)

• Avoid driving or other activities requiring alertness

• Avoid alcohol ingestion or CNS depressants

• Do not discontinue medication abruptly after long-term use

MONITORING PARAMETERS

• CBC, serum folate, vitamin D (if on long-term therapy)

• PT in patients receiving anticoagulants, LFTs

• Mental status, vital signs

---

butalbital compound
(byoo-tal′bih-tall)
Rx: Butalbital/ acetaminophen/caffeine: Amaphen, Americet, Endolor, Esgic, Ezol, Fioricet, Fiorpap, Geone, Medigesic, Repan, Tencet; **Butalbital/ acetaminophen/caffeine with codeine:** Ezol III, Fioricet w/codeine; **Butalbital/ acetaminophen:** Bancap, Phrenilin, Phrenilin Forte, Sedapap-10, Triaprin; **Butalbital/aspirin/ caffeine:** Farbital, Fiorgen PF, Fiorinal, Fiormor Fiortal Fortabs; **Butalbital/ aspirin/caffeine with codeine:** Fiorinal w/codeine
Chemical Class: Barbituric acid derivative
Therapeutic Class: Nonnarcotic analgesic
DEA Class: Schedule III (aspirin-containing products)

CLINICAL PHARMACOLOGY
Mechanism of Action: Combines the analgesic properties of acetaminophen, aspirin, and caffeine with the anxiolytic and muscle relaxant properties of butalbital
INDICATIONS AND USES: Tension (muscle contraction) headache
DOSAGE
Adult
• PO 1-2 tabs q4h as needed, max 6 tabs/day
💲 **AVAILABLE FORMS/COST OF THERAPY**
Butalbital/Acetaminophen/Caffeine
• Cap, Gel—Oral: 50 mg/325 mg/40 mg, 100's: **$7.95-$156.65**

• Tab, Uncoated—Oral: 50 mg/325 mg/40 mg, 30's: **$8.00-$164.98**
• With Codeine Cap, Gel—Oral: 50 mg/325 mg/40 mg/30 mg, 100's: **$124.50-$163.56**
Butalbital/Aspirin/Caffeine
• Cap, Gel—Oral: 50 mg/325 mg/40 mg, 100's: **$37.13-$78.04**
• Tab, Uncoated—Oral: 325 mg/50 mg/40 mg, 100's: **$4.46-$79.40**
• With Codeine Cap, Gel—Oral: 50 mg/325 mg/ 40 mg/ 30 mg, 100's: **$93.61-$163.56**
CONTRAINDICATIONS: Porphyria
PRECAUTIONS: History of drug abuse, elderly, children
PREGNANCY AND LACTATION: Pregnancy category C (category D if used for prolonged periods or in high doses at term); excretion into breast milk unknown (see also aspirin, acetaminophen, and caffeine)
SIDE EFFECTS/ADVERSE REACTIONS
(see also aspirin, acetaminophen, and caffeine)
CNS: Chronic daily headache, depression, *dizziness, drowsiness,* lightheadedness, mental confusion
GI: Flatulence, nausea, vomiting
INTERACTIONS
Drugs
❷ *Oral anticoagulants:* Barbiturates inhibit the hypoprothrombinemic response to oral anticoagulants; fatal bleeding episodes have occurred when barbiturates were discontinued in patients stabilized on an anticoagulant (see also aspirin, acetaminophen, and caffeine)
SPECIAL CONSIDERATIONS
PATIENT/FAMILY EDUCATION
• May cause psychological and/or physical dependence
• May cause drowsiness, use caution driving or operating machinery
• Avoid alcohol and other CNS depressants

butenafine

(byoo-ten′a-feen)
Rx: Mentax
Chemical Class: Benzylamine derivative
Therapeutic Class: Antifungal

CLINICAL PHARMACOLOGY
Mechanism of Action: Blocks the biosynthesis of ergosterol, an essential component of fungal cell membranes; fungicidal
Pharmacokinetics
TOP: Slight transdermal absorption; peak 6-15 hr; excreted in urine (metabolites)
INDICATIONS AND USES: Interdigital tinea pedis (athlete's foot); tinea cruris
Antifungal spectrum usually includes:
Epidermophyton floccosum, Trichophyton mentagrophytes, Trichophyton rubrum
DOSAGE
Adult and Child >12 yr
• TOP cover affected and immediately surrounding skin qd for 2-4 wk
$ **AVAILABLE FORMS/COST OF THERAPY**
• Cre—Top: 1%, 15, 30 g: **$29.56**/15 g
PRECAUTIONS: Sensitivity to allylamine antifungals (cross-reactivity possible)
PREGNANCY AND LACTATION: Pregnancy category B
SIDE EFFECTS/ADVERSE REACTIONS
SKIN: Burning, contact dermatitis, erythema, irritation, itching, stinging

SPECIAL CONSIDERATIONS
• Good cutaneous absorption, prolonged skin retention, and fungicidal activity are potential advantages. Comparative trials with other agents necessary

butoconazole

(byoo-toe-ko´na-zole)
OTC: Femstat-3
Chemical Class: Imidazole derivative
Therapeutic Class: Antifungal

CLINICAL PHARMACOLOGY
Mechanism of Action: Alteration of the fungal cell membrane, which allows leakage of essential intracellular components
Pharmacokinetics
VAG: 5.5% of dose absorbed, peak plasma levels at 24 hr, $t_{1/2}$ 21-24 hr
INDICATIONS AND USES: Local treatment of vulvovaginal candidiasis
DOSAGE
Adult
• VAG 1 applicator hs $\times$ 3 days (nonpregnant), 6 days (2nd and 3rd trimester pregnancy)
S AVAILABLE FORMS/COST OF THERAPY
• Cre—Vag: 2%, 3 $\times$ 5 g applicators: **$14.42**
PREGNANCY AND LACTATION: Pregnancy category C; excretion into breast milk unknown
SIDE EFFECTS/ADVERSE REACTIONS
GU: Burning, discharge, finger itching, rash, soreness, stinging, swelling, vulvovaginal itching

butorphanol

(byoo-tor´fa-nole)
Rx: Stadol
Chemical Class: Synthetic opiate derivative—morphinian congener
Therapeutic Class: Narcotic agonist-antagonist analgesic

CLINICAL PHARMACOLOGY
Mechanism of Action: Analgesia via μ subclass opiate receptor binding in CNS; μ receptors mediate morphinelike supraspinal analgesia, euphoria, and respiratory and physical depression; narcotic antagonist activity is approximately 30 $\times$ pentazocine or 1/40 naloxone
Pharmacokinetics
IM: Onset 10-30 min, peak ½ hr, duration 3-4 hr
IV: Onset 1 min, peak 5 min, duration 2-4 hr
PR: Onset slow, duration 4-6 hr
NASAL: Onset 15 min, peak 30-60 min 80% protein bound; extensively metabolized by liver, excreted by kidneys (reduce dose to 75% for CrCl 10-50 ml/min, to 50% for CrCl <10 ml/min); $t_{1/2}$ 2½-3½ hr
INDICATIONS AND USES: Moderate to severe pain, including postoperative analgesia; preoperative or preanesthetic medication, as a supplement to balanced anesthesia; relief of pain during labor
DOSAGE
Adult
NOTE: 2 mg IM is equivalent to 10 mg morphine
• IV 0.5-2 mg q3-4h prn; NASAL 1 mg (1 spray in one nostril); may repeat in 60-90 minutes if adequate pain relief is not achieved; initial 2-dose sequence outlined above may be repeated in 3-4 hr as needed;

depending on the severity of the pain, an initial dose of 2 mg (1 spray in each nostril) may be given

• *Geriatric:* Half the usual dose at twice the usual interval

§ AVAILABLE FORMS/COST OF THERAPY

• Aer, Spray—Nasal: 10 mg/ml, 2.5 ml: **$60.53-$97.76**

• Inj, Sol—IM, IV: 1 mg/ml, 1 ml: **$4.63-$24.27**; 2 mg/ml, 1 ml: **$8.02-$26.60**

CONTRAINDICATIONS: Narcotic addiction (may precipitate withdrawal), CHF, MI

PRECAUTIONS: Hypotension, addictive personality, head injuries, increased intracranial pressure, respiratory depression, hepatic disease, renal disease, child <18 yr

PREGNANCY AND LACTATION: Pregnancy category B; crosses placenta; excreted in breast milk, though probably clinically insignificant

SIDE EFFECTS/ADVERSE REACTIONS

CNS: Asthenia/lethargy, confusion, dizziness (19%), drowsiness (43%), drug abuse and dependence, *euphoria,* hallucinations, *headache, sedation*

CV: Bradycardia, hypertension, hypotension, palpitations

EENT: Blurred vision, diplopia, *epistaxis, miosis, nasal congestion, nasal irritation, sinus congestion* (nasal spray), tinnitus

GI: Anorexia, constipation, cramps, *dry mouth,* increased amylase, *nausea, vomiting*

GU: Dysuria, increased urinary output, urinary retention

RESP: Pulmonary hypertension, ***respiratory depression***

SKIN: Bruising, *diaphoresis,* flushing, pruritus, rash, urticaria

INTERACTIONS

Drugs

• *Nasal vasoconstrictors:* Slower onset of action of butorphanol (nasal spray)

SPECIAL CONSIDERATIONS

• Chronic use can precipitate withdrawal symptoms of anxiety, agitation, mood changes, hallucinations, dysphoria, weakness, and diarrhea

• Although not classified as a controlled substance by the FDA, prolonged use can result in habituation and drug-seeking behavior

• 2 mg=1 spray in each nostril

---

cabergoline

(kab-er'go-leen)

Rx: Dostinex

Chemical Class: Synthetic ergoline derivative

Therapeutic Class: Antiparkinson's agent, dopaminergic

CLINICAL PHARMACOLOGY

Mechanism of Action: D_2 receptor agonist; inhibits prolactin

Pharmacokinetics

PO: Well absorbed, peak 0.5-4 hr, $t_{1/2}$ 63-68 hr; extensively metabolized to inactive metabolites, excreted mostly in feces, <14% in urine; 41% protein bound

INDICATIONS AND USES: Hyperprolactinemia, Parkinson's disease,* inhibition of lactation,* prolactinomas acromegaly,* polycystic ovary syndrome*

DOSAGE

Adult

• PO 0.25 mg 2 × per wk; increase by 0.25 mg 2 × per wk to desired prolactin level or 1 mg 2 × per wk

§ AVAILABLE FORMS/COST OF THERAPY

• Tab—Oral: 0.5 mg, 8's: **$262.95**

CONTRAINDICATIONS: Sensitivity to ergot derivatives, uncontrolled hypertension, pregnancy-induced hypertension

PREGNANCY AND LACTATION: Pregnancy category B; unknown if excreted in breast milk

SIDE EFFECTS/ADVERSE REACTIONS

CNS: Confusion, *dizziness (25%)*, dyskinesias, *fatigue, headache (43%)*, somnolence, vertigo, visual hallucinations

CV: Edema, orthostatic hypotension

EENT: Nasal stuffiness

GI: Abdominal pain, *constipation (16%), nausea (45%)*, vomiting

SPECIAL CONSIDERATIONS

• More potent with longer half-life than bromocriptine or pergolide, allowing for less frequent dosing

• Initial treatment produces dramatic response; as disease progresses response duration decreases

---

caffeine

(kaf′een)

OTC: Caffedrine, No-Doz, QuickPep, Stay Awake, Vivarin

Chemical Class: Xanthine derivative

Therapeutic Class: Analeptic; CNS stimulant

CLINICAL PHARMACOLOGY

Mechanism of Action: Increases calcium permeability in sarcoplasmic reticulum; promotes accumulation of cAMP; competitively blocks adenosine receptors; stimulates the CNS; produces diuresis; relaxes bronchial smooth muscle

Pharmacokinetics

PO: Onset 15 min, peak ½-1 hr; metabolized by liver, less than 5% excreted unchanged by kidneys; crosses placenta; $t_{1/2}$ 3-4 hr

INDICATIONS AND USES: Respiratory depression associated with overdose (IM); aid in staying awake and restoring mental alertness; adjuvant with analgesics; neonatal apnea*; headaches associated with spinal puncture,* orthostatic hypotension*

DOSAGE

Adult

• PO 100-200 mg q4h prn; Sus Action 200 mg q3-4h; IM 250-500 mg

Child

• *Neonatal apnea:* IV/IM/PO 5-10 mg/kg loading dose followed by 2.5-5 mg/kg qd; adjust maintenance dose based on response and serum levels

⑤ AVAILABLE FORMS/COST OF THERAPY

• Inj, Sol—IM, IV: 125 mg/ml, 2 ml: **$9.70-$34.95** (Rx only)

• Tab—Oral: 100 mg, 60's: **$5.81**; 200 mg, 30's: **$1.85**

• Tab, Sus Action—Oral: 200 mg, 16's: **$2.33**

PRECAUTIONS: Dysrhythmias, Gilles de la Tourette's disorder, psychologic disorders, depression (large parenteral doses can cause further depression in an already depressed patient), ulcers, diabetes mellitus

PREGNANCY AND LACTATION: Pregnancy category B; amounts in breast milk after maternal ingestion of caffeinated beverages not clinically significant; accumulation can occur in heavy-using mothers

SIDE EFFECTS/ADVERSE REACTIONS

CNS: Aggressiveness, dizziness, headache, *hyperactivity, insomnia*, irritability, mild delirium, *restless-*

---

ness, scintillating scotoma, *stimulation, talkativeness,* tinnitus, tremors, twitching

CV: **Dysrhythmias,** extrasystole, palpitations, tachycardia

GI: Anorexia, diarrhea, gastric irritation, nausea, vomiting

GU: Diuresis

METAB: Hyperglycemia

SKIN: Hyperesthesia

INTERACTIONS

Drugs

🔳 *β-adrenergic agents:* Enhanced beta-adrenergic stimulating effects

🔳 *Cimetidine:* Impairs caffeine metabolism resulting in excessive CNS or cardiovascular effects

🔳 *Clozapine:* Caffeine inhibits CYP1A2, with elevations of clozapine levels

🔳 *Contraceptives, oral:* Impair caffeine metabolism resulting in excessive CNS or cardiovascular effects

🔳 *Disulfiram:* Impairs caffeine metabolism resulting in excessive CNS or cardiovascular effects

🔳 *Fluroquinolone antibiotics:* Increases caffeine concentrations and may enhance its side effects

🔳 *Fluconazole:* Increased caffeine concentrations

🔳 *Mexiletine:* 30%-50% reduction in caffeine clearance; potentially increased risk of CNS or cardiovascular effects

🔳 *Phenylpropanolamine:* Additive effects

🔳 *Phenytoin:* Induced hepatic metabolism of caffeine; decreased caffeine effects

🔳 *Pipemidic acid:* Produces a large increase in caffeine concentrations and may increase side effects

🔳 *Terbinafine:* Impairs caffeine metabolism resulting in excessive CNS or cardiovascular effects

🔳 *Theophylline:* Caffeine reduces theophylline clearance by 30%; may affect serum theophylline levels

Labs

• *False positive elevations:* Serum uric acid levels, urine levels of VMA, catecholamines, 5-hydroxyindoleacetic acid

SPECIAL CONSIDERATIONS

PATIENT/FAMILY EDUCATION

• Gradual taper if used long-term to prevent withdrawal syndrome, especially headache

• Most authorities believe caffeine and other analeptics should not be used in overdose with CNS depressants and recommend other supportive therapy

---

calcifediol

(kal-si-fe-dye´ole)

Rx: Calderol

Chemical Class: Sterol derivative

Therapeutic Class: Vitamin D analog

CLINICAL PHARMACOLOGY

Mechanism of Action: Same as 25-hydroxy-vitamin D; product of first metabolic step to biologic activity; relatively inactive before renal hydroxylation to calcitriol; increases intestinal absorption of calcium; increases renal tubular absorption of phosphate; increases rate of accretion and resorption of minerals in bone; regulates calcium homeostasis

Pharmacokinetics

PO: Peak 4 hr, duration 15-20 days; rapid absorption from small intestine; activated in kidneys, stored in liver and fat; excreted via bile in feces; $t_{1/2}$ 12-22 days

---

* = non-FDA-approved use

INDICATIONS AND USES: Management of metabolic bone disease or hypocalcemia in patients on chronic renal dialysis

DOSAGE

Adult

• PO 300-350 µg q wk divided into qd or qod doses, may increase q4 wk

§ **AVAILABLE FORMS/COST OF THERAPY**

• Cap, Elastic—Oral: 20 µg, 60's: **$64.56**; 50 µg, 60's: **$140.38**

CONTRAINDICATIONS: Hyperphosphatemia, hypercalcemia, vitamin D toxicity

PRECAUTIONS: Renal calculi, CV disease

PREGNANCY AND LACTATION: Pregnancy category C; excreted in breast milk and may cause infant hypercalcemia

SIDE EFFECTS/ADVERSE REACTIONS

CNS: Drowsiness, fever, headache, lethargy, vertigo

CV: **Dysrhythmias**

EENT: Conjunctivitis, photophobia, rhinorrhea, tinnitus

GI: Anorexia, constipation, cramps, diarrhea, dry mouth, jaundice, metallic taste, nausea, vomiting

GU: Hematuria, hypercalciuria, hyperphosphatemia, polyuria

MS: Arthralgia, decreased bone development, myalgia

SPECIAL CONSIDERATIONS

PATIENT/FAMILY EDUCATION

• Adequate dietary calcium is necessary for clinical response to vitamin D therapy

MONITORING PARAMETERS

• Blood Ca, P determinations must be made every 2 wk or more frequently if necessary

• Vitamin D levels also helpful, although less frequently

• Height and weight in children

calcipotriene

(kal-sip'oh-tri-een)

Rx: Dovonex

Chemical Class: Synthetic vitamin D_3 analog

Therapeutic Class: Antipsoriatic

CLINICAL PHARMACOLOGY

Mechanism of Action: Vitamin D_3 receptors occur in many parts of the body, including keratinocytes; the scaly red patches of psoriasis are caused by abnormal growth and production of keratinocytes; calcipotriene regulates skin cell production and development

Pharmacokinetics

TOP: 6% of applied dose absorbed systemically (mostly converted to inactive metabolites within 24 hr); transported in blood bound to specific plasma proteins; recycled via the liver and excreted in the bile; systemic disposition expected to be similar to the naturally occurring vitamin

INDICATIONS AND USES: Treatment of moderate plaque psoriasis

DOSAGE

Adult

• TOP apply thin layer to affected skin qd or bid

§ **AVAILABLE FORMS/COST OF THERAPY**

• Cre—Top: 0.005%, 30, 60, 100, 120 g: **$46.73**/30 g

• Oint—Top: 0.005%, 30, 60, 100, 120 g: **$46.73**/30 g

• Sol—Top: 0.005%, 60 ml: **$104.25**

CONTRAINDICATIONS: Demonstrated hypercalcemia, evidence of vitamin D toxicity, use on the face

PRECAUTIONS: Elderly, children

PREGNANCY AND LACTATION: Pregnancy category C

---

italic = common side effects   ***bold italic*** = life-threatening reactions

SIDE EFFECTS/ADVERSE REACTIONS

METAB: Hypercalcemia

SKIN: Burning, dermatitis, dry skin, erythema, folliculitis, hyperpigmentation, *itching,* peeling, rash, skin atrophy, *skin irritation (10% to 15%);* worsening of psoriasis (including development of facial/scalp psoriasis)

SPECIAL CONSIDERATIONS
MONITORING PARAMETERS

• Serum calcium (if elevated discontinue therapy until normal calcium levels are restored); topical administration can yield systemic effects with excessive use

---

calcitonin (salmon)
(kal-si-toe′nin)
Rx: Salmon: Calcimar, Miacalcin (nasal)
Chemical Class: Polypeptide hormone
Therapeutic Class: Hypercalcemia antidote; antiosteoporotic

CLINICAL PHARMACOLOGY

Mechanism of Action: Decreases bone resorption calcitriol (1,25-dihydroxycholecalciferol)and blood calcium levels; increases deposits of calcium in bones; analgesic effect thought to be related to prostaglandin inhibition

Pharmacokinetics

IM/SC: Onset 15 min, peak 4 hr, duration 8-24 hr; metabolized by kidneys, excreted as inactive metabolites

INTRANASAL: 7.5% bioavailability

INDICATIONS AND USES: Hypercalcemia; postmenopausal osteoporosis; Paget's disease; analgesia secondary to vertebral fracture*

DOSAGE

Skin test (salmon calcitonin): 1 unit/0.1 mg (0.1 ml of 10 IU/ml dilution) intradermally; observe for 15 min for significant erythema

Adult

• *Osteoporosis:* Salmon SC/IM 100 IU qd; intranasal 200 IU qd alternating nostrils

• *Hypercalcemia:* Salmon IM 4-8 IU/kg q6-12h

• *Paget's disease:* Human SC 50-100 IU mg/day initially; maintenance range 50 IU bid to 25-50 IU 2-3×/week; Salmon SC/IM 100 IU qd initially; usual maintenance 50 IU qd or qod

• *Analgesic doses:* Same as above, salmon 100 IU SC/IM qd × 2-4 wk, then 50 IU qod three times weekly as maintenance (effect should be noticeable within 2 wk)

🔲 **AVAILABLE FORMS/COST OF THERAPY**

• Inj, Sol—IM, SC: 200 IU/ml, 2 ml: **$31.35-$53.40** (salmon)

• Spray, Sol—Nasal: 200 IU/metered dose, 14 doses/2 ml: **$68.99**

CONTRAINDICATIONS: Hypersensitivity (skin test recommended for salmon calcitonin), children

PRECAUTIONS: Hypocalcemia

PREGNANCY AND LACTATION: Pregnancy category C; inhibits lactation in animals

SIDE EFFECTS/ADVERSE REACTIONS

CNS: Chills, dizziness, flushing, headache, tetany, weakness

CV: Chest pressure

EENT: Bleeding (nasal), dryness, itching, nasal irritation, redness, *rhinitis*

GI: Abdominal pain, anorexia, diarrhea, epigastric pain, nausea, salty taste, vomiting

GU: Diuresis

MS: Swelling, tingling of hands

---

* = non-FDA-approved use

RESP: Dyspnea

SKIN: Edema of feet, flushing, pruritus of ear lobes, rash

SPECIAL CONSIDERATIONS
PATIENT/FAMILY EDUCATION

• Before first dose of new bottle of nasal spray pump must be activated by holding upright and pumping nozzle 6 times until a faint spray is emitted

• Human calcitonin for injection (Cibacalcin) Novartis, pharmaceutical orphan drug

---

calcitriol

(kal-si-trye′ole)

Rx: Calcijex, Rocaltrol

Chemical Class: Sterol derivative

Therapeutic Class: Vitamin D analog; antiosteoporotic

CLINICAL PHARMACOLOGY

Mechanism of Action: 1,25-(OH)$2D_3$ (calcitriol), the active form of vitamin D_3; active in regulation of the absorption of calcium from the gastrointestinal tract and its utilization in the body; increases renal tubular resorption of phosphate

Pharmacokinetics

PO: Peak 3-6 hr, duration 3-5 days, $t_{1/2}$ 3-6 hr, rapid oral absorption; metabolized and excreted via bile in feces, 4%-6% excreted in urine

INDICATIONS AND USES: Hypocalcemia and resultant metabolic bone disease in patients on chronic renal dialysis; hypoparathyroidism and pseudohypoparathyroidism; osteoporosis*(congenital, steroid induced, postmenopausal); osteitis fibrosa; osteodystrophy; osteomalacia

DOSAGE
Adult

• *Hypocalcemia:* PO 0.25 μg qd; may increase by 0.25 μg/day q4-8wk; maintenance 0.25-1 μg qd; IV 0.5 μg three times weekly (can be administered through the catheter at the end of dialysis)

• *Hypoparathyroidism/pseudohypoparathyroidism:* PO 0.25 μg qd; may be increased by 0.25 μg/day q2-4wk; maintenance 0.25-2 μg qd

• *Osteoporosis:* 0.25 μg qd

Child >1 yr

• *Hypoparathyroidism/pseudohypoparathyroidism:* PO 0.25 μg qd; may be increased q2-4 wk; maintenance 0.25-0.75 μg qd

💲 AVAILABLE FORMS/COST OF THERAPY

• Cap, Elastic—Oral: 0.25 μg, 100's: **$120.95-$139.99**; 0.5 μg, 100's: **$193.38-$223.83**

• Inj, Sol—IV: 1 μg/ml, 1 ml: **$6.90-$14.60**; 2 μg/ml, 1 ml: **$12.71**

CONTRAINDICATIONS: Hyperphosphatemia, hypercalcemia, vitamin D toxicity

PRECAUTIONS: Renal calculi, CV disease

PREGNANCY AND LACTATION: Pregnancy category C; may be excreted in breast milk

SIDE EFFECTS/ADVERSE REACTIONS

CNS: Drowsiness, fever, headache, lethargy, vertigo

GI: Anorexia, constipation, cramps, diarrhea, dry mouth, *jaundice*, metallic taste, nausea, vomiting

GU: Hematuria, hypercalciuria, hyperphosphatemia, polyuria

MS: Arthralgia, decreased bone development, myalgia

INTERACTIONS
Drugs

3 *Thiazide diuretics:* Hypercalcemia

---

3 *Verapamil:* Hypercalcemia may inhibit the activity of verapamil

SPECIAL CONSIDERATIONS
PATIENT/FAMILY EDUCATION
• Adequate dietary calcium is necessary for clinical response to vitamin D therapy

MONITORING PARAMETERS
• Blood Ca and P determinations must be made every week until stable, or more frequently if necessary
• Vitamin D levels also helpful, although less frequently
• Height and weight in children

---

calcium salts

Rx: Calcium acetate: PhosLo
OTC: *Calcium carbonate:* Amitone, Cal-Carb Forte, Calci-Chew, Calci-Mix, Caltrate 600, Chooz, Florical, Maalox, Mallamint, Mylanta, Nephro-Calci, Os-Cal 500, Oysco 500, Oyst-Cal 500, Oyster Calcium, Rolaids, Titralac, Tums, Tums Ex; *Calcium citrate:* Citracal; *Calcium glubionate:* Neo-Calglucon; *Tricalcium phosphate:* Posture
Combinations
  Rx: with cholecalciferol (Os-Cal-D)
  OTC: with sodium fluoride (Caltrate, Florical)
Therapeutic Class: Antacid; antiosteoporotic; phosphate adsorbent (acetate)

CLINICAL PHARMACOLOGY
Mechanism of Action: Neutralizes gastric acidity; acetate salt binds phosphate in GI tract, increases elimination; caution needed for maintenance of nervous, muscular, skeletal, enzyme reactions, normal cardiac contractility, coagulation of blood; effects secretory activity of endocrine, exocrine glands

Pharmacokinetics
PO: 30% absorbed (variably) depending on demand; absorption vitamin D dependent; bioavailability not significantly different between different salts
IV: Rapid increase in serum levels, with return to pre-drug level within 30 min-2 hr; 80% excreted in the feces as insoluble salts, urinary excretion accounts for the remaining 20%

INDICATIONS AND USES: Prevention and treatment of hypocalcemia, hypermagnesemia, hypoparathyroidism, osteoporosis; neonatal tetany; cardiac toxicity caused by hyperkalemia; cardiac arrest (adjunct); lead colic; hyperphosphatemia; vitamin D deficiency; hyperacidity (antacid); calcium antagonist toxicity; hypertension during pregnancy

DOSAGE
U.S. RDA is:
Adults: 1000-1500 mg
Children: <4 yr: 800 mg
Infants: 600 mg
Adult
• Calcium acetate
Hyperphosphatemia: PO initial, 1334 mg (2 tabs) with meals; increase gradually to bring phosphate below 6 mg/dl (usually 3-4 tabs per meal)
• Calcium carbonate
Hyperphosphatemia: 1-17 g qd in divided doses
Hypocalcemia (replenish electrolytes): PO 1.25 g (500 mg Ca^{++}) 4-6 per day, chewed with water
Antacid: PO tabs 500 mg-1 g (250-500 mg Ca^{++}) 1 and 3 hr pc, hs prn; Susp 1.25 g (500 mg Ca^{++}), 1 and 3 hr pc, hs prn
Hypertension in pregnancy: 500 mg tid during third trimester

• Calcium chloride

Hypocalcemia (replenish electrolytes): IV 500 mg-1 g (6.8-13.6 mEq Ca^{++}) q1-3 days as indicated by serum calcium levels; give at <1 ml/min

Cardiotonic: IV 500 mg-1 g (6.8-13.6 mEq Ca^{++}); give at <1 ml/min; Intraventricular 200-800 mg (2.72-9.6 mEq Ca^{++}) inj as single dose

• Calcium citrate

Hypocalcemia (replenish electrolytes): PO: 950 mg-1.9 g (200-400 mg Ca^{++}) tid-qid, pc

• Calcium glubionate

Hypocalcemia (replenish electrolytes): 5.4 g (345 mg Ca^{++}) tid-qid

• Calcium gluceptate

Hypocalcemia (replenish electrolytes): IM 440 mg-1.1 g (1.8-4.5 mEq Ca^{++}); IV 1.1-4.4 g (1.8-4.5 mEq Ca^{++}), slowly (rate not to exceed 2 ml/min)

• Calcium gluconate

Hypocalcemia, hyperkalemia, hypermagnesemia (replenish electrolytes): PO 11 g (1 g Ca^{++})/day in divided doses; IV 1 g (4.72 mEq Ca^{++}) at 0.5 ml/min (10% sol)

• Calcium lactate

Hypocalcemia: PO 325 mg-1.3 g (1 g Ca^{++}/day) tid with meals

• Tribasic calcium phosphate

Hypocalcemia: PO 1.6 mg (600 mg Ca^{++}) bid after meals

Child

• Calcium chloride: IV 25 mg/kg over several min

• Calcium glubionate

Infants up to 1 yr PO 1.8 g (115 mg Ca^{++}) 5× daily before meals

Children 1-4 yr PO 3.6 g (230 mg Ca^{++}) tid, ac

Children > 4 yr PO; see adult dose

• Calcium gluceptate

Newborn

Hypocalcemia: IM 440 mg-1.1 g (1.8-4.5 mEq Ca^{++}); IV 440 mg-1.1 g (1.8-4.5 mEq Ca^{++}) as single dose, rate not to exceed 2 ml/min

Exchange transfusions in newborns: IV 110 mg (approx. 0.45 mEq Ca^{++}) after every 100 ml of blood transfused

• Calcium gluconate: PO 500 mg/kg/day in divided doses, pc

• Calcium lactate: PO 500 mg/kg/day in divided doses

💲 AVAILABLE FORMS/COST OF THERAPY

Calcium Acetate

• Inj, Sol—IV: 0.5 mEq/ml, 10 ml: **$0.89**

• Tab, Uncoated—Oral: 667 mg, 200's: **$18.50-$29.45**

• Gelcap—Oral: 667 mg, 200's: cost not available

Calcium Carbonate (mg of calcium)

• Susp—Oral: 1250 mg (500 mg Ca)/5 ml, 500 ml: **$9.50**

• Tab, Uncoated, Chewable—Oral: 500 mg, 100's: **$2.10-$3.25**; 600 mg, 60's: **$1.75-$6.20**; 750 mg (300 mg Ca), 96's: **$2.50-$5.10**; 1000 mg, 72's: **$2.72-$4.11**; 1250 mg (500 mg Ca), 100's: **$8.94-$10.60**

• Tab, Uncoated—Oral: 650 mg (260 mg Ca), 60's: **$2.93-$11.65**; 1250 mg (500 mg Ca), 60's: **$1.89-$12.46**

Calcium Chloride

• Inj, Sol—IV: 10%, 10 ml: **$5.33-$13.45**

Calcium Citrate (mg of calcium)

• Tab—Oral: 950 mg (200 mg Ca), 100's: **$3.00-$6.88**

Calcium Glubionate (mg of calcium)

• Syr—Oral: 1800 mg (115 mg Ca)/5 ml, 480 ml: **$17.95-$29.34**

Calcium Gluceptate

• Inj, Sol—IM: 220 mg (90 mg Ca)/5 ml, 5 ml: **$2.43**

Calcium Gluconate (mg of calcium)

• Inj, Sol—IV: 10%, 10 ml: **$1.29-$1.70**

• Tab—Oral: 500 mg (45 mg Ca), 100's: **$14.94**; 650 mg (58.5 mg Ca), 100's: **$4.25**; 1000 mg (90 mg Ca), 100's: **$26.70**

Calcium Lactate (mg of calcium)

• Tab—Oral: 325 mg (42.25 mg Ca), 100's: **$1.50-$2.25**; 650 mg (84.5 mg Ca), 100's: **$0.99-$7.30**

Tribasic Calcium Phosphate (mg of calcium)

• Tab—Oral: 1565.2 mg (600 mg Ca), 60's: **$7.97**

CONTRAINDICATIONS: Hypercalcemia, hypercalciuria, hyperparathyroidism, bone tumors, digitalis toxicity, ventricular fibrillation, renal calculi, sarcoidosis, renal insufficiency (tribasic calcium phosphate)

PRECAUTIONS: Elderly, fluid restriction, decreased GI motility, GI obstruction, dehydration

PREGNANCY AND LACTATION: Pregnancy category C; some oral supplemental calcium may be excreted in breast milk (chloride, gluconate, unknown); concentrations not sufficient to produce an adverse effect in neonates

SIDE EFFECTS/ADVERSE REACTIONS

CV: Bradycardia, *cardiac arrest, dysrhythmias,* heart block, hemorrhage, hypotension, rebound hypertension, shortened Q-T

GI: Anorexia, constipation, diarrhea, eructation, flatulence, nausea, obstruction, rebound hyperacidity, vomiting

GU: Renal dysfunction, *renal failure,* renal stones

METAB: Hypercalcemia (drowsiness, lethargy, muscle weakness, headache, constipation, *coma,* anorexia, nausea, vomiting, polyuria, thirst); metabolic alkalosis; milk-alkali syndrome (nausea, vomiting, disorientation, headache)

MISC: Burning at IV site, extravasation, necrosis, pain, severe venous thrombosis

INTERACTIONS

Drugs

3 *Calcium channel blockers:* Calcium administration (especially parenteral) may inhibit calcium channel blocker activity

3 *Digoxin, digitoxin:* Elevated calcium concentrations associated with acute digitalis toxicity

3 *Doxycycline, Tetracycline:* Cotherapy with a tetracycline and a divalent or trivalent cation can reduce the serum concentration and efficacy of tetracyclines

3 *Iron:* Some calcium antacids reduce the GI absorption of iron; inhibition of the hematological response to iron has been reported

3 *Itraconazole, Ketoconazole:* Antacids containing calcium may reduce antifungal concentrations

3 *Quinidine:* Calcium antacids capable of increasing urine pH may increase serum quinidine concentrations

3 *Quinolones:* Reduced bioavailability of quinolone antibiotics

3 *Sodium polystyrene sulfonate resin:* Combined use with calcium-containing antacid may result in systemic alkalosis

3 *Thiazides:* Large doses of calcium with thiazides may lead to milk-alkali syndrome

Labs

• *False increase:* Chloride, green color, benzodiazepine (false positive)

• *False decrease:* Magnesium, oxylate, lipase

SPECIAL CONSIDERATIONS

• Percentage elemental calcium content of various calcium salts: calcium acetate (25), calcium carbonate (40), calcium chloride (27.2), calcium citrate (21), calcium glu-

C

bionate (6.5), calcium gluceptate (8.2), calcium gluconate (9.3), calcium lactate (13), tricalcium phosphate, (39)

MONITORING PARAMETERS
• Serum calcium or serum ionized calcium concentrations (ionized calcium concentrations are preferable to determine free and bound calcium, especially with concurrent low serum albumin)
• Alternatively, ionized calcium can be estimated using the following rule: Total serum calcium will fall by 0.8 mg/dL for each 1.0 g/dL decrease in serum albumin concentration

---

candesartan

(kan-de-sar´-tan)
Rx: Atacand
Chemical Class: Angiotensin II receptor antagonist
Therapeutic Class: Antihypertensive

CLINICAL PHARMACOLOGY
Mechanism of Action: Antihypertensive (inhibition of vasoconstriction and aldosterone secretion), smooth muscle hypoproliferative, and cardioprotective effects are attributable to selective blockade of angiotensin II (AT1) receptors found throughout the cardiovascular and renal systems; effects independent of angiotensin II synthesis
Pharmacokinetics
PO: Onset 2-4 hrs; peak 6-8 hrs; majority of antihypertensive response to a fixed-dose is manifested in 2 wk; full impact present after 4 wk;
oral bioavailability 15%, unaffected by meals; >99% protein bound; apparent clearance 0.20-0.25 L/h/kg; candesartan cilexetil, the esterified pro-drug of candesartan completely

metabolized during absorption from the intestinal wall (peak metabolite levels 3-4 hrs), 33% renal excreted; 67% recovered in feces; $t_{1/2}$ 5-7 hrs

INDICATIONS AND USES: Hypertension, CHF (left ventricular dysfunction*), myocardial infarction*, diabetic nephropathy*

DOSAGE
Adult and child >16 yr
• Hypertension: PO 8-32 mg qd

🆂 AVAILABLE FORMS/COST OF THERAPY
• Tab, Uncoated—Oral: 4 mg, 30's: **$37.50**; 8 mg, 30's: **$37.26**; 16 mg, 100's: **$125.00**; 32 mg, 100's: **$175.00**

CONTRAINDICATIONS: Primary hyperaldosteronism; bilateral renal artery stenosis

PRECAUTIONS: Hypovolemic patients (salt and/or volume depleted; diuretic therapy) at greater risk of symptomatic hypotension; concurrent potassium-sparing diuretics, potassium-laden salt substitutes, or other potassium-sparing medications, bilateral renal artery stenosis; aortic or mitral valve stenosis; hypertrophic cardiomyopathy; severe hepatic dysfunction/cholestasis

PREGNANCY AND LACTATION: Pregnancy category C (1st trimester) and D (2nd and 3rd trimester)

SIDE EFFECTS/ADVERSE REACTIONS
CNS: Anxiety, depression, dizziness (2.4%), drowsiness, fatigue (1.4%), headache (3.8%), lightheadedness, parethesia, vertigo
CV: Flushing, palpitations, tachycardia
EENT: Epistaxis
MS: Back pain, myalgia (1.9%)
RESP: Cough (1.8-6.5%), upper respiratory infection
SKIN: Facial edema, angioedema, diaphoresis
MISC: Angioedema

---

italic = common side effects   ***bold italic*** = life-threatening reactions

INTERACTIONS
Drugs

Ⓑ *Cimetidine:* Increased levels of candesartan

Ⓑ *Fluconazole:* Decreased conversion to active metabolite (CYP2C9 inhibition), loss of antihypertensive effects

❷ *Lithium:* Increased renal lithium reabsorption at the proximal tubular site due to the natriuresis associated with the inhibition of aldosterone secretion; increased risk of lithium toxicity

Ⓑ *Phenobarbital:* Decreased levels of candesartan

Ⓑ *Rifampin:* Induced metabolism of losartan and metabolite, resulting in a decrease in the area under the concentration-time curve (AUC) and half-life of both compounds and reduced losartan efficacy

SPECIAL CONSIDERATIONS

• Potentially as or more effective than angiotensin-converting enzyme inhibitors, without cough; no evidence for reduction in morbidity and mortality as first-line agents in hypertension yet; whether they provide the same cardiac and renal protection also still tentative; like ACE inhibitors, less effective in black patients

PATIENT/FAMILY EDUCATION

• Call your clinician immediately if the following side effects are noted: wheezing; lip, throat or face swelling; hives or rash

MONITORING PARAMETERS

• Baseline electrolytes, urinalysis, blood urea nitrogen and creatinine with recheck at 2-4 wk after initiation (sooner in volume-depleted patients); monitor sitting BP; watch for symptomatic hypotension, particularly in volume-depleted patients

---

capreomycin
(kap-ree-oh-mye′sin)
Rx: Capastat
Chemical Class: S. capreolus derivative
Therapeutic Class: Antituberculosis agent

CLINICAL PHARMACOLOGY

Mechanism of Action: Inhibits RNA synthesis, decreases mycobacterial replication

Pharmacokinetics

IM: Peak 1-2 hr, $t_{1/2}$ 4-6 hr (prolonged with decreased renal function); excreted in urine unchanged (small amount in bile)

INDICATIONS AND USES: Pulmonary tuberculosis caused by *Mycobacterium tuberculosis* after failure or intolerability with primary medications; use concurrently with other antituberculars

DOSAGE
Adult

• IM 1 g or 13.9 mg/kg (not to exceed 20 mg/kg/day) qd × 2-4 mo, then 1 g 2-3×/wk × 18-24 mo, not to exceed 20 mg/kg/day; *must* be given with another antitubercular medication; dosage reduction necessary with declining renal function, as follows (dose in mg/kg/day designed to achieve steady state levels of 10 mg/L: if CrCl = 50 ml/min, give 7 mg/kg q24h; if CrCl = 20 ml/min, give 3.6 mg/kg q24h; if CrCl = 10 ml/min, give 2.4 mg/kg q24h; if CrCl = 0 ml/min, give 1.3 mg/kg q24h)

Child

• 15-30 mg/kg qd, though safety and efficacy not established

Ⓢ AVAILABLE FORMS/COST OF THERAPY

• Inj, Sol—IM: 1 g/vial: **$25.54**

PRECAUTIONS: Renal disease, hearing impairment, hepatic disease, myasthenia gravis, Parkinsonism

PREGNANCY AND LACTATION: Pregnancy category C; breast milk excretion is unknown; however, problems in humans have not been documented (poorly absorbed from GI tract)

SIDE EFFECTS/ADVERSE REACTIONS

CNS: Fever, headache, hearing loss, neuromuscular blockade, tinnitus, vertigo

EENT: Deafness, *ototoxicity* (11%), tinnitus

GU: Albuminuria, alkalosis, decreased CrCl, hematuria, hypokalemia, increased BUN, ***nephrotoxicity*** (36%), proteinuria, ***tubular necrosis***

HEME: Eosinophilia, leukocytosis, ***leukopenia***

SKIN: Irritation, pain, rash, sterile abscess at injection site; urticaria

INTERACTIONS

Drugs

■ *Amphotericin B, Cephalosporins, Cyclosporine, Methoxyflurane:* Additive nephrotoxicity risk

■ *Carboplatin:* Additive ototoxicity

❷ *Ethacrynic acid:* Additive ototoxicity

❷ *Neuromuscular blocking agents:* Potentiate the respiratory suppression produced by neuromuscular blocking agents

■ *Oral anticoagulants:* Enhanced hypoprothrombinemic response

SPECIAL CONSIDERATIONS

• When used in renal insufficiency or pre-existing auditory impairment, risks of additional 8th-nerve impairment or renal injury should be weighed against the benefits of therapy

MONITORING PARAMETERS

• Electrolytes, BUN, creatinine weekly

• Blood levels of drug

• Audiometric testing before, during, after treatment

---

capsaicin

(cap-say′sin)

OTC: Zostrix, Zostrix HP

Chemical Class: Alkaloid derivative of Solanaceae plant family

Therapeutic Class: Topical analgesic

CLINICAL PHARMACOLOGY

Mechanism of Action: Early counterirritant properties, then depletes substance P in sensory neurons

Pharmacokinetics

TOP: Therapeutic effect in 14-28 days

INDICATIONS AND USES: Relief of pain in postherpetic neuralgia, diabetic neuropathy, rheumatoid arthritis, osteoarthritis, mastectomy,* psoriasis*

DOSAGE

Adult and Child ≥2 yr

• *TOP:* Apply 3-5 times/day, less frequent application not effective; continue for 3-5 months, some pts may require lifelong therapy

💲 **AVAILABLE FORMS/COST OF THERAPY**

• Cre—Top: 0.025%, 20, 45, 60 g: **$5.70-$13.04**/60 g; 0.075%, 30, 45, 60 g: **$8.05-$35.62**/60 g

• Gel—Top: 0.025%, 60 g: **$4.37-$6.13**; 0.05%, 60 g: **$5.37**

• Lot—Top: 0.025%, 60 ml: **$9.00**; 0.075% 60 ml: **$10.20**

CONTRAINDICATIONS: Application to damaged skin

SIDE EFFECTS/ADVERSE REACTIONS

CNS: Neurotoxicity

SKIN: Burning, itching, local discomfort

SPECIAL CONSIDERATIONS

• Pretreatment with topical lidocaine 5% ointment may relieve burning

PATIENT/FAMILY EDUCATION

• Wash hands following use

---

captopril

(cap-toe-pril)

Rx: Capoten

Combinations

  Rx: with hydrochlorothiazide (Capozide)

Chemical Class: Sulfhydryl-containing angiotensin-converting enzyme (ACE) inhibitor

Therapeutic Class: Antihypertensive

CLINICAL PHARMACOLOGY

Mechanism of Action: Antihypertensive, hypoproliferative, and cardioprotective effects atributable to competitive inhibition of angiotensin-converting enzyme (ACE) yielding decreased plasma concentrations of angiotensin II, plasma aldosterone concentrations, systemic vascular resistance, blood pressure, preload, and afterload, not accompanied by changes in heart rate, pressor sensitivity to exogenous norepinephrine, or baroreceptor sensitivity

Pharmacokinetics

PO: Peak 1 hr (presence of food reduces absorption by 3%-40%), duration 2-6 hr, metabolized by liver, excreted in urine (40%-50% unchanged); $t_{1/2}$ <2-3 hr crosses placenta; excreted in breast milk

INDICATIONS AND USES: Hypertension (essential, malignant,* renovascular, associated with pheochromocytoma,* scleroderma*), CHF (left ventricular dysfunction), MI (left ventricular salvage), erythrocytosis,* diabetic and non-diabetic nephropathy, retinopathy with diabetes, hepatorenal syndrome,* polycythemia vera,* Bartter's syndrome,* aldosteronism,* cystinuria,* rheumatoid arthritis,* Kaposi's sarcoma*

DOSAGE

Adult

• *Hypertension:* PO initial: 6.25 mg-12.5 mg tid [patients with low blood pressure, hyponatremia (<130 mEq/L), hypovolemia, or those on diuretics]; others 25 mg tid; increase every 1-2 weeks to 50 mg tid; usual maintenance range 25-150 tid; max 450 mg/day

• *Congestive heart failure* (left ventricular dysfunction): PO 3.125-6.25 mg tid (for patients pretreated with diuretics, hypotensive, hypovolemic, or hyponatremic); others 12.5 mg bid-tid; may increase to 50 mg bid-tid (as systolic blood pressure will allow, i.e., >100 mm Hg), generally given with digitalis and diuretics; maximum daily doses, 450 mg/day

• *Myocardial infarction* (left ventricular salvage): PO initial dose of 6.25 mg (to minimize excessive or symptomatic hypotensive responses) given within 3 days of MI; if tolerated, 12.5 mg tid, with titration over the next few days to a goal of 50 mg tid as maintenance

• *Diabetic nephropathy:* PO 50 mg bid or 25 mg tid

Child

• *Hypertension:* PO initial dose, 0.01 mg-0.25 mg/kg q12h (infants); 0.-0.5 mg tid (older children); maintenance dose, 2 mg/kg/dose bid-tid

---

* = non-FDA-approved use

• *Congestive heart failure* (left ventricular dysfunction): PO initial 2.5 mg/kg/dose, increasing to 3.5 mg/kg/dose, usually tid, with diuretics and digoxin

$ AVAILABLE FORMS/COST OF THERAPY

• Tab, Uncoated—Oral: 12.5 mg, 100's: **$53.67-$120.94**; 25 mg, 100's: **$5.76-$110.29**; 50 mg, 100's: **$7.67-$187.46**; 100 mg, 100's: **$129.95-$249.71**

PRECAUTIONS: History of anaphylaxis, renal insufficiency (<30 ml/min), hypotension (CHF, elderly, volume depletion—diuretics, dialysis, cirrhosis), aortic stenosis, hyperkalemia (potassium supplements, potassium-sparing diuretics, renal disease, diabetes), neutropenia (autoimmune diseases, collagen vascular, febrile illness, immunosuppressant drug therapy), proteinuria, renal artery stenosis, surgery/anesthesia (excessive hypotension, correctable with fluids)

PREGNANCY AND LACTATION: Pregnancy category C (1st trimester) and D (2nd and 3rd trimesters—fetal and neonatal hypotension, neonatal skull hypoplasia, anuria, reversible or irreversible renal failure, death, oligohydramnios); excreted into breast milk in small amounts; compatible with breast feeding

SIDE EFFECTS/ADVERSE REACTIONS

CNS: Chills, fever

CV: Chest pain, hypotension, palpitations, postural hypotension, tachycardia

GI: Loss of taste

GU: Acute reversible renal failure, dysuria, frequency, impotence, nephrotic syndrome, nocturia, oliguria, polyuria, proteinuria

HEME: **Agranulocytosis, neutropenia**

METAB: Hyperkalemia, hyponatremia

RESP: Angioedema, **bronchospasm,** *cough,* dyspnea

SKIN: Rash

INTERACTIONS

Drugs

❷ *Allopurinol:* Increased risk of hypersensitivity reactions including Stevens-Johnson syndrome, skin eruptions, fever, and arthralgias

❸ *α-blockers:* Possible exaggerated "first dose" response

❸ *Aspirin:* Reduced hemodynamic effects of captopril; less likely at doses <236 mg qd

❸ *Azathioprine:* Increased myelosuppression

❸ *Cyclosporine:* Increased nephrotoxicity

❸ *Indomethacin:* Inhibits the antihypertensive response to ACE inhibition; other NSAIDs probably have similar effect

❸ *Insulin:* ACE inhibitors enhance insulin sensitivity; hypoglycemia possible

❸ *Iron:* Increased risk of systemic reaction (GI symptoms, hypotension) with parenteral iron

❸ *Lithium:* Increased risk of lithium toxicity

❸ *Loop diuretics:* Initiation of ACE inhibition therapy with concurrent intensive diuretic therapy may cause significant hypotension, renal insufficiency

❸ *Mercaptopurine:* Increased risk of neutropenia

❸ *Potassium, Potassium-sparing diuretics:* ACE inhibition tends to increase potassium; increased risk of hyperkalemia in predisposed patients

❸ *Trimethoprim:* Additive risk of hyperkalemia, especially in patient predisposed to renal insufficiency

italic = common side effects · **bold italic** = life-threatening reactions

Labs
• ACE inhibition can account for approximately 0.5mEq/L rise in serum potassium
• Blood in urine: Decreased reactivity with occult blood test
• Fructosamine: Captopril interferes with assay increasing serum fructosamine
• Ketones in urine: False positive dip-sticks
• *False positive:* Urine acetone

SPECIAL CONSIDERATIONS
PATIENT/FAMILY EDUCATION
• Caution with salt substitutes containing potassium chloride
• Rise slowly to sitting/standing position to minimize orthostatic hypotension
• Dizziness, fainting, lightheadedness may occur during 1st few days of therapy
• May cause altered taste perception or cough; persistent dry cough usually does not subside unless medication is stopped; notify clinician if these symptoms persist

MONITORING PARAMETERS
• BUN, creatinine, potassium within 2 wk after initiation of therapy (increased levels may indicate acute renal failure)

---

carbamazepine

(kar-ba-maz'e-peen)
Rx: Atretol, Carbatrol, Epitol, Tegretol, Tegretol-XR
Chemical Class: Iminostilbene derivative
Therapeutic Class: Anticonvulsant; antineuralgic; antimanic; antipsychotic

---

CLINICAL PHARMACOLOGY
Mechanism of Action: Anticonvulsant action by inhibition of influx of sodium ions across nerve cell membrane in motor cortex, reducing polysynaptic response and blocking posttetanic potentiation; antineuralgic may involve $GABA_B$ receptors, which may be linked to calcium channels; antimanic/antipsychotic effects on neurotransmitter modulator systems

Pharmacokinetics
PO: Anticonvulsant onset varies hours to days; antineuralgic onset 8-72 hr; antimanic onset 7-10 days; peak concentrations: susp 1.5 hr; tabs 4-5 hr; therapeutic serum concentrations 4-12 µg/ml; absorption slow (suspension faster than tablets); metabolized by liver (autoinduction); excreted in urine and feces; crosses placenta; excreted in breast milk; $t_{1/2}$ variable 14-16 hr after repeated dosing

INDICATIONS AND USES: Tonic-clonic, complex-partial, mixed seizures; trigeminal neuralgia, glossopharyngeal neuralgia; manic depressive disorder,* chronic neurogenic pain syndromes,* diabetes insipidus (central),* alcohol withdrawal,* psychotic disorders,* restless legs syndrome*

DOSAGE
Adult
• *Seizures:* PO 200 mg bid; may be increased by 200 mg/day in divided doses q6-8h; maintenance 800-1200 mg/day; max 1200 mg/day
• *Trigeminal neuralgia:* PO 100 mg bid; may increase 100 mg q12h until pain subsides; not to exceed 1.2 g/day; maintenance is 200-400 mg bid
• *Antidiuretic:* 300-600 mg/day, as sole therapy; 200-400 mg/day, if concurrent with other antidiuretic agents
• *Antipsychotic:* PO 200-400 mg/day divided tid-qid; max 1600 mg/day

Child <12 yr
• *Seizures:* PO 10-20 mg/kg/day in 2-3 divided doses

$ AVAILABLE FORMS/COST OF THERAPY
• Cap, Sus Action—Oral: 200 mg, 120's: **$49.00**; 300 mg, 120's: **$77.83**
• Susp—Oral: 100 mg/5 ml, 450 ml: **$24.39-$36.40**
• Tab, Uncoated—Oral: 200 mg, 100's: **$20.64-$56.63**
• Tab, Chewable—Oral: 100 mg, 100's: **$17.40-$31.85**
• Tab, Sus Action—Oral: 100 mg, 100's: **$27.26**; 200 mg, 100's: **$56.53**; 400 mg, 100's: **$98.79**

CONTRAINDICATIONS: Hypersensitivity to tricyclic antidepressants, bone marrow depression, concomitant use of MAO inhibitor

PRECAUTIONS: Glaucoma, hepatic disease, renal disease, cardiac disease, psychosis, child <6 yr

PREGNANCY AND LACTATION: Pregnancy category C; concentration in milk approximately 60% of maternal plasma concentration; compatible with breast feeding

SIDE EFFECTS/ADVERSE REACTIONS
CNS: Ataxia, confusion, dizziness, *drowsiness,* fatigue, hallucinations, headache, paralysis
CV: Aggravation of coronary artery disease, **CHF,** hypertension, hypotension
EENT: Blurred vision, conjunctivitis, diplopia, dry mouth, nystagmus, tinnitus
GI: Abdominal pain, anorexia, *constipation, diarrhea,* enzymes, glossitis, hepatitis, increased liver enzymes, *nausea,* stomatitis, vomiting
GU: Albuminuria, frequency, glycosuria, impotence, urinary retention
HEME: **Agranulocytosis, aplastic anemia,** eosinophilia, leukocytosis, **neutropenia, thrombocytopenia**

RESP: Pulmonary hypersensitivity (fever, dyspnea, pneumonitis)
SKIN: Rash, **Stevens-Johnson syndrome,** urticaria

INTERACTIONS
Drugs
3 *Acetaminopen:* Enhanced hepatotoxic potential; reduced acetaminophen response
3 *Antidepressants, tricyclic:* Carbamazepine reduces serum concentrations of imipramine and probably other cyclic antidepressants
3 *Benzodiazepines (alprazolam, diazepam, midazolam, triazolam):* Metabolized by CYP3A4; enzyme induced by carbamazepine; reduced benzo effect
2 *Calcium channel blockers:* Verapamil and diltiazem reduce the metabolism of carbamazepine leading to increased carbamazepine toxicity when these CCBs are added to chronic carbamazepine therapy; enzyme induction by carbamazepine can reduce the bioavailability of CCBs that undergo extensive 1st-pass hepatic clearance, like felodipine (94% reduction)
3 *Cimetidine:* Transient (1 week) increases in carbamazepine levels
3 *Corticosteroids:* Carbamazepine reduces levels and therapeutic effect
3 *Cyclosporine:* Carbamazepine reduces cyclosporine blood levels
2 *Danazol:* Increases carbamazepine levels with toxicity expected
3 *Doxycycline:* Carbamazepine reduces doxycycline levels and antibiotic effects
3 *Erythromycin, clarithromycin:* Increased carbamazepine levels
3 *Ethinyl Estradiol, Oral contraceptives:* Carbamazepine-induced metabolic induction may lead to menstrual irregularities and unplanned pregnancies

---

italic = common side effects   ***bold italic*** = life-threatening reactions

3 *Felbamate:* Reductions in carbamazepine levels and increases in 10,11-epoxide metabolite, along with decreased felbamate concentrations

3 *Fluoxetine, fluvoxamine:* Inhibits carbamazepine metabolism, increased levels and risk of toxicity

3 *Isoniazid:* Increases carbamazepine levels with increased risk of toxicity

3 *Isotretinoin:* Reduced carbamazepine bioavailability

3 *Lamotrigine:* Increased carbamazepine metab and risk of toxicity; carbamazepine reduces lamotrigine levels

3 *Lithium:* Increased potential for neurotoxicity with normal lithium concentrations; reverses carbamazepine-induced leukopenia; additive antithyroidal effects

3 *Mebendazole:* Carbamazepine decreases mebendazole levels, significant only when large doses given

3 *Methadone:* Carbamazepine reduces levels and therapeutic effect

3 *Metronidazole:* Increases carbamazepine concentrations with toxicity

3 *Neuroleptics:* Reduced concentration of and therapeutic response to these agents when used with carbamazepine

3 *Omeprazole:* May increase carbamazepine concentrations

3 *Oral anticoagulants:* Decreased prothrombin time

3 *Phenytoin:* Concurrent use reduces serum concentrations of both

2 *Propoxyphene:* Increases carbamazepine levels

3 *Theophylline:* Carbamazepine reduces levels and therapeutic effect

3 *Thyroid:* Carbamazepine reduces levels and therapeutic effect

3 *Valproic acid:* Valproic acid can increase, decrease, or have no effect on carbamazepine, monitor serum levels; carbamazepine decreases levels of valproic acid

Labs

• *Chloride, serum:* falsely elevated at elevated carbamazepine concentrations

• *Thyroxine (T_4), free serum:* Falsely elevated by certain test methods

• *Tri-iodothyronine (T_3), free serum:* Falsely decreased by certain test methods

• *T_3 uptake:* Carbamazepine interference falsely increases assay

• *Uric acid, serum:* High carbamazepine levels falsely decrease uric acid

SPECIAL CONSIDERATIONS
PATIENT/FAMILY EDUCATION

• Caution about driving and other activities that require alertness, at least initially

• Drug may turn urine pink to brown

MONITORING PARAMETERS

• CBC—aplastic anemia and agranulocytosis have been reported 5-8× greater than in the general public

• Liver function test

• Serum drug levels (therapeutic 4-12 µg/ml) during initial treatment

---

* = non-FDA-approved use

carbamide peroxide

(kar'ba-mide per-ox'ide)

OTC: *Otic:* Debrox, Murine Ear Drops

OTC: *Oral:* Gly-Oxide Liquid, Orajel Perioseptic, Proxigel

Chemical Class: Urea compound and hydrogen peroxide

Therapeutic Class: Cerumenolytic; topical oral anti-inflammatory

CLINICAL PHARMACOLOGY

Mechanism of Action: Foaming action facilitates removal of impacted cerumen; releases oxygen on contact with mouth tissues to provide cleansing effects, reduced inflammation, pain relief, and inhibition of odor-causing bacteria

INDICATIONS AND USES: Impacted cerumen, prevention of cerumenosis; oral inflammation (canker sores, denture irritation, irritated gums)

DOSAGE

Adult and Child

• INSTILL 5-10 gtt affected ear bid × 3-4 days

• PO Place several gtts of undiluted solution on affected area qid (expectorate after 2-3 min); gently massage gel on affected area qid

$ **AVAILABLE FORMS/COST OF THERAPY**

• Gel—Oral: 10%, 36 g: **$11.09**

• Liq—Oral: 10%, 15, 30, 60 ml: **$2.40-$8.28**/60 ml; 15%, 13.3 ml: **$3.98**

• Sol—Otic: 6.5%, 15, 30, 180 ml: **$0.90-$8.68**/15 ml

CONTRAINDICATIONS: Otic surgery, perforated eardrum; children <3 yr (PO)

PREGNANCY AND LACTATION: Pregnancy category C

SIDE EFFECTS/ADVERSE REACTIONS

EENT: Irritation in ear, itching, redness

carbenicillin

(car-ben'a-sill-in)

Rx: Geocillin

Chemical Class: Semi-synthetic penicillin derivative

Therapeutic Class: Antibiotic

CLINICAL PHARMACOLOGY

Mechanism of Action: Inhibits bacterial wall synthesis, bactericidal

Pharmacokinetics

PO: Peak urine concentration within 3 hr (therapeutic concentrations *only* in urine)

Rapidly absorbed PO from the small intestine (40% bioavailable), distributed to bile, 50% protein bound; $t_{1/2}$ 1-1.5 hr; excreted in the urine (85%-90% unchanged); crosses placenta

INDICATIONS AND USES: Acute and chronic infections of the upper and lower urinary tract and in asymptomatic bacteriuria, prostatitis

Antibacterial spectrum usually includes:

• Gram-negative organisms: *Neisseria gonorrhoeae, Enterobacter* sp., *Enterococcus faecalis, E. coli, Haemophilus influenzae, Klebsiella* sp., *Pseudomonas aeruginosa, Serratia* sp.

• Anaerobes: *Bacteroides* sp.

DOSAGE

Adult

• *UTI:* PO 382-764 mg q6h (use high doses for infections due to *Pseudomonas* and enterococci)

• *Prostatitis:* 764 mg q6h

$ AVAILABLE FORMS/COST OF THERAPY

• Tab, Uncoated—Oral: 382 mg, 100's: **$221.76**

PRECAUTIONS: Severe renal impairment (CrCl < 10 ml/min will not achieve therapeutic levels)

PREGNANCY AND LACTATION: Pregnancy category B

SIDE EFFECTS/ADVERSE REACTIONS

CNS: Headache

EENT: Itchy eyes

GI: Bad taste, diarrhea, flatulence, glossitis, mild SGOT elevations, nausea, vomiting

GU: Vaginitis

HEME: Eosinophilia, *bone marrow suppression*

SKIN: Hypersensitivity reactions (skin rash, urticaria, pruritus)

INTERACTIONS

Drugs

3 *Aminoglycosides:* Chemically inactivated by carbenicillin

3 *Methotrexate:* Increased methotrexate serum concentration

3 *Probenecid:* Increased penicillin concentrations

Labs

• *Albumin:* Decreased serum concentrations

• *Amino acids:* Increased urine

• *Bilirubin:* Increased serum bilirubin levels

• *Gentamicin:* 25% increase in serum level

• *Glucose:* False positive using Clinitest

• *Protein:* Increased serum levels

• *Triglycerides:* Increased serum levels

SPECIAL CONSIDERATIONS

NOTE: When high and rapid blood and urine levels of antibiotic are indicated, alternative parenteral therapy should be used

---

carbidopa and levodopa

(kar-bee-doe'pa; lee-voe-doe'pa)

Rx: Sinemet, Sinemet CR

Chemical Class: Catecholamine precursor

Therapeutic Class: Antiparkinson's agent; antidyskinetic

CLINICAL PHARMACOLOGY

Mechanism of Action: Symptoms of Parkinson's disease are related to depleted dopamine in the corpus striatum; carbidopa inhibits peripheral decarboxylation of levodopa; thus, more levodopa is made available for transport to brain and conversion to dopamine, which replenishes dopamine in the corpus striatum

Pharmacokinetics

PO: Peak concentration, 0.7 hr (tabs), 2.4 hr (Sus Action), absorption rapid and complete within 2-3 hr (tabs); gradual and continuous over 4-6 hr (Sus Action); widely distributed, 36% protein bound, $t_{1/2}$ 1-2 hr; excreted in urine (metabolites)

INDICATIONS AND USES: Parkinson's disease, restless legs syndrome,* phenylketonuria,* psoriasis,* shingles,* sleep behavior disorder,* swallowing disorders,* tardive dyskinesia,* vitiligo*

DOSAGE

Adult

• Sinemet

PO 1 tab of 25 mg carbidopa/100 mg levodopa tid or 10 mg/100 mg tid-qid; increase by 1 tab qd-qod prn until dosage of 8 tabs/day is reached; provide at least 70-100 mg of carbidopa/day

• Sinemet CR

PO 1 tab bid at intervals of not < 6 hr; usual dose is 2-8 tabs/day in divided

---

doses at intervals of 4-8 hr while awake; allow at least 3 days between dosage adjustments

• *Restless legs:* PO 1 tab 25 mg/100 mg qhs

$ **AVAILABLE FORMS/COST OF THERAPY**

• Tab, Uncoated—Oral: 10 mg/100 mg, 100's: **$52.10-$82.69**; 25 mg/100 mg, 100's: **$26.05-$93.36**; 25 mg/250 mg, 100's: **$71.30-$118.96**

• Tab, Sus Action—Oral: 25 mg/100 mg, 100's: **$89.60-$104.59**; 50 mg/200 mg, 100's: **$170.70-$201.16**

CONTRAINDICATIONS: Narrow-angle glaucoma, undiagnosed skin lesions

PRECAUTIONS: Renal disease, cardiac disease, hepatic disease, respiratory disease, MI with dysrhythmias, convulsions, peptic ulcer

PREGNANCY AND LACTATION: Pregnancy category C; should not be given to nursing mothers

SIDE EFFECTS/ADVERSE REACTIONS

CNS: Agitation, anxiety, confusion, dizziness, *fatigue,* hallucination, *hand tremors, headache,* hypomania, *insomnia, involuntary choreiform movements, nightmares, numbness,* psychosis, severe depression, *twitching, weakness*

CV: Hypertension, *orthostatic hypotension,* palpitation, tachycardia

EENT: Blurred vision, dilated pupils, diplopia

GI: Abdominal distress, anorexia, bitter taste, constipation, diarrhea, *dry mouth, dysphagia, flatulence, nausea, vomiting*

GU: Dark urine, incontinence, urinary retention

*HEME: **Agranulocytosis, hemolytic anemia, leukopenia***

METAB: Weight change

SKIN: Alopecia, rash, sweating

INTERACTIONS

Drugs

🔳 *Benzodiazepines:* May exacerbate Parkinsonism in patients receiving levodopa; inhibits antiparkinsonian effects of levodopa

🔳 *Food:* High protein diets inhibit the efficacy of levodopa

🔳 *Iron (oral):* Reduces levodopa bioavailability by 50%

🔳 *MAOIs:* May result in hypertensive response

🔳 *Methionine:* Inhibits the clinical response to levodopa

❷ *Neuroleptics:* Phenothiazines block dopamine receptors, can produce extrapyramidal symptoms, and inhibit the antiparkinsonian effect of levodopa

🔳 *Phenytoin:* May inhibit the antiparkinsonian effect of levodopa

🔳 *Pyridoxine:* Inhibits the antiparkinsonian effect of levodopa; concurrent carbidopa negates the interaction

🔳 *Spiramycin:* Reduces the plasma concentration of levodopa, with reduction of antiparkinson efficacy

🔳 *Tacrine:* May inhibit the effect of levodopa in Parkinsons patients; dosage adjustments may be required

Labs

• *Acid phosphatase:* Increased serum acid phosphatase

• *Amino acids:* Increased urine amino acids

• *Aspartate aminotransferase:* Increased serum aspartate aminotransferase

• *Bilirubin:* Decreased serum bilirubin at concentrations of 15 mg/dL (Kodak Ektachem systems 2083); increased bilirubin at concentrations above 80 mg/dL (methods of Jendrassik and Grof) and below 5 mg/dL (Kodak Ektachem systems 2083)

---

italic = common side effects   ***bold italic*** = life-threatening reactions

• *Bilirubin, conjugated:* Decreased serum levels by 0.3 mg/dL at therapeutic levels of levodopa; minimally increased serum levels at markedly elevated levodopa concentrations (i.e., >60 mg/dL)

• *Catecholamines:* Increased plasma catecholamines, reported as epinephrine and norepinephrine

• *Cholinesterase:* Increased serum cholinesterase activity

• *Sputum:* Brown discoloration reported

• *Creatinine:* Increased serum creatinine

• *Creatinine clearance:* Increased urinary creatinine clearance (Jaffe method)

• *Ferric chloride test:* False positive

• *Glucose:* Decreases serum glucose as measured by GODPERID method, Ames Seralyzer, and glucose oxidase method; increased serum glucose by alkaline ferricyanide procedure, Technicon SMA method, and glucokinase method of Scott; false negative urine glucose (inhibits glucose oxidase method)

• *Guaiacols Spot test:* False negative

• *Hydroxy-methoxymandelic acid:* Increased urinary levels

• *Lithium:* Positive bias on serum lithium levels measured with Kodak Ektachem systems 2083

• *Triglycerides:* Lowered triglyceride levels measured by GPOPAP method

• *Urea nitrogen:* Decreases BUN

• *Uric acid:* Lowers serum urate levels as measured by uricase PAP method

SPECIAL CONSIDERATIONS
• Caution with use until after MAO inhibitors have been discontinued for 2 wk
• If previously on levodopa, discontinue for at least 8 hr before change to carbidopa and levodopa

PATIENT/FAMILY EDUCATION
• Limit protein taken with drug
• Arise slowly from a reclining position

carboprost
(kar´boe-prost)
Rx: Hemabate
Chemical Class: Prostaglandin F2α
Therapeutic Class: Abortifacient; uterine stimulant; antihemorrhagic (postpartum and postabortal uterine bleeding)

CLINICAL PHARMACOLOGY
Mechanism of Action: Stimulates uterine contractions, GI and vascular smooth muscle
Pharmacokinetics
IM: Peak 30 min; mean abortion time 16 hr; metabolized in lungs, liver; excreted in urine (metabolites)

INDICATIONS AND USES: Postpartum hemorrhage due to uterine atony that has not responded to conventional methods of management; abortion between 13-20 wk gestation as calculated from the 1st day of the last normal menstrual period and in the following conditions related to 2nd trimester abortion:

• Failure of expulsion of the fetus during the course of treatment by another method

• Premature rupture of membranes using intrauterine methods with loss of drug and insufficient or absent uterine activity

• Requirement of a repeat intrauterine instillation of drug for expulsion of the fetus

• Inadvertent or spontaneous rupture of membranes in the presence of a previable fetus and absence of adequate activity for expulsion

DOSAGE

Adult

• *Abortion:* IM 250 µg, then 250 µg q1½-3½ hr; may increase to 500 µg if no response; not to exceed 12 mg total dose or continuous administration for >2 days

• *Refractory postpartum uterine bleeding:* IM 250 µg single inj (75% response); selected cases, multiple dosing at intervals of 15 to 90 min; max dose 2 mg (total)

$ **AVAILABLE FORMS/COST OF THERAPY**

• Inj, Sol—IM: 250 µg/ml, 1 ml: **$3.14-$52.96**

CONTRAINDICATIONS: Severe pulmonary, cardiac, or hepatic disease, acute PID

PRECAUTIONS: Asthma, anemia, jaundice, diabetes mellitus, seizure disorders, past uterine surgery

PREGNANCY AND LACTATION: Pregnancy category C; any dose which produces increased uterine tone could put the embryo or fetus at risk.

SIDE EFFECTS/ADVERSE REACTIONS

CNS: Chills, fever, headache

CV: Chest pain, ***dysrhythmias***

GI: Diarrhea, nausea, vomiting

GU: Endometritis, uterine/vaginal pain

RESP: Coughing, dyspnea, wheezing

SPECIAL CONSIDERATIONS

• Antiemetic, analgesic, and antidiarrheal medications should be considered concurrently to counter adverse GI effects

• In the treatment of uterine atony, IV oxytocin, uterine massage and IM methylergonovine (unless contraindicated) should be used before carboprost

carisoprodol

(kar′i-so-pro′dol)

Rx: Soma, Vanadom

Combinations

> **Rx:** with aspirin (Soma Compound); with aspirin and codeine (Soma Compound with Codeine)

Chemical Class: Meprobamate congener

Therapeutic Class: Skeletal muscle relaxant

CLINICAL PHARMACOLOGY

Mechanism of Action: Muscle relaxation by blocking interneuronal activity in the descending reticular formation and spinal cord; produces sedation

Pharmacokinetics

PO: Onset ½ hr, duration 4-6 hr; metabolized by liver, excreted in urine; $t_{1/2}$ 8 hr

INDICATIONS AND USES: Adjunct to rest, physical therapy, and other measures for the relief of discomfort associated with acute, painful, musculoskeletal conditions; does not directly relax tense skeletal muscles

DOSAGE

Adult and Child >12 yr

• PO 350 mg tid-qid (take last dose hs)

$ **AVAILABLE FORMS/COST OF THERAPY**

• Tab, Uncoated—Oral: 350 mg, 100's: **$7.45-$334.07**

CONTRAINDICATIONS: Hypersensitivity (including related compounds such as meprobamate, mebutamate, or tybamate), child <12 yr, intermittent porphyria

PRECAUTIONS: Renal disease, hepatic disease, addictive personality, elderly

---

italic = common side effects   ***bold italic*** = life-threatening reactions

PREGNANCY AND LACTATION: Pregnancy category C; crosses placenta; excreted in breast milk (2-4× maternal plasma)

SIDE EFFECTS/ADVERSE REACTIONS

CNS: Agitation, ataxia, depression, *dizziness, drowsiness,* headache, insomnia, irritability, syncope, tremor, vertigo, *weakness*

CV: Facial flushing, postural hypotension, tachycardia

EENT: Diplopia, temporary loss of vision

GI: Epigastric discomfort, hiccups, *nausea,* vomiting

SKIN: Eosinophilia, erythema multiforme, facial flushing, fever, fixed drug eruptions, pruritus, rash

SPECIAL CONSIDERATIONS
• Caution when used in addiction-prone individuals
• Abused on the street in conjunction with narcotics

PATIENT/FAMILY EDUCATION
• Abrupt cessation may precipitate mild withdrawal symptoms such as abdominal cramps, insomnia, chills, headache, and nausea

---

carteolol

(kar-tee'oe-lole)

Rx: Cartrol, Ocupress
Chemical Class: Nonselective β-adrenergic blocker with intrinsic sympathomimetic activity
Therapeutic Class: Antihypertensive; antiglaucoma agent

CLINICAL PHARMACOLOGY
Mechanism of Action: Nonselective β-adrenergic blocker with intrinsic sympathomimetic activity

Pharmacokinetics
PO: Onset 1-2 hr, peak 2-4 hr, duration 8-12 hr, food slows absorption but does not lower total absorption; metabolized by liver (metabolites inactive); excreted in urine, bile; crosses placenta; $t_{1/2}$ 6-8 hr

INDICATIONS AND USES: Chronic open-angle glaucoma, hypertension

DOSAGE

Adult
• *Hypertension:* PO 2.5-10 mg qd; in renal impairment: CrCl 20-60 ml/min, dosage interval is 48 hr; CrCl <20 ml/min, dosage interval is 72 hr
• *Chronic open-angle glaucoma:* Ophth sol, 1%, 1 gtt in affected eye bid

⑤ AVAILABLE FORMS/COST OF THERAPY
• Sol—Ophth: 1%, 5, 10, 15 ml: **$37.06-$56.11**/10 ml
• Tab, Plain Coated—Oral: 2.5 mg, 100's: **$106.88**; 5 mg, 100's: **$131.88**

CONTRAINDICATIONS: Hypersensitivity to β-blockers, heart block (2nd or 3rd degree), sinus bradycardia, overt CHF, bronchial asthma

PRECAUTIONS: Major surgery, diabetes mellitus, renal disease, thyroid disease, COPD, well-compensated heart failure, nonallergic bronchospasm; exacerbation of angina or MI may occur following abrupt discontinuation of β-blockers; ophth carteolol may be absorbed systemically; adverse reactions found with systemic administration may occur with ophth administration

PREGNANCY AND LACTATION: Pregnancy category C; excreted in breast milk

---

SIDE EFFECTS/ADVERSE REACTIONS

CNS: Anxiety, catatonia, decreased concentration, depression, dizziness, drowsiness, *fatigue (7%),* headache, insomnia, lethargy, mental changes, nightmares, paresthesia

CV: **AV block,** bradycardia, chest pain, **CHF,** orthostatic hypotension, palpitations, peripheral vascular insufficiency, **ventricular dysrhythmias**

EENT: Double vision; dry, burning eyes; sore throat, tinnitus, visual changes

GI: Anorexia, constipation, diarrhea, dry mouth, flatulence, nausea, vomiting

GU: Dysuria, ejaculatory failure, impotence, urinary retention

HEME: **Agranulocytosis, thrombocytopenic purpura (rare)**

MS: Arthralgia, joint pain, muscle cramps

RESP: **Bronchospasm,** dyspnea, nasal stuffiness, pharyngitis, wheezing

SKIN: Alopecia, fever, pruritus, rash, urticaria

MISC: Decreased exercise tolerance, facial swelling, Raynaud's syndrome, weight change

INTERACTIONS

Drugs

🔳 *Adenosine:* Increased risk of bradycardic response

🔳 *Amiodarone:* Increased bradycardic effect of carteolol

🔳 *Antacids:* Decreased absorption of oral carteolol

🔳 *Antidiabetics:* Carteolol reduces response to hypoglycemia (sweating excepted)

🔳 *Antipyrine:* Many β-blockers increase serum concentrations of antipyrine; though antipyrine is not used therapeutically, this interaction has implications by other drugs whose metabolism is similarly inhibited

🔳 *Barbiturates, Rifampin:* Enhanced carteolol metabolism

🔳 *Bupivacaine:* Potentiates cardiodepression and heart block

🔳 *Cimetidine, Propafenone, Propoxyphene, Quinidine:* Decreased carteolol metabolism

🔳 *Cocaine:* β-Blockade increases angina-inducing potential of cocaine

🔳 *Contrast media:* Increased risk of anaphylaxis

🔳 *Digoxin, digitoxin:* Bradycardia potentiated

🔳 *Dipyridamole:* Bradycardia

🔳 *Epinepherine:* Enhanced pressor response resulting in hypertension and bradycardia

🔳 *Fluoxetine:* Fluoxetine may reduce hepatic metabolism; increased β-blocking activity

🔳 *Isoproterenol:* Reduced effectiveness of isoproterenol in the treatment of asthma

🔳 *Neuroleptics:* Decreased carteolol metabolism; decreased neuroleptic metabolism

🔳 *Nonsteroidal anti-inflammatory drugs:* Reduced antihypertensive effect

🔳 *Physostigmine:* Additive bradycardia

🔳 *Prazosin, Terazosin:* Enhanced 1st-dose response to prazosin

🔳 *Tacrine:* Additive bradycardia

🔳 *Theophylline:* Decreased metabolism of theophylline

SPECIAL CONSIDERATIONS

• Does not alter serum cholesterol or triglycerides

PATIENT/FAMILY EDUCATION

• Do not stop drug abruptly; taper over 2 wk

• Do not use OTC products containing α-adrenergic stimulants (nasal decongestants, cold remedies) unless directed by physician

---

italic = common side effects   ***bold italic*** = life-threatening reactions

carvedilol

(kar-vea'die-lole)

Rx: Coreg

Chemical Class: Nonselective β-adrenergic blocker; peripheral α-adrenergic blocker

Therapeutic Class: Antihypertensive; congestive heart failure agent

CLINICAL PHARMACOLOGY

Mechanism of Action: PO: Competitive β-adrenergic and α-adrenergic antagonist; produces negative inotropic and chronotropic responses; slows AV nodal conduction; decreases heart rate; decreases myocardial oxygen consumption; antiarrhythmic effects (class II); reduction in platelet aggregation and blood viscosity; suppression of renin release; inhibition of central sympathetic outflow; decreases presynaptic receptor neurotransmitter release; no intrinsic sympathomimetic; moderate membrane stabilizing activity; high lipid solubility

Pharmacokinetics

PO: Extensive first pass metabolism, 25% to 35% bioavailable; beta blocker effects seen in 30-60 min; terminal elimination $t_{1/2}$ 7-10 hrs; 98% protein bound; extensive hepatic metabolism, metabolite 13 times more potent beta blocker than parent drug, <2% excreted unchanged in urine; metabolites excreted in bile and feces

INDICATIONS AND USES: Hypertension, congestive heart failure, angina pectoris,* arrhythmias,* doxorubicin-induced cardiomyopathy,* nitrate tolerance,* postmyocardial infarction,* anxiety*

DOSAGE

Adult and child >16 yr

• *Angina pectoris:* PO 25-50 mg

• *Congestive heart failure:* PO: 3.125 mg bid × 2 wk; if tolerated, double dose q2wk to the highest tolerated dose (max 25 mg bid for patients <85 kg; 50 mg bid for patients >85 kg). Administration with food slows absorption and reduces risk of postural hypotension

• *Hypertension:* PO 6.25 mg bid; adjust dose upward to 12.5 mg, then 25 mg bid every 1-2 wk as tolerated (max 50 mg daily)

$ **AVAILABLE FORMS/COST OF THERAPY**

• Tab, Coated—Oral: 3.125, 6.25, 12.5, 25 mg, 100's, all: **$172.24**

CONTRAINDICATIONS: Bronchial asthma, cardiogenic shock, overt cardiac failure, second and third degree AV block, severe sinus bradycardia, clinically manifest hepatic impairment

PRECAUTIONS: Anesthesia/surgery (myocardial depression), avoid abrupt withdrawal, bronchospastic airways, congestive heart failure, diabetes mellitus, hyperthyroidism/thyrotoxicosis, concurrent clonidine (discontinue several days prior to withdrawal of clonidine), peripheral vascular disease, renal disease, Prinzmetal's variant angina

PREGNANCY AND LACTATION: Pregnancy category C; increased spontaneous abortion in animal studies; highly lipophilic with a large volume of distribution, may accumulate in human breast milk; monitor infant closely

SIDE EFFECTS/ADVERSE REACTIONS

CNS: Dizziness

CV: **AV block,** bradycardia (2%), **CHF,** postural hypotension (1.8%), syncope (0.1%)

GI: Elevated LFTs (1.1%)

RESP: **Bronchospasm**

---

* = non-FDA-approved use

INTERACTIONS
Drugs
❸ *α-1 adrenergic blockers:* Potential enhanced first dose response (marked initial drop in blood pressure, particularly on standing)

❸ *Amiodarone:* Symptomatic bradycardia and sinus arrest; AV node refractory period prolonged and sinus node automaticity decreased, especially patients with bradycardia, sick sinus syndrome, or partial AV

❸ *Benzodiazepines:* Increased benzodiazepine activity

❸ *Catecholamine-depleting agents:* Reserpine, MAOIs; hypotension or bradycardia possible

❸ *Cimetidine:* Via inhibition of hepatic metabolism, cimetidine increases many β-blocker serum concentrations

❸ *Clonidine:* Withdrawal of clonidine abruptly may exaggerate the hypertension due to unopposed alpha stimulation; safer than other beta-blockers, however

❸ *Cyclosporin:* Increased trough cyclosporin concentrations

❸ *CYP2D6 inhibitors:* Quinidine, fluoxetine, paroxetine, propafenone; increased levels of carvedilol

❸ *Digoxin:* Additive prolongation of atrioventricular (AV) conduction time

❸ *Dihydropyridine calcium channel blockers:* Severe hypotension or impaired cardiac performance; most prevalent with impaired left ventricular function, cardiac arrhythmias, or aortic stenosis

❸ *Diltiazem:* Potentiates beta-adrenergic effects; hypotension, left ventricular failure, and AV conduction disturbances problematic in elderly, patients with left ventricular dysfunction, aortic stenosis, or with large doses of either drug

❸ *Hypoglycemic agents:* Masked hypoglycemia, hyperglycemia

❸ *Nonsteroidal antiinflammatory drugs:* Reduced antihypertensive effect

❸ *Rifampin:* 70% decrease in carvedilol concentrations

❸ *Verapamil:* Potentiates beta-adrenergic effects; hypotension, left ventricular failure, and AV conduction disturbances problematic in elderly, patients with left ventricular dysfunction, aortic stenosis, or with large doses of either drug

SPECIAL CONSIDERATIONS
PATIENT/FAMILY EDUCATION
• Do not discontinue abruptly; may require taper; rapid withdrawal may produce rebound hypertension or angina
• Careful monitoring essential when initiating therapy to detect and correct worsening symptoms of heart failure
• If heart rate drops below 55 beats per minute, reduce dosage
• Initiate therapy with 3.125 mg dosage to decrease risk of synocope
• Take with food
• Avoid driving, hazardous tasks during initiation of therapy
• Response less in African-Americans

MONITORING PARAMETERS
• Angina: Reduction in nitroglycerin usage; frequency, severity, onset, and duration of angina pain; heart rate.
• Arrhythmias: Heart rate
• Congestive heart failure: Functional status, cough, dyspnea on exertion, paroxysmal nocturnal dyspnea, exercise tolerance, and ventricular function
• Hypertension: Blood pressure
• Postmyocardial infarction: Left ventricular function, lower resting heart rate

---

italic = common side effects   ***bold italic*** = life-threatening reactions

• Toxicity: Blood pressure, blood glucose, bronchospasm, hypotension, bradycardia, depression, confusion, hallucination, sexual dysfunction

cascara sagrada

(kas-kar'a)

OTC: Cascara Sagrada, Cascara Aromatic
Chemical Class: Anthraquinone derivative
Therapeutic Class: Stimulant laxative

CLINICAL PHARMACOLOGY
Mechanism of Action: Direct chemical irritation in colon; increases propulsion of stool
Pharmacokinetics
PO: Peak 6-12 hr, only slightly absorbed; metabolized by liver, excreted by kidneys and in feces
INDICATIONS AND USES: Constipation; bowel or rectal preparation for surgery or examination
DOSAGE
Adult
• PO 325 mg (1 tab) or 5 ml of fluid extract qd prn
Child
• Age 2-12 yr: PO ½ adult dose; Age <2 yr: PO ¼ adult dose
$ **AVAILABLE FORMS/COST OF THERAPY**
• Sol (aromatic fluid)—Oral: 480 ml: **$16.29**
• Sol (fluid extract)—Oral: 120, 480 ml: **$12.00-$16.51**/480 ml
• Tab—Oral: 150 mg, 60's: **$5.53**; 325 mg, 100's: **$1.24-$4.72**
CONTRAINDICATIONS: GI bleeding, obstruction, appendicitis, acute surgical abdomen
PRECAUTIONS: CHF, abdominal pain, nausea/vomiting, alcoholism (aromatic form)

PREGNANCY AND LACTATION: Pregnancy category C; excreted in breast milk
SIDE EFFECTS/ADVERSE REACTIONS
GI: Anorexia, cramps, diarrhea, melanosis coli, *nausea, vomiting*
GU: Discoloration of urine (pink, red, brown)
METAB: Alkalosis, hypocalcemia, hypokalemia
MS: Tetany
INTERACTIONS
Labs
• *Increase:* Color of urine (brown-acid; yellow-pink- alkaline); porphobilinogen; urobiligen
SPECIAL CONSIDERATIONS
• Stimulant laxatives are habit forming
• Long term use may lead to colonic atony

castor oil

OTC: Emulsoil, Purge
Chemical Class: Fatty acid ester
Therapeutic Class: Stimulant laxative

CLINICAL PHARMACOLOGY
Mechanism of Action: Increases motor activity of small intestine and colon; causes fluid secretion in colon
Pharmacokinetics
PO: Peak effect 2-3 hr; ester hydrolyzed in small intestine and partially absorbed
INDICATIONS AND USES: Constipation; bowel preparation for surgery or examination
DOSAGE
Adult
• PO LIQ 15-60 ml

Child
• Age >2 yr: PO LIQ 5-15 ml; Age <2 yr: PO LIQ 1.25-7.5 ml

$ AVAILABLE FORMS/COST OF THERAPY
• Liq—Oral: 95% oil, 60 ml: **$1.80-$2.55**
• Oil—Oral: 30, 60, 120, 480 ml: **$0.75-$1.99**/60 ml

CONTRAINDICATIONS: Fecal impaction, GI bleeding, appendicitis, intestinal obstruction

PRECAUTIONS: Abdominal pain, nausea/vomiting, laxative dependence; colonic atony from prolonged use

PREGNANCY AND LACTATION: Pregnancy category X; excreted in breast milk

SIDE EFFECTS/ADVERSE REACTIONS
GI: Anorexia, colon irritation, *cramps,* diarrhea, flatus, *nausea,* rebound constipation, *vomiting*
METAB: Alkalosis; fluid or electrolyte imbalance; hypokalemia

SPECIAL CONSIDERATIONS
• Stimulant laxatives are habit forming
• Long-term use may lead to colonic atony

---

cefaclor
(sef'a-klor)
Rx: Ceclor, Ceclor CD
Chemical Class: Cephalosporin (2nd generation)
Therapeutic Class: Antibiotic

CLINICAL PHARMACOLOGY
Mechanism of Action: Inhibits bacterial cell wall synthesis, bactericidal

Pharmacokinetics
PO: Peak ½-1 hr (15 μg/ml after 500 mg), $t_{1/2}$ 36-54 min; 25% bound by plasma proteins; 60%-85% elimi-nated unchanged in urine in 8 hr; crosses placenta; when taken with food, peak concentration is 50%-75% of that when taken fasting; serum $t_{1/2}$ slightly prolonged in renal insufficiency; $t_{1/2}$ 2.3-2.8 hr if anephric; hemodialysis shortens $t_{1/2}$ by 25%-30%

INDICATIONS AND USES: Pharyngitis, tonsillitis, otitis media, bronchitis, pneumonia, skin and urinary tract infections caused by susceptible organisms
Antibacterial spectrum usually includes:
• Gram-positive organisms: *S. pneumoniae, S. pyogenes, S. aureus*
• Gram-negative organisms: *H influenzae, Moraxella catarrhalis, E. coli, P. mirabilis, Klebsiella* sp.
• Anaerobes: *Peptococci, Peptostreptococci*
• β-lactamase-producing strains of the above pathogens are usually susceptible

DOSAGE
Adult
• PO 250-500 mg q8h, double dose in serious infections and pneumonia
Child >1 mo
• PO 20-40 mg/kg qd in divided doses q8h, not to exceed 1 g/day (use higher dose in serious infections and otitis media)

$ AVAILABLE FORMS/COST OF THERAPY
• Cap, Gel—Oral: 250 mg, 100's: **$184.80-$242.86**; 500 mg, 100's: **$364.52-$440.55**
• Powder, Reconst—Oral: 125 mg/5 ml, 75, 150 ml: **$14.20-$37.20**/150 ml; 187 mg/5 ml, 50, 100 ml: **$26.65-$41.28**/100 ml; 250 mg/5 ml, 75, 150 ml: **$28.50-$68.53**/150 ml; 375 mg/5 ml, 50, 100 ml: **$48.27-$56.38**/100 ml
• Tab, Sus Action—Oral: 375 mg, 60's: **$264.89**; 500 mg, 100's: **$379.30**

---

italic = common side effects   ***bold italic*** = life-threatening reactions

CONTRAINDICATIONS: Infants <1 mo

PRECAUTIONS: Hypersensitivity to penicillins, renal disease

PREGNANCY AND LACTATION: Pregnancy category B; excreted in breast milk

SIDE EFFECTS/ADVERSE REACTIONS

CNS: Chills, dizziness, fever, headache, paresthesia, weakness

GI: Abdominal pain, anorexia, bleeding, diarrhea, glossitis, increased LFTs, nausea, ***pseudomembranous colitis,*** vomiting

GU: Candidiasis, ***nephrotoxicity,*** vaginitis

HEME: **Bone marrow suppression** eosinophilia, ***hemolytic anemia,*** lymphocytosis, thrombocytosis

RESP: Dyspnea

SKIN: Dermatitis, rash, urticaria

MISC: Serum sickness-like syndrome

INTERACTIONS

Drugs

3 *Aminoglycosides:* Additive nephrotoxicity

3 *Loop diuretics:* Increased nephrotoxicity

2 *Warfarin:* Hypoprothrombinemic response enhanced

Labs

• *Creatinine:* Analytical increases and decreases depending on assay

SPECIAL CONSIDERATIONS

• Last choice 2nd generation cephalosporin given relative decreased activity against *S. pneumonia* and increased side effects

---

cefadroxil
(sef-a-drox'ill)
Rx: Duricef
Chemical Class: Cephalosporin (1st generation)
Therapeutic Class: Antibiotic

CLINICAL PHARMACOLOGY

Mechanism of Action: Inhibits bacterial cell wall synthesis; bactericidal

Pharmacokinetics

PO: Peak 1-1½ hr; measurable levels persist for 12 hr; 90% excreted unchanged in urine within 24 hr; $t_{1/2}$ 1-2 hr; 20% bound by plasma proteins

INDICATIONS AND USES: Infections of the urinary tract and skin caused by susceptible organisms; pharyngitis and tonsilitis caused by Group A β-hemolytic streptococci Antibacterial spectrum usually includes:

• Gram-negative bacilli: *E. coli, P. mirabilis, Klebsiella*

• Gram-positive organisms: *S. pneumoniae, S. pyogenes, S. aureus*

DOSAGE

Adult

• PO 1-2 g qd or q12h, give a loading dose of 1 g initially; dosage reduction appropriate in renal impairment (CrCl <50 ml/min)

Child

• PO 30 mg/kg/day

$ **AVAILABLE FORMS/COST OF THERAPY**

• Cap—Oral: 500 mg, 100's: **$284.65-$455.00**

• Powder, Reconst—Oral: 125 mg/5 ml, 50, 100 ml: **$17.11-$25.99**/100 ml; 250 mg/5 ml, 50, 100 ml: **$29.38-$36.84**/100 ml; 500 mg/5 ml, 50, 75, 100 ml: **$44.48-$51.00**/100 ml

• Tab, Uncoated—Oral: 1 g, 100's: **$697.11**

CONTRAINDICATIONS: Infants <1 mo

PRECAUTIONS: Hypersensitivity to penicillins

PREGNANCY AND LACTATION: Pregnancy category B; low concentrations in milk

SIDE EFFECTS/ADVERSE REACTIONS

CNS: Chills, dizziness, fever, headache, paresthesia, weakness

GI: Abdominal pain, *anorexia,* bleeding; *diarrhea,* glossitis, increased LFTs, nausea, ***pseudomembranous colitis,*** vomiting

GU: Candidiasis, ***nephrotoxicity,*** proteinuria, pruritus, vaginitis

HEME: ***Bone marrow suppression, eosinophilia, hemolytic anemia,*** lymphocytosis

RESP: Dyspnea

SKIN: Dermatitis, rash, urticaria

INTERACTIONS

Drugs

3 *Aminoglycosides:* Additive nephrotoxicity

3 *Loop diuretics:* Increased nephrotoxicity

SPECIAL CONSIDERATIONS

• No clinical advantage over less expensive cephalexin

---

cefamandole

(sef-a-man′dole)

Rx: Mandol

Chemical Class: Cephalosporin (2nd generation)

Therapeutic Class: Antibiotic

CLINICAL PHARMACOLOGY

Mechanism of Action: Inhibits bacterial wall synthesis; bactericidal

Pharmacokinetics

IM/IV: Peak 1-1½ hr, $t_{1/2}$, ½-1 hr; 60%-75% bound by plasma proteins; distributed to pleura, joint fluids, bile, and bone; 85% excreted by kidneys over 8 hr

INDICATIONS AND USES: Infections of the lower respiratory tract, urinary tract, skin and skin structure, bone, and joints; peritonitis, septicemia, and presurgical prophylactic therapy caused by susceptible organisms

Antibacterial spectrum usually includes:

• Gram-positive organisms: *S. pneumoniae, S. aureus* (penicillinase and non-penicillinase-producing), β-hemolytic streptococci, *S. epidermidis, S. pyogenes*

• Gram-negative organisms: *H. influenzae, Klebsiella* sp., *P. mirabilis, E. coli, Proteus* sp., *Enterobacter* sp.

• Anaerobes: *Peptostreptococcus, Peptococcus* sp., *Clostridium* sp.

DOSAGE

Adult

• IM/IV 500 mg-1g q4-8h, may give up to 2 g q4h for severe infections; 1 or 2 g IM/IV ½-1 hr prior to surgery, followed by 1 or 2 g q6h after surgery for 24-48 hr for prophylaxis

• Dosage reduction indicated in severe renal impairment (CrCl <5 ml/min): 1 g q12h

Child >1 mo

• IM/IV 50-150 mg/kg/day in divided doses q4-8h, not to exceed adult dose; 50 to 100 mg/kg/day in equally divided doses ½-1 hr before surgery and q6h for 24-48 hr after surgery for prophylaxis

$ **AVAILABLE FORMS/COST OF THERAPY**

• Inj, Dry-Sol—IM, IV: 1 g/vial: **$0.90-$9.73**; 2 g/vial: **$18.13-$18.80**

CONTRAINDICATIONS: Infants <1 mo

---

italic = common side effects   ***bold italic*** = life-threatening reactions

PRECAUTIONS: Hypersensitivity to penicillins, renal disease; hypoprothrombinemia

PREGNANCY AND LACTATION: Pregnancy category B; low milk concentrations

SIDE EFFECTS/ADVERSE REACTIONS

CNS: Chills, dizziness, fever, headache, paresthesia, weakness

GI: Abdominal pain, anorexia, **bleeding;** *diarrhea,* glossitis, increased LFTs, *nausea,* **pseudomembranous colitis,** transient hepatitis and cholestatic jaundice, *vomiting*

GU: Candidiasis, **nephrotoxicity,** vaginitis

HEME: **Bone marrow suppression,** eosinophilia, **hemolytic anemia, hypoprothrombinemia,** lymphocytosis

RESP: Dyspnea

SKIN: Dermatitis, maculopapular rash, urticaria

MISC: Thrombophlebitis (rare)

INTERACTIONS

Drugs

❸ *Aminoglycosides:* Potential additive nephrotoxicity

❸ *Ethanol:* Disulfiram-like reactions secondary to acetaldehyde accumulation

❸ *Loop diuretics:* Increased nephrotoxicity

❷ *Oral anticoagulants:* Additive hypoprothrombinemia

Labs

• *Creatinine:* Increases and decreases depending assay

• *Erythromycin:* False positive

• *Metronidazole:* Interferes with assay

SPECIAL CONSIDERATIONS

• Caution with alcohol; disulfiram reaction possible

MONITORING PARAMETERS

• If severe diarrhea occurs, pseudomembranous colitis should be considered

• Bleeding: ecchymosis, bleeding gums, hematuria, stool guaiac daily

---

cefazolin

(sef-a´zoe-lin)

Rx: Ancef, Kefzol

Chemical Class: Cephalosporin (1st generation)

Therapeutic Class: Antibiotic

CLINICAL PHARMACOLOGY

Mechanism of Action: Inhibits bacterial cell wall synthesis; bactericidal

Pharmacokinetics

IM: Peak ½-2 hr

IV: Peak 10 min, $t_{1/2}$ 1½-2¼ hr; distribution (70%-86% protein bound) to bile; without obstructive biliary disease, bile levels can exceed serum levels by up to 5 ×; with obstructive biliary disease, bile levels considerably lower than serum levels; to synovial fluid, comparable to levels reached in serum at about 4 hr after administration; eliminated unchanged in urine

INDICATIONS AND USES: Infections of the lower respiratory tract, urinary tract, biliary tract, and genitourinary tract; infections of the skin and skin structure, bones and joints; endocarditis, prostatitis, surgical prophylaxis, septicemia

Antibacterial spectrum usually includes:

• Gram-positive organisms: *S. pneumoniae, S. pyogenes, S. aureus*

• Gram-negative bacilli: *E. coli, P. mirabilis, Klebsiella sp, H. influenzae*

DOSAGE

Adult

• *Life-threatening infections:* IM/IV 1-2 g q6h

• *Mild/moderate infections:* IM/IV 250-500 mg q8h

• *Surgical prophylaxis:* IM/IV 1 g ½-1 hr prior to surgery then 500 mg-1 g q6-8 hr × 24 hr postoperatively

• Dosage reduction appropriate in renal impairment (CrCl <50 ml/min)

Child >1 mo

• *Life-threatening infections:* IM/IV 100 mg/kg in 3-4 equal doses

• *Mild/moderate infections:* IM/IV 25-50 mg/kg in 3-4 equal doses

$ AVAILABLE FORMS/COST OF THERAPY

• Inj, Dry-Sol—IM, IV: 500 mg/vial: **$1.04-$5.32**; 1 g/vial: **$0.28-$13.32**

CONTRAINDICATIONS: Infants <1 mo

PRECAUTIONS: Hypersensitivity to penicillins, renal disease

PREGNANCY AND LACTATION: Pregnancy category B; low milk concentrations

SIDE EFFECTS/ADVERSE REACTIONS

CNS: Chills, dizziness, fever, headache, paresthesia, weakness

GI: Abdominal pain, anorexia, **bleeding;** *diarrhea,* glossitis, increased LFTs, nausea, vomiting, ***pseudomembranous colitis***

GU: Candidiasis, ***nephrotoxicity,*** pruritus, vaginitis

HEME: **Bone marrow suppression,** eosinophilia, **hemolytic anemia,** lymphocytosis

SKIN: Dermatitis, rash, urticaria

INTERACTIONS

Drugs

3 *Aminoglycosides:* Additive nephrotoxicity

3 *Ethanol:* Disulfiram-like reaction

3 *Chloramphenicol:* Inhibits antibacterial activity of cefazolin

3 *Loop diuretics:* Increased nephrotoxicity

❷ *Oral Anticoagulants:* Additive hypoprothrombinemia

---

cefdinir

(sef'di-neer)

Rx: Omnicef
Chemical Class: Cephalosporin (3rd generation)
Therapeutic Class: Antibiotic

CLINICAL PHARMACOLOGY
Mechanism of Action: Inhibits bacterial cell wall synthesis; bactericidal

Pharmacokinetics
PO: Peak 2-4 hr, t½ 1.7 hr, not significantly metabolized, excreted by kidney

INDICATIONS AND USES: Infections of the upper and lower respiratory tract (community acquired pneumonia, sinusitis, bronchitis, pharyngitis, tonsillitis); skin and skin structure due to susceptible organisms

Antibacterial spectrum usually includes:

• Gram-positive organisms: *Staphylococcus aureus* (not MRSA), *Streptococcus pyogenes, Streptococcus pneumoniae* (penicillin-susceptible strains only), Viridans group *streptococci*

• Gram-negative organisms: *Haemophilius influenzae, Moraxella catarrhalis, E. coli, Klebsiella pneumoniae, Proteus mirabilis*

DOSAGE

Adult and Child >16 yr

• *Upper respiratory infections:* PO 600 mg q24h × 10 days

• *Lower respiratory infections, skin/skin structure infections:* PO 300 mg q12h × 10 days

• *Renal failure:* CrCl <30 ml/min, 300 mg qd

---

italic = common side effects   ***bold italic*** = life-threatening reactions

Child >6 mo

• PO 14 mg/kg q24h to max 600 mg qd (qd dosing not studied in skin infections, 7 mg/kg q12h recommended)

• *Renal failure:* CrCl <30 ml/min, 7 mg/kg qd (max 300 mg)

$ AVAILABLE FORMS/COST OF THERAPY

• Cap—Oral: 300 mg, 60's: **$235.71**

• Susp—Oral: 125 mg/5 ml, 60, 100 ml: **$61.57/100 ml**

PRECAUTIONS: Hypersensitivity to penicillins, renal disease

PREGNANCY AND LACTATION: Pregnancy category B, not detected in human milk after administration of single 600 mg dose

SIDE EFFECTS/ADVERSE REACTIONS

CNS: Headache

GI: **Pseudomembranous colitis,** red stools (not significant, formed by a complex of cefdinir and iron), *diarrhea* (16%), nausea, dyspepsia, flatulence, elevated LFTs

GU: Monilial vaginitis, *renal failure*

HEME: **Bone marrow suppression**

SKIN: **Stevens-Johnson syndrome**

INTERACTIONS

Drugs

⬛ *Antacids, iron:* Interference with cefdinir absorption, take antibiotic 2 hr before or after (can be administered with iron fortified infant formula)

⬛ *Probenecid:* Inhibits cefdinir excretion

⬛ *Live typhoid vaccine:* Interference with immune response to vaccine, give vaccine at least 24 hr after last dose

Labs

• *False positive:* Urine ketones using nitroprusside method, urine glucose using Clinitest, Benedict's or Fehling's solution, direct Coomb's

SPECIAL CONSIDERATIONS

• May be taken without regard to food

• More active *in vitro* against *S. aureus* and *Enterococcus faecalis* than cefixime, but less active against some enterobacteraceae

---

cefditoren pivoxil

(seff-di-tore´en pi-vox´il)

Rx: Spectracef

Chemical Class: Cephalosporin (3rd generation)

Therapeutic Class: Antibiotic

CLINICAL PHARMACOLOGY

Mechanism of Action: Inhibits bacterial cell wall synthesis; bactericidal

Pharmacokinetics

PO: A prodrug hydrolyzed by esterases during absorption to active cefditoren, absorption enhanced by fatty meal, peak 1.5-3 hr, $t_{1/2}$ 1.3-2 hr, excreted by kidney

INDICATIONS AND USES: Mild to moderate infections caused by susceptible organisms

Antibacterial spectrum usually includes:

• Gram-positive organisms: *Staphylococcus aureus* (not MRSA), *Streptococcus pneumoniae* (penicillin susceptible strains), *Streptococcus pyogenes*

• Gram-negative organisms: *Haemophilus influenzae, Haemophilus parainfluenzae, Moraxella catarrhalis*

DOSAGE

Adult and Child >12 yr

• PO 200-400 mg bid

• *Renal failure:* CrCl 30-49 ml/min/1.73 m² max dose 200 mg bid; CrCl <30 ml/min/1.73 m² max dose 200 mg qd

$ AVAILABLE FORMS/COST OF THERAPY

• Tab, Coated—Oral: 200 mg, 60's: **$98.25**

CONTRAINDICATIONS: Carnitine deficiency or inborn errors of metabolism that result in carnitine deficiency (cefditoren causes renal excretion of carnitine), milk protein hypersensitivity (tablets contain sodium caseinate, a milk protein)

PRECAUTIONS: Renal insufficiency, penicillin hypersensitivity

PREGNANCY AND LACTATION: Pregnancy category B, excreted into breast milk

SIDE EFFECTS/ADVERSE REACTIONS

CNS: Headache

GI: **Pseudomembranous colitis, diarrhea** (11-14%), nausea, abdominal pain, dyspepsia, elevated LFTs

GU: Vaginal moniliasis

HEME: Increased prothrombin time, **bone marrow suppression**

SKIN: **Stevens-Johnson syndrome**

INTERACTIONS

Drugs

3 *Antacids, H₂ blockers:* Reduced absorption of cefditoren

3 *Probenecid:* Decreased cefditoren excretion

Labs

• *False positive:* Urine glucose (Benedict's or Fehling's solution or Clinitest tablets)

• *False negative:* Urine, plasma glucose (glucose oxidase or hexokinase methods)

SPECIAL CONSIDERATIONS

• Older oral cephalosporins preferred; no more efficacious than 2nd generation oral cephalosporins, no advantage over penicillin in strep pharyngitis

• Not recommended for prolonged therapy as carnitine deficiency may result

PATIENT/FAMILY EDUCATION

• Take with meals

---

cefepime

(sef'e-peem)

Rx: Maxipime

Chemical Class: Cephalosporin (4th generation)

Therapeutic Class: Antibiotic

CLINICAL PHARMACOLOGY

Mechanism of Action: Inhibits bacterial cell wall synthesis; bactericidal

Pharmacokinetics

IV/IM: Peak 30 min (IV), peak 2 hr (IM); $t_{1/2}$ 2 h; 20% protein bound; excreted in breast milk; metabolites excreted renally

INDICATIONS AND USES: Infections of the urinary (including pyelonephritis) and lower respiratory (pneumonia) tracts and skin and skin structure infections, including cases associated with bacteremia caused by susceptible organisms, empiric monotherapy for febrile neutropenia in pediatric patients

Antibacterial spectrum usually includes:

• Gram-positive organisms: *S. pnemoniae, S. aureus* (methicillin-susceptible strains only), *S. pyogenes* (Group A streptococci), *S. epidermidis* (methicillin-susceptible strains only), *S. saprophyticus, S. agalactiae* (Group B streptococci)

• Gram-negative organisms: *E. coli, K. pneumoniae, P. mirabilis, Pseudomonas aeruginosa, Enterobacter* sp., *Acinetobacter calcoaceticus, Citrobacter diversus, C. freundii, Haemophilus influenzae* (including β-lactamase-producing strains), *Klebsiella oxytoca, Moraxella catarrhalis* (including β-lactamase-producing strains), *Morganella*

---

italic = common side effects   ***bold italic*** = life-threatening reactions

morganii, Proteus vulgaris, Providencia retteri, P. stuartii, Serratia marcescens

DOSAGE

Adult

• *Uncomplicated or complicated urinary tract infection:* 0.5-2 g IV/IM q12h × 7-10 days

• *Pneumonia:* 1-2 g IV q12h × 10 days

• *Moderate to severe skin and skin structure infections:* 2 g IV q12h × 10 days

NOTE: IM route appropriate only for mild to moderate urinary tract infection; doses above appropriate for concurrent bacteremia

• *Maintenance dosing with renal impairment:* If CrCl > 60 ml/min, usual dosing; CrCl 30-60 ml/min, usual dose given q24h; CrCl 11-29 ml/min, ½ usual dose given q24h; CrCl ≤10 ml/min, ¼ usual dose given q24h

Child 2 mo-16 yr

• ≤40 kg: 50 mg/kg IV q12h (q8h for febrile neutropenia) × 7-10 days

🛇 AVAILABLE FORMS/COST OF THERAPY

• Inj—IV/IM: 500 mg/vial: **$8.00**; 1 g/ml vial: **$15.30-$17.05**; 2 g/ml vial: **$30.36-$34.51**

PRECAUTIONS: Hypersensitivity to penicillins, decreased prothrombin activity

PREGNANCY AND LACTATION: Pregnancy category B; excreted into breast milk in very low concentrations (0.5 μg/ml)

SIDE EFFECTS/ADVERSE REACTIONS

CNS: Encephalopathy (in renally impaired without dosage reduction), *seizures*

CV: Thrombophlebitis

EENT: Oral candidiasis

GI: Abdominal cramps, diarrhea, hepatic dysfunction including cholestasis, nausea, *pseudomembranous colitis,* vomiting

GU: Renal dysfunction, *nephrotoxicity,* vaginitis

HEME: Bone marrow suppression, hemolytic anemia, *hemorrhage,* hypoprothrombinemia

SKIN: Erythema multiforme, Stevens-Johnson syndrome, toxic epidermal necrolysis

MISC: Serum sickness-like reactions

INTERACTIONS

Drugs

🖪 *Aminoglycosides:* Additive nephrotoxicity

🖪 *Loop diuretics:* Increased nephrotoxicity

❷ *Oral anticoagulants:* Potential increase in hypoprothrombinemic response to oral anticoagulants

Labs

• *False positive:* Positive direct Coombs test, positive urine glucose test (copper reduction method, i.e., Clinitest)

SPECIAL CONSIDERATIONS

• Broad spectrum, 4th generation cephalosporin demonstrating a low potential for resistance due to lack of β-lactamase induction and low potential for selection of resistant mutant strains; as effective as ceftazidime and cefotaxime in comparative trials; twice daily dosing may add economic advantage

---

* = non-FDA-approved use

cefixime

(sef-ix'ime)

Rx: Suprax
Chemical Class: Cephalosporin
(3rd generation)
Therapeutic Class: Antibiotic

CLINICAL PHARMACOLOGY
Mechanism of Action: Inhibits bacterial cell wall synthesis; bactericidal

Pharmacokinetics
PO: Peak 1 hr, $t_{1/2}$ 3-4 hr; 65% bound by plasma proteins; 50% eliminated unchanged in urine; crosses placenta

INDICATIONS AND USES: Infections of the upper and lower respiratory tract (including pharyngitis, tonsillitis), otitis media, genitourinary tract (including uncomplicated UTI and gonorrhea, cervical, and urethral due to *N. gonorrhoeae*)
Antibacterial spectrum usually includes:
• Gram-positive organisms: *S. pneumoniae, S. pyogenes*
• Gram-negative organisms: *E. coli, P. mirabilis, Klebsiella; H. influenzae, M. catarrhalis, Neisseria gonorrhoeae*
• Anaerobes: *Peptostreptococcus, Peptococcus* sp.

DOSAGE
Adult
• PO 400 mg qd as a single dose or 200 mg q12h; for uncomplicated cervical/urethral GC infections, single 400 mg oral dose
Child <50 kg or <12 yr
• PO 8 mg/kg/day as a single dose or 4 mg/kg q12h

$ **AVAILABLE FORMS/COST OF THERAPY**
• Susp—Oral: 100 mg/5 ml, 50. 75, 100 ml: **$36.51-$39.70**/50 ml

• Tab, Plain Coated—Oral: 200 mg, 100's: **$408.61**; 400 mg, 100's: **$800.81**
CONTRAINDICATIONS: Infants <6 mo
PRECAUTIONS: Hypersensitivity to penicillins
PREGNANCY AND LACTATION: Pregnancy category B; excreted in breast milk
SIDE EFFECTS/ADVERSE REACTIONS

CNS: Chills, confusion, dizziness, fatigue, fever, headache, lethargy, paresthesia
GI: Anorexia, ***bleeding;*** diarrhea, dysgeusia, flatulence, glossitis, heartburn, increased LFTs; nausea, ***pseudomembranous colitis,*** vomiting
GU: Candidiasis, ***nephrotoxicity,*** proteinuria, pruritus, vaginitis
HEME: ***Bone marrow suppression*** eosinophilia, ***hemolytic anemia,*** lymphocytosis
RESP: ***Bronchospasm,*** dyspnea
SKIN: ***Exfoliative dermatitis,*** rash, urticaria
INTERACTIONS
Drugs
3 *Aminoglycosides:* Additive nephrotoxicity
3 *Loop diuretics:* Increased nephrotoxicity
2 *Oral anticoagulants:* Enhanced hypoprothrombinemia
Labs
• *Cefotaxime:* Interferes with assay
• *Creatinine:* Increases or decreases depending on assay
SPECIAL CONSIDERATIONS
• No *S. aureus* coverage

---

italic = common side effects   ***bold italic*** = life-threatening reactions

cefmetazole

(sef-met'a-zole)
Rx: Zefazone
Chemical Class: Cephalosporin
(2nd generation)
Therapeutic Class: Antibiotic
NOTE: Removed from the market
voluntarily by manufacturer

CLINICAL PHARMACOLOGY
Mechanism of Action: Inhibition of
bacterial cell wall synthesis; bactericidal
Pharmacokinetics
IV: Peak, 86 μg/ml after 1 g INF; 68%
bound by plasma proteins; excreted
by kidneys; $t_{1/2}$ 1-3 hr
INDICATIONS AND USES: Infections of the lower respiratory tract,
urinary tract, skin and skin structure,
bones and joints; septicemia, intra-
abdominal infections, uncomplicated gonorrhea, perioperative prophylaxis
Antibacterial spectrum usually includes:
• Gram-positive organisms: *S.
pneumoniae, S. pyogenes, S. agalactiae, S. aureus*
• Gram-negative organisms: *H. influenzae, E. coli, Proteus, Klebsiella, Morganella Morganii, Providencia stuartii, Neisseria gonorrhoeae*
• Anaerobes: *B. fragilis, Clostridium* sp.
DOSAGE
Adult
• *Uncomplicated gonorrhea:* Single
dose IM 1 g (with 1 g of probenecid
given by mouth at the same time or
up to ½ hour before)
• *UTI:* IV 2 g q12h
• *Mild to moderate infections:* IV 2 g
q8h
• *Severe to life-threatening infections:* IV 2 g q6h

• *Perioperative prophylaxis:* For
vaginal hysterectomy, abdominal
hysterectomy, cesarean section, colorectal surgery, or cholecystectomy
(high risk) in adults, 2 g given as a
single dose 30-90 min before surgery or 1 g doses given 30-90 min
before surgery and repeated 8 and 16
hr later (if surgery lasts more than 4
hours, the preoperative dose should
be repeated)
Dosage reduction appropriate with
impaired renal function
💲 AVAILABLE FORMS/COST OF THERAPY
• Inj, Lyphl-Sol—IV: 1 g/vial:
$7.19; 2 g/vial: **$14.32**
CONTRAINDICATIONS: Infants
<1 mo
PRECAUTIONS: Hypersensitivity
to penicillins
PREGNANCY AND LACTATION:
Pregnancy category B; trace milk
concentrations
SIDE EFFECTS/ADVERSE REACTIONS
CNS: Chills, confusion, dizziness,
fatigue, fever, headache, lethargy,
paresthesia
EENT: Periorbital edema
GI: Anorexia, *bleeding;* diarrhea
(4%), flatulence, glossitis, heartburn, increased AST, ALT, bilirubin,
LDH, alk phosphatase; nausea,
pain, *pseudomembranous colitis,*
vomiting
GU: Candidiasis, increased BUN,
nephrotoxicity, proteinuria, pruritus, *renal failure,* vaginitis
HEME: Agranulocytosis, anemia,
*eosinophilia, hemolytic anemia,
leukopenia,* lymphocytosis, *neutropenia, pancytopenia, thrombocytopenia*
SKIN: Angioedema, erythema, *exfoliative dermatitis,* pruritus, rash,
thrombophlebitis, urticaria

* = non-FDA-approved use

MISC: Pain and/or swelling at inj site, phlebitis, superinfection, thrombophlebitis

INTERACTIONS

Drugs

3 *Aminoglycosides:* Additive nephrotoxicity

3 *Chloramphenicol:* Inhibits antibacterial activity of cefmetazole

2 *Oral anticoagulants:* Additive hypoprothrombinemia; enhanced anticoagulation effect

---

cefonicid

(se-fon′i-sid)

Rx: Monocid

Chemical Class: Cephalosporin (2nd generation)

Therapeutic Class: Antibiotic

CLINICAL PHARMACOLOGY

Mechanism of Action: Inhibits bacterial cell wall synthesis; bactericidal

Pharmacokinetics

IV: Peak 5 min

IM: Peak 1 hr, t₁/₂ 4½ hr; 98% protein bound; although reaches therapeutic levels in bile, levels lower than those seen with other cephalosporins, and amounts released into the GI tract are minute; *not* metabolized, 99% excreted unchanged in the urine in 24 hr

INDICATIONS AND USES: Infections of the lower respiratory and urinary tracts; skin and skin structure infections, septicemia, bone and joint infections, preoperative prophylaxis

Antibacterial spectrum usually includes:

• Gram-positive organisms: *S. aureus, S. epidermidis S. pneumoniae, S. pyogenes* Gram-negative organisms: *E. coli, K. pneumoniae, Providencia rettgeri, Proteus vulgaris,* *Morganella morganii, Proteus mirabilis, H. influenzae, Moraxella catarrhalis, K. oxytoca, Enterobacter aerogenes, N. gonorrhoeae* Anaerobes: *C. perfringens, Peptostreptococcus anaerobius, Peptococcus magnus, C. freundii, C. diversus, Fusobacterium* sp.

DOSAGE

Adult

• IM/IV 1-2 g/24 hr (divide in two doses if giving 2 g)

• *Perioperative prophylaxis:* IV 1 g 1 hr prior to procedure

Dosage reduction appropriate in renal impairment (CrCl <50 ml/min)

$ AVAILABLE FORMS/COST OF THERAPY

• Inj, Lyphl-Sol—IM, IV: 1 g: **$27.10**

CONTRAINDICATIONS: Infants <1 mo

PRECAUTIONS: Hypersensitivity to penicillins, renal disease

PREGNANCY AND LACTATION: Pregnancy category B; excreted in breast milk in low concentrations

SIDE EFFECTS/ADVERSE REACTIONS

CNS: Chills, dizziness, fever, headache, paresthesia, weakness

GI: Abdominal pain, anorexia, **bleeding,** *diarrhea;* glossitis, increased LFTs, *nausea, vomiting*

GU: Candidiasis, **nephrotoxicity,** vaginitis

HEME: **Bone marrow suppression,** anemia, eosinophilia, **hemolytic anemia,** lymphocytosis

SKIN: Dermatitis, rash, urticaria

INTERACTIONS

Drugs

3 *Aminoglycosides:* Additive nephrotoxicity

3 *Chloramphenicol:* Inhibits the antibacterial activity of cefonicid

3 *Loop diuretics:* Increased nephrotoxicity

---

italic = common side effects   ***bold italic*** = life-threatening reactions

cefoperazone

(sef-oh-per´a-zone)
Rx: Cefobid
Chemical Class: Cephalosporin
(3rd generation)
Therapeutic Class: Antibiotic

CLINICAL PHARMACOLOGY
Mechanism of Action: Inhibits bacterial cell wall synthesis; bactericidal
Pharmacokinetics
IV: Peak 5 min, duration 6-8 hr
IM: Peak 1-2 hr, duration 6-8 hr
$t_{1/2}$ 2 hr; 70%-75% eliminated unchanged in bile, 20%-30% unchanged in urine
INDICATIONS AND USES: Infections of the lower respiratory tract, urinary tract, skin; bone infections, septicemia, peritonitis, PID caused by susceptible organisms
Antibacterial spectrum usually includes:
• Gram-positive organisms: *S. aureus,* (penicillinase and non-penicillinase-producing strains), *S. epidermidis, Streptococcus pneumoniae, S. pyogenes,* Group A β-hemolytic streptococci, *S. agalactiae,* Group B β-hemolytic streptococci, *Enterococcus, Streptococcus faecalis, S. faecium, S. durans*
• Gram-negative organisms: *H. influenzae, E. coli, Proteus mirabilis, P. vulgaris, Klebsiella, Enterobacter, Serratia, Citrobacter, Morganella morganii, N. gonorrhoeae, Providencia, Pseudomonas aeruginosa*
• Anaerobes: *Peptococcus* and *Peptostreptococcus, Clostridium* sp., *Bacteroides* sp.
DOSAGE
Adult
• *Mild/moderate infections:* IM/IV 1-2 g q12h

• *Severe infections:* IM/IV 6-12 g/day divided in 2-4 equal doses
• *Hepatic disease or biliary obstruction:* Doses >4 g/day generally not necessary
Child
• Neonates 50 mg/kg/dose q12h; children 100-150 mg/kg/day divided q8-12h, up to 12 g/day
§ AVAILABLE FORMS/COST OF THERAPY
• Inj, Sol—IM, IV: 1 g: **$17.57**; 2 g: **$35.14**; 10 g: **$157.29**
CONTRAINDICATIONS: Infants <1 mo
PRECAUTIONS: Hypersensitivity to penicillins
PREGNANCY AND LACTATION: Pregnancy category B; low concentrations excreted in human milk
SIDE EFFECTS/ADVERSE REACTIONS
CNS: Chills, dizziness, fever, headache, paresthesia, weakness
GI: Abdominal pain, *anorexia, bleeding; diarrhea,* glossitis, increased LFTs; *nausea, pseudomembranous colitis,* vomiting
GU: Candidiasis, **nephrotoxicity,** proteinuria, vaginitis
HEME: **Bone marrow suppression,** anemia, **bleeding,** eosinophilia, **hemolytic anemia, hypoprothrombinemia,** leukopenia, lymphocytosis,
RESP: Dyspnea
SKIN: Dermatitis, rash, urticaria
INTERACTIONS
Drugs
❸ *Aminoglycosides:* Increased risk of nephrotoxicity
❸ *Ethanol:* Disulfiram-like reactions
❸ *Loop diuretics:* Increased nephrotoxicity
❷ *Oral anticoagulants:* Via hypoprothrombinemia, may enhance anticoagulant effects

Labs
• *Creatinine:* Increased serum values
SPECIAL CONSIDERATIONS
• No dose adjustment necessary in renal failure when usual doses are administered
PATIENT/FAMILY EDUCATION
• Avoid alcohol during and for 3 days after use

---

cefotaxime

(sef-oh-taks'eem)
Rx: Claforan
Chemical Class: Cephalosporin (3rd generation)
Therapeutic Class: Antibiotic

CLINICAL PHARMACOLOGY
Mechanism of Action: Inhibits bacterial cell wall synthesis; bactericidal.
Pharmacokinetics
IV: Onset 5 min
IM: Onset 30 min, $t_{1/2}$ 1 hr; 35%-65% protein bound; 40%-65% is eliminated unchanged in urine in 24 hr, 25% metabolized to active and inactive metabolites
INDICATIONS AND USES: Infections of the lower respiratory tract, genitourinary tract (including UTI, uncomplicated gonorrhea, PID, endometritis, pelvic cellulitis), skin and skin structure, bone and joints, CNS, intra-abdominal infections; perioperative prophylaxis (e.g., abdominal or vaginal hysterectomy, gastrointestinal and genitourinary tract surgery)
Antibacterial spectrum usually includes:
• Gram-positive organisms: Group A streptococci, *S. pneumoniae, S. pyogenes, Staphylococcus aureus* (penicillinase and non-penicillinase producing), *Enterococcus* sp., *S. epidermidis*
• Gram-negative organisms: *E. coli, Klebsiella* sp., *H. influenzae* (including ampicillin-resistant strains), *H. parainfluenzae, P. mirabilis, S. marcescens, Enterobacter* sp., indole-positive *Proteus, Citrobacter* sp., *Morganella morganii, Providencia rettgeri, N. gonorrhoeae* (including penicillinase-producing strains), *N. meningitidis*
• Anaerobes: *Bacteroides* sp. (including *Bacteroides fragilis*), *Clostridium* sp., *Peptostreptococcus* sp., *Peptococcus* sp., *Fusobacterium* sp.
DOSAGE
Adult
• IM/IV 1-2 g q8-12h
• *Severe infections:* IM/IV 2 g q4h; not to exceed 12 g/day
• *Uncomplicated gonorrhea:* 1 g IM
• *Perioperative prophylaxis:* IM/IV 1 g 30-90 min prior to start of surgery, followed by doses at 6 and 12 hr postsurgery
Dosage reduction appropriate for severe renal impairment (CrCl <10 ml/min)
Child
• Neonates: 0-1 wk of age 50 mg/kg IV q12h; 1-4 wk of age 50 mg/kg IV q8h (it is not necessary to differentiate between premature and normal gestational-age infants)
• Infants and children (1 mo to 12 yr): <50 kg 50-180 mg/kg IM or IV divided into 4-6 equal doses; >50 kg the usual adult dosage should be used; max daily dosage should not exceed 12 g
⑤ AVAILABLE FORMS/COST OF THERAPY
• Inj, Dry-Sol—IM, IV: 0.5 g/vial: **$8.62**; 1 g/vial: **$10.60**; 2 g/vial: **$21.17**
PRECAUTIONS: Hypersensitivity to penicillins

---

italic = common side effects   ***bold italic*** = life-threatening reactions

PREGNANCY AND LACTATION: Pregnancy category B; low milk concentrations

SIDE EFFECTS/ADVERSE REACTIONS

CNS: Chills, dizziness, fever, headache, paresthesia, weakness

GI: Abdominal pain, *anorexia, bleeding; diarrhea,* glossitis, increased AST, ALT, bilirubin, LDH, alk phosphatase; *nausea,* pain, *pseudomembranous colitis, vomiting*

GU: Candidiasis, proteinuria, pruritus, vaginitis, *nephrotoxicity*

HEME: **Bone marrow suppression,** eosinophilia, **hemolytic anemia,** lymphocytosis

SKIN: Dermatitis, induration (IM), inflammation (IV), pain, rash, urticaria

INTERACTIONS

Drugs

❸ *Aminoglycosides:* Additive nephrotoxicity

❸ *Chloramphenicol:* Inhibits antibacterial activity of cidal-cefotaxime

❷ *Oral anticoagulants:* Hypoprothrombinemia

Labs

• *False serum increases:* Albumin, alkaline phosphatase, calcium ceftriaxone cholesterol, creatine kinase, creatinine, glucose, iron, iron saturation, metronidazole, potassium, sodium, tetracycline, trimethoprim

• *False serum decreases:* Ammonia, amylase, chloride, γ-glutamyltransferase (GGT), lactate dehydrogenase, magnesium, phosphate, potassium, urea nitrogen, uric acid

• *False positive:* Clindamycin, colistin, erythromycin, polymyxin

---

cefotetan
(sef'oh-tee-tan)
Rx: Cefotan
Chemical Class: Cephamycin (structurally related to cephalosporins, 2nd generation)
Therapeutic Class: Antibiotic

CLINICAL PHARMACOLOGY

Mechanism of Action: Inhibits bacterial cell wall synthesis; bactericidal

Pharmacokinetics

IM: Peak 1 hr, $t_{1/2}$ 3-5 hr; 88% bound by plasma proteins; wide distribution; no active metabolites, 50%-80% eliminated unchanged in urine over 24 hr

INDICATIONS AND USES: Infections of the lower respiratory tract, urinary tract, skin and skin structure; intra-abdominal, gynecologic, bone and joint infections, as well as perioperative prophylaxis of susceptible organisms

Antibacterial spectrum usually includes:

• Gram-positive organisms: *Streptococcus pneumoniae, S. pyogenes, Staphylococcus aureus* (penicillinase- and non-penicillinase-producing strains), *S. epidermidis*

• Gram-negative organisms: *E. coli, Klebsiella* sp., *Proteus* sp., *H. influenzae* (including ampicillin-resistant strains), *Serratia marcescens, Shigella, N. gonorrhoeae*

• Anaerobes: *Peptococcus* sp; *Peptostreptococcus* sp., *Bacteroides* sp. (excluding *B. distasonis, B. ovatus, B. thetaiotaomicron*), *Fusobacterium* sp.

DOSAGE

Adult

• IV/IM 1-2g q12h, may increase to 3 g q12 hr for life-threatening infections

---

• *Perioperative prophylaxis:* IV 1-2 g ½-1 hr before surgery
• *Renal failure:* Give usual dose q24 hr for CrCl of 10-30 ml/min; q48 hr for CrCl <10 ml/min

Child
• IV/IM 20-40 mg/kg q12h

§ AVAILABLE FORMS/COST OF THERAPY
• Inj, Dry-Sol—IM, IV: 10 g: **$118.32**
• Inj, Lyphl-Sol—IM, IV: 1 g/vial: **$12.17-$13.19**; 2 g/vial: **$23.89-$25.86**

CONTRAINDICATIONS: Infants <1 mo

PRECAUTIONS: Hypersensitivity to penicillins, renal disease

PREGNANCY AND LACTATION: Pregnancy category B; small amounts excreted into breast milk

SIDE EFFECTS/ADVERSE REACTIONS
CNS: Chills, dizziness, fever, headache, paresthesia, weakness
CV: Hypotension
GI: Abdominal pain, *anorexia,* **bleeding;** *diarrhea,* glossitis, increased LFTs, *nausea,* **pseudomembranous colitis,** *vomiting*
GU: Candidiasis, **nephrotoxicity,** proteinuria, vaginitis
HEME: **Bone marrow suppression,** eosinophilia, **hypoprothrombinemia,** lymphocytosis
SKIN: Dermatitis, **exfoliative dermatitis,** pruritus, rash, thrombophlebitis, urticaria

INTERACTIONS
Drugs
3 *Aminoglycosides:* Additive nephrotoxicity
3 *Ethanol:* Disulfiram-like reaction
3 *Chloramphenicol:* Inhibits antibacterial activity of cidal-cefotetan
2 *Oral anticoagulants:* Additive hypoprothrombinemia; enhanced anticoagulant effects

SPECIAL CONSIDERATIONS
PATIENT/FAMILY EDUCATION
• Avoid alcohol during and for 3 days after use

---

cefoxitin
(se-fox'i-tin)
Rx: Mefoxin
Chemical Class: Cephamycin (structurally related to cephalosporins, 2nd generation)
Therapeutic Class: Antibiotic

CLINICAL PHARMACOLOGY
Mechanism of Action: Inhibits bacterial cell wall synthesis; bactericidal
Pharmacokinetics
IV: Peak 5 min
IM: Peak 20-30 min
$t_{1/2}$ 1 hr; 55%-75% bound by plasma proteins; passes into pleural and joint fluids and is detectable in antibacterial concentrations in bile; 85% eliminated unchanged in urine; crosses blood-brain barrier

INDICATIONS AND USES: Infections of the lower respiratory tract, urinary tract, skin and skin structure; gynecologic, intra-abdominal, bone, and joint infections as well as perioperative prophylaxis of susceptible organisms; septicemia; uncomplicated gonorrhea
Antibacterial spectrum usually includes:
• Gram-positive organisms: *Streptococcus pneumoniae, S. pyogenes, Staphylococcus aureus* (penicillinase- and nonpenicillinase- producing strains), *S. epidermidis*
• Gram-negative organisms: *E. coli, Klebsiella* sp., *Proteus* sp., *H. influenzae* (including ampicillin-resistant strains), *N. gonorrhoeae, Morganella morganii, Providencia* sp.

---

italic = common side effects   ***bold italic*** = life-threatening reactions

• Anaerobes: *Peptococcus* sp., *Peptostreptococcus* sp., *Bacteroides* sp. (excluding *B. distasonis, B. ovatus, B. thetaiotaomicron*).

DOSAGE
Adult
• IM/IV 1-2 g q6-8h
• *Uncomplicated gonorrhea:* 2 g IM as single dose with 1 g PO probenecid
• *Severe infections:* IM/IV 2 g q4h or 3 g q6h
• *Perioperative prophylaxis:* IM/IV 2 g 30-60 min prior to surgery, then 2 g q6h × 24 hr
Dose reduction appropriate in renal impairment (CrCl <50 ml/min)
Child ≥ 3 mo
• IM/IV 80 to 160 mg/kg of body weight per day divided into 4-6 equal doses, not to exceed 12 g/day

$ AVAILABLE FORMS/COST OF THERAPY
• Inj, Dry-Sol—IM, IV: 1 g: **$10.44-$28.13**; 2 g: **$20.85-$56.25**; 10 g: **$104.44-$112.50**

PRECAUTIONS: Hypersensitivity to penicillins, renal disease

PREGNANCY AND LACTATION: Pregnancy category B; low milk concentrations

SIDE EFFECTS/ADVERSE REACTIONS
CNS: Chills, dizziness, fever, headache, paresthesia,weakness
CV: Hypotension
GI: Abdominal pain, anorexia, **bleeding;** *diarrhea,* glossitis, increased LFTs; *nausea,* **pseudomembranous colitis,** *vomiting*
GU: Candidiasis, **nephrotoxicity**, proteinuria, vaginitis
HEME: **Bone marrow suppression,** eosinophilia, **hemolytic anemia, hypoprothrombinemia,** lymphocytosis
SKIN: Dermatitis, **exfoliative dermatitis,** pruritus, rash, thrombophlebitis, urticaria

INTERACTIONS
Drugs
3 *Aminoglycosides:* Additive nephrotoxicity
3 *Chloramphenicol:* Inhibits antibacterial activity of cidal-cefoxitin
2 *Oral anticoagulants:* Additive hypoprothrombinemia, enhanced anticoagulant effects
Labs
• *False serum increases:* Creatinine (serum and urine), cefuroxime, gentamicin, metronidazole, potassium, tetracycline
• *False urine increases:* 17-hydroxycorticosteroids
• *False serum decreases:* Creatine clearance
• *False positive:* Polymyxin

cefpodoxime
(sef-pod´ox-ime)
Rx: Vantin
Chemical Class: Cephalosporin (2nd generation)
Therapeutic Class: Antibiotic

CLINICAL PHARMACOLOGY
Mechanism of Action: Inhibits bacterial cell wall synthesis; bactericidal
Pharmacokinetics
PO: Peak 2-3 hr; absorbed as prodrug; de-esterified to its active metabolite, cefpodoxime (approximately 50% of the administered dose is systemically absorbed); minimal metabolism; $t_{1/2}$ 2-3 hr; 25% bound by plasma proteins; 30% eliminated unchanged in urine in 12 hr

INDICATIONS AND USES: Infections of the upper and lower respiratory tract, skin and skin structure, urinary tract; sexually transmitted diseases (uncomplicated urethral and cervical gonorrhea)

---

* = non-FDA-approved use

Antibacterial spectrum usually includes:

• Gram-positive organisms: *Streptococcus pneumoniae, S. pyogenes, Staphylococcus aureus* (including penicillinase-producing strains), *S. saprophyticus*

• Gram-negative organisms: *H. influenzae* (some β-lactamase-producing strains), *N. gonorrhoeae* (including penicillinase-producing strains), *Moraxella catarrhalis, E. coli, Klebsiella pneumoniae, Proteus mirabilis*

DOSAGE

Adult

• *Pneumonia:* 200 mg q12h for 14 days

• *Uncomplicated gonorrhea:* 200 mg single dose

• *Skin and skin structure:* 400 mg q12h for 7-14 days

• *Pharyngitis and tonsillitis:* 100 mg q12h for 10 days

• *Uncomplicated UTI:* 100 mg q12h for 7 days

• *Renal failure:* Increase dosing interval to q24h for CrCl <30 ml/min

Child 5-12 yr

• *Acute otitis media:* 10 mg/kg q24h for 10 days (max 400 mg/dose)

• *Pharyngitis/tonsillitis:* 5 mg/kg q12h (max 100 mg/dose) for 10 days

🛇 AVAILABLE FORMS/COST OF THERAPY

• Susp—Oral: 50 mg/5 ml, 50, 75, 100 ml: **$40.70**/100 ml; 100 mg/5 ml, 50, 75, 100 ml: **$77.43**/100 ml

• Tab, Uncoated—Oral: 100 mg, 100's: **$343.55**; 200 mg, 100's: **$453.63**

CONTRAINDICATIONS: Infants

PRECAUTIONS: Hypersensitivity to penicillins, renal disease

PREGNANCY AND LACTATION: Pregnancy category B; excreted into breast milk; average 2% of serum levels at 4 hr following 200 mg dose

SIDE EFFECTS/ADVERSE REACTIONS

CNS: Chills, dizziness, fatigue, fever, headache, lethargy, paresthesia

GI: Anorexia, **bleeding;** *diarrhea,* glossitis, increased LFTs; *nausea,* **pseudomembranous colitis,** *vomiting*

GU: Candidiasis, **nephrotoxicity,** *vaginitis*

HEME: **Bone marrow suppression,** eosinophilia, **hemolytic anemia,** lymphocytosis

RESP: Dyspnea

SKIN: Dermatitis, rash, urticaria

INTERACTIONS

Drugs

🖪 *Aminoglycosides:* Additive nephrotoxicity

🖪 *Antacids:* Reduced bioavailability and serum cefpodoxime levels

🖪 *H₂-blockers (cimetidine, famotidine, nizatidine, ranitidine), Proton pump inhibitors (lansoprazole, omeprazole):* Reduced bioavailability and serum cefpodoxime levels

🖪 *Loop diuretics:* Increased nephrotoxicity

SPECIAL CONSIDERATIONS

• Reserve use for otitis media to infections that fail to respond to less expensive agents (e.g., amoxicillin, co-trimoxazole)

• Suspension tastes very bitter

---

cefprozil

(sef-pro′zil)

Rx: Cefzil

Chemical Class: Cephalosporin (2nd generation)

Therapeutic Class: Antibiotic

CLINICAL PHARMACOLOGY

Mechanism of Action: Inhibits bacterial cell wall synthesis; bactericidal

---

Pharmacokinetics

PO: Peak serum and urine concentration 1.5 and 4 hr; 95% absorbed (no food effect observed); plasma protein binding 36%; t$_{1/2}$ 1.3 hr

INDICATIONS AND USES: Infections of the upper and lower respiratory tract (pharyngitis, tonsillitis, otitis media, secondary bacterial infection of acute bronchitis, acute bacterial exacerbation of chronic bronchitis); skin and skin structure due to susceptible organisms

Antibacterial spectrum usually includes:

• Gram-positive organisms: *Staphylococcus aureus* (including penicillinase-producing strains), *Streptococcus pneumoniae, S. pyogenes*
• Gram-negative organisms: *Moraxella catarrhalis, H. influenzae* (including penicillinase-producing strains)

DOSAGE

Adult

• *Upper respiratory infections:* PO 500 mg qd × 10 days
• *Lower respiratory infections:* PO 500 mg bid × 10 days
• *Skin/skin structure infections:* PO 250-500 mg q12h or 500 mg qd × 10 days
• *Renal disease:* Decrease dose by 50% in patients with CrCl <30 ml/min

Child 6 mo-12 yr

• *Upper respiratory tract infections:* PO 7.5 mg/kg q12h × 10 days
• *Otitis media:* PO 15 mg/kg q12h × 10 days
• *Skin/skin structure infections:* PO 20 mg/kg qd × 10 days

💲 AVAILABLE FORMS/COST OF THERAPY

• Susp—Oral: 125 mg/5 ml, 50, 75, 100 ml: **$32.65-$37.25**/100 ml; 250 mg/5 ml, 50, 75, 100 ml: **$59.16-$67.46**/100 ml

• Tab, Uncoated—Oral: 250 mg, 100's: **$387.83-$389.66**; 500 mg, 100's: **$793.73**

PRECAUTIONS: Elderly, hypersensitivity to penicillins

PREGNANCY AND LACTATION: Pregnancy category B; excreted into breast milk in low concentratons

SIDE EFFECTS/ADVERSE REACTIONS

CNS: Chills, dizziness, fever, headache, paresthesia, weakness
GI: Abdominal pain, anorexia, ***bleeding;*** diarrhea, flatulence, glossitis, increased LFTs; ***pseudomembranous colitis,*** vomiting
GU: Candidiasis, genitoanal pruritus, hematuria, ***nephrotoxicity,*** vaginitis
HEME: ***Bone marrow suppression,*** eosinophilia, ***hemolytic anemia,*** lymphocytosis
SKIN: Dermatitis, rash, urticaria
RESP: Dyspnea

INTERACTIONS

Drugs

3 *Aminoglycosides:* Additive nephrotoxicity
3 *Loop diuretics:* Increased nephrotoxicity

SPECIAL CONSIDERATIONS

• Reserve use for otitis media to infections that fail to respond to less expensive agents (e.g., amoxicillin, co-trimoxazole)
• Suspension contains phenylalanine 28 mg/5 ml

---

* = non-FDA-approved use

ceftazidime

(sef-taz'i-deem)

Rx: Ceptaz, Fortaz, Tazicef, Tazidime

Chemical Class: Cephalosporin (3rd generation)

Therapeutic Class: Antibiotic

CLINICAL PHARMACOLOGY

Mechanism of Action: Inhibits bacterial cell wall synthesis; bactericidal

Pharmacokinetics

IM: Peak 1 hr, <10% bound to plasma proteins; 80% eliminated unchanged in urine; $t_{1/2}$ 1.9 hr

INDICATIONS AND USES: Infections of the lower respiratory tract, urinary tract, skin and skin structure; bone and joint, gynecological, intra-abdominal infections; septicemia; meningitis caused by susceptible organisms

Antibacterial spectrum usually includes:

• Gram-positive organisms: *Streptococcus pneumoniae, S. pyogenes,* Group B streptococci, *Staphylococcus aureus*

• Gram-negative organisms: *H. influenzae, E. coli, E. aerogenes, P. aeruginosa, P. mirabilis, P. vulgaris, Klebsiella, Citrobacter, Enterobacter, Salmonella, Shigella, Acinetobacter, Neisseria, Serratia*

DOSAGE

Adult

• IV/IM 1 g q8-12h

• *Uncomplicated UTI:* IM/IV 250 mg q12h

• *Complicated UTI:* IM/IV 500 mg q8-12h

• *Bone and joint infections:* IV 2 g q12h

• *Severe infections/meningitis:* IV 2 g q8h

• *Renal disease:* Decrease dose or increase dosing interval in patients with CrCl <30 ml/min

Child 1 mo-12 yr

• IV 30-50 mg/kg q8h, not to exceed 6 g/day

• Neonates 0-4 wk

• IV 30 mg/kg q12h

💲 AVAILABLE FORMS/COST OF THERAPY

• Inj, Dry-Sol—IV, IM: 500 mg/vial: **$7.11-$7.41**; 1 g/vial: **$1.42-$19.15**; 2 g/vial: **$28.45-$41.24**; 6 g/vial: **$82.91-$118.56**

PRECAUTIONS: Hypersensitivity to penicillins, renal disease, children

PREGNANCY AND LACTATION: Pregnancy category B; excreted in human milk in low concentrations

SIDE EFFECTS/ADVERSE REACTIONS

CNS: Chills, dizziness, fever, headache, paresthesia, weakness

GI: Anorexia, ***bleeding;*** diarrhea, glossitis, increased LFTs, nausea ***pseudomembranous colitis,*** vomiting

GU: Candidiasis, ***nephrotoxicity,*** proteinuria, vaginitis

HEME: ***Bone marrow suppression,*** eosinophilia, ***hemolytic anemia,*** lymphocytosis

RESP: Dyspnea

SKIN: Dermatitis, rash, urticaria

INTERACTIONS

Drugs

3 *Aminoglycosides:* Additive nephrotoxicity

3 *Chloramphenicol:* Inhibition of the antibacterial activity of ceftazidime

3 *Loop diuretics:* Increased nephrotoxicity

SPECIAL CONSIDERATIONS

• Especially useful for infections due to *Pseudomonas aeruginosa* (with or without an aminoglycoside)

---

italic = common side effects   ***bold italic*** = life-threatening reactions

ceftibuten

(cef'te-bute-in)

Rx: Cedax

Chemical Class: Cephalosporin
(3rd generation, oral)

Therapeutic Class: Antibiotic

CLINICAL PHARMACOLOGY

Mechanism of Action: Inhibits bacterial cell wall synthesis; bactericidal

Pharmacokinetics

PO: C_{max} 15 µg/ml 2.6 hr after 400 mg adult dose, 13.4 µg/ml 2 hr after 9 mg/kg pediatric dose; well absorbed (80% bioavailability), capsule and suspension equal; widely distributed, 65%-77% protein bound; renal excretion; $t_{1/2}$ 1.53-2.5 hr

INDICATIONS AND USES: Pharyngitis, tonsillitis, otitis media, acute bacterial exacerbation of chronic bronchitis, gonococcal urethritis* Antibacterial spectrum usually includes:

• Gram-positive organisms: *Streptococcus pyogenes, S. pneumoniae* (penicillin susceptible strains only)

• Gram-negative organisms: Enterobacter sp., *E. coli, Klebsiella* sp., *Morganella morganii, Proteus* sp., *Providencia* sp., *Salmonella* sp., *Serratia* sp., *Haemophilus influenzae, Neisseria* sp., *Moraxella catarrhalis*

DOSAGE

Adult

• PO 400 mg qd × 10 days

• *Renal failure:* CrCl 30-49 ml/min, 4.5 mg/kg or 200 mg qd; CrCl 5-29 ml/min, 2.25 mg/kg or 100 mg qd

Child <12 yr

• PO 9 mg/kg, up to 400 mg qd × 10 days

🟦 AVAILABLE FORMS/COST OF THERAPY

• Cap, Gel—Oral: 400 mg, 100's: **$741.40**

• Powder, Reconst—Oral: 90 mg/5 ml, 30, 60, 120 ml: **$38.55**/60 ml; 180 mg/5 ml, 30, 60 ml: **$98.87**/60 ml

PRECAUTIONS: Hypersensitivity to penicillins, renal disease

PREGNANCY AND LACTATION: Pregnancy category B; excreted into breast milk in negligible concentrations

SIDE EFFECTS/ADVERSE REACTIONS

CNS: Chills, dizziness, fever, headache, paresthesia, weakness

GI: Abdominal pain, anorexia, *bleeding,* diarrhea, glossitis, nausea, *pseudomembranous colitis,* vomiting

GU: Candidiasis, *nephrotoxicity,* proteinuria, vaginitis

HEME: **Bone marrow suppression,** anemia, eosinophilia, *hemolytic anemia,* lymphocytosis, thrombocytosis

RESP: Dyspnea

SKIN: Dermatitis, rash, urticaria

INTERACTIONS

Drugs

🔳 *Aminoglycosides:* Additive nephrotoxicity

🔳 *Loop diuretics:* Increased nephrotoxicity

SPECIAL CONSIDERATIONS

• Comparable to many other oral cephalosporins; may produce higher serum levels and better penetration, but unsubstantiated

• Clinical application as alternative in respiratory tract infections

• Recommend empty stomach administration for the suspension

---

* = non-FDA-approved use

ceftizoxime

(sef-ti-zox′eem)
Rx: Cefizox
Chemical Class: Cephalosporin
(3rd generation)
Therapeutic Class: Antibiotic

CLINICAL PHARMACOLOGY
Mechanism of Action: Inhibits bacterial cell wall synthesis; bactericidal
Pharmacokinetics
IM: Peak 1 hr, 30% bound by plasma proteins; not metabolized, eliminated unchanged in urine in 24 hr; crosses placenta; $t_{1/2}$ 1.7 hr
INDICATIONS AND USES: Infections of the skin and skin structures, bone and joints, lower respiratory tract, urinary tract; gonorrhea, pelvic inflammatory disease, septicemia, meningitis, intra-abdominal infections caused by susceptible organisms
Antibacterial spectrum usually includes:
• Gram-positive organisms: *Streptococcus pneumoniae, S. pyogenes, S. agalactiae, Staphylococcus aureus, S. epidermis*
• Gram-negative organisms: *Acinetobacter, H. influenzae, E. coli, E. aerogenes, P. mirabilis, P. vulgaris, Providencia rettgeri, P. aeruginosa, Serratia, Klebsiella, Enterobacter, Morganella morganii, N. gonorrhoeae*
• Anaerobes: *Bacteroides* sp., *Peptococcus, Peptostreptococcus*
DOSAGE
Adult
• IM/IV 1-2 g q8-12h, may give up to 2g q4h in life-threatening infections
• *PID:* IV 2 g q8h
• *Uncomplicated   gonorrhea:*
Single, 1 g IM dose

Dosage reduction appropriate in renal impairment (CrCl < 50 ml/min)
Child ≥6 mo
• 150-200 mg/kg/day divided q6-8h
💲 AVAILABLE FORMS/COST OF THERAPY
• Inj, Sol—IV: 500 mg/vial: **$67.50**; 1 g/vial: **$12.81**; 2 g/vial: **$24.00**
CONTRAINDICATIONS: Infants <1 mo
PRECAUTIONS: Hypersensitivity to penicillins, renal disease
PREGNANCY AND LACTATION: Pregnancy category B; excreted in human milk in low concentrations
SIDE EFFECTS/ADVERSE REACTIONS
CNS: Dizziness, fever, headache, paresthesia
GI: Abdominal pain, anorexia, ***bleeding;*** diarrhea, glossitis, increased LFTs; nausea, ***pseudomembranous colitis,*** vomiting
GU: Candidiasis, proteinuria, pruritus, vaginitis, **nephrotoxicity**
HEME: ***Bone marrow suppression,*** eosinophilia, ***hemolytic anemia***
RESP: Dyspnea
SKIN: Dermatitis, rash, urticaria
INTERACTIONS
Drugs
3 *Aminoglycosides:* Additive nephrotoxicity
3 *Loop diuretics:* Increased nephrotoxicity

ceftriaxone

(sef-try-ax′one)
Rx: Rocephin
Chemical Class: Cephalosporin
(3rd generation)
Therapeutic Class: Antibiotic

CLINICAL PHARMACOLOGY
Mechanism of Action: Inhibits bacterial cell wall synthesis; bactericidal

---

italic = common side effects   ***bold italic*** = life-threatening reactions

Pharmacokinetics

IV: Peak 30 min (123 µg/ml for 1 g)
IM: Peak 1.5-4 hr (83 µg/ml for 1 g)
90% bound by plasma proteins;
35%-60% eliminated unchanged in
urine, remainder secreted in bile;
crosses placenta; elimination $t_{1/2}$ 7.2
hr, prolonged in elderly, liver disease (9 hr), and renal disease (CrCl
<16 ml/min 15 hr, CrCl 16-60
ml/min 11-12 hr.)

INDICATIONS AND USES: Infections of the lower respiratory tract,
urinary tract, skin, bone, joint; intra-
abdominal infections; septicemia;
meningitis caused by susceptible organisms; localized and disseminated gonococcal infections including pelvic inflammatory disease;
surgical prophylaxis

Antibacterial spectrum usually includes:

• Gram-positive organisms: *Streptococcus pneumoniae, S. pyogenes,
Staphylococcus aureus*

• Gram-negative organisms: *H. influenzae, E. coli, E. aerogenes, E.
cloacae, P. mirabilis, P. vulgaris,
Serratia marcescens, Providencia
rettgeri, Klebsiella* sp., *Citrobacter*
sp., *Salmonella* sp. (including *S.
typhi), Shigella* sp., *Acinetobacter*
sp., *Neisseria* sp.; some strains of
Pseudomonas aeruginosa

• Anaerobes: *B. fragilis, B. bivivus,
B. melaninogenicus, Peptostreptococcus* sp.

DOSAGE

Adult

• *Infections of the lower respiratory
tract, urinary tract, skin, bone, joint;
intra-abdominal infections; septicemia:* IM/IV 1-2 g qd

• *Uncomplicated gonorrhea:* IM
125 mg as single dose plus 1 g
azithromycin PO or doxycycline
100 mg PO bid × 7 days

• *Meningitis:* IM/IV 100 mg/kg/day
in equal doses q12h; not to exceed 4
g qd

• *Surgical prophylaxis:* IV 1 g ½-2
hr preop

Child

• *Acute otitis media:* IM 50 mg/kg
(max 1 g) as a single dose

• *Infections of the lower respiratory
tract, urinary tract, skin, bone, joint;
intra-abdominal infections; septicemia:* IM/IV 50-75 mg/kg/day in
equal doses q12h; not to exceed 2 g
qd

• *Meningitis:* IM/IV 100 mg/kg/day
in equal doses q12h; not to exceed 4
g qd

$ AVAILABLE FORMS/COST OF THERAPY

• Inj, Dry-Sol—IM, IV: 250
mg/vial: **$14.92-$16.48**; 500
mg/vial: **$27.05-$29.87**; 1 g/vial:
$35.28-$52.76; 2 g/vial: **$91.98-
$104.21**

PRECAUTIONS: Hypersensitivity
to penicillins, renal disease

PREGNANCY AND LACTATION:
Pregnancy category B; excreted in
breast milk

SIDE EFFECTS/ADVERSE REACTIONS

CNS: Chills, dizziness, fever, headache, paresthesia, weakness

GI: Abdominal pain, anorexia,
bleeding; diarrhea, glossitis, increased LFTs; nausea, ***pseudomembranous colitis,*** vomiting

GU: Candidiasis, ***nephrotoxicity,***
vaginitis

HEME: **Bone marrow suppression,**
eosinophilia, **hemolytic anemia,**
lymphocytosis, thrombocytosis

RESP: Dyspnea

SKIN: Dermatitis; induration or tenderness at injection site; rash, urticaria

---

* = non-FDA-approved use

INTERACTIONS
Drugs
3 *Aminoglycosides:* Additive nephrotoxicity

3 *Loop diuretics:* Increased nephrotoxicity

2 *Warfarin:* Hypoprothrombinemic response enhanced

SPECIAL CONSIDERATIONS
• Meningitis the only indication requiring bid dosing; qd sufficient for all other indications in adults

• Often administered in acute care settings for dubious indications due to long $t_{1/2}$, avoid overuse

---

cefuroxime
(sef-yoor-ox′eem)

Rx: Zinacef, Kefurox (as sodium), Ceftin (as axetil)
Chemical Class: Cephalosporin (2nd generation)
Therapeutic Class: Antibiotic

CLINICAL PHARMACOLOGY
Mechanism of Action: Inhibits bacterial cell wall synthesis; bactericidal

Pharmacokinetics
PO: Peak level 2 hr (7 µg/ml after 500 mg); absorption greater after food (absolute bioavailability increases from 37% to 52%); bioavailability of susp 91% of tab; peak plasma concentration for susp 71% of peak plasma concentration for tab

IV: Peak 30 min

IM: Peak 15-60 min; 33%-50% bound by plasma proteins; 70%-100% eliminated unchanged in urine; crosses placenta, blood-brain barrier; not metabolized; $t_{1/2}$ 1-2 hr

INDICATIONS AND USES: Pharyngitis, tonsillitis, otitis media, bronchitis, pneumonia, infections of the skin and urinary tract, localized and disseminated gonococcal infections, bone or joint infections, septicemia, or meningitis caused by susceptible organisms; treatment of early Lyme's disease

Antibacterial spectrum usually includes:

• Gram-positive organisms: *Streptococcus pneumoniae, S. pyogenes, Staphylococcus aureus*

• Gram-negative organisms: *H. influenzae, H. parainfluenzae, Moraxella catarrhalis* (including ampicillin- and cephalothin-resistant strains), *E. coli, P. mirabilis, Neisseria* sp., *Klebsiella* sp.

• Anaerobes: *Peptococcus* and *Peptostreptococcus* sp.; β-lactamase-producing strains of these pathogens are usually susceptible

DOSAGE
Adult
• *Pharyngitis, tonsillitis, bronchitis, skin infections:* PO (tab) 250-500 mg q12h

• *UTI:* PO (tab) 125-250 mg q12h

• *Uncomplicated gonorrhea:* PO 1000 mg single dose; IM 1.5 g single dose, 2 sites, with 1g PO probenecid

• *Early Lyme disease:* PO 500 mg bid × 20 days.

• *Uncomplicated urinary tract infections, skin infections, disseminated gonococcal infections, uncomplicated pneumonia:* IM/IV 750 mg-1.5 g q8h

• *Bone and joint infections:* IM/IV 1.5 g q8h

• *Surgical prophylaxis:* IV 1.5 g ½-1 hr preop

• *Severe infections including meningitis:* IM/IV 1.5 g q6h; may give up to 3 g q8h for bacterial meningitis

• *Dosage in renal impairment:* CrCl >20 ml/min, use 750 mg-1.5 g q8h; CrCl 10-20 ml/min, use 750 mg q12h; CrCl <10 ml/min, use 750 mg q24h; since cefuroxime sodium is dialyzable, patients on hemodialysis should be given a further dose at the end of the dialysis

Child

• *Pharyngitis, tonsillitis, bronchitis:* Age >12 yr PO (tab) 250-500 mg q12h; age 3 mo-12 yr PO (susp) 20 mg/kg/day, divided bid, max dose 500 mg daily

• *Skin infections:* Age >12 yr PO (tab) 250-500 mg q12h; age 3 mo-12 yr PO (susp) 30 mg/kg/day, divided bid, max dose 1000 mg daily

• *Otitis media:* Age >12 yr PO (tab) 250 mg bid, age 3 mo-12 yr PO (susp) 30 mg/kg/day, divided bid, max dose 1000 mg daily

• *Uncomplicated urinary tract infections, skin infections, disseminated gonococcal infections, uncomplicated pneumonia:* Age >3 mo IM/IV 50-100 mg/kg qd (not to exceed the max adult dosage) in equally divided doses q8h

• *Bone and joint infections:* Age >3 mo IM/IV 150 mg/kg qd (not to exceed the max adult dosage) in equally divided doses q8h

• *Severe infections including meningitis:* Age >3 mo IM/IV 50-100 mg/kg qd in equally divided doses q6-8h; may give up to 200-240 mg/kg/day IV in divided doses for bacterial meningitis

S **AVAILABLE FORMS/COST OF THERAPY**

• Inj, Dry-Sol—IM; IV: 750 mg/vial: **$6.40-$7.79**; 1.5 g/vial: **$12.42-$23.90**

• Powder, Reconst—Oral: 125 mg/5 ml, 50, 100, 200 ml: **$36.08**/100 ml; 250 mg/5 ml, 50, 100 ml: **$58.51**/100 ml

• Tab, Coated—Oral: 125 mg, 60's: **$129.07**; 250 mg, 60's: **$241.80**; 500 mg, 60's: **$401.82**

CONTRAINDICATIONS: Infants <1 mo

PRECAUTIONS: Hypersensitivity to penicillins, renal disease, history of GI disease, colitis

PREGNANCY AND LACTATION: Pregnancy category B; excreted in breast milk

SIDE EFFECTS/ADVERSE REACTIONS

CNS: Chills, dizziness, fever, headache, paresthesia, weakness

GI: Abdominal pain, anorexia, ***bleeding;*** diarrhea, glossitis, increased LFTs; nausea, ***pseudomembranous colitis,*** vomiting

GU: Candidiasis, ***nephrotoxicity,*** vaginitis

HEME: ***Bone marrow suppression,*** eosinophilia, ***hemolytic anemia,*** lymphocytosis, thrombocytosis

RESP: Dyspnea

SKIN: Rash, urticaria

INTERACTIONS

Drugs

3 *Aminoglycosides:*   Additive nephrotoxicity

3 *Antacids, H_2-blockers, omeprazole, lansoprazole:* Decreased absorption of cefuroxime axetil

3 *Loop diuretics:* Increased nephrotoxicity

SPECIAL CONSIDERATIONS

• Oral tabs and oral susp not bioequivalent

• Take with food

• Alternative to amoxicillin or co-trimoxazole for resistant upper respiratory pathogens; expensive, but bid dosing

---

* = non-FDA-approved use

celecoxib

(sel-eh-cox'ib)
Rx: Celebrex
Chemical Class: Cyclooxyge-
nase-2 (COX-2) inhibitor
Therapeutic Class: Nonsteroi-
dal antiinflammatory drug
(NSAID)

CLINICAL PHARMACOLOGY
Mechanism of Action: Suppression
of production of prostaglandin E₂ at
inflammation sites via inhibition of
the cyclooxygenase-2 (COX-2) isoform. COX-2 is the inducible isoform, responsible for production of
the inflammatory prostaglandins.
Nonsteroidal   antiinflammatory
drug (NSAID) (analgesic, antipyretic, antiinflammatory)
Pharmacokinetics
PO: Peak about 3 hr; food enhanced
bioavailability; 97% bound to
plasma protein; extensively metabolized by liver (via CYP450 2C9-3
inactive metabolites), excreted in
urine (27%) and feces (57%); t₁/₂
9-10 hr; crosses placenta
INDICATIONS AND USES: Signs
and symptoms of osteoarthritis and
rheumatoid arthritis, moderate to severe pain, primary dysmenorrhea,
reduce number of adenomatous colorectal polyps in familial adenomatous polyposis, dental pain*
DOSAGE
Adult and Child >16 yr
• *Osteoarthritis:* PO 200 mg qd or
100 mg bid
• *Rheumatoid arthritis:* PO 100-200
mg bid
• *Acute pain and primary dysmenorrhea:* 400 mg initially, additional
200 mg prn on first day, 200 mg bid
prn subsequent days
• *Familial adenomatous polyposis:*
400 mg bid with food

• *Dosage in hepatic impairment:*
Child-Pugh Class II hepatic impairment, reduce dose by 50%
**💲 AVAILABLE FORMS/COST
OF THERAPY**
• Cap—Oral: 100 mg, 100's:
$149.00; 200 mg, 100's: **$257.00**
CONTRAINDICATIONS: Documented allergic-type reaction to sulfonamides, rhinitis, urticaria,
asthma, or allergic reactions to aspirin or other antiinflammatory agents
PRECAUTIONS: Late pregnancy
(premature closure of ductus arteriosus), liver dysfunction, hypertension, congestive heart failure, previous history of gastrointestinal ulceration, bleeding, or perforation, renal
dysfunction, concurrent use of warfarin
PREGNANCY AND LACTATION:
Pregnancy category C; breast milk
secretion, unknown
**SIDE EFFECTS/ADVERSE REAC-
TIONS**
CNS: Dizziness, headache
CV: Fluid retention, peripheral
edema
EENT: Hypersensitivity reactions in
aspirin-sensitive asthma patients
GI: Dyspepsia, diarrhea, abdominal
pain, flatulence, ulcer, ***gastrointestinal bleed,*** LFT elevations
*GU: **Acute renal failure***
*RESP: Upper respiratory tract infec-
tion,* sinusitis, pharyngitis, rhinitis
INTERACTIONS
Drugs
3 *Diuretics:* Potential reduction of
both diuretic and antihypertensive
effects of loop and thiazide diuretics
3 *ACE-inhibitors:* May reduce antihypertensive effect of ACE-inhibitors
3 *Fluconazole:* Two-fold increase
in celecoxib plasma concentration
due to inhibition of CYP2C9
3 *Lithium:* Steady-state lithium
plasma levels increased 18%

3 *Warfarin:* Bleeding events reported, predominantly in elderly; increases in PT possible

SPECIAL CONSIDERATIONS

• COX-2 specific inhibition good choice for patients with inflammatory conditions who are at high risk of gastrointestinal adverse effects (e.g., older than 60 years, history of peptic ulcer disease, prolonged, high-dose NSAID therapy, concurrent use of corticosteroids or anticoagulants)

MONITORING PARAMETERS

• Rheumatoid arthritis—Decreased acute phase reactants (ESR, C-reactive protein), pain relief, reduction in number of swollen joints, improved range of motion, less fatigue, functional capacity, structural damage, maintenance of normal lifestyle
• Osteoarthritis—Decreased pain and stiffness of affected joints
• Toxicity—Initial hemogram, fecal occult blood, then q 6-12 mo; electrolytes and renal function tests q 6-12 mo; LFT's q 6-12 mo in high-risk patients; query patient for dyspepsia, nausea, vomiting, right upper abdominal pain, anorexia, fatigue, jaundice, edema, weight gain, decreased urine output

---

cellulose sodium phosphate

Rx: Calcibind
Chemical Class: Phosphorylated cellulose
Therapeutic Class: Hypercalciuria

CLINICAL PHARMACOLOGY

Mechanism of Action: Decreases hypercalciuria by binding with calcium in bowel; reduces urinary calcium by approximately 50 mg/5 g qd of CSP

Pharmacokinetics
Not absorbed

INDICATIONS AND USES: Absorptive hypercalciuria type I with recurrent calcium oxalate or calcium phosphate renal stones

DOSAGE

Adult

• PO 15 g qd in divided doses with each meal, then 10 g qd (5 g with supper, 2.5 g with each remaining meal) when 24 hr urine Ca excretion <150 mg; for each 15 g qd of CSP, give 1.5 g magnesium gluconate bid (at least 1 hr before or after a dose of CSP)

$ **AVAILABLE FORMS/COST OF THERAPY**

• Powder, Reconst—Oral: 2.5 g/scoop, 300 g: **$103.13**

CONTRAINDICATIONS: Hyperparathyroidism, hypomagnesemia, enteric hyperoxaluria, metabolic bone disease, hypocalcemia

PRECAUTIONS: CHF, ascites, liver disease, children <16, elderly

PREGNANCY AND LACTATION: Pregnancy category C

SIDE EFFECTS/ADVERSE REACTIONS

GI: Anorexia, diarrhea, dyspepsia, nausea
GU: Hyperoxaluria, hyperphosphaturia, hypomagnesuria
METAB: Depletion of trace metals (copper, zinc, iron), hypomagnesemia

SPECIAL CONSIDERATIONS
PATIENT/FAMILY EDUCATION

• Suspend each dose of CSP powder in glass of water, soft drink or fruit juice
• Injest within 30 min of a meal

MONITORING PARAMETERS

• Serum Ca, Mg, copper, zinc, iron, parathyroid hormone, CBC every 3 to 6 mo

---

• Serum parathyroid hormone should be obtained at least once between the 1st 2 wk to 3 mo of treatment

---

cephalexin

(sef-a-lex'in)

Rx: Biocef, Keflex, Keftab
Chemical Class: Cephalosporin (1st generation)
Therapeutic Class: Antibiotic

CLINICAL PHARMACOLOGY
Mechanism of Action: Inhibits bacterial cell wall synthesis; bactericidal
Pharmacokinetics
PO: Peak 1 hr (15 μg/ml after 500 mg), duration 6-8 hr, 5%-15% bound by plasma proteins; 90%-100% eliminated unchanged in urine within 8 hr; crosses placenta; $t_{1/2}$ 30-72 min; may be given without regard to meals
INDICATIONS AND USES: Pharyngitis, tonsillitis, otitis media, bronchitis, pneumonia, skin, bone and urinary tract infections caused by susceptible organisms
Antibacterial spectrum usually includes:
• Gram-positive organisms: *Streptococcus pneumoniae, S. pyogenes, Staphylococcus aureus*
• Gram-negative organisms: *H. influenzae, E. coli, P. mirabilis, Moraxella catarrhalis, Klebsiella* sp.
DOSAGE
Adult
• *Bronchitis, pneumonia, urinary tract infections:* PO 250-500 mg q6h
• *Pharyngitis, tonsillitis, cystitis, mild to moderate skin infections:* PO 500 mg q12h
• *Severe infections:* PO 500 mg-1 g q6h

• *Dosage in renal impairment:* CrCl 11-40 ml/min, max adult dose 500 mg q8-12h; CrCl 5-10 ml/min, max adult dose 250 mg q12h; CrCl <5 ml/min, max adult dose 250 mg q12-24h
Child
• *Bronchitis, pneumonia, urinary tract infections:* PO 25-50 mg/kg/day in 4 equal doses
• *Pharyngitis, tonsillitis, cystitis, mild to moderate skin infections:* Age >15 yr PO 500 mg q12h; age >1 yr PO 25-50 mg/kg/day in 2 equal doses
• *Severe infections:* PO 50-100 mg/kg/day in 4 equal doses
• *Otitis media:* PO 75-100 mg/kg/day in 4 equal doses
$ AVAILABLE FORMS/COST OF THERAPY
• Cap, Gel—Oral: 250 mg, 100's: **$15.80-$141.67**; 500 mg, 100's: **$25.00-$337.20**
• Powder, Reconst—Oral: 125 mg/5 ml, 100, 200 ml: **$3.78-$21.00**/100 ml; 250 mg/5 ml, 100, 200 ml: **$5.69-$32.99**/100 ml
• Tab, Plain Coated—Oral: 500 mg, 100's: **$206.59-$317.27**
CONTRAINDICATIONS: Infants <1 mo
PRECAUTIONS: Hypersensitivity to penicillins, renal disease
PREGNANCY AND LACTATION: Pregnancy category B; excreted in breast milk
SIDE EFFECTS/ADVERSE REACTIONS
CNS: Chills, dizziness, fever, headache, paresthesia, weakness
GI: Abdominal pain, anorexia, ***bleeding;*** *diarrhea,* glossitis, increased LFTs, nausea, ***pseudomembranous colitis,*** vomiting
GU: Candidiasis, ***nephrotoxicity,*** proteinuria, pruritus, vaginitis

---

italic = common side effects   **bold italic** = life-threatening reactions

HEME: **Bone marrow suppression,** eosinophilia, **hemolytic anemia,** lymphocytosis, thrombocytosis
RESP: Dyspnea
SKIN: Dermatitis, rash, urticaria
MISC: Serum sickness-like syndrome

INTERACTIONS
Drugs
3 *Aminoglycosides:* Additive nephrotoxicity
3 *Loop diuretics:* Increased nephrotoxicity
Labs
• *Increase:* Urinary amino acids
• *False positive:* Urine glucose with Benedict's, Fehlings, Clinitest
• *Decrease:* Urine leukocytes

SPECIAL CONSIDERATIONS
• 1st generation oral cephalosporin of choice

---

cephalothin
(sef-a-loe'thin)
Rx: Keflin
Chemical Class: Cephalosporin (1st generation)
Therapeutic Class: Antibiotic

CLINICAL PHARMACOLOGY
Mechanism of Action: Inhibits bacterial wall synthesis; bactericidal
Pharmacokinetics
IM: Peak 0.5 hr; 65%-80% bound by plasma proteins; excreted by the kidneys (inhibited by probenecid); $t_{1/2}$ ½-1 hr

INDICATIONS AND USES: Infections of the respiratory tract, skin and skin structures, genitourinary tract, gastrointestinal tract, bones and joints; endocarditis, septicemia; perioperative prophylaxis for contaminated or potentially contaminated procedures

Antibacterial spectrum usually includes:
• Gram-positive organisms: Group A β-hemolytic streptococci, staphylococci (including coagulase-positive, coagulase-negative, and penicillinase-producing strains [not MRSA]); *Streptococcus pneumoniae*
• Gram-negative organisms: *Haemophilus influenzae, Escherichia coli, Klebsiella* sp., *Proteus mirabilis, Salmonella* sp., *Shigella* sp.

DOSAGE
Adult
• IM/IV 500 mg-1 g q4-6h
• *Uncomplicated gonorrhea:* IM 2 g as single dose
• *Severe infections:* IM/IV 1-2 g q4h Dosage reduction indicated in renal impairment (CrCl <50 ml/min)
• *Preoperative:* IV 1-2 g ½-1 hrs prior to procedure
Child
• IM/IV 14-27 mg/kg q4h or 20-40 mg/kg q6h

🛇 AVAILABLE FORMS/COST OF THERAPY
• Inj, Dry-Sol—IM, IV: 1 g/vial: **$3.42-$3.99**; 2 g/vial: **$6.84-$7.41**
• Inj, Premix—IV: 1 g/50 ml: **$10.08**; 2 g/50 ml: **$14.30**

PRECAUTIONS: Hypersensitivity to penicillins, renal disease
PREGNANCY AND LACTATION: Pregnancy category B; excreted into breast milk in low concentrations; no adverse effects have been observed

SIDE EFFECTS/ADVERSE REACTIONS
CNS: Chills, dizziness, fever, headache, paresthesia, weakness
GI: Abdominal pain, anorexia, **bleeding; diarrhea,** glossitis, increased LFTs; nausea, **pseudomembranous colitis,** vomiting
GU: Candidiasis, **nephrotoxicity,** proteinuria, pruritus, vaginitis

---

* = non-FDA-approved use

HEME: **Bone marrow suppression,** eosinophilia, **hemolytic anemia,** lymphocytosis
RESP: Dyspnea
SKIN: Dermatitis, rash, urticaria

INTERACTIONS
Drugs
🛇 Aminoglycosides: Additive nephrotoxicity
🛇 Furosemide: Increased nephrotoxicity

Labs
• False positive: Urinary protein; urinary glucose by Benedict's or Fehling's solution, Clinitest tabs
• False increase: Creatinine (serum, urine), urinary 17-KS
• False decrease: Urine leukocytes

---

cephapirin

(sef-a-peer'in)
Rx: Cefadyl
Chemical Class: Cephalosporin (1st generation)
Therapeutic Class: Antibiotic

CLINICAL PHARMACOLOGY
Mechanism of Action: Inhibits bacterial cell wall synthesis; bactericidal

Pharmacokinetics
IM: Peak 30 min, 44-50% bound by plasma proteins; metabolized in liver, 40%-70% eliminated unchanged in urine; $t_{1/2}$ 21-47 min

INDICATIONS AND USES: Infections of the respiratory tract, skin and skin structures, urinary tract; septicemia; endocarditis; osteomyelitis; perioperative prophylaxis for contaminated or potentially contaminated procedures

Antibacterial spectrum usually includes:

• Gram-positive organisms: Group A β-hemolytic streptococci, staphylococci (including coagulaseposi-

tive, coagulase-negative, and penicillinase-producing strains [not MRSA]); Streptococcus pneumoniae

• Gram-negative organisms: Haemophilus influenzae, Escherichia coli, Klebsiella sp., Proteus mirabilis

DOSAGE
Adult
• IM/IV 500 mg-1 g q4-6h, maximum 12 g/day
• Preoperative: IV/IM 1-2 g ½-1 hr prior to surgery
• Renal function impairment (serum creatinine >5 mg/dl): IM/IV 7.5-15 mg/kg q12h
Child
• IM/IV 40-80 mg/kg/day divided q6h

💲 **AVAILABLE FORMS/COST OF THERAPY**
• Inj, Dry-Sol—IM; IV: 1 g/vial: **$1.64**

PRECAUTIONS: Hypersensitivity to penicillins, renal disease, prolonged use, colitis

PREGNANCY AND LACTATION: Pregnancy category B; excreted into breast milk in low concentrations; no adverse effects have been observed

SIDE EFFECTS/ADVERSE REACTIONS
CNS: Chills, dizziness, fever, headache, paresthesia, weakness
GI: Abdominal pain, anorexia, **bleeding; diarrhea,** glossitis, increased LFTs; nausea, **pseudomembranous colitis,** vomiting
GU: Candidiasis, **nephrotoxicity,** proteinuria, pruritus, vaginitis
HEME: **Bone marrow suppression,** eosinophilia, **hemolytic anemia,** lymphocytosis
RESP: Dyspnea
SKIN: Dermatitis, rash, urticaria

---

italic = common side effects   ***bold italic*** = life-threatening reactions

INTERACTIONS
Drugs
3 *Aminoglycosides:* Additive nephrotoxicity

3 *Loop diuretics:* Increased nephrotoxicity

SPECIAL CONSIDERATIONS
• No advantage over cefazolin; price should guide usage of 1st generation cephalosporins

---

cephradine
(sef'ra-deen)

Rx: Velosef

Chemical Class: Cephalosporin (1st generation)

Therapeutic Class: Antibiotic

CLINICAL PHARMACOLOGY
Mechanism of Action: Inhibits bacterial cell wall synthesis; bactericidal

Pharmacokinetics
PO: Peak 1 hr

IM: Peak 1 hr

8%-17% bound to plasma proteins; 80%-90% eliminated unchanged in urine; $t_{1/2}$ 0.75-1.5 hr

INDICATIONS AND USES: Infections of the respiratory tract, skin and skin structure, urinary tract; otitis media; osteomyelitis

Antibacterial spectrum usually includes:

• Gram-positive organisms: Group A β-hemolytic streptococci, staphylococci (including penicillinase-producing strains [not MRSA]); *Streptococcus pneumoniae*

• Gram-negative organisms: *Escherichia coli, Proteus mirabilis, Klebsiella* spp., *Hemophilus influenzae*

DOSAGE
Adult
• *Skin, respiratory infections:* PO 250 mg q6h or 500 mg q12h

• *Lobar pneumonia:* PO 500 mg q6h or 1g q12h

• *UTI:* PO 500 mg q12 (up to 1 g q6h may be administered for severe infections)

• *Renal function impairment:* PO CrCl 5-20 ml/min 250 mg q6h; CrCl <5 ml/min 250 mg q12h

Child >9 mo
• PO 25-50 mg/kg/day divided q6h or q12h

• *Otitis media:* PO 75-100 mg/kg/day divided q6h or q12h; max 4g/day

§ AVAILABLE FORMS/COST OF THERAPY
• Cap, Gel—Oral: 250 mg, 100's: **$30.00-$98.81**; 500 mg, 100's: **$52.00-$209.05**

• Powder, Reconst—Oral:: 125 mg/5 ml, 100, 200 ml: **$4.25-$10.14**/100 ml; 250 mg/5 ml, 100, 200 ml: **$7.98-$20.33**/100 ml

PRECAUTIONS: Hypersensitivity to penicillins, renal disease

PREGNANCY AND LACTATION: Pregnancy category B; excreted into breast milk in low concentrations; no adverse effects have been observed

SIDE EFFECTS/ADVERSE REACTIONS
CNS: Chills, dizziness, fever, headache, paresthesia, weakness

GI: Abdominal pain, anorexia, **bleeding; diarrhea,** glossitis, increased LFTs; nausea, **pseudomembranous colitis,** vomiting

GU: Candidiasis, **nephrotoxicity,** proteinuria, pruritus, vaginitis

HEME: **Bone marrow suppression,** eosinophilia, **hemolytic anemia,** lymphocytosis

RESP: Dyspnea

SKIN: Dermatitis, rash, urticaria

INTERACTIONS
Drugs
3 *Aminoglycosides:* Additive nephrotoxicity

3 *Loop diuretics:* Increased nephrotoxicity

SPECIAL CONSIDERATIONS

• No advantage over cephalexin; cost should be major consideration for selection of first generation cephalosporins

---

cetirizine

(si-tear'a-zeen)
Rx: Zyrtec
Chemical Class: Piperazine derivative
Therapeutic Class: Antihistamine

CLINICAL PHARMACOLOGY

Mechanism of Action: Decreases allergic response by blocking histamine at H_1-receptors; negligible anticholinergic and antiserotonergic activity; negligible brain penetration and interaction with cerebral H_1-receptors

Pharmacokinetics

PO: Peak 1 hr; rapid absorption reduced by food; 93% protein bound; 70% excreted by kidneys (primarily as unchanged drug, 10% in feces); $t_{1/2}$ 8.3 hr

INDICATIONS AND USES: Seasonal and perennial allergic rhinitis; chronic idiopathic urticaria

DOSAGE

Adult

• PO 5-10 mg qd prn; reduce dose to 5 mg qd for patients with decreased renal function (CrCl <30) and in hepatically impaired patients

Child ≥6 yr

• PO 5-10 mg qd prn

$ **AVAILABLE FORMS/COST OF THERAPY**

• Syrup—Oral: 5 mg/5 ml, 480 ml: **$119.12**
• Tab, Coated—Oral: 5, 10 mg, 100's: **$203.83**

PRECAUTIONS: Activities requiring mental alertness; coadministration with alcohol and other CNS depressants

PREGNANCY AND LACTATION: Pregnancy category B; excreted into breast milk

SIDE EFFECTS/ADVERSE REACTIONS

CNS: Anorexia, confusion, depression, fatigue, headache, insomnia, nervousness, paresthesia, *somnolence*

CV: **Cardiac failure,** flushing, hypertension, palpitation, tachycardia

EENT: Deafness, earache, epistaxis, ototoxicity, rhinitis, tinnitus

GI: Diarrhea, dry mouth, dyspepsia, flatulence, increased appetite, increased salivation, nausea, vomiting

GU: Breast pain, cystitis, dysmenorrhea, dysuria, hematuria, polyuria, urinary retention

METAB: Dehydration, diabetes mellitus, thirst

MS: Arthralgia, arthritis, arthrosis, muscle weakness, myalgia

RESP: Bronchospasm, coughing, dyspnea

MISC: Lymphadenopathy

SPECIAL CONSIDERATIONS

• H_1 antagonist with minimal effect on CNS; no affinity for other receptors
• Very potent antihistamine
• Kinetics allow qd dosing and do not have cytochrome P-450 drug interactions
• Effective versus itching

---

italic = common side effects   ***bold italic*** = life-threatening reactions

cevimeline

(sev-im'el-ine)
Rx: Evoxac
Chemical Class: Oxathiolane derivative
Therapeutic Class: Salivation stimulant

CLINICAL PHARMACOLOGY

Mechanism of Action: Cholinergic agonist which binds to muscarinic receptors; increases secretion of salivary glands

Pharmacokinetics

PO: Peak 1.5-2 hr (delayed by administration with food); <20% bound to plasma proteins, extensively bound to tissues; metabolized by liver (CYP 2D6 and CYP 3A3/4), excreted in urine (84% of dose after 24 hr); $t_{1/2}$ 5 hr

INDICATIONS AND USES: Symptoms of dry mouth in patients with Sjögren's Syndrome

DOSAGE

Adult
• PO 30 mg tid

💲 AVAILABLE FORMS/COST OF THERAPY
• Cap, Gel—Oral: 30 mg, 100's: **$143.06**

CONTRAINDICATIONS: Uncontrolled asthma; acute iritis; angle-closure glaucoma

PRECAUTIONS: Cardiovascular disease; controlled asthma, chronic bronchitis, COPD; history of nephrolithiasis or cholelithiasis; children

PREGNANCY AND LACTATION: Pregnancy category C; excretion into breast milk unknown, use caution in nursing mothers

SIDE EFFECTS/ADVERSE REACTIONS

CNS: Headache, depression
CV: Peripheral edema, chest pain
EENT: Rhinitis, conjunctivitis, abnormal vision, eye pain, ear ache, salivary gland pain, salivary gland enlargement, sialoadenitis, ulcerative stomatitis
GI: Nausea, diarrhea, excessive salivation, abdominal pain, vomiting, constipation, dry mouth, gastroesophageal reflux
GU: Vaginitis
HEME: Anemia
MS: Arthralgia, skeletal pain, myalgia, leg cramps
RESP: Coughing
SKIN: Pruritus, skin disorder, rash
MISC: Excessive sweating, fatigue, insomnia, hot flushes, tremor, hypertonia, fever, anorexia, vertigo, hiccup, hyporeflexia, hypoesthesia

INTERACTIONS

Drugs

3 *Beta-blockers:* Increased possibility of cardiac conduction disturbances

3 *Parasympathomimetics:* Additive pharmacologic effects

3 *Antimuscarinics:* Potential interference with desirable antimuscarinic effects

SPECIAL CONSIDERATIONS
PATIENT/FAMILY EDUCATION

• May cause visual disturbance, use caution driving at night or performing hazardous activities in reduced lighting

• Ensure adequate fluid intake to prevent dehydration, especially if drug causes excessive sweating

charcoal, activated

(char'coal)

OTC: *Oral caps:* CharcoCaps
Oral tablets: Charco Plus DS
Oral Suspensions (activated):
Actidose-Aqua, Liqui-Char,
CharcoAide
Combinations
  OTC: with simethicone
  (Charcoal Plus, Flatulex);
  with sorbitol (Actidose with
  sorbitol)
Chemical Class: Carbon
Therapeutic Class: Antiflatu-
lent; antidote (activated);
antidiarrheal

CLINICAL PHARMACOLOGY

Mechanism of Action: Adsorbent,
detoxicant, soothing agent; reduces
volume of intestinal gas; binds poi-
sons, toxins, irritants in GI tract;
bound toxins inactive until excreted

Pharmacokinetics

PO: Insoluble in water; excreted in
feces

INDICATIONS AND USES: Flatulence; emergency treatment in most
poisonings; dyspepsia, abdominal
distention; deodorant in wounds; diarrhea

DOSAGE

Adult

• *Flatulence/dyspepsia:* PO 520-
975 mg pc up to 4.16 g/day

• *Poisoning:* PO 25-100 g (or 1 g/kg
or approximately 10 × the amount
of poison ingested; may give 20-40
g q6h for 1-2 days in severe poisoning

Child <1 yr

• *Poisoning:* 1 g/kg as single dose

Child 1-12 yr

• *Poisoning:* 25-50 g as single dose

**$ AVAILABLE FORMS/COST
OF THERAPY**

• Cap—Oral: 260 mg, 100's: **$2.00**

• Susp (activated)—Oral: 15 g/75
ml, 75, 150 ml: **$3.60**/75 ml; 25
g/120 ml: **$4.50-$7.61**

• Tab—Oral: 250 mg, 125's: **$7.43**

• Tab, enteric coated—Oral: 250
mg, 125's: **$13.56**

CONTRAINDICATIONS: Unconsciousness, semiconsciousness;
poisoning with cyanide, mineral acids, alkalies

PRECAUTIONS: Absence of bowel
sounds

SIDE EFFECTS/ADVERSE REAC-
TIONS

GI: Black stools, constipation, diarrhea, nausea, vomiting

INTERACTIONS

Drugs

❷ *Digitalis glycosides:* Reduced
digoxin levels; less effect on digitoxin

SPECIAL CONSIDERATIONS

• Administer activated charcoal for
adsorption in emergency management of poisonings as a slurry with
water, a saline cathartic, or sorbitol

chenodiol

(kee-noe-dye'ole)

Rx: Chenix
Chemical Class: Chenodeoxy-
cholic acid
Therapeutic Class:
Cholelitholytic

CLINICAL PHARMACOLOGY

Mechanism of Action: Suppresses
hepatic synthesis of cholesterol and
cholic acid, replacing cholic acid
with drug metabolite; contributes to
biliary cholesterol desaturation and
gradual dissolution of radiolucent
cholesterol gallstones; has no effects
on radiopaque (calcified) gallstones
or on radiolucent bile pigment
stones

italic = common side effects   ***bold italic*** = life-threatening reactions

Pharmacokinetics

PO: Extensive enterohepatic recirculation; 80% excreted in feces as metabolite

INDICATIONS AND USES: Dissolution of gallstones in patients with radiolucent stones in well-opacifying gallbladders, in whom effective surgery would be undertaken except for the presence of increased surgical risk due to systemic disease or age (the likelihood of successful dissolution is far greater if the stones are floatable or small)

DOSAGE

Adult

• PO 250 mg bid for 2 wk, then increased by 250 mg/day, not to exceed 16 mg/kg/day

⑤ AVAILABLE FORMS/COST OF THERAPY

• Tab, Plain Coated—Oral: 250 mg, 100's: **$107.98**

CONTRAINDICATIONS: Hepatic disease, bile duct abnormalities, biliary GI fistula

PRECAUTIONS: Children, atherosclerosis, elderly, colon cancer

PREGNANCY AND LACTATION: Pregnancy category X; excretion into breast milk unknown; use extreme caution in nursing mothers

SIDE EFFECTS/ADVERSE REACTIONS

GI: Absence of taste, *biliary pain,* cramps; *diarrhea,* dyspepsia, dysphagia, fecal urgency, flatulence, heartburn, hepatotoxicity, increased ALT, AST, LDH (50% of patients); *nausea,* vomiting

*HEME: **Leukopenia***

METAB: Increased total and LDL-cholesterol

SPECIAL CONSIDERATIONS

• Comparative trials of ursodiol and chenodiol show equivalent efficacy; ursodiol associated with less adverse effects, hence preferred

MONITORING PARAMETERS

• Monthly aminotransferase levels for 3 mo then q3 mo

• Serum cholesterol, cholecystogram or ultrasonogram, CBC

---

chloral hydrate

(klor-al hye′drate)

Rx: Aquachloral, Noctec

Chemical Class: Halogenated alcohol

Therapeutic Class: Sedative/hypnotic

DEA Class: Schedule IV

CLINICAL PHARMACOLOGY

Mechanism of Action: CNS depressant effects are due to active metabolite trichloroethanol: hypnotic doses produce mild cerebral depression and quiet deep sleep with little or no "hangover"; slight blood pressure and respiration depression; uncertain effects on REM sleep

Pharmacokinetics

PO: Onset 30 min-1 hr, duration 4-8 hr

PR: Onset slow, duration 4-6 hr

Metabolized by liver to trichloroethanol, excreted by kidneys and feces; $t_{1/2}$ (trichloroethanol) 8-11 hr

INDICATIONS AND USES: Nocturnal sedation, preoperative sedation, sedation prior to EEG evaluations; adjunct to opiates and analgesics in postoperative care and pain control; alcohol withdrawal

DOSAGE

Adult

• *Sedation:* PO/PR 250 mg tid pc

• *Hypnotic:* PO/PR 500 mg-1 g ½ hr before bedtime or ½ hr before surgery; max 2 g/day

Child

• *Sedative:* PO 8 mg/kg tid; not to exceed 500 mg tid

---

* = non-FDA-approved use

• *Hypnotic:* PO/PR 50 mg/kg in one dose; not to exceed 1 g

§ AVAILABLE FORMS/COST OF THERAPY

• Cap, Gel—Oral: 500 mg, 100's: **$7.31**
• Supp—Rect: 325 mg, 12's: **$29.13**; 500 mg, 100's: **$125.00-$213.50**; 650 mg, 12's: **$39.75**
• Syr—Oral: 500 mg/5 ml, 480 ml: **$9.41-$13.79**

CONTRAINDICATIONS: Severe renal disease, hepatic disease, or cardiac disease; gastritis

PRECAUTIONS: Cardiac disease, GI conditions, acute intermittant porphyria, history of drug abuse, tartrazine sensitivity, elderly

PREGNANCY AND LACTATION: Pregnancy category C; excreted into breast milk; may cause mild drowsiness in infant, otherwise compatible with breast feeding

SIDE EFFECTS/ADVERSE REACTIONS

CNS: Ataxia, disorientation, dizziness, *drowsiness,* hallucinations (rare), hangover (rare), headache, lightheadedness, mental confusion, nightmares, paranoia, somnambulism, stimulation

GI: Diarrhea, flatulence, gastric irritation, nausea, unpleasant taste, vomiting

HEME: Eosinophilia, **leukopenia**

SKIN: Eczematoid dermatitis, erythema, hives, rash, scarlatiniform exanthems, urticaria

INTERACTIONS

Drugs

❸ *Ethanol:* Additive CNS-depressant effects

❸ *Warfarin:* Transient increase in the hypoprothrombinemic response to warfarin

Labs

• *Interference:* Urine catecholamines, urinary 17-hydroxycorticosteroids

• *False positive:* Urine glucose (Benedict's reagent)
• *False increase:* Serum urea nitrogen, vitamin B_{12}

SPECIAL CONSIDERATIONS

• Not as effective as benzodiazepines, loses much of effectiveness for inducing and maintaining sleep after 2 weeks of use
• Frequently used preoperatively or preprocedurally in children because less paradoxical excitement (not confirmed by well-controlled studies)

PATIENT/FAMILY EDUCATION

• May cause GI upset, recommend administration with full glass of water or fruit juice, dilute syrup in a half glass of water or fruit juice

---

chloramphenicol
(klor-am-fen´i-kole)

Rx: *Systemic:* Chloromycetin
Ophthalmic: Chloromycetin
Ophthalmic, Chloroptic;
Otic: Chloromycetin Otic
Combinations

  Rx: Topical: with desoxyribonuclease and fibrinolysin (Elase-Chloromycetin); Ophthalmic: Hydrocortisone acetate and polymixin B sulfate (Opthocort); hydrocortisone acetate (Chloromycetin Hydrocortisone)

Chemical Class: Dichloroacetic acid derivative
Therapeutic Class: Antibiotic

CLINICAL PHARMACOLOGY
Mechanism of Action: Reversibly binds to 50S ribosomal subunits of susceptible organisms, thus inhibiting protein synthesis

italic = common side effects   ***bold italic*** = life-threatening reactions

Pharmacokinetics

PO/IV: Peak 1-2 hr, duration 8 hr; 60% bound to plasma proteins; $t_{1/2}$ 1.5-4 hr; conjugated in liver, excreted in urine (up to 15% as free drug) and feces (in neonates, 6%-80% of drug excreted unchanged in the urine; $t_{1/2}$ 10-24 hr)

INDICATIONS AND USES: *Systemic:* Meningitis, paratyphoid fever, Q fever, rickettsial pox, Rocky Mountain spotted fever, septicemia, typhoid fever, typhus infections; serious infections due to organisms resistant to other less toxic antibiotics or when its penetration into the site of infection is clinically superior to other antibiotics to which the organisms are sensitive; *ophthalmic:* superficial ocular infections involving the conjunctiva or cornea (use only in serious infections for which less toxic drugs are ineffective or contraindicated); *otic:* superficial infections involving the external auditory canal; *topical:* infected skin lesions Antibacterial spectrum usually includes:

• Gram-positive organisms: *Streptococcus pneumoniae* and other streptococci
• Gram-negative organisms: *Haemophilus influenzae, Neisseria meningitidis, Salmonella, Proteus mirabilis, Pseudomonas mallei, P. cepacia, Vibrio cholerae, Francisella tularensis, Yersinia pestis, Brucella, Shigella*
• Anaerobes: *Prevotella melaningogenica, B. fragilis, Clostridium, Fusobacterium, Veillonella*
• Other: *Rickettsia, Chlamydia,* and *Mycoplasma*

DOSAGE

Adult

• PO/IV 50-100 mg/kg/day divided q6h, max 4 g/day; OPHTH apply 1 gtt or small amount of ointment q3-6h, increase interval between applications after 48 hr; OTIC instill 2-3 gtt into the ear tid; TOP apply daily

Child

• *Meningitis:* IV 75-100 mg/kg/day divided q6h; max dose 4 g/day
• *Other infections:* IV 50-75 mg/kg/day divided q6h; max 4 g/day

Neonates

• IV 20 mg/kg loading dose, maintenance dose based on postnatal age (given 12 hr after loading dose); ≤7 days or ≤2000 g 25 mg/kg/day q24h; >7 days and >2000 g 50 mg/kg/day q12h

💲 **AVAILABLE FORMS/COST OF THERAPY**

• Cap—Oral: 250 mg, 100's: **$26.80-$125.43**; Oint—Ophth: 1%, 3.5 g: **$8.99-$14.94**
• Inj, Lyphl-Sol—IV: 1 g: **$6.25-$10.67**
• Oint—Ophth: 1%, 3.5 g: **$1.65-$20.52**
• Oint—Top: 1% with deoxyribonuclease and fibrinolysin, 30 g: **$40.80**
• Sol—Ophth: 0.5%, 2.5, 7.5, 15 ml: **$2.70-$27.69**/15 ml
• Sol—Otic: 5 mg/ml, 15 ml: **$27.68**

CONTRAINDICATIONS: Trivial infections, prophylaxis

PRECAUTIONS: Neonates (use in reduced dosages to avoid "gray baby syndrome" toxicity), repeated courses, prolonged therapy, impaired hepatic or renal function, acute intermittent porphyria, G-6-PD deficiency, bone marrow depression (drug induced)

PREGNANCY AND LACTATION: Pregnancy category C; use caution at term due to potential for "gray baby syndrome" toxicity; excreted into breast milk; milk levels are too low to precipitate the "gray baby syndrome," but a theoretical risk does exist for bone marrow depression

SIDE EFFECTS/ADVERSE REACTIONS

CNS: Confusion, delirium, headache, mild depression, peripheral neuropathy

CV: ***"Gray baby syndrome" in newborns (failure to feed, pallor, cyanosis, abdominal distention, irregular respiration, vasomotor collapse)***

EENT: Irritation in ear (otic preparations), itching, optic neuritis (prolonged therapy); overgrowth of nonsusceptible organisms (ophthalmic preparations); poor corneal wound healing, temporary visual haze

GI: Diarrhea, enterocolitis, glossitis, *nausea, vomiting*

HEME: ***Aplastic anemia, granulocytopenia, hypoplastic anemia, thrombocytopenia***

SKIN: Angioedema, burning, contact dermatitis, itching, rash, stinging, urticaria

INTERACTIONS

Drugs

🔳 *Barbiturates:* Increased serum barbiturate concentrations; reduced serum chloramphenicol concentrations

🔳 *Ceftazidime:* Inhibited antibacterial activity

🔳 *Cimetidine:* Increased risk of myelosuppression

🔳 *Penicillins:* Inhibited antibacterial activity of penicillins

🔳 *Phenytoin:* Predictable increases in serum phenytoin concentrations, toxicity has occurred

🔳 *Rifampin:* Reduced chloramphenicol concentrations

🔳 *Sulfonylureas:* Increased hypoglycemic effects of tolbutamide and chlorpropamide

❷ *Warfarin:* Enhanced hypoprothrombinemic response to warfarin and possibly other oral anticoagulants

Labs

• *False positive:* Urine glucose (copper reduction)
• *False decrease:* Serum folate, serum urea nitrogen, serum uric acid
• *False increase:* 17-ketosteroids, CSF protein, serum protein, serum urea nitrogen

SPECIAL CONSIDERATIONS

• Because of severe adverse effects (e.g. aplastic anemia) not indicated for less serious infections; aplastic anemia reported with topical use

MONITORING PARAMETERS

• CBC with platelets and reticulocytes before and frequently during therapy (discontinue drug if bone marrow depression occurs); serum iron and iron-binding globulin saturation may also be useful
• Serum drug level (peak 10-20 µg/ml, trough 5-10 µg/ml) weekly (more often in impaired hepatic, renal systems)
• Early signs of "gray baby syndrome" (cyanosis, abdominal distension, irregular respiration, failure to feed), ***drug should be discontinued immediately***

---

chlordiazepoxide
(klor-dye-az-e-pox′ide)
Rx: Libritabs, Librium, Mitran, Resposans-10
Combinations
  Rx: with amitriptyline (Limbitrol DS 10-25); with clidinium (Clindex, Librax)
Chemical Class: Benzodiazepine
Therapeutic Class: Anxiolytic
DEA Class: Schedule IV

CLINICAL PHARMACOLOGY

Mechanism of Action: CNS depressants via facilitation of inhibitory GABA at benzodiazepine receptor sites (BZ_1 associated with sleep; BZ_2—associated with memory, motor, sensory, and cognitive function); effects include muscle relaxation (spinal cord), anticonvulsant activity (brain stem), ataxia (cerebellum), emotional behavior (limbic and cortical areas), and anxiolytic effects (separate from general CNS depression); other effects include sedative, appetite-stimulating, and weak analgesic actions

Pharmacokinetics

PO: Onset 30 min, peak ½-4 hr

IM: Slow erratic absorption and lower peak plasma levels than oral or IV administration

Metabolized by liver to active metabolites, excreted by kidneys; $t_{½}$ 5-30 hr

INDICATIONS AND USES: Anxiety disorders, acute alcohol withdrawal, preoperative apprehension and anxiety; familial, senile, or essential action tremors*; tension headache,* panic disorders*

DOSAGE

Adult

• *Mild anxiety:* PO 5-10 mg tid-qid
• *Severe anxiety:* PO 20-25 mg tid-qid; IM/IV 50-100 mg initially, then 25-50 mg tid-qid prn
• *Preoperative apprehension and anxiety:* PO 5-10 mg tid-qid on days before surgery; IM 50-100 mg 1 hr before surgery
• *Acute alcohol withdrawal:* PO/IM/IV 50-100 mg initially; repeat in 2-4 hr prn; not to exceed 300 mg/day

Geriatric or debilitated patients

• PO 5 mg bid-qid

Child >6 yr

• PO 5 mg bid-qid, not to exceed 10 mg bid-tid

§ AVAILABLE FORMS/COST OF THERAPY

• Cap, Gel—Oral: 5 mg, 100's: **$0.94-$66.41**; 10 mg, 100's: **$1.11-$96.54**; 25 mg, 100's: **$1.34-$165.56**
• Inj, Conc, w/buf—IM, IV: 100 mg/ampul, 5 ml: **$20.34**

CONTRAINDICATIONS: Narrow-angle glaucoma, psychosis

PRECAUTIONS: Elderly, debilitated, hepatic disease, renal disease, long-term use, history of drug abuse

PREGNANCY AND LACTATION: Pregnancy category D; excreted into breast milk; drug and metabolites may accumulate to toxic levels in nursing infant

SIDE EFFECTS/ADVERSE REACTIONS

CNS: Anterograde amnesia, anxiety, ataxia, *confusion,* depression, dizziness, *drowsiness,* fatigue, hallucinations, headache, hysteria, insomnia, psychosis, slurred speech, stimulation, tremor

CV: Bradycardia, hypertension, hypotension, orthostatic hypotension, *shock,* tachycardia

EENT: Auditory disturbances, blurred vision, mydriasis, nystagmus

GI: Anorexia, constipation, diarrhea, dry mouth, nausea, vomiting

GU: Changes in libido, incontinence, menstrual irregularities, urinary retention

SKIN: Dermatitis, hair loss, hirsutism, itching, rash, urticaria

INTERACTIONS

Drugs

§ *Cimetidine:* Increased plasma levels of chlordiazepoxide and/or active metabolites

§ *Disulfiram:* Increased serum chlordiazepoxide concentrations

§ *Ethanol:* Enhanced adverse psychomotor side effects of benzodiazepines

---

* = non-FDA-approved use

3 *Fluconazole, itraconazole, ketoconazole:* Increased chlordiazepoxide concentrations

3 *Levodopa:* Potential for exacerbation of Parkinsonism in patients taking levodopa

Labs

• *False increase:* Urine 5-HIAA, urine 17-ketogenic steroids
• *False decrease:* Urine 17-ketogenic steroids
• *False positive:* Urine pregnancy tests

SPECIAL CONSIDERATIONS

• No advantage over diazepam; poor choice for elderly patients
• Do not use for everyday stress or use longer than 4 mo
• Do not discontinue medication abruptly after long-term use

---

chloroquine

(klor'oh-kwin)

Rx: Aralen

Chemical Class: Synthetic 4-aminoquinoline derivative
Therapeutic Class: Antimalarial; amebicide

CLINICAL PHARMACOLOGY

Mechanism of Action: Inhibits parasite replication via an interaction with DNA transcription

Pharmacokinetics

PO: Peak 1-6 hr, rapidly and completely absorbed; 55% protein bound; deposited in brain, spinal cord, liver, spleen, kidney, lungs, and leukocytes (from $30 \times$ -$70 \times$ the plasma concentration); metabolized in the liver, excretion slow (enhanced via acidification of urine) in urine, feces; crosses placenta; $t_{1/2}$ 3-5 days

INDICATIONS AND USES: Prophylaxis and treatment of acute attacks of malaria caused by susceptible strains, including *P. vivax, P. malariae, P. ovale, P. falciparum* (some strains); extraintestinal amebiasis

DOSAGE

NOTE: The dosage of chloroquine is often expressed or calculated as the base: 500 mg tab of chloroquine phosphate is equivalent to 300 mg base; 50 mg of chloroquine hydrochloride is equivalent to 40 mg base

Adult

• *Malaria suppression:* PO 300 mg (base)/wk on same day of wk; treatment should begin 1-2 wk before exposure and for 4 wk after; if treatment begins after exposure, 600 mg (base) in 2 divided doses 6 hr apart
• *Acute attack:* PO 600 mg (base) initial dose followed by 300 mg 6-8 hr later, then 300 mg on each of 2 consecutive days (total dose 1.5 g in 3 days); IM 160-200 mg initially, repeat in 6 hr if necessary; begin oral therapy as soon as possible and continue for 3 days until 1.5 g of base has been administered
• *Extraintestinal amebiasis:* IM 200-250 mg qd (HCl) up to 12 days, then substitute or resume PO administration as soon as possible; PO 600 mg (base) qd for 2 days, then 300 mg qd for 2-3 wk

Child

• *Malaria suppression:* PO 5 mg/kg/wk on same day of wk, not to exceed 300 mg (base); treatment should begin 1-2 wk before exposure and for 4 wk after; if treatment begins after exposure, 10 mg/kg (base) in 2 divided doses 6 hr apart
• *Acute attack:* PO 10 mg/kg (base) initial dose (do not exceed 600 mg) followed by 5 mg/kg 6-8 hr later (do not exceed 300 mg) then 5 mg/kg (do not exceed 300 mg) on each of 2 consecutive days (total dose 25 mg/kg in 3 days)

💲 AVAILABLE FORMS/COST OF THERAPY

• Inj, Sol—IV, IM (Hydrochloride): 50 mg/ml, 5 ml: **$20.72**
• Tab, Uncoated—Oral (Phosphate salt): 250 mg (150 mg base), 100's: **$17.50-$189.75**; 500 mg (300 mg base), 100's: **$101.25-$131.53**

CONTRAINDICATIONS: Retinal field changes, porphyria

PRECAUTIONS: Children, blood dyscrasias, severe GI disease, neurologic disease, alcoholism, hepatic disease, G-6-PD deficiency, psoriasis, eczema, lactation

PREGNANCY AND LACTATION: Pregnancy category C; excreted into breast milk; average infant consumption, considered safe;

NOTE: Doesn't protect infant against malaria

SIDE EFFECTS/ADVERSE REACTIONS

CNS: Fatigue, headache, psychosis, *seizures,* stimulation
CV: Asystole with syncope, ECG changes, *heart block,* hypotension
EENT: Blurred vision, *corneal changes,* corneal edema, deafness, *difficulty focusing,* photophobia, *retinal changes,* tinnitus, vertigo
GI: Anorexia, cramps, diarrhea, *nausea, vomiting*
HEME: Agranulocytosis, hemolytic anemia, leukopenia, thrombocytopenia
SKIN: Eczema, *exfoliative dermatitis,* lichen planus-like eruptions, pigmentary changes, pruritus, skin eruptions

INTERACTIONS

Drugs

🔳 *Chlorpromazine:* Increased chlorpromazine concentrations
🔳 *Cyclosporine:* Elevates cyclosporine levels, toxicity possible
🔳 *Methotrexate:* Decreased methotrexate levels

🔳 *Praziquantel:* Decreased praziquantel absorption

SPECIAL CONSIDERATIONS

• Certain strains of *P. falciparum* have become resistant to chloroquine

MONITORING PARAMETERS

• Ophthalmic examinations (visual acuity, slit lamp, funduscopic, visual fields) and CBC if long-term treatment or drug dosage >150 mg/day

---

chlorothiazide
(klor-oh-thye′a-zide)
Rx: Diachlor, Diurigen, Diuril
Combinations
  Rx: with methyldopa (Aldoclor); with reserpine (Chloroserp, Diaserp, Diupres)
Chemical Class: Sulfonamide derivative
Therapeutic Class: Thiazide diuretic; antihypertensive

CLINICAL PHARMACOLOGY

Mechanism of Action: Inhibits reabsorption of sodium and chloride in cortical thick ascending limb of the loop of Henle and the early distal tubules, increasing the urinary excretion of sodium and chloride; sulfonamide moiety provides some carbonic anhydrase inhibition activity; other actions: increased potassium and bicarbonate excretion; decreased calcium excretion; uric acid retention; antihypertensive action dependent on sodium depletion, drop in peripheral vascular resistance, and reduction in extracellular volume

Pharmacokinetics
PO: Poor oral absorption (33%); onset 2 hr, peak 4 hr, duration 6-12 hr

---

IV: Onset 15 min, maximal action 30 min

Eliminated unchanged by the kidneys; crosses placenta, but not blood-brain barrier; excreted in breast milk; $t_{1/2}$ 45-120 min

INDICATIONS AND USES: Edema (CHF, hepatic cirrhosis, nephrotic syndrome, acute glomerulonephritis, corticosteroid and estrogen therapy; hypertension; calcium nephrolithiasis*; prevention of osteoporosis*; diabetes insipidus

DOSAGE

NOTE: Equivalent hydrochlorothiazide dose: 50 mg-500 mg.

Adult

• *Edema:* PO/IV 500 mg-1 g/day in 1-2 divided doses

• *Hypertension:* PO 500 mg-1 g/day in 1-2 divided doses; max 2 g/day in divided doses

Child

• *Diuresis/hypertension:* PO 10-20 mg/kg/day in 2 divided doses, not to exceed 375 mg per day in infants up to 2 yr of age or 1 g per day in children 2 to 12 yr of age; infants less than 6 mo of age, up to 30 mg/kg/day in 2 divided doses; IV use generally not recommended

$ AVAILABLE FORMS/COST OF THERAPY

• Inj—IV: 500 mg: **$10.13**

• Susp—Oral: 250 mg/5 ml, 237 ml: **$12.26**

• Tab, Uncoated—Oral: 250 mg, 100's: **$3.32-$16.81**; 500 mg, 100's: **$7.24-$26.69**

CONTRAINDICATIONS: Anuria, renal decompensation

PRECAUTIONS: Fluid and electrolyte imbalance (including sodium, potassium, magnesium, calcium), renal disease, hepatic disease, gout, COPD, lupus erythematosus, diabetes mellitus, hyperparathyroidism, vomiting, diarrhea, elevated cholesterol/triglycerides

PREGNANCY AND LACTATION: Pregnancy category C; therapy for preexisting hypertension can be continued throughout pregnancy with minimal risk; initiating for simple edema not recommended; few unequivocal indications for diuretic therapy in pregnancy except for pulmonary edema or congestive heart failure; excreted in low concentrations in breast milk; compatible with breast feeding

SIDE EFFECTS/ADVERSE REACTIONS

CNS: Anxiety, depression, *dizziness,* drowsiness, fatigue, headache, paresthesia, weakness

CV: Arrhythmias, irregular pulse, orthostatic hypotension, palpitations, volume depletion

EENT: Blurred vision

GI: Anorexia, constipation, cramps, diarrhea, GI irritation, hepatitis, *nausea,* pancreatitis, *vomiting*

GU: Frequency, glucosuria, polyuria, uremia, impotence, decreased libido

HEME: **Agranulocytosis, aplastic anemia, hemolytic anemia, leukopenia, neutropenia, thrombocytopenia**

METAB: Hypercalcemia, *hyperglycemia, hyperuricemia,* hypochloremia, *hypokalemia,* hypomagnesemia, lipid abnormalities (increased total and LDL cholesterol, triglycerides) hyponatremia, hypophosphatemia, increased creatinine, BUN

SKIN: Fever, photosensitivity, purpura, rash, urticaria

INTERACTIONS

Drugs

❷ *Angiotensin-converting enzyme inhibitors:* Risk of postural hypotension when added to ongoing diuretic therapy; more common with loop diuretics; first-dose hypotension possible in patients with so-

---

italic = common side effects   ***bold italic*** = life-threatening reactions

dium depletion or hypovolemia caused by diuretics or sodium restriction; hypotensive response is usually transient; hold diuretic day of first dose

🔢 *Calcium (high doses):* Risk of milk-alkali syndrome; monitor for hypercalcemia

🔢 *Carbenoxolone:* Additive potassium wasting; severe hypokalemia

🔢 *Cholestyramine/colestipol:* Reduced serum concentrations of thiazide diuretics

🔢 *Corticosteroids:* Concomitant therapy may result in excessive potassium loss

🔢 *Diazoxide:* Hyperglycemia

🔢 *Digitalis glycosides:* Diuretic-induced hypokalemia may increase the risk of digitalis toxicity

🔢 *Hypoglycemic agents:* Thiazide diuretics tend to increase blood glucose, may increase dosage requirements of antidiabetic drugs

🔢 *Lithium:* Increases serum lithium concentrations; toxicity may occur

🔢 *Methotrexate:* Increased bone marrow suppression

🔢 *Nonsteroidal antiinflammatory drugs:* Concurrent use may reduce diuretic and antihypertensive effects

Labs

• *Interference:* Urine 17-hydroxy-corticosteroids

• False decrease: urine estriol

SPECIAL CONSIDERATIONS

• Doses above 250 mg provide no further blood pressure reduction, but are more likely to induce metabolic disturbance (i.e., hypokalemia, hyperuricemia, etc.)

• May protect against osteoporotic hip fractures

• Loop diuretics or metolazone more effective if CrCl <40-50 ml/min

PATIENT/FAMILY EDUCATION

• Will increase urination temporarily (approximately 3 wk); take early in the day to prevent sleep disturbance

• May cause sensitivity to sunlight; avoid prolonged exposure to the sun and other ultraviolet light

• May cause gout attacks; notify clinician if sudden joint pain occurs

MONITORING PARAMETERS

• Weight, urine output, serum electrolytes, BUN, creatinine, CBC, uric acid, glucose, lipids

---

chloroxine

(klor-ox'ine)

Rx: Capitrol

Chemical Class: Hydroxyquinoline derivative

Therapeutic Class: Antiseborrheic

CLINICAL PHARMACOLOGY

Mechanism of Action: Presumed reduction in scaling via effects on mitotic activity; antibacterial and antifungal role in seborrheic dermatitis speculated as *S. aureus* and *Pityrosporon* spp. are often present in increased numbers

INDICATIONS AND USES: Dandruff and mild to moderately severe seborrheic dermatitis

DOSAGE

Adult

• TOP rub into wet scalp, allow to remain for 3 min before rinse, repeat; 2 treatments/wk usually sufficient

💲 **AVAILABLE FORMS/COST OF THERAPY**

• Shampoo—Top: 110 ml: **$22.26**

CONTRAINDICATIONS: Acute inflammation

PRECAUTIONS: External use only, avoid contact with eyes

---

* = non-FDA-approved use

PREGNANCY AND LACTATION:
Pregnancy category C; excretion into breast milk unknown

SIDE EFFECTS/ADVERSE REACTIONS

SKIN: Discoloration of light-colored (blond, gray, bleached) hair, irritation and burning

SPECIAL CONSIDERATIONS
PATIENT/FAMILY EDUCATION
• Improvement may not occur for 14 days

---

chlorphenesin

(klor-fen´e-sin)
Rx: Maolate
Chemical Class: Carbamate derivative
Therapeutic Class: Skeletal muscle relaxant

CLINICAL PHARMACOLOGY
Mechanism of Action: Unknown; related to central sedative properties; does not directly relax muscle or depress nerve conduction

Pharmacokinetics
PO: Onset ½ hr, peak 1-2 hr, duration 4-6 hr; metabolized by liver, excreted in urine; crosses placenta; $t_{1/2}$ 4 hr

INDICATIONS AND USES: Adjunct for relieving pain in acute, painful musculoskeletal conditions

DOSAGE
Adult
• PO 800 mg tid; maintenance 400 mg qid, not to exceed 8 wk of therapy

$ AVAILABLE FORMS/COST OF THERAPY
• Tab, Uncoated—Oral: 400 mg, 50's: **$39.58**

PRECAUTIONS: Renal disease, hepatic disease, addictive personality, elderly, hypersensitivity to FD&C Yellow No. 5 (tartrazine), aspirin hypersensitivity

PREGNANCY AND LACTATION:
Pregnancy category C; excreted in breast milk (large amounts), safety not established

SIDE EFFECTS/ADVERSE REACTIONS

CNS: Confusion, depression, *dizziness, drowsiness,* headache, insomnia, tremor, *weakness*
CV: Postural hypotension, tachycardia
EENT: Diplopia, temporary loss of vision
GI: Hiccups, *nausea,* vomiting
HEME: ***Blood dyscrasias***
SKIN: Facial flushing, fever, pruritus, rash

SPECIAL CONSIDERATIONS
PATIENT/FAMILY EDUCATION
• Avoid concurrent alcohol, other CNS depressants, hazardous activities if drowsiness/dizziness occurs

---

italic = common side effects   ***bold italic*** = life-threatening reactions

chlorpheniramine

(klor-fen-eer'a-meen)

Rx: Chlor-Phen, Prohist-8
OTC: Aller-Chlor,
Chlo-Amine, Chlorate,
Chlor-Trimeton, Pfeiffer's
Allergy, Teldrin
Combinations
  Rx: with hydrocodone (Tussionex); with phenylephrine
    and pyrilamine (Rynaton);
    with phenylpropanolamine
    (Ornade, Resaid S.R.); with
    pseudoephedrine (Deconamine, Fedahist)
  OTC: with phenylpropanolamine (Allerhist Maximum
    Strength, Contac 12-Hour
    Capsules, Triaminic Syrup)
    with pseudoephedrine
    (Chlor-Trimeton, Dorcol
    Children's Cold Formula
    Liquid, Fedahist)
Chemical Class: Alkylamine
derivative
Therapeutic Class: Antihistamine

CLINICAL PHARMACOLOGY
Mechanism of Action: Decreases
allergic response by blocking histamine at H_1-receptors
Pharmacokinetics
PO: Onset 20-60 min, duration 8-12
hr; detoxified in liver; excreted by
kidneys   (metabolites/unchanged
drug); $t_{1/2}$ 20-24 hr
INDICATIONS AND USES: Perenial
and seasonal allergic rhinitis (PO);
allergic reactions to blood and
plasma, adjunctive anaphylactic
therapy (parenteral)

DOSAGE
Adult
• PO 2-4 mg tid-qid, not to exceed 36
mg/day; Sus Action 8-12 mg bid-tid,
not to exceed 36 mg/day; IM/IV/SC
5-40 mg/day
Child
• 2-5 yr: PO 1 mg q6h, not to exceed
6 mg/day
• 6-12 yr: PO 2 mg q4-6h, not to exceed 12 mg/day; Sus Action 8 mg hs
or qd (not recommended for child
<6 yr)
$ **AVAILABLE FORMS/COST
    OF THERAPY**
• Cap, Gel, Sus Action—Oral: 8 mg,
100's: **$6.25-$12.98**; 12 mg, 100's:
$4.20-$14.60
• Inj, Sol—IV: 10 mg/ml, 1 ml:
$0.40
• Syr—Oral: 2 mg/5 ml, 120, 480
ml: **$1.19-$3.60/120 ml**
• Tab, Uncoated—Oral: 4 mg,
100's: **$0.68-$16.12**
• Tab, Chewable—Oral: 2 mg, 96's:
$14.80
• Tab, Sus Action—Oral: 8 mg,
100's: **$19.60-$114.84**; 12 mg,
100's: **$35.78**
CONTRAINDICATIONS: Acute
asthma attack, lower respiratory
tract disease
PRECAUTIONS: Increased intraocular pressure (angle-closure
glaucoma), renal disease, cardiac
disease, hypertension, bronchial
asthma, seizure disorder, stenosed
peptic ulcers, hyperthyroidism, prostatic hypertrophy, bladder neck obstruction, elderly
PREGNANCY AND LACTATION:
Pregnancy category B
SIDE EFFECTS/ADVERSE REACTIONS
CNS: Anxiety, confusion, *dizziness,
drowsiness,* euphoria, fatigue, neuritis, paresthesia, poor coordination
EENT: Blurred vision, dilated pupils,
dry nose, throat; tinnitus

GI: Anorexia, diarrhea, *dry mouth,* nausea

GU: Dysuria, frequency, *retention*

HEME: Agranulocytosis, hemolytic anemia, thrombocytopenia

RESP: Chest tightness, increased thick secretions, wheezing

SKIN: Photosensitivity

SPECIAL CONSIDERATIONS

• More potent antihistamine than nonsedating agents (e.g., fexofenidine), good first-line choice for allergic rhinitis

PATIENT/FAMILY EDUCATION

• Tolerance develops to sedation with chronic use

---

chlorpromazine

(klor-proe′ma-zeen)

Rx: Thorazine
Chemical Class: Aliphatic phenothiazine derivative
Therapeutic Class: Antipsychotic; antiemetic

CLINICAL PHARMACOLOGY

Mechanism of Action: Dopamine receptor antagonist, with higher affinity for D_2 over D_1 receptors, and variable selectivity among the cortical dopamine tracts; also activity on nondopaminergic sites, i.e., cholinergic, alpha$_1$-adrenergic and histamine receptors (explaining side effects); standard phenothiazine, with high incidence of sedation and orthostatic hypotension, moderate risk of extrapyramidal and anticholinergic effects

Pharmacokinetics

PO: Absorption variable, onset erratic 30-60 min, duration 4-6 hr

PO-ER: Onset 30-60 min, peak unknown, duration 10-12 hr

IM: Well absorbed, peak 15-20 min, duration 4 to 8 hr

IV: Onset 5 min, peak 10 min, duration unknown

REC: Onset erratic, duration 3 hr Widely distributed; metabolized by liver, excreted in urine (metabolites); crosses placenta; 95% bound to plasma proteins; elimination $t_{1/2}$ 10-30 hr

INDICATIONS AND USES: Psychotic disorders, mania, schizophrenia, anxiety; intractable hiccups; nausea, vomiting; preoperatively for relaxation; acute intermittent porphyria; behavioral problems in children; adjunct in treatment of tetanus; treatment of 'angel dust' psychosis,* migraine headaches (IM/IV)*

DOSAGE

Adult

• *Psychosis:* PO 10 mg tid-qid or 25 mg bid-tid, increase by 20-50 mg semiweekly, maintenance 200-800 mg/day; IM 25 mg, may repeat dose of 25-50 mg in 1 hr prn, increase gradually over several days up to 400 mg q4-6h in severe cases, substitute PO when possible

• *Nausea and vomiting:* PO 10-25 mg q4-6h prn; IM 25-50 mg q3h prn; Rect 50-100 mg q6-8h prn, not to exceed 400 mg/day; IV 25-50 mg qd-qid

• *Intractable hiccups:* PO 25-50 mg tid-qid; IM 25-50 mg (use only if PO dose does not work); IV 25-50 mg in 500-1000 ml saline (only for severe hiccups)

• *Intermittent porphyria:* PO 25-50 mg tid-qid; IM 25 mg tid-qid

• *Tetanus:* IM 25-50 mg tid-qid; IV 25-50 mg

Child

• Not to exceed 40 mg/day (<5 yr) or 75 mg/day (5-12 yr)

• *Psychosis:* PO 0.5 mg/kg q4-6h prn; IM 0.5 mg/kg q6-8h; Rect 1 mg/kg q6-8h

---

italic = common side effects   ***bold italic*** = life-threatening reactions

• *Nausea and vomiting:* PO 0.55 mg/kg q4-6h prn, IM 0.55 mg/kg q6-8h prn; Rect 1.1 mg/kg: q6-8h prn; IV 0.55 mg/kg q6-8h

$ AVAILABLE FORMS/COST OF THERAPY

• Cap, Sus Action—Oral: 30 mg, 50's: **$59.55**; 75 mg, 50's: **$80.00**; 150 mg, 50's: **$107.85**

• Conc—Oral: 30 mg/ml, 120 ml: **$5.31-$17.66**; 100 mg/ml, 240 ml: **$20.12-$192.20**

• Inj, Sol—IM, IV: 25 mg/ml, 1 ml: **$1.50-$8.32**

• Supp—Rect: 25 mg, 12's: **$47.19**; 100 mg, 12's: **$59.75**

• Tab, Plain Coated—Oral: 10 mg, 100's: **$4.74-$42.50**; 25 mg, 100's: **$3.00-$62.81**; 50 mg, 100's: **$4.00-$75.40**; 100 mg, 100's: **$7.00-$92.60**; 200 mg, 100's: **$10.00-$117.65**

CONTRAINDICATIONS: Circulatory collapse, liver damage, cerebral arteriosclerosis, coronary disease, severe hypertension/hypotension, blood dyscrasias, coma, child <2 yr, brain damage, bone marrow depression, alcohol and barbiturate withdrawal

PRECAUTIONS: Seizure disorders, hypertension, hepatic disease, cardiac disease, elderly (orthostasis upon arising), COPD

PREGNANCY AND LACTATION: Pregnancy category C; enters breast milk in small concentrations; report of drowsy and lethargic infant who consumed milk with 92 ng/ml concentration

SIDE EFFECTS/ADVERSE REACTIONS

CNS: Extrapyramidal symptoms (pseudoparkinsonism, akathisia, dystonia), headache, **seizures,** tardive dyskinesia

CV: **Cardiac arrest,** ECG changes, hypertension, *orthostatic hypotension,* tachycardia

EENT: Blurred vision, dry eyes, glaucoma

GI: Anorexia, constipation, diarrhea, dry mouth, jaundice, nausea, vomiting, weight gain

GU: Amenorrhea, breast engorgement, enuresis, gynecomastia, impotence, urinary frequency, urinary retention

HEME: **Agranulocytosis,** anemia, **leukocytosis, leukopenia**

RESP: Dyspnea, **laryngospasm,** respiratory depression

SKIN: Dermatitis, photosensitivity, *rash*

MISC: **Neuroleptic malignant syndrome (NMS)**

INTERACTIONS

Drugs

🔳 *Amodiaquine, chloroquine, sulfadoxine-pyrimethamine:* Increased chlorpromazine concentrations

🔳 *Anticholinergics:* May inhibit neuroleptic response; excess anticholinergic effects

🔳 *Antidepressants:* Potential for increased therapeutic and toxic effects from increased levels of both drugs

🔳 *Barbiturates:* Decreased neuroleptic levels

🔳 *Clonidine, guanadrel, granethidine:* Severe hypotensive episodes possible

🔳 *Epinephrine:* Blunted pressor response to epinephrine

🔳 *Ethanol:* Additive CNS depression

❷ *Levodopa:* Inhibited antiparkinsonian effect of levodopa

🔳 *Lithium:* Lowered levels of both drugs, rarely neurotoxicity in acute mania

🔳 *Narcotic analgesics:* Hypotension and increased CNS depression

🔳 *Orphenadrine:* Lower neuroleptic concentrations, excessive anticholinergic effects

---

* = non-FDA-approved use

3 *Propranolol:* Increased plasma levels of both drugs with accentuated responses

Labs

• *False decrease:* 5-HIAA, vitamin B_{12}
• *Interference:* 17-ketogenic steroids
• *False increase:* Urine bilirubin, cholesterol, urine porphobilinogen, CSF protein, urine protein
• *False positive:* Ferric chloride test, guiacols spot test, phenylketones

SPECIAL CONSIDERATIONS
PATIENT/FAMILY EDUCATION

• Orthostasis on rising, especially in elderly
• Avoid hot tubs; hot showers, tub baths
• Meticulous oral hygiene; frequent rinsing of mouth, sugarless gum for dry mouth
• Use a sunscreen and sunglasses
• Urine may turn pink or red

---

chlorpropamide
(klor-pro´pa-mide)
Rx: Diabinese
Chemical Class: Sulfonylurea (first generation)
Therapeutic Class: Oral hypoglycemic

CLINICAL PHARMACOLOGY
Mechanism of Action: Decreases blood sugar via stimulation of insulin secretion and increased tissue responsiveness to insulin; initial hypoglycemic effects due to stimulation of pancreatic islets (dependent upon functioning β-cells); extrapancreatic effect predominantly due to inhibition of hepatic glucose production, but may also facilitate improved insulin-insulin receptor binding

Pharmacokinetics
PO: Onset 1 hr. peak 3-6 hr. duraton 60 hr; completely absorbed by GI route; 90%-95% plasma protein bound; metabolized in liver, excreted in urine (metabolites and unchanged drug); $t_{1/2}$ 36 hr

INDICATIONS AND USES: Diabetes mellitus, type 2, neurogenic diabetes insipidus*

DOSAGE
Adult
• PO 100-250 mg qd initially, then 100-500 mg maintenance according to response, max 750 mg/day

S **AVAILABLE FORMS/COST OF THERAPY**
• Tab, Uncoated—Oral: 100 mg, 100's: **$3.75-$43.66**; 250 mg, 100's: **$4.95-$92.28**

CONTRAINDICATIONS: Diabetes mellitus, type 1; ketoacidosis
PRECAUTIONS: Elderly, cardiac disease, thyroid disease, renal disease, hepatic disease, severe hypoglycemic reactions
PREGNANCY AND LACTATION: Pregnancy category D; inappropriate for use during pregnancy due to inadequate for blood glucose control, potential for prolonged neonatal hypoglycemia, and risk of congenital abnormalities; insulin is the drug of choice for control of blood sugars during pregnancy; breast milk reported at 17% of plasma; the potential for neonatal hypoglycemia dictates caution in nursing mothers

SIDE EFFECTS/ADVERSE REACTIONS

CNS: Dizziness, drowsiness, fatigue, *headache,* tinnitus, vertigo, *weakness*
GI: Anorexia, **cholestatic jaundice,** diarrhea, **hepatotoxicity,** hunger, nausea, vomiting

---

italic = common side effects   ***bold italic*** = life-threatening reactions

HEME: **Agranulocytosis, aplastic anemia, hemolytic anemia, leukopenia, pancytopenia, thrombocytopenia**

METAB: Hepatic porphyria, hypoglycemia, hyponatremia, syndrome of inappropriate antidiuretic hormone release

SKIN: Allergic reactions, eczema, erythema multiforme, **exfoliative dermatitis,** photo-sensitivity, pruritus, rash, urticaria

INTERACTIONS

Drugs

3 *Anabolic steroids:* Chloramphenicol, Fibric acid derivatives, MAOIs, Salicylates, Sulfonamides: Enhanced hypoglycemic effect

▲ *Ethanol:* Altered glycemic control, most commonly hypoglycemia; disulfiram-like reaction may occur

3 *Halofenate:* Increased sulfonylurea concentrations

❷ *NSAIDs:* Enhanced hypoglycemic effect

3 *Thiazide diuretics:* Increased glucose concentrations, may increase dose requirements

Labs

• *False increase:* Serum calcium

SPECIAL CONSIDERATIONS

PATIENT/FAMILY EDUCATION

• Multiple drug interactions, including alcohol and salicylates

• Symptoms of hypoglycemia: tingling lips/tongue, nausea, confusion, fatigue, sweating, hunger, visual changes (spots)

• Due to potential for prolonged hypoglycemia, other sulfonylureas should be considered before trying chlorpropamide (especially in the elderly)

MONITORING PARAMETERS

• Self-monitored blood glucose; glycosolated hemoglobin q 3-6 mo

---

chlorthalidone

(klor-thal´i-doan)

Rx: Hygroton, Thalitone

Combinations

Rx: with atenolol (Tenoretic); with clonidine (Combipres, Chlorpres); with reserpine (Demi-Regroton, Regroton)

Chemical Class: Phthalimidine derivative

Therapeutic Class: Thiazide diuretic; antihypertensive

CLINICAL PHARMACOLOGY

Mechanism of Action: Inhibits reabsorption of sodium and chloride in cortical thick ascending limb of the loop of Henle and the early distal tubules, increasing the urinary excretion of sodium and chloride; sulfonamide moiety provides some carbonic anhydrase inhibition activity; other actions: increased potassium and bicarbonate excretion; decreased calcium excretion; uric acid retention; antihypertensive action dependent on sodium depletion, drop in peripheral vascular resistance, and reduction in extracellular volume

Pharmacokinetics

PO: Absorption, 65%; onset 2 hr, peak 6 hr, duration 48-72 hr, excreted unchanged by kidneys; crosses placenta; $t_{1/2}$ 51-89 hr

INDICATIONS AND USES: Edema (CHF, hepatic cirrhosis, nephrotic syndrome, acute glomerulonephritis and corticosteroid and estrogen therapy); hypertension; calcium nephrolithiasis*; osteoporosis*; diabetes insipidus prevention

DOSAGE

NOTE: Equivalent hydrochlorothiazide dose: 50 mg-50 mg

---

* = non-FDA-approved use

Adult
• PO 15-100 mg/day or 100 mg every other day

Child
• PO 2 mg/kg 3×/wk

§ AVAILABLE FORMS/COST OF THERAPY
• Tab, Uncoated—Oral: 15 mg, 100's: **$69.78-$84.78**; 25 mg, 100's: **$5.50-$90.85**; 50 mg, 100's: **$6.45-$92.61**; 100 mg, 100's: **$8.45-$148.86**

CONTRAINDICATIONS: Anuria, renal decompensation

PRECAUTIONS: Fluid and electrolyte imbalance (including sodium, potassium, magnesium, calcium), renal disease, hepatic disease, gout, COPD, lupus erythematosus, diabetes mellitus, hyperparathyroidism, vomiting, diarrhea, elevated cholesterol/triglycerides

PREGNANCY AND LACTATION: Pregnancy category B; therapy for preexisting hypertension can be continued throughout pregnancy with minimal risk; initiating for simple edema not recommended; few unequivocal indications for diuretic therapy in pregnancy except for pulmonary edema or congestive heart failure; compatible with breast feeding

SIDE EFFECTS/ADVERSE REACTIONS

CNS: Anxiety, depression, *dizziness,* drowsiness, *fatigue,* headache, paresthesia, *weakness*

CV: Irregular pulse, orthostatic hypotension, palpitations, volume depletion

EENT: Blurred vision

GI: Anorexia, constipation, cramps, diarrhea, GI irritation, hepatitis, *nausea,* pancreatitis, *vomiting*

GU: Frequency, glucosuria, impotence, polyuria, **uremia**

HEME: **Agranulocytosis, aplastic anemia, hemolytic anemia, leukopenia, neutropenia, thrombocytopenia**

METAB: Lipid abnormalities (increased total and LDL-cholesterol, triglycerides), Gout, hypercalcemia, hyperglycemia, hyperuremia, hypochloremia, *hypokalemia,* hypomagnesemia, hyponatremia, increased creatinine, BUN

SKIN: Fever, photosensitivity, purpura, rash, urticaria

INTERACTIONS

Drugs

❷ *Angiotensin-converting enzyme inhibitors:* Risk of postural hypotension when added to ongoing diuretic therapy; more common with loop diuretics; first dose hypotension possible in patients with sodium depletion or hypovolemia due to diuretics or sodium restriction; hypotensive response is usually transient; hold diuretic day of first dose

❸ *Calcium:* Increased risk of milk-alkali syndrome

❸ *Carbenoxolone:* Additive potassium wasting, severe hypokalemia

❸ *Cholestyramine, Colestipol:* Reduced absorption

❸ *Corticosteroids:* Concomitant therapy may result in excessive potassium loss

❸ *Diazoxide:* Hyperglycemia

❸ *Digitalis glycosides:* Diuretic-induced hypokalemia increases risk of digitalis toxicity

❸ *Hypoglycemic agents:* Increased dosage requirements due to increased glucose levels

❸ *Lithium:* Increased lithium levels, potential toxicity

❸ *Methotrexate:* Increased risk of bone marrow depression

❸ *Nonsteroidal antiinflammatory drugs:* Concurrent use may reduce diuretic and antihypertensive effects

Labs
• False decrease: urine esriol

SPECIAL CONSIDERATIONS
• Doses above 25 mg provide no further blood pressure reduction, but are more likely to induce metabolic disturbance (i.e., hypokalemia, hyperuricemia, etc.)
• May protect against osteoporotic hip fractures
• Loop diuretics or metolazone more effective if CrCl <40-50 ml/min

PATIENT/FAMILY EDUCATION
• Will increase urination temporarily (approximately 3 wk); take early in the day to prevent sleep disturbance
• May cause sensitivity to sunlight; avoid prolonged exposure to the sun and other ultraviolet light
• May cause gout attacks; notify clinician if sudden joint pain occurs

MONITORING PARAMETERS
• Weight, urine output, serum electrolytes, BUN, creatinine, CBC, uric acid, glucose, lipids

---

chlorzoxazone
(klor-zox′a-zone)
Rx: Parafon Forte DSC, Remular-S
Chemical Class: Benzoxazole derivative
Therapeutic Class: Skeletal muscle relaxant

CLINICAL PHARMACOLOGY
Mechanism of Action: Inhibition of multisynaptic reflex arcs involved in producing and maintaining skeletal muscle spasm of varied etiology at the level of the spinal cord and subcortical areas of the brain; mode of action may be related to sedative properties

Pharmacokinetics
PO: Onset 30 min, peak 1-2 hr, duration 6 hr; metabolized in liver, excreted in urine (glucuronide metabolites); $t_{1/2}$ 1 hr

INDICATIONS AND USES: Adjunct to rest and physical therapy for the relief of discomfort associated with acute, painful musculoskeletal conditions; does not directly relax tense skeletal muscles

DOSAGE
Adult
• PO 250-750 mg tid-qid
Child
• PO 20 mg/kg/day in divided doses bid-tid

$ AVAILABLE FORMS/COST OF THERAPY
• Tab, Uncoated—Oral: 250 mg, 100's: **$5.25-$62.35**; 500 mg, 100's: **$9.25-$145.66**

CONTRAINDICATIONS: Impaired hepatic function

PRECAUTIONS: Lactation, hepatic disease, elderly

PREGNANCY AND LACTATION: Pregnancy category C

SIDE EFFECTS/ADVERSE REACTIONS

CNS: Dizziness, drowsiness, headache, insomnia, malaise, stimulation

GI: Anorexia, constipation, diarrhea, **gastrointestinal bleeding, hepatotoxicity,** jaundice, *nausea,* vomiting

GU: Urine discoloration

HEME: Anemia, **granulocytopenia**

SKIN: Angioedema, ecchymoses, petechiae, pruritus, rash

SPECIAL CONSIDERATIONS
PATIENT/FAMILY EDUCATION
• Potential for psychologic dependency

---

cholestyramine

(koe-less-tir′a-meen)

Rx: Questran, Questran Light

Chemical Class: Bile acid sequestrant

Therapeutic Class: Antilipemic

CLINICAL PHARMACOLOGY

Mechanism of Action: Absorbs, combines with bile acids to form insoluble complex that is excreted via feces; loss of bile acids lowers cholesterol levels

Pharmacokinetics

PO: Excreted in feces, max effect in 2 wk

INDICATIONS AND USES: Primary hypercholesterolemia, pruritus associated with partial biliary obstruction, diarrhea caused by excess bile acid or *Clostridium difficile* toxin,* digitalis toxicity*

DOSAGE

Adult

• PO 4 g 1-6 × daily (recommended schedule is bid), not to exceed 32 g/day

Child

• PO 240 mg/kg/day in 3 divided doses

💲 AVAILABLE FORMS/COST OF THERAPY

• Powder—Oral: 4 g/9 g, 60 pkts: **$41.86-$131.80**; 378 g: **$35.34-$57.73** (Questran)

• Powder, Reconst—Oral: 4 g/5 g, 60 pkts: **$35.35-$132.53**; 210 g: 210 g/214 g: **$32.69-$52.05**/210 g (Questran Light)

CONTRAINDICATIONS: Complete biliary obstruction

PRECAUTIONS: Children, constipation

PREGNANCY AND LACTATION: Pregnancy category C

SIDE EFFECTS/ADVERSE REACTIONS

CNS: Dizziness, drowsiness, headache, tinnitus, vertigo

GI: Abdominal pain, constipation, fecal impaction, flatulence, hemorrhoids, *nausea,* peptic ulcer, steatorrhea, vomiting

MS: Joint pain, muscle

SKIN: Irritation of perianal area, tongue, skin; rash

HEME: Bleeding, decreased protime, decreased vitamin A, D, K, red cell folate content, hyperchloremic acidosis

INTERACTIONS

Drugs

3 *Acetaminophen, Amiodarone, Corticosteroids, Diclofenac, Digitalis glycosides, Furosemide, Methotrexate, Metronidazole, Thiazide diuretics, Thyroid hormones, Valproic acid:* Cholestyramine reduces interacting drug concentrations and probably subsequent therapeutic response

3 *Oral anticoagulants:* Inhibition of hypoprothrombinemic response; colestipol might be less likely to interact

SPECIAL CONSIDERATIONS

• Avoid use in patients with elevated triglycerides

PATIENT/FAMILY EDUCATION

• Give all other medications 1 hr before or 4 hr after cholestyramine to avoid poor absorption

• Mix drug with applesauce or noncarbonated beverage (2-6 oz), let stand for 2 min; do not take dry

---

choline magnesium trisalicylate
(koe´leen mag-nees´ee-um tri-sal´eh-cye´late)

Rx: CMT, Trilisate, Tricosal, Trisalcid
Chemical Class: Salicylate derivative
Therapeutic Class: Nonnarcotic analgesic; NSAID

CLINICAL PHARMACOLOGY
Mechanism of Action: Inhibits prostaglandin synthesis; analgesic, anti-inflammatory, antipyretic actions
Pharmacokinetics
PO: Onset 15-30 min, peak 1.5-2 hrs, rapid absorption; metabolized by liver; excreted by kidneys
INDICATIONS AND USES: Mild to moderate pain, rheumatoid arthritis, osteoarthritis, related rheumatic disorders

DOSAGE
NOTE: Each 500 mg of choline magnesium trisalicylate contains 500 mg of salicylate (equivalent to 650 mg aspirin); dosage based on total salicylate content
Adult
• PO 1-4.5 g of salicylate daily in single dose or in 2-3 divided doses (based on response, tolerance, and serum salicylate concentration)
Child
• PO 50 mg/kg/day divided into 2 doses

🛈 AVAILABLE FORMS/COST OF THERAPY
• Liq—Oral: 500 mg/5 ml, 240 ml: **$27.00-$31.97**
• Tab, Uncoated—Oral: 500 mg, 100's: **$25.00-$96.85**; 750 mg, 100's: **$30.00-$120.23**; 1000 mg, 100's: **$38.00-$155.02**

CONTRAINDICATIONS: GI bleeding, bleeding disorders, children <3 yr, vitamin K deficiency, children with flu-like symptoms
PRECAUTIONS: Anemia, hepatic disease, renal disease, Hodgkin's disease, lactation
PREGNANCY AND LACTATION: Pregnancy category C; excreted into breast milk
SIDE EFFECTS/ADVERSE REACTIONS
CNS: Coma, confusion, dizziness, drowsiness, flushing, hallucinations, headache, *seizures,* stimulation
CV: Pulmonary edema, rapid pulse
EENT: Hearing loss, tinnitus
GI: Anorexia, *diarrhea,* GI bleeding, *heartburn,* hepatitis, *nausea, vomiting*
*HEME: **Agranulocytosis, hemolytic anemia,*** increased pro-time (transient), *leukopenia, neutropenia, thrombocytopenia*
METAB: Hypoglycemia, hypokalemia, hyponatremia
RESP: Hyperpnea, wheezing
SKIN: Bruising, *rash,* urticaria
INTERACTIONS
Labs
• *False increase:* Serum bicarbonate, CSF protein, serum theophylline
• *False decrease:* Urine cocaine, urine estrogen, serum glucose, urine 17-hydroxycorticosteroids, urine opiates
• *False positive:* Ferric chloride test
SPECIAL CONSIDERATIONS
• Consider for patients with GI intolerance to aspirin or patients in whom interference with normal platelet function by aspirin or other NSAIDs is undesirable
PATIENT/FAMILY EDUCATION
• Solution may be mixed with fruit juice just before administration; do not mix with antacid

---

* = non-FDA-approved use

MONITORING PARAMETERS
• Liver and renal function studies, stool for occult blood and hct if long-term therapy

---

choline salicylate
(koe'leen sa-lis'i-late)
OTC: Arthropan
Chemical Class: Salicylate derivative
Therapeutic Class: Nonnarcotic analgesic; NSAID

CLINICAL PHARMACOLOGY
Mechanism of Action: Inhibits prostaglandin synthesis; analgesic, anti-inflammatory, antipyretic actions
Pharmacokinetics
PO: Onset 15-30 min, rapid absorption; metabolized by liver, excreted by kidneys
INDICATIONS AND USES: Mild to moderate pain, rheumatoid arthritis, osteo-arthritis, related rheumatic disorders
DOSAGE
NOTE: Dosage based on total salicylate content
Adult
• *Arthritis:* PO 870-1740 mg (5-10 ml) up to qid
• *Pain/fever:* PO 870 mg (5 ml) q3-4h prn (max 6 × /day)
Child
• PO 50 mg/kg/day in 2 divided doses for children weighing up to 37 kg and 2250 mg/day for larger children
§ AVAILABLE FORMS/COST OF THERAPY
• Liq—Oral: 870 mg/5 ml, 480 ml: **$45.73**
CONTRAINDICATIONS: GI bleeding, bleeding disorders, children <3 yr, vitamin K deficiency, children with flu-like symptoms

PRECAUTIONS: Anemia, hepatic disease, renal disease, Hodgkin's disease
PREGNANCY AND LACTATION: Pregnancy category C; excreted into breast milk
SIDE EFFECTS/ADVERSE REACTIONS
CNS: Coma, confusion, dizziness, drowsiness, flushing, hallucinations, headache, *seizures,* stimulation
CV: Pulmonary edema, rapid pulse
EENT: Hearing loss, tinnitus
GI: Anorexia, *diarrhea,* **GI bleeding,** *heartburn,* hepatitis, *nausea, vomiting*
HEME: **Agranulocytosis, hemolytic anemia,** increased pro-time (transient), **leukopenia, neutropenia, thrombocytopenia**
METAB: Hypoglycemia, hypokalemia, hyponatremia
RESP: Hyperpnea, wheezing
SKIN: Bruising, *rash,* urticaria
INTERACTIONS
Labs
• *False increase:* Serum bicarbonate, CSF protein, serum theophylline
• *False decrease:* Urine cocaine, urine estrogen, serum glucose, urine 17-hydroxycorticosteroids, urine opiates
• *False positive:* Ferric chloride test
SPECIAL CONSIDERATIONS
• Consider for patients with GI intolerance to aspirin or patients in whom interference with normal platelet function by aspirin or other NSAIDs is undesirable
MONITORING PARAMETERS
• Liver and renal function studies, stool for occult blood and hct if long-term therapy

---

italic = common side effects   ***bold italic*** = life-threatening reactions

ciclopirox

(sye-kloe-peer'ox)
Rx: Loprox, Penlac
Chemical Class: N-hydroxypy-ridinone derivative
Therapeutic Class: Topical antifungal

CLINICAL PHARMACOLOGY
Mechanism of Action: Interferes with fungal cell membrane, which increases permeability, which allows leaking of intracellular material
Pharmacokinetics
TOP: 1.3% absorbed systematically; $t_{1/2}$ 1.7 hr; excreted via kidneys
INDICATIONS AND USES: Topical dermal infections (tinea cruris, tinea corporis, tinea pedis, tinea versicolor, cutaneous candidiasis) caused by susceptible organisms; mild to moderate onychomycosis due to Trichophyton rubrum (nail lacquer)
Antifungal spectrum usually includes: *Trichophyton mentagrophytes, Epidermophyton floccosum, Trichophyton rubrum, Microsporum canis, Candida albicans, Malassezia furfur*
DOSAGE
Adult
• *Cream, gel, lotion:* TOP apply bid
• *Nail lacquer:* TOP apply qd evenly over entire nail plate, when possible apply to nail bed, hyponychium, and under surface of nail plate; daily applicaton should be applied over previous coat; remove every 7 days with alcohol and file away loose nail material and trim nails
Child >10 yr
• *Cream, gel, lotion:* TOP apply bid

$ AVAILABLE FORMS/COST OF THERAPY
• Cre—Top: 1%, 15, 30, 90 g: **$22.20**//30 g
• Gel—Top: 1%, 30, 45 g: **$31.82**/30 g
• Lotion—Top: 1%, 30, 60 ml: **$46.50**/60 ml
• Sol—Top, Nail Laquer: 8%, 3.3, 6.6 ml: **$59.94**/3.3 ml
PREGNANCY AND LACTATION: Pregnancy category B; excretion into breast milk unknown
SIDE EFFECTS/ADVERSE REACTIONS
SKIN: Burning, pain, pruritus, rash, stinging, urticaria
SPECIAL CONSIDERATIONS
• Use of nail lacquer requires monthly removal of the unattached, infected nails by a health care professional; in clinical trials <12% of patients achieved a clear or almost clear nail
PATIENT/FAMILY EDUCATION
• *Cream/gel/lotion:*
• Continue medication for several days after condition clears
• Consult prescriber if no improvement after 4 wk of treatment
• *Nail lacquer:*
• 48 weeks of daily applications considered full treatment, may take 6 mo before see improvement

cidofovir

(ci-dah'fo-veer)
Rx: Vistide
Chemical Class: Acyclic purine nucleoside analog
Therapeutic Class: Antiviral

CLINICAL PHARMACOLOGY
Mechanism of Action: Metabolite (cidofovir diphosphate) inhibits viral DNA viral polymerase at intrac-

ellular concentrations 50- to 1000-fold lower than those required to inhibit cellular DNA synthesis

Pharmacokinetics

IV: Peak serum levels 12 μg/ml following 5 mg/kg INF; concurrent PO high dose probenecid/saline hydration doubles peak levels; minimal protein binding or hepatic systemic metabolism; intracellularly, phosphorylated to active diphosphate form (independent of virus infection); V_d, 300 ml/kg (steady state); $t_{1/2}$ 2.5 hr; 70% urinary excretion; no accumulation with weekly dosing

INDICATIONS AND USES: Cytomegalovirus retinitis in AIDS patients who are unresponsive to, intolerant to, or have relapsed on IV foscarnet or ganciclovir

DOSAGE

Adult

• *Cytomegalovirus retinitis in AIDS patients:* 5 mg/kg IV weekly for 2 wk (induction); 5 mg/kg IV every other week until retinitis progression or therapy-limiting toxicity; (see Special Considerations section); probenecid coadministration considered mandatory; for patients with renal insufficiency, schedule is same but dose reduced: CrCl 41-55 ml/min: 2 mg/kg; CrCl 30-40 ml/min: 1.5 mg/kg; CrCl 20-29 ml/min: 1.0 mg/kg; CrCl ≤19 ml/min: 0.5 mg/kg

💲 AVAILABLE FORMS/COST OF THERAPY

• Inj, Sol—IV: 75 mg/ml; 5 ml: **$846.00**

CONTRAINDICATIONS: Severe hypersensitivity to probenecid or sulfa drugs

PRECAUTIONS: Renal impairment (should administer probenecid/saline hydration concurrently to prevent nephrotoxicity), myelosuppression; do not give within 7 days of drugs listed in Drug Interactions section

PREGNANCY AND LACTATION: Pregnancy category C

SIDE EFFECTS/ADVERSE REACTIONS

GI: Dyspepsia (with probenecid)

GU: **Nephrotoxicity** (proximal tubular dysfunction), **renal insufficiency (29%)**

HEME: **Neutropenia**

SKIN: Rash (with probenecid)

INTERACTIONS

Drugs

🛡 *Aminoglycosides:* Additive nephrotoxicity

🛡 *Amphotericin B:* Additive nephrotoxicity

🛡 *Foscarnet:* Additive nephrotoxicity

🛡 *Pentamidine:* Additive nephrotoxicity (IV route only)

SPECIAL CONSIDERATIONS

• Concurrent high-dose probenecid plus saline hydration reduces nephrotoxicity; procedure: probenecid 2 g 3 hr prior to INF, then 1 g at 2 and 8 hr after INF; normal saline 1000 ml over 1 hr immediately prior to INF

MONITORING PARAMETERS

• Renal function, urinalysis (especially serum creatinine and urine protein prior to each dose), and blood chemistry (to include serum uric acid, phosphate, and bicarbonate), white counts with differential during intravenous therapy

cilostazol

(sil-os´tah-zol)

Rx: Pletal
Chemical Class: Quinolinone derivative
Therapeutic Class: Hemorheologic agent

CLINICAL PHARMACOLOGY

Mechanism of Action: Inhibits cAMP phosphodiesterase III; increases levels of cAMP in platelets and blood vessels resulting in vasodilation and inhibition of platelet aggregation

Pharmacokinetics

PO: Peak plasma concentration 3 to 4 hr, duration 48 hr; extensively metabolized by liver, primarily through CYP3A4 and to a lesser extent CYP2C19; 74% renally excreted in urine, 20% in feces; $t_{\frac{1}{2}}$ 11-13 hr (parent compound and active metabolites)

INDICATIONS AND USES: Intermittent claudication, percutaneous transluminal coronary angioplasty,* coronary stent implantation,* graft vs. host disease*

DOSAGE

Adult and child >16 yr

• *Intermittent claudication:* PO 100 mg bid, consider a decrease in dose to 50 mg bid if coadministration with a CYP3A4 or CYP2C19 inhibitor

🔢 AVAILABLE FORMS/COST OF THERAPY

• Tab, Coated—Oral: 50 mg, 60's: **$93.71**; 100 mg, 60's: **$98.40**

CONTRAINDICATIONS: Congestive heart failure

PRECAUTIONS: Congestive heart failure (several drugs with this pharmacologic effect have caused decreased survival compared with placebo in patients with class III-IV CHF), cardiovascular lesions, children

PREGNANCY AND LACTATION: Pregnancy category C; excreted in breast milk

SIDE EFFECTS/ADVERSE REACTIONS

CNS: Dizziness, vertigo, *headache*
CV: Palpitations, tachycardia, *peripheral edema*
GI: Abnormal stool, diarrhea, dyspepsia, flatulence, nausea
MS: Back pain, myalgia
RESP: Cough, pharyngitis, rhinitis
MISC: Infection

INTERACTIONS

Drugs

🔳 *Diltiazem:* Increase cilostazol concentrations

🔳 *Erythromycin, azole antifungals, fluoxetine, nefazodone, and sertraline:* as CYP3A4 or CYP2C19 inhibitors, may increase cilostazol levels; clinical effects unknown

🔳 *Omeprazole:* Increase cilostazol concentrations

🔳 *Foods: Grapefruit juice:* Increases cilostazol levels; *High fat:* increases absorption of cilostazol (80% increase of Cmax, 25% increase of AUC)

SPECIAL CONSIDERATIONS

• Cilostazol has been shown, in a multicenter, randomized, double-blind study (DPPARA 2), to be superior to pentoxifylline for treatment of claudication symptoms

PATIENT/FAMILY EDUCATION

• Take ½ hr before meal or 2 hr after meal

MONITORING PARAMETERS

• Beneficial effects usually seen in 2 to 4 wk, may take up to 12 wk

---

* = non-FDA-approved use

cimetidine

(sye-met´i-deen)

Rx: Tagamet

OTC: Tagamet HB

Chemical Class: Imidazole derivative

Therapeutic Class: Gastrointestinal antiulcer agent

CLINICAL PHARMACOLOGY

Mechanism of Action: Competitive, reversible inhibitor of histamine at gastric H_2-receptors; reduces gastric acid secretion

Pharmacokinetics

IM/IV: Onset 10 min, peak ½ hr, duration 4-5 hr

PO: Peak 1-1½ hr

Well absorbed (PO, IM); 30%-40% metabolized by liver (sulfoxide, major metabolite), excreted in urine (75% unchanged after 24 hr); $t_{1/2}$ 1½-2 hr

INDICATIONS AND USES: Short-term treatment of duodenal and benign gastric ulcers; maintenance therapy for duodenal ulcer; erosive gastroesophageal reflux disease (GERD); prevention of upper gastrointestinal bleeding in critically ill patients; treatment of pathological hypersecretory conditions (i.e., Zollinger-Ellison syndrome, systemic mastocytosis, multiple endocrine adenomas); heartburn, acid indigestion, and sour stomach (OTC only); as part of a multiple-drug regimen to eradicate *Helicobacter pylori* in the treatment of peptic ulcer*; chronic viral warts in children,* chronic idiopathic urticaria (in combination with H_1-receptor antagonists)*

DOSAGE

Adult and child >16 yr

• *Treatment:* PO 300 mg qid with meals, hs or 400 mg bid or 800 mg hs × 8 wk; after 8 wk give 300-400 mg hs dose only; IV bolus 300 mg/20 ml 0.9% NaC1 over 1-2 min q6h; IV INF 300 mg/50 ml D_5W over 15-20 min q6h; continuous IV INF 37.5 mg/hr (900 mg/day); IM 300 mg q6h, not to exceed 2400 mg/day

• *Prophylaxis of duodenal ulcer:* 400 mg hs

• *GERD:* PO 1600 mg/day (800 mg bid or 400 mg qid) for 12 wk

• *Pathologic hypersecretory states:* PO 300 mg qid; increase prn; do not exceed 2400 mg/day

• *Heartburn, acid indigestion, sour stomach (OTC only):* PO 200 mg (2 tabs) up to bid prn

AVAILABLE FORMS/COST OF THERAPY

• Inj, Sol—IM, IV: 150 mg/2 ml: **$1.41-$3.32**

• Inj, Sol—IV: 300 mg/50 ml, 50 ml: **$6.25-$11.16**

• Liq—Oral: 300 mg/5 ml, 240, 480 ml: **$161.81-$172.99**/480 ml

• Tab, Coated—Oral: 200 mg, 12's: **$5.70** (OTC); 200 mg, 100's: **$65.69-$96.55**; 300 mg, 100's: **$16.75-$111.40**; 400 mg, 100's: **$125.85-$167.66**; 800 mg, 100's: **$220.00-$600.00**

PRECAUTIONS: Organic brain syndrome, hepatic disease, renal disease, elderly

PREGNANCY AND LACTATION: Pregnancy category B; excreted into breast milk and may accumulate; theoretically, adversely affects the nursing infant's gastric acidity, inhibits drug metabolism, and produces CNS stimulation—all not reported; compatible with breast feeding

---

italic = common side effects   ***bold italic*** = life-threatening reactions

SIDE EFFECTS/ADVERSE REACTIONS

CNS: Anxiety, confusion, depression, dizziness, headache, psychosis, *seizures,* tremors, weakness

CV: Bradycardia, tachycardia

GI: Abdominal cramps, diarrhea, jaundice, paralytic ileus

GU: Galactorrhea, gynecomastia, impotence; increase in BUN, creatinine

HEME: **Agranulocytosis, aplastic anemia, neutropenia, thrombocytopenia**

SKIN: Alopecia, **exfoliative dermatitis,** flushing, rash, sweating, urticaria

INTERACTIONS

Drugs

🔢 *Amiodarone, benzodiazepines; calcium channel blockers; amiodarone; cyclic antidepressants; carbamazepine; carmustine; chloramphenicol; cisapride; citalopram; clozapine; diltiazem; femoxidine; flecanide; glyburide; glipizide; labetolol; lidocaine; lomustine; melphalan; metoprolol; narcotic analgesics; moricizine; N-acetylprocainamide; nicotine; phenytoin; peridolol; praziquantel; procainamide; propafinone; propranolol; quinidine; tacrine; theophylline; tolbutamide:* Increased concentrations of interacting drugs with potential for toxicity

🔢 *Ketoconazole, cefpodoxime, cefuroxime:* Reduced concentrations of interacting drugs

❷ *Warfarin:* Increased concentrations of interacting drugs with potential for toxicity

Labs

• *False positive:* Hemoccult

SPECIAL CONSIDERATIONS

• Generic formulations offer less costly alternative for patients not at risk for drug interactions

PATIENT/FAMILY EDUCATION

• Stagger doses of cimetidine and antacids

---

cinoxacin

(sin-ox′a-sin)

Rx: Cinobac

Chemical Class: Quinolone derivative

Therapeutic Class: Antibiotic

CLINICAL PHARMACOLOGY

Mechanism of Action: Interferes with the enzyme DNA gyrase needed for the synthesis of bacterial DNA; bactericidal

Pharmacokinetics

PO: Peak 2 hr, duration 6-8 hr, excreted in urine (unchanged/inactive metabolites); $t_{1/2}$ 1½ hr

INDICATIONS AND USES: Infections of the urinary tract caused by susceptible organisms

Antibacterial spectrum usually includes: *E. coli, Klebsiella, Enterobacter, P. mirabilis, P. vulgaris, M. morganii, Serratia, Citrobacter*

DOSAGE

Adult and Child >12 yr

• PO 1 g/day in 2-4 divided doses × 1-2 wk

• *Preventive therapy:* PO 250 mg qhs for up to 5 mo

🔢 **AVAILABLE FORMS/COST OF THERAPY**

• Cap, Gel—Oral: 250 mg, 40's: **$59.60**; 500 mg, 50's: **$77.60-$134.51**

CONTRAINDICATIONS: Anuria, CNS damage

PRECAUTIONS: Renal disease, hepatic disease

PREGNANCY AND LACTATION: Pregnancy category B

SIDE EFFECTS/ADVERSE REACTIONS

CNS: Agitation, confusion, *dizziness, headache,* insomnia
EENT: Blurred vision, sensitivity to light, tinnitus, visual disturbances
GI: Abdominal cramps, anorexia, diarrhea, *nausea, vomiting*
SKIN: Edema, photosensitivity, pruritus, rash, urticaria

---

ciprofloxacin

(sip-ro-floks′a-sin)
Rx: Ciloxan (ophthalmic), Cipro
Chemical Class: Fluoroquinolone derivative
Therapeutic Class: Antibiotic

CLINICAL PHARMACOLOGY
Mechanism of Action: Interferes with the enzyme DNA gyrase, needed for the synthesis of bacterial DNA; bactericidal
Pharmacokinetics
PO: Peak 1-2 hr; 60%-85% bioavailable PO with minimal 1st pass; widely distributed; 30%-50% excreted in urine as active drug, 20%-40% of dose excreted in feces (biliary excretion); $t_{1/2}$ 4 hr; metabolites less active

INDICATIONS AND USES: Infections of the lower respiratory tract, skin and skin structure, bone and joints, urinary tract, external auditory canal*; uncomplicated gonorrhea; typhoid fever; chronic prostatitis; intra-abdominal infections (in combination with metronidazole); infectious diarrhea; empirical therapy in febrile neutropenia (IV); superficial ocular infections caused by susceptible organisms (ophthalmic)
Antibacterial spectrum usually includes:

• Gram-positive organisms: *Enterococcus faecalis,* (many strains are only moderately susceptible), *Staphylococcus aureus, S. epidermidis, Streptococcus pneumoniae* (minimally)
• Gram-negative organisms: *Campylobacter jejuni, Citrobacter diversus, C. freundii, Enterobacter cloacae, Escherichia coli, H. influenzae, H. parainfluenzae, Klebsiella pneumoniae, Morganella morganii, Proteus mirabilis, P. vulgaris, Providencia rettgeri, P. stuartii, Pseudomonas aeruginosa, Serratia marcescens, Shigella flexneri, S. sonnei, Neisseria gonorrhoeae*
• Most strains of *Pseudomonas cepacia* and some strains of *Pseudomonas maltophilia* are resistant to ciprofloxacin as are most anaerobic bacteria, including *Bacteroides fragilis* and *Clostridium difficile*

DOSAGE
Adult
• *Uncomplicated UTI:* PO 100-250 mg q12h; IV 200 mg q12h × 7 days
• *Complicated/severe urinary tract infections:* PO 500 mg q12h × 14 days; IV 400 mg q12h
• *Respiratory, skin, bone, and joint infections:* (Bone and joint infections may require treatment for 4 to 6 wk or longer) PO 500-750 mg q12h × 7-14 days
• *Infectious diarrhea:* 500 mg q12h × 5-7 days
• *Uncomplicated gonorrhea:* PO 500 mg as a single dose, plus doxycycline 100 mg bid or other agent active against chlamydia
• *Typhoid fever:* PO 500 mg q12h
• *Ocular:* 1 gtt 5-6 times/day
• *Renal impairment:* CrCl 10-50 ml/min 50% of dose; CrCl <10 ml/min 30% of dose

💲 AVAILABLE FORMS/COST OF THERAPY

• Inj, Sol—IV: 200 mg/100 ml, 1's: **$15.61**; 400 mg/200 ml, 1's: **$31.25**
• Oint—Ophth: 0.3%, 3.5 g: **$42.25**
• Sol—Ophth: 0.3%, 2.5, 5, 10 ml: **$32.95-$39.12**/5 ml
• Sus—Oral: 250 mg/5 ml, 100 ml: **$88.14**; 500 mg/5 ml, 100 ml: **$103.19**
• Tab, Uncoated—Oral: 100 mg, 6's: **$16.83**; 250 mg, 100's: **$385.00**; 500 mg, 100's: **$515.85**; 750 mg, 100's: **$432.70**

PRECAUTIONS: Children (arthropathy in juvenile animals), renal disease, excessive sunlight, caution with known or suspected CNS disorders

PREGNANCY AND LACTATION: Pregnancy category C; appears in breast milk at levels similar to serum; allow 48 hr to elapse after last dose, before resuming breast feeding

SIDE EFFECTS/ADVERSE REACTIONS

CNS: Chills, depression, dizziness, fatigue, fever, hallucinations, headache, insomnia, nightmares, restlessness
EENT: Blurred vision, tinnitus
GI: Abdominal pain/discomfort, nausea, constipation; diarrhea, dysphagia, flatulence, heartburn, increased ALT, AST; oral candidiasis, vomiting
SKIN: Flushing, photosensitivity, pruritus, rash, urticaria

INTERACTIONS

Drugs
🔢 *Aluminum:* Reduced absorption of ciprofloxacin; do not take within 4 hr of dose
🔢 *Antacids:* Reduced absorption of ciprofloxacin; do not take within 4 hr of dose
🔢 *Antipyrine:* Inhibits metabolism of antipyrine; increased plasma antipyrine level
🔢 *Caffeine:* Inhibits metabolism of caffeine; increased plasma caffeine level
🔢 *Calcium:* Reduced absorption of ciprofloxacin; do not take within 4 hr of dose
🔢 *Diazepam:* Inhibits metabolism of diazepam; increased plasma diazepam level
🔢 *Didanosine:* Markedly reduced absorption of ciprofloxacin; take ciprofloxacin 2 hr before didanosine
🔢 *Foscarnet:* Coadministration increases seizure risk
🔢 *Iron:* Reduced absorption of ciprofloxacin; do not take within 4 hr of dose
🔢 *Magnesium:* Reduced absorption of ciprofloxacin; do not take within 4 hr of dose
🔢 *Metoprolol:* Inhibits metabolism of metoprolol; increased plasma metoprolol level
🔢 *Pentoxifylline:* Inhibits metabolism of pentoxifylline; increased plasma pentoxifylline level
🔢 *Phenytoin:* Inhibits metabolism of phenytoin; increased plasma phenytoin level
🔢 *Propranolol:* Inhibits metabolism of propranolol; increased plasma propranolol level
🔢 *Ropinirole:* Inhibits metabolism of ropinirole; increased plasma ropinirole level
🔢 *Sodium bicarbonate:* Reduced absorption of ciprofloxacin; do not take within 4 hr of dose
🔢 *Sucralfate:* Reduced absorption of ciprofloxacin; do not take within 4 hr of dose
🔢 *Theobromine:* Inhibits metabolism of theobromine; increased plasma theobromine level

---

* = non-FDA-approved use

3 *Theophylline:* Inhibits metabolism of theophylline; cut maintenance theophylline dose in half during therapy with ciprofloxacin

3 *Warfarin:* Inhibits metabolism of warfarin; increases hypoprothrombinemic response to warfarin

3 *Zinc:* Reduced absorption of ciprofloxacin; do not take within 4 hr of dose

Labs
• *False increase:* Urine coproporphyrin I, coproporphyrin III, urine porphyrins

SPECIAL CONSIDERATIONS
• Reserve use for UTI to documented pseudomonal infection or complicated UTI
• Considered 1st-line therapy for otitis externa in diabetic patients

---

citalopram
(sy-tal′oh-pram)
Rx: Celexa
Chemical Class: Bicyclic phthalane derivative
Therapeutic Class: Selective serotonin reuptake inhibitor antidepressant

---

CLINICAL PHARMACOLOGY
Mechanism of Action: Inhibitor of CNS neuronal uptake of serotonin (5HT); no significant activity for histaminergic, alpha or beta adrenergic, muscarinic, or dopaminergic

Pharmacokinetics
PO: Peak serum concentrations 2 to 4 hr; bioavailability 80%, unaffected by meals, metabolized by liver enzymes CYP3A4 and CYP2C19. Primary metabolite is desmethylcitalopram, which is active but less selective and less potent than parent drug; 20% (12% un-changed) excreted in urine, significant elimination in feces; $t_{1/2}$ 33 to 37 hr

INDICATIONS AND USES: Major depressive disorder, diabetic neuropathy,* obsessive-compulsive disorder,* panic disorder,* poststroke emotional lability,* premenstrual dysphoria syndrome,* alcohol abuse,* dementia*

DOSAGE
Adult and child >16 yr
• *Depression:* 20-60 mg qd
• *Alcohol abuse:* 40 mg qd
• *Diabetic neuropathy:* 40 mg qd
• *Poststroke emotional lability:* 20 mg qd if patient <66 yr old

Dosage in renal failure
• No adjustment needed

Dosage in hepatic insufficiency
• 20 mg qd, may increase to 40 mg qd in unresponsive patients

Dosage in geriatric patients
• *Depression:* 20 mg qd, may increase to 40 mg qd in unresponsive patients
• *Dementia:* 20-30 mg qd
• *Poststroke emotional lability:* 10 mg qd in patients >66 yr old

AVAILABLE FORMS/COST OF THERAPY
• Sol—Oral: 10 mg/5 ml, 120, 240 ml: **$53.60**/120 ml
• Tab, Coated—Oral: 10 mg, 100's: **$215.58**; 20 mg, 100's: **$224.70**; 40 mg, 100's: **$234.48**

CONTRAINDICATIONS: Concurrent use of MAOIs or use within 2 wk of discontinuation of MAOIs

PRECAUTIONS: Hepatic insufficiency, cardiovascular disease, seizure disorders, suicidal tendencies, mania, children and adolescence (no clinical data)

---

italic = common side effects   ***bold italic*** = life-threatening reactions

PREGNANCY AND LACTATION:
Pregnancy category C; breast feeding: unknown, 2 cases of infants experiencing excessive somnolence, decreased feeding, and weight loss have been reported

SIDE EFFECTS/ADVERSE REACTIONS

CNS: Migraine, parethesia, somnolence, impaired concentration, fatigue, drowsiness, sleep disturbance, confusion, restlessness, *amnesia, apathy, **suicidal attempt,*** **seizures**

CV: Hypotension, postural hypotension, palpitations

EENT: Visual changes

GI: Nausea, vomiting, xerostomia, taste perversion, constipation, dyspepsia, anorexia, increased appetite, flatulence

GU: Polyuria, dysuria, amenorrhea, *abnormal ejaculation* (>5%)

MS: Myalgia

RESP: Cough

SKIN: Increased sweating, rash

INTERACTIONS

Drugs

❷ *Buspirone:* Increased risk of serotonin syndrome

❸ *Cimetidine:* Increased levels of desmethylcitalopram via inhibition of CYP2D6 by cimetidine

❸ *Imipramine:* Increased bioavailability and half-life of desipramine (the major metabolite of imipramine) via inhibition of CYP2D6 by citalopram

▲ *MAOIs, dexfenfluramine, sibutramine:* increased risk of sertonin syndrome

❸ *Metoprolol:* May increase levels of metoprolol, but no clinically significant changes in blood pressure or heart rate have been observed

❸ *Naratriptan, rizatriptan, sumatriptan, zolmatriptan:* Increased risk of weakness, hyperreflexia, and incoordination

SPECIAL CONSIDERATIONS
• No clinical advantage over other SSRIs

PATIENT/FAMILY EDUCATION
• Therapeutic response may take 5 to 6 wk; most commonly taken once daily in the afternoon or evening

---

clarithromycin

(clare-i-thro-mye′sin)
Rx: Biaxin, Biaxin XL
Chemical Class: Macrolide derivative
Therapeutic Class: Antibiotic

CLINICAL PHARMACOLOGY
Mechanism of Action: Binds to 50S ribosomal subunits of susceptible bacteria and suppresses protein synthesis

Pharmacokinetics
PO: Peak 2-4 hr; 65% bound to plasma proteins; extensively metabolized in liver (14-OH metabolite twice as active as parent compound vs *Haemophilus influenzae*); $t_{1/2}$ 3-7 hr (metabolite 5-7 hr); Sus Action TAB: lower and later peak but equivalent 24 hr AUCs, 30% lower AUC under fasting conditions, Peak 5-9 hr

INDICATIONS AND USES: Infections of upper and lower respiratory tract, pharyngitis, tonsilitis, otitis media, maxillary sinusitis, acute bacterial exacerbation of chronic bronchitis, community-acquired pneumonia, skin and skin structure infection, skin and skin structures; disseminated mycobacterial infections due to *Mycoplasma avium* and *M. intracellulare* eradication of *Helicobacter pylori* associated with active duodenal ulcer disease (in combination with omeprazole and metronidazole)

Antibacterial spectrum usually includes:

• Gram-positive organisms: *Staphylococcus aureus, Streptococcus pneumoniae, S. pyogenes, S. agalactiae,* streptococci (Groups C, F, G), Viridans group streptococci, *Listeria monocytogenes*

• Gram-negative organisms: *Haemophilus influenzae, Moraxella catarrhalis, Bordetella pertussis, Campylobacter jejuni, Legionella pneumophila, Neisseria gonorrhoeae, Pasteurella multocida*

• Anaerobes: *Clostridium perfringens, Peptococcus niger, Propionibacterium acnes, Bacteriodes melaninogenicus*

• Other organisms: *Mycoplasma pneumoniae, M. avium* complex (MAC) consisting of *M. avium* and *M. intracellulare; Chlamydia trachomatis, H. pylori*

DOSAGE
Adult
• *Acute maxillary sinusitis:* PO 500 mg bid × 14 days; Sus Action PO 1000 mg qd × 14 days

• *Acute exacerbation of chronic bronchitis:* (due to *Haemophilus*) PO 500 mg bid × 7-14 days; Sus Action PO 1000 mg qd × 7 days; (due to *Moraxella, S. pneumoniae*) PO 250 mg bid × 7-14 days; Sus Action PO 1000 mg qd × 7 days

• *Mycobacterial infections:* PO 500 mg bid × 7-14 days; Sus Action PO 1000 mg qd × 7 days

• *Other infections:* PO 250 mg bid for 7-14 days

• *H. pylori:* PO 500 mg bid × 10 days (with omeprazole 20 mg bid and amoxicillin 1 g bid)

Dosing adjustment in renal impairment (CrCl <30 ml/min): decrease dose by 50% or double dosing interval

Child
• 15 mg/kg/day divided q12h × 10 days

• *Mycobacterial infections:* PO 7.5 mg/kg bid, do not exceed 500 mg bid

▣ AVAILABLE FORMS/COST OF THERAPY
• Powder, Reconst—Oral: 125 mg/5 ml, 50, 100 ml: **$27.85**/100 ml; 250 mg/5 ml, 50, 100 ml: **$48.95**/100 ml

• Tab, Coated—Oral: 250, 500 mg, 60's: **$248.57**

• Tab, Coated, Sust Action—Oral: 500 mg, 60's: **$275.26**

CONTRAINDICATIONS: Concomitant administration with pimozide, cisapride, or terfenadine (QT prolongation)

PRECAUTIONS: Renal impairment, children, pregnancy use only if no other alternative

PREGNANCY AND LACTATION: Pregnancy category C; excretion into breast milk unknown; use caution in nursing mothers

SIDE EFFECTS/ADVERSE REACTIONS
CNS: Headache, psychosis

GI: Abdominal pain, abnormal taste, anorexia, *diarrhea,* heartburn, ***hepatotoxicity, nausea,*** stomatitis, ***vomiting,*** less GI symptoms reported with Sus Action TAB

GU: Moniliasis, vaginitis

SKIN: Pruritus, rash, urticaria

INTERACTIONS
Drugs
🖪 *Alfentanil:* Prolonged anesthesia and respiratory depression

🖪 *Alprazolam:* Increased plasma alprazolam concentration

🖪 *Amprenavir:* Plasma concentrations of clarithromycin may be increased by amprenavir; plasma concentrations of amprenavir may be increased by clarithromycin

⚠ *Astemizole:* QT prolongation and life-threatening dysrhythmia

❸ *Atorvastatin:* Increased plasma atorvastatin concentration with risk of rhabdomyolysis

❸ *Bromocriptine:* Increased bromocriptine concentration with toxicity

❸ *Buspirone:* Increased plasma buspirone concentration

❸ *Carbamazepine:* Markedly increased plasma carbamazepine concentrations

⚠ *Cisapride:* QT prolongation and life-threatening dysrhythmia

❷ *Clozapine:* Increased plasma clozapine concentrations

❸ *Colchicine:* Potential colchicine toxicity

❸ *Cyclosporine:* Increased plasma cyclosporine concentrations

❸ *Diazepam:* Increased plasma concentration of diazepam

❸ *Digoxin:* Reduced bacterial flora may increase plasma digoxin concentrations

❸ *Disopyramide:* Increased plasma disopyramide concentrations

❷ *Ergotamine:* Potential for ergotism

❸ *Ethanol:* Ethanol reduces plasma clarithromycin concentration

❸ *Felodipine:* Increased plasma felodipine concentrations

❸ *Food:* Food may increase or decrease the bioavailability of clarithromycin

❸ *Indinavir:* Plasma concentrations of clarithromycin may be increased by indinavir; plasma concentrations of indinavir may be increased by clarithromycin

❸ *Itraconazole:* Increased plasma itraconazole concentration

❸ *Lovastatin:* Increased plasma lovastatin concentration with risk of rhabdomyolysis

❸ *Methylprednisolone:* Increased plasma methylprednisolone concentrations

❸ *Midazolam:* Increased plasma concentration of midazolam

❸ *Nelfinavir:* Plasma concentrations of clarithromycin may be increased by nelfinavir; plasma concentrations of nelfinavir may be increased by clarithromycin

❸ *Penicillin:* Decreased activity of penicillin

⚠ *Pimozide:* QT prolongation and life-threatening dysrhythmia

❸ *Phenytoin:* Increased plasma phenytoin concentrations

❸ *Quinidine:* Increased plasma concentration of quinidine

❸ *Rifabutin:* Increased plasma rifabutin concentrations

❸ *Ritonavir:* Plasma concentrations of clarithromycin may be increased by ritonavir, plasma concentrations of ritonavir may be increased by clarithromycin

❸ *Saquinavir:* Plasma concentrations of clarithromycin may be increased by saquinavir; plasma concentrations of saquinavir may be increased by clarithromycin

❸ *Sildenafil:* Increased plasma sildenafil concentration

❷ *Simvastatin:* Increased plasma simvastatin concentration with risk of rhabdomyolysis

❸ *Tacrolimus:* Increased plasma tacrolimus concentration

⚠ *Terfenadine:* QT prolongation and life-threatening dysrhythmia

❸ *Theophylline:* Increased plasma theophylline concentration

❸ *Triazolam:* Increased plasma triazolam concentration

❸ *Valproic acid:* Increased plasma valproic acid concentration

❸ *Warfarin:* Markedly increased hypoprothrombinemic response to warfarin

* = non-FDA-approved use

3 *Zafirlukast:* Reduced plasma zafirlukast concentration probably by reducing bioavailability

3 *Zopiclone:* Increased plasma zopiclone concentration

SPECIAL CONSIDERATIONS

PATIENT/FAMILY EDUCATION

• Take Sus Action TAB with food, immediate release and granules without regard to food

• Do NOT refrigerate suspension

---

clemastine

(klem′as-teen)

Rx: Tavist

OTC: Tavist-1, Antihist-I

Combinations

  OTC: with phenylpropanolamine (Tavist D)

Chemical Class: Ethanolamine derivative

Therapeutic Class: Antihistamine

CLINICAL PHARMACOLOGY

Mechanism of Action: Decreases allergic response by blocking histamine at H_1-receptors

Pharmacokinetics

PO: Peak 5-7 hr, duration 10-12 hr; metabolized by liver, excreted by kidneys

INDICATIONS AND USES: Perennial and seasonal allergic rhinitis; uncomplicated allergic skin manifestations of urticaria and angioedema

DOSAGE

Adult and Child >12 yr

• PO 1.34-2.68 mg bid-tid, not to exceed 8.04 mg/day

$ **AVAILABLE FORMS/COST OF THERAPY**

• Syr—Oral: 0.67 mg/5 ml, 120, 480 ml: **$16.50-$31.44**/120 ml

• Tab, Uncoated—Oral: 1.34 mg, 16's: **$2.80-$6.88** (OTC); 2.68 mg, 100's: **$72.50-$134.74**

CONTRAINDICATIONS: Narrow-angle glaucoma, bladder neck obstruction

PRECAUTIONS: Liver disease, elderly, increased intraocular pressure, hyperthyroidism, cardiovascular disease, hypertension, urinary retention, renal disease, stenosed peptic ulcers

PREGNANCY AND LACTATION: Pregnancy category C; excreted into breast milk; may cause drowsiness and irritability in nursing infant; use with caution during breast feeding

SIDE EFFECTS/ADVERSE REACTIONS

CNS: Anxiety, confusion, *dizziness, drowsiness,* euphoria, fatigue, neuritis, paresthesia, poor coordination

CV: Hypotension, palpitations, tachycardia

EENT: Blurred vision, dry nose, throat; mydriasis, nasal stuffiness, tinnitus

GI: Anorexia, *constipation,* diarrhea, *dry mouth,* nausea, vomiting

GU: Dysuria, frequency, impotence, retention

HEME: **Agranulocytosis, hemolytic anemia, thrombocytopenia**

RESP: Chest tightness, increased thick secretions, wheezing

SKIN: Photosensitivity, rash, urticaria

SPECIAL CONSIDERATIONS

• No advantage over loratadine or cetirizine; lower doses associated with less sedation and efficacy

---

clidinium
(kli-din'ee-um)
Rx: Quarzan
Combinations
Rx: with chlordiazepoxide
(Clindex, Librax)
Chemical Class: Synthetic quaternary ammonium derivative
Therapeutic Class: Anticholinergic; gastrointestinal antispasmodic; gastrointestinal antiulcer agent (adjunct)

CLINICAL PHARMACOLOGY
Mechanism of Action: Inhibits gastrointestinal motility and diminishes gastric acid secretion
Pharmacokinetics
PO: Onset 1 hr, duration 3 hr; ionized, excreted in urine
INDICATIONS AND USES: Peptic ulcer disease (in combination with other drugs); functional GI disorders (diarrhea, pylorospasm, hypermotility, neurogenic colon)*; irritable bowel syndrome (spastic colon, mucous colitis)*; acute enterocolitis,* ulcerative colitis,* diverticulitis,* mild dysenteries,* pancreatitis,* splenic flexure syndrome*
DOSAGE
Adult
• PO 2.5-5 mg tid-qid ac, hs (use lower dose for elderly or debilitated patients)
§ AVAILABLE FORMS/COST OF THERAPY
• Cap, Gel—Oral: 2.5 mg, 100's: **$20.02**; 5 mg, 100's: **$27.28**
CONTRAINDICATIONS: Narrow-angle glaucoma, obstructive uropathy (e.g., bladder neck obstruction due to prostatic hypertrophy), obstructive disease of the GI tract (e.g., pyloroduodenal stenosis), paralytic ileus, intestinal atony, unstable cardiovascular status in acute hemorrhage, severe ulcerative colitis, toxic megacolon complicating ulcerative colitis, myasthenia gravis
PRECAUTIONS: Hyperthyroidism, coronary artery disease, dysrhythmias, CHF, ulcerative colitis, hypertension, hiatal hernia, hepatic disease, renal disease, urinary retention, prostatic hypertrophy, elderly
PREGNANCY AND LACTATION: Pregnancy category C; excretion into breast milk unknown, although would be expected to be minimal due to quaternary structure (see also atropine)
SIDE EFFECTS/ADVERSE REACTIONS
CNS: Anxiety, confusion, dizziness, drowsiness, hallucination, headache, insomnia, stimulation (especially in elderly), weakness
CV: Palpitations, tachycardia
EENT: Blurred vision, cycloplegia, increased ocular tension, mydriasis, photophobia
GI: Absence of taste, *constipation, dry mouth,* dysphagia, heartburn, nausea, paralytic ileus, vomiting
GU: Hesitancy, impotence, *retention*
SKIN: Allergic reactions, anhidrosis, fever, pruritus, rash, urticaria
SPECIAL CONSIDERATIONS
• Adjunctive agent; no significant effect on ulcer disease alone
PATIENT/FAMILY EDUCATION
• Avoid driving or other hazardous activities until stabilized on medication
• Avoid alcohol or other CNS depressants; will enhance sedating properties of this drug

* = non-FDA-approved use

clindamycin

(klin-da-mye'sin)

Rx: Cleocin, Cleocin T, Cleocin vaginal cream, Cleocin vaginal ovules, Clinda-Derm

Chemical Class: Lincomycin derivative

Therapeutic Class: Antibiotic

CLINICAL PHARMACOLOGY

Mechanism of Action: Inhibits bacterial protein synthesis by preferentially binding to the 50S ribosomal subunit

Pharmacokinetics

PO: Peak 45 min, duration 6 hr

IM: Peak 3 hr, duration 8-12 hr

VAG: Peak 16 hr (total 5% systemic absorption)

90% bound to plasma proteins; metabolized in liver, excreted in urine, bile, feces as active/inactive metabolites; $t_{1/2}$ 2.5 hr

INDICATIONS AND USES: Infections of the respiratory tract (e.g., empyema, anaerobic pneumonitis, lung abscess), skin and soft tissues, female pelvis and genital tract; septicemia; intra-abdominal infections (e.g., peritonitis, abscess); bone and joint infections; CNS toxoplasmosis in AIDS patients (in combination with pyrimethamine)*; *Pneumocystis carinii* pneumonia (in combination with primaquine)*; *Chlamydia trachomatis* infections in women*; acne vulgaris (top formulations); rosacea (top formulations)*; bacterial vaginosis (vag formulations)

Antibacterial spectrum usually includes:

• Gram-positive organisms: *Staphylococcus aureus, S. epidermidis* (penicillinase and non-penicilli-nase-producing strains), streptococci (except *Str. faecalis*), pneumococci

• Anaerobes: *Bacteroides* spp. (including *B. fragilis* and *B. melaninogenicus*), *Fusobacterium, Propionibacterium, Eubacterium, Actinomyces* spp., *Peptococcus, Peptostreptococcus, Clostridium perfringens, C. tetani, Veillonella*

DOSAGE

Adult

• PO 150-450 mg q6-8h, not to exceed 1.8 g/day; IM/IV 1.2-1.8 g/day in 2-4 divided doses, not to exceed 4.8 g/day; VAG cream insert 1 applicatorful qhs for 3 or 7 days in non-pregnant and for 7 days in pregnant patients; VAG suppositories insert 1 ovule qhs for 3 days in non-pregnant patients; TOP apply bid

Child

• PO 10-30 mg/kg/d divided q6h; IM/IV 25-40 mg/kg/d divided q6-8h; TOP apply bid

§ AVAILABLE FORMS/COST OF THERAPY

• Cap, Gel—Oral: 75 mg, 100's: **$114.80**; 150 mg, 100's: **$59.00-$211.94**; 300 mg, 100's: **$371.71-$422.40**

• Cre—Vag: 2%, 40 g: **$43.16-$45.32**

• Gel—Top: 1%, 30, 60 g: **$27.52-$35.89**/30 g

• Granule, Reconst—Oral: 75 mg/5 ml, 100 ml: **$21.91**

• Inj, Sol—IM, IV: 150 mg/ml, 2 ml: **$7.58-$11.34**

• Lotion—Top: 1%, 60 ml: **$44.68**

• Sol—Top: 1%, 30, 60 ml: **$17.94-$40.76**/60 ml

• Supp—Vag: 100 mg, 3's: **$42.36**

• Swab, Medicated—Top: 1%, 60's: **$39.42-$47.31**

CONTRAINDICATIONS: Regional enteritis, ulcerative colitis, antibiotic-associated colitis

---

PRECAUTIONS: History of GI disease, liver disease, renal disease, atopic individuals, tartrazine sensitivity (75 and 150 mg caps), elderly, prolonged therapy; pregnancy (vag suppositories)

PREGNANCY AND LACTATION: Pregnancy category B; excreted into breast milk; compatible with breast feeding

SIDE EFFECTS/ADVERSE REACTIONS

GI: Abdominal pain, anorexia, *diarrhea,* increased AST, ALT, bilirubin, alk phosphatase; jaundice, *nausea,* **pseudomembranous colitis,** *vomiting,* weight loss

GU: Urinary frequency, vaginitis, vulvar irritation

HEME: **Agranulocytosis,** eosinophilia, **leukopenia, thrombocytopenia**

SKIN: Abscess at inj site, erythema, pain, pruritus, rash, urticaria

INTERACTIONS

Drugs

3 *Food:* Decreased clindamycin concentrations with diet foods containing sodium cyclamate

2 *Kaolin-pectin:* Decreased clindamycin concentrations

Labs

• *False increase:* Serum theophylline

SPECIAL CONSIDERATIONS

• Most active antibiotic against anaerobes

• Preferred topical antiacne antibiotic

PATIENT/FAMILY EDUCATION

• Avoid intercourse and use of vaginal products (tampons, douches) when using the vag cream or suppositories

• Vag cream contains mineral oil and vag suppositories contain an oleaginous base which may weaken rubber or latex products such as condoms or diaphragms, avoid use within 72 hr following treatment with vag cream or suppositories

---

clioquinol

(klee-oh-kwee′nole)
Combinations
  Rx: with hydrocortisone (Ala-Quin, Corque, Dek-Quin); with hydrocortisone and pramoxine (1 + 1 − F)
Chemical Class: Halogenated hydroxyquinoline
Therapeutic Class: Topical anti-infective

CLINICAL PHARMACOLOGY

Mechanism of Action: Increases cell membrane permeability in susceptible organisms by binding sterols; decreases potassium, sodium, and nutrients in cell; inhibits the growth of various mycotic organisms such as Microsporons, Trichophytons, and *Candida albicans* and gram positive cocci such as staphylococci and enterococci

Pharmacokinetics

Some absorbed through the skin; excreted in urine (conjugated form), the rest excreted slowly

INDICATIONS AND USES: Inflamed conditions of the skin such as eczema, athlete's foot, other fungal infections

DOSAGE

Adult

• Top apply to affected area bid-tid, not for use >1 wk

$ AVAILABLE FORMS/COST OF THERAPY

Clioquinol/Hydrocortisone

• Cre—Top: 3%/0.5%, 15, 30 g: **$1.50**/15 g; 3%/1%, 20, 30 g: **$1.50-$6.50**/20 g

• Oint—Top: 3%/1%, 20 g: **$1.44-$4.28**

CONTRAINDICATIONS: Lesions of the eye, tuberculosis of the skin, most viral skin lesions (including herpes simplex, vaccinia, varicella), children <2 yr of age, diaper rash

PRECAUTIONS: Sensitized skin, deep or puncture wounds, serious burns

PREGNANCY AND LACTATION: Pregnancy category C; excretion into breast milk unknown

SIDE EFFECTS/ADVERSE REACTIONS

CNS: Neurotoxicity with systemic use

SKIN: Burning, contact dermatitis, dry skin, erythema, pruritus, rash, redness, staining of hair and skin, stinging, urticaria

SPECIAL CONSIDERATIONS

• Potential neurotoxicity with absorption (with occlusion); since other agents without this toxicity exist, questionable utility

---

clobetasol

(klo-bet′a-sol)

Rx: Cormax, Embeline E, Temovate, Temovate E
Chemical Class: Synthetic glucocorticoid
Therapeutic Class: Topical corticosteroid, very high potency

CLINICAL PHARMACOLOGY
Mechanism of Action: Depresses formation, release, and activity of endogenous mediators of inflammation, such as prostaglandins, kinins, histamine, liposomal enzymes, and the complement system resulting in decreased edema, erythema, and pruritus

Pharmacokinetics
Absorbed through the skin (increased by inflammation and occlusive dressings); metabolized primarily in the liver

INDICATIONS AND USES: Psoriasis, eczema, contact dermatitis, pruritus (usually reserved for severe dermatoses that have not responded to less potent formulation)

DOSAGE
Adult and Child >12 yr
• TOP apply to affected area bid, rub completely into skin

§ AVAILABLE FORMS/COST OF THERAPY
• Cre—Top: 0.05%, 15, 30, 45, 60 g: **$25.45-$47.40**/30 g
• Foam—Top: 0.05%, 50, 100 g: **$73.10**/50 g
• Gel—Top: 0.05%, 15, 30, 60 g: **$31.85-$43.86**/30 g
• Oint—Top: 0.05%, 15, 30, 45, 60 g: **$25.45-$43.86**/30 g
• Sol—Top: 0.05%, 25, 50 ml: **$39.60-$69.85**/50 ml

CONTRAINDICATIONS: Fungal infections; use on face, groin, or axilla

PRECAUTIONS: Viral infections, bacterial infections, children, prolonged use

PREGNANCY AND LACTATION: Pregnancy category C; unknown whether top application could result in sufficient systemic absorption to produce detectable amounts in breast milk (systemic corticosteroids are secreted into breast milk in quantities not likely to have detrimental effects on infant)

SIDE EFFECTS/ADVERSE REACTIONS

SKIN: Acne, allergic contact dermatitis, atrophy, burning, dryness, folliculitis, hypertrichosis, hypopigmentation, irritation, itching, miliaria, perioral dermatitis, secondary infection, striae

---

italic = common side effects   ***bold italic*** = life-threatening reactions

MISC: Potential for systemic absorption and reversible HPA axis suppression (more likely with occlusive dressings, prolonged administration, application to large surface areas, liver failure, and in children)

SPECIAL CONSIDERATIONS

• No demonstrated superiority over other high-potency agents; cost should govern use

PATIENT/FAMILY EDUCATION

• Apply sparingly only to affected area

• Avoid contact with the eyes

• Do not put bandages or dressings over treated area unless directed by clinician

• Do not use on weeping, denuded, or infected areas

• Discontinue drug, notify clinician if local irritation or fever develops

---

clocortolone

(klo-kort'o-lone)
Rx: Cloderm
Chemical Class: Synthetic glucocorticoid
Therapeutic Class: Topical corticosteroid, intermediate potency

---

CLINICAL PHARMACOLOGY

Mechanism of Action: Depresses formation, release, and activity of endogenous mediators of inflammation, such as prostaglandins, kinins, histamine, liposomal enzymes, and the complement system resulting in decreased edema, erythema, and pruritus

Pharmacokinetics

Absorbed through the skin (increased by inflammation and occlusive dressings); metabolized primarily in the liver

INDICATIONS AND USES: Psoriasis, eczema, contact dermatitis, pruritus

DOSAGE

Adult and Child

• TOP apply to affected area tid or qid, rub completely into skin

§ **AVAILABLE FORMS/COST OF THERAPY**

• Cre—Top: 0.1%, 15, 45 g: **$16.25-$20.25**/15 g

CONTRAINDICATIONS: Fungal infections; use on face, groin, or axilla

PRECAUTIONS: Viral infections, bacterial infections, children

PREGNANCY AND LACTATION: Pregnancy category C; unknown whether top application could result in sufficient systemic absorption to produce detectable amounts in breast milk (systemic corticosteroids are secreted into breast milk in quantities not likely to have detrimental effects on infant)

SIDE EFFECTS/ADVERSE REACTIONS

SKIN: Acne, allergic contact dermatitis, atrophy, burning, dryness, folliculitis, hypertrichosis, hypopigmentation, irritation, itching, miliaria, perioral dermatitis, secondary infection, striae

MISC: Systemic absorption of topical corticosteroids has produced reversible HPA axis suppression (more likely with occlusive dressings, prolonged administration, application to large surface areas, liver failure, and in children)

SPECIAL CONSIDERATIONS

• No demonstrated superiority over other low-potency agents; cost should govern use

PATIENT/FAMILY EDUCATION

• Apply sparingly only to affected area

• Avoid contact with the eyes

• Do not put bandages or dressings over treated area unless directed by clinician
• Discontinue drug, notify clinician if local irritation or fever develops
• Do not use on weeping, denuded, or infected areas

---

clofazimine

(kloe-faz′i-meen)
Rx: Lamprene
Chemical Class: Iminophenazine dye
Therapeutic Class: Leprosy, *Mycobacterium avium* complex

CLINICAL PHARMACOLOGY
Mechanism of Action: Binds to mycobacterial DNA and inhibits growth; also exerts anti-inflammatory properties in controlling erythema nodosum leprosum reactions; precise mechanisms of action are unknown
Pharmacokinetics
PO: Deposited in fatty tissue and reticuloendothelial system, $t_{1/2}$ 70 days; small amount excreted in feces, sputum, sweat

INDICATIONS AND USES: Lepromatous leprosy (including dapsone-resistant lepromatous leprosy and lepromatous leprosy complicated by erythema nodosum leprosum); combination therapy with other anti-infectives in *Mycobacterium avium-intracellulare* (MAC) infections*

DOSAGE
Adult
• *Dapsone-resistant leprosy:* PO 100 mg qd in combination with 1 or more other antileprosy drugs for 3 yr, followed by monotherapy with 100 mg clofazamine qd

• *Dapsone-sensitive multibacillary leprosy:* PO 50-100 mg qd in combination with 2 or more other antileprosy drugs for 2 yr, followed by single-drug therapy with an appropriate agent
• *Erythema nodosum leprosum:* PO 100-200 mg qd for up to 3 mo or longer, then taper dose to 100 mg qd when possible
• *MAC infections:* PO 100 mg qd-tid in combination with other mycobacterial agents
Child
• *Leprosy:* PO 1 mg/kg q24h in combination with dapsone and rifampin

$ **AVAILABLE FORMS/COST OF THERAPY**
• Cap, Elastic—Oral: 50 mg, 100's: **$19.61**

PRECAUTIONS: Children, abdominal pain, diarrhea, depression
PREGNANCY AND LACTATION: Pregnancy category C; excreted into breast milk; do not administer to nursing mother unless clearly indicated

SIDE EFFECTS/ADVERSE REACTIONS
CNS: Dizziness, drowsiness, fatigue, giddiness, headache, neuralgia
EENT: Conjunctival and corneal pigmentation; dry, burning, itching, irritated eyes
GI: Abdominal/epigastric pain, anorexia, constipation, diarrhea, enlarged liver, eosinophilic enteritis, *GI intolerance,* hepatitis, jaundice, nausea, taste disorder, vomiting, weight loss
HEME: Eosinophilia
METAB: Hypokalemia
SKIN: Acneiform eruptions, *dryness,* erythroderma, *ichthyosis,* monilial cheilosis, phototoxicity, *pigmentation (pink to brownish black),* pruritus, rash

---

italic = common side effects   ***bold italic*** = life-threatening reactions

INTERACTIONS
Labs
• *Increase:* Albumin, bilirubin, AST
SPECIAL CONSIDERATIONS
• Use in conjunction with other anti-leprosy agents to prevent development of resistance
PATIENT/FAMILY EDUCATION
• May discolor skin from pink to brownish black, as well as discoloring the conjunctivae, lacrimal fluid, sweat, sputum, urine, and feces; skin discoloration may take several mo or yr to disappear after discontinuation of therapy

---

clofibrate
(kloe-fye´brate)
Rx: Atromid-S
Chemical Class: Fibric acid derivative
Therapeutic Class: Antilipemic

CLINICAL PHARMACOLOGY
Mechanism of Action: Acts to lower elevated serum lipids by reducing the very low-density lipoprotein fraction rich in triglycerides; serum cholesterol may be decreased, particularly in those patients whose cholesterol elevation is due to the presence of intermediate-density lipoprotein (IDL) as a result of Type III hyperlipoproteinemia
Pharmacokinetics
PO: Peak 2-6 hr; >90% bound to plasma proteins; metabolized in liver, excreted in urine; $t_{1/2}$ 18-22 hr
INDICATIONS AND USES: Primary dysbetalipoproteinemia (Type III hyperlipidemia); Type IV and V hyperlipidemia (in patients at risk of abdominal pain and pancreatitis)
DOSAGE
Adult
• PO 2 g/day in 4 divided doses

💲 AVAILABLE FORMS/COST OF THERAPY
• Cap, Elastic—Oral: 500 mg, 100's: **$20.00-$115.41**
CONTRAINDICATIONS: Severe hepatic or renal disease, primary biliary cirrhosis
PRECAUTIONS: Peptic ulcer
PREGNANCY AND LACTATION: Pregnancy category C; animal data suggest that the drug is excreted into breast milk; use caution in nursing mothers
SIDE EFFECTS/ADVERSE REACTIONS
CNS: Dizziness, drowsiness, fatigue, headache, weakness
CV: Angina, **dysrhythmias,** thrombophlebitis
GI: Abdominal distress, bloating, cholelithiasis, diarrhea, dyspepsia, flatulence, hepatomegaly, increased liver enzymes, *nausea,* stomatitis, vomiting, weight gain
GU: Decreased libido, dysuria, hematuria, impotence, oliguria, proteinuria
HEME: Anemia, bleeding, eosinophilia, **leukopenia**
MS: Arthralgias, *myalgias*
SKIN: Alopecia, dry hair and skin, pruritus, rash, urticaria
MISC: Polyphagia
INTERACTIONS
Drugs
3 *Antidiabetics:* Enhanced effect of oral hypoglycemic drugs in some patients
3 *Furosemide:* Enhanced effects of both drugs in patients with hypoalbuminemia
2 *Lovastatin:* Increased risk of myopathy
2 *Oral anticoagulants:* Increased hypoprothrombinemic response to warfarin and possibly other oral anticoagulants; serious bleeding episodes have occurred

SPECIAL CONSIDERATIONS

• No evidence substantiates a beneficial effect from clofibrate on cardiovascular mortality (a 36% increase in incidence of noncardiovascular deaths was reported in one study)

• Fibric acid derivatives only as alternative lipid-lowering drugs; clofibrate alternative to gemfibrozil

---

clomiphene

(kloe'mi-feen)

Rx: Clomid, Milophene, Serophene

Chemical Class: Nonsteroidal antiestrogenic

Therapeutic Class: Ovulation stimulant

CLINICAL PHARMACOLOGY

Mechanism of Action: Decreases the number of cytoplasmic estrogenic receptors, stimulating the secretion of luteinizing hormone (LH), follicle-stimulating hormone (FSH), and gonadotropins, which in turn stimulate the maturation and endocrine activity of the ovarian follicle and the subsequent development and function of the corpus luteum

Pharmacokinetics

PO: Metabolized in liver, excreted in feces

INDICATIONS AND USES: Ovulatory dysfunction in patients desiring pregnancy who have normal liver function, good levels of endogenous estrogen (reduced levels are less favorable but do not preclude successful therapy), and whose partners have adequate sperm; male infertility*

DOSAGE

Adult

• *Ovulatory failure:* PO 50 mg qd for 5 days beginning on day 5 of cycle; may be repeated at dosage of 100 mg until conception occurs or 3 cycles of therapy have been completed

• *Male infertility:* PO 25 mg qd for 25 days with 5 days rest, or 100 mg every Monday, Wednesday, and Friday

💲 AVAILABLE FORMS/COST OF THERAPY

• Tab, Uncoated—Oral: 50 mg, 100's: **$207.60-$304.49**

CONTRAINDICATIONS: Hepatic disease, undiagnosed vaginal bleeding

PRECAUTIONS: Hypertension, depression, seizure disorder, diabetes mellitus, ovarian cyst, polycystic ovary syndrome, uterine fibroids

PREGNANCY AND LACTATION: Pregnancy category X; each new course of drug should be started only after pregnancy has been excluded

SIDE EFFECTS/ADVERSE REACTIONS

CNS: Dizziness, insomnia, lightheadedness, nervousness

CV: Vasomotor flushing

EENT: Blurred vision, diplopia, photophobia

GI: Abdominal pain, bloating, constipation, nausea, vomiting

GU: Abnormal uterine bleeding, breast pain, frequency, multiple ovulation, oliguria, *ovarian enlargement,* polyuria, ***ovarian hyperstimulation syndrome***

SKIN: Alopecia, dermatitis, rash, urticaria

SPECIAL CONSIDERATIONS

• Though gonadotropin therapy is more effective for inducing ovulation, expense and time requirements warrant clomiphene trial

---

italic = common side effects **bold italic** = life-threatening reactions

PATIENT/FAMILY EDUCATION
• Risk of multiple births increased—is approx 8% (7% twins, <1% triplets or greater)
• Record basal body temperature to determine whether ovulation has occurred; if ovulation can be determined (there is a slight decrease in temperature, then a sharp increase for ovulation), attempt coitus 3 days before and qod until after ovulation
• Prolonged use may increase the risk of ovarian cancer

---

clomipramine
(klom-ip′ra-meen)
Rx: Anafranil
Chemical Class: Tertiary amine
Therapeutic Class: Antiobsessional; tricyclic antidepressant

CLINICAL PHARMACOLOGY
Mechanism of Action: Inhibits the reuptake of serotonin (5-HT) norepinephrine and amine blocking activity, moderate and very high, respectively
Pharmacokinetics
PO: Peak 4.7 hr; extensively bound to tissue and plasma proteins, demethylated in liver; active metabolites excreted in urine; $t_{1/2}$ 32 hr (parent compound), 69 hr (metabolite)
INDICATIONS AND USES: Obsessive-compulsive disorder (OCD), depression,* anxiety disorders*
DOSAGE
Adult
• *OCD:* PO 25 mg hs, increase gradually over 4 wk to a dose of 75-250 mg/day in divided doses; after titration, the entire dose may be given hs
• *Depression:* PO 50-150 mg/day in a single or divided dose
• *Anxiety/agoraphobia:* PO 25-75 mg/day

Child
• PO 25 mg hs, increase gradually over several wk to 3 mg/kg/day or 100 mg, whichever is smaller
🔣 AVAILABLE FORMS/COST OF THERAPY
• Cap, Gel—Oral: 25 mg, 100's: **$75.00-$118.13**; 50 mg, 100's: **$101.13-$159.22**; 75 mg, 100's: **$113.33-$209.59**
CONTRAINDICATIONS: Administration within 14 days of MAOI therapy, acute recovery period following MI
PRECAUTIONS: Seizure disorder, suicidal patients, elderly, cardiac disease
PREGNANCY AND LACTATION: Pregnancy category C; withdrawal symptoms, including jitteriness, tremor, and seizures have been reported in neonates whose mothers had taken clomipramine until delivery; has been found in human milk; use caution in nursing mothers
SIDE EFFECTS/ADVERSE REACTIONS
CNS: Abnormal dreaming, agitation, anxiety, confusion, depersonalization, depression, *dizziness,* emotional lability, *headache,* hypertonia, impaired concentration, increased appetite, *insomnia,* irritability, *libido change,* memory impairment, migraine, myoclonus, *nervousness,* panic reaction, paresthesia, psychosomatic disorder, *somnolence,* speech disorder, *tremor,* weight gain, yawning
CV: Bradycardia, **dysrhythmia,** pallor, palpitations, postural hypotension, syncope, tachycardia
EENT: Abnormal vision, tinnitus
GI: Abdominal pain, anorexia, constipation, diarrhea, dry mouth, dyspepsia, dysphagia, esophagitis, flatulence, *nausea,* tooth disorder, ulcerative stomatitis, vomiting

---

* = non-FDA-approved use

GU: Ejaculation disorder, impotence, urinary retention
MS: Arthralgia, back pain, myalgia
RESP: **Bronchospasm,** coughing, pharyngitis, rhinitis, sinusitis
SKIN: Abnormal skin odor, acne, dermatitis, dry skin, increased sweating, pruritus, rash, urticaria

INTERACTIONS

Drugs

🔢 *Barbiturates:* Reduced serum concentrations of cyclic antidepressants

❷ *Bethanidine:* Reduced antihypertensive effect of bethanidine

🔢 *Carbamazepine:* Reduced cyclic antidepressant serum concentrations

❷ *Clonidine:* Reduced antihypertensive response to clonidine; enhanced hypertensive response with abrupt clonidine withdrawal

🔢 *Debrisoquin:* Inhibited antihypertensive response of debrisoquin

❷ *Epinephrine:* Markedly enhanced pressor response to IV epinephrine

🔢 *Ethanol:* Additive impairment of motor skills; abstinent alcoholics may eliminate cyclic antidepressants more rapidly than nonalcoholics

🔢 *Fluoxetine, fluvoxamine, grapefruit juice:* Marked increases in cyclic antidepressant plasma concentrations

🔢 *Guanethidine:* Inhibited antihypertensive response to guanethidine

⚠ *MAOIs:* Excessive sympathetic response, mania, or hyperpyrexia possible

❷ *Moclobemide:* Potential association with fatal or non-fatal serotonin syndrome

🔢 *Neuroleptics:* Increased therapeutic and toxic effects of both drugs

❷ *Norepinephrine:* Markedly enhanced pressor response to norepinephrine

❷ *Phenylephrine:* Enhanced pressor response to IV phenylephrine

🔢 *Propoxyphene:* Enhanced effect of cyclic antidepressants

🔢 *Quinidine:* Increased cyclic antidepressant serum concentrations

SPECIAL CONSIDERATIONS

PATIENT/FAMILY EDUCATION

• Beneficial effects may take 2-3 wk
• Use caution while driving or during other activities requiring alertness; may cause drowsiness
• Avoid alcohol and other CNS depressants
• Do not discontinue abruptly

---

clonazepam

(kloe-na'zi-pam)
Rx: Klonopin
Chemical Class: Benzodiazepine
Therapeutic Class: Anticonvulsant; anxiolytic
DEA Class: Schedule IV

CLINICAL PHARMACOLOGY

Mechanism of Action: CNS depressants via facilitation of inhibitory GABA at benzodiazepine receptor sites (BZ_1—associated with sleep; BZ_2—associated with memory, motor, sensory, and cognitive function); effects include muscle relaxation (spinal cord), anticonvulsant activity (brain stem), ataxia (cerebellum), emotional behavior (limbic and cortical areas), and anxiolytic effects (separate from general CNS depression); anticonvulsant activity: suppresses the spike and wave discharge in absence seizures (petit mal) and decreases the frequency, amplitude, duration, and spread of discharge in minor motor seizures

---

italic = common side effects   ***bold italic*** = life-threatening reactions

Pharmacokinetics

PO: Peak 1-3 hr; 88% bound to plasma proteins; metabolized by liver, CYP3A, (principal metabolite is inactive), excreted in urine; $t_{1/2}$ 18-50 hr

INDICATIONS AND USES: Lennox-Gastaut syndrome (petit mal variant), akinetic and myoclonic seizures, absence seizures (petit mal) in patients who have failed to respond to succinimides; anxiety; panic disorder; restless legs*, Parkinsonian dysarthria*, multifocal tic disorders*, acute manic episodes of bipolar affective disorder*, deafferentation pain syndromes*, schizophrenia (adjunctive therapy)*

DOSAGE

Adult

• *Seizure disorders:* PO 1.5 mg/day in 3 divided doses

• *Panic disorder:* PO 0.25 mg bid initially, may be increased 0.125-0.25 mg bid q 3 days until response or side effects, target 1 mg/day, max 4 mg/day

Child <10 yr or <30 kg

• PO 0.01-0.03 mg/kg/day in 2-3 divided doses, not to exceed 0.05 mg/kg/day, may be increased 0.25-0.5 mg q3d until desired response, not to exceed 0.1-0.2 mg/kg/day

$ **AVAILABLE FORMS/COST OF THERAPY**

• Tab, Uncoated—Oral: 0.125 mg, 100's: **$72.37**; 0.25 mg, 100's: **$76.19**; 0.5 mg, 100's: **$70.69-$88.30**; 1 mg, 100's: **$81.04-$100.70**; 2 mg, 100's: **$112.41-$139.54**

CONTRAINDICATIONS: Severe liver disease, acute narrow-angle glaucoma

PRECAUTIONS: COPD, impaired renal function, abrupt discontinuation (may precipitate withdrawal), status epilepticus, elderly

PREGNANCY AND LACTATION: Pregnancy category D; increased risk of congenital malformations, episodes of prolonged apnea, hypothermia in newborn reported; excreted into breast milk, breast feeding not recommended

SIDE EFFECTS/ADVERSE REACTIONS

CNS: Ataxia, behavioral changes, confusion, dizziness, *drowsiness,* headache, insomnia, slurred speech, suicidal tendencies, tremor

CV: Bradycardia, hypotension, palpitations

EENT: Abnormal eye movements, blurred vision, diplopia, nystagmus

GI: Anorexia, constipation, diarrhea, gastritis, nausea, polyphagia, sore gums, xerostomia

GU: Dysuria, enuresis, nocturia, urinary retention

HEME: Anemia, eosinophilia, *leukocytosis, thrombocytopenia*

RESP: Congestion, dyspnea, respiratory depression

SKIN: Rash

INTERACTIONS

Drugs

3 *CNS depressants:* Alcohol, narcotics, barbiturates, anxiolytics, phenothiazine, thioxanthene and butyrophenone antipsychotics, MAOIs, tricyclic antidepressants; CNS depression potentiated

3 *CYP3A inducers:* Phenytoin, carbamazepine, phenobarbital; decreased serum clonazepam concentrations

3 *Disulfiram:* Increased serum clonazepam concentrations

3 *Oral antifungals:* Decreased serum clonazepam concentrations, use cautiously

3 *Valproic acid:* Increased occurrence of absence seizures

* = non-FDA-approved use

SPECIAL CONSIDERATIONS

• Up to 30% of patients have shown a loss of anticonvulsant activity, often within 3 mo of administration; dosage adjustment may reestablish efficacy

PATIENT/FAMILY EDUCATION

• Do not take more than prescribed amount, may be habit-forming
• Avoid driving, activities that require alertness; drowsiness may occur
• Avoid alcohol ingestion or other CNS depressants
• Do not discontinue medication abruptly after long-term use

MONITORING PARAMETERS

• Although relationship between serum concentrations and seizure control is not well established, proposed therapeutic concentrations are 20-80 ng/ml; potentially toxic concentrations >80 ng/ml
• Close attention to seizure frequency is important in order to detect the emergence of tolerance

---

clonidine

(klon'ih-deen)

Rx: Catapres, Catapres-TTS, Duraclon
Combinations
  Rx: with chlorthalidone
    (Chlorpres, Combipress)
Chemical Class: Imidazoline derivative
Therapeutic Class: Antihypertensive, centrally acting sympathoplegic

---

CLINICAL PHARMACOLOGY

Mechanism of Action: Centrally active antihypertensive: stimulates central α_2-adrenergic receptors resulting in reduced sympathetic outflow from the CNS to the heart, kidneys, and peripheral vasculature; decreases systolic and diastolic blood pressure and pulse; chronic therapy associated with only mild reductions or no change in cardiac output; plasma renin activity is unchanged or mildly reduced

Pharmacokinetics

PO: Bioavailability 65%-95%, peak effect 3-5 hr; duration 6-10 hr

TOP: Therapeutic plasma levels 2-3 days after initial application, drug released at constant rate for approximately 7 days; following removal, plasma levels persist for 8 hr then decline slowly over several days

Metabolized in liver, excreted in urine (22% unchanged); $t_{1/2}$ 6-23 hr

INDICATIONS AND USES: Hypertension, alcohol withdrawal,* diabetic diarrhea,* Gilles de la Tourette syndrome,* hypertensive urgencies,* menopausal flushing,* opiate detoxification,* postherpetic neuralgia,* smoking cessation,* ulcerative colitis*; in combination with opiates for severe pain in cancer patients (epidural), surgery,* labor,* hyperhydrosis, spinal cord injury spasticity, chorea, akathisia, restless leg syndrome, hemodynamic stabilization preoperatively,* postoperative shivering,* atropine/neostigmine tachycardia*

DOSAGE

Adult

• PO 0.1 mg bid initially, increase 0.1-0.2 mg/day if needed, max 2.4 mg/day (minimize sedation by giving majority of daily dose hs); TOP apply patch to hairless area of intact skin on upper arm or torso once q7d, rotate sites, start with TTS-1 (0.1 mg/24 hr) and increase after 1-2 wk if needed (using >2 TTS-3 systems usually does not improve efficacy)
• *Severe cancer pain:* 30 μg/hr via continuous epidural infusion; use caution with infusion rates >40 μg/hr

---

italic = common side effects   ***bold italic*** = life-threatening reactions

Child
• PO 5-25 µg/kg/day in divided doses q6h, increase at 5-7 day intervals

💲 AVAILABLE FORMS/COST OF THERAPY

• Film, cont rel—Percutaneous: 0.1 mg/24 hr, 12's: **$136.80**; 0.2 mg/24 hr, 12's: **$230.31**; 0.3 mg/24 hr, 4's: **$106.50**
• Inj—Epidural: 100 µg/ml, 10 ml: **$58.06**
• Tab, Uncoated—Oral: 0.1 mg, 100's: **$3.00-$83.19**; 0.2 mg, 100's: **$3.38-$103.62**; 0.3 mg, 100's: **$4.20-$159.70**

PRECAUTIONS: Severe coronary insufficiency, recent MI, cerebrovascular disease, chronic renal failure, abrupt discontinuation (PO)

PREGNANCY AND LACTATION: Pregnancy category C; secreted into breast milk; hypotension has not been observed in nursing infants, although clonidine was found in the serum of the infants

SIDE EFFECTS/ADVERSE REACTIONS

Less severe with transdermal systems

CNS: Agitation, anxiety, delirium, depression, *dizziness,* dreams or nightmares, *drowsiness,* hallucinations, headache, insomnia, nervousness, restlessness, *sedation*

CV: Bradycardia, **CHF, dysrhythmias,** orthostatic hypotension, palpitations, Raynaud's phenomenon, rebound hypertension, tachycardia

GI: Anorexia, *constipation, dry mouth,* nausea, parotid pain, transient LFT elevations, vomiting

GU: Impotence, loss of libido, nocturia, urinary retention

METAB: Gynecomastia, transient elevation of blood glucose, weight gain

MS: Cramps of the lower limbs, fatigue, muscle or joint pain, weakness

SKIN: Alopecia, angioedema, hair thinning, pruritus, rash, transient localized skin reactions (TOP), urticaria

INTERACTIONS

Drugs

3 *β-blockers:* Rebound hypertension from clonidine withdrawal exacerbated by noncardioselective β-blockers

2 *Cyclic antidepressants:* Cyclic antidepressants may inhibit the antihypertensive response to clonidine

3 *Cyclosporine, tacrolimus:* Increased cyclosporine or tacrolimus concentrations

3 *Insulin:* Diminished symptoms of hypoglycemia

3 *Neuroleptics, nitroprusside:* Severe hypotension possible

Labs

• Growth hormone-stimulation test

SPECIAL CONSIDERATIONS
PATIENT/FAMILY EDUCATION

• Avoid hazardous activities, since drug may cause drowsiness
• Do not discontinue oral drug abruptly or withdrawal symptoms may occur (anxiety, increased BP, headache, insomnia, increased pulse, tremors, nausea, sweating)
• Response may take 2-3 days if drug is given transdermally
• Do not use OTC (cough, cold, or allergy) products unless directed by clinician
• Rise slowly to sitting or standing position to minimize orthostatic hypotension, especially elderly
• Dizziness, fainting, lightheadedness may occur during 1st few days of therapy
• May cause dry mouth; use hard candy, saliva product, or frequent rinsing of mouth

---

* = non-FDA-approved use

MONITORING PARAMETERS
• Blood pressure (posturally), blood glucose in patients with diabetes mellitus, confusion, mental depression

---

clopidogrel

(clo-pid′o-grill)
Rx: Plavix
Chemical Class: Thienopyridine
Therapeutic Class: Platelet aggregation inhibitor

CLINICAL PHARMACOLOGY
Mechanism of Action: Selectively and irreversibly inhibits ADP-induced platelet aggregation by inhibiting the binding of ADP to its receptors on platelets, thereby affecting ADP-dependent activation of the glycoprotein IIb/IIIa complex, the major site of platelet-fibrinogen binding
Pharmacokinetics
PO: Peak 1 hr; (significant antiaggregating activity in 2 hr); steady-state effect on bleeding time (1-2 × baseline), 3-7 days; following discontinuation, baseline values return in 5 days; 50% absorbed (PO); clopidogrel is a prodrug that is activated by hepatic metabolism (CYP1A), to the major circulating metabolite, a carboxylic acid derivative, which is a CYP2C9 inhibitor; metabolite excreted in both feces and urine; $t_{1/2}$ of major metabolite, 8 hr

INDICATIONS AND USES: Reduction of atherosclerotic events (myocardial infarction, stroke, and vascular death) in patients with atherosclerosis documented by recent stroke, myocardial infarction, or established peripheral arterial disease; prevention of thrombosis following intracoronary stent placement*

DOSAGE
Adult
• PO 75 mg qd (no dosage adjustments for elderly patients or those with renal impairment)

💲 AVAILABLE FORMS/COST OF THERAPY
• Tab, Film-Coated—Oral: 75 mg, 90's: **$289.15**

CONTRAINDICATIONS: Active pathological bleeding; coagulation disorders; patients receiving anticoagulants or other antiplatelet agents

PRECAUTIONS: Previous hypersensitivity or other untoward effects related to ticlopidine; hypertension; hepatic or renal impairment; history of bleeding or hemostatic disorders; history of drug-related hematologic disorders; patients scheduled for major surgery; pregnancy

PREGNANCY AND LACTATION: Pregnancy category B; excreted into breast milk in rats

SIDE EFFECTS/ADVERSE REACTIONS
CNS: Dizziness, headache, ***intracranial bleeding***
CV: Hypertension
GI: Abdominal pain, diarrhea, dyspepsia, ***GI ulceration and hemorrhage,*** nausea
GU: Liver enzyme elevation
HEME: Neutropenia (uncommon), prolonged bleeding time, purpura
SKIN: Pruritus, rash, urticaria

INTERACTIONS
Drugs
❸ *Fluvastatin:* Inhibition of hepatic metabolism (CYP2C9) of fluvastatin with increased risk of myositis; *in vitro* data
❸ *Nonsteroidal antiinflammatory agents:* Increased bleeding risk

---

italic = common side effects   ***bold italic*** = life-threatening reactions

3 *Phenytoin:* Inhibition of hepatic metabolism (CYP2C9) of phenytoin and increased risk of toxicity; *in vitro* data

3 *Tamoxifen:* Inhibition of hepatic metabolism (CYP2C9) and increased tamoxifen effects; *in vitro* data

3 *Tolbutamide:* Inhibition of hepatic metabolism (CYP2C9) of tolbutamide with increased risk of hypoglycemia; *in vitro* data

3 *Torsemide:* Inhibition of hepatic metabolism (CYP2C9) of torsemide with enhanced diuretic effects; *in vitro* data; increased bleeding risk

3 *Warfarin:* Inhibition of hepatic metabolism (CYP2C9) of warfarin with enhanced hypoprothrombinemic effects; *in vitro* data; increased bleeding risk

SPECIAL CONSIDERATIONS
• Comparative studies indicate that the drug is at least effective as aspirin; comparisons with ticlopidine lacking, however, no frequent CBC monitoring necessary
• Should probably replace ticlopidine as an aspirin alternative
• 28 × the cost of an equivalent supply of aspirin

PATIENT/FAMILY EDUCATION
• Inform clinician of signs and symptoms of bleeding, prior to surgery, dental work; inform clinician of sore throat, fever, etc. (consider neutropenia)

clorazepate
(klor-az′e-pate)
Rx: Gen-Xene, Tranxene, Tranxene-SD
Chemical Class: Benzodiazepine
Therapeutic Class: Antianxiety agent; anticonvulsant
DEA Class: Schedule IV

CLINICAL PHARMACOLOGY
Mechanism of Action: CNS depressant via facilitation of inhibitory GABA at benzodiazepine receptor sites (BZ_1—associated with sleep; BZ_2—associated with memory, motor, sensory, and cognitive function); effects include muscle relaxation (spinal cord), anticonvulsant activity (brain stem), ataxia (cerebellum), emotional behavior (limbic and cortical areas), and anxiolytic effects (separate from general CNS depression)
Pharmacokinetics
PO: Onset 15 min, peak 1-2 hr, duration 4-6 hr; metabolized by liver to active metabolites, excreted by kidneys; $t_{1/2}$ 30-100 hr

INDICATIONS AND USES: Anxiety disorders, acute alcohol withdrawal, partial seizures (adjunctive therapy)
DOSAGE
Adult
• *Anxiety:* PO 7.5-15 mg bid-qid or as single qhs dose of 15-22.5 mg; lower doses may be indicated for elderly or debilitated patients
• *Alcohol withdrawal:* PO 30 mg initially, then 15 mg bid-qid on 1st day; gradually decrease dose over subsequent days
• *Seizure disorders:* PO 7.5 mg tid; may increase by 7.5 mg/wk or less; not to exceed 90 mg/day

---

* = non-FDA-approved use

Child 9-12 yr
• *Seizure disorders:* PO 3.75-7.5 mg bid; increase by 3.75 mg at weekly intervals; max 60 mg/day in 2-3 divided doses

$ AVAILABLE FORMS/COST OF THERAPY
• Tab, Uncoated—Oral: 3.75 mg, 100's: **$6.38-$181.76**; 7.5 mg, 100's: **$7.13-$226.14**; 15 mg, 100's: **$39.00-$306.80**
• Tab, Uncoated, Sus Action—Oral: 11.25 mg, 100's: **$480.98**; 22.5 mg, 100's: **$616.00**

CONTRAINDICATIONS: Narrow-angle glaucoma, psychosis
PRECAUTIONS: Elderly, debilitated, hepatic disease, renal disease, long-term use, history of drug abuse
PREGNANCY AND LACTATION: Pregnancy category D; excreted into breast milk; drug and metabolites may accumulate to toxic levels in nursing infant

SIDE EFFECTS/ADVERSE REACTIONS

CNS: Anterograde amnesia, anxiety, ataxia, *confusion,* depression, dizziness, *drowsiness,* fatigue, hallucinations, headache, hysteria, insomnia, psychosis, slurred speech, stimulation, tremor
CV: Bradycardia, **cardiovascular collapse,** hypertension, hypotension, orthostatic, tachycardia
EENT: Auditory disturbances, blurred vision, mydriasis, nystagmus
GI: Anorexia, constipation, diarrhea, dry mouth, nausea, vomiting
GU: Changes in libido, incontinence, menstrual irregularities, urinary retention
SKIN: Dermatitis, hair loss, hirsutism, itching, rash, urticaria

INTERACTIONS
Drugs
3 *Cimetidine:* Increased plasma levels of clorazepate and/or active metabolites
3 *Disulfiram:* Increased serum clorazepate concentrations
3 *Ethanol:* Enhanced adverse psychomotor side effects of benzodiazepines
3 *Rifampin:* Reduced serum clorazepate concentrations

SPECIAL CONSIDERATIONS
• Do not use for everyday stress or for longer than 4 mo
• No advantage over diazepam
PATIENT/FAMILY EDUCATION
• Do not discontinue medication abruptly after long-term use

---

clotrimazole
(kloe-trim′a-zole)
Rx: Topical: Lotrimin, Mycelex
Oral: Mycelex
Vaginal: Mycelex-G, Mycelex Twin Pack
OTC: Topical: Gynix Lotrimin AF, Mycelex OTC
Vaginal: Gyne-Lotrimin, Mycelex 7, Femcare
Combinations
  Rx: with betamethasone dipropionate (Lotrisone)
Chemical Class: Imidazole derivative
Therapeutic Class: Topical antifungal

CLINICAL PHARMACOLOGY
Mechanism of Action: Broad-spectrum antifungal agent that inhibits growth of pathogenic dermatophytes, yeasts, and *Malassezia furfur;* exhibits fungistatic and fungicidal activity against isolates of *Trichophyton rubrum, T. mentagro-*

---

phytes, *Epidermophyton floccosum, Microsporum canis,* and *Candida* sp., including *C. albicans;* interferes with fungal DNA replication by binding sterols in fungal cell membrane, which increases permeability and causes leaking of cell nutrients

Pharmacokinetics

Well absorbed following oral administration, eliminated mainly as inactive metabolites; minimally absorbed following top and vag administration

INDICATIONS AND USES: Tinea pedis, tinea cruris, tinea corporis, tinea versicolor; *C. albicans* infection of the vagina, vulva, throat, mouth

DOSAGE

Adult and Child >3 yr

• PO 10 mg troche dissolved slowly 5 × /day; TOP apply bid

Adult and Child >12 yr

• VAG 100 mg qhs for 7 days or 200 mg qhs for 3 days or 500 mg × 1 or 5 g (1 applicatorful) of 1% VAG cream qhs for 7-14 days

§ AVAILABLE FORMS/COST OF THERAPY

• Cre—Top: 1%, 15, 30, 45 g: **$5.44-$29.21**/30 g
• Cre—Vag: 1%, 45, 90 g: **$5.94-$23.69**/45 g
• Lotion—Top: 1%, 30 ml: **$32.35**
• Sol—Top: 1%, 10, 30 ml: **$15.52-$30.94**/30 ml
• Tab, Uncoated, Sus Action—Vag: 100 mg, 7's: **$6.49-$12.00**; 200 mg, 3's: **$9.00-$10.26**; 500 mg, 1's: **$13.88-$15.40**
• Troche—Buccal: 10 mg, 70's: **$73.26-$96.36**

PREGNANCY AND LACTATION: Pregnancy category B; excretion in breast milk unknown

SIDE EFFECTS/ADVERSE REACTIONS

GI: Abdominal cramps, bloating
GU: Dyspareunia, urinary frequency

SKIN: Blistering, burning, peeling, rash, skin fissures, stinging, urticaria

INTERACTIONS

Drugs

3 *Cyclosporine, Tacrolimus:* Clotrimazole troche administration may increase cyclosporine or tacrolimus concentrations

---

cloxacillin

(klox-a-sill'in)
Chemical Class: Isoxazolyl penicillin derivative, (penicillinase-resistant)
Therapeutic Class: Antibiotic

CLINICAL PHARMACOLOGY
Mechanism of Action: Inhibits bacterial wall synthesis; bactericidal
Pharmacokinetics
PO: Peak 1 hr, duration 6 hr, $t_{1/2}$ 30-60 min; metabolized in liver, excreted in urine and bile

INDICATIONS AND USES: Infections of the respiratory tract, skin and skin structure, bones and joints Antibacterial spectrum usually includes:
• Gram-positive organisms: most gram-positive aerobic cocci, *Staphylococcus aureus, S. epidermidis* (except methicillin-resistant strains)

DOSAGE

Adult
• PO 250-500 mg q6h

Child
• PO 50-100 mg/kg/day in divided doses q6h, max 4 g/day

§ AVAILABLE FORMS/COST OF THERAPY
• Cap, Gel—Oral: 250 mg, 100's: **$14.11-$37.96**; 500 mg, 100's: **$27.78-$79.63**

• Powder, Reconst—Oral: 125 mg/5 ml,100, 200 ml: **$5.24-$11.04/200 ml**

PRECAUTIONS: Hypersensitivity to cephalosporins, prolonged or repeated therapy

PREGNANCY AND LACTATION: Pregnancy category B

SIDE EFFECTS/ADVERSE REACTIONS

CNS: Anxiety, depression, fever, hallucinations, headache, twitching

GI: Abdominal pain, colitis, *diarrhea;* glossitis, increased AST, ALT; *nausea, vomiting*

GU: Hematuria, vaginitis

HEME: **Bone marrow depression,** eosinophilia, increased bleeding time

SKIN: Rash, urticaria

INTERACTIONS

Drugs

❸ *Tetracyclines:* Possible inhibition of antibacterial activity of penicillins

Labs

• *False increase:* Urine amino acids
• *Interference:* 17-ketosteroids

SPECIAL CONSIDERATIONS

• Sodium content of 250 mg cap = 0.6 mEq; sodium content of 125 mg susp = 0.24 mEq

---

clozapine

(klo′za-peen)

Rx: Clozaril

Chemical Class: Dibenzodiazepine derivative

Therapeutic Class: Antipsychotic

CLINICAL PHARMACOLOGY

Mechanism of Action: Serotonin 5-HT$_2$ > dopamine (D$_2$)-receptor antagonist; activity at several neurotransmitter systems: selective antagonist at limbic dopamine receptors (D$_1$, D$_2$, D$_4$, D$_5$) and serotonin receptors (5-HT$_2$, 5-HT$_6$, 5-HT$_7$); antagonism at alpha$_1$-adrenergic receptors; and activity at muscarinic, histamine H$_1$, or nicotinic receptors; high sedation and anticholinergic effects; moderate orthostatic hypotension and weight gain; minimal extrapyramidal symptoms

Pharmacokinetics

PO: Peak 2.5 hr; 95% protein bound; completely metabolized by the liver (CYP2D6, 3A4, 1A2), excreted in urine and feces (metabolites); t$_{1/2}$ 8-12 hr

INDICATIONS AND USES: Severely ill schizophrenic patients who fail to respond adequately to standard antipsychotic drug treatment

DOSAGE

Adult

• PO 12.5 mg qd-bid initially, increase by 25-50 mg/day to achieve a target range of 300-450 mg/day after 2 wk; increase prn by no more than 100 mg in 2 wk intervals; do not exceed 900 mg/day; use lowest dose to control symptoms

🅢 **AVAILABLE FORMS/COST OF THERAPY**

• Tab, Uncoated—Oral: 25 mg, 100's: **$135.96-$316.95**; 100 mg, 100's: **$122.35-$352.26**

NOTE: Available only through patient management system, combining WBC testing, patient monitoring, pharmacy and drug distribution services, all linked to compliance with required safety monitoring (1-800-448-5938)

CONTRAINDICATIONS: Myeloproliferative disorders, uncontrolled epilepsy, history of clozapine-induced agranulocytosis or severe granulocytopenia, severe CNS depression, comatose states, narrow-angle glaucoma

---

PRECAUTIONS: Cardiovascular disease, pulmonary disease, elderly, prostatic enlargement, hepatic disease, renal disease, general anesthesia, seizure disorders

PREGNANCY AND LACTATION: Pregnancy category B; may be excreted in breast milk, avoid breast feeding during clozapine therapy

SIDE EFFECTS/ADVERSE REACTIONS

CNS: Agitation, akathisia, akinesia, anxiety, ataxia, confusion, depression, disturbed sleep, *dizziness, drowsiness,* epileptiform movements, fatigue, headache, hyperkinesia, hypokinesia, insomnia, lethargy, myoclonic jerks, nightmares, restlessness, rigidity, *sedation, **seizures,*** slurred speech, syncope, tremor, *vertigo,* weakness

CV: Angina, cardiac abnormality, chest pain, ECG change, hypertension, hypotension, *tachycardia*

EENT: Blurred vision

GI: Abdominal discomfort, anorexia, constipation, diarrhea, dry mouth, heartburn, LFT abnormality, nausea, *salivation,* vomiting

GU: Abnormal ejaculation; incontinence; urinary urgency, frequency, retention

HEME: **Agranulocytosis,** eosinophilia, **leukopenia, neutropenia**

SKIN: Rash

MISC: Fever, weight gain

INTERACTIONS

Drugs

3 *Carbamazepine, phenytoin, primadone, valproic acid:* Considerable reduction in plasma clozapine concentrations

3 *Cimetidine, clarithromycin, troleandomycin:* Increased serum clozapine concentrations

3 *Digitoxin:* Increased serum digitoxin concentrations due to protein-binding displacement

3 *Diazepam:* Isolated cases of cardiorespiratory collapse have been reported

3 *Epinephrine:* Reversed pressor effects of epinephrine

2 *Erythromycin:* Increased serum clozapine concentrations

3 *Fluoxetine:* Modest elevation of serum clozapine concentrations

2 *Fluvoxamine:* Marked increase in plasma clozapine concentrations and side effects; increased risk of leukocytosis

3 *Paroxetine:* Modest elevation of serum clozapine concentrations

3 *Quinidine:* Increased serum clozapine concentrations possible

3 *Sertraline:* Modest elevation of serum clozapine concentrations

3 *Type 1C antiarrhythmics:* Propafenone, flecainide, encainide; increased serum clozapine concentration possible

3 *Warfarin:* Increased serum warfarin concentrations due to protein-binding displacement

SPECIAL CONSIDERATIONS

• The risk of agranulocytosis and seizures limits use to patients who have failed to respond or were unable to tolerate treatment with appropriate courses of standard antipsychotics

• Advise patients to report immediately the appearance of lethargy, weakness, fever, sore throat, malaise, mucous membrane ulceration, or other possible signs of infection

• Patients cannot be reinitiated on clozapine if WBC counts fall below 2000/mm^3 or ANC falls below 1000/mm^3 during clozapine therapy

MONITORING PARAMETERS

• WBC at baseline and then q wk for first 6 mo, every other week thereafter if WBC counts maintained (WBC ≥3000/mm^3, ANC

≥1500/mm³); WBC counts q wk for at least 4 weeks after discontinuation

• Blood pressure, LFTs

---

codeine

(koe'deen)

Combinations

Rx: with acetaminophen (Tylenol no. 2, Tylenol no. 3, Tylenol no. 4); with aspirin (Empirin no. 3, Empirin no. 4)

OTC: with guaifenesin (Robitussin AC); with APAP (Capital, Aceta); with APAP butalbital, caffeine (Fioricet, Phenaphen); with aspirin (Fiorinal)

Chemical Class: Natural opium alkaloid; phenanthrene derivative

Therapeutic Class: Narcotic analgesic; antitussive

DEA Class: Schedule II (combinations: Schedule III or Schedule V [Elixir])

CLINICAL PHARMACOLOGY

Mechanism of Action: Narcotic agonist with activity at μ-receptors (supraspinal analgesia, euphoria, respiratory and physical depression, miosis, and reduced GI motility), κ-receptors (pentazocine-like spinal analgesia, sedation, and miosis), and Δ-receptors (dysphoria, psychotomimetic effects [e.g., hallucinations], and respiratory and vasomotor stimulation caused by drugs with antagonist activity); compared to morphine, less analgesia, constipation, respiratory depression, sedation, emesis, and physical dependence; more antitussive effect

Pharmacokinetics

IM: Onset 10-30 min, peak 30-60 min

PO: Onset 30-60 min, peak 60-90 min

Metabolized in liver to morphine, excreted in urine (unchanged and metabolites); $t_{1/2}$ 2½-3½ hr

INDICATIONS AND USES: Mild to moderate pain, antitussive

DOSAGE

Adult

• *Analgesia:* PO/IM/SC 15-60 mg q4h prn

• *Antitussive:* PO 10-20 mg q4-6h; not to exceed 120 mg/day

Child

• *Analgesia:* PO/IM/SC 0.5-1 mg/kg/dose q4-6h prn, max 60 mg/dose

• *Antitussive:* PO 1-1.5 mg/kg/day in divided doses q4-6h prn; max 60 mg/dose

⑤ AVAILABLE FORMS/COST OF THERAPY

• Inj, Sol—IM, SC: 15 mg/ml, 2 ml: **$0.87**; 30 mg/ml, 2 ml: **$0.90**; 60 mg/ml, 1 ml: **$1.28**

• Sol—Oral: 15 mg/5 ml, 500 ml: **$35.78**

• Tab, Uncoated—Oral: 15 mg, 100's: **$37.41**; 30 mg, 100's: **$40.27-$50.13**; 60 mg, 100's: **$73.77-$95.58**

PRECAUTIONS: Head injury, increased intracranial pressure, acute abdominal conditions, elderly, severe impairment of hepatic or renal function, hypothyroidism, Addison's disease, prostatic hypertrophy, urethral stricture, history of drug abuse

PREGNANCY AND LACTATION: Pregnancy category C (category D if used for prolonged periods or in high doses at term); use during labor produces neonatal respiratory de-

---

pression; passes into breast milk in very small amounts; compatible with breast feeding

SIDE EFFECTS/ADVERSE REACTIONS

CNS: Agitation, dependency, dizziness, *drowsiness,* lethargy, restlessness, *sedation*

CV: Bradycardia, orthostatic hypotension, palpitations, tachycardia

GI: Anorexia, constipation, nausea, vomiting

GU: Urinary retention

RESP: Respiratory depression

SKIN: Flushing, rash, urticaria

INTERACTIONS

Drugs

■ *Barbiturates:* Additive respiratory and CNS depressant effects

■ *Antihistamines, chloral hydrate, glutethimide, methocarbamol:* Enhanced depressant effects

■ *Cimetidine:* Increased respiratory and CNS depression

■ *Ethanol:* Additive CNS effects

❷ *Quinidine:* Inhibited analgesic effect of codeine

Labs

• *Increase:* Urine morphine

• False elevatons of amylase and lipase

SPECIAL CONSIDERATIONS
PATIENT/FAMILY EDUCATION

• Minimize nausea by administering with food and remain lying down following dose

• Do not administer agonist/antagonist analgesics (i.e., pentazocine, nalbuphine, butorphanol, dezocine, buprenorphine) to patient who has received a prolonged course of codeine (a pure agonist). In opioid-dependent patients, mixed agonist/antagonist analgesics may precipitate withdrawal symptoms

---

colchicine

(kol'chi-seen)

Rx: Colsalide

Combinations

Rx: with probenicid (Proben-C, Colbenemid)

Chemical Class: Colchicum autumnale alkaloid

Therapeutic Class: Antigout agent

CLINICAL PHARMACOLOGY

Mechanism of Action: Antiinflammatory: decreases leukocyte motility, phagocytosis, and lactate production; binds to microtubular protein; interferes with mitotic spindles in granulocytes; prevents release of glycoprotein that causes joint pain and inflammation

Pharmacokinetics

PO: Peak ½-2 hr, $t_{1/2}$ 20 min V_d = 2L/kg; deacetylated in liver; excreted in feces

INDICATIONS AND USES: Gouty arthritis (prevention, treatment), amyloidosis,* aphthous stomatitis,* pseudogout,* Behçet's syndrome,* familial Mediterranean fever,* alcoholic cirrhosis*

DOSAGE

Adult

• *Prevention of gouty arthritis:* PO 0.5-1.8 mg qd depending on severity; IV 0.5-1 mg qd-bid

• *Treatment of gouty arthritis:* PO 0.5-1.2 mg, then 0.5-1.2 mg q1h, until pain decreases or side effects occur; IV 2 mg over 2-5 min, then 0.5 mg q6h, not to exceed 4 mg/day; no colchicine should be given by any route for at least 7 days after a full course of IV therapy (4 mg)

■ **AVAILABLE FORMS/COST OF THERAPY**

• Inj, Sol—IV: 1 mg/2 ml, 2 ml: **$5.04**

---

* = non-FDA-approved use

• Tab, Uncoated—Oral: 0.5 mg, 100's: **$39.64**; 0.6 mg, 100's: **$3.95-$30.36**

CONTRAINDICATIONS: Serious GI, renal, hepatic, cardiac disorders; blood dyscrasias

PRECAUTIONS: Elderly, lactation, children; may induce ileal vitamin B_{12} malabsorption; extravasation may lead to shock

PREGNANCY AND LACTATION: Pregnancy category D (known teratogen)

SIDE EFFECTS/ADVERSE REACTIONS

CNS: Peripheral neuritis

GI: Anorexia, cramps, *diarrhea, malaise,* metallic taste, *nausea, vomiting*

GU: Azotemia, hematuria, oliguria, reversible azoospermia

HEME: **Agranulocytosis, aplastic anemia, pancytopenia, thrombocytopenia**

MS: Myopathy (more common in persons with renal impairment)

SKIN: Alopecia, dermatitis, erythema, pruritus, purpura

INTERACTIONS

Drugs

3 *Cyclosporine, tacrolimus:* Increased serum level of cyclosporine or tacrolimus

3 *Erythromycin, clarithromycin, troleandomycin:* Potential for severe colchicine toxicity

Labs

• *Interference:* Urinary 17-hydroxycorticosteroids

SPECIAL CONSIDERATIONS
MONITORING PARAMETERS

• CBC, platelets, reticulocytes before and during therapy (q3mo)

---

coleselevam

(koh-le-sev'e-lam)

Rx: WelChol

Chemical Class: Hydrophilic, nonabsorbed polymer

Therapeutic Class: Bile acid binding resin, bile acid sequestrant

---

CLINICAL PHARMACOLOGY

Mechanism of Action: Bile acid binding in the intestine, impedes absorption, depleting the bile acid pool; hepatic enzymes upregulate to increase the conversion of cholesterol to bile acids, increasing the clearance of LDL-cholesterol; percentage of change in lipid parameters: LDL-cholesterol (-15%); total cholesterol (-10%); HDL-cholesterol (3%), TG (10%)

Pharmacokinetics

PO: Hydrophilic, water-soluble polymer that is not hydrolyzed by digestive enzymes and is not absorbed

INDICATIONS AND USES: Primary hypercholesterolemia (Fredrickson Type IIa - primarily elevated LDL-cholesterol)

DOSAGE

Adult

• 3 tablets bid with meals; max dose 7 tablets/day

$ **AVAILABLE FORMS/COST OF THERAPY**

• Tab, coated off-white—Oral: 625 mg, 180's: **$147.65**

CONTRAINDICATIONS: Bowel obstruction, hypersensitivity

PRECAUTIONS: TG levels >300 mg/dL; conditions with increased susceptibility to vitamin K or fat soluble vitamin deficiencies

---

italic = common side effects   ***bold italic*** = life-threatening reactions

PREGNANCY AND LACTATION: Pregnancy category B (no harm in animal studies, but no adequate and well-controlled studies in pregnant women; no expected excretion into breast milk

SIDE EFFECTS/ADVERSE REACTIONS

CNS: Asthenia

GI: Abdominal pain, constipation, diarrhea, dyspepsia, flatulence, nausea

INTERACTIONS

• Although no drug interactions have been documented, binding to drugs given concomitantly may be significantly impacted; drug where small differences in serum level may be significant should be monitored closely

SPECIAL CONSIDERATIONS

• Combination colesevelam and an HMG-CoA reductase inhibitor is effective in further lowering serum total cholesterol and LDL-cholesterol levels beyond that achieved by either agent alone

• Take tablets with a liquid, and with a meal

PATIENT/FAMILY EDUCATION

• Tablets should be taken with a liquid, and with a meal

MONITORING PARAMETERS

• Plasma lipids

---

colestipol

(koe-les'ti-pole)

Rx: Colestid

Chemical Class: Bile acid sequestrant

Therapeutic Class: Antilipemic

CLINICAL PHARMACOLOGY

Mechanism of Action: Combines with bile acids to form insoluble complex that is excreted through feces; increased fecal loss of bile acids leads to increased oxidation of cholesterol to bile acids, increased hepatic uptake of LDLs, and decreased serum LDL levels; serum triglyceride levels may increase or remain unchanged

Pharmacokinetics

PO: Not absorbed; excreted in feces

INDICATIONS AND USES: Primary hypercholesterolemia, xanthomas, pruritus due to biliary obstruction,* diarrhea due to bile acids*

DOSAGE

Adult

• PO 5-30 g qd in 2-4 divided doses, ac and hs; increase dose by 5 g at 1-2 mo intervals

💲 **AVAILABLE FORMS/COST OF THERAPY**

• Granule—Oral: 5 g/scoop, 500 g: **$112.33**

• Packet—Oral: 5 g/pkt, 90's: **$76.91**

• Packet—Oral: 5 g/7.5 g pkt, 60's: **$115.11**

• Tab, Uncoated—Oral: 1 g, 120's: **$57.65**

CONTRAINDICATIONS: Biliary obstruction

PRECAUTIONS: Lactation; children; bleeding disorders; may prevent absorption of fat-soluble vitamins such as A, D, E, and K; prolonged use may lead to the development of hyperchloremic acidosis;

PREGNANCY AND LACTATION: Pregnancy category B

SIDE EFFECTS/ADVERSE REACTIONS

CNS: Dizziness, headache

GI: Abdominal pain, constipation, fecal impaction, flatulence, hemorrhoids, nausea, peptic ulcer, steatorrhea, vomiting

HEME: **Bleeding**

METAB: Decreased vitamin A, D, E, K absorption; hyperchloremic acidosis

SKIN: Irritation of perianal area, rash

---

* = non-FDA-approved use

INTERACTIONS
Drugs
3 *Acetaminophen, Amiodarone, Corticosteroids, Diclofenac, Digitalis glycosides, Furosemide, Methotrexate, Metronidazole, Thiazide diuretics, Thyroid hormones, Valproic acid:* Cholestyramine reduces interacting drug concentrations and probably subsequent therapeutic response

3 *Oral anticoagulants:* Inhibition of hypoprothrombinemic response; colestipol might be less likely to interact

SPECIAL CONSIDERATIONS
• Bile acid sequestrant choice should be based on cost and patient acceptability
• Give all other medications 1 hr before colestipol or 4 hr after colestipol to avoid poor absorption

contraceptives, oral (combined)
Rx: *Monophasic:* Alesse, Brevicon, Demulen 1/35, Demulen 1/50, Desogen, Genora 0.5/35, Genora 1/35, Genora 1/50, Jenest-28, Levite, Levlen, Levora, Loestrin Fe 1/20, Loestrin Fe 1.5/30, Lo/Ovral, Low-Ogestrel, Modicon, Necon 1/50, Nelova 0.5/35, Nelova 1/35, Nelova 1/50, Nordette, Norethin 1/35, Norethin 1/50, Norinyl 1+35, Norinyl 1+50, Ortho-Cept, Ortho-Cyclen, Ortho-Novum 1/35, Ortho-Novum 1/50, Ovcon-35, Ovcon-50, Ovral, Preven, Zovia 1/35E, Zovia 1/50E

Rx: *Biphasic:* Necon 10/11, Ortho-Novum10/11, Mircette

Rx: *Triphasic:* Ortho-Novum 7/7/7, Ortho Tri-Cyclen, Tri-Levlen, Tri-Norinyl, Triphasil

Chemical Class: Synthetic estrogen/progestin combinations
Therapeutic Class: Contraceptives

CLINICAL PHARMACOLOGY
Mechanism of Action: Inhibit ovulation by suppressing the gonadotropins, FSH and LH; alter cervical mucus (inhibiting sperm penetration) and endometrium (reducing likelihood of implantation)
Pharmacokinetics
Estrogens
PO: Ethinyl estradiol (EE) peak 1.3 hr; mestranol demethylated to ethinyl estradiol (slight delay in subsequent peak, 1.9 hr); 98% bound to plasma proteins; metabolized in

liver; excreted in urine and bile; undergoes some enterohepatic recirculation; $t_{1/2}$ 13-27 hr

Progestins

PO: Bound both to albumin (79%-95%) and sex hormone-binding globulin; metabolized in liver, excreted in urine and bile; $t_{1/2}$ norethindrone 5-14 hr, levonorgestrel 11-45 hr; desogestrel metabolite 38+20 hr, norgestimate metabolite 12-30 hr

INDICATIONS AND USES: Prevention of pregnancy; emergency contraception (postcoital contraception or "morning after" pill)*; dysmenorrhea*; dysfunctional uterine bleeding,* endometriosis*

DOSAGE

Adult and Adolescent

• *21-day regimen:* PO 1 tab qd for 21 days beginning (a) 1st Sunday after menstruation begins or (b) day 5 of cycle, or (c) day 1 of cycle (consult instructions on dispensers or packs); no tabs are taken for next 7 days (withdrawal flow will normally occur about 3 days following last tab)

• *28-day regimen:* PO 1 tab qd for 28 days continuously beginning (a) 1st Sunday after menstruation begins, or (b) day 5 of cycle, or (c) day 1 of cycle (consult instructions on dispensers or packs); start new pack of tabs after completing 28-day course

• *Emergency contraception:* 2 doses, 1st dose within 72 hr of unprotected intercourse; 2nd dose 12 hr later:

FORMULATION	TABLETS/DOSE
Norgestrel 0.5 mg + ethinyl estradiol 50 µg (Ovral)	2
Levonorgestrel 0.15 mg or norgestrel 0.3 mg + ethinyl estradiol 30 µg (Nordette, Lo/Ovral, Levlen, Levora)	4
Levonorgestrel 0.25 mg + ethinyl estradiol 0.05 mg (Preven)	2

• Norgestrel-only regimens preferred because of less nausea and vomiting with equal efficacy (see Norgestrel)

§ AVAILABLE FORMS/COST OF THERAPY

EE/Desogestrel

• 0.02 mg EE/0.01 mg EE/0.15 mg desogestrel: 28's: **$31.48** (Mircette)

• 0.03 mg/0.15 mg: 28's: **$4.10-$34.14** (Desogen, Ortho-Cept)

EE/Ethynodiol Diacetate

• 0.035 mg/1 mg: 28's: **$29.29-$34.69** (Demulen 1/35, Zovia 1/35E)

• 0.05 mg/1 mg: 28's: **$32.64-$37.10** (Demulen 1/50, Zovia 1/50E)

EE/Levonorestrel

• 0.02 mg/0.1 mg/: 28's: **$28.14-$32.95** (Alesse, Levite)

• 0.03 mg/0.05, 0.075, 0.125 mg: 28's: **$25.82-$30.34** (Tri-Levlen, Triphasil)

• 0.03 mg/0.15 mg: 28's: **$24.07-$34.49** (Levora, Nordette, Levlen)

• 0.05 mg/0.25 mg: 4's: **$12.50** (Preven)

EE/Norethindrone Acetate

• 0.02 mg/1 mg: 28's: **$28.65-$30.85** (Loestrin Fe 1/20)

• 0.03 mg/1.5 mg: 28's: **$28.94-$31.15** (Loestrin Fe 1.5/30)

EE/Norethindrone

• 0.035 mg/0.4 mg: 28's: **$31.76** (Ovcon-35)

• 0.035 mg/0.5 mg: 28's: **$12.53-$37.24** (Nelova 0.5/35E, Brevicon, Modicon, Genora 0.5/35)

• 0.035 mg/0.5, 0.75, 1 mg: 28's: **$31.45** (Ortho-Novum 7/7/7)

• 0.035 mg/0.5, 1 mg: 28's: **$15.00-$37.24** (Necon 10/11, Ortho-Novum 10/11, Jenest-28)

• 0.035 mg/0.5, 1, 0.5 mg: 28's: **$27.01** (Tri-Norinyl)

---

* = non-FDA-approved use

• 0.035 mg/1 mg: 28's: **$12.00-$34.14** (Norinyl 1+35, Genora 1/35, Nelova 1/35E, Ortho-Novum 1/35, N.E.E. 1/35, Norethin 1/35E)

• 0.05 mg/1 mg: 28's: **$34.91** (Ovcon-50)

EE/Norgestimate

• 0.035 mg/0.18, 0.215, 0.25 mg: 28's: **$33.81** (Ortho Tri-Cyclen)

• 0.035 mg/0.25 mg: 28's: **$34.14** (Ortho-Cyclen)

EE/Norgestrel

• 0.03 mg/0.3 mg: 28's: **$39.35-$34.04** (Lo/Ovral, Low-Ogestrel)

• 0.05 mg/0.5 mg: 28's: **$22.46-$50.10** (Ogestrel, Ovral)

Mestranol/Norethindrone

• 0.05 mg/1 mg: 28's: **$12.54-$34.14** (Genora 1/50, Nelova 1/50M, Necon 1/50, Ortho-Novum 1/50, Norinyl 1/50)

CONTRAINDICATIONS: Thrombophlebitis, thromboembolic disorders, history of deep vein thrombophlebitis, cerebrovascular disease, MI, CAD, known or suspected breast carcinoma or estrogen-dependent neoplasia, carcinoma of endometrium; hepatic adenomas, carcinomas; past or present angina pectoris, undiagnosed abnormal vaginal bleeding, cholestatic jaundice

PRECAUTIONS: Hypertension, gallbladder disease, CHF, diabetes mellitus, depression, migraine headache, seizure disorders, hepatic disease, family history of breast or endometrial cancer, history of thromboembolic disorders, uterine fibroids, hypertriglyceridemia, hypercalcemia, cigarette smoking (especially >35 yr)

PREGNANCY AND LACTATION: Pregnancy category X; may decrease quantity and quality of breast milk

SIDE EFFECTS/ADVERSE REACTIONS

CNS: Depression, migraine headache, emotional lability

CV: ***Arterial thromboembolism, pulmonary embolism, CVA, MI,*** hypertension, venous thrombosis edema

EENT: Contact lens intolerance, ***retinal thrombosis***

GI: Nausea and vomiting, gallbladder disease, bloating, benign hepatic tumors ***mesenteric thrombosis***

GU: Breakthrough bleeding (80% resolve in 3 mo), *spotting,* amenorrhea, change in cervical secretions, breast enlargement, breast tenderness

METAB: Hyperglycemia, hypertriglyceridemia, hypercalcemia, vitamin B-6 deficiency

SKIN: Melasma

INTERACTIONS

Drugs

🔢 *Barbiturates, carbamazepine, griseofulvin, phenytoin, penicillins, rifampin; rifabutin, ritonavir, tetracyclines:* Reduced efficacy of oral contraceptives

🔢 *Corticosteroids:* Enhanced effect of corticosteroids

🔢 *Cyclosporine:* Elevated cyclosporine concentrations

🔢 *Grapefruit juice:* Increased ethinyl estradiol concentration

⚠ *Smoking:* Increased risk of oral contraceptive-induced adverse cardiovascular events

❷ *Warfarin:* Increased risk of thromboembolic disease with oral contraceptives

Labs

• *False positive:* Serum antinuclear antibodies

SPECIAL CONSIDERATIONS

PATIENT/FAMILY EDUCATION

• Take at same time each day with food

---

italic = common side effects   ***bold italic*** = life-threatening reactions

• Notify clinician if breakthrough bleeding/spotting lasts more than a few days or persists in the 3rd cycle
• Use additional methods of birth control until after the 1st week of administration in the initial cycle or for entire cycle if diarrhea or vomiting occurs
• Does not protect against sexually transmitted diseases (provide condoms additionally where appropriate)
• Notify clinician immediately of severe headache, chest pain, abdominal pain, eye pain or blurred vision, calf pain
• Take a missed pill as soon as remembered, use backup contraception for remainder of cycle

MONITORING PARAMETERS
• Blood pressure

---

corticotropin (ACTH)

(kor-ti-koe-troe′pin)
Rx: Acthar Gel, H.P.
Chemical Class: Adrenocorticotropic hormone
Therapeutic Class: Adrenal corticosteroid

CLINICAL PHARMACOLOGY
Mechanism of Action: Stimulates adrenal cortex to produce cortisol, corticosterone, several weakly androgenic steroids, and, to a limited extent, aldosterone

Pharmacokinetics
IV/IM/SC: Onset <1 hr; duration 2-4 hr, repository form has duration up to 3 days; plasma $t_{1/2}$ <20 min; excreted in urine; cortisol response dependent on total dose and total time of administration

INDICATIONS AND USES: Testing adrenocortical function; conditions in which the anti-inflammatory effect of glucocorticoids is desired;

ACTH has no advantage over glucocorticoids except perhaps in multiple sclerosis and dermatomyositis/polymyositis

DOSAGE
Adult
• *Testing of adrenocortical function:* IM/SC up to 80 U in divided doses qid; IV 10-25 U in 500 ml D_5W given over 8 hr
• *Anti-inflammatory:* SC/IM 40 U in divided doses qid or 40 U q12-24h (gel/repository form)
• *Acute exacerbations of multiple sclerosis:* IM 80-120 U qd (gel/repository form) for up to 3 wk
Child
• *Anti-inflammatory:* SC/IM 1.6 U/kg in divided doses qid or 0.8 U/kg q12-24h (gel/repository form)

$ AVAILABLE FORMS/COST OF THERAPY
• Inj, Lyphl-Sol—IM, SC: 25 U/vial, 1's: **$21.82**; 40 U/vial, 1's: **$33.43**
• Inj, Repos Gel: 80 U/ml, 5 ml: **$16.50-$49.98**

CONTRAINDICATIONS: Systemic fungal infections, smallpox vaccination, ocular herpes simplex, primary adrenocortical insufficiency/hyperfunction

PRECAUTIONS: Latent TB, recent significant intercurrent illness or surgery, scleroderma, osteoporosis, CHF, hypertension, hepatic disease, peptic ulcer disease, hyperthyroidism, childbearing-age women, psychiatric disorders, myasthenia gravis, posterior subcapsular cataracts, systemic infection

PREGNANCY AND LACTATION: Pregnancy category C; monitor infants with significant *in utero* exposure for hyperadrenalism. Unknown if excreted in breast milk

---

* = non-FDA-approved use

SIDE EFFECTS/ADVERSE REACTIONS

CNS: Behavioral changes, depression, dizziness, euphoria, headache, insomnia, mood swings, pseudotumor cerebri, psychosis, *seizures*

CV: **CHF,** hypertension

EENT: Increased intraocular pressure, posterior subcapsular cataracts

GI: Nausea, **pancreatitis,** peptic ulcer, ulcerative esophagitis, vomiting

METAB: Calcium loss, Cushingoid symptoms, growth retardation in children, hyperglycemia, hypokalemic alkalosis, menstrual irregularities, negative nitrogen balance due to protein catabolism, sodium retention

MS: Arthralgia, aseptic necrosis of femoral and humeral heads, compression fractures, muscle atrophy, myalgia, osteoporosis, steroid myopathy, weakness

SKIN: Acne, ecchymoses, hirsutism, hyperpigmentation, *impaired wound healing,* petechiae, rash, suppression of skin test reactions, sweating, urticaria

INTERACTIONS

Labs

• *False increase:* 11-hydroxycorticosteroids

SPECIAL CONSIDERATIONS

• May mask infections

• Intercurrent illness may require increased corticosteroids

• Drug-induced adrenocorticoid insufficiency may be minimized by gradual systemic dosage reduction; relative insufficiency may exist for up to 1 yr after discontinuation; therefore, be prepared to supplement in situations of stress

cortisone

(kor′ti-sone)

Rx: Cortone

Chemical Class: Glucocorticoid

Therapeutic Class: Systemic corticosteroid

CLINICAL PHARMACOLOGY

Mechanism of Action: Decreases inflammation by depressing migration of polymorphonuclear leukocytes and activity of endogenous mediators of inflammation; has many profound metabolic effects, possesses mineralocorticoid activity

Pharmacokinetics

PO: Peak 2 hr, duration 1½ days

IM: Absorbed slowly over 24-48 hr

INDICATIONS AND USES: Antiinflammatory or immunosuppressive agent in the treatment of a variety of diseases of hematologic, allergic, inflammatory, neoplastic and autoimmune origin; in replacement doses for primary or secondary adrenocortical insufficiency

DOSAGE

Adult

• PO 25-300 mg qd or q2d, titrated to patient response

AVAILABLE FORMS/COST OF THERAPY

• Tab, Uncoated—Oral: 5 mg, 50's: **$11.38**; 10 mg, 100's: **$42.05**; 25 mg, 100's: **$3.34-$94.10**

CONTRAINDICATIONS: Systemic fungal infections

PRECAUTIONS: Psychosis, diabetes mellitus, glaucoma, osteoporosis, seizure disorders, ulcerative colitis (intestinal perforation), latent tuberculosis or amebiasis (reactivation of disease), hypertension, CHF, myasthenia gravis (if used with anti-cholinesterase agents), renal disease, esophagitis, peptic ulcer

PREGNANCY AND LACTATION: Pregnancy category C; excreted in breast milk

SIDE EFFECTS/ADVERSE REACTIONS

CNS: Behavioral changes, depression, dizziness, euphoria, headache, insomnia, mood swings, pseudotumor cerebri, psychosis, *seizures*

CV: CHF, embolism, hypertension, thrombophlebitis

EENT: Fungal infections, increased intraocular pressure, posterior subcapsular cataracts

GI: Intestinal perforation, nausea, *pancreatitis,* peptic ulcer, ulcerative esophagitis, vomiting

HEME: Thrombocytopenia

METAB: Calcium loss, Cushingoid symptoms, growth retardation in children, hyperglycemia, hypokalemic alkalosis, menstrual irregularities, negative nitrogen balance due to protein catabolism, sodium retention

MS: Arthralgia, aseptic necrosis of femoral and humeral heads, compression fractures, muscle atrophy, myalgia, osteoporosis, steroid myopathy, weakness

SKIN: Acne, ecchymoses, hirsutism, hyperpigmentation, *impaired wound healing,* petechiae, rash, suppression of skin test reactions, sweating, urticaria

INTERACTIONS

Drugs

3 *Aminoglutethamide:* Enhanced elimination of corticosteroids; marked reduction in corticosteroid response; increased clearance of prednisone; doubling of dose may be necessary

3 *Antidiabetics:* Increased blood glucose

3 *Barbiturates, carbamazepine:* Reduced serum concentrations of corticosteroids; increased clearance of prednisone

3 *Cholestyramine, colestipol:* Possible reduced absorption of corticosteroids

3 *Cyclosporine:* Possible increased concentration of both drugs, seizures

3 *Erythromycin, troleandomycin, clarithromycin, ketoconazole:* Possible enhanced steroid effect

3 *Estrogens, oral contraceptives:* Enhanced effects of corticosteroids

3 *Isoniazid:* Reduced plasma concentrations of isoniazid

3 *IUDs:* Inhibition of inflammation may decrease contraceptive effect

3 *NSAIDs:* Increased risk GI ulceration

3 *Rifampin:* Reduced therapeutic effect of corticosteroids; may reduce hepatic clearance of prednisone

3 *Salicylates:* Subtherapeutic salicylate concentrations possible

SPECIAL CONSIDERATIONS

• Increased dose of rapidly acting corticosteroids may be necessary in patient subjected to unusual stress

• May mask infections

• Do not give live virus vaccines to patients on prolonged therapy

• Patients on chronic steroid therapy should wear medical bracelet

• Drug-induced adrenocorticoid insufficiency may be minimized by gradual systemic dosage reduction; relative insufficiency may exist for up to 1 yr after discontinuation

• Symptoms of adrenal insufficiency include: nausea, fatigue, anorexia, hypotension, hypoglycemia, fever

MONITORING PARAMETERS

• Serum K and glucose

• Growth in children on prolonged therapy

• Edema, blood pressure, CHF, mental status, weight

---

cosyntropin
(koe-sin-troe´pin)
Rx: Cortrosyn
Chemical Class: ACTH derivative
Therapeutic Class: Adrenal corticosteroid

CLINICAL PHARMACOLOGY
Mechanism of Action: Stimulates adrenal cortex to produce cortisol; cosyntropin contains the first 24 of the 39 amino acids of natural ACTH; 0.25 mg of cosyntropin stimulates the adrenal cortex maximally and to the same extent as 25 units of natural ACTH
Pharmacokinetics
IV/IM: Onset 5 min, peak 1 hr, duration 2-4 hr
INDICATIONS AND USES: Testing adrenocortical function
DOSAGE
Adult
• IM/IV 0.25 mg
Child
• IM/IV age >2 yr 0.25 mg; age <2 yr 0.125 mg
§ AVAILABLE FORMS/COST OF THERAPY
• Inj, Dry-Sol—IM, IV: 0.25 mg: **$18.37**
PREGNANCY AND LACTATION: Pregnancy category C
SIDE EFFECTS/ADVERSE REACTIONS
SKIN: Flushing, pruritus, rash, urticaria
SPECIAL CONSIDERATIONS
MONITORING PARAMETERS
• Check plasma cortisol levels at baseline and 30-60 min after drug is administered; normal adrenal function indicated by an increase of at least 70 µg/L or a measured level of 20 µg

---

co-trimoxazole (sulfamethoxazole and trimethoprim)
(koe-trye-mox´a-zole)
Rx: Bactrim, Bethaprim, Cotrim, Comoxol, Septra, Sulfatrim, Uroplus
Chemical Class: Sulfonamide derivative (sulfamethoxazole); dihydrofolate reductase inhibitor (trimethoprim)
Therapeutic Class: Antibiotic

CLINICAL PHARMACOLOGY
Mechanism of Action: The combination blocks 2 consecutive steps in the bacterial biosynthesis of essential nucleic acids and proteins
Pharmacokinetics
PO: Rapidly absorbed, peak 1-4 hr; $t_{1/2}$ (SMX) 10-12 hr, (TMP) 8-11 hr; excreted in urine (metabolites and unchanged); 70% (SMX), 44% (TMP) bound to plasma proteins
INDICATIONS AND USES: Infections of the urinary tract, otitis media, acute exacerbation of chronic bronchitis, enteritis, *Pneumocystis carinii* pneumonia (treatment and prophylaxis), traveler's diarrhea, cholera,* salmonella-type infections,* nocardiosis,* prostatitis*
Antibacterial spectrum usually includes:
• Gram-positive organisms: *Streptococcus pneumoniae, Staphylococcus aureus,* Group A β-hemolytic streptococci (some strains may not respond to co-trimoxazole in tonsillopharyngeal infections), *Nocardia*
• Gram-negative organisms: *Acinetobacter, Enterobacter, Escherichia coli, Klebsiella pneumoniae, Pro-*

---

teus mirabilis, Salmonella, Shigella, H. influenzae, H. ducreyi, N. gonorrhoeae, indole-positive *Proteus* (70% of isolates), *Providencia* and *Serratia* (50% of isolates)

• Protozoa: *Pneumocystis carinii*

DOSAGE

Adult

• *UTIs, shigellosis, acute exacerbations of chronic bronchitis, acute otitis media:* PO 160 mg TMP/800 mg SMX q12h for 10-14 days (3 days for uncomplicated cystitis in otherwise healthy females, 5 days for shigellosis); IV 8-10 mg TMP/kg/day in 2-4 divided doses q6, 8, or 12h for up to 14 days (5 days for shigellosis)

• *Traveler's diarrhea:* PO 160 mg TMP/800 mg SMX q12h for 5 days

• *Pneumocystis carinii pneumonitis:* PO 20 mg TMP/kg/day divided q6h for 14 days; IV 15-20 mg TMP/kg/day divided q6-8h for 14 days

• *Pneumocystis carinii pneumonia prophylaxis:* PO 160 mg TMP/800 mg SMX qd or 3 × /wk

Dosage adjustment for impaired renal function: CrCl >30 ml/min, usual regimen; CrCl 15-30 ml/min, ½ usual regimen; CrCl <15 ml/min, not recommended

Child >2 mo

• *UTIs, shigellosis, and acute otitis media:* PO 8 mg TMP/kg/day divided q12h (1 ml/kg susp divided q12h)

• *Pneumocystis carinii pneumonitis:* PO/IV 15-20 mg TMP/kg/day divided q6h for 14 days

$ AVAILABLE FORMS/COST OF THERAPY

• Inj, Conc-Sol—IV: 80 mg SMX/16 mg TMP/5 ml: **$3.93-$6.47**

• Susp—Oral: 200 mg SMX/40 mg TMP/5 ml, 100, 150, 200, 480 ml: **$6.33-$21.54**/200 ml

• Tab, Uncoated—Oral: 400 mg SMX/80 mg TMP, 100's: **$7.88-$102.49**; 800 mg SMX/160 mg TMP, 100's: **$9.09-$161.48**

CONTRAINDICATIONS: Megaloblastic anemia due to folate deficiency, infants <2 mo

PRECAUTIONS: Streptococcal pharyngitis, elderly patients receiving diuretics, renal and hepatic function impairment, possible folate deficiency (elderly, chronic alcoholics, anticonvulsant therapy, malabsorption syndrome, malnutrition), G-6-PD deficiency

PREGNANCY AND LACTATION: Pregnancy category C; **do not use at term,** may cause kernicterus in the neonate; not recommended in the neonatal nursing period because sulfonamides excreted in breast milk may cause kernicterus

SIDE EFFECTS/ADVERSE REACTIONS

CNS: Anxiety, aseptic meningitis, ataxia, chills, depression, fatigue, hallucinations, headache, insomnia, *seizures,* vertigo

GI: Abdominal pain, anorexia, diarrhea, glossitis, hepatitis, *nausea,* pancreatitis, *pseudomembranous enterocolitis,* stomatitis, *vomiting*

GU: Crystalluria, *renal failure, toxic nephrosis*

HEME: Agranulocytosis, eosinophilia, *hemolytic anemia, leukopenia, methemoglobinemia, neutropenia, thrombocytopenia*

RESP: Cough, shortness of breath

SKIN: Dermatitis, erythema, pain and inflammation at inj site; *photosensitivity, rash, Stevens-Johnson syndrome,* urticaria

MISC: Drug fever

INTERACTIONS

Drugs

3 *Dapsone:* Increased dapsone and trimethoprim concentrations

---

3 *Disulfiram, metronidazole:* Cotrimoxazole contains 10% ethanol, disulfiram reaction possible

3 *Methotrexate:* Elevated methotrexate concentrations and toxicity

3 *Oral anticoagulants:* Enhanced hypoprothrombinemic response to warfarin and possibly other oral anticoagulants

3 *Oral hypoglycemics:* Increased potential for hypoglycemia

3 *Phenytoin:* Increased phenytoin concentrations

Labs

• *False increase:* Creatinine (due to interference with assay), urobilinogen, urine protein, plasma α-aminonitrogen

• *False positive:* Urinary glucose test

• *False decrease:* Serum creatine kinase

SPECIAL CONSIDERATIONS

• Pay special attention to complaints of skin rash, especially those involving mucous membranes (could signify early Stevens-Johnson syndrome), sore throat, mouth sores, fever, or unusual bruising or bleeding

MONITORING PARAMETERS

• Baseline and periodic CBC for patients on long-term or high-dose therapy

cromolyn

(kroe′moe-lin)

Rx: *Inhalation* Intal

Rx: *Opthalmic* Crolom, Opticrom

Rx: *Oral* Gastrocrom

OTC: *Nasal* Nasalcrom

Chemical Class: Mast cell stabilizer

Therapeutic Class: Antiasthmatic, inhaled antiinflammatory, nasal antiinflammatory, ophthalmic antiinflammatory

CLINICAL PHARMACOLOGY

Mechanism of Action: Stabilizes membrane of the sensitized mast cell

Pharmacokinetics

Absorption: 1% of oral dose, 0.03% of ophthalmic dose, 8% of inhalation dose; after inhalation, peak level 15 min, elimination $t_{1/2}$ 80 min; excreted unchanged in feces

INDICATIONS AND USES: Allergic rhinitis; allergic conjunctivitis; bronchial asthma; prevention of acute bronchospasm induced by environmental pollutants or exercise; systemic mastocytosis; prevention of food allergy

DOSAGE

Adult

• *Allergic conjunctivitis:* Ophth sol 1-2 gtt 4-6 times/day; 1 gtt approx. 1.6 mg cromolyn sodium

• *Allergic rhinitis:* Nasal sol 1 spray each nostril tid-qid

• *Bronchial asthma:* INH 2 puffs qid via MDI or 20 mg qid via nebulization

• *Exercise-induced bronchospasm:* INH 2 puffs via MDI or 20 mg via nebulization 10-15 min but <1 hr before exercise

---

italic = common side effects   ***bold italic*** = life-threatening reactions

• *Systemic mastocytosis:* PO 200 mg qid; 30 min before meals and at bedtime
Child
• *Allergic conjunctivitis:* Age >2 yr ophth sol 1-2 gtt 4-6 times/day
• *Allergic rhinitis:* Age >6 yr nasal sol 1 spray each nostril tid-qid
• *Exercise-induced bronchospasm:* Age 2-5 yr 20 mg qid via nebulization; age >5 yr INH 2 puffs qid via MDI 10-15 min but <1 hr before exercise
• *Bronchial asthma:* Age 2-5 yr 20 mg qid via nebulization; age >5 yr INH 2 puffs qid via MDI or 20 mg qid via nebulization
• *Systemic mastocytosis:* Age <2 yr PO 5 mg/kg qid; age 2-12 yr PO 100 mg qid; 30 min before meals and at bedtime

🔒 **AVAILABLE FORMS/COST OF THERAPY**
• Aer, Spray—INH: 800 μg/spray, 8.1 g, 112 sprays: **$49.00-$58.24**; 800 μg/spray, 14.2 g, 200 sprays: **$77.95-$81.85**
• Cap—Oral: 100 mg, 100's: **$94.10**
• Concentrate—Oral: 20 mg/ml, 96's: **$180.80**
• Sol—INH: 10 mg/ml, 2 ml 60's: **$21.15-$67.36**
• Sol—Nasal: 5.2 mg/spray, 100 sprays: **$8.74-$23.62**
• Sol—Ophth: 4%, 10 ml: **$36.47-$54.08**
• Sol—Oral: 20 mg/ml, 5 ml: **$1.88**
CONTRAINDICATIONS: Status asthmaticus
PRECAUTIONS: Renal disease, hepatic disease, child <5 yr, because of propellants in MDI caution in coronary artery disease or history of cardiac arrhythmias
PREGNANCY AND LACTATION: Pregnancy category B; excretion in breast milk unknown

SIDE EFFECTS/ADVERSE REACTIONS
CNS: Dizziness, headache, neuritis
EENT: Burning eyes, cough, *hoarseness,* nasal burning, nasal congestion, nasal stinging, throat irritation
GI: Anorexia, *bitter taste,* diarrhea, dry mouth, nausea, vomiting
GU: Dysuria, frequency
MS: Joint pain or swelling
RESP: Cough
SPECIAL CONSIDERATIONS
PATIENT/FAMILY EDUCATION
• Therapeutic effect in asthma may take up to 4 wk

---

crotamiton
(kroe-tam′i-ton)
Rx: Eurax
Chemical Class: Synthetic chloroformate salt
Therapeutic Class: Scabicide

CLINICAL PHARMACOLOGY
Mechanism of Action: Toxic to *Sarcoptes scabiei*
Pharmacokinetics
Active topically; systemic absorption after topical use is unknown
INDICATIONS AND USES: Scabies in adults, scabies in children,* pruritic skin
DOSAGE
Adult and Child
• TOP (cre, lotion), massage into skin of entire body from chin down; repeat application 24 hr later
🔒 **AVAILABLE FORMS/COST OF THERAPY**
• Cre—Top: 10%, 60 g: **$12.72**
• Lotion—Top: 10%, 60, 454 ml: **$14.84/60 ml**
CONTRAINDICATIONS: Inflammation, abrasions, or breaks in skin or mucous membranes
PRECAUTIONS: Children

PREGNANCY AND LACTATION:
Pregnancy category C

SIDE EFFECTS/ADVERSE REACTIONS

SKIN: Contact dermatitis, irritation, itching, rash

SPECIAL CONSIDERATIONS
PATIENT/FAMILY EDUCATION

• 60 g is sufficient for 2 applications/adult

• Reapply locally during 48 hr treatment period after handwashing, etc

• A cleansing bath should be taken 48 hr after the last application

• After treatment, use topical corticosteroids to decrease contact dermatitis, antihistamines for pruritus; pruritus may continue for 4-6 wk

---

cyanocobalamin (vitamin B$_{12}$)

(sye-an-oh-koe-bal'a-min)
Rx: Cyanoject, Cyomin
Chemical Class: Synthetic B complex vitamin
Therapeutic Class: Vitamin supplement; blood modifier

CLINICAL PHARMACOLOGY
Mechanism of Action: Needed for nucleoprotein and myelin synthesis, protein and carbohydrate metabolism, normal growth, normal erythropoiesis

Pharmacokinetics
PO: Irregularly absorbed from the distal small gut; requires intrinsic factor but can be overcome with dosage increases (i.e., mean absorption rate of oral cyanocobalamin by patients with pernicious anemia is 1.2%; daily cobalamin turnover rate is about 2 µg/day, so oral doses of 100-250 µg are sufficient); peak 8-12 hr
IM: Peak 1 hr

Stored in liver, kidneys, stomach; 50%-90% excreted in urine; crosses placenta

INDICATIONS AND USES: Vitamin B$_{12}$ deficiency, pernicious anemia, vitamin B$_{12}$ malabsorption syndrome, Schilling test; increased requirements with pregnancy, thyrotoxicosis, hemolytic anemia, hemorrhage, renal and hepatic disease; prevention and treatment of cyanide toxicity associated with nitroprusside*

DOSAGE
Adult
• *Deficiency:* PO 250 µg qd × 5-10 days, maintenance 250-500 µg qd; IM/SC 30-100 µg qd 5-10 days, maintenance 100-200 µg IM qmo

• *Pernicious anemia/malabsorption syndrome:* IM 100-1000 µg qd × 2 wk, then 100-1000 µg IM qmo

• *Schilling test:* IM 1000 µg in one dose

Child
• *Deficiency:* Total IM/SC dose is 1-5 mg given in single 100 µg doses qd over 2 or more wk; maintenance 60 µg IM qmo or more

• *Pernicious anemia/malabsorption syndrome:* IM 100-500 µg qd over 2 wk, then 60 µg IM/SC qmo

• *Schilling test:* IM 1000 µg in one dose

$ AVAILABLE FORMS/COST OF THERAPY

• Inj, Sol—IM, IV, SC: 1000 µg/ml: **$0.09-$2.36**

• Tab—Oral: 100   µg,   100's: **$1.30-$4.50**;   250   µg,   100's: **$1.89-$3.90**;   500   µg,   100's: **$2.40-$5.85**; 1000 µg, 100's: **$4.91-$10.50**

• Tab—SL: 2500 µg, 50's: **$5.76**

CONTRAINDICATIONS: Optic nerve atrophy

PREGNANCY AND LACTATION: Pregnancy category C; excreted in breast milk in concentrations that approximate the mother's serum; compatible with breast feeding

SIDE EFFECTS/ADVERSE REACTIONS

CNS: Flushing, optic nerve atrophy

CV: **CHF,** peripheral vascular thrombosis, **pulmonary edema**

GI: Diarrhea

METAB: Hypokalemia

SKIN: Itching, pain at injection site, rash

SPECIAL CONSIDERATIONS

• Recommended dietary allowance: 0.5-2.6 µg/day depending on age and status (i.e., more during pregnancy and lactation)

• Nutritional sources: egg yolks, fish, organ meats, dairy products, clams, oysters

MONITORING PARAMETERS

• CBC with reticulocyte count after 1st wk of therapy

---

cyclandelate

(sye-klan´da-late)

Rx: Cyclandelate

Therapeutic Class: Peripheral vasodilator

CLINICAL PHARMACOLOGY

Mechanism of Action: Musculotropic; acts directly to relax vascular smooth muscle; no significant adrenergic-stimulating or adrenergic-blocking actions

Pharmacokinetics

PO: Onset 15 min, peak 1½ hr, duration 4 hr

INDICATIONS AND USES: Possibly effective: intermittent claudication, thrombophlebitis (to control associated vasospasm and muscular ischemia), Raynaud's phenomenon, ischemic cerebrovascular disease, arteriosclerosis obliterans, nocturnal leg cramps, dementia of cerebrovascular origin,* memory disorders,* migraine prophylaxis,* vertigo,* tinnitus and visual disturbances attributable to chronic cerebrovascular insufficiency,* diabetic peripheral polyneuropathy*

DOSAGE

Adult

• PO 200 mg qid, not to exceed 400 mg qid, maintenance dose is 400-800 mg/day in 2-4 divided doses

§ AVAILABLE FORMS/COST OF THERAPY

• Cap—Oral: 200 mg, 100's: **$5.25-$15.51**; 400 mg, 100's: **$7.00-$20.50**

PRECAUTIONS: Glaucoma, recent MI, hypertension, severe obliterative coronary artery or cerebrovascular disease ("steal" syndrome, diseased areas compromised by vasodilatory effects elsewhere)

PREGNANCY AND LACTATION: Pregnancy category C

SIDE EFFECTS/ADVERSE REACTIONS

CNS: Dizziness, headache, paresthesias, weakness

CV: Tachycardia

GI: Eructation, heartburn, nausea

HEME: Increased bleeding time (rare)

SKIN: Flushing, sweating

---

* = non-FDA-approved use

cyclobenzaprine

(sye-kloe-ben′za-preen)

Rx: Flexeril
Chemical Class: Tricyclic amine
Therapeutic Class: Skeletal muscle relaxant

CLINICAL PHARMACOLOGY

Mechanism of Action: Reduction of tonic somatic motor activity in the brain stem, producing skeletal muscle relaxant activity without interfering with muscle function; effects similar to tricyclic antidepressants

Pharmacokinetics
PO: Onset 1 hr, peak 3-8 hr, duration 12-24 hr, $t_{1/2}$ 1-3 days; metabolized by liver, excreted in urine

INDICATIONS AND USES: Adjunct to rest and physical therapy for relief of muscle spasm and pain in musculoskeletal conditions; fibrositis syndrome*

DOSAGE

Adult
• PO 10 mg tid × 1 wk (range 20-40 mg/day), max 60 mg/day, use should not exceed 3 wk

§ AVAILABLE FORMS/COST OF THERAPY
• Tab, Coated—Oral: 10 mg, 100's: **$7.40-$120.13**

CONTRAINDICATIONS: Acute recovery phase of MI, dysrhythmias, heart block, CHF, child <12 yr, intermittent porphyria, thyroid disease

PRECAUTIONS: History of urinary retention, angle-closure glaucoma, increased intraocular pressure, patients taking anticholinergic medication, addictive personality, elderly; lowers seizure threshold

PREGNANCY AND LACTATION: Pregnancy category B; no data available, but closely related tricyclic antidepressants are excreted into breast milk

SIDE EFFECTS/ADVERSE REACTIONS

CNS: Asthenia, confusion, depression, *dizziness, drowsiness,* headache, insomnia, nervousness, paresthesia, tremor, *weakness*
CV: **Dysrhythmias,** postural hypotension, tachycardia
EENT: Diplopia, temporary loss of vision
GI: Constipation, *dry mouth,* dyspepsia, hiccups, *nausea,* unpleasant taste, vomiting
GU: Change in libido, frequency, urinary retention
SKIN: Facial flushing, fever, pruritus, rash, sweating

INTERACTIONS

Drugs
3 *Droperidol, fluoxetine:* A patient receiving cyclobenzaprine and fluoxetine developed ventricular tachycardia and fibrillation after droperidol was added; relative contribution of each drug to the adverse effect unclear
2 *MAOIs:* Hyperpyretic crisis, severe convulsions, and deaths have occurred in patients receiving closely related tricyclic antidepressants and MAOIs; separate use by 14 days

Labs
• *Interference:* Serum amitriptyline assay

SPECIAL CONSIDERATIONS
• Avoid use in elderly due to anticholinergic side effects

PATIENT/FAMILY EDUCATION
• Use caution with alcohol, other CNS depressants
• Avoid with hazardous activities if drowsiness or dizziness occur

---

italic = common side effects   ***bold italic*** = life-threatening reactions

cyclophosphamide
(sye-kloe-foss'fa-mide)
Rx: Cytoxan, Neosar
Chemical Class: Synthetic nitrogen mustard
Therapeutic Class: Antineoplastic

CLINICAL PHARMACOLOGY
Mechanism of Action: Active metabolites alkylate DNA, RNA, thus interfering with growth of susceptible, rapidly proliferating malignant cells (mechanism is thought to involve cross-linking of tumor cell DNA); activity is not cell cycle phase specific
Pharmacokinetics
PO: Bioavailability >75%
IV: Peak, 2-3 hr (as metabolites)
Metabolized by liver, excreted in urine (5%-25% unchanged); $t_{1/2}$ 3-12 hr; 60% bound to plasma proteins
INDICATIONS AND USES: Malignant disease: Used concurrently or sequentially with other antineoplastic drugs for lymphomas, leukemias, and other malignancies
Nonmalignant disease: Biopsy proven "minimal change" nephrotic syndrome in children; severe rheumatic conditions* (Wegener's granulomatosis, steroid-resistant vasculitides, progressive rheumatoid arthritis, systemic lupus erythematosus, polyarteritis nodosa, polymyositis); multiple sclerosis*
DOSAGE
Adult
• *Malignant disease:* PO initially 1-5 mg/kg/day, maintenance is 1-5 mg/kg/day; IV initially 40-50 mg/kg in divided doses over 2-5 days, maintenance 10-15 mg/kg q7-10 days, or 3-5 mg/kg q3 days

Child
• *Malignant disease:* PO/IV 2-8 mg/kg or 60-250 mg/m^2 in divided doses for 6 or more days; maintenance 10-15 mg/kg q7-10 days or 30 mg/kg q3-4wk; dose should be reduced by half when bone marrow depression occurs
• *Nephrotic syndrome:* PO 2.5 to 3 mg/kg/day × 60-90 days
$ AVAILABLE FORMS/COST OF THERAPY
• Inj, Lyphl-Sol—IV: 1, 2 g/vial: **$49.33-$51.42**/1 g; 100, 200 mg/vial: **$10.20-$11.42**/100 mg
• Tab, Uncoated—Oral: 25 mg, 100's: **$203.22-$235.21**; 50 mg, 100's: **$341.68-$431.66**
CONTRAINDICATIONS: Suppressed bone marrow function
PRECAUTIONS: Radiation therapy
PREGNANCY AND LACTATION: Pregnancy category D; excreted in breast milk; contraindicated because of potential for adverse effects relating to immune suppression, growth, and carcinogenesis
SIDE EFFECTS/ADVERSE REACTIONS
CNS: Dizziness, headache
CV: **Cardiotoxicity** (high doses)
GI: Colitis, *diarrhea,* **hepatotoxicity,** *nausea, vomiting, weight loss*
GU: Amenorrhea, azoospermia, hematuria, hemorrhagic cystitis, neoplasms, *ovarian fibrosis, sterility,*
HEME: **Leukopenia, myelosuppression, pancytopenia, thrombocytopenia**
METAB: Syndrome of inappropriate antidiuretic hormone (SIADH)
RESP: Fibrosis
SKIN: Alopecia, dermatitis
INTERACTIONS
Drugs
3 *Allopurinol:* Increased cyclophosphamide toxicity

3 *Digoxin:* Decreased digoxin absorption from tablets; Lanoxicaps and elixir not affected

3 *Succinylcholine:* Prolonged neuromuscular blockade

3 *Warfarin:* Inhibited hypoprothrombinemic response to warfarin

SPECIAL CONSIDERATIONS
MONITORING PARAMETERS
• CBC, differential, platelet count qwk; withhold drug if WBC is <4000 or platelet count is <75,000
• Renal function studies: BUN, UA, serum uric acid; urine CrCl before, during therapy
• I&O; report fall in urine output ≤30 ml/hr

---

cycloserine
(sye-kloe-ser´een)

Rx: Seromycin
Chemical Class: Streptomyces orchidaceus product
Therapeutic Class: Antituberculosis agent; antibiotic

CLINICAL PHARMACOLOGY
Mechanism of Action: Inhibits cell wall synthesis in susceptible strains of gram-positive and gram-negative bacteria and in *Mycobacterium tuberculosis*

Pharmacokinetics
PO: Peak 4-8 hr, therapeutic levels 25-30 µg/ml, blood levels <30 µg/ml minimizes toxicity; 65% excreted unchanged in urine, remaining metabolized to unknown substances; crosses placenta

INDICATIONS AND USES: Pulmonary and extrapulmonary tuberculosis (like all antituberculosis drugs, cycloserine should be administered in conjunction with other effective chemotherapy and not as the sole therapeutic agent); acute UTI caused by susceptible strains of gram-positive and gram-negative bacteria, especially *Enterobacter* spp. and *E. coli* (when more conventional therapy has failed and when the organism has been demonstrated to be susceptible to the drug)

DOSAGE
Adult
• PO 250 mg q12h × 2 wk, then 250 mg q8h × 2 wk, then 250 mg q6h if there are no signs of toxicity; not to exceed 1 g/day

Child
• PO 10-20 mg/kg/day q12h (max 0.75-1 g); individualize doses

§ AVAILABLE FORMS/COST OF THERAPY
• Cap, Gel—Oral: 250 mg, 40's: **$141.71-$167.40**

CONTRAINDICATIONS: Seizure disorders, severe renal disease, alcoholism (chronic), depression, severe anxiety, psychosis

PRECAUTIONS: Children, mild renal impairment, anemia

PREGNANCY AND LACTATION: Pregnancy category C; excreted into breast milk (72% of serum levels); compatible with breast feeding

SIDE EFFECTS/ADVERSE REACTIONS
CNS: Aggression, anxiety, confusion, depression, drowsiness, headache, lethargy, psychosis, *seizures,* tremors
CV: CHF
HEME: Leukocytosis, megaloblastic anemia, vitamin B$_{12}$, folic acid deficiency
SKIN: Dermatitis, photosensitivity

INTERACTIONS
Drugs
3 *Isoniazid:* Increased risk of CNS toxicity

SPECIAL CONSIDERATIONS
• L-enantiomer (1-cycloserine) in Gaucher's disease (Orphan Drug)
• Pyridoxine may prevent neurotoxicity (200-300 mg/day)

---

italic = common side effects   ***bold italic*** = life-threatening reactions

PATIENT/FAMILY EDUCATION
• Avoid concurrent alcohol
MONITORING PARAMETERS
• Mental status closely and liver function tests qwk

---

cyclosporine

(sye-kloe-spor'in)
Rx: Neoral, Sandimmune, SangCya
Chemical Class: Cyclic peptide
Therapeutic Class: Immuno-suppressant

CLINICAL PHARMACOLOGY
Mechanism of Action: Produces immunosuppression by inhibiting T-lymphocytes (mainly T-helper cells, but T-suppressor cells may also be suppressed); also inhibits lymphokine production and release including interleukin-2; does not cause bone marrow suppression

Pharmacokinetics
PO: Variable bioavailability (4%-89%), peak 3.5 hr; 90% protein bound (lipoproteins); $t_{1/2}$ (terminal) 25 hr; metabolized in liver (mixed function oxidase enzymes) to 17 metabolites, only 0.1% left unchanged; excretion primarily biliary-feces, 0.1% excreted in urine

INDICATIONS AND USES: PO/IV prophylaxis of organ rejection in kidney, liver, and heart allogeneic transplants in conjunction with adrenal corticosteroids; prophylaxis of organ rejection in pancreas, bone marrow, and heart/lung transplantation.* Also used (at dosage 1-10 mg/kg/day) in: severe psoriasis; alopecia areata*; aplastic anemia*; atopic dermatitis*; Behçet's disease*; biliary cirrhosis*; Crohn's disease*; dermatomyositis*; Graves' ophthalmopathy*; insulin-dependent diabetes mellitus*; lupus nephritis*; multiple sclerosis*; myasthenia gravis*; nephrotic syndrome*; pemphigus and pemphigoid*; polymyositis*; psoriatic arthritis*; pulmonary sarcoidosis*; pyoderma gangrenosum*; rheumatoid arthritis*; ulcerative colitis*; uveitis*; Orphan Drug status: ophth keratoconjunctivitis sicca with Sjogren's syndrome; graft rejection following keratoplasty; corneal-melting syndromes (i.e., Mooren's ulcer)

DOSAGE
Adult and Child
• PO 15 mg/kg several hr before surgery, then daily for 2 wk, reduce dosage by 2.5 mg/kg/wk to 5-10 mg/kg/day (adjust based on blood levels); IV 5-6 mg/kg several hr before surgery, then daily, switch to PO form as soon as possible

$ **AVAILABLE FORMS/COST OF THERAPY**
Neoral
• Cap, Elastic—Oral: 25 mg, 30's: **$47.76**; 100 mg, 30's: **$190.85**
• Sol—Oral, for micro emulsion: 100 mg/5 ml, 50 ml: **$346.70**
Sandimmune
• Cap (soft gel), for micro emulsion: 25 mg, 30's: **$54.26**; 100 mg, 30's: **$185.16-$216.64**
• Inj, Sol—IV: 50 mg/ml, 5 ml: **$303.73**
• Sol—Oral: 100 mg/ml, 50 ml: **$308.40-$350.66**

CONTRAINDICATIONS: Hypersensitivity to Cremophor EL (Sandimmune dosage forms)
PRECAUTIONS: Renal disease, hepatic disease, concurrent nephrotoxic drugs; anaphylaxis possible with 1st IV dose; malabsorption syndromes
PREGNANCY AND LACTATION: Pregnancy category C; excreted into breast milk, avoid nursing.

---

* = non-FDA-approved use

SIDE EFFECTS/ADVERSE REACTIONS

CNS: Headache, tremors

CV: Hypertension (50% of renal transplants; most cardiac transplants)

GI: Diarrhea, *gum hyperplasia,* hepatotoxicity, nausea, *oral Candida,* pancreatitis, vomiting

GU: Albuminuria, hematuria, proteinuria, ***renal failure***

*HEME: **Leukopenia***

METAB: Hypomagnesemia (related to neurotoxicity)

SKIN: Acne, *hirsutism,* rash

INTERACTIONS

Drugs

🔳 *Allopurinol, amiodarone, chloroquine, clarithromycin, clonidine, clotrimazole, oral contraceptives, erythromycin, fluconazole, griseofulvin, itraconazole, ketoconazole, miconazole, ticlopidine:* Increased cyclosporine levels, potential for toxicity

🔳 *Aminoglycosides, amphotericin B, colchicine, enalapril, melphalan, sulfonamides:* Additive nephrotoxicity with cyclosporine

❷ *Anabolic steroids:* Increased cyclosporine levels, potential for toxicity

🔳 *Barbiturates, carbamazepine, nafcillin, pyrazinamide, phenytoin, sulfonamides:* Reduced cyclosporine levels, potential for therapeutic failure

🔳 *Calcium channel blockers:* Diltiazem, verapamil increase cyclosporine levels; isradipine, nifedipine, nitrendipine do not interact

🔳 *Cisapride, metoclopramide:* Increased bioavailability and serum levels of single-dose cyclosporine

🔳 *Digitalis glycosides:* Cyclosporine in patients stabilized on digitalis leads to increased levels and potential toxicity

🔳 *Doxorubicin, imipenem:* CNS toxicity

🔳 *HMG-CoA reductase inhibitors:* Increased risk of reversible myopathy

🔳 *Methotrexate:* Increased toxicity of both agents

🔳 *NSAIDs:* Increased risk of cyclosporine nephrotoxicity

❷ *Rifampin:* Reduced cyclosporine levels, potential for therapeutic failure

SPECIAL CONSIDERATIONS

• Neoral has increased bioavailability compared to Sandimmune (do NOT use interchangeably)

PATIENT/FAMILY EDUCATION

• Oral sol may be mixed with milk, chocolate milk, or orange juice to improve palatability. Do not mix with grapefruit juice (increased cyclosporine levels).

MONITORING PARAMETERS

• Renal function studies: BUN, creatinine q mo during treatment, 3 mo after treatment

• Liver function studies and serum levels during treatment

• Blood level monitoring: maintenance of 24-hr trough levels of 250-800 ng/ml (whole blood, RIA) or 50-300 ng/ml (plasma, RIA) should minimize side effects and rejection events

cyproheptadine
(si-proe-hep'ta-deen)
Rx: Periactin
Chemical Class: Piperidine derivative
Therapeutic Class: Antihistamine

CLINICAL PHARMACOLOGY
Mechanism of Action: Decreases allergic response by blocking histamine at H_1-receptors; also a serotonin antagonist
Pharmacokinetics
PO: Duration 4-6 hr; metabolized in liver, excreted by kidneys (40% unchanged)
INDICATIONS AND USES: Perennial and seasonal allergic rhinitis, vasomotor rhinitis, allergic conjunctivitis; allergic skin manifestations of urticaria and angioedema; cold urticaria; dermatographism; adjunctive anaphylactic therapy; appetite stimulant*; cluster headaches*; SSRI-induced sexual dysfunction*
DOSAGE
Adult
• PO 4 mg tid-qid, not to exceed 0.5 mg/kg/day
Child
• PO (0.25 mg/kg/day); 2-6 yr 2 mg bid-tid, not to exceed 12 mg/day; 7-14 yr 4 mg bid-tid, not to exceed 16 mg/day
$ AVAILABLE FORMS/COST OF THERAPY
• Syr—Oral: 2 mg/5 ml, 480 ml: **$6.72-$32.86**
• Tab, Uncoated—Oral: 4 mg, 100's: **$2.93-$50.89**
CONTRAINDICATIONS: Acute asthma attack, lower respiratory tract disease

PRECAUTIONS: Increased intraocular pressure due to closed-angle glaucoma, renal disease, cardiac disease, bronchial asthma, seizure disorder, stenosed peptic ulcers, prostatic hypertrophy, bladder neck obstruction, elderly
PREGNANCY AND LACTATION: Pregnancy category B; excreted in breast milk
SIDE EFFECTS/ADVERSE REACTIONS
CNS: Anxiety, confusion, *dizziness, drowsiness,* euphoria, fatigue, neuritis, paresthesia, poor coordination
CV: Hypotension, palpitations, tachycardia
EENT: Blurred vision, dilated pupils; dry nose, throat, mouth; nasal stuffiness; tinnitus
GI: Anorexia, *constipation,* diarrhea, dry mouth, nausea, vomiting, weight gain
GU: Dysuria, frequency, *retention*
RESP: Chest tightness, increased thick secretions, wheezing
SKIN: Photosensitivity, rash, urticaria
MISC: Increased appetite
INTERACTIONS
Drugs
3 *Fluoxetine:* Potential for worsening of depression when cyproheptadine added to fluoxetine therapy
Labs
• *False positive:* Urine tricyclic antidepressant assay

---

* = non-FDA-approved use

dalteparin
(doll'teh-pare-in)
Rx: Fragmin
Chemical Class: Depolymerized heparin derivative (low molecular weight heparin)
Therapeutic Class: Anticoagulant

CLINICAL PHARMACOLOGY
Mechanism of Action: Enhances the inhibition of Factor Xa and thrombin by binding to and accelerating antithrombin activity; preferentially inhibits Factor Xa; activated partial thromboplastin time (PTT) not affected
Pharmacokinetics
SC: Peak activity 4 hr; renal elimination $t_{1/2}$ 1.47-2.5 hr (prolonged in renal failure)
INDICATIONS AND USES: Prophylaxis against deep vein thrombosis (DVT), which may lead to pulmonary embolism (PE), in patients undergoing abdominal surgery who are at risk for thromboembolic complications and following hip replacement surgery (>40 yr of age, obese, undergoing surgery under general anesthesia lasting longer than 30 min, malignancy, history of DVT or PE); unstable angina/non-Q-wave MI; treatment of venous thromboembolism*
DOSAGE
Adult
• Prevention of DVT, abdominal surgery: SC 2,500 IU qd starting 1-2 hr prior to surgery and for 5-10 days postoperatively; high-risk patients (e.g., malignancy) should receive 5,000 IU the evening before surgery, then qd for 5-10 days postoperatively

• Prevention of DVT, hip replacement surgery: SC 2,500 IU within 2 hr before surgery, 2nd dose of 2,500 IU in evening of the day of surgery (≥6 hr after 1st dose), omit 2nd dose if surgery performed in evening; on 1st postoperative day begin 5,000 IU SC qd for 5-10 days; alternatively 5,000 IU can be administered evening prior to surgery followed by 5,000 IU qd for 5-10 days starting the evening of surgery
• Treatment of DVT: SC 200 IU/kg qd or 100 IU/kg q12h; initiate warfarin therapy concurrently and continue dalteparin for a minimum of 5 days and until therapeutic oral anticoagulant effect has been achieved (INR 2-3)
• Unstable angina/non-Q-wave MI: SC 120 IU/kg (max 10,000 IU) q12h with PO ASA (75-165 mg qd); continue until patient clinically stabilized (5-8 days)
💲 **AVAILABLE FORMS/COST OF THERAPY**
• Sol—SC: 2500 anti-Factor Xa/0.2 ml: **$15,303.95**; 5000 anti-Factor Xa/0.2 ml: **$24.90**; 10,000 anti-Factor Xa/10ml: **$428.00**
CONTRAINDICATIONS: Active major bleeding, thrombocytopenia associated with positive *in vitro* tests for antiplatelet antibody in the presence of dateparin, known hypersensitivity to pork products
PRECAUTIONS: History of heparin-induced thrombocytopenia; severe uncontrolled hypertension, bacterial endocarditis, congenital or acquired bleeding disorders, active ulceration and angiodysplastic gastrointestinal disease; hemorrhagic stroke or shortly after brain, spinal, or ophthalmological surgery; bleeding diathesis, thrombocytopenia or platelet defects; severe liver or kidney insufficiency; hypertensive or

diabetic retinopathy; recent gastrointestinal bleeding; neuraxial anesthesia

PREGNANCY AND LACTATION: Pregnancy category B

SIDE EFFECTS/ADVERSE REACTIONS

HEME: Hemorrhage, ***thrombocytopenia***

SKIN: Pain at injection site, skin necrosis

INTERACTIONS

Drugs

🔲 *Aspirin:* Increased risk of hemorrhage

🔲 *Oral anticoagulants:* Additive anticoagulant effects

SPECIAL CONSIDERATIONS

• Cannot be used interchangeably (unit for unit) with unfractionated heparin or other low molecular weight heparins

MONITORING PARAMETERS

• CBC with platelets, stool occult blood, urinalysis

• Monitoring aPTT is not required

---

danaparoid

(da-nap´ar-oid)

Rx: Organan

Chemical Class: Low-molecular weight heparinoid consisting of heparan sulfate, dermatan sulfate and chondroitin sulfate

Therapeutic Class: Anticoagulant

CLINICAL PHARMACOLOGY

Mechanism of Action: Inactivates factor Xa via a catalytic effect on antithrombin activity; factor IIa inhibition also occurs, but is substantially less than that seen with unfractionated heparin (anti-Xa/anti-IIa ratio >20:1 compared to 1:1 with unfractionated heparin); has only minor effects on platelet function

Pharmacokinetics

SC: Peak anti-Xa activity 2-5 hr, bioavailability approaches 100%; not metabolized in liver; renal excretion accounts for up to 50% of total plasma clearance of anti-Xa activity; elimination $t_{1/2}$ based on plasma anti-Xa activity 18-28 hr

INDICATIONS AND USES: Prevention of deep vein thrombosis (DVT) in patients undergoing elective total hip replacement surgery; heparin-induced thrombocytopenia*

DOSAGE

Adult

• SC 750 anti-Xa units bid for 7-10 days with the first dose given 1-4 hr prior to surgery; postoperative dose should not be given sooner than 2 hr after surgery

• Heparin-induced thrombocytopenia: IV 2,250 U bolus (1,500 U if <60 kg; 3,000 U if 75-90 kg; 3,750 U if >90 kg), followed by 400 U/hr for 4 hr, then 300 U/hr for 4 hr, then 150-200 U/hr to maintain anti-Xa levels between 0.5-0.8 U/ml; continue until platelet counts recover

💲 **AVAILABLE FORMS/COST OF THERAPY**

• Inj, Sol—SC: 750 U/0.6 ml: **$129.41-$140.19**

CONTRAINDICATIONS: Hypersensitivity to sulfites; severe hemorrhagic diathesis (hemophilia and idiopathic thrombocytopenic purpura); cerebrovascular hemorrhage or other active hemorrhagic states (except disseminated intravascular coagulation); positive *in vitro* aggregation test in presence of danaparoid in patients with Type II thrombocytopenia; hypersensitivity to pork products

---

PRECAUTIONS: Previous hypersensitivity to unfractionated heparin or low-molecular weight heparins; thrombocytopenia; recent childbirth; peptic ulcer disease; severe uncontrolled hypertension; diabetic retinopathy; acute bacterial endocarditis; renal impairment; liver disease; recent lumbar puncture; vasculitis; neuraxial analgesia

PREGNANCY AND LACTATION: Pregnancy category B

SIDE EFFECTS/ADVERSE REACTIONS

CV: Chest pain, ECG changes, tachycardia

HEME: Hemorrhage, ***thrombocytopenia***

SKIN: Injection site hematoma, pain at injection site, rash, wound infection

INTERACTIONS

Drugs

3 *Aspirin:* Increased risk of hemorrhage

3 *Oral anticoagulants:* Additive anticoagulant effects

SPECIAL CONSIDERATIONS

• Offers advantage over low-molecular weight heparins for the management of heparin-induced thrombocytopenia

• Does not offer a significant advantage over unfractionated heparin with respect to bleeding complications for any indication

MONITORING PARAMETERS

• CBC with platelets, stool occult blood, urinalysis

• Monitoring aPTT is not required

danazol
(da′na-zole)
Rx: Danocrine
Chemical Class: Ethisterone derivative
Therapeutic Class: Androgen

D

CLINICAL PHARMACOLOGY

Mechanism of Action: Suppresses the pituitary-ovarian axis; depresses the output of follicle-stimulating hormone (FSH) and luteinizing hormone (LH); possesses weak androgenic activity; decreases immunoglobulin levels

Pharmacokinetics

PO: Peak 2 hr; extensively metabolized in liver, excreted in urine; $t_{1/2}$ 4½ hr

INDICATIONS AND USES: Endometriosis amenable to hormonal management; reduction of nodularity, pain, and tenderness in fibrocystic breast disease; prevention of attacks of hereditary angioedema (cutaneous, abdominal, laryngeal); precocious puberty*; gynecomastia*; menorrhagia*; idiopathic immune thrombocytopenia*; lupus-associated thrombocytopenia*; autoimmune hemolytic anemia*

DOSAGE

Adult

• *Endometriosis:* PO initially 400 mg bid to achieve rapid response and amenorrhea; decrease to dose sufficient to maintain amenorrhea (100-200 mg bid) for 3-9 mo

• *Fibrocystic breast disease:* PO 100-400 mg/day in 2 divided doses

• *Hereditary angioedema:* PO initially 200 mg bid-tid; decrease dose by 50% or less at 1-3 mo intervals to lowest effective dose; if attack occurs, increase dose by up to 200 mg/day

---

italic = common side effects   ***bold italic*** = life-threatening reactions

$ **AVAILABLE FORMS/COST OF THERAPY**

• Cap, Gel—Oral: 50 mg, 100's: **$133.22-$159.86**; 100 mg, 100's: **$199.88-$249.46**; 200 mg, 100's: **$286.00-$415.67**

CONTRAINDICATIONS: Undiagnosed abnormal genital bleeding; markedly impaired hepatic, renal, or cardiac function; porphyria, pregnancy

PRECAUTIONS: Breast cancer, long-term use, epilepsy, migraine; cardiac, renal, or hepatic dysfunction

PREGNANCY AND LACTATION: Pregnancy category X may result in androgenic effects in the fetus; initiate therapy during menstruation or rule out pregnancy prior to initiating therapy in women of child-bearing potential; contraindicated during breast feeding

SIDE EFFECTS/ADVERSE REACTIONS

CNS: Dizziness, emotional lability, fatigue, headache, nervousness, sleep disorders, tremor

CV: Elevated blood pressure

GI: Constipation, hepatic dysfunction (doses >400 mg/day), nausea, vomiting, ***pancreatitis***

GU: Clitoral hypertrophy, hematuria, pelvic pain, testicular atrophy, menstrual irregularities (spotting, amenorrhea, cycle disturbances), vaginal dryness

METAB: Decreased HDL, increased LDL

SKIN: Acne, edema, flushing, *mild hirsutism, oily skin or hair,* sweating

MISC: Changes in libido, decrease in breast size, deepening of the voice, glucose intolerance, weight gain

INTERACTIONS

Drugs

❷ *Carbamazepine:* Predictably increases serum carbamazepine concentrations, toxicity possible

❷ *Cyclosporine:* Increased serum cyclosporine concentrations, toxicity possible

❸ *HMG-CoA reductase inhibitors (lovastatin, pravastatin):* Myositis risk increased

❷ *Oral anticoagulants:* Enhanced hypoprothrombinemic response

❷ *Tacrolimus:* Increased tacrolimus concentrations, toxicity possible

Labs

• *False decrease:* Plasma cortisol, serum testosterone, serum thyroxine

• *False increase:* Plasma cortisol, serum testosterone

SPECIAL CONSIDERATIONS

• Useful for palliative treatment of moderate to severe endometriosis or infertility due to endometriosis and for those whom alternative hormonal therapy is ineffective, intolerable, or contraindicated

• Drug of choice for treating all types of hereditary angioedema except for children or pregnant women where fibrolytic inhibitors (aminocaproic acid) may be preferred

• Breast pain should be treated conservatively (analgesics, supportive bra). Hormonal therapy is not innocuous. Symptoms usually return after discontinuation

• Ovarian function usually returns within 60-90 days after discontinuation

PATIENT/FAMILY EDUCATION

• Use nonhormonal contraceptive measures during therapy; discontinue use if pregnancy is suspected

MONITORING PARAMETERS

• Potassium, blood sugar, urine glucose during long-term therapy

dantrolene

(dan'troe-leen)

Rx: Dantrium

Chemical Class: Hydantoin derivative

Therapeutic Class: Skeletal muscle relaxant; malignant hyperthermia antidote

CLINICAL PHARMACOLOGY

Mechanism of Action: Reduces contraction of skeletal muscle by a direct action on excitation-contraction coupling, apparently by decreasing the amount of calcium released from the sarcoplasmic reticulum

Pharmacokinetics

PO: Peak 5 hr, highly protein bound, metabolized in liver, excreted in urine (metabolites and unchanged drug); $t_{1/2}$ 8 hr

INDICATIONS AND USES: Control of spasticity resulting from upper motor neuron disorders such as spinal cord injury, stroke, cerebral palsy, or multiple sclerosis; malignant hyperthermia (prevention of initial and recurrent episodes, treatment of crises); exercise-induced muscle pain*; neuroleptic malignant syndrome*; heatstroke*

DOSAGE

Adult

• *Spasticity:* PO 25 mg qd × 7 days then 25 mg tid × 7 days, increase to 50 mg tid × 7 days then 100 mg tid; may dose qid, max 400 mg/day

• *Malignant hyperthermia:* PO 4-8 mg/kg/day in 3-4 divided doses 1-2 days prior to surgery, last dose given 3-4 hr preoperatively; postoperatively use same dose for 1-3 days to prevent recurrence; IV 1 mg/kg may repeat prn to a cumulative dose of 10 mg/kg for acute episodes; 2.5 mg/kg 15-60 min before surgery for prevention

Child

• *Spasticity:* PO 0.5 mg/kg qd x 7 days then 0.5 mg/kg tid x 7 days, increase to 1 mg/kg tid x 7 days then 2 mg/kg tid; may dose qid, max 400 mg/day

• *Malignant hyperthermia:* Same as adult

💲 AVAILABLE FORMS/COST OF THERAPY

• Cap, Gel—Oral: 25 mg, 100's: **$100.80**; 50 mg, 100's: **$151.00**; 100 mg, 100's: **$187.81**

• Inj, Sol—IV: 20 mg, 1's: **$71.10**

CONTRAINDICATIONS: Active hepatic disease, muscle spasm resulting from rheumatic disorders

PRECAUTIONS: Age >35 yr and females (increased risk for hepatotoxicity), long-term use, impaired pulmonary function, severely impaired cardiac function, history of previous liver disease

PREGNANCY AND LACTATION: Pregnancy category C; do not use in nursing women

SIDE EFFECTS/ADVERSE REACTIONS

CNS: Disorientation, *dizziness, drowsiness, fatigue,* headache, insomnia, nervousness, paresthesias, *seizures,* tremors, *weakness*

CV: Chest pain, erratic blood pressure, palpitations

EENT: Blurred vision, mydriasis, nasal congestion

GI: Abdominal pain, anorexia, constipation, *diarrhea,* dry mouth, dysphasia, *GI bleeding, hepatotoxicity,* increased AST and alk phosphatase, *nausea,* vomiting

GU: Crystalluria, hematuria, impotence, nocturia, urinary frequency, urinary incontinence, urinary retention

RESP: Pleural effusion, ***pulmonary edema***

SKIN: Acne-like rash, photosensitivity, pruritus, rash, sweating, urticaria

INTERACTIONS

Drugs

3 *Calcium channel blockers:* Rare cases of CV collapse with concomitant use of dantrolene and verapamil; calcium channel blockers and dantrolene use not recommended during management of malignant hyperthermia

3 *CNS depressants:* Increased drowsiness

3 *Estrogen:* Possible increased hepatotoxicity in females >35 yr on estrogen therapy

3 *Vecuronium:* Dantrium may potentiate vecuronium-induced neuromuscular block

SPECIAL CONSIDERATIONS

• Use carefully where spasticity is utilized to sustain upright posture and balance in locomotion or to obtain or maintain increased function

• Discontinue after 6 wk if improvement does not occur

• Use lowest dose possible (hepatotoxicity dose-related)

PATIENT/FAMILY EDUCATION

• IV therapy may decrease grip strength and increase weakness of leg muscles, especially walking down stairs

• Caution driving or operating hazardous machinery

MONITORING PARAMETERS

• Baseline and periodic LFTs (AST, ALT, alk phosphatase, total bilirubin)

---

dapsone

(dap′sone)

Rx: Dapsone

Chemical Class: Sulfone

Therapeutic Class: Leprostatic; antiprotozoal

CLINICAL PHARMACOLOGY

Mechanism of Action: Competitive antagonist of para-aminobenzoic acid (PABA); prevents normal bacterial utilization of PABA for the synthesis of folic acid

Pharmacokinetics

PO: Rapid, complete absorption; 73% bound to plasma proteins; metabolized in liver, excreted in urine and bile; $t_{1/2}$ 25-31 hr

INDICATIONS AND USES: All forms of leprosy (Hansen's disease) except for cases of proven dapsone resistance; dermatitis herpetiformis; *Pneumocystis carinii* pneumonia (PCP) in HIV-infected patients (in combination with trimethoprim)*; alternative to co-trimoxazole for PCP prophylaxis (alone or in combination with pyrimethamine)*; prevention of the 1st episode of toxoplasmosis in HIV-infected patients (in combination with pyrimethamine)*; treatment of relapsing polychondritis*; prophylaxis of malaria*; brown recluse spider bites*

DOSAGE

Adult

• *Leprosy:* PO 50-100 mg qd for 3-10 yr (addition of rifampin 600 mg qd for the 1st 6 mo is recommended)

• *Dermatitis herpetiformis:* PO 50 mg qd initially; increase to 300 mg qd or higher to achieve full control; reduce dosage to minimum level as soon as possible

• *PCP prophylaxis:* PO 50-100 mg qd

---

* = non-FDA-approved use

Child
• *Leprosy:* PO 1-2 mg/kg/day; max 100 mg/day

$ AVAILABLE FORMS/COST OF THERAPY
• Tab, Uncoated—Oral: 25 mg, 100's: **$19.46**; 100 mg, 100's: **$20.34**

PRECAUTIONS: Renal disease, hepatic disease, G-6-PD deficiency, anemia, severe cardiopulmonary disease, methemoglobin reductase deficiency

PREGNANCY AND LACTATION: Pregnancy category C; extensive, but uncontrolled, experience and 2 published surveys in pregnant women have not shown increases in the risk for fetal abnormalities if administered during all trimesters; excreted in breast milk, hemolytic reactions can occur in neonates, discontinue nursing or discontinue drug; alternatively, some authors have suggested infants should be kept with mothers infected with leprosy, and breast feeding during drug therapy encouraged

SIDE EFFECTS/ADVERSE REACTIONS

CNS: Headache, insomnia, paresthesia, peripheral neuropathy, psychosis, vertigo
EENT: Blurred vision, optic neuritis, photophobia, tinnitus
GI: Abdominal pain, anorexia, nausea, vomiting
GU: **Nephrotic syndrome**, proteinuria, **renal papillary necrosis**
HEME: **Agranulocytosis, aplastic anemia, hemolytic anemia** (dose related)
SKIN: Drug-induced systemic lupus erythematosis, photosensitivity

INTERACTIONS
Drugs
3 *Didanosine:* Higher failure rate in pneumocystis infections, possibly due to inhibited dissolution of dapsone in stomach; administer dapsone 2-3 hr before didanosine
3 *Probenecid:* Increased serum dapsone concentrations, clinical importance not established
3 *Rifampin:* Reduced serum dapsone concentrations; increased methemoglobin concentrations
3 *Trimethoprim:* Increased serum dapsone concentrations; increased trimethoprim concentrations

SPECIAL CONSIDERATIONS
• Use in conjunction with either rifampin or clofazimine to prevent development of drug resistance and reduce infectiousness of patient with leprosy more quickly

PATIENT/FAMILY EDUCATION
• Full therapeutic effects on leprosy may not occur for several mo; compliance with dosage schedule, duration is necessary

MONITORING PARAMETERS
• CBC weekly for the 1st mo, qmo for 6 mo, and semiannually thereafter
• Periodic LFTs

---

darbepoetin alfa
(dar-beh-poe′ee-tin)
Rx: Aranesp
Chemical Class: Amino acid glycoprotein
Therapeutic Class: Hematopoetic agent

CLINICAL PHARMACOLOGY
Mechanism of Action: Produced by recombinant DNA technology in the hamster ovary and similar to endogenous erythropoietin; induces red blood cell production by stimulating

---

committed erythroid progenitor cells; induces bone marrow release of reticulocytes into bloodstream where they mature to erythrocytes

Pharmacokinetics

SC: Peak 24-72 hr, $t_{1/2}$ 27-89 hr

IV: $t_{1/2}$ 21 hr

Steady-state levels achieved in 4 wk with once weekly dosing; clinical response in 2-6 weeks

INDICATIONS AND USES: Anemia in patients with chronic renal failure

DOSAGE

Adult and Child >16 yr

• *CRF:* SC/IV 0.45 µg/kg once weekly; target dose to response (see monitoring parameters); maintenance dosage may be lower than this, especially in predialysis patients; some patients have been treated with SC dose every 2 weeks

• Estimated starting doses (µg/wk) based on previous erythropoietin (U/wk) dose:

<2,500 U: 6.25 µg

2,500-4,999 U: 12.5 µg

5,000-10,999 U: 25 µg

11,000-17,999 U: 40 µg

18,000-33,999 U: 60 µg

34,000-89,999 U: 100 µg

90,000 U: 200 µg

Child

• Safety and efficacy not established

$ AVAILABLE FORMS/COST OF THERAPY

• Inj, Sol—IV, SC: 200 µg/vial: **$997.50**; 100 µg/vial: **$498.75**; 60 µg/vial: **$299.25**; 40 µg/vial: **$199.50**; 25 µg/vial: **$124.69**

CONTRAINDICATIONS: Uncontrolled hypertension; hypersensitivity to mammalian cell-derived products or to human albumin (one formulation)

PRECAUTIONS: Seizure disorder, vascular disease, history of thrombosis

PREGNANCY AND LACTATION: Pregnancy category C, unknown if excreted in human milk

SIDE EFFECTS/ADVERSE REACTIONS

CNS: **Seizures,** *headache, dizziness*

CV: Hypertension (23%), *hypotension* (22%), *peripheral edema,* **CHF**, *chest pain,* **cardiac arrhythmia**

GI: Nausea, vomiting (15%), *diarrhea* (16%), *abdominal pain,* constipation

HEME: Thrombosis

MS: Myalgia (21%), *arthralgia, back pain*

RESP: Dyspnea (12%), *cough*

SKIN: Pain at injection site, pruritus

MISC: Fever, infection

SPECIAL CONSIDERATIONS

• Two formulations available, one containing polysorbate 80, the other containing human albumin; a theoretical risk for Creutzfeldt-Jakob disease exists with the albumin formulation but is considered extremely remote

• Advantage over erythropoietin is decreased frequency of dosing

PATIENT/FAMILY EDUCATION

• Educate about blood pressure monitoring

• Proper instruction for home administration if deemed appropriate

MONITORING PARAMETERS

• Hematocrit/hemoglobin weekly for 4 weeks or until stable; if Hb increases >1.0 g/dL in any 2 week period, decrease dose (possible increased seizure risk); target Hb level to not exceed 12 g/L

• Serum ferritin, transferrin saturation; supplemental iron recommended if ferritin <100 µg/L or transferrin saturation <20%

• If lack of response or failure to maintain response occur, check for causative factors (e.g., folate or vitamin B_{12} deficiency, occult blood loss, malignancy)
• Blood pressure

---

deferoxamine
(de-fer-ox´a-meen)
Rx: Desferal
Chemical Class: Siderochrome
Therapeutic Class: Heavy metal antidote (aluminum, iron)

CLINICAL PHARMACOLOGY
Mechanism of Action: Chelates iron by forming a stable complex that prevents iron from entering into further chemical reactions; readily chelates free serum iron, iron from ferritin and hemosiderin, but not from transferrin; does not combine with iron from cytochromes and hemoglobin
Pharmacokinetics
Rapidly metabolized by plasma enzymes, excreted in urine; iron chelate excreted renally giving urine a red color, some chelate also excreted in bile; $t_{1/2}$ 1 hr
INDICATIONS AND USES: Acute iron intoxication; promotion of iron excretion in patients who have secondary iron overload from multiple transfusions; aluminum accumulation in bone in renal failure patients,* aluminum-induced dialysis encephalopathy*
DOSAGE
Adult
• *Acute iron intoxication:* IM 1 g stat, then 0.5 g q4h for 2 doses, additional doses of 0.5 g q4-12h prn, max 6 g/day; IV infuse at a rate ≤15 mg/kg/hr, dosage the same as IM max 6 g/day (use only in cardiovascular collapse)

• *Chronic iron overload:* IM 0.5-1 g/day; SC via portable pump INF 1-2 g/day over 8-12 hr; IV give 2 g with, but separate from, each unit of blood at a rate ≤15 mg/kg/hr
Child
• *Acute iron intoxication:* IM 90 mg/kg q8h, max 6 g/day; IV 15 mg/kg/hr, max 6 g/day
• *Chronic iron overload:* IV 15 mg/kg/hr, max 6 g/day; SC via portable pump INF 20-40 mg/kg/day over 8-12 hr
$ AVAILABLE FORMS/COST OF THERAPY
• Inj, Sol—IM, IV, SC: 500 mg: **$15.53**
CONTRAINDICATIONS: Severe renal disease or anuria
PREGNANCY AND LACTATION: Pregnancy category C; excretion into breast milk unknown; use caution in nursing mothers
SIDE EFFECTS/ADVERSE REACTIONS
CV: Hypotension (with rapid IV inj), tachycardia
GI: Abdominal cramps, diarrhea
EENT: Blurred vision, cataracts, ototoxicity
MS: Leg cramps
SKIN: Erythema, pain at inj site, pruritus, urticaria
SPECIAL CONSIDERATIONS
• Acute iron intoxication:
• Deferoxamine indicated if:
• Free serum iron present
• Patient symptomatic
• Serum iron >350 µg/dL
PATIENT/FAMILY EDUCATION
• May turn urine red
MONITORING PARAMETERS
• Visual acuity tests, slit-lamp examinations, funduscopy, and audiometry are recommended periodically in patients treated for prolonged periods of time
• BUN, creatinine, CrCl
• Serum iron levels

---

italic = common side effects   ***bold italic*** = life-threatening reactions

delavirdine

(deh-la'ver-deen)
Rx: Rescriptor
Chemical Class: Arylpipera-
zine derivative
Therapeutic Class: Nonnucleoside reverse transcriptase
inhibitor

CLINICAL PHARMACOLOGY
Mechanism of Action: Inhibits
DNA- and RNA-directed polymerase function of HIV-1 by allos-
teric inhibition
Pharmacokinetics
PO: Well-absorbed, peak 1 hr; 99%
protein bound; does not penetrate
CSF; metabolized by cytochrome
P450 3A enzyme system, inhibits its
own metabolism causing reduced
clearance at higher doses; $t_{1/2}$ 7 hr at
daily dose of 1200 mg; 44% of dose
excreted in feces, 51% of dose excreted in urine; inhibits CYP3A and
CYP2C9

INDICATIONS AND USES: Combi-
nation therapy for HIV-1
DOSAGE
Adult and Child >12 yr
• PO: 400 mg tid
• For latest treatment guidelines, see
www.hivatis.org
$ **AVAILABLE FORMS/COST
OF THERAPY**
• Tab, Uncoated—Oral: 100 mg,
360's: **$282.96-$316.35**; 200 mg,
180's: **$292.02-$316.35**
CONTRAINDICATIONS: Concur-
rent use of rifampin
PRECAUTIONS: Children, hepatic
disease
PREGNANCY AND LACTATION:
Pregnancy category C, teratogenic
in rats; excreted in breast milk at
high concentrations

**SIDE EFFECTS/ADVERSE REAC-
TIONS**
CNS: Confusion, depression, dizzi-
ness, *headache,* insomnia, somno-
lence
CV: Bradycardia, tachycardia
EENT: Epistaxis, gingivitis, pharyn-
gitis, rhinitis
GI: Diarrhea, dyspepsia, increased
alkaline phosphatase, ALT, AST;
nausea (11%)
GU: Breast enlargement, menorrhagia, nephrolithiasis, proteinuria
HEME: **Anemia (79%), leukopenia
(16%), thrombocytopenia (42%)**
METAB: Hyperkalemia
MS: Increased CPK, myalgia
RESP: Cough, dyspnea
SKIN: **Rash (45%),** pruritus
MISC: Fatigue
INTERACTIONS
Drugs
3 *Aluminum:* Antacids reduce GI
absorption of delavirdine by 50% if
taken at same time; separate doses
by at least 1 hr
3 *Antacids:* Antacids reduce GI absorption of delavirdine by 50% if
taken at same time; separate doses
by at least 1 hr
▲ *Astemizole:* Delavirdine increases astemizole plasma level;
coadministration contraindicated
3 *Barbiturates:* Barbiturates decrease plasma delavirdine levels
3 *Benzodiazepines:* Delavirdine
increases benzodiazepine plasma
levels by inhibiting hepatic metabolism
3 *Calcium:* Antacids reduce GI absorption of delavirdine by 50% if
taken at same time; separate doses
by at least 1 hr
3 *Carbamazepine:* Carbamazepine decreases plasma delavirdine
levels
❷ *Cimetidine:* Cimetidine reduces
GI absorption of delavirdine; coadministration not recommended

❷ *Cisapride:* Delavirdine increases cisapride plasma level; coadministration not recommended

❸ *Clarithromycin:* Delavirdine increases clarithromycin plasma levels; clarithromycin increases delavirdine plasma levels

❸ *Dapsone:* Delavirdine increases dapsone plasma level

❸ *Didanosine:* Delavirdine reduces didanosine absorption; didanosine reduces delavirdine absorption; separate doses by at least 1 hr

❷ *Ergotamines:* Delavirdine increases ergotamine plasma level; coadministration not recommended

❷ *Famotidine:* Famotidine reduces GI absorption of delavirdine; coadministration not recommended

❸ *Fluoxetine:* Fluoxetine increases delavirdine levels by inhibiting hepatic metabolism

❸ *Indinavir:* Delavirdine increases indinavir AUC by 40%; reduce indinavir dose to 600 mg tid

❷ *Lansoprazole:* Lansoprazole reduces GI absorption of delavirdine; coadministration not recommended

❷ *Lovastatin:* Delavirdine increases lovastatin plasma level; coadministration not recommended

❸ *Magnesium:* Antacids reduce GI absorptioin of delavirdine by 50% if taken at same time; separate doses by at least 1 hr

❷ *Midazolam:* Delavirdine increases midazolam plasma level; coadministration not recommended

❸ *Nelfinavir:* Delavirdine increases nelfinavir AUC by 100%; nelfinavir reduces delavirdine AUC by 50%; no data on dose adjustment

❷ *Nizatidine:* Nizatidine reduces GI absorption of delavirdine; coadministration not recommended

❸ *Nifedipine:* Delavirdine increases nifedipine plasma level

❷ *Omeprazole:* Omeprazole reduces GI absorption of delavirdine; coadministration not recommended

❸ *Phenytoin:* Phenytoin decreases plasma delavirdine level

❷ *Quinidine:* Delavirdine increases quinidine plasma level

❷ *Ranitidine:* Ranitidine reduces GI absorption of delavirdine; coadministration not recommended

❷ *Rifabutin:* Rifabutin decreases plasma delavirdine level; coadministration not recommended

▲ *Rifampin:* Rifampin decreases plasma delavirdine level; coadministration contraindicated

❸ *Ritonavir:* Delavirdine increases ritonavir AUC by 70%; no data on dose adjustment

❷ *Saquinavir:* Delavirdine increases saquinavir AUC by 5-fold; additive hepatic toxicity possible; adjust Fortovase dose to 800 mg tid

❷ *Simvastatin:* Delavirdine increases simvastatin plasma level; coadministration not recommended

❸ *Sodium bicarbonate:* Antacids reduce GI absorption of delavirdine by 50% if taken at same time; separate doses by at least 1 hr

▲ *Terfenadine:* Delavirdine increases terfenadine plasma level; coadministration contraindicated

❷ *Triazolam:* Delavirdine increases triazolam plasma level; coadministration not recommended

❸ *Warfarin:* Delavirdine increases warfarin effect

SPECIAL CONSIDERATIONS
PATIENT/FAMILY EDUCATION
• May take without regard to food; patients with achlorhydria should take with acidic beverage (orange or cranberry juice); may cause alcohol intolerance
MONITORING PARAMETERS
• CBC, hepatic, and renal function

demeclocycline
(dem-e-kloe-sye′kleen)
Rx: Declomycin
Chemical Class: Tetracycline derivative
Therapeutic Class: Antibiotic

CLINICAL PHARMACOLOGY
Mechanism of Action: Inhibits protein synthesis by binding with the 30S and possibly the 50S ribosomal subunit(s) of susceptible bacteria; may also cause alterations in the cytoplasmic membrane; bacteriostatic

Pharmacokinetics
PO: Peak 3-6 hr, $t_{1/2}$ 10-17 hr; excreted in urine; 65%-91% bound to serum protein

INDICATIONS AND USES: Chronic hyponatremia associated with the syndrome of inappropriate antidiuretic hormone (SIADH) secretion*; Rocky Mountain spotted fever, typhus fever, Q fever, rickettsialpox, tick fevers, *Mycoplasma pneumoniae,* psittacosis and ornithosis, lymphogranuloma venereum and granuloma inguinale, relapsing fever, chancroid, infections of the respiratory and urinary tract, syphilis and yaws, Vincent's infection, acute intestinal amebiasis (adjunct to amebicides), trachoma, inclusion conjunctivitis, severe acne

Antibacterial spectrum usually includes:
• Gram-positive organisms: *Bacillus anthracis, Actinomyces israelii, Arachnia propionica, Clostridium perfringens, C. tetani, Listeria monocytogenes, Nocardia, Propionibacterium acnes*
• Gram-negative organisms: *Bartonella bacilliformis, Bordetella pertussis, Brucella, Calymmatobacterium granulomatis, Campylobacter fetus, Francisella tularensis,* *Haemophilus ducreyi, H. influenzae, Legionella pneumophilia, Leptotrichia buccalis, Neisseria gonorrhoeae, N. meningitidis, Pasteurella multocida, Pseudomonas pseudomallei, P. mallei, Shigella, Spirillum minus, Streptobacillus moniliformis, Vibrio cholerae, V. parahaemolyticus, Yersinia enterocolitica, Y. pestis* Other organisms: *Rickettsia akari, R. prowazeki, R. rickettsii, R. tsutsugamushi, R. typhi, Coxiella burnetii, Chlamydia trachomatis, C. psittaci, Mycoplasma hominis, M. pneumoniae, Ureaplasma urealyticum, Borrelia recurrentis, Leptospira, Treponema pallidum, T. pertenue*

DOSAGE
Adult
• PO 150 mg q6h or 300 mg q12h
• *Gonorrhea:* PO 600 mg, then 300 mg q12h for 4 days; total 3 g
• *SIADH:* PO 600-1200 mg/day in divided doses

Child >8 yr
• PO 6-12 mg/kg/day in divided doses q6-12h

🔣 AVAILABLE FORMS/COST OF THERAPY
• Tab, Plain Coated—Oral: 150 mg, 100's: **$506.29**; 300 mg, 48's: **$442.20**

CONTRAINDICATIONS: Children <8 yr

PRECAUTIONS: Renal disease, hepatic disease, nephrogenic diabetes insipidus, exposure to direct sunlight, outdated products

PREGNANCY AND LACTATION: Pregnancy category D; problems associated with use of the tetracyclines during or around pregnancy include adverse effects on fetal teeth and bones, maternal liver toxicity, and congenital defects; excreted into breast milk in low concentrations; use caution in nursing mothers

---

* = non-FDA-approved use

SIDE EFFECTS/ADVERSE REACTIONS

CNS: Fever, headache, paresthesia
CV: Pericarditis
GI: Abdominal cramps, abdominal pain, anorexia, *diarrhea,* dysphagia, enterocolitis, epigastric burning, flatulence, glossitis, hepatotoxicity, *nausea,* oral candidiasis, ***pseudomembranous colitis,*** stomatitis, vomiting
GU: Nephrogenic diabetes insipidus, ***nephrotoxicity,*** polydipsia, polyuria
HEME: Eosinophilia, ***hemolytic anemia, neutropenia, thrombocytopenia***
SKIN: ***Exfoliative dermatitis,*** *photosensitivity,* pruritus, rash, urticaria
MISC: Decreased calcification of deciduous teeth, angioedema, pseudotumor cerebri (adults) and bulging fontanels (infants)

INTERACTIONS

Drugs

3 *Antacids:* Reduced serum concentration of demeclocycline; take 2 hr before or 6 hr after antacids containing aluminum, calcium, or magnesium

2 *Bismuth:* Reduced serum concentration of demeclocycline; do not coadminister

3 *Calcium:* See antacids

3 *Cholestyramine:* Reduced serum concentration of demeclocycline; take 2 hr before or 3 hr after cholestyramine

3 *Colestipol:* Reduced serum concentration of demeclocycline; take 2 hr before or 3 hr after colestipol

3 *Digoxin:* Demeclocycline may increase serum digoxin levels

3 *Food:* Reduced serum concentration of demeclocycline; take 2 hr before or 3 hr after food

3 *Iron:* Reduced serum concentration of demeclocycline; take 2 hr before or 3 hr after iron

3 *Magnesium:* See antacids

2 *Methoxyflurane:* Demeclocycline enhances nephrotoxicity of methoxyflurane

3 *Oral contraceptives:* Contraceptive failure may occur rarely; mechanism unknown

3 *Penicillins:* Demeclocycline may reduce penicillin efficacy

3 *Warfarin:* Demeclocycline may increase effect of warfarin

3 *Zinc:* Reduced serum concentration of demeclocycline; take 2 hr before or 3 hr after zinc

Labs

• *False increase:* Urinary catecholamines

SPECIAL CONSIDERATIONS

• No advantages over other tetracyclines as anti-infective; higher incidence of phototoxicity; active against water intoxication and SIADH

PATIENT/FAMILY EDUCATION

• Sunscreen does not seem to decrease photosensitivity
• Avoid milk products; take with full glass of water on an empty stomach 1 hr before meals or 2 hr after meals

MONITORING PARAMETERS

• LFTs during prolonged administration

---

desipramine

(dess-ip'ra-meen)
Rx: Norpramin, Pertofrane
Chemical Class: Dibenzazepine derivative: secondary amine
Therapeutic Class: Tricyclic Antidepressant

CLINICAL PHARMACOLOGY

Mechanism of Action: Inhibits the reuptake of norepinephrine and serotonin (amine blocking activity, very high and moderate, respectively) at the presynaptic neuron, prolonging neuronal activity; inhibits histamine and acetylcholine activity; mild peripheral vasodilator effects and possible "quinidine-like" actions

Pharmacokinetics

PO: Peak 2-4 hr; therapeutic response 2-4 wk; metabolized by liver, excreted by kidneys; $t_{1/2}$ 14-62 hr

INDICATIONS AND USES: Depression, facilitation of cocaine withdrawal,* eating disorders,* panic attacks*

DOSAGE

Adult

• PO 25 mg/day in single or divided doses initially, increase by 25 mg q3-5 days to 100-200 mg/day, max 300 mg/day

Geriatric/Adolescent

• PO 25-100 mg/day, doses >150 mg/day not recommended

Child 6-12 yr

• PO 10-30 mg/day or 1-5 mg/kg/day in divided doses, max 5 mg/kg/day

$ AVAILABLE FORMS/COST OF THERAPY

• Tab, Plain Coated—Oral: 10 mg, 100's: **$15.90-$120.00**; 25 mg, 100's: **$16.80-$69.66**; 50 mg, 100's: **$25.28-$156.15**; 75 mg, 100's: **$53.15-$198.75**; 100 mg, 100's: **$84.77-$261.16**; 150 mg, 50's: **$109.50-$189.21**

CONTRAINDICATIONS: Acute recovery phase of MI; concurrent use of MAOIs

PRECAUTIONS: Suicidal patients, convulsive disorders, prostatic hypertrophy, psychiatric disease, severe depression, increased intraocular pressure, narrow-angle glaucoma, urinary retention, cardiac disease, hepatic or renal disease, hyperthyroidism, electroshock therapy, elective surgery, elderly, abrupt discontinuation

PREGNANCY AND LACTATION: Pregnancy category C; excreted into breast milk; effect on the nursing infant unknown, but may be of concern

SIDE EFFECTS/ADVERSE REACTIONS

CNS: Anxiety, confusion (especially in elderly), *dizziness,* EPS (elderly), fatigue, headache, increased psychiatric symptoms, insomnia, memory impairment, nervousness, nightmares, panic, stimulation, tremors, weakness

*CV: **Dysrhythmias,*** ECG changes, hypertension, *orthostatic hypotension,* palpitations, syncope, tachycardia

EENT: Blurred vision, mydriasis, nasal congestion, ophthalmoplegia, tinnitus

GI: Constipation, cramps, *dry mouth,* epigastric distress, hepatitis, increased appetite, jaundice, nausea, paralytic ileus, stomatitis, vomiting

GU: Urinary retention

HEME: **Agranulocytosis,** eosinophilia, **leukopenia, thrombocytopenia**

METAB: Weight gain

SKIN: Photosensitivity, pruritus, rash, sweating, urticaria

INTERACTIONS

Drugs

3 *Barbiturates:* Reduced serum concentrations of cyclic antidepressants

2 *Bethanidine:* Reduced antihypertensive effect of bethanidine

3 *Carbamazepine:* Reduced serum concentrations of cyclic antidepressants

3 *Cimetidine:* Increased serum concentrations of cyclic antidepressants

❷ *Clonidine:* Reduced antihypertensive effect of clonidine; enhanced hypertensive response with abrupt clonidine withdrawal

▣ *Debrisoquin:* Reduced antihypertensive effect of debrisoquin

▣ *Diltiazem:* Increased serum concentrations of cyclic antidepressants

❷ *Epinephrine:* Markedly enhanced pressor response to IV epinephrine

▣ *Ethanol:* Additive impairment of motor skills; abstinent alcoholics may eliminate cyclic antidepressants faster than nonalcoholics

▣ *Fluoxetine:* Marked increases in serum concentrations of cyclic antidepressants

▣ *Fluvoxamine:* Marked increases in serum concentrations of cyclic antidepressants

❷ *Guanabenz, guanethidine:* Reduced antihypertensive effect

▣ *Guanadrel, guanfacine:* Reduced antihypertensive effect

▣ *Indinavir:* Increase in serum concentrations of cyclic antidepressants

▣ *Lithium:* Increased risk of neurotoxicity

❷ *Moclobemide:* Potential association with fatal or nonfatal serotonin syndrome

❷ *MAOIs:* Excessive sympathetic response, manias, or hyperpyrexia possible

▣ *Neuroleptics:* Increased therapeutic and toxic effects of both drugs

❷ *Norepinephrine:* Markedly enhanced pressor response to IV norepinephrine

▣ *Paroxetine:* Marked increases in serum concentrations of cyclic antidepressants

▣ *Propoxyphene:* Increased serum concentrations of cyclic antidepressants

▣ *Quinidine:* Increased serum concentrations of cyclic antidepressants

▣ *Rifampin:* Reduced serum concentrations of cyclic antidepressants

▣ *Ritonavir:* Marked increases in serum concentrations of cyclic antidepressants

▣ *Sulfonylureas:* Cyclic antidepressants may increase hypoglycemic effect

SPECIAL CONSIDERATIONS

• Equally effective as other tricyclic antidepressants for depression; fewer anticholinergic effects than tertiary amines, less orthostasis, and mild stimulatory property

PATIENT/FAMILY EDUCATION

• Therapeutic effects may take 4-6 wk

• Use caution in driving or other activities requiring alertness

• Avoid alcohol and other CNS depressants

• Do not discontinue abruptly after long-term use

MONITORING PARAMETERS

• Determination of desipramine plasma concentrations is not routinely recommended but may be useful in identifying toxicity, drug interactions, or noncompliance (adjustments in dosage should be made according to clinical response not plasma concentrations); therapeutic level is 50-200 ng/ml

---

desloratadine

(des-loer-at'ah-deen)

Rx: Clarinex
Chemical Class: Piperidine derivative
Therapeutic Class: Antihistamine

CLINICAL PHARMACOLOGY

Mechanism of Action: Decreases allergic response by blocking histamine at H_1-receptors; provides antihistamine action without sedation

Pharmacokinetics
PO: Peak 3 hr; 82-87% bound to plasma proteins, does not readily cross the blood brain barrier; extensively metabolized to 3-hydroxy-desloratadine, and active metabolite; excreted equally in urine and feces as metabolic products; $t_{1/2}$ 27 hr

INDICATIONS AND USES: Relief of nasal and non-nasal symptoms of seasonal allergic rhinitis

DOSAGE
Adult and Child >12 yr
• PO 5 mg qd
• In patients with liver or renal impairment, a starting dose of 5 mg qod is recommended

🔟 **AVAILABLE FORMS/COST OF THERAPY**
• Tab, Film-Coated—Oral: 5 mg, 100's: **$219.17**

CONTRAINDICATIONS: Hypersensitivity to loratadine

PRECAUTIONS: Increased intraocular pressure, hepatic disease, renal insufficiency, children <12 yr

PREGNANCY AND LACTATION: Pregnancy category C; passes into breast milk, use caution in nursing mothers

SIDE EFFECTS/ADVERSE REACTIONS
CNS: Somnolence, dizziness
EENT: Pharyngitis, dry throat
GI: Dry mouth, nausea
MS: Myalgia
MISC: Fatigue, influenza-like symptoms

SPECIAL CONSIDERATIONS
• Major metabolite of loratadine
• Intranasal corticosteroids are preferred therapy unless allergy symptoms are mild and infrequent
• Reserve for patients unable to tolerate sedating antihistamines like chlorpheniramine

PATIENT/FAMILY EDUCATION
• May be taken without regard to meals

---

desmopressin
(des-moe-press'in)
Rx: DDAVP, Stimate
Chemical Class: Synthetic arginine vasopressin analog
Therapeutic Class: Antihemophilic; hemostatic; antidiuretic

CLINICAL PHARMACOLOGY
Mechanism of Action: A posterior pituitary hormone analog; has ADH activity (promotes renal tubular reabsorption of water); less vascular or GI smooth muscle constriction than natural vasopressin; causes increase in plasma factor VIII levels, which increases platelet aggregation

Pharmacokinetics
NASAL: Onset 1 hr, peak 1-2 hr, duration 8-20 hr, terminal $t_{1/2}$ 76 min

INDICATIONS AND USES: Primary nocturnal enuresis (intranasal only); neurogenic diabetes insipidus; spontaneous, trauma-induced or prevention of perioperative bleeding in patients with hemophilia A with factor VIII levels >5%; spontaneous, trauma-induced, or prevention of perioperative bleeding in patients with von Willebrand's disease (Type I); determination of the capacity of the kidneys to concentrate urine; chronic autonomic failure (e.g., nocturnal polyuria, overnight weight loss, morning postural hypotension)*

DOSAGE
Adult
• *Central diabetes insipidus:* Nasal (via rhinal tube) 0.1-0.4 ml qd, as a single or divided dose; most adults require 0.2 ml qd in 2 divided doses; the AM and PM doses should be separately adjusted for an adequate diurnal rhythm of water turnover; PO 0.05 bid, titrate to optimum

---

* = non-FDA-approved use

therapeutic dose (range, 0.1-1.2 mg divided 2 or 3 × daily; IV/SC 0.5-1 ml/day in 2 divided doses, adjusted separately for an adequate diurnal rhythm of water turnover; when switching from intranasal to IV the comparable antidiuretic dose is ¹⁄₁₀ the intranasal dose

• *Hemophilia A and von Willebrand's disease (Type I):* IV 0.3 µg/kg diluted in 50 ml NS infused slowly over 15-30 min, 30 min before procedure; intranasal 300 µg (stimate only; use 2 hr before surgical procedure)

Child

• *Primary nocturnal enuresis:* Nasal (>6yr) initially 20 µg or 0.2 ml sol qhs; may increase up to 40 µg qhs prn; decrease to 10 µg qhs if the patient has shown a response to 20 µg. PO 0.2 mg initially at hs, titrate for response to maximum dose of 0.6 mg

• *Central diabetes insipidus:* Nasal (via rhinal tube) (3 mo-12 yr) 0.05 to 0.3 ml qd, either as single dose or divided into 2 doses; PO 0.05 mg qd; titrate with fluid restriction

• *Hemophilia A and von Willebrand's disease (Type I):* IV 0.3 mg/kg diluted in 50 ml NS (>10 kg) or 10 ml NS (≤10 kg) infused slowly over 15-30 min, 30 min before procedure; intranasal 300 µg (> 50 kg) or 150 µg (≤50 kg) (stimate only; use 2 hr before surgical procedure)

🅢 **AVAILABLE FORMS/COST OF THERAPY**
• Inj, Sol—IV; SC: 4 µg/ml, 10 ml: **$145.20-$270.00**; 15 µg/ml, 10 ml: **$972.00**
• Sol—Nasal: 0.1 mg/ml, 2 ml: **$85.06**
• Spray—Nasal: 10 µg/inh, 2.5, 5, 30 ml: **$121.56-$161.06**/5 ml; 0.15 mg/inh, 2 ml: **$575.00**

• Tab—Oral: 0.1 mg, 100's: **$246.50**; 0.2 mg, 100's: **$303.00**

CONTRAINDICATIONS: Type IIB von Willebrand's disease

PRECAUTIONS: Coronary artery disease, hypertensive cardiovascular disease, elderly, children: bleeding disorders, proven safe and effective for age ≥ 3 months (parenteral) or ≥11 months (Stimate intranasal)

PREGNANCY AND LACTATION: Pregnancy category B (no uterotonic action at antidiuretic doses); compatible with breast feeding

SIDE EFFECTS/ADVERSE REACTIONS

CNS: Drowsiness, flushing, headache, lethargy, ***seizures***

CV: Increased blood pressure

EENT: Congestion, nasal irritation, rhinitis

GI: Cramps, heartburn, nausea

GU: Vulvar pain

SPECIAL CONSIDERATIONS
• Though useful in the treatment of children with enuresis, relapse following discontinuation is common; conservative therapy preferred long-term; desmopressin best used intermittently (e.g., overnight with friend)

PATIENT/FAMILY EDUCATION
• Nasal tube delivery system is supplied with a flexible calibrated plastic tube (rhinyle); draw sol into the rhinyle, insert 1 end of tube into nostril, blow on the other end to deposit sol deep into nasal cavity
• Ingest only enough water to satisfy thirst (especially elderly and children)

MONITORING PARAMETERS
• Diabetes insipidus: Urine volume and osmolality, plasma osmolality

---

• Hemophilia A: Determine factor VIII coagulant activity before injecting desmopressin for hemostasis; if activity is <5% of normal, do not rely on desmopressin

• Von Willebrand's disease: Assess levels of factor VIII coagulant, factor VIII antigen, and ristocetin cofactor; skin bleeding time may also be helpful

---

desonide
(dess'oh-nide)
Rx: Delomide, DesOwen, Tridesilon
Chemical Class: Synthetic glucocorticoid
Therapeutic Class: Topical corticosteroid, low potency

CLINICAL PHARMACOLOGY
Mechanism of Action: Depresses formation, release, and activity of endogenous mediators of inflammation such as prostaglandins, kinins, histamine, liposomal enzymes, and the complement system resulting in decreased edema, erythema, and pruritus
Pharmacokinetics
Absorbed through the skin (increased by inflammation and occlusive dressings); metabolized primarily in the liver
INDICATIONS AND USES: Psoriasis, eczema, contact dermatitis, pruritus, superficial bacterial infections of the external auditory canal (otic preparation)
DOSAGE
Adult and Child
• TOP apply to affected area bid-tid, rub completely into skin; OTIC instill 3-4 gtt tid-qid or insert wick saturated with solution and allow to remain *in situ*

🛇 AVAILABLE FORMS/COST OF THERAPY
• Cre—Top: 0.05%, 15, 60, 90 g: **$7.96-$20.31**/15 g
• Lotion—Top: 0.05%, 60, 120 ml: **$33.44**/60 ml
• Oint—Top: 0.05%, 15, 60 g: **$9.95-$20.31**/15 g
CONTRAINDICATIONS: Fungal infections
PRECAUTIONS: Viral infections, bacterial infections, children; use on face, genitals, axilla
PREGNANCY AND LACTATION: Pregnancy category C; unknown whether top application could result in sufficient systemic absorption to produce detectable amounts in breast milk (systemic corticosteroids are secreted into breast milk in quantities not likely to have detrimental effects on infant)
SIDE EFFECTS/ADVERSE REACTIONS
SKIN: Acne, allergic contact dermatitis, atrophy, burning, dryness, folliculitis, hypertrichosis, hypopigmentation, irritation, itching, miliaria, perioral dermatitis, secondary infection, striae
MISC: Systemic absorption of topical corticosteroids has produced reversible HPA axis suppression (more likely with occlusive dressings, prolonged administration, application to large surface areas, liver failure, and in children)
SPECIAL CONSIDERATIONS
PATIENT/FAMILY EDUCATION
• Apply sparingly only to affected area
• Avoid contact with the eyes
• Do not put bandages or dressings over treated area unless directed by clinician
• Discontinue drug and notify clinician if local irritation or fever develops

---

* = non-FDA-approved use

• Do not use on weeping, denuded, or infected areas

---

desoximetasone
(des-ox-i-met´a-sone)
Rx: Topicort, Topicort LP
Chemical Class: Synthetic glucocorticoid
Therapeutic Class: Topical corticosteroid, intermediate potency (0.05% cream), high potency (0.05% gel, 0.25% cream, ointment)

CLINICAL PHARMACOLOGY
Mechanism of Action: Depresses formation, release, and activity of endogenous mediators of inflammation such as prostaglandins, kinins, histamine, liposomal enzymes, and the complement system resulting in decreased edema, erythema, and pruritus
Pharmacokinetics
Absorbed through the skin (increased by inflammation and occlusive dressings), metabolized primarily in the liver
INDICATIONS AND USES: Psoriasis, eczema, contact dermatitis, pruritus
DOSAGE
Adult and Child
• Top apply to affected area bid-tid, rub completely into skin
$ AVAILABLE FORMS/COST OF THERAPY
• Cre—Top: 0.05%, 15, 60 g: **$9.00-$21.68**/15 g; 0.25%, 15, 60, 120 g: **$11.90-$28.73**/15 g
• Gel—Top: 0.05%, 15, 60 g: **$18.44-$24.95**/15 g
• Oint—Top: 0.25%, 15, 60 g: **$15.41-$49.83**/15 g
CONTRAINDICATIONS: Fungal infections; use on face, groin, or axilla

PRECAUTIONS: Viral infections, bacterial infections, children
PREGNANCY AND LACTATION: Pregnancy category C; it is unknown whether topical application could result in sufficient systemic absorption to produce detectable amounts in breast milk (systemic corticosteroids are secreted into breast milk in quantities not likely to have any detrimental effects on infant)
SIDE EFFECTS/ADVERSE REACTIONS
HEME: Leukocytosis
METAB: Reduced glucose tolerance
SKIN: Acne, allergic contact dermatitis, atrophy, burning, dryness, folliculitis, hypertrichosis, hypopigmentation, irritation, itching, miliaria, perioral dermatitis, secondary infection, striae
MISC: Reversible HPA axis suppression (more likely with occlusive dressings, prolonged administration, application to large surface areas, liver failure, or use in children)
SPECIAL CONSIDERATIONS
• Potent, fluorinated topical corticosteroid with comparable efficacy to fluocinonide, diflorasone, amcinonide, betamethasone, dipropionate, and halcinonide; cost should govern use
PATIENT/FAMILY EDUCATION
• Apply sparingly only to affected area
• Avoid contact with the eyes
• Do not put bandages or dressings over treated area unless directed by clinician
• Discontinue drug, notify clinician if local irritation or fever develops
• Do not use on weeping, denuded, or infected areas

---

italic = common side effects   ***bold italic*** = life-threatening reactions

desoxyribonuclease
(des-oxy-ribe-o-new´clee-ase)
Rx: Elase
Combinations
　Rx: with chloramphenicol;
　　Elase-Chloromycetin
Chemical Class: Lytic enzyme
Therapeutic Class: Debriding
agent; irrigating agent

CLINICAL PHARMACOLOGY
Mechanism of Action: Purulent exudates consist largely of fibrinous material and nucleoprotein; desoxyribonuclease attacks the DNA and fibrinolysin attacks principally the fibrin of blood clots and fibrinous exudates

INDICATIONS AND USES: Top— Debriding agent in general surgical wounds, ulcerative lesions (trophic, decubitus, stasis, arteriosclerotic), 2nd and 3rd degree burns, circumcision, episiotomy; intravaginal— cervicitis (benign, postpartum, and postconization) and vaginitis; irrigating agent—infected wounds (abscesses, fistulae, and sinus tracts), otorhinolaryngologic wounds, superficial hematomas (except when the hematoma is adjacent to or within adipose tissue)

DOSAGE
Adult
• *General topical use:* Apply thin layer of ointment and cover with petrolatum gauze or other nonadherant dressing, change qd-tid; sol may be applied topically as a liquid, wet dressing, or spray by using a conventional atomizer
• *Wet dressing:* Mix 1 vial of powder with 10-50 ml saline and saturate strips of fine-mesh gauze or unfolded sterile gauze sponge with sol; pack ulcerated area with gauze, al-low to dry (approximately 6-8 hr), then remove dried gauze; repeat tid-qid
• *Intravaginal:* Apply 5 g of ointment deep into vagina qhs for 5 applications
• *Abscesses, empyema cavities, fistulae, sinus tracts, or SC hematomas:* Prepare sol by reconstituting contents of each vial of powder with 10 ml isotonic saline; drain and replace sol at 6-10 hr intervals

§ AVAILABLE FORMS/COST OF THERAPY
• Oint—Top: 10, 30 g: **$15.61-$23.99**/10 g
PRECAUTIONS: History of sensitivity to bovine material
SIDE EFFECTS/ADVERSE REACTIONS
SKIN: Local hyperemia

SPECIAL CONSIDERATIONS
• Successful enzymatic debridement depends on the following factors: surgical removal of any dense, dry eschar prior to administration; enzyme must be in constant contact with the substrate; periodic removal of accumulated necrotic debris; secondary closure or skin grafting as soon as possible after optimal debridement

PATIENT/FAMILY EDUCATION
• Frequency of application is more important than amount of ointment used
• Do not use sol more than 24 hr after reconstitution

dexamethasone

(dex-a-meth'a-sone)

Rx: Ophthalmic: Ak-Dex
Ophthalmic, Maxidex,
Ocumed Systemic:

Rx: Cortastat, Dalalone D.P.,
Decadron, Decaject,
Dexasone L.A., Dexone LA,
Solurex, Dalalone,
Dexasone, Dexone
Combinations

Rx: with neomycin, (Neo-
Decadron, Ak-Neo-Dex);
with neomycin and poly-
mixin B (Dexacidin,
Maxitrol, Dexasporin); with
tobramycin (Tobradex);
with lidocaine (Decadron
with Xylocaine)

Chemical Class: Synthetic glucocorticoid

Therapeutic Class: Systemic
corticosteroid; ophthalmic corticosteroid

CLINICAL PHARMACOLOGY

Mechanism of Action: Decreases
inflammation by depressing migration of polymorphonuclear leukocytes and activity of endogenous
mediators of inflammation. Has
many profound metabolic effects,
does not possess mineralocorticoid
activity

Pharmacokinetics

PO: Peak 1-2 hr

IM: Peak 8 hr

Metabolized in liver, excreted in
urine and bile; biologic $t_{1/2}$ 36-54 hr

INDICATIONS AND USES: *Ophthalmic:* Steroid-responsive inflammatory conditions of the palbebral
and bulbar conjunctiva, lid, cornea,
and anterior segment of the globe;
corneal injury

Systemic: Anti-inflammatory or immunosuppressant agent in the treatment of a variety of diseases of hematologic, allergic, inflammatory,
neoplastic, and autoimmune origin;
acute mountain sickness*; anti-
emetic*; bacterial meningitis (to decrease incidence of hearing loss)*;
diagnosis of depression*; hirsut-
ism*; prevention of neonatal respiratory distress syndrome (by administration to mother)*

DOSAGE

Adult

• *Anti-inflammatory:*   PO/IM/IV
0.75-9 mg/day in divided doses
q6-12h; IM 8-16 mg q1-3 wk (acetate)

• *Cerebral edema:* IV 10 mg loading
dose, then 4 mg IM/IV q6h

• *Shock:* IV 1-6 mg/kg or 40 mg
q2-6h (phosphate)

• *Prophylaxis during premature labor* (to prevent infant respiratory
distress due to immature lungs): 6
mg q12h × 4 doses

• *Intralesional:* 0.8-1.6 mg (acetate)

• *Intra-articular and soft tissue:*
4-16 mg q1-3 wk (acetate); large
joints 2-4 mg (phosphate); small
joints 0.8-1 mg (phosphate); bursae
2-3 mg (phosphate); tendon sheaths
0.4-1 mg (phosphate); soft tissue infiltration 2-6 mg (phosphate); ganglia 1-2 mg (phosphate)

• *Ophth:* Instill 1 gtt into conjunctival sac q1-4h depending on condition; apply ¼ in ribbon of oint to
lower conjunctival sac tid-qid; reduce frequency of administration
once a favorable response is obtained

Child 6-12 yr

• *Anti-inflammatory:*   PO/IM/IV
0.08-0.3 mg/kg/day or 2.5-10
mg/m²/day in divided doses q6-12h

• *Bacterial meningitis (>2 mo):* IV 0.6 mg/kg/day divided q6h for 1st 4 days of antibiotic treatment; initiate with 1st dose of antibiotic

• *Cerebral edema:* PO/IM/IV 1-2 mg/kg loading dose, then 1-1.5 mg/kg/day (max 16 mg/day) in divided doses q4-6h

• *Physiologic replacement:* PO/IM/IV 0.03-0.15 mg/kg/day or 0.6-0.75 mg/m²/day in divided doses q6-12h

• *Ophth:* Same as adult

🛢 AVAILABLE FORMS/COST OF THERAPY

• Elixir—Oral: 0.5 mg/5 ml, 60, 100, 120, 240 ml: **$6.50-$18.29**/100 ml

• Inj, Sol (phosphate): 24 mg/ml, 5 ml: **$117.21**

• Inj, Sol (phosphate)—IM, IV: 4 mg/ml, 5 ml: **$1.38-$29.54**; 10 mg/ml, 10 ml: **$4.94-$28.54**

• Inj, Susp—Intra-articular; IM (acetate): 8 mg/ml, 5 ml: **$3.79-$56.40**; 16 mg/ml, 5 ml: **$25.00**

• Oint—Ophth: 0.05%, 3.5 g: **$1.65-$7.25**

• Sol—Ophth: 0.1%, 5 ml: **$1.95-$19.45**

• Sol—Oral: 1 mg/ml, 30 ml: **$17.30**

• Susp—Ophth: 0.1%, 5, 15 ml: **$32.65**/5 ml

• Tab, Uncoated—Oral: 0.25 mg, 100's: **$4.05-$11.05**; 0.5 mg, 100's: **$6.15-$64.90**; 0.75 mg, 100's: **$2.05-$77.92**; 1 mg, 100's: **$28.90**; 1.5 mg, 100's: **$8.25-$76.00**; 2 mg, 100's: **$56.60-$59.00**; 4 mg, 100's: **$22.55-$214.00**; 6 mg, 100's: **$98.88-$193.80**

CONTRAINDICATIONS: Systemic fungal infections; (ophth): acute superficial herpes simplex keratitis and other viral diseases of the cornea and conjunctiva; fungal diseases of ocular structures; ocular TB; following uncomplicated removal of a superficial corneal foreign body

PRECAUTIONS: Psychosis, cerebral malaria, elderly, AIDS, latent tuberculosis or amebiasis (reactivation of disease), diabetes mellitus, glaucoma, osteoporosis, ulcerative colitis (intestinal perforation), CHF, myasthenia gravis, renal disease, esophagitis, peptic ulcer, hypertension; (ophth): infections of the eye, glaucoma

PREGNANCY AND LACTATION: Pregnancy category C; used in patients with premature labor at about 24-36 wk gestation to stimulate fetal lung maturation; excreted in breast milk, could suppress infant's growth and interfere with endogenous corticosteroid production

SIDE EFFECTS/ADVERSE REACTIONS

CNS: Depression, headache, *mood changes, seizures,* vertigo

*CV: **CHF**,* hypertension, tachycardia, ***thromboembolism,*** thrombophlebitis

EENT: Blurred vision, cataracts, *dryness,* epistaxis, increased intraocular pressure, localized infections of nose and pharynx with *C. albicans, nasal irritation,* nasal septum perforation, rebound congestion, sneezing, sore throat, *stinging* (nasal); cataracts, decreased acuity, glaucoma exacerbation, increased intraocular pressure, increased probability of corneal infection, optic nerve damage, poor corneal wound healing, stinging, transient burning (ophth)

GI: Abdominal distention, diarrhea, ***GI hemorrhage,*** increased appetite, *nausea, **pancreatitis***

GU: Hypercalciuria

METAB: Cushingoid state, decreased glucose tolerance, decreased T₄, growth suppression in children, *HPA suppression,* hyperglycemia

MS: Aseptic necrosis of femoral and humeral heads, fractures, myopathy, osteoporosis, weakness

SKIN: Acne, bruising, ecchymosis, petechiae, poor wound healing, striae, suppression of skin test reactions, thin fragile skin

INTERACTIONS
Drugs
■ *Aminoglutethamide:* Enhanced elimination of corticosteroids; marked reduction in corticosteroid response; increased clearance of dexamethasone; doubling of dose may be necessary

■ *Antidiabetics:* Increased blood glucose

■ *Barbiturates, carbamazepine:* Reduced serum concentrations of corticosteroids; increased clearance of dexamethasone

■ *Cholestyramine, colestipol:* Possible reduced absorption of corticosteroids

■ *Cyclosporine:* Possible increased concentration of both drugs, seizures

■ *Erythromycin, troleandomycin, clarithromycin, ketoconazole:* Possible enhanced steroid effect

■ *Estrogens, oral contraceptives:* Enhanced effects of corticosteroids

■ *Isoniazid:* Reduced plasma concentrations of isoniazid

■ *IUDs:* Inhibition of inflammation may decrease contraceptive effect

■ *NSAIDs:* Increased risk GI ulceration

■ *Rifampin:* Reduced therapeutic effect of corticosteroids; may reduce hepatic clearance of prednisone

■ *Salicylates:* Subtherapeutic salicylate concentrations possible

Labs
• *False negative:* Skin allergy tests

SPECIAL CONSIDERATIONS
• Signs of adrenal insufficiency include fatigue, anorexia, nausea, vomiting, diarrhea, weight loss, weakness, dizziness, and low blood sugar; drug induced secondary adrenocorticoid insufficiency and low blood sugar; drug-induced adrenocorticoid insufficiency may be minimized by gradual systemic dosage reduction; relative insufficiency may exist for up to 1 yr after discontinuation, therefore, be prepared to supplement in situations of stress
• May mask infections
• Do not give live virus vaccines to patients on prolonged therapy
• Patients on chronic steroid therapy should wear medical alert bracelet

MONITORING PARAMETERS
• Potassium and blood sugar during long-term therapy
• Observe growth and development of children on prolonged therapy
• Check lens and intraocular pressure frequently during prolonged use of ophthalmic preparations

---

dexchlorpheniramine
(dex´klor-fen-eer´a-meen)
Rx: Polaramine
Combinations
   Rx: with guaifenesin, pseudoephedrine (Polaramine Expectorant)
Chemical Class: Alkylamine derivative
Therapeutic Class: Antihistamine

CLINICAL PHARMACOLOGY
Mechanism of Action: Decreases allergic response by blocking histamine at H_1 receptors

---

Pharmacokinetics

PO: Onset 20-60 min, peak 3 hr, duration 8-12 hr; protein binding 60%-70%; detoxified in liver; excreted by kidneys (metabolites/free drug); $t_{1/2}$ 20-24 hr

INDICATIONS AND USES: Perennial and seasonal allergic rhinitis; vasomotor rhinitis, allergic conjunctivitis; allergic skin manifestations of urticaria and angioedema; dermatographism; adjunctive anaphylactic therapy

DOSAGE

Adult

• PO 2-6 mg q6h prn; Sus Action 4-6 mg bid prn

Child

• PO age 6-11 yr 1 mg q6h; age 2-5 yr 0.5 mg q6h

§ AVAILABLE FORMS/COST OF THERAPY

• Syr—Oral: 2 mg/5ml, 480 ml: **$13.15-$42.36**

• Tab, Uncoated—Oral: 2 mg, 100's: **$57.31**

• Tab, Sus Action—Oral: 4 mg, 100's: **$29.95-$82.97**; 6 mg, 100's: **$40.95-$115.96**

CONTRAINDICATIONS: Acute asthma attack, lower respiratory tract disease

PRECAUTIONS: History of bronchial asthma, increased intraocular pressure secondary to angle-closure glaucoma; hyperthyroidism, cardiovascular disease, hypertension due to atropine-like actions, elderly

PREGNANCY AND LACTATION: Pregnancy category B

SIDE EFFECTS/ADVERSE REACTIONS

CNS: Anxiety, confusion, *dizziness, drowsiness,* euphoria, fatigue, neuritis, paresthesia, poor coordination

EENT: Blurred vision, dilated pupils, dry nose, throat; tinnitus

GI: Anorexia, diarrhea, dry mouth, nausea

GU: Dysuria, frequency, *retention*

HEME: **Agranulocytosis, hemolytic anemia, thrombocytopenia**

RESP: Chest tightness, increased thick secretions, wheezing

SKIN: Photosensitivity

INTERACTIONS

Labs

• *False negative:* Skin allergy tests

SPECIAL CONSIDERATIONS

• Active dextro-isomer of chlorpheniramine

---

dextroamphetamine

(dex-troe-am-fet´a-meen)

Rx: Dexedrine, Dextrostat

Chemical Class: D-β-phenylisopropylamine

Therapeutic Class: CNS stimulant

DEA Class: Schedule II

CLINICAL PHARMACOLOGY

Mechanism of Action: Sympathomimetic amines with CNS stimulant activity; increases release of norepinephrine and dopamine in cerebral cortex and reticular activating system; promotes norepinephrine release from peripheral adrenergic nerve terminals; peripheral alpha and beta activity includes elevation of systolic and diastolic blood pressures and weak bronchodilator and respiratory stimulation action; heart rate reflexly slowed at standard doses, arrhythmias with overdose

Pharmacokinetics

PO: Onset 30 min, peak 1-3 hr, duration 4-20 hr; metabolized by liver, urine excretion pH dependent (greater excretion with acidic urine); crosses placenta; $t_{1/2}$ 10-30 hr

INDICATIONS AND USES: Narcolepsy, attention deficit disorder with hyperactivity, exogenous obesity*

---

* = non-FDA-approved use

D

DOSAGE
Adult
• *Narcolepsy:* PO 5-60 mg/day in divided doses
• *Obesity:* PO 10-15 mg qd (Sus Action) in AM or 5-30 mg/day in divided doses of 5-10 mg, administer 30-60 min ac
Child
• *Narcolepsy:* Age >12 yr PO 10 mg qd increasing by 10 mg qd at weekly intervals; age 6-12 yr PO 5 mg qd increasing by 5 mg/wk (max 60 mg qd)
• *Obesity:* Age >12 yr PO same as adult
• *Attention deficit disorder:* Age >6 yr PO 5 mg qd-bid increasing by 5 mg qd at weekly intervals; age 3-6 yr PO 2.5 mg qd increasing by 2.5 mg qd at weekly intervals (max dose 40 mg/day)
• Sus Action forms may be used for qd dosage

$ **AVAILABLE FORMS/COST OF THERAPY**
• Cap, Gel, Sus Action—Oral: 5 mg, 100's: **$87.75**; 10 mg, 100's: **$109.30**; 15 mg, 100's: **$139.78**
• Tab, Uncoated—Oral: 5 mg, 100's: **$23.96-$24.55**; 10 mg, 100's: **$45.98**

CONTRAINDICATIONS: Hyperthyroidism, hypertension, glaucoma, drug abuse, cardiovascular disease, anxiety, within 14 days of taking MAOIs
PRECAUTIONS: Tourette syndrome, child <3 yr; amphetamines have a high abuse potential
PREGNANCY AND LACTATION: Pregnancy category C; excreted in breast milk

SIDE EFFECTS/ADVERSE REACTIONS
CNS: **Addiction,** aggressiveness, chills, *dependence,* dizziness, dysphoria, headache, *hyperactivity, insomnia,* irritability, *restlessness,* stimulation, *talkativeness,* tremor
CV: Cardiomyopathy, decrease in heart rate, **dysrhythmias,** hypertension, *palpitations, tachycardia*
GI: Anorexia, constipation, diarrhea, dry mouth, metallic taste, weight loss
GU: Change in libido, impotence
SKIN: Urticaria

INTERACTIONS
Drugs
3 *Antacids:* Decreased urinary excretion of dextroamphetamine
3 *Furazolidone:* Hypertensive reactions
3 *Guanadrel, Guanethidine:* Antihypertensive effect inhibited by dextroamphetamine
⚠ *MAOIs:* Severe hypertensive reactions possible
❷ *Selegiline:* Severe hypertensive reactions possible
3 *Sodium bicarbonate:* May inhibit dextroamphetamine excretion
Labs
• *False positive:* Urine amino acids

SPECIAL CONSIDERATIONS
• Use for obesity should be reserved for patients failing to respond to alternative therapy; weigh the limited benefit against the substantial risk of addiction and dependence

PATIENT/FAMILY EDUCATION
• Tolerance or dependency is common
• Avoid OTC preparations unless approved by clinician
• Do not crush or chew Sus Action dosage forms

---

italic = common side effects   ***bold italic*** = life-threatening reactions

dextromethorphan

(dex-troe-meth-or′fan)

OTC: Benylin DM, Children's Hold, Delsym, Hold DM, Pertussin, Robitussin Cough Calmers, Robitussin Pediatric, Scott-Tussin DM Cough Chaser, Sucrets Cough Control, Suppress, Trocal, Vicks Formula 44 Combinations

    OTC: with benzocaine (Spec T, Vicks Formula 44 cough control discs, Vicks cough silencers); with guaifenesin (Robitussin DM)

Chemical Class: Levorphanol derivative

Therapeutic Class: Antitussive

CLINICAL PHARMACOLOGY
Mechanism of Action: Depresses cough center in medulla

Pharmacokinetics
PO: Onset 15-30 min, duration 3-6 hr

INDICATIONS AND USES: Nonproductive cough

DOSAGE
Adult
• PO 10-20 mg q4h or 30 mg q6-8h, not to exceed 120 mg/day
• PO Sus Action liq 60 mg bid, not to exceed 120 mg/day

Child
• PO: Age 6-12 yr 5-10 mg q4h, not to exceed 60 mg/day; age 2-6 yr 2.5-5 mg q4h, not to exceed 30 mg/day; Sus Action liq: Age 6-12 yr 30 mg bid, not to exceed 60 mg/day; age 2-5 yr 15 mg bid, not to exceed 30 mg/day

$ AVAILABLE FORMS/COST OF THERAPY
• Liq, Sus Action—Oral: 30 mg/5 ml, 90 ml: **$5.56-$6.62**

• Loz—Oral: 2.5 mg, 20's: **$1.92**; 5 mg, 16's: **$2.56**
• Syr—Oral: 3.5 mg/5 ml, 120 ml: **$2.76**; 7.5 mg/5 ml, 60 ml: **$2.26**; 15 mg/5 ml, 120 ml: **$2.51**

PRECAUTIONS: Chronic, persistent, or productive cough; nausea, vomiting; fever; persistent headache

PREGNANCY AND LACTATION: Pregnancy category C

SIDE EFFECTS/ADVERSE REACTIONS
CNS: Dizziness
GI: Nausea

INTERACTIONS
Drugs
▲ *Isocarboxazid, MAOIs, Phenelzine:* Increased risk of toxicity due to dextromethorphan

3 *Quinidine, terbinafine:* Reduced hepatic metabolism of dextromethorphan

3 *Fluoxetine:* Case report of a patient on fluoxetine developing visual hallucinations when she began to take dextromethorphan; causality not established

2 *Sibutramine:* Increased risk of serotonin syndrome

---

dezocine

(dez′o-seen)

Rx: Dalgan

Chemical Class: Synthetic opiate derivative—aminotetralin series

Therapeutic Class: Narcotic agonist-antagonist analgesic

CLINICAL PHARMACOLOGY
Mechanism of Action: Analgesia via μ subclass opiate receptor binding in CNS; μ receptors mediate morphine-like supraspinal analgesia, euphoria, and respiratory and

physical depression; narcotic antagonist activity is greater than pentazocime

Pharmacokinetics

IM: Onset 30 min, peak 50-90 min, duration 2-4 hr

IV: Onset 10 min, peak 30 min, duration 2-4 hr

Metabolized by liver, excreted by kidneys; may cross placenta

INDICATIONS AND USES: Severe pain

DOSAGE

NOTE: 10 mg parenteral dose equivalent to 10 mg morphine

Adult

• IM 5-20 mg q3-6h, not to exceed 120 mg/day; IV 2.5-10 mg q2-4h

$ **AVAILABLE FORMS/COST OF THERAPY**

• Inj, Sol—IM, IV: 5 mg/ml, 1 ml: **$8.54**; 10 mg/ml, 1 ml: **$9.58**; 15 mg/ml, 1 ml: **$8.40**

PRECAUTIONS: Patients physically dependent on narcotics (may precipitate withdrawal), addictive personality, increased intracranial pressure, respiratory depression, hepatic disease, renal disease, child <18 yr, elderly, biliary surgery, COPD, sulfite sensitivity

PREGNANCY AND LACTATION: Pregnancy category C

SIDE EFFECTS/ADVERSE REACTIONS

CNS: Anxiety, confusion, delirium, dependency, depression, dizziness, drowsiness, headache, sedation, sleep disturbances, slurred speech

CV: Chest pain, edema, hypertension, hypotension, pallor, pulse irregularity, thrombophlebitis

EENT: Blurred vision, diplopia

GI: Abdominal pain, anorexia, constipation, cramps, diarrhea, dry mouth, nausea, vomiting

GU: Urinary frequency, hesitancy, retention

RESP: Hiccups, ***respiratory depression***

SKIN: Chills, inj site reactions, pruritus, rash, sweating

---

diazepam

(dye-az'e-pam)

Rx: Diastat, Diastat-Pediatric, Valium, Valrelease

Chemical Class: Benzodiazepine

Therapeutic Class: Anxiolytic; sedative/hypnotic; anesthesia adjunct; skeletal muscle relaxant; anticonvulsant

DEA Class: Schedule IV

CLINICAL PHARMACOLOGY

Mechanism of Action: CNS depressants via facilitation of inhibitory GABA at benzodiazepine receptor sites (BZ_1—associated with sleep; BZ_2—associated with memory, motor, sensory, and cognitive function); effects include muscle relaxation (spinal cord), anticonvulsant activity (brain stem), ataxia (cerebellum), emotional behavior (limbic and cortical areas), and anxiolytic effects (separate from general CNS depression); other effects include sedative, appetite-stimulating, and weak analgesic actions

Pharmacokinetics

PO: Rapidly absorbed, onset 15-45 min, peak 0.5-1½ hr, duration 2-3 hr

IM: Absorption slow and erratic (deltoid muscle optimal site), onset 15-30 min, peak 0.5-1½ hr, duration 1-1½ hr

IV: Onset 1-3 min, duration 15 min

Metabolized by liver, excreted by kidneys, crosses the blood-brain barrier; $t_{1/2}$ 20-50 hr

PR: Onset 5-15 min, peak 1.5 hr

INDICATIONS AND USES: Anxiety, acute alcohol withdrawal, adjunctive anesthesia; amnesia in cardioversion, endoscopic procedures, etc.; conscious sedation, insomnia, status epilepticus, adjunct in seizure disorders; skeletal muscle spasm relaxation; epilepsy in patients taking stable drug regimens who require intermittent use of diazepam to control episodic increased seizure frequency (rectal viscous solution only); tremor,* tension headache,* panic disorder*

DOSAGE

Adult

• *Anxiety/convulsive disorders:* PO 2-10 mg tid-qid

• *Sedative-hypnotic, alcohol withdrawal:* PO 10 mg tid-qid, tapered prn

• *Skeletal muscle relaxant:* PO 2-10 mg tid-qid

• *Status epilepticus:* IV bolus 5-20 mg infused at a rate of 2 mg/min, may repeat q5-10 min, not to exceed 60 mg; may repeat in 30 min if seizures reappear

• *Adjunct for epilepsy:* PR 0.2 mg/kg prn

Geriatric

• 2-2.5 mg qd-bid, titrated prn

Child

• IV bolus 0.1-0.3 mg/kg (over 3 min); may repeat q15 min × 2 doses

• *Tetanic muscle spasms:* Infants >30 days to <5 yr IM/IV 1-2 mg to 5-10 mg q3-4h prn

• *Anxiety/convulsive disorders:* >6 mo PO 1-2.5 mg tid-qid (0.04-0.2 mg/kg tid-qid prn)

• *Adjunct for epilepsy:* PR: age 2-5 yr 0.5 mg/kg prn; age 6-11 yr 0.3 mg/kg prn; age ≥ 12 yr 0.2 mg/kg prn

$ AVAILABLE FORMS/COST OF THERAPY

• Inj, Sol—IM, IV: 5 mg/ml, 2 ml: **$0.63-$7.63**

• Sol—Oral: 5 mg/ml, 30 ml: **$23.52**

• Sol, viscous—Rectal: 5 mg/ml, 2.5, 5, 10, 15, 20 mg, 2's: **$159.90** (with rectal delivery system)

• Tab—Uncoated—Oral: 2 mg, 100's: **$3.00-$65.51**; 5 mg, 100's: **$3.38-$101.90**; 10 mg, 100's: **$3.75-$171.55**

CONTRAINDICATIONS: Narrow-angle glaucoma, psychosis

PRECAUTIONS: Elderly, debilitated, hepatic disease, renal disease, children, low serum albumin

PREGNANCY AND LACTATION: Pregnancy category D; drug and metabolite enter breast milk; lethargy and loss of weight in nursing infant have been reported

SIDE EFFECTS/ADVERSE REACTIONS

CNS: Anxiety, confusion, depression, *dizziness, drowsiness,* fatigue, hallucinations, headache, insomnia, stimulation, tremors, withdrawal syndrome

CV: ECG changes, hypotension; *orthostatic hypotension,* tachycardia, venous thrombosis, phlebitis, local irritation, swelling, and vascular impairment following IV inj into small veins on hand

EENT: Blurred vision, mydriasis, tinnitus

GI: Anorexia, constipation, diarrhea, dry mouth, increased ALT/AST, nausea, vomiting

RESP: **Respiratory depression**

SKIN: Dermatitis, itching, rash

INTERACTIONS

Drugs

🔢 *Carbamazepine:* Markedly reduces effect of oral diazepam; parenteral diazepam less affected

🔢 *Cimetidine:* Inhibits hepatic metabolism of diazepam

🔢 *Ciprofloxacin:* Inhibits hepatic metabolism of diazepam; may also competitively inhibit gamma amino butyric acid receptors

* = non-FDA-approved use

❷ *Clarithromycin:* Inhibits hepatic metabolism of diazepam

3 *Clozapine:* Additive respiratory and cardiovascular depression

3 *Delavirdine:* Inhibits hepatic metabolism of diazepam

3 *Disulfiram:* Inhibits hepatic metabolism of diazepam

3 *Erythromycin:* Inhibits hepatic metabolism of diazepam

3 *Ethanol:* Additive CNS effects

3 *Fluconazole:* Inhibits hepatic metabolism of diazepam

3 *Fluoxetine:* Inhibits hepatic metabolism of diazepam

3 *Fluvoxamine:* Inhibits hepatic metabolism of diazepam

3 *Isoniazid:* Inhibits hepatic metabolism of diazepam

3 *Itraconazole:* Inhibits hepatic metabolism of diazepam

3 *Ketoconazole:* Inhibits hepatic metabolism of diazepam

3 *Levodopa:* May reduce anti-Parkinsonian effect

3 *Metoprolol:* Inhibits hepatic metabolism of diazepam

3 *Omeprazole:* Inhibits hepatic metabolism of diazepam

3 *Phenytoin:* Markedly reduces effect of oral diazepam; parenteral diazepam less affected

3 *Quinolones:* Inhibits hepatic metabolism of diazepam; may also competitively inhibit gamma amino butyric acid receptors

3 *Rifampin:* Markedly reduces effect of diazepam

3 *Troleandomycin:* Inhibits hepatic metabolism of diazepam

Labs
• *Increase:* Urine 5-HIAA

SPECIAL CONSIDERATIONS
• Flumazenil (Mazicon), a benzodiazepine receptor antagonist is indicated for complete or partial reversal of the sedative effects of benzodiazepines

PATIENT/FAMILY EDUCATION
• Avoid driving, activities that require alertness; drowsiness may occur
• Avoid alcohol, other psychotropic medications unless prescribed by clinician

---

diazoxide
(dye-az-ox′ide)
Rx: Hyperstat (IV), Proglycem (PO)
Chemical Class: Benzothiadiazine derivative
Therapeutic Class: Antihypertensive; antihypoglycemic

CLINICAL PHARMACOLOGY
Mechanism of Action: Vasodilates arteriolar smooth muscle by direct relaxation; reduction in blood pressure with concomitant increases in heart rate, cardiac output; decreases release of insulin from β-cells in pancreas, resulting in an increase in blood glucose

Pharmacokinetics
PO: Onset 1 hr, duration 8 hr
IV: Onset 1-2 min, peak 5 min, duration 3-12 hr
$t_{1/2}$ 20-36 hr; excreted slowly in urine; crosses blood-brain barrier, placenta

INDICATIONS AND USES: Hypertensive crisis when urgent decrease of diastolic pressure required; increase blood glucose levels in hyperinsulinism

DOSAGE
Adult
• *Hypertension:* IV bolus 1-3 mg/kg rapidly up to a max of 150 mg in a single inj; dose may be repeated at 5-15 min intervals until desired response is achieved; give IV in 30 sec or less

---

italic = common side effects   ***bold italic*** = life-threatening reactions

• *Hypoglycemia:* PO initial 1 mg/kg q8h, adjusted prn according to response; maintenance 3-8 mg/kg/day given bid-tid (max 15 mg/kg/day)

Child

• *Hypertension:* IV bolus 1-2 mg/kg rapidly; administration same as adult; not to exceed 150 mg

• *Hypoglycemia:* PO initial 3.3 mg/kg q8h, adjusted prn; maintenance 8-15 mg/kg/day given bid-tid

$ AVAILABLE FORMS/COST OF THERAPY

• Cap—Oral: 50 mg, 100's: **$160.09**
• Inj, Sol—IV: 15 mg/ml, 20 ml: **$134.81**
• Susp—Oral: 50 mg/ml, 30 ml: **$154.70**

CONTRAINDICATIONS: Hypersensitivity to thiazides, sulfonamides; hypertension associated with aortic coarctation or AV shunt; pheochromocytoma; dissecting aortic aneurysm; functional hypoglycemia

PRECAUTIONS: Tachycardia; fluid, electrolyte imbalances; lactation; impaired cerebral or cardiac circulation; gout; diabetes mellitus

PREGNANCY AND LACTATION: Pregnancy category C

SIDE EFFECTS/ADVERSE REACTIONS

CNS: Anxiety, blurred vision, confusion, dizziness, EPS, euphoria, headache, insomnia, malaise, paresthesia, sleepiness, TIAs, weakness

CV: Angina pectoris, edema, hypotension, palpitations, rebound hypertension, ***supraventricular tachycardia,*** T-wave changes

EENT: Cataracts, diplopia, lacrimation, ring scotoma, subconjunctival hemorrhage, tinnitus

GI: Changes in ability to taste, dry mouth, nausea, vomiting

GU: Decreased urinary output, hematuria, increased BUN, reversible nephrotic syndrome

HEME: Decreased hemoglobin/hematocrit, ***thrombocytopenia***

METAB: Hyperglycemia, hyperuricemia

SKIN: Hypertrichosis, rash

MISC: Breast tenderness, allergic reactions

INTERACTIONS

Drugs

3 *Carboplatin, cisplatin:* Increased risk of nephrotoxicity

3 *Hydralazine:* Severe hypotensive reactions

3 *Phenytoin:* Decreased phenytoin levels in children, probably due to enhanced metabolism

3 *Thiazide diuretics:* Hyperglycemia

SPECIAL CONSIDERATIONS

• Often administered concurrently with a diuretic to prevent congestive heart failure due to fluid retention

• Oral susp dosage form produces higher concentration than cap form

• Hyperglycemia transient (24-48 hr) after IV administration

• If not effective within 2-3 wk of treatment of hypoglycemia, reevaluate

---

dibucaine

(dye'byoo-kane)

OTC: Nupercainal

Chemical Class: Amide derivative

Therapeutic Class: Topical anesthetic

CLINICAL PHARMACOLOGY

Mechanism of Action: Inhibits nerve impulses from sensory nerves

Pharmacokinetics

TOP: Onset up to 15 min, duration 3-4 hr, readily systemically absorbed through traumatized or

abraded skin; hepatic and some renal biotransformation; renally excreted as metabolites

INDICATIONS AND USES: Pruritus, pain, sunburn, toothache, rectal pain and irritation, dermatitis (e.g., poison ivy), minor wounds

DOSAGE

Adult and Child

• TOP apply qid as needed

$ AVAILABLE FORMS/COST OF THERAPY

• Cre—Top: 0.5%, 45 g: **$3.24**
• Oint—Top: 1%, 30, 60 g: **$1.05-$4.49**/30 g

CONTRAINDICATIONS: Infants <1 yr, application to large areas

PRECAUTIONS: Child <6 yr, sepsis, denuded skin

PREGNANCY AND LACTATION: Pregnancy category C; excretion into breast milk unknown

SIDE EFFECTS/ADVERSE REACTIONS

SKIN: Irritation, rash, sensitization

SPECIAL CONSIDERATIONS

• Cross-sensitivity between amide derivatives and ester anesthetics or pramoxine has not been reported

---

dichlorphenamide

(die-klor-fen′a-mide)

Rx: Daranide

Chemical Class: Sulfonamide derivative

Therapeutic Class: Antiglaucoma agent

CLINICAL PHARMACOLOGY

Mechanism of Action: Carbonic anhydrase inhibition reduces rate of aqueous humor formation, decreasing intraocular pressure; inhibits hydrogen ion secretion in renal tubule with increased secretion of sodium, potassium, bicarbonate, water

Pharmacokinetics

PO: Onset 1 hr, peak effect 2-4 hr, duration 6-12 hr

INDICATIONS AND USES: Glaucoma, open-angle and angle-closure

DOSAGE

Adult

• PO 100-200 mg initially, then 100 mg q12h to response; maintenance 25-50 mg qd-tid

$ AVAILABLE FORMS/COST OF THERAPY

• Tab, Uncoated—Oral: 50 mg, 100's: **$63.69**

CONTRAINDICATIONS: Hepatic insufficiency, renal failure, adrenocortical insufficiency, hyperchloremic acidosis, hypokalemia, hyponatremia, impaired alveolar ventilation (pulmonary disease, edema, infection, or obstruction)

PRECAUTIONS: Hypokalemia when cirrhosis is present or during concomitant use of steroids or ACTH; respiratory acidosis

PREGNANCY AND LACTATION: Pregnancy category C; safety in lactation not established

SIDE EFFECTS/ADVERSE REACTIONS

CNS: Ataxia, confusion, depression, disorientation, dizziness, drowsiness, *fatigue,* headache, lassitude, *malaise,* nervousness, *paresthesias of the extremities,* **seizures,** tremor, *weakness*

EENT: Myopia, tinnitus

GI: Anorexia, constipation, *diarrhea,* hepatic insufficiency, melena, *nausea, taste alteration, vomiting*

GU: Decreased libido, glycosuria, hematuria, impotence, phosphaturia, renal calculi, renal colic, *urinary frequency*

HEME: **Blood dyscrasias**

METAB: Hyperglycemia, *hypokalemia*

MS: Flaccid paralysis

---

italic = common side effects   ***bold italic*** = life-threatening reactions

RESP: Acidosis (shortness of breath, troubled breathing)

SKIN: Photosensitivity, pruritus, rash, ***Stevens-Johnson syndrome,*** skin eruptions, urticaria

MISC: Fever, hypersensitivity, weight loss

INTERACTIONS

Drugs

🔳 *Flecainide:* Increased serum flecainide levels

🔳 *Methenamine compounds:* Alkalinization of urine decreases antibacterial effects

🔳 *Mexiletine:* Increased serum mexiletine levels

🔳 *Phenytoin:* Increased risk of osteomalacia

🔳 *Primadone:* Case reports suggest decreased serum primadone levels with a similar drug

🔳 *Quinidine:* Alkalinization of urine increases quinidine serum levels

❷ *Salicylates:* Increased serum levels of carbonic anhydrase inhibitors, CNS toxicity

SPECIAL CONSIDERATIONS

• Usually most successful when given in combination with miotics (e.g., pilocarpine)

• If quick relief of angle-closure glaucoma does not occur, surgery may be mandatory

PATIENT/FAMILY EDUCATION

• May cause drowsiness

---

diclofenac

(dye-kloe′fen-ak)

Rx: Potassium: Cataflam

Sodium: Voltaren, Voltaren XR, Solarze

Combinations

  Rx: with misoprostol (Arthotec)

Chemical Class: Phenylacetic acid derivative

Therapeutic Class: NSAID with analgesic and antipyretic activity

CLINICAL PHARMACOLOGY

Mechanism of Action: Reversible cyclooxygenase (i.e., prostaglandin synthetase) inhibitor; nonselectively decreases the formation of both prostaglandins and thromboxone A_2; variable effects on lipoxygenase synthesis and subsequent leukotriene production; antiinflammatory, antipyretic, and analgesic activity; inhibits platelet aggregation

Pharmacokinetics

PO: Time to peak, sodium salt 2-3 hr, potassium salt 30 min; $t_{1/2}$ 2 hr, synovial $t_{1/2}$ 3 × longer

Completely absorbed (oral), 99.7% bound to plasma proteins; metabolized in liver, 50% bioavailable after 1st pass, excreted in urine and bile

OPHTH: Limited systemic absorption

INDICATIONS AND USES: Actinic keratosis (topically), ankylosing spondylitis, biliary colic,* cataract removal—inflammation (ophth), cataract removal—mydriasis* (ophth), prevention of cognitive decline,* prevention of colon cancer,* corneal abrasion,* dysmenorrhea, erythermalgia,* fever,* gouty arthritis,* headache,* keratitis,* myalgia,* osteoarthritis, pain—mild to moderate

---

DOSAGE

Adult

• *Osteoarthritis:* PO 100-150 mg/day in divided doses (50 mg bid-tid or 75 mg bid), Sus Action TAB 100 mg qd

• *Rheumatoid arthritis:* PO 100-200 mg/day in divided doses (50 mg tid-qid or 75 mg bid), Sus Action TAB 100 mg qd may increase to bid if benefits >risks

• *Ankylosing spondylitis:* PO 100-125 mg/day; give 25 mg qid and 25 mg hs if needed

• *Pain, dysmenorrhea:* PO 50 mg immediate-release tid; loading dose (100 mg) useful in some patients

• *Postoperative/cataracts:* Ophth 1 gtt qid, starting 24 hr after surgery for 2 wk

• *Actinic keratoses:* Gel apply to lesion areas bid, 0.5 g gel for each 5 cm × 5 cm lesion site, duration 60-90 days

💲 AVAILABLE FORMS/COST OF THERAPY

Diclofenac Sodium

• Sol—Ophth: 0.1%, 5 ml: **$34.38-$49.81**

• Tab, Sus Action—Oral: 100 mg, 100's: **$281.24-$375.45**

• Tab, Enteric Coated—Oral: 25 mg, 100's: **$44.30-$79.53**; 50 mg, 100's: **$86.13-$154.49**; 75 mg, 100's: **$104.31-$187.09**

• Gel—Topical: 3%, 25, 50 g: **$93.75**/50 g

Diclofenac Potassium

• Tab, Uncoated—Oral: 50 mg, 100's: **$155.19-$230.38**

CONTRAINDICATIONS: Bronchospasm, nasal polyps, angioedema precipitated by aspirin or other NSAIDs

PRECAUTIONS: History of GI ulceration, bleeding, or perforation; renal dysfunction, hypertension or cardiac conditions aggravated by fluid retention and edema, history of liver dysfunction, history of coagulation

PREGNANCY AND LACTATION: Pregnancy category B; excreted in breast milk

SIDE EFFECTS/ADVERSE REACTIONS

CNS: Anxiety, confusion, depression, dizziness, drowsiness, fatigue, insomnia, muscle weakness, nervousness, paresthesia, tremors

CV: **CHF, dysrhythmias,** fluid retention, hypertension, hypotension, palpitations, peripheral edema, tachycardia

EENT: Blurred vision; hearing loss, tinnitus; Ophth: anterior chamber reaction, burning, elevated intraocular pressure, irritation, keratitis, ocular allergy

GI: Anorexia, cholestatic hepatitis, constipation, cramps, diarrhea, dry mouth, flatulence, **GI bleeding,** jaundice, *nausea,* peptic ulcer, *vomiting*

GU: Azotemia, cystitis, dysuria, hematuria, **nephrotoxicity,** oliguria, UTI

HEME: **Blood dyscrasias,** bruising, epistaxis

RESP: **Bronchospasm,** dyspnea, hemoptysis, **laryngeal edema,** pharyngitis, rhinitis, shortness of breath

SKIN: Alopecia, erythema, petechiae, photosensitivity, pruritus, purpura, rash, sweating

INTERACTIONS

Drugs

3 *Aminoglycosides:* Reduced clearance with elevated aminoglycoside levels and potential for toxicity (especially indomethacin in premature infants; other NSAIDs probably)

3 *Anticoagulants:* Excessive hypoprothrombinemia, decreased platelet aggregation with increased risk of GI bleeding

---

italic = common side effects   ***bold italic*** = life-threatening reactions

❸ *Antihypertensives (alpha blockers, angiotension-converting enzyme inhibitors, angiotensin II receptor blockers, beta blockers, diuretics):* Inhibition of antihypertensive and other favorable hemodynamic effects

❸ *Corticosteroids:* Increased risk of GI ulceration

❸ *Cyclosporine:* Increased nephrotoxicity risk

❸ *Digoxin:* Increased serum digoxin concentrations

❸ *Lithium:* Decreased clearance of lithium (mediated via prostaglandins) resulting in elevated serum lithium levels and risk of toxicity

❷ *Methotrexate:* Decreased renal secretion of methotrexate resulting in elevated methotrexate levels and risk of toxicity

❸ *Phenylpropanolamine:* Possible acute hypertensive reaction

❸ *Potassium-sparing diuretics:* Additive hyperkalemia potential

❷ *Triamterene:* Acute renal failure reported with addition of indomethacin; caution with other NSAIDs

Labs
• *Increase:* Serum AST, plasma cortisol, plasma glucose (oxidase-peroxidase method)

SPECIAL CONSIDERATIONS
• No significant advantage over other NSAIDs; cost should govern use

MONITORING PARAMETERS
• Initial hemogram and fecal occult blood test within 3 mo of starting regular chronic therapy; repeat every 6-12 mo (more frequently in high-risk patients (>65 years, peptic ulcer disease, concurrent steroids or anticoagulants); electrolytes, creatinine, and BUN within 3 mo of starting regular chronic therapy; repeat every 6-12 mo

• Complete healing of actinic keratoses may not be evident for up to 30 days post cessation of therapy

---

dicloxacillin
(dye-klox′a-sill-in)
Rx: Dycill, Dynapen
Chemical Class: Penicillin derivative (penicillinase-resistant)
Therapeutic Class: Antibiotic

CLINICAL PHARMACOLOGY
Mechanism of Action: Inhibits bacterial wall synthesis, bactericidal
Pharmacokinetics
PO: Peak 1 hr, duration 4-6 hr, $t_{1/2}$ 30-60 min; absorption stable to acid; concurrent food decreases absorption; 98% plasma protein bound; excreted unchanged in urine

INDICATIONS AND USES: Infections of the bone and localized skin and skin structure caused by susceptible organisms

Antibacterial spectrum usually includes:
• Gram-positive organisms: *Staphylococcus aureus, Streptococcus pyogenes, S. viridans, S. faecalis, S. bovis, S. pneumoniae,* including those producing penicillinase

DOSAGE
Adult
• PO 125-500 mg q6h
Child
• PO 12.5-25 mg/kg in divided doses q6h, max 4 g/day

§   AVAILABLE FORMS/COST OF THERAPY
• Cap, Gel—Oral: 250 mg, 100's: **$33.98-$93.95**; 500 mg, 100's: **$59.43-$179.00**
• Powder, Reconst—Oral: 62.5 mg/5 ml, 100, 200 ml: **$16.69/200 ml**

PRECAUTIONS: Hypersensitivity to cephalosporins; asthma, eczema, mononucleosis (rash)

PREGNANCY AND LACTATION: Pregnancy category B; penicillins are excreted into breast milk in low concentrations; compatible with breast feeding

SIDE EFFECTS/ADVERSE REACTIONS

CNS: Anxiety, coma, depression, hallucinations, lethargy, *seizures,* twitching

GI: Abdominal pain, colitis, *diarrhea,* glossitis, increased AST, ALT; *nausea,* **pseudomembranous colitis,** *vomiting*

GU: Glomerulonephritis, hematuria, *moniliasis,* oliguria, proteinuria, *vaginitis*

HEME: **Bone marrow depression,** increased bleeding time

INTERACTIONS

Drugs

3 *Macrolide antibiotics, chloramphenicol, tetracyclines:* Possible inhibition of antibacterial activity of penicillins

3 *Methotrexate:* Potentiation of methotrexate toxicity

3 *Oral contraceptives:* Possible impaired contraceptive efficacy

3 *Warfarin:* Reduced hypoprothrombinemic response

Labs

• *False increase:* Nafcillin level

SPECIAL CONSIDERATIONS
PATIENT/FAMILY EDUCATION

• Should be taken with water 1 hr before or 2 hr after meals on an empty stomach

---

dicumarol

(die-coom′er-all)
Rx: Dicumarol
Chemical Class: Coumarin derivative
Therapeutic Class: Oral anticoagulant

CLINICAL PHARMACOLOGY
Mechanism of Action: Interferes with hepatic synthesis of vitamin K-dependent clotting factors, causing depression in the activity of factors II, VII, IX, X and proteins C and S in a dose-dependent manner; has no direct effect on established thrombus, but prevents further extension of formed clot

Pharmacokinetics
PO: Onset of action 1-5 days; duration of action 2-10 days; slow and incomplete absorption; >99% plasma protein bound, metabolized by hepatic microsomal enzymes; excreted as inactive metabolites in the urine and feces; t½ 1-4 days

INDICATIONS AND USES: Prophylaxis and treatment of deep venous thrombosis and pulmonary thromboembolism; prophylaxis of embolism associated with atrial fibrillation, MI, cardioversion of chronic atrial fibrillation, prosthetic heart valves*; cerebral embolism*

DOSAGE
Adult
• PO 25-200 mg/d, as indicated by INR determinations

$ AVAILABLE FORMS/COST OF THERAPY
• Tab, Uncoated—Oral: 25 mg, 100's: **$12.78**

CONTRAINDICATIONS: Pregnancy; hemorrhagic tendencies; recent or contemplated surgery of the eye or CNS, or surgery resulting in large, open surfaces; bleeding from

---

the GI, respiratory, or GU tract; threatened abortion; aneurysm; ascorbic acid deficiency; polyarthritis; severe uncontrolled or malignant hypertension; severe renal or hepatic disease; pericarditis and pericardial effusion; subacute bacterial endocarditis; visceral carcinoma; following procedures with potential for uncontrollable bleeding; history of warfarin-induced skin necrosis; uncooperative patient

PRECAUTIONS: Trauma, infection, renal insufficiency, hypertension, vasculitis, indwelling catheters, severe diabetes, active tuberculosis, postpartum, protein C deficiency, hepatic insufficiency, elderly, children, hyperthyroidism, hypothyroidism, CHF, polyarteritis, deverticulitis, antibiotic therapy, malnutrition

PREGNANCY AND LACTATION: Pregnancy category D; no adverse effect or any change in PT have been noted in nursing infants; compatible with breast feeding for normal full-term infants

SIDE EFFECTS/ADVERSE REACTIONS

CV: Systemic cholesterol microembolization (purple toe syndrome)

GI: Diarrhea, intestinal obstruction from submucosal or intramural hemorrhage, mouth ulcers, nausea, paralytic ileus, sore mouth

GU: Red-orange urine

*HEME: **Hemorrhage***

METAB: Adrenal insufficiency, pyrexia

SKIN: Alopecia, dermatitis, ***exfoliative dermatitis, skin necrosis,*** urticaria

INTERACTIONS

• Drug interactions involving dicumarol similar to those involving warfarin; refer to warfarin drug interaction section

SPECIAL CONSIDERATIONS

• Warfarin is the coumarin anticoagulant of choice

MONITORING PARAMETERS

• Dosage of anticoagulants must be individualized and adjusted according to INR determinations; it is recommended that INR determinations be performed prior to initiation of therapy, at 24-hr intervals while maintenance dosage is being established, then once or twice weekly for the following 3-4 wks, then at 1-4 wk intervals for the duration of treatment

• Maintain INR at 2-3 (2.5-3.5 for mechanical valves, recurrent systemic thromboembolism)

---

dicyclomine
(dye-sye′kloe-meen)
Rx: Bentyl, Dicyclocot
Chemical Class: Synthetic tertiary amine
Therapeutic Class: Gastrointestinal antispasmodic; anticholinergic

---

CLINICAL PHARMACOLOGY

Mechanism of Action: Inhibits muscarinic actions of acetylcholine at postganglionic parasympathetic neuroeffector sites

Pharmacokinetics

PO: Onset 1-2 hr, duration 3-4 hr; metabolized by liver; $t_{1/2}$ 9-10 hr; excreted in urine

INDICATIONS AND USES: Functional bowel/irritable bowel syndrome; adjunctive treatment of peptic ulcer disease,* infant colic*

DOSAGE

Adult

• PO 10-40 mg tid-qid prn; IM 20 mg q4-6h prn

Child >2 yr

• PO 10 mg tid-qid prn

---

* = non-FDA-approved use

Child 6 mo-2 yr
- PO 5 mg tid-qid prn

🅂 **AVAILABLE FORMS/COST OF THERAPY**
- Cap, Gel—Oral: 10 mg, 100's: **$1.60-$33.99**
- Inj, Sol—IM: 10 mg/ml, 2 ml: **$3.20-$17.43**
- Syr—Oral: 10 mg/5 ml, 480 ml: **$37.76**
- Tab, Uncoated—Oral: 20 mg, 100's: **$1.60-$48.50**

CONTRAINDICATIONS: Narrow-angle glaucoma, GI obstruction, myasthenia gravis, paralytic ileus, GI atony, toxic megacolon

PRECAUTIONS: Hyperthyroidism, coronary artery disease, dysrhythmias, CHF, ulcerative colitis, hypertension, hiatal hernia, hepatic disease, renal disease, urinary retention, prostatic hypertrophy, small children, Down Syndrome

PREGNANCY AND LACTATION: Pregnancy category B; single case report of apnea in nursing infant; avoid in nursing women

SIDE EFFECTS/ADVERSE REACTIONS

CNS: Anxiety, *coma* (child <3 mo), *confusion,* dizziness, drowsiness, hallucination; headache, insomnia, *seizures, stimulation in elderly,* weakness

CV: Palpitations, tachycardia

EENT: Blurred vision, cycloplegia, increased ocular tension, mydriasis, photophobia

GI: Absence of taste, *constipation, dry mouth,* dysphagia, heartburn, nausea, paralytic ileus, vomiting

GU: Hesitancy, impotence, *retention*

SKIN: Allergic reactions, anhidrosis, fever, pruritus, rash, urticaria

INTERACTIONS

Drugs

🔋 *Amantadine, Tricyclic antidepressants, MAOIs, H₁-antihistamines:* Increased anticholinergic effects

🔋 *Phenothiazines, Levodopa, Ketoconazole:* Decreased therapeutic effects

SPECIAL CONSIDERATIONS
- Not for intravenous use

---

didanosine (ddI)

(dye-dan′o-seen)

Rx: Videx, Videx EC
Chemical Class: Nucleoside analog
Therapeutic Class: Antiretroviral

CLINICAL PHARMACOLOGY

Mechanism of Action: Nucleoside analog, incorporates into viral DNA, leading to chain termination; interferes with viral replication by inhibiting reverse transcriptase

Pharmacokinetics

PO: Peak 0.5-1 hr, 2 hr (enteric coated); $t_{1/2}$ 1.6 hr; acid labile (administration with meal decreases peak concentrations and AUC); bioavailability variable, average 30%; extensive metabolism; renal elimination accounts for 50%; no accumulation reported

INDICATIONS AND USES: HIV infections in adults and children

DOSAGE

Adult

- PO ≥60 kg, 200 mg bid or 400 mg qd; 250 mg buffered powder bid; 400 mg qd delayed-release capsules; <60 kg, 125 mg bid or 250 mg qd; 167 mg buffered powder bid; 250 mg qd delayed-release capsules; 2 tab of appropriate strength

---

italic = common side effects   ***bold italic*** = life-threatening reactions

should be taken at each dose for adequate buffering to prevent gastric degradation

• For latest treatment guidelines see www.hivatis.org

• *Renal impairment:*

• CrCl 30-59 ml/min: ≥60 kg, PO 100 mg bid or 200 mg qd; 100 mg bid buffered powder; 200 mg qd Sus Action cap; <60 kg, PO 75 mg bid or 150 mg qd; 100 mg bid buffered powder; 125 mg qd Sus Action cap

• CrCl 10-29 ml/min: ≥60 kg, PO 150 mg qd; 167 mg qd buffered powder; 125 mg qd Sus Action cap; <60 kg, PO 100 mg qd; 100 mg qd buffered powder; 125 mg qd Sus Action cap

• CrCl <10 ml/min: ≥60 kg, PO 100 mg qd; 100 mg qd buffered powder; 125 mg qd Sus Action cap; <60 kg, PO 75 mg qd; 100 mg qd buffered powder; Sus Action cap not suitable for patients <60 kg and CrCl <10 ml/min

Child

• PO 1.1-1.4 m^2, 100 mg tab bid, or 125 mg pedi powder bid; 0.8-1 m^2, 75 mg tab bid, or 94 mg pedi powder bid; 0.5-0.7 m^2, 50 mg tab bid, or 62 mg pedi powder bid; <0.4 m^2, 25 mg tab bid, or 31 mg pedi powder bid

• For latest treatment guidelines see www.hivatis.org

💲 AVAILABLE FORMS/COST OF THERAPY

• Cap, Sus Action—Oral: 125 mg, 30's: **$92.91**; 200 mg, 30's: **$148.65**; 250 mg, 30's: **$185.81**; 400 mg, 30's: **$297.30**

• Packet—Oral: 100 mg, 30's: **$65.57**; 167 mg, 30's: **$105.58**; 250 mg, 30's: **$163.95**

• Sol—Oral: 20 mg/ml, 100 ml: **$38.13**; 40 mg/ml, 100 ml: **$83.25**

• Tab, Chewable—Oral: 25 mg, 60's: **$28.32**; 50 mg, 30's: **$63.23**; 100 mg, 60's: **$82.50-$131.15**; 150 mg, 60's: **$132.97-$196.75**; 200 mg, 60's: **$247.69**

PRECAUTIONS: Renal, hepatic disease, children, sodium-restricted diets, elevated amylase, hyperuricemia, pre-existing peripheral neuropathy, history of pancreatitis (risk of recurrence 30%; consider stopping ddI permanently for patients with ddI-induced pancreatitis), alcohol consumption; morbid obesity, hypertriglyceridemia, cholelithiasis, phenylketonuria (chewable tablets contain phenylalanine)

PREGNANCY AND LACTATION: Pregnancy category B; unknown if excreted in breast milk; discontinuation of breast feeding recommended

SIDE EFFECTS/ADVERSE REACTIONS

CNS: Abnormal thinking, anxiety, asthenia, chills, CNS depression, confusion, dizziness, fever, hypertonia, insomnia, pain, *peripheral neuropathy (34%)*, **seizures**

CV: **CHF, dysrhythmia,** hypertension, palpitation, syncope, vasodilation

EENT: Ear pain, epistaxis, optic neuritis, otitis, photophobia, retinal depigmentation, visual impairment

GI: Abdominal pain, constipation, *diarrhea (34%),* dry mouth, dyspepsia, flatulence, **hepatic failure (rare),** melena, nausea, oral thrush, **pancreatitis (7%),** stomatitis, taste perversion, vomiting

GU: Hyperuricemia

HEME: **Anemia, granulocytopenia, leukopenia, thrombocytopenia**

METAB: Lactic acidosis

MS: Arthritis, muscular atrophy, myalgia, myopathy

RESP: **Bronchospasm,** cough, dyspnea, hypoventilation, pneumonia, sinusitis

SKIN: Alopecia, ecchymosis, hemorrhage, petechiae, pruritus, rash, sweating

INTERACTIONS
Drugs

▲ *Allopurinol:* Increased plasma didanosine concentrations; coadministration not recommended

■ *Dapsone:* Buffering compound may inhibit dissolution of dapsone in the stomach

■ *Delavirdine:* Decreased plasma delavirdine concentrations; give ddI 1 hr after delavirdine

■ *Food:* Reduced bioavailability

■ *Ganciclovir:* Increased ddI concentrations

■ *Indinavir:* Decreased plasma indinavir concentrations; give ddI 1 hr after indinavir

■ *Itraconazole, ketoconazole:* Alkalinization of stomach by didanosine reduces the solubility and absorption of antifungal

■ *Methadone:* Decreased plasma didanosine concentrations

■ *Quinolones:* Decreased concentrations after binding to the aluminum and magnesium ions in the didanosine buffering compound

❷ *Stavudine:* Increased risk of pancreatitis

■ *Tetracyclines:* Decreased antibiotic concentrations after binding to calcium ions in ddI buffering compound

SPECIAL CONSIDERATIONS
MONITORING PARAMETERS
• Amylase, lipase, ophthalmologic examinations
• Suspend use until pancreatitis excluded if patient develops nausea, abdominal pain
• Tablets contain 264.5 mg sodium, packets 1380 mg sodium
• Administer on empty stomach

dienestrol
(dye-en-ess′trole)
Rx: Ortho Dienestrol
Chemical Class: Nonsteroidal synthetic estrogen derivative
Therapeutic Class: Estrogen

D

CLINICAL PHARMACOLOGY
Mechanism of Action: Synthetic estrogen substitute; acts on female GU tract and reproductive system
Pharmacokinetics
TOP: 50% systemic absorption (better than non-vaginal estrogen products); distributed mainly to adipose tissue; primarily hepatic degradation; excreted in urine

INDICATIONS AND USES: Atrophic vaginitis, kraurosis vulvae

DOSAGE
Adult
• VAG CRE 1 applicatorful 1-2 × /day for 2 wk, then ½ dose or every other day for 2 wk, then 1 application 2-3 × weekly as maintenance

⑤ AVAILABLE FORMS/COST OF THERAPY
• Cre—Vag: 0.01%, 78 g: **$28.14-$34.00**

CONTRAINDICATIONS: Breast cancer, estrogen-dependent neoplasia, thromboembolic disorders, reproductive cancer, genital bleeding (abnormal, undiagnosed)

PRECAUTIONS: Hypertension, asthma, blood dyscrasias, gallbladder disease, CHF, diabetes mellitus, bone disease, depression, migraine headache, convulsive disorders, hepatic disease, renal disease, family history of cancer of the breast or reproductive tract

PREGNANCY AND LACTATION: Pregnancy category X; no reports of adverse effects on nursing infant; may reduce milk volume and decrease nitrogen and protein content

---

italic = common side effects   **bold italic** = life-threatening reactions

SIDE EFFECTS/ADVERSE REACTIONS

CNS: Depression, dizziness, headache, migraines, ***stroke***

CV: Edema, elevated blood pressure, ***pulmonary embolism, MI,*** thromboembolism, thrombophlebitis

EENT: Contact lens intolerance, increased corneal lens curvature

GI: Anorexia, cramps, diarrhea, gall-bladder disease, increased appetite, increased weight, *nausea,* ***pancreatitis,*** vomiting

GU: Amenorrhea, breakthrough bleeding, breast changes, cervical eversion, dysmenorrhea, ***endometrial cancer,*** endometrial hyperplasia

SKIN: Chloasma, dermatitis, erythema nodosum/multiforme, melasma, photosensitivity

INTERACTIONS

Drugs

❷ *Anticoagulants:* Possible altered hypoprothrombinemic response

❸ *Corticosteroids:* Estrogen can decrease clearance and increase therapeutic and toxic effects of corticosteroids

❸ *Cyclosporine:* Increased risk of toxicity

---

diethylpropion

(die-ethyl-prop´ion)

Rx: Tenuate

Chemical Class: Phenethylamine derivative

Therapeutic Class: Anorexiant

DEA Class: Schedule IV

CLINICAL PHARMACOLOGY

Mechanism of Action: Alters adrenergic control of nerve impulse transmission in the appetite control center of the hypothalamus; decreases hunger

Pharmacokinetics

PO: Duration 4 hr

PO-SUS REL: Duration 10-14 hr

Metabolized by liver; excreted by kidneys; $t_{1/2}$ 1-3½ hr

INDICATIONS AND USES: Treatment adjunct in exogenous obesity

DOSAGE

Adult

• PO 25 mg tid 1 hr ac or 75 mg controlled release qd midmorning

🅂 **AVAILABLE FORMS/COST OF THERAPY**

• Tab, Uncoated—Oral: 25 mg, 100's: **$4.75-$59.97**

• Tab, Uncoated, Sus Action—Oral: 75 mg, 100's: **$45.88-$132.56**

CONTRAINDICATIONS: Hyperthyroidism, hypertension, glaucoma, angina pectoris, drug abuse, cardiovascular disease, children <12 yr, severe arteriosclerosis, agitated states

PRECAUTIONS: Convulsive disorders (increased risk of seizures)

PREGNANCY AND LACTATION: Pregnancy category B; excreted in breast milk; no reports of adverse effects

SIDE EFFECTS/ADVERSE REACTIONS

CNS: Anxiety, confusion, depression, dizziness, dysphoria, euphoria, fatigue, headache, *hyperactivity,* incoordination, insomnia, malaise, *restlessness,* tremors

CV: ***Dysrhythmias,*** ECG changes, hypertension, *palpitations,* pulmonary hypertension, *tachycardia*

EENT: Blurred vision, eye irritation, mydriasis

GI: Anorexia, constipation, diarrhea, dry mouth, nausea, pain, unpleasant taste, vomiting

GU: Change in libido, dysuria, impotence, menstrual irregularities, polyuria, urinary frequency

HEME: ***Bone marrow depression***

SKIN: Erythema, rash, urticaria

MISC: Chills, ecchymosis, excessive sweating, fever, flushing, hair loss, muscle/chest pain

INTERACTIONS

Labs

• *False positive:* Urine cocaine, diazepam, methaqualone, phencyclidine

SPECIAL CONSIDERATIONS

• Tolerance to anorectic effects may develop within weeks; cross-tolerance is almost universal

• Measure the limited usefulness against the inherent risks (habituation) of this agent

• Most patients will eventually regain weight lost during use of this product

---

diethylstilbestrol

(dye-eth-il-stil-bess´trole)

Rx: Stilphostrol
(diphosphonate salt)
Chemical Class: Nonsteroidal synthetic estrogen derivative
Therapeutic Class: Antineoplastic

CLINICAL PHARMACOLOGY

Mechanism of Action: Increases cellular synthesis of DNA, RNA, and various proteins in responsive tissues of the female reproductive tract affects release of pituitary gonadotropins

Pharmacokinetics

Primarily hepatic metabolism and renal excretion

INDICATIONS AND USES: Postcoital contraception*; inoperable breast and prostatic cancer

DOSAGE

Adult

• *Postcoital contraception:* PO 25 mg bid × 5 days, starting within 72 hr of intercourse

• *Prostatic cancer:* PO 1-3 mg qd initially, may then be reduced to 1 mg qd; IV 0.25-1 g qd × 5 days, then 1-2 × /wk; (diphosphate form) PO 50-200 mg tid, max 1 g/day

• *Breast cancer:* PO 15 mg qd

§ AVAILABLE FORMS/COST OF THERAPY

• Tab, Uncoated—Oral: 1 mg, 100's: **$9.91**; 5 mg, 100's: **$26.40**
Diphosphonate Salt

• Inj, Sol—IV: 250 mg/5 ml, 1's: **$15.17**

• Tab—Oral: 50 mg, 50's: **$91.99**

CONTRAINDICATIONS: Breast cancer (except in selected patients being treated for metastatic disease), active thromboembolic disorders, known or suspected estrogen-dependent neoplasia, undiagnosed abnormal genital bleeding, pregnancy

PRECAUTIONS: Hypertension, gallbladder disease, CHF, diabetes mellitus, seizure disorders, hepatic disease, uterine fibroids, hypertriglyceridemia, family history of breast or endometrial cancer, hypercalcemia

PREGNANCY AND LACTATION: Pregnancy category X; increased incidence of vaginal and cervical carcinoma in female offspring exposed *in utero;* may reduce quantity and quality of milk

SIDE EFFECTS/ADVERSE REACTIONS

CNS: Depression, migraine headache, emotional lability

CV: **Arterial thromboembolism, pulmonary embolism, CVA, MI,** hypertension, venous thrombosis, edema

EENT: Contact lens intolerance, **retinal thrombosis**

GI: Nausea and vomiting, gallbladder disease, bloating, benign hepatic tumors, **mesenteric thrombosis**

---

italic = common side effects   ***bold italic*** = life-threatening reactions

GU: Breakthrough bleeding, spotting, amenorrhea, change in cervical secretions, breast enlargement, breast tenderness, testicular atrophy
METAB: Hyperglycemia, hypertriglyceridemia, hypercalcemia
SKIN: Melasma

INTERACTIONS

Drugs

▣ *P450 inducers (e.g., rifampin, barbiturates):* Decreased estrogen levels

▣ *Corticosteroids:* Increased steroid effect

▣ *Phenytoin:* Loss of seizure control, decreased estrogen levels

▣ *Warfarin:* Theoretical increased risk thromboembolism

SPECIAL CONSIDERATIONS
PATIENT/FAMILY EDUCATION

• Nausea, especially in the morning is primarily central in origin, but solid food often provides some relief

---

diflorasone

(die-floor´a-sone)
Rx: Florone, Florone E, Maxiflor, Psorcon, Psorcon E
Chemical Class: Synthetic glucocorticoid
Therapeutic Class: Topical corticosteroid, very high potency (0.05% ointment), high potency (0.05% cream, emollient base ointment)

CLINICAL PHARMACOLOGY
Mechanism of Action: Depresses formation, release, and activity of endogenous mediators of inflammation such as prostaglandins, kinins, histamine, liposomal enzymes, and the complement system resulting in decreased edema, erythema, and pruritus

Pharmacokinetics
Absorbed through the skin (increased by inflammation and occlusive dressings); metabolized primarily in the liver
INDICATIONS AND USES: Psoriasis, eczema, contact dermatitis, pruritus
DOSAGE
Adult and Child
• Apply to affected area bid, rub completely into skin
Ⓢ **AVAILABLE FORMS/COST OF THERAPY**
• Cre—Top: 0.05%, 15, 30, 60 g: **$43.19-$66.74**/30 g
• Oint—Top: 0.05%, 15, 30, 60 g: **$36.09-$69.45**/30 g
CONTRAINDICATIONS: Fungal infections; use on face, groin, or axilla
PRECAUTIONS: Viral infections, bacterial infections, children
PREGNANCY AND LACTATION: Pregnancy category C; unknown whether topical application could result in sufficient systemic absorption to produce detectable amounts in breast milk (systemic corticosteroids are secreted into breast milk in quantities not likely to have detrimental effects on infant)
SIDE EFFECTS/ADVERSE REACTIONS
SKIN: Acne, allergic contact dermatitis, atrophy, burning, dryness, folliculitis, hypertrichosis, hypopigmentation, irritation, itching, miliaria, perioral dermatitis, secondary infection, striae
MISC: Reversible HPA axis suppression (more likely with occlusive dressings, prolonged administration, application to large surface areas, liver failure, or use in children)
SPECIAL CONSIDERATIONS
• No demonstrated superiority over other high-potency agents; cost should govern use

---

* = non-FDA-approved use

PATIENT/FAMILY EDUCATION
• Apply sparingly only to affected area
• Avoid contact with the eyes
• Do not put bandages or dressings over treated area unless directed by clinician
• Discontinue drug, notify clinician if local irritation or fever develops
• Do not use on weeping, denuded, or infected areas

---

diflunisal
(dye-floo'ni-sal)
Rx: Dolobid
Chemical Class: Salicylate derivative
Therapeutic Class: NSAID with analgesic and antipyretic activity

---

CLINICAL PHARMACOLOGY
Mechanism of Action: Reversible cyclooxygenase inhibitor; nonselectively decreases the formation of both prostaglandins and thromboxane A_2; variable effects on lipoxygenase synthesis and subsequent leukotriene production; antiinflammatory, antipyretic, and analgesic activity; inhibits platelet aggregation
Pharmacokinetics
PO: Peak 2-3 hr, onset 1 hr, >99% bound to plasma proteins, $t_{1/2}$ 8-12 hr (dose dependent); excreted mainly in urine as glucuronide conjugates
INDICATIONS AND USES: Osteoarthritis, rheumatoid arthritis, ankylosing spondylitis,* prevention of cognitive decline,* pain—mild to moderate, migraine headache,* tendonitis,* dysmenorrhea*

DOSAGE
Adult
• *Mild to moderate pain:* PO 500-1000 mg initially, then 250-500 mg q8-12h
• *Osteoarthritis/rheumatoid arthritis:* PO 500-1000 mg/day in 2 divided doses; max 1500 mg/day

$ AVAILABLE FORMS/COST OF THERAPY
• Tab, Plain Coated—Oral: 250 mg, 100's: **$87.25-$98.65**; 500 mg, 100's: **$58.33-$129.23**

PRECAUTIONS: History of GI ulceration, bleeding, or perforation; renal dysfunction, hypertension or cardiac conditions aggravated by fluid retention and edema, history of liver dysfunction, children with fever (potential association with Reye's syndrome)

PREGNANCY AND LACTATION: Pregnancy category C; use during 3rd trimester not recommended due to effects on fetal cardiovascular system (closure of ductus arteriosus); excreted into breast milk in concentrations 2%-7% those in maternal plasma; use caution in nursing mothers

SIDE EFFECTS/ADVERSE REACTIONS
CNS: Confusion, dizziness, flushing, hallucinations, headache, insomnia, paresthesias, somnolence, stimulation, vertigo
CV: Chest pain, palpitations
EENT: Blurred vision, corneal deposits, decreased acuity
GI: Abnormal LFTs, anorexia, constipation, *diarrhea,* flatulance, **GI bleeding, GI pain,** heartburn, hepatitis, *nausea,* vomiting
GU: Uricosuria
HEME: **Agranulocytosis, thrombocytopenia**
RESP: Dyspnea

SKIN: Dry mucous membranes, erythema multiforme, ***exfoliative dermatitis,*** photosensitivity, pruritus, *rash,* ***Stevens-Johnson syndrome,*** stomatitis, sweating, ***toxic epidermal necrolysis,*** urticaria

INTERACTIONS

Drugs

3 *Aminoglycosides:* Reduced clearance with elevated aminoglycoside levels and potential for toxicity

3 *Anticoagulants:* Excessive hypoprothrombinemia, decreased platelet aggregation with increased risk of GI bleeding

3 *Antihypertensives (alpha blockers, angiotensin-converting enzyme inhibitors, angiotensin II receptor blockers, beta blockers, diuretics):* Inhibition of antihypertensive and other favorable hemodynamic effects

3 *Corticosteroids:* Increased risk of GI ulceration

3 *Cyclosporine:* Increased nephrotoxicity risk

3 *Lithium:* Decreased clearance of lithium (mediated via prostaglandins) resulting in elevated serum lithium levels and risk of toxicity

3 *Methotrexate:* Decreased renal secretion of methotrexate resulting in elevated methotrexate levels and risk of toxicity

3 *Phenylpropanolamine:* Possible acute hypertensive reaction

3 *Potassium-sparing diuretics:* Additive hyperkalemia potential

3 *Triamterene:* Acute renal failure reported with addition of indomethacin; caution with other NSAIDs

Labs

• *False increase:* Serum salicylate
• *False decrease:* T_4, T_3 uptake

SPECIAL CONSIDERATIONS

• No significant advantage over other NSAIDs; cost should govern use

MONITORING PARAMETERS

• Initial hemogram and fecal occult blood test within 3 mo of starting regular chronic therapy; repeat every 6-12 mo (more frequently in high-risk patients (> 65 years, peptic ulcer disease, concurrent steroids or anticoagulants); electrolytes, creatinine, and BUN within 3 mo of starting regular chronic therapy; repeat every 6-12 mo

---

digitoxin

(di-ji-tox'in)

Rx: Crystodigin
Chemical Class: Digitalis derivative
Therapeutic Class: Antidysrhythmic; cardiac glycoside

CLINICAL PHARMACOLOGY

Mechanism of Action: Increases influx of calcium ions into intracellular cytoplasm, resulting in increased cardiac muscle contractility (positive inotropic effect); decreases SA and AV node conduction (negative chronotropic effect)

Pharmacokinetics

PO: Onset 1-4 hr, peak 8-12 hr, $t_{1/2}$ 168-192 hr, 90%-97% bound to plasma proteins; metabolized by the liver, excreted via the kidneys (metabolites)

INDICATIONS AND USES: Congestive heart failure (CHF), atrial fibrillation, atrial flutter, paroxysmal atrial tachycardia (PAT), cardiogenic shock

---

DOSAGE
Adult
• Loading dose PO (rapid) 0.6 mg, followed by 0.4 mg, then 0.2 mg at q4-6h intervals; (slow) 0.2 mg bid for 4 days; maintenance dose PO 0.05-0.3 mg qd. Dosage reduction not needed in renal function impairment
Child
• Loading dose PO <1 yr 0.045 mg/kg, 1-2 yr 0.04 mg/kg, >2 yr 0.03 mg/kg divided into 3, 4, or more portions with >6 hr between doses; maintenance dose PO 1/10 loading dose

⑤ AVAILABLE FORMS/COST OF THERAPY
• Tab, Uncoated—Oral: 0.1 mg, 100's: **$5.57**

CONTRAINDICATIONS: Ventricular tachycardia, ventricular fibrillation

PRECAUTIONS: Hypokalemia, hypomagnesemia, hypercalcemia, hypothyroidism, severe pulmonary disease, sick sinus syndrome, hepatic disease, acute MI, AV block, elderly, Wolff-Parkinson-White syndrome

PREGNANCY AND LACTATION: Pregnancy category C; passes readily to fetus; excretion into breast milk unknown; digoxin, a related cardiac glycoside, is considered compatible with breast feeding

SIDE EFFECTS/ADVERSE REACTIONS
CNS: Anorexia, apathy, confusion, delirium, disorientation, drowsiness, EEG abnormalities, hallucinations, headache, mental depression, neuralgia, psychosis, restlessness, *seizures,* weakness
*CV: **Atrial fibrillation, AV block,** bradycardia, premature ventricular contractions (PVCs), **ventricular fibrillation, ventricular tachycardia***
EENT: Visual disturbances (blurred, yellow or green vision, halo effect)

GI: Abdominal discomfort, *diarrhea,* **hemorrhagic necrosis of the intestines,** *nausea, vomiting*
HEME: Eosinophilia, **thrombocytopenia**
SKIN: Rash

INTERACTIONS
Drugs
③ *Alprazolam, amiodarone, diltiazem, verapamil, bepridil, nitrendipine, quinidine, carvedilol, cyclosporine, erythromycin and tetracyclines (change in bacterial flora causing effect may persist for months), hydroxychloroquine, NSAIDs, azole antifungals, omeprazole, lansoprazole, propafenone, quinine, spironolactone, tacrolimus:* Increased digitalis levels
③ *Amphotericin B diuretics:* Enhanced digitalis toxicity secondary to drug-induced hypokalemia
③ *Beta-blockers:* Potentiation of bradycardia
③ *Calcium (IV):* Digitalis toxicity
❷ *Charcoal:* Reduced digitalis levels
③ *Cholestyramine, Kaolo-pectin (digoxin tablets only), neomycin, penicillamine, rifampin, sulfasalazine:* Reduced digitalis levels
③ *Metoclopramide, cisapride:* Reduced digitalis levels by slowly dissolving digoxin tablets only (Lanoxin tablets and capsules not affected)
③ *Succinylcholine:* Increased arrhythmias
Labs
• *False increase:* Urine 17-hydroxycorticosteroids

SPECIAL CONSIDERATIONS
• When digitalis indicated digoxin is 1st line drug because of its shorter $t_{1/2}$ and faster clearance in the event toxicity develops
• Rule out digitalis toxicity if nausea, vomiting, arrhythmias develop

• Listed adverse effects are mostly signs of toxicity

MONITORING PARAMETERS

• Heart rate and rhythm, periodic ECGs

• Serum potassium, magnesium, calcium, creatinine

• Serum digitoxin levels when compliance, effectiveness, or systemic availability is questioned or toxicity suspected; therapeutic range 9-25 ng/ml

---

digoxin

(di-jox'in)

Rx: Lanoxicaps, Lanoxin

Chemical Class: Digitalis glycoside

Therapeutic Class: Antidysrhythmic; cardiac glycoside

CLINICAL PHARMACOLOGY

Mechanism of Action: Increases influx of calcium ions into intracellular cytoplasm, resulting in increased cardiac muscle contractility (positive inotropic effect); decreases SA and AV node conduction (negative chronotropic effect)

Pharmacokinetics

IV: Onset 5-30 min, peak 1-5 hr

PO: Onset 30-120 min, peak 2-6 hr, $t_{1/2}$ 30-40 hr, 20%-25% bound to plasma proteins; excreted mainly by kidneys

INDICATIONS AND USES: Congestive heart failure in patients receiving diuretics or diuretics and ACE inhibitors (CHF), control of ventricular response rate in atrial fibrillation, atrial flutter, paroxysmal atrial tachycardia (PAT), cardiogenic shock

DOSAGE

Administer IV slowly over 5 min; IM route not recommended due to local irritation, pain, and tissue damage

Adult

• Loading dose (give ½ total dose initially, then ¼ total dose in each of 2 subsequent doses at 8-12 hr intervals); IV 0.5-1 mg; PO 0.75-1.5 mg; maintenance dose IV 0.1-0.4 mg qd; PO 0.125-0.5 mg qd

Child >10 yr

• Loading dose (administered as for adult); IV 8-12 µg/kg; PO 10-15 µg/kg; maintenance dose IV 2-3 µg/kg qd; PO 2.5-5 µg/kg qd

Child 5-10 yr

• Loading dose (administered as for adult); IV 15-30 µg/kg; PO 20-35 µg/kg; maintenance dose IV 4-8 µg/kg divided q12h; PO 5-10 µg/kg divided q12h

Child 2-5 yr

• Loading dose (administered as for adult); IV 25-35 µg/kg; IV 30-40 µg/kg; maintenance dose IV 6-9 µg/kg divided q12h; PO 7.5-10 µg/kg divided q12h

Child 1-24 mo

• Loading dose (administered as for adult); IV 30-50 µg/kg; PO 35-60 µg/kg; maintenance dose IV 7.5-12 µg/kg divided q12h; PO 10-15 µg/kg divided q12h

Full term infant

• Loading dose (administered as for adult); IV 20-30 µg/kg; PO 25-35 µg/kg; maintenance dose IV 5-8 µg/kg divided q12h; PO 6-10 µg/kg divided q12h

Preterm infant

• Loading dose (administered as for adult); IV 15-25 µg/kg; PO 20-30 µg/kg; maintenance dose: IV 4-6 µg/kg divided q12h; PO 5-7.5 µg/kg divided q12h

$ AVAILABLE FORMS/COST OF THERAPY

• Cap, Elastic—Oral: 0.05 mg, 100's: **$14.34-$28.08**; 0.1 mg, 100's: **$30.64**; 0.2 mg, 100's: **$35.64**

• Elixir—Oral: 0.05 mg/ml, 60 ml: **$9.63-$35.04**

• Inj, Sol—IM, IV: 0.1 mg/ml, 1 ml: **$5.42-$6.96**; 0.25 mg/ml, 2 ml: **$2.34-$2.99**

• Tab, Uncoated—Oral: 0.125 mg, 100's: **$4.44-$34.19**; 0.25 mg, 100's: **$2.00-$30.07**; 0.5 mg, 100's: **$18.02-$25.00**

CONTRAINDICATIONS: Ventricular tachycardia, ventricular fibrillation

PRECAUTIONS: Hypokalemia, hypomagnesemia, hypercalcemia, hypothyroidism, severe pulmonary disease, sick sinus syndrome, hepatic disease, acute MI, AV block, elderly, Wolff-Parkinson-White syndrome

PREGNANCY AND LACTATION: Pregnancy category C, passes readily to fetus; excreted into breast milk; considered compatible with breast feeding

SIDE EFFECTS/ADVERSE REACTIONS

CNS: Anorexia, apathy, confusion, delirium, disorientation, drowsiness, EEG abnormalities, hallucinations, headache, mental depression, neuralgia, psychosis, restlessness, **seizures,** weakness

CV: **Atrial fibrillation, AV block,** bradycardia, premature ventricular contractions (PVCs), **ventricular fibrillation, ventricular tachycardia**

EENT: Visual disturbances (blurred, yellow or green vision, halo effect)

GI: Abdominal discomfort, *diarrhea,* **hemorrhagic necrosis of the intestines,** *nausea, vomiting*

HEME: Eosinophilia, **thrombocytopenia**

SKIN: Rash

INTERACTIONS

Drugs

3 *Alprazolam, amiodarone, diltiazem, verapamil, bepridil, nitrendipine, quinidine, carvedilol, cyclosporine, erythromycin and tetracyclines (change in bacterial flora causing effect may persist for months), hydroxychloroquine, NSAIDs, azole antifungals, omeprazole, lansoprazole, propafenone, quinine, spironolactone, tacrolimus:* Increased digoxin levels

3 *Amphotericin B diuretics:* Enhanced digitalis toxicity secondary to drug-induced hypokalemia

3 *Beta-blockers:* Potentiation of bradycardia

3 *Calcium (IV):* Digitalis toxicity

2 *Charcoal:* Reduced digitalis levels

3 *Cholestyramine, Kaolo-pectin (digoxin tablets only) neomycin, penicillamine, rifampin, sulfasalazine:* Reduced digitalis levels

3 *Cyclophosphamide:* Impaired digoxin (especially tablets) absorption; digitoxin not affected

3 *Metoclopramide, cisapride:* Reduced digitalis levels by slowly dissolving digoxin tablets only (Lanoxin tablets and capsules not affected)

3 *Succinylcholine:* Increased arrhythmias

Labs

• *False increase:* Urine 17-hydroxycorticosteroids

SPECIAL CONSIDERATIONS

• Preferred digitalis glycoside

• Rule out digitalis toxicity if nausea, vomiting, arrhythmias develop

• Listed adverse effects are mostly signs of toxicity

MONITORING PARAMETERS

• Heart rate and rhythm, periodic ECGs

---

italic = common side effects   **bold italic** = life-threatening reactions

• Serum potassium, magnesium, calcium, creatinine

• Serum digoxin levels when compliance, effectiveness, or systemic availability is questioned or toxicity suspected

• Obtain serum drug concentrations at least 8-12 hr after a dose (preferably prior to next scheduled dose); therapeutic range 0.5-2.0 ng/ml

---

digoxin immune Fab

Rx: Digibind
Chemical Class: Antibody fragment
Therapeutic Class: Digoxin antidote

CLINICAL PHARMACOLOGY

Mechanism of Action: Antibody fragments bind to free digoxin to reverse digoxin toxicity by not allowing digoxin to bind to sites of action; derived from sheep antibodies

Pharmacokinetics

IV: Onset of improvement in signs and symptoms of digoxin toxicity 30 min, $t_{1/2}$ 15-20 hr, antigen binding fragment digoxin complex accumulates in the blood and is excreted by the kidneys

INDICATIONS AND USES: Potentially life-threatening digoxin intoxication (has also been used successfully to treat life-threatening digitoxin overdose)

DOSAGE

Adult

• IV dose (mg) = dose ingested (mg) × 0.8 × 66.7; if digoxin liq cap or digitoxin used, do not multiply ingested dose by 0.8; if ingested amount is unknown, give 800 mg IV. Alternatively, calculate the equimolar dose required from the total amount of digoxin (or digitoxin) in the patient's body. An estimate of the total body load can be made from a serum level: For digoxin body load in mg = serum digoxin concentration × 0.56 × weight in kg/1000. Each 40 mg vial will bind 0.6 mg of digoxin or digitoxin; calculate the number of vials required by dividing body load in mg by 0.6 mg/vial; dose (in number of vials) = body load (mg)/0.6 mg/vial

$ AVAILABLE FORMS/COST OF THERAPY

• Inj, Conc-Sol—IV: 40 mg/vial, 1's: **$400.00-$758.24**

PRECAUTIONS: Children, cardiac disease, renal disease, allergy to ovine products

PREGNANCY AND LACTATION: Pregnancy category C; excretion into breast milk unknown; use caution in nursing mothers

SIDE EFFECTS/ADVERSE REACTIONS

METAB: Hypokalemia

MISC: Hypersensitivity (anaphylaxis, fever)

INTERACTIONS

Labs

• *Interference:* Immunoassay digoxin

SPECIAL CONSIDERATIONS

MONITORING PARAMETERS

• Potassium, serum digoxin level prior to therapy

• Continuous ECG monitoring

---

* = non-FDA-approved use

dihydroergotamine
(dye-hye-droe-er-got′a-meen)
Rx: D.H.E. 45, Migranol (nasal)
Chemical Class: Ergot alkaloid
Therapeutic Class: Antimigraine agent

CLINICAL PHARMACOLOGY
Mechanism of Action: Causes vasoconstriction of dilated cranial blood vessels associated with vascular headaches, with a concomitant decrease in the amplitude of pulsations
Pharmacokinetics
IM: Onset 15-30 min
IV: Onset within a few min
NASAL: Onset 60 min
Ninety percent bound to plasma proteins, $t_{1/2}$ (terminal) 21-32 hr; metabolized by liver, excreted in urine and bile
INDICATIONS AND USES: Prevent or abort vascular headaches including migraine and cluster headaches
DOSAGE
Adult
• IM 1 mg at first sign of headache, repeat at 1 hr intervals prn, do not exceed 3 mg/attack or 6 mg/wk; IV 1 mg at first sign of headache, repeat in 1 hr prn, do not exceed 2 mg/attack or 6 mg/wk
• NASAL 1 spray in each nostril at first sign of headache, may repeat in 15 min prn; max 6 sprays/day
§ AVAILABLE FORMS/COST OF THERAPY
• Inj, Sol—IM, IV: 1 mg/ml, 1 ml: **$16.61**
• Spray—Nasal: 0.5 mg/inh, 4 ml: **$85.08**

CONTRAINDICATIONS: Pregnancy, peripheral vascular disease, hepatic or renal impairment, coronary artery disease, uncontrolled hypertension, sepsis
PRECAUTIONS: Prolonged administration, excessive dosage
PREGNANCY AND LACTATION: Pregnancy category X; likely excreted into breast milk; ergotamine has caused symptoms of ergotism (e.g., vomiting, diarrhea) in the infant; excessive dosage or prolonged administration may inhibit lactation
SIDE EFFECTS/ADVERSE REACTIONS
CV: Chest pain, coronary vasoconstriction (large doses), increase or decrease in blood pressure, transient tachycardia or bradycardia
GI: Nausea (10%), vomiting
MISC: Itching, localized edema, muscle pain in the extremities, numbness and tingling of fingers and toes, weakness in the legs
INTERACTIONS
Drugs
❷ *Clarithromycin, erythromycin (not azithromycin or dirithromycin):* Increased ergotism (hypertention and ischemia)
❷ *Nitroglycerin:* Enhanced ergot effect, decreased antianginal effects
❷ *Sibutramine:* Increased risk of serotonin syndrome
SPECIAL CONSIDERATIONS
• Considered alternative abortive acute migraine agent; nasal spray less effective than triptans
PATIENT/FAMILY EDUCATION
• Initiate therapy at 1st sign of attack
• Prolonged use may lead to withdrawal headaches

---

italic = common side effects   ***bold italic*** = life-threatening reactions

dihydrotachysterol

(dye-hye-droe-tak-iss'ter-ole)

Rx: DHT, Hytakerol

Chemical Class: Sterol derivative

Therapeutic Class: Vitamin D analog; antiosteoporotic

CLINICAL PHARMACOLOGY

Mechanism of Action: Stimulates intestinal calcium absorption and mobilization of bone calcium in the absence of parathyroid hormone and of functioning renal tissue; also increases renal phosphate excretion

Pharmacokinetics

PO: Onset 2 wk; hydroxylated in the liver to 25-hydroxydihydrotachysterol, the major circulating active form of the drug; excreted in bile

INDICATIONS AND USES: Treatment of acute, chronic, and latent forms of postoperative tetany; idiopathic tetany; hypoparathyroidism; pseudohypoparathyroidism*; familial hypophosphatemia*; renal osteodystrophy in chronic renal failure*; osteoporosis (with calcium and flouride)*

DOSAGE

Adult

• PO 0.75-2.5 mg/day for 4 days initially, then 0.2-1.75 mg/day as required for normal serum calcium levels; average dose 0.6 mg qd

Child

• PO 1-5 mg/day for 4 days initially, then 0.5-1.5 mg/day as required for normal serum calcium levels

Neonate

• PO 0.05-0.1 mg/day

§ AVAILABLE FORMS/COST OF THERAPY

• Cap, Gel—Oral: 0.125 mg, 50's: **$154.09**

• Sol—Oral: 0.2 mg/ml, 30 ml: **$38.79**

• Tab, Uncoated—Oral: 0.125 mg, 50's: **$49.36**; 0.2 mg, 100's: **$100.28**; 0.4 mg, 50's: **$90.00**

CONTRAINDICATIONS: Hypercalcemia and hypervitaminosis D

PRECAUTIONS: Renal stones, renal failure, heart disease

PREGNANCY AND LACTATION: Pregnancy category A (category D if used in doses above the recommended daily allowance); excretion into breast milk unknown; vitamin D is excreted into breast milk in limited amounts; considered compatible with breast feeding, however, serum calcium levels of the infant should be monitored if the mother is receiving pharmacologic doses

SIDE EFFECTS/ADVERSE REACTIONS

CNS: Amnesia, ataxia, coma, depression, disorientation, drowsiness, fever, hallucinations, headache, lethargy, syncope, vertigo

CV: Cardiovascular failure

EENT: Tinnitus

GI: Anorexia, constipation, cramps, diarrhea, dry mouth, jaundice, metallic taste, nausea, vomiting

GU: Hematuria, hypercalciuria, hyperphosphatemia, polyuria, *renal failure*

MS: Arthralgia, decreased bone development, hypotonia, myalgia, weakness

SPECIAL CONSIDERATIONS

• Vitamin D analog of choice for prevention and treatment of renal osteodystrophy; less expensive than calcitriol

PATIENT/FAMILY EDUCATION

• Compliance with dosage instructions, diet (evaluate vitamin D ingested in fortified foods, maintain adequate calcium intake) is essential

MONITORING PARAMETERS

• Serum Ca^{++} and phosphate

---

* = non-FDA-approved use

• If adverse reactions occur rule out hypercalcemia, worsening renal function

---

dihydroxyaluminum sodium carbonate
(dye-hye-drox´ee-a-loom´-a-nim)
OTC: Rolaids
Chemical Class: Aluminum product
Therapeutic Class: Antacid

CLINICAL PHARMACOLOGY
Mechanism of Action: Neutralizes gastric acidity, reduces pepsin
Pharmacokinetics
PO: Onset 20-40 min; excreted in feces
INDICATIONS AND USES: Symptomatic relief of gastroesophageal reflux, acid indigestion; hyperacidity associated with peptic ulcer, gastritis, peptic esophagitis, gastric hyperacidity, hiatal hernia
DOSAGE
Adult
• PO chew 1-2 tab prn
§ AVAILABLE FORMS/COST OF THERAPY
• Tab, Chewable—Oral: 334 mg, 150's: **$1.72-$2.99**
PRECAUTIONS: Elderly, fluid restriction, decreased GI motility, GI obstruction, dehydration, renal disease, sodium-restricted diets
PREGNANCY AND LACTATION: Pregnancy category C
SIDE EFFECTS/ADVERSE REACTIONS
GI: Anorexia, *constipation,* fecal impaction
METAB: Hypercalciuria, hypophosphatemia
MISC: Aluminum intoxication, osteomalacia

INTERACTIONS
Drugs
§ *Allopurinol, beta blockers, ateviridine, cefpodoxime and cefuroxime (not cefetamet or cefixime), quinolones, tetracyclines, iron, isoniazid, ketoconazole and itraconazole (not fluconazole), penicillamine:* Decreased absorption
§ *Glipizide, glyburide:* Enhanced gastric absorption, monitor for hypoglycemia
§ *Lithium:* Lower lithium concentrations
§ *Methenamine:* Interference with urinary antibacterial activity if urine pH >5.5
§ *Salicylates:* Lower serum concentrations from reduced renal tubular reabsorption
§ *Sympathomimetic amines, flecainide, tocainide, mexiletine, quinidine, quinine:* Decreased elimination secondary to increased urine pH, increased drug effects (large doses only)
§ *Vitamin C:* Increased aluminum absorption
SPECIAL CONSIDERATIONS
PATIENT/FAMILY EDUCATION
• Thoroughly chew tab before swallowing, follow with a glass of water
• May impair absorption of many drugs; take other drugs 2 hr before or 4-6 hr after antacid
• May cause premature dissolution of enteric coated tablets
• Stools may appear white or speckled

---

diltiazem

(dil-tye´a-zem)
Rx: Cardizem, Cardizem CD, Cardizem SR, Dilacor XR, Diltia XT, Tiamate, Tiazac
Combinations
   Rx: with enalapril (Teczem)
Chemical Class: Benzothiazepine
Therapeutic Class: Calcium channel blocker: Antianginal; antihypertensive; antidysrhythmic (class IV)

CLINICAL PHARMACOLOGY
Mechanism of Action: Inhibits calcium ion influx across cell membrane during cardiac depolarization; produces relaxation of coronary vascular smooth muscle; dilates coronary arteries; slows SA/AV node conduction times, dilates peripheral arteries; hemodynamics: decreases myocardial contractility; no effect or increases cardiac output; decreases peripheral vascular resistance

Pharmacokinetics
PO: Peak serum conc 2-4 hr
PO-SUS REL: Peak serum conc 6-11 hr
PO QD CAP: Peak serum conc 10-14 hr
$t_{1/2}$ 4-6 hr, 70-80% bound to plasma proteins; rapid absorption; bioavailability 47%; Vd 1.7 L/kg; metabolized by liver, excreted in urine (96% as metabolites)

INDICATIONS AND USES: *Oral:* Angina pectoris due to coronary artery spasm, chronic stable angina, essential hypertension (SR only); Also prevention of reinfarction of non-Q-wave MI,* tardive dyskinesia,* Raynaud's syndrome,* migraine headache prophylaxis*

* = non-FDA-approved use

Parenteral: Atrial fibrillation or flutter (IV), paroxysmal supraventricular tachycardia (IV).
DOSAGE
Adult
• Immed Rel PO 30 mg qid, gradually increase to 180-360 mg/day divided tid-qid until optimal response is obtained; Sus Action (Cardizem SR) PO 60-120 mg bid, adjust at 14 day intervals until optimal response obtained, optimum range 240-350 mg/day; Sus Action (Cardizem CD, Dilacor XR) once daily cap PO 180-240 mg qd, max 540 mg/day; IV 0.25 mg/kg as a bolus over 2 min (a second 0.35 mg/kg bolus dose may be administered after 15 min if response is inadequate), then continuous INF of 5-15 mg/hr for up to 24 hr; conversion from IV to PO, start PO approximately 3 hr after bolus dose; PO (mg/day) = 10 × {[rate (mg/hr) × 3] + 3};3 mg/hr = 120 mg/day; 5 mg/hr = 180 mg/day; 7 mg/hr = 240 mg/day; 11 mg/hr = 360 mg/day

AVAILABLE FORMS/COST OF THERAPY
• Cap, Gel, Sus Action—Oral: 60 mg, 100's: **$29.60-$101.09**; 90 mg, 100's: **$79.20-$115.50**; 120 mg, 100's: **$103.15-$150.57**; 180 mg, 100's: **$48.10-$119.08**; 240 mg, 100's: **$112.95-$165.59**; 300 mg, 100's: **$258.93-$292.59**; 360 mg, 100's: **$263.91**; 420 mg, 90's: **$227.19**
• Inj, Sol—IV: 5 mg/ml, 5 ml: **$10.20-$12.00**
• Tab, Plain Coated—Oral: 30 mg, 100's: **$11.87-$54.91**; 60 mg, 100's: **$12.53-$90.73**; 90 mg, 100's: **$20.42-$121.18**; 120 mg, 100's: **$99.00-$158.62**
CONTRAINDICATIONS: Sick sinus syndrome or 2nd or 3rd degree heart block (except with a functioning pacemaker), hypotension <90 mm

Hg systolic, acute MI with pulmonary congestion, atrial fibrillation or atrial flutter associated with an accessory bypass tract such as in WPW syndrome or short PR syndrome (IV), ventricular tachycardia (IV)

PRECAUTIONS: CHF, hypotension, hepatic injury, children, impaired renal or hepatic function

PREGNANCY AND LACTATION: Pregnancy category C; excreted into breast milk in concentrations that may approximate those in maternal serum; use caution in nursing mothers

SIDE EFFECTS/ADVERSE REACTIONS

CNS: Abnormal dreams, amnesia, depression, *dizziness,* gait abnormality, hallucinations, *headache,* insomnia, nervousness, paresthesia, personality change, somnolence, tremor

CV: Angina, **arrhythmia, AV block (1st degree), AV block (2nd or 3rd degree),** bradycardia, bundle branch block, **congestive heart failure,** *edema,* flushing, hypotension, palpitations, syncope, tachycardia

GI: Anorexia, constipation, diarrhea, dysgeusia, dyspepsia, GERD; mild elevations of LFTs; *nausea,* thirst, vomiting, weight increase

METAB: Metabolic acidosis

SKIN: Petechiae, photosensitivity, pruritus, rash, urticaria

INTERACTIONS

Drugs

🔳 *Alpha blockers:* Additive increased antihypertensive effect

🔳 *Amiodarone:* Cardiotoxicity with bradycardia and decreased cardiac output

🔳 *Antipyrine:* Increased antipyrine concentrations

🔳 *Aspirin:* Enhanced antiplatelet activity

🔳 *Azole antifungals:* Possible increased calcium channel blocker effects

🔳 *Beta-blockers:* Inhibition of metabolism of propranolol and metoprolol (not atenolol); additive effects on cardiac conduction and hypotension

❷ *Carbamazepine:* Increase in carbamazepine toxicity

🔳 *Cyclosporine, tacrolimus:* Increased blood concentrations, renal toxicity

🔳 *Digitalis glycosides:* Reduced elimination, increased digitalis levels, toxicity

🔳 *Ecainide:* Increased ecainide levels

🔳 *Erythromycin, troleandomycin:* Increased levels calcium channel blocker

🔳 *Fentanyl:* Severe hypotension or increased fluid volume requirements

🔳 *H₂-receptor antagonists:* Serum diltiazem concentrations increased

🔳 *Lithium:* Neurotoxicity

🔳 *Neuromuscular blockers:* Prolonged blockade by vecuronium and pancuronium

🔳 *Nitroprusside:* Enhanced hypotension

🔳 *Phenobarbital:* Reduced calcium channel blocker concentration

🔳 *Phenytoin:* Increased phenytoin levels

🔳 *Rifampin:* Decreased diltiazem concentrations

🔳 *Tricyclic antidepressants:* Increased TCA levels

Labs

• *False positive:* Urine ketones

---

italic = common side effects   ***bold italic*** = life-threatening reactions

dimenhydrinate
(dye-men-hye´dri-nate)
Rx: Hydrate
OTC: Calm-X, Dramamine, Triptone
Chemical Class: Ethanolamine derivative
Therapeutic Class: Antihistamine; antivertigo agent

CLINICAL PHARMACOLOGY
Mechanism of Action: Has a depressant action on hyperstimulated labyrinthine function; antiemetic effects may be due to diphenhydramine moiety (dimenhydrinate is a mixture of diphenhydramine and 8-chlorotheophylline)
Pharmacokinetics
PO: Onset 15-30 min
IM: Onset 20-30 min
Duration 3-6 hr; metabolized in liver, excreted in urine
INDICATIONS AND USES: Prevention and treatment of motion sickness; Meniere's disease,* other vestibular disturbances*
DOSAGE
Adult
• PO 50-100 mg q4-6h, do not exceed 400 mg/day; IM/IV 50 mg prn
Child 6-12 yr
• PO 25-50 mg/q6-8h, do not exceed 150 mg/day; IM 1.25 mg/kg or 37.5 mg/m² qid, do not exceed 300 mg/day
Child 2-6 yr
• PO 12.5-25 mg q6-8h, do not exceed 75 mg/day
§ AVAILABLE FORMS/COST OF THERAPY
• Inj, Sol—IM, IV: 50 mg/ml, 10 ml: **$1.69-$12.48**
• Liq—Oral: 12.5 mg/4 ml, 120, 480 ml: **$12.48**/480 ml
• Tab, Uncoated—Oral: 50 mg, 100's: **$0.77-$21.13**

• Tab, Chewable—Oral: 50 mg, 24's: **$6.35**
CONTRAINDICATIONS: Neonates (IV products may contain benzyl alcohol)
PRECAUTIONS: Children, prostatic hypertrophy, stenosing peptic ulcer, pyloroduodenal obstruction, bladder neck obstruction, narrow-angle glaucoma, cardiac dysrhythmias, elderly, children <2 yr
PREGNANCY AND LACTATION: Pregnancy category B; has been used for the treatment of hyperemesis gravidarum; small amounts are excreted into breast milk; use caution in nursing mothers
SIDE EFFECTS/ADVERSE REACTIONS
CNS: Confusion, dizziness, *drowsiness,* excitation, headache, heaviness and weakness of hands, insomnia (especially in children), lassitude, nervousness, restlessness, tingling, vertigo
CV: Palpitations, tachycardia
EENT: Blurring of vision, diplopia, nasal stuffiness
GI: Anorexia, constipation, diarrhea, *dry mouth,* epigastric distress, nausea, vomiting
GU: Difficult or painful urination
HEME: **Hemolytic anemia**
SKIN: Drug rash, photosensitivity, urticaria
SPECIAL CONSIDERATIONS
PATIENT/FAMILY EDUCATION
• For prevention of motion sickness administer at least 30 min before exposure to motion

* = non-FDA-approved use

dimercaprol
(dye-mer-kap'role)

Rx: BAL in Oil, British Anti-Lewisite

Chemical Class: Dithiol derivative

Therapeutic Class: Heavy metal antidote (arsenic, gold, mercury, lead)

CLINICAL PHARMACOLOGY

Mechanism of Action: Promotes excretion of heavy metals by chelation, increasing urinary and fecal elimination of the metals

Pharmacokinetics

IM: Peak 30-60 min; metabolism and excretion are complete within 4 hr, excretion via urine and feces

INDICATIONS AND USES: Treatment of arsenic, gold, and mercury poisoning; acute lead poisoning (in conjunction with calcium edetate disodium)

DOSAGE

Adult and Child

• *Mild arsenic and gold poisoning:* IM 2.5 mg/kg/dose q6h for 2 days, then q12h on 3rd day, then qd thereafter for 10 days

• *Severe arsenic and gold poisoning:* IM 3 mg/kg/dose q4h for 2 days, then q6h on 3rd day, then q12h thereafter for 10 days

• *Mercury poisoning:* IM 5 mg/kg initially followed by 2.5 mg/kg/dose qd-bid for 10 days

• *Lead poisoning:* IM 4 mg/kg alone for first dose, then 3-4 mg/kg/dose with calcium edetate disodium administered at a separate site q4h for 5-7 days

⑤ AVAILABLE FORMS/COST OF THERAPY

• Inj, Sol—IM: 100 mg/ml, 3 ml: **$74.76**

CONTRAINDICATIONS: Hepatic insufficiency (except postarsenical jaundice); iron, cadmium, or selenium poisoning; severe renal disease

PRECAUTIONS: Acute renal insufficiency, G-6-PD deficiency, acidic urine, hypertension

PREGNANCY AND LACTATION: Pregnancy category D; use only in life-threatening poisoning

SIDE EFFECTS/ADVERSE REACTIONS

CNS: Anxiety, headache

CV: Rise in blood pressure, tachycardia

EENT: Burning sensation in the lips, mouth and throat; conjunctivitis, lacrimation, blepharal spasm; feeling of constriction in the throat; rhinorrhea

GI: Abdominal pain, *nausea,* salivation, *vomiting*

GU: Burning sensation in the penis

SKIN: Sweating

SPECIAL CONSIDERATIONS

• Administer by deep IM injection only

MONITORING PARAMETERS

• Blood pressure, pulse

• BUN, Cr, urine pH (alkaline urinary pH decreases renal damage)

• Specific heavy metal levels

dinoprostone (PGE$_2$)
(dye-noe-prost'one)

Rx: Cervidil, Prepidil Gel, Prostin E$_2$

Chemical Class: Prostaglandin

Therapeutic Class: Abortifacient; uterine stimulant

CLINICAL PHARMACOLOGY

Mechanism of Action: Stimulates uterine contractions, GI and vascular smooth muscle

---

italic = common side effects   ***bold italic*** = life-threatening reactions

Pharmacokinetics
Onset 20 min (more rapid from gel form); metabolized in spleen, kidney, lungs, excreted in urine

INDICATIONS AND USES: Abortion during 2nd trimester, benign hydatidiform mole, expulsion of uterine contents in fetal deaths to 28 wk, missed abortion, cervical ripening, labor induction

DOSAGE
Adult
• *Abortifacient:* Vag supp (Prostin E$_2$)—20 mg high into vagina, repeat q3-5h until abortion occurs, max 240 mg
• *Cervical ripening:* Gel (Prepidil)—administer contents of 1 syringe (0.5 mg) into cervical canal just below the internal os, repeat in 6 hr prn, max 1.5 mg/24 hr; Insert (Cervidil)—Place transversely in posterior fornix of vagina; remove after 12 hr

§ AVAILABLE FORMS/COST OF THERAPY
• Gel—Cervical: 0.5 mg/3 g: **$97.96**
• Insert—Vag: 0.3 mg/hr: **$202.74**
• Supp—Vag: 20 mg, 1's: **$135.06**

CONTRAINDICATIONS: SUPP: Acute PID; cardiac, pulmonary, renal, or hepatic disease; viable fetus; GEL: History of major uterine surgery (including C-section with vertical uterine scar), cephalopelvic disproportion, grand multiparae (≥6 previous term pregnancies), non-vertex presentation, hyperactive or hypertonic uterine patterns, fetal distress, obstetric emergencies favoring surgical intervention, placenta previa or unexplained vaginal bleeding, vasa previa, active herpes genitalia

PRECAUTIONS: Asthma, glaucoma, hepatic/renal function impairment, hypotension, hypertension, cardiovascular disease, anemia, jaundice, diabetes, epilepsy, chorioamnionitis, cervicitis, infected endocervical lesions, acute vaginitis, previous C-section with transverse uterine scar, ruptured membranes

PREGNANCY AND LACTATION: Pregnancy category C; complete any failed attempts at pregnancy termination by some other means

SIDE EFFECTS/ADVERSE REACTIONS

CNS: Chills, dizziness, fever, *headache*
CV: Hypertension (transient)
EENT: Blurred vision
GI: Diarrhea, nausea, vomiting
GU: Vaginal pain, vaginismus, vaginitis, vulvitis
HEME: Transient leukocytosis
MS: Joint swelling, leg cramps, weakness
SKIN: Rash, skin color changes

INTERACTIONS
Drugs
• *Oxytoxin:* Augmented activity, use sequentially not concurrently (6-12 hr after gel, 30 min after removal of insert)

SPECIAL CONSIDERATIONS
• Do not place gel above level of internal os; use 20 mm endocervical catheter if no effacement present; 10 mm catheter if cervix 50% effaced
• May use small amount water soluble lubricant with insert; do not use insert without retrieval system

PATIENT/FAMILY EDUCATION
• Remain supine for 10-15 min (vag supp), 15-30 min (gel), 2h (insert)

MONITORING PARAMETERS
• Blood pressure, fetal monitor (for cervical ripening)

---

* = non-FDA-approved use

diphenhydramine
(dye-fen-hye´dra-meen)

Rx: Banaril, Benadryl, Dytuss, Hyrexin, Tusstat, Tuxadryl

OTC: Allermax, Banophen, Banophen Caplets, Belix, Benadryl 25, Benylin Cough, Bydramine Cough, Diphen Cough, Dormarex 2, Genahist, Gen-D-phen, Hydramine Cough, Nidryl, Nordryl Cough, Phendry, Uni-Bent Cough

Combinations

   OTC: with acetaminophen (Excedrin PM, Extra Strength Tylenol PM, Sominex Pain Relief, Unisom with Pain Relief); with calamine (Caladryl)

Chemical Class: Ethanolamine derivative

Therapeutic Class: Antihistamine; antivertigo agent; antipruritic; hypnotic; antianaphylactic (adjunct); antiparkinson's agent

---

CLINICAL PHARMACOLOGY
Mechanism of Action: Decreases allergic response by blocking histamine at H_1-receptors

Pharmacokinetics
PO: Peak 2-4 hr, 78% bound to plasma proteins; metabolized in the liver; $t_{1/2}$ 2-8 hr

INDICATIONS AND USES: Perennial and seasonal allergic rhinitis; vasomotor rhinitis; allergic conjunctivitis; symptomatic relief of common cold; allergic and non-allergic pruritic symptoms; uncomplicated allergic skin manifestations of urticaria and angioedema; adjunctive therapy of anaphylactic reactions; motion sickness; sleep aid; parkinsonism (including drug-induced); cough suppressant; acute dystonic reactions

DOSAGE
Adult
• PO/IM/IV 15-50 mg q4h, do not exceed 400 mg/day; for sleep PO 50 mg at hs; TOP apply prn

Child
• PO/IM/IV 5 mg/kg/day or 150 mg/m^2/day divided q6-8h, do not exceed 300 mg/day

💲 AVAILABLE FORMS/COST OF THERAPY
• Cap, Gel—Oral: 25 mg, 100's: **$1.04-$21.69**; 50 mg, 100's: **$1.12-$29.25**
• Cream—Top: 2%, 15 g: **$2.93-$11.05**
• Elixir—Oral: 12.5 mg/5 ml, 480 ml: **$2.40-$15.50**
• Inj, Sol—IM, IV: 10 mg/ml, 30 ml: **$2.00-$8.25**; 50 mg/ml, 1 ml: **$1.03-$2.94**
• Spray—Top: 2%, 60 ml: **$4.57-$4.74**

CONTRAINDICATIONS: Narrow-angle glaucoma, bladder neck obstruction

PRECAUTIONS: Liver disease, elderly, increased intraocular pressure, hyperthyroidism, cardiovascular disease, hypertension, urinary retention, renal disease, stenosed peptic ulcers

PREGNANCY AND LACTATION: Pregnancy category C; excreted into breast milk; although levels are not thought to be sufficiently high after therapeutic doses to affect the infant, the manufacturer considers the drug contraindicated in nursing mothers due to the increased sensitivity of newborn or premature infants to antihistamines

---

italic = common side effects   ***bold italic*** = life-threatening reactions

SIDE EFFECTS/ADVERSE REACTIONS

CNS: Anxiety, confusion, *dizziness, drowsiness,* euphoria, fatigue, neuritis, paresthesia, poor coordination
CV: Palpitations, tachycardia
EENT: Blurred vision, dilated pupils, *dry nose, throat,* nasal stuffiness, tinnitus
GI: Anorexia, *constipation,* diarrhea, *dry mouth,* nausea, vomiting
GU: Dysuria, frequency, impotence, retention
HEME: **Bone marrow suppression, hemolytic anemia**
RESP: Chest tightness, increased thick secretions, wheezing
SKIN: Photosensitivity, rash, urticaria; topical preparations can sensitize the skin

INTERACTIONS

Drugs

3 *Anticholinergics:* Possible enhanced anticholinergic, CNS effects

Labs

• *False negative:* Skin allergy tests
• *False positive:* Urine methadone, serum and urine tricyclic antidepressant

---

diphenoxylate and atropine

(dye-fen-ox′i-late)

Rx: Lomocot, Lomotil, Lonox. Vi-Atro, Motofen (difenoxin and atropine)
Chemical Class: Meperidine analog
Therapeutic Class: Antidiarrheal
DEA Class: Schedule V, Schedule IV (Motofen)

CLINICAL PHARMACOLOGY

Mechanism of Action: Direct effect on circular smooth muscle of the bowel that prolongs GI transit time; available only in combination with atropine sulfate (to discourage deliberate overdosage); lacks analgesic activity

Pharmacokinetics

PO: Onset 1 hr, peak 2 hr, duration 3-4 hr; metabolized in liver, excreted in bile and urine; difenoxin is the principal active metabolite of diphenoxylate

INDICATIONS AND USES: Diarrhea, reduction of ileostomy discharge

DOSAGE

Adult

• diphenoxylate PO 5 mg (2 tab or 10 ml) qid, then taper dose as tolerated; difenoxin PO 2 mg (2 tab) initially, then 1 mg (1 tab) after each loose stool or q3-4h prn, max 8 mg (8 tab)/24 hr

Child 2-12 yr

• PO, Sol 0.3-0.4 mg/kg qd in 4 divided doses; difenoxin not recommended in children <12 yr

$ AVAILABLE FORMS/COST OF THERAPY

• Sol—Oral: 2.5 mg diphenoxylate/0.025 mg atropine/5 ml, 60 ml: **$6.28-$19.86**
• Tab, Uncoated—Oral: 2.5 mg diphenoxylate/0.025 mg atropine, 100's: **$3.15-$67.21**
• Tab, Uncoated—Oral: 1 mg difenoxin/0.025 mg atropine, 100's: **$17.53-$62.20**

CONTRAINDICATIONS: Obstructive jaundice, diarrhea associated with pseudomembranous enterocolitis or enterotoxin-producing bacteria; child <2 yr (difenoxin only)

PRECAUTIONS: Age <2 yr (diphenoxylate), acute ulcerative colitis (may induce toxic megacolon), severe hepatorenal disease, fluid and electrolyte imbalances, Down's syndrome

PREGNANCY AND LACTATION:
Pregnancy category C; excreted in breast milk

SIDE EFFECTS/ADVERSE REACTIONS

CNS: Fatigue, *dizziness, drowsiness,* depression, insomnia, restlessness

EENT: Dry mouth, blurred vision

GI: Abdominal pain or distention, constipation, ileus, *nausea,* vomiting

SKIN: Rash (hypersensitivity)

INTERACTIONS

Drugs

❷ *MAOIs:* Possible hypertensive crisis

❸ *Barbiturates, tranquilizers, narcotics, alcohol:* Potentiation of effects

SPECIAL CONSIDERATIONS

• Equally effective as codeine or loperamide

PATIENT/FAMILY EDUCATION

• Prolonged use not recommended

• Drowsiness or dizziness may occur; use caution when driving or operating dangerous machinery

---

dipyridamole

(dye-peer-id′a-mole)

Rx: Persantine

Combinations

  Rx: with aspirin (Aggrenox)

Chemical Class: Substituted pyrimidine derivative

Therapeutic Class: Coronary vasodilator, antiplatelet agent

CLINICAL PHARMACOLOGY

Mechanism of Action: Inhibits platelet adhesion, likely by inhibiting thromboxane A_2 formation and inhibiting phosphodiesterase

Pharmacokinetics

PO: Onset 30 min, peak 2-2½ hr, duration 6 hr

IV: Onset 1 min, peak 7 min, duration 30 min

Protein binding 91%-99%, conjugated in liver to glucuronide, excreted in bile, undergoes enterohepatic recirculation

INDICATIONS AND USES: Adjunct to warfarin to prevent thromboembolic complications of cardiac valve replacement; adjunct to aspirin to prevent coronary bypass graft occlusion* or transient ischemic attack*; as diagnostic aid in thallium myocardial perfusion imaging for the evaluation of CAD; to reduce the risk of stroke in patients who have had transient ischemia of the brain or completed ischemic stroke caused by thrombosis (Aggrenox)

DOSAGE

Adult

• Adjunct to warfarin therapy: PO 75-100 mg qid

• *Diagnostic aid in myocardial perfusion studies:* IV 0.14 mg/kg/min for 4 min, max dose 60 mg

Child

• *Inhibition of platelet adhesion:* PO 3-6 mg/kg/day in 3 divided doses

🖫 **AVAILABLE FORMS/COST OF THERAPY**

• Inj, Sol—IV: 5 mg/ml, 10 ml: **$27.60-$157.80**

• Tab, Coated—Oral: 25 mg, 100's: **$3.75-$51.59**; 50 mg, 100's: **$7.28-$80.60**; 75 mg, 100's: **$9.75-$107.81**

PRECAUTIONS: Ischemic heart disease, bleeding disorders, hypotension

PREGNANCY AND LACTATION: Pregnancy category C; excreted in breast milk

SIDE EFFECTS/ADVERSE REACTIONS

CNS: Dizziness, headache

GI: Abdominal distress, anorexia, diarrhea, nausea, vomiting

SKIN: Flushing, rash

INTERACTIONS

Drugs

🔳 *Adenosine:* Increased concentrations of adenosine, potentiates adenosine's pharmacologic effects

🔳 *Beta blockers:* Additive bradycardia

SPECIAL CONSIDERATIONS

• Contributes little to the effect of aspirin alone

---

dirithromycin

(die-rith-ro-my'sin)

Rx: Dynabac

Chemical Class: Macrolide antibiotic

Therapeutic Class: Antibiotic

CLINICAL PHARMACOLOGY

Mechanism of Action: Bacteriostatic via reversible binding to 50S ribosomal unit, thereby impairing protein synthesis

Pharmacokinetics

PO: Peak 4 hr; rapidly absorbed and converted by nonenzymatic hydrolysis to the microbiologically active compound erythromycylamine; 15%-32% protein bound; good tissue penetration into upper and lower respiratory tract and prostate; nonenzymatic hydrolysis to inactive metabolites; fecal and renal elimination; $t_{1/2}$ 44 hr

INDICATIONS AND USES: Infections of upper (including otitis media, pharyngitis, tonsillitis) and lower respiratory tract, skin and skin structure caused by susceptible organisms

Antibacterial spectrum usually includes:

• Gram-positive organisms: *Streptococcus pneumonia, Staphylococcus aureus, Str. pyogenes*

• Gram-negative organisms: *Legionella, Moraxella catarrhalis*

• Anerobes: *P. acnes*

• *Other: Mycoplasma pneumonia, Chlamydia trachomatis*

DOSAGE

Adult (Child >12 yr)

• PO 500 mg qd for 7-14 days

🔳 **AVAILABLE FORMS/COST OF THERAPY**

• Tab, Enteric Coated—Oral: 250 mg, 60's: **$112.50-$232.07**

PRECAUTIONS: Hepatic insufficiency

PREGNANCY AND LACTATION: Pregnancy category C; excreted into rodent breast milk; no human data

SIDE EFFECTS/ADVERSE REACTIONS

CNS: Asthenia, dizziness, headache

GI: Abdominal pain, diarrhea, dyspepsia, gas, *nausea,* vomiting

INTERACTIONS

Drugs

🔳 *Penicillins:* Dirithromycin may inhibit antibacterial activity of penicillins

SPECIAL CONSIDERATIONS

• Long $t_{1/2}$ and higher tissue concentrations allow qd dosing; however, the improved antimicrobial activity against *H.influenzae* and lower incidence of GI adverse effects have not been realized with this agent; Azithromycin probably best choice pending further comparisons

PATIENT/FAMILY EDUCATION

• Take with food or within 1 hr of having eaten

---

* = non-FDA-approved use

disopyramide

(dye-soe-peer'a-mide)
Rx: Norpace, Norpace CR
Chemical Class: Substituted pyramide derivative
Therapeutic Class: Antidys-rhythmic (class IA)

D

CLINICAL PHARMACOLOGY
Mechanism of Action: Lengthens effective refractory period of the atrium and ventricle; decreases conduction velocity; has minimal effect on effective refractory period of the AV node; decreases the disparity in refractoriness between infarcted and adjacent normal myocardium; anticholinergic actions

Pharmacokinetics
PO: Peak 30 min-3 hr, duration 6-12 hr, $t_{1/2}$ 4-10 hr; metabolized in liver, excreted unchanged in urine (50%) and feces (10%); crosses placenta; protein binding concentration dependent (50%-65% at plasma levels of 2-4 µg/ml)

INDICATIONS AND USES: Life-threatening ventricular dysrhythmias such as sustained ventricular tachycardia; supraventricular tachycardia*

DOSAGE
Adult
• PO 100-200 mg q6h; in renal dysfunction, if CrCl 30-40 ml/min, dose should be 100 mg q8h, if CrCl 15-30 ml/min, dose should be 100 mg q12h, if CrCl <15 ml/min, dose should be 100 mg q24h; may give loading dose of 300 mg for rapid effect; PO (Sus Action CAP) 200-300 mg q12h; not recommended in renal dysfunction

Child
• PO age 12-18 yr: 6-15 mg/kg/day in divided doses q6h; age 4-12 yr: 10-15 mg/kg/day in divided doses q6h; age 1-4 yr: 10-20 mg/kg/day in divided doses q6h; age <1 yr: 10-30 mg/kg/day in divided doses q6h

💲 AVAILABLE FORMS/COST OF THERAPY
• Cap, Gel—Oral: 100 mg, 100's: **$13.50-$78.71**; 150 mg, 100's: **$19.43-$92.95**
• Cap, Gel, Sus Action—Oral: 100 mg, 100's: **$57.56-$94.78**; 150 mg, 100's: **$93.24-$114.75**

CONTRAINDICATIONS: 2nd or 3rd degree block, cardiogenic shock, CHF (uncompensated), sick sinus syndrome, QT prolongation

PRECAUTIONS: Children, diabetes mellitus, renal disease, hepatic disease, myasthenia gravis, narrow-angle glaucoma, cardiomyopathy, conduction abnormalities (including accessory pathways)

PREGNANCY AND LACTATION: Pregnancy category C; excreted in breast milk

SIDE EFFECTS/ADVERSE REACTIONS
CNS: Anxiety, depression, *dizziness,* fatigue, *headache,* insomnia, paresthesias, psychosis

CV: Angina, **AV block,** *bradycardia,* **cardiac arrest, CHF,** chest pain, edema, *hypotension,* increased QRS or QT duration, PVCs, syncope, tachycardia

EENT: Blurred vision; dry nose, throat, eyes; narrow-angle glaucoma

GI: Anorexia, *constipation (11%),* diarrhea, *dry mouth (32%),* flatulence, nausea, vomiting

GU: Hesitancy (14%), impotence, *retention,* urinary frequency, urgency

HEME: **Agranulocytosis,** anemia (rare), **thrombocytopenia**

METAB: Hypoglycemia

MS: Pain in extremities, weakness

SKIN: Pruritus, rash, urticaria

---

italic = common side effects   ***bold italic*** = life-threatening reactions

INTERACTIONS
Drugs
🟦 *Barbiturates, phenytoin, rifampin:* Reduced disopyramide level via induction

🟦 *Beta blockers:* Enhanced negative inotropy

🟦 *Clarithromycin, erythromycin, troleandromycin:* Macrolide increased disopyramide-serum concentration resulting in dysrhythmias

🟦 *Lidocaine:* Arrhythmias or heart failure in predisposed patients

🟦 *Potassium, potassium-sparing diuretics:* Increased potassium concentration can enhance disopyramide effects on myocardial conduction

Labs
• *Increase:* Liver enzymes, lipids, BUN, creatinine
• *Decrease:* Hgb/hct, blood glucose

SPECIAL CONSIDERATIONS
• Due to potential for prodysrhythmic effects, use for asymptomatic PVCs or lesser dysrhythmias should be avoided

MONITORING PARAMETERS
• Monitor ECG closely; if PR, QRS, or QT interval increase by 25%, stop drug
• Therapeutic plasma levels are 2-4 µg/ml

---

disulfiram
(dye-sul′fi-ram)
Rx: Antabuse
Chemical Class: Thiuram derivative
Therapeutic Class: Alcohol deterrent

CLINICAL PHARMACOLOGY
Mechanism of Action: Blocks oxidation of alcohol at acetaldehyde stage; accumulation of acetaldehyde produces disulfiram–alcohol reaction

Pharmacokinetics
PO: Onset 12 hr, effect lasts up to 2 wk; oxidized by liver; metabolites excreted by kidney, 20% excreted unchanged in feces

INDICATIONS AND USES: Adjunctive treatment of chronic alcoholism

DOSAGE
Adult
• PO 250-500 mg qd for 1-2 wk, then 125-500 mg qd until fully socially recovered

💲 **AVAILABLE FORMS/COST OF THERAPY**
• Tab, Uncoated—Oral: 250 mg, 100's: **$6.50-$140.40**; 500 mg, 50's: **$11.95-$74.25**

CONTRAINDICATIONS: Alcohol intoxication, psychoses, cardiovascular disease; recent use of metronidazole, isoniazid, paraldehyde, alcohol, or alcohol-containing preparations (e.g., cough syrups, tonics); patients with history of rubber contact dermatitis should be evaluated for hypersensitivity to thiuram derivatives before receiving

PRECAUTIONS: Hypothyroidism, hepatic disease, diabetes mellitus, seizure disorders, nephritis, stroke

PREGNANCY AND LACTATION: Pregnancy category X; excreted in breast milk

---

SIDE EFFECTS/ADVERSE REACTIONS

CNS: Dizziness, *drowsiness,* fatigue, *headache,* neuritis, peripheral neuropathy, psychosis, restlessness, ***seizures,*** sweating, tremors

GI: Anorexia, ***hepatotoxicity,*** metallic or garlic-like taste, nausea, severe thirst, vomiting

METAB: Increased cholesterol

SKIN: Dermatitis, rash, urticaria

MISC: ***Disulfiram–alcohol reaction: flushing, sweating, headache, nausea, vomiting, chest pain, palpitations, dyspnea, tachycardia, confusion, and hypotension (reactions may occur with blood ethanol level as low as 5-10 mg/dl)***

INTERACTIONS

Drugs

🔳 *Benzodiazepines (clonazepam, clorazepate, diazepem, flurazepam, halazepam, prazepam, triazolam):* Increased serum concentrations of these drugs

🔳 *Cocaine:* Substantial increase in plasma cocaine levels and cardiovascular effects

🔳 *Co-trimoxazole:* IV co-trimoxazole contains 10% ethanol; ethanol intolerance possible

⚠ *Ethanol:* Severe ethanol intolerance; warn patients to avoid all forms of ethanol

❷ *Isoniazid:* Use with disulfiram promotes encephalopathy

🔳 *Metronidazole:* Use with disulfiram promotes encephalopathy

❷ *Oral anticoagulants:* Increased hypoprothromburemic response to oral anticoagulants

🔳 *Phenytoin:* Increased phenytoin levels, toxicity possible

🔳 *Theophylline:* Increased theophylline levels, toxicity possible

🔳 *Tranylcypromine:* Case report of delirium in one patient

SPECIAL CONSIDERATIONS
PATIENT/FAMILY EDUCATION

• Disulfiram–alcohol reaction may occur for 2 wk after last dose
• May occur with external use of alcohol-containing products (i.e., liniments)
• Do not administer 1st dose until patient has abstained from alcohol for at least 12 hr

D

dobutamine

(doe-byoo′ta-meen)
Rx: Dobutrex
Chemical Class: Synthetic catecholamine
Therapeutic Class: β-Adrenergic agonist: sypathomimetic

CLINICAL PHARMACOLOGY

Mechanism of Action: Direct acting positive inotropic agent via β-adrenoceptor agonism producing additional mild chronotropic, hypertensive, arrhythmogenic and vasodilative effects; does not release endogenous nonepinepherine; in patients with depressed cardiac function, increases cardiac output, without increased heart rate; systemic vascular resistance is usually decreased

Pharmacokinetics

IV: Onset 1-2 min, peak 10 min, $t_{1/2}$ 2 min; metabolized in liver (inactive metabolites); metabolites excreted in urine

INDICATIONS AND USES: Short-term treatment of adults with cardiac decompensation due to depressed myocardial contractility; diagnostic aid for ischemic heart disease*

DOSAGE

Adult

• IV INF 2.5-15 μg/kg/min, max dose 40 μg/kg/min

---

italic = common side effects   ***bold italic*** = life-threatening reactions

$ AVAILABLE FORMS/COST OF THERAPY

• Inj, Dry-Sol—IV: 12.5 mg/ml, 20 ml: **$5.63-$51.88**

CONTRAINDICATIONS: Hypertrophic cardiomyopathy, uncontrolled atrial fibrillation or flutter (unless a digitalis preparation is used prior to starting therapy with dobutamine)

PRECAUTIONS: Children, hypertension, sulfite sensitivity (preparation may contain sulfite)

PREGNANCY AND LACTATION: Pregnancy category C; excreted in breast milk

SIDE EFFECTS/ADVERSE REACTIONS

CNS: Anxiety, dizziness, headache, paresthesia

CV: Angina, *dysrhythmia,* hypertension, palpitations, *PVCs, tachycardia*

GI: Heartburn, nausea, vomiting

METAB: Hypokalemia

MS: Leg cramps

INTERACTIONS

Drugs

• *Sodium bicarbonate:* Alkalinizing substances inactivate dobutamine

SPECIAL CONSIDERATIONS
MONITORING PARAMETERS

• Continuously monitor ECG, BP, and PCWP

docusate
(dok'yoo-sate)

OTC: Sodium; Colace, Dioeze, Diocto, DOK, DOSS DSS, Modane Soft, Regulax SS

OTC: *Calcium;* Sulfolax, Surfak Stool Softener Combinations

OTC: with senna concentrate (Senokot-S); with phenolphthalein (Doxidan); with casanthranol (Peri-Colace); with cascara sagrada (Nature's Remedy)

Chemical Class: Anionic surfactant

Therapeutic Class: Stool softener; laxative

CLINICAL PHARMACOLOGY

Mechanism of Action: Detergent activity; facilitates admixture of fat and water to soften stool

Pharmacokinetics

PO: Onset 24-72 hr, absorbed to some extent in duodenum and jejunum; excreted in bile

INDICATIONS AND USES: Constipation associated with hard, dry stools; stool softener in patients who should avoid straining during defecation; cerumenolytic*

DOSAGE

Adult

• *Laxative/stool softener:* PO 50-400 mg/day in 1-4 divided doses

• *Cerumenolytic:* Fill ear canal with liquid; produces substantial ear wax disintegration in 15 min, complete disintegration after 24 hr

Child <3 yr

• PO 10-40 mg/day in 1-4 divided doses

Child 3-6 yr

• PO 20-60 mg/day in 1-4 divided doses

Child 6-12 yr
• PO 40-150 mg/day in 1-4 divided doses

$ AVAILABLE FORMS/COST OF THERAPY
• Cap, Softgel—Oral: 50 mg, 100's: **$2.95-$22.88**; 100 mg, 100's: **$1.40-$17.68**; 250 mg, 100's: **$1.83-$21.75**
• Liq—Oral: 150 mg/15 ml, 480 ml: **$7.33-$99.46**
• Syr—Oral: 60 mg/15 ml, 480 ml: **$2.00-$20.11**

CONTRAINDICATIONS: Obstruction, fecal impaction, nausea/vomiting, acute abdominal pain, concomitant use of mineral oil

PREGNANCY AND LACTATION: Pregnancy category C; no reports linking use of docusate with congenital defects have been located; diarrhea has been reported in 1 infant exposed to docusate while breast feeding, but relationship between symptom and drug is unknown

SIDE EFFECTS/ADVERSE REACTIONS
EENT: Throat irritation
GI: Anorexia, bitter taste, cramps, diarrhea, nausea
SKIN: Rash

SPECIAL CONSIDERATIONS
PATIENT/FAMILY EDUCATION
• Drink plenty of water during administration

dofetilide
(doe-fet'ill-ide)
Rx: Tikosyn
Chemical Class: Methanesulfonanilide derivative
Therapeutic Class: Antiarrhythmic: potassium channel blocker (class III antiarrhythmic)

D

CLINICAL PHARMACOLOGY
Mechanism of Action: Class III antiarrhythmic (i.e., selective potassium channel blocker); prolongs the duration of action potential, then, refractoriness by delaying the membrane repolarizatioin; ECG changes include prolongation of the QT and QTc intervals without change in the QRS interval; no effect on cardiac output, stroke volume index, or systemic vascular resistance; dose-dependent negative chronotropic effects but lacks negative inotropic activity

Pharmacokinetics
PO: Peak serum levels within 2-3 hr; bioavailability near 100%, unaffected by food; Vd 3L/kg; 60%-70% protein bound; 50% hepatic metabolism (CYP3A4); 50% unchanged recovered in urine; t½ 10 hr

INDICATIONS AND USES: Maintenance of normal sinus rhythm (delay in time to recurrence of atrial fibrillation/atrial flutter) in patients with atrial fibrillation/atrial flutter of greater than one wk duration who have been converted to normal sinus rhythm; conversion of atrial fibrillation and atrial flutter to normal sinus rhythm

DOSAGE
Adult
NOTE: 1) Dofetilide therapy must be initiated in a setting capable of providing continuous ECG monitoring

---

italic = common side effects   ***bold italic*** = life-threatening reactions

and management of serious ventricular arrhythmias; 2) Pretherapy anticoagulation should be initiated and continued after conversion according to customary medical practice; 3) Pretherapy ECG for determination of QTc <400 msec (500 msec with ventricular conduction abnormalities); 4) Pretherapy creatinine clearance calculation

• PO: initial dose 125-500 µg bid depending on calculated creatinine clearance; for calculated creatinine clearance >60 ml/min, use initial dose of 500 µg bid; 40-60 ml/min, 250 µg bid; 20-40 ml/min, 125 µg; dofetilide is contraindicated when calculated creatinine clearance is <20 ml/min

• PO continuation dosing 2-3 hr post initial dose, redetermine QTc: 1) if QTc >15% increase from baseline or 2) if QTc >400 msec, adjust dose as follows: if starting dose (based on CrCl) is 500 µg bid, adjusted dose for QTc prolongation is 250 µg bid; if starting dose is 250 µg bid, adjusted dose is 125 µg bid; if starting dose is 125 µg bid, adjusted dose is 125 µg bid

§ AVAILABLE FORMS/COST OF THERAPY

• Cap—Oral: 125 µg, 250 µg, 500 µg, 60's, all: **$108.00**

CONTRAINDICATIONS: Congenital or acquired long QT syndromes; baseline QTc >440 msec (500 msec in patients with ventricular conduction abnormalities); renal impairment (calculated creatinine clearance <20 ml/min)

PRECAUTIONS: Ventricular arrhythmia, renal impairment, hypokalemia

PREGNANCY AND LACTATION: Pregnancy category C; no information on the presence of dofetilide in breast milk; breast feeding while on dofetilide not advised

SIDE EFFECTS/ADVERSE REACTIONS

CNS: Headache, dizziness, insomnia, cerebral ischemia, cerebrovascular accident, facial paralysis, flaccid paralysis, migraine, paresthesia, syncope

CV: **Ventricular arrhythmias, including torsades de pointes,** *ventricular fibrillation, ventricular tachycardia, AV block, bundle branch block,* **heart block,** chest pain, bradycardia, edema, myocardial infarction

GI: Nausea, diarrhea, abdominal pain, liver damage

MS: Back pain

RESP: Respiratory tract infection, dyspnea, flu syndrome, angioedema, cough

SKIN: Rash

INTERACTIONS

Drugs

3 *Amiloride:* May compete with dofetilide for renal cationic secretion and subsequently increase dofetilide levels

2 *Cimetidine:* Increases dofetilide levels by 13%-58%, dose dependent

2 *Ketoconazole and other azole antifungals:* Increases dofetilide levels by 53%-97% by inhibition of CYP3A4

3 *Metformin:* May compete with dofetilide for renal cationic secretion and subsequently increase dofetilide levels

2 *Sulfamethoxazole:* Increases dofetilide AUC by 93% and Cmax by 103%

3 *Triamterene:* May compete with dofetilide for renal cationic secretion and subsequently increase dofetilide levels

2 *Trimethoprim:* Increases dofetilide AUC by 93% and Cmax by 103%

* = non-FDA-approved use

❷ *Verapamil:* Increases dofetilide levels by 42% and increased risk of torsade de pointes

❸ *Other potential drug interactions:* Macrolide antibiotics, protease inhibitors, serotonin reuptake inhibitors, amiodarone, cannabinoids, diltiazem, grapefruit juice, nefazodone, norfloxacin, quinine, zafirlukast: potential to increase dofetilide concentrations via inhibition of CYP3A4

SPECIAL CONSIDERATIONS
MONITORING PARAMETERS
• ECG, QTc intervals, renal function

---

dolasetron
(doe-lass'eh-tron)
Rx: Anzemet
Chemical Class: Nonbenzamide
Therapeutic Class: Antiemetic

CLINICAL PHARMACOLOGY
Mechanism of Action: Selectively blocks the action of serotonin at $5-HT_3$ receptors; cytotoxic chemotherapy appears to be associated with release of serotonin from enterochromaffin cells of the small intestine which may stimulate vagal afferents through $5-HT_3$ receptors initiating the vomiting reflex

Pharmacokinetics
IV: Peak <1 hr (active metabolite)
PO: Peak 1½ hr, bioavailability 59%
Rapidly metabolized to active metabolite which is 50 times more potent than parent compound; excreted in urine (45%-68%) and feces (25%); $t_{1/2}$ approximately 10 min (parent drug) and 8 hr (active metabolite)

INDICATIONS AND USES: Prevention of nausea and vomiting associated with emetogenic cancer chemotherapy; prevention and treatment of postoperative nausea and vomiting; radiotherapy-induced nausea and vomiting*

DOSAGE
Adult
• Chemotherapy: IV 1.8 mg/kg 30 min prior to chemotherapy; PO 100 mg as a single dose administered 1 hr prior to chemotherapy
• Postoperative: IV 12.5 mg as a single dose 15 min before cessation of anesthesia or when nausea and vomiting present; PO 100 mg 2 hr prior to surgery

Child (2-16 yr)
• Chemotherapy: IV 1.8 mg/kg 30 min prior to chemotherapy (100 mg max); PO 1.8 mg/kg 1 hr prior to chemotherapy (100 mg max)
• Postoperative: IV 0.35 mg/kg as a single dose 15 min before cessation of anesthesia or when nausea and vomiting present; PO 1.2 mg/kg within 2 hr before surgery (100 mg max)

🛇 AVAILABLE FORMS/COST OF THERAPY
• Inj—IV: 100 mg/vial: **$180.38**
• Tab—Oral: 50 mg, 5's: **$249.00-$299.59**; 100 mg, 5's: **$366.54-$397.09**

PRECAUTIONS: Hypertension, CAD, dysrhythmias, cardiac conduction defects, CHF, seizure disorder

PREGNANCY AND LACTATION: Pregnancy category B; excretion in breast milk unknown, use caution in nursing mothers

SIDE EFFECTS/ADVERSE REACTIONS
CNS: Dizziness, headache, lightheadedness
CV: ECG changes, hypertension, hypotension
EENT: Blurred vision
GI: Constipation, diarrhea, elevated transaminases, *increased appetite*
MISC: Chills, fever

---

italic = common side effects   ***bold italic*** = life-threatening reactions

SPECIAL CONSIDERATIONS
• No obvious advantage over other agents in this class (ondansetron, granisetron)

---

donepezil
(dah-nep´eh-zil)
Rx: Aricept
Chemical Class: Piperidine derivative
Therapeutic Class: Antidementia agent; cholinergic

CLINICAL PHARMACOLOGY
Mechanism of Action: Enhances cholinergic function by increasing the concentration of acetylcholine through reversible inhibition of its hydrolysis by acetylcholinesterase; does not appear to alter the course of the underlying dementing process
Pharmacokinetics
PO: Peak plasma concentration 3-4 hr; bioavailibility, 100%; 96% bound to plasma proteins; extensively metabolized to 4 major metabolites (2 are active), excreted mainly in urine (unchanged and metabolites); $t_{1/2}$ 70 hr
INDICATIONS AND USES: Mild to moderate dementia of the Alzheimer's type
DOSAGE
Adult
• PO 5 mg hs; may increase to 10 mg hs after 4-6 wk (higher dose has not been shown to provide a significantly greater clinical benefit for most patients and may increase cholinergic adverse events)
§ AVAILABLE FORMS/COST OF THERAPY
• Tab—Film-coated: 5 mg, 10 mg, 30's, all: **$473.09**
PRECAUTIONS: Sick sinus syndrome or other supraventricular cardiac conduction conditions, history of peptic ulcer disease, bladder outflow obstruction, seizure disorder, asthma/COPD
PREGNANCY AND LACTATION:
Pregnancy category C
SIDE EFFECTS/ADVERSE REACTIONS
CNS: Abnormal dreams, depression, dizziness, *fatigue,* headache, *insomnia,* somnolence
CV: Syncope
GI: Anorexia, *diarrhea, nausea, vomiting*
GU: Frequent urination
HEME: Ecchymosis
METAB: Weight decrease
MS: Arthritis, *muscle cramps*
INTERACTIONS
Drugs
⊠ *Fluvoxamine:* Possible increase in fluvoxamine levels
SPECIAL CONSIDERATIONS
• Clinicians were unable to notice improvement in the majority of patients in clinical trials; advantages over tacrine include qd dosing and apparent lack of liver toxicity
MONITORING PARAMETERS
• Close monitoring for clinical improvement and periodic reassessment of need for continued therapy

---

dopamine
(doe´pa-meen)
Rx: Intropin
Chemical Class: Synthetic catecholamine
Therapeutic Class: α- and β-adrenergic sympathomimetic; vasosuppressor

---

CLINICAL PHARMACOLOGY
Mechanism of Action: Stimulates both adrenergic and dopaminergic receptors in a dose-dependent manner; low doses (1-5 µg/kg/min) stimulate mainly dopaminergic re-

ceptors producing renal and mesenteric vasodilation; intermediate doses (5-15 µg/kg/min) stimulate both dopaminergic and β₁-adrenergic receptors producing cardiac stimulation and renal vasodilation; large doses (>15 µg/kg/min) stimulate α-adrenergic receptors producing vasoconstriction and increases in peripheral vascular resistance and blood pressure

Pharmacokinetics

IV: Onset 5 min, duration <10 min; metabolized in plasma, kidneys, and liver by MAO (75% to inactive metabolites, 25% to norepinephrine); t₁/₂ 2 min

INDICATIONS AND USES: Correction of hemodynamic imbalances in shock syndromes (e.g. MI, trauma, septicemia, renal failure, CHF); COPD*; CHF*; respiratory distress syndrome (RDS) in infants*

DOSAGE

Adult and Child

• IV INF 1-20 µg/kg/min, titrated to desired response; do not exceed 50 µg/kg/min

$ AVAILABLE FORMS/COST OF THERAPY

• Inj, Conc-Sol—IV: 40 mg/ml, 5 ml: **$0.84-$11.16**; 80 mg/ml, 5 ml: **$1.24-$8.31**; 160 mg/ml, 5 ml: **$1.10-$8.14**

CONTRAINDICATIONS: Pheochromocytoma, uncorrected tachydysrhythmia or ventricular fibrillation

PRECAUTIONS: Hypovolemia, arterial embolism, occlusive vascular disease, abrupt discontinuation, sulfite sensitivity, concurrent use of MAOIs

PREGNANCY AND LACTATION: Pregnancy category C; because dopamine is indicated only in life-threatening situations, chronic use would not be expected; no data available regarding use in breast feeding

SIDE EFFECTS/ADVERSE REACTIONS

CNS: Headache

CV: Aberrant conduction, *anginal pain,* bradycardia, *ectopic beats,* hypertension, *palpitation, tachycardia, vasoconstriction,* widened QRS complex

EENT: Dilated pupils (high doses)

GI: Nausea, vomiting

GU: Azotemia

RESP: Dyspnea

SKIN: Gangrene (high doses for prolonged periods of time), necrosis, piloerection, tissue sloughing with extravasation

INTERACTIONS

Drugs

🔳 *Ergot alkaloids:* Gangrene has been reported

🔳 *Phenytoin:* Increased risk of hypotension with IV phenytoin administration

Labs

• *False increase:* Urine amino acids; urine catecholamines; serum creatinine

• *False decrease:* Serum creatinine

SPECIAL CONSIDERATIONS

• *Dilute before use if not prediluted;* antidote for extravasation: infiltrate area as soon as possible with 10-15 ml NS containing 5-10 mg phentolamine

MONITORING PARAMETERS

• Urine flow, cardiac output, blood pressure, pulmonary wedge pressure

dornase alfa

(door′nace al′fa)

Rx: Pulmozyme

Chemical Class: Recombinant human deoxyribonuclease I
Therapeutic Class: Mucolytic

CLINICAL PHARMACOLOGY

Mechanism of Action: Hydrolyzes DNA in sputum of cystic fibrosis (CF) patients and reduces sputum viscoelasticity

Pharmacokinetics

INH: Does not produce significant elevations in serum DNase concentrations; no accumulation of serum DNase has been noted; following nebulization, enzyme levels are measurable in sputum within 15 min and decline rapidly thereafter

INDICATIONS AND USES: Cystic fibrosis (as an adjunct to standard therapies to reduce the frequency of respiratory infections requiring parenteral antibiotics and to improve pulmonary function)

DOSAGE

Adult and Child ≥5 yr

• NEB 2.5 mg qd; some patients (age >21, forced vital capacity (FVC) >70%) may benefit from bid administration

$ **AVAILABLE FORMS/COST OF THERAPY**

• Sol—INH: 1 mg/ml, 2.5 ml: **$34.37**

PRECAUTIONS: Safety and efficacy have not been demonstrated in children <5 yr or patients with FVC <40% of predicted

PREGNANCY AND LACTATION: Pregnancy category B; excretion into breast milk unknown; however, since serum levels of DNase have not been shown to increase above endogenous levels, little drug would be expected to be excreted into breast milk

SIDE EFFECTS/ADVERSE REACTIONS

Most events likely reflected sequelae of the underlying lung disease

CNS: Asthenia, fever

CV: Chest pain

EENT: Conjunctivitis, laryngitis, *pharyngitis, voice alteration*

GI: Abdominal pain, gallbladder disease, intestinal obstruction, liver disease, pancreatic disease

METAB: Diabetes mellitus, weight loss

MS: Flu-like syndrome

RESP: Apnea, bronchiectasis, change in sputum, cough increase, dyspnea, hemoptysis, hypoxia, lung function decrease, nasal polyps, rhinitis, sinusitis, sputum increase, wheeze

SKIN: Rash

SPECIAL CONSIDERATIONS

• Safety and efficacy have been demonstrated only with the following nebulizers and compressors: disposable jet nebulizer *Hudson T Updraft II,* disposable jet nebulizer *Marquest Acorn II* in conjunction with a *Pulmo-Aide* compressor, and reusable *PARI LC Jet+* nebulizer in conjunction with the *PARI PRONEB* compressor

PATIENT/FAMILY EDUCATION

• Must be stored in refrigerator at 2-8°C and protected from strong light (keep refrigerated when transporting and do not leave at room temp for >24 hr)

• Do not dilute or mix with other drugs in nebulizer

doxapram

(dox'a-pram)
Rx: Dopram
Chemical Class: Monohydrated pyrrolidinone derivative
Therapeutic Class: Analeptic

CLINICAL PHARMACOLOGY

Mechanism of Action: Respiratory stimulation through activation of peripheral carotid chemoreceptors; with higher doses medullary respiratory centers are stimulated

Pharmacokinetics

IV: Onset 20-40 sec, peak 1-2 min, duration 5-10 min; metabolized by liver, metabolites excreted by kidneys; $t_{1/2}$ 2.4-4.1 hr

INDICATIONS AND USES: Chronic obstructive pulmonary disease (COPD) associated with acute hypercapnia (temporary measure in hospitalized patients); postanesthesia respiratory stimulation; drug-induced CNS depression; apnea of prematurity resistant to methylxanthines*

DOSAGE

Adult

• *Postanesthetic respiratory stimulation:* IV inj 0.5-1 mg/kg, not to exceed 1.5 mg/kg total as a single inj, or 2 mg/kg total when given as multiple inj at 5 min intervals; IV INF 250 mg in 250 ml sol, initiate at 5 mg/min until response satisfactory, then maintain at 1-3 mg/min to sustain desired effect; recommended total dose 4 mg/kg

• *Drug-induced CNS depression:* IV inj priming dose of 2 mg/kg, repeated in 5 min, repeat q1-2h till patient awakes; IV INF priming dose of 2 mg/kg, if no response continue supportive measures and repeat priming dose in 1-2 hr, if some respiratory stimulation occurs infuse 1 mg/ml sol at 1-3 mg/min, not to exceed 3 g/day

• *COPD:* IV INF 1-2 mg/min, not to exceed 3 mg/min; do not infuse for longer than 2 hr

Child

• *Apnea of prematurity:* IV 2.5-3 mg/kg loading dose, followed by continuous INF of 1 mg/kg/hr; titrate to lowest rate at which apnea is controlled; do not exceed 2.5 mg/kg/hr

$ AVAILABLE FORMS/COST OF THERAPY

• Inj, Sol—IV: 20 mg/ml, 20 ml: **$40.61-$92.74**

CONTRAINDICATIONS: Seizure disorders; severe hypertension, bronchial asthma, dyspnea, or cardiac disorders; pneumothorax; pulmonary embolism; pulmonary fibrosis, conditions resulting in constriction of chest wall, muscles of respiration, or alveolar expansion; head injury; incompetence of ventilatory mechanism due to muscle paresis; flail chest

PRECAUTIONS: Bronchial asthma, pheochromocytoma, severe tachycardia, dysrhythmias, hypertension, children

PREGNANCY AND LACTATION: Pregnancy category B; excretion into breast milk unknown

SIDE EFFECTS/ADVERSE REACTIONS

CNS: Apprehension, bilateral Babinski, clonus, disorientation, dizziness, *headache,* hyperactivity, increased deep tendon reflexes, involuntary movements, pyrexia, *seizures*

CV: Chest pain, **dysrhythmias,** flushing, lowered T waves, *mild to moderate increase in blood pressure,* phlebitis, tightness in chest, *variations in heart rate*

---

italic = common side effects   ***bold italic*** = life-threatening reactions

EENT: **Laryngospasm,** pupillary dilation

GI: Desire to defecate, diarrhea, nausea, vomiting

GU: Proteinuria, spontaneous voiding, urinary retention

HEME: Decreased Hgb, hct, or RBC; decreased WBC in patients with pre-existing leukopenia; hemolysis (with rapid infusion)

RESP: **Bronchospasm,** cough, dyspnea, hiccups, rebound hypoventilation, tachypnea

SKIN: Local skin irritation with extravasation

INTERACTIONS
Drugs

3 *Anesthetics, inhalation:* Sensitized myocardium at risk of arrhythmia; delay administration of doxapram 10 min

2 *MAO Inhibitors:* Additive pressor effect

SPECIAL CONSIDERATIONS
MONITORING PARAMETERS

• Baseline ABG then q30 min (for use in COPD)

---

doxazosin
(dox-ay′zoe-sin)
Rx: Cardura
Chemical Class: Quinazoline derivative
Therapeutic Class: α_1-adrenergic blocker: antihypertensive; symptomatic benign prostatic hypertrophy

CLINICAL PHARMACOLOGY
Mechanism of Action: Selectively blocks postsynaptic α_1-adrenergic receptors; dilates both arterioles and veins, reducing peripheral vascular resistance and blood pressure; no reflex tachycardia or changes in renin release; blockade of α_1-adrenoceptors in bladder neck and prostate relaxes smooth muscle, improving urine flow rates in benign prostatic hypertrophy

Pharmacokinetics
PO: Onset 2 hr, peak 2-3 hr; 98% bound to plasma proteins; extensively metabolized in liver, excreted via bile, feces, and urine; $t_{1/2}$ 22 hr

INDICATIONS AND USES: Hypertension, benign prostatic hyperplasia

DOSAGE
Adult

• PO 1 mg qd, increasing to 16 mg qd if required; usual range 4-16 mg/day

§ **AVAILABLE FORMS/COST OF THERAPY**

• Tab, Uncoated—Oral: 1 mg, 100's: **$92.33-$109.18**; 2 mg, 100's: **$92.33-$116.59**; 4 mg, 100's: **$96.92-$114.60**; 8 mg, 100's: **$101.78-$120.34**

PRECAUTIONS: Children, hepatic disease

PREGNANCY AND LACTATION: Pregnancy category C; may accumulate in breast milk; use caution in nursing mothers

SIDE EFFECTS/ADVERSE REACTIONS

CNS: Anxiety, asthenia, ataxia, depression, *dizziness,* fever, *headache,* hypertonia, insomnia, nervousness, paresthesia, somnolence

CV: Chest pain, **dysrhythmia,** edema, flushing, palpitations, postural hypotension, tachycardia

EENT: Abnormal vision, tinnitus, vertigo

GI: Abdominal discomfort, constipation, diarrhea, dry mouth, flatulence, nausea, vomiting

GU: Incontinence, polyuria

MS: Arthralgia, myalgia

RESP: Dyspnea

SKIN: Pruritus, rash

INTERACTIONS
Drugs
■ *ACE inhibitors:* Increased potential for first dose hypotension

■ *Indomethacin:* Decreased hypotensive effect of doxazosin

■ *Verapamil, nifedipine:* Enhanced hypotensive effects of both drugs

■ *β-adrenergic blockers:* Exaggerated first-dose response

Labs
• False positive urinary metabolites of norepinephrine and VMA

• No effect on prostate specific antigen (PSA)

SPECIAL CONSIDERATIONS
• The doxazosin arm of the ALLHAT study was stopped early; the doxazosin group had a 25% greater risk of combined cardiovascular disease events which was primarily accounted for by a doubled risk of CHF vs the chlorthalidone group; doxazosin was also found to be less effective at controlling systolic BP an average of 3 mm Hg; may want to consider primary antihypertensives in addition to alpha blockers for BPH symptoms

• Use as a single antihypertensive agent limited by tendency to cause sodium and water retention and increased plasma volume

PATIENT/FAMILY EDUCATION
• Alert patient to the possibility of syncopal and orthostatic symptoms, especially with 1st dose ("1st-dose syncope")

• Initial dose should be administered at bedtime in the smallest possible dose

doxepin
(dox'eh-pin)

Rx: *Systemic:* Adapin, Sinequan; *Topical:* Zonalon
Chemical Class: Dibenzoxepin derivative: tertiary amine
Therapeutic Class: Tricyclic antidepressant; topical antipruritic

CLINICAL PHARMACOLOGY
Mechanism of Action: Inhibits reuptake of norepinephrine and serotonin (blocking activity slight and moderate, respectively) at the presynaptic neuron prolonging neuronal activity; inhibits histamine and acetylcholine activity; mild peripheral vasodilator effects and possible "quinidine-like" actions on cardiac conduction; moderate anticholinergic and orthostatic hypotensive, high sedative side effects

Pharmacokinetics
PO: Metabolized by liver to desmethyldoxepin (active), excreted by kidneys, $t_{1/2}$ 8-24 hr; 80%-85% bound to plasma proteins

INDICATIONS AND USES: Depression, anxiety, chronic pain,* peptic ulcer disease,* panic disorder,* dermatologic disorders,* pruritus associated with atopic dermatitis and lichen simplex chronicus (top formulation)

DOSAGE
Adult
• PO 50-75 mg/day in divided doses, may increase to 300 mg/day or may give daily dose hs; TOP apply thin film of cream qid for up to 8 days

Adolescents
• PO 25-50 mg/day in single or divided doses, gradually increase to 100 mg/day

---

🅂 AVAILABLE FORMS/COST OF THERAPY

• Cre—Top: 5%, 30, 45 g: **$21.82-$34.54**/30 g
• Cap, Gel—Oral: 10 mg, 100's: **$9.05-$125.62**; 25 mg, 100's: **$10.50-$53.78**; 50 mg, 100's: **$14.75-$75.68**; 75 mg, 100's: **$29.90-$125.54**; 100 mg, 100's: **$21.00-$136.88**; 150 mg, 100's: **$52.45-$231.71**
• Conc—Oral: 10 mg/ml, 120 ml: **$13.00-$31.32**

CONTRAINDICATIONS: Urinary retention, narrow-angle glaucoma, acute recovery phase of MI, concurrent use of MAOIs

PRECAUTIONS: Suicidal patients, seizure disorders, prostatic hypertrophy, psychiatric disease, severe depression, increased intraocular pressure, cardiac disease, hepatic disease, renal disease, hyperthyroidism, electroshock therapy, elective surgery, elderly, abrupt discontinuation, children

PREGNANCY AND LACTATION: Pregnancy category C (top formulation is category B); paralytic ileus has been observed in an infant exposed to doxepin and chlorpromazine at term; excreted into breast milk (as well as active metabolite); effect on nursing infant unknown, but may be of concern

SIDE EFFECTS/ADVERSE REACTIONS

CNS: Anxiety, confusion (especially in elderly), *dizziness, drowsiness,* extrapyramidal symptoms (elderly), fatigue, headache, increased psychiatric symptoms, insomnia, memory impairment, nervousness, nightmares, panic, stimulation, tremors, weakness

CV: **Dysrhythmias,** ECG changes, hypertension, *orthostatic hypotension,* palpitations, syncope, tachycardia

EENT: Blurred vision, mydriasis, nasal congestion, ophthalmoplegia, tinnitus

GI: Constipation, cramps, diarrhea, *dry mouth,* epigastric distress, hepatitis, increased appetite, jaundice, nausea, *paralytic ileus,* stomatitis, vomiting

GU: Urinary retention

HEME: **Agranulocytosis,** eosinophilia, *leukopenia, thrombocytopenia*

SKIN: Burning or stinging at application site, crackling (TOP), *dryness or tightness of skin,* edema, irritation, paresthesias, photosensitivity; pruritus, *pruritus or eczema exacerbation,* rash, scaling, sweating, tingling, urticaria

INTERACTIONS

Drugs

🛐 *Barbiturates:* Reduced serum concentrations of cyclic antidepressants

❷ *Bethanidine:* Reduced antihypertensive effect of bethanidine

🛐 *Carbamazepine:* Reduced cyclic antidepressant serum concentrations

❷ *Clonidine:* Reduced antihypertensive response to clonidine; enhanced hypertensive response with abrupt clonidine withdrawal

🛐 *Debrisoquin:* Inhibited antihypertensive response of debrisoquin

❷ *Epinephrine:* Markedly enhanced pressor response to IV epinephrine

🛐 *Ethanol:* Additive impairment of motor skills; abstinent alcoholics may eliminate cyclic antidepressants more rapidly than non-alcoholics

🛐 *Fluoxetine, flluvoxamine, grapefruit juice:* Marked increases in cyclic antidepressant plasma concentrations

🛐 *Guanethidine:* Inhibited antihypertensive response to guanethidine

❷ *Moclobemide:* Potential association with fatal or non-fatal serotonin syndrome

⚠ *MAOIs:* Excessive sympathetic response, mania, or hyperpyrexia possible

❸ *Neuroleptics:* Increased therapeutic and toxic effects of both drugs

❷ *Norepinephrine:* Markedly enhanced pressor response to norepinephrine

❷ *Phenylephrine:* Enhanced pressor response to IV phenylephrine

❸ *Propoxyphene:* Enhanced effect of cyclic antidepressants

❸ *Quinidine:* Increased cyclic antidepressant serum concentrations

SPECIAL CONSIDERATIONS

• Equally effective as other tricyclic antidepressants for depression; distinguishing characteristics include: sedative, anxiolytic, antihistaminic properties

PATIENT/FAMILY EDUCATION

• Therapeutic effects may take 4-6 wk

• Do not discontinue abruptly after long-term use

• If drowsiness occurs with top application, decrease surface area being treated or number of daily applications

MONITORING PARAMETERS

• CBC; ECG; mental status: mood, sensorium, affect, suicidal tendencies

doxycycline
(dox-i-sye′kleen)

Rx: Atridox, Doryx, Doxy, Doxy Caps, Doxychel Hyclate, Periostat, Vibramycin, Vibra-Tabs

Chemical Class: Tetracycline derivative

Therapeutic Class: Antibiotic

CLINICAL PHARMACOLOGY

Mechanism of Action: Inhibits protein synthesis by binding with the 30S and possibly the 50S ribosomal subunit(s) of susceptible organisms

Pharmacokinetics

PO: Peak 1.5-4 hr, food decreases absorption approximately 20%; 90% bound to plasma proteins; not metabolized in liver, partially inactivated in the GI tract by chelate formation; $t_{1/2}$ 15-26 hr; excreted in urine (23%) and feces (30%)

INDICATIONS AND USES: Rocky Mountain spotted fever; typhus fever and the typhus group; Q fever; rickettsialpox; tick fevers caused by Rickettsiae; respiratory tract infections; lymphogranuloma venereum; psittacosis (ornithosis); trachoma; inclusion conjunctivitis; uncomplicated urethral, endocervical, or rectal infections in adults; nongonococcal urethritis; relapsing fever; chancroid; plague; tularemia; cholera; *Campylobacter fetus* infections; brucellosis; bartonellosis; granuloma inguinale; malaria prophylaxis, acne, periodontitis subgingival scaling and root planing in adults Antibacterial spectrum usually includes:

• Gram-positive organisms: *Streptococcus pyogenes* (44% of strains found to be resistant), *Str. pneumoniae* (74% of strains found to be resistant), enterococcus group (*Str. faecalis* and *Str. faecium*), α-hemolytic streptococci (viridans group)

• Gram-negative organisms: *Neisseria gonorrhoeae, Calymmatobacterium granulomatis, Haemophilus ducreyi, H. influenzae, Yersinia pestis, Francisella tularensis, Vibrio cholera, Bartonella bacilliformis, Brucella* spp.

• Other organisms: Rickettsiae, *Clostridium* spp., *Chlamydia psittaci, C. trachomatis, Fusobacterium fusiforme, Actinomyces* spp., *Mycoplasma pneumoniae, Bacillus anthracis, Ureaplasma urealyticum, Propionibacterium acnes, Borrelia recurrentis, Entamoeba* spp., *Treponema pallidum, T. pertenue, Balantidium coli, Plasmodium falciparum*

DOSAGE

Adult

• PO/IV 100-200 mg/day in 1-2 divided doses

Child ≥ 8 yr

• PO/IV 2-5 mg/kg/day in 1-2 divided doses; do not exceed 200 mg/day

§ AVAILABLE FORMS/COST OF THERAPY

Doxycycline Calcium

• Syr—Oral: 50 mg/5ml, 480 ml: **$201.23**

Doxycycline Hyclate

• Cap—Oral: 20 mg, 100's: **$80.94-$85.00**

• Cap, Gel—Oral: 50 mg, 50's: **$6.30-$110.39**; 100 mg, 50's: **$12.71-$367.08**

• Cap, Gel, Coated Pellets—Oral: 75 mg, 60's: **$155.99**; 100 mg, 50's: **$83.63-$146.82**

• Inj, Sol—IV: 100 mg/vial: **$16.70**; 200 mg/vial: **$37.24**

• Powder, Reconst—Oral: 25 mg/5 ml, 60 ml: **$13.26**

• Tab, Plain Coated—Oral: 100 mg, 100's: **$55.44**

Doxycycline Monohydrate

• Cap, Gel—Oral: 50 mg, 100's: **$118.74-$145.12**; 100 mg, 100's: **$213.23**

• Tab, Plain Coated—Oral: 50 mg, 50's: **$145.12**; 100 mg, 50's: **$118.46**

CONTRAINDICATIONS: Children <8 yr

PRECAUTIONS: Hepatic disease, prolonged or repeated therapy

PREGNANCY AND LACTATION: Pregnancy category D; excreted into breast milk; theoretical possibility for dental staining seems remote because serum levels in infant undetectable

SIDE EFFECTS/ADVERSE REACTIONS

CNS: Fever, headache, paresthesia

CV: Pericarditis

GI: Abdominal cramps, abdominal pain, anorexia, *diarrhea,* enterocolitis, epigastric burning, flatulence, glossitis, hepatotoxicity, *nausea, pseudomembranous colitis,* stomatitis, vomiting

GU: Azotemia, increased BUN, polydipsia, polyuria

HEME: Eosinophilia, **hemolytic anemia, neutropenia, thrombocytopenia**

SKIN: **Exfoliative dermatitis,** highly irritating (avoid extravasation), *photosensitivity,* pruritus, rash, urticaria

MISC: Angioedema, bulging fontanels (infants), decreased calcification of deciduous teeth, pseudotumor cerebri (adults)

INTERACTIONS

Drugs

3 *Antacids:* Reduced serum concentration and efficacy of doxycycline

3 *Barbiturates:* Reduced serum doxycycline concentrations

3 *Bismuth:* Reduced bioavailability of doxycycline

🖻 *Calcium:* See antacids

🖻 *Carbamazepine:* Reduced serum doxycycline concentrations

🖻 *Cholestyramine; colestipol:* Reduced serum concentration of doxycycline; take 2 hr before or 3 hr after resin dose

🖻 *Ethanol:* Chronic ethanol ingestion may reduce the serum concentrations of doxycycline

🖻 *Iron:* Reduced serum concentration and efficacy of doxycycline

🖻 *Magnesium:* See antacids

🖻 *Oral contraceptives:* Potential for decreased efficacy of oral contraceptives

🖻 *Penicillins:* Doxycycline may reduce penicillin efficacy

🖻 *Phenytoin:* Reduced serum doxycycline concentrations

🖻 *Warfarin:* Potential for enhanced hypoprothrombinenic response to warfarin

🖻 *Zinc:* Reduced serum concentration of doxycycline; take 2 hr before or 3 hr after zinc

SPECIAL CONSIDERATIONS
• Tetracycline of choice due to broad spectrum, long $t_{1/2}$, superior tissue penetration, and excellent oral absorption

PATIENT/FAMILY EDUCATION
• Do not take with antacids, iron products
• Take with food

dronabinol

(droe-nab'i-nol)

Rx: Marinol
Chemical Class: Synthetic cannabinoid derivative
Therapeutic Class: Antiemetic, appetite stimulant
DEA Class: Schedule II

D

CLINICAL PHARMACOLOGY
Mechanism of Action: Central sympathomimetic and neural cannabinoid receptor activity mediate effect; tachyphylaxis and tolerance develop to psychological effects but not appetite stimulant effect

Pharmacokinetics
PO: Onset 30-60 min, peak effect 2-4 hr, duration of psychoactive effect 4-6 hr, appetite stimulant effect 24 hr; absorption 90%; highly lipid soluble; 97% protein bound; metabolized in liver; metabolites and drug excreted in bile (85%) and urine (15%); metabolites detected in urine for 5 wk after single dose

INDICATIONS AND USES: Nausea related to cancer chemotherapy not responsive to conventional agents; appetite stimulant in AIDS-related anorexia

DOSAGE
Adult
• *Antiemetic:* PO 5 mg/m^2 1-3 hr before chemotherapy, then q2-4h up to 6 doses qd; max dose 15 mg/m^2
• *Appetite stimulant:* PO 2.5 mg bid, 1 hr ac; max dose 20 mg qd

💲 **AVAILABLE FORMS/COST OF THERAPY**
• Cap, Elastic—Oral: 2.5 mg, 100's: **$335.16**; 5 mg, 100's: **$663.05**; 10 mg, 60's: **$826.55**

CONTRAINDICATIONS: Hypersensitivity to any cannabinoid or sesame oil

---

italic = common side effects   ***bold italic*** = life-threatening reactions

PRECAUTIONS: Children, history of abuse or dependence

PREGNANCY AND LACTATION: Pregnancy category C; excreted in breast milk

SIDE EFFECTS/ADVERSE REACTIONS

CNS: Abnormal thinking, *anxiety,* ataxia, confusion, depersonalization, *difficulty concentrating, dizziness, euphoria (24%),* hallucination, *mood change,* somnolence

CV: Orthostatic hypotension, palpitations, tachycardia, vasodilation

EENT: Change in vision, dry mouth, rhinitis, sinusitis, tinnitus

GI: Diarrhea, nausea, vomiting

MS: Myalgias

RESP: Cough

SKIN: Sweating

SPECIAL CONSIDERATIONS

• May have additive sedative or behavioral effects with CNS depressants

• Use caution escalating the dose because of increased frequency of adverse reactions at higher doses

---

droperidol

(droe-per'i-dole)

Rx: Inapsine

Combinations

   Rx: with fentanyl (Innovar)

Chemical Class: Butyrophenone derivative

Therapeutic Class: Antiemetic; sedative; anesthesia adjunct

CLINICAL PHARMACOLOGY

Mechanism of Action: Alters the action of dopamine at subcortical levels in CNS to produce sedation; produces mild α-adrenergic blockade, peripheral vascular dilation, and reduction of pressor effect of epinephrine

Pharmacokinetics

IV/IM: Onset 3-10 min (full effect may not be apparent for 30 min), duration 2-4 hr; metabolized in liver, excreted in urine and feces; $t_{1/2}$ 2.2 hr

INDICATIONS AND USES: Premedication for surgery; induction, maintenance in general anesthesia; antiemetic in cancer chemotherapy*

DOSAGE

Adult

• *Adjunct to general anesthesia:* IV 2.5 mg/10 kg given with analgesic or general anesthetic

• *Premedication for surgery:* IM 2.5-10 mg 30-60 min preoperatively

• *Maintaining general anesthesia:* IV 1.25-2.5 mg

Child 2-12 yr

• *Adjunct to general anesthesia:* IV 1-1.5 mg/10 kg, titrated to response needed

• *Premedication for surgery:* IM 1-1.5 mg/10 kg 30-60 min preoperatively

$ AVAILABLE FORMS/COST OF THERAPY

• Inj, Sol—IM, IV: 2.5 mg/ml, 2 ml: **$1.05-$5.31**

CONTRAINDICATIONS: Known or suspected QT prolongation

PRECAUTIONS: Elderly, cardiovascular disease (hypotension, bradydysrhythmias), renal disease, liver disease, Parkinson's disease, child <2 yr

Electrolyte imbalance particularly hypokalemia and hypomagnesemia, pheochromocytoma

PREGNANCY AND LACTATION: Pregnancy category C; has been used to promote analgesia for cesarean section patients without affecting respiration of the newborn; excretion into breast milk unknown, use caution in nursing mothers

---

* = non-FDA-approved use

NOTE: Has been used as a continuous IV infusion for hyperemesis gravidarum during the 2nd and 3rd trimesters without apparent fetal harm

SIDE EFFECTS/ADVERSE REACTIONS

CNS: Akathisia, chills, dizziness, *drowsiness,* dystonia, hallucinations, shivering

*CV: **QT prolongation, torsade de pointes, cardiac arrest, ventricular tachycardia,*** hypertension, *hypotension*

EENT: Oculogyric crisis

MS: Muscular rigidity

*RESP: **Apnea, bronchospasm, respiratory arrest, respiratory depression***

INTERACTIONS

Drugs

⚠ *Arrhythmogenic agents:* Any drug known to prolong QT interval should not be used with droperidol; class I or III antiarrhythmics, antimalarials, calcium channel blockers (bepridil, isradipine, nicardipine), neuroleptics (haloperidol, pimozide, thioridazine), antidepressants (desimipramine, venlafaxine)

❷ *Diuretics, laxatives:* Hypokalemia or hypomagnesemia may precipitate QT prolongation

❸ *CNS depressants:* Additive or potentiating effects with droperidol; barbiturates, tranquilizers, opioids

SPECIAL CONSIDERATIONS

MONITORING PARAMETERS

• QT prolongation has occurred in patients with no known CV disease and with doses at or below recommended doses

• Baseline ECG, blood pressure, heart rate, respiratory rate

dyphylline

(dye'fi-lin)

Rx: Dilor, Dylix, Lufyllin, Neothylline

Combinations

Rx: with guaifenesin (Dilex-G, Dilor-G, Lufyllin-GG); with ephedrine, guaifenesin, phenobarbital (Lufyllin-EPG)

Chemical Class: Xanthine derivative

Therapeutic Class: Antiasthmatic, bronchodilator; COPD agent

CLINICAL PHARMACOLOGY

Mechanism of Action: Possesses the peripheral vasodilator and bronchodilator actions characteristic of theophylline (approximately 1/10th as potent as theophylline); has diuretic and myocardial stimulant effects

Pharmacokinetics

PO: Bioavailability 68%-82%, peak 1 hr; not metabolized to theophylline; 83% excreted unchanged in urine, $t_{1/2}$ 2 hr

INDICATIONS AND USES: Bronchial asthma, bronchospasm in chronic bronchitis and emphysema

DOSAGE

Adult

• PO up to 15 mg/kg q6h; IM 250-500 mg q6h (administer by slow IM inj; do not administer IV), not to exceed 15 mg/kg/dose

💲 **AVAILABLE FORMS/COST OF THERAPY**

• Elixir—Oral: 100 mg/15 ml, 480 ml: **$29.88-$67.10**; 160 mg/5 ml, 480 ml: **$34.91**

• Inj, Sol—IM: 250 mg/ml, 2 ml: **$4.84**

• Tab, Uncoated—Oral: 200 mg, 100's: **$12.81-$167.75**; 400 mg, 100's: **$13.71-$258.65**

CONTRAINDICATIONS: Concurrent use with other xanthine preparations

PRECAUTIONS: Severe cardiac disease, hypertension, hyperthyroidism, acute myocardial injury, peptic ulcer, CHF, children

PREGNANCY AND LACTATION: Pregnancy category C; excreted into breast milk, compatible with breast feeding

SIDE EFFECTS/ADVERSE REACTIONS

CNS: Anxiety, dizziness, headache, *insomnia,* light-headedness, muscle twitching, *restlessness, seizures*

CV: Dysrhythmias, flushing, hypotension, *palpitations, sinus tachycardia*

GI: Anorexia, dyspepsia, epigastric pain, *nausea, vomiting*

RESP: Tachypnea

SKIN: Flushing, urticaria

MISC: Albuminuria, dehydration, fever, hyperglycemia

INTERACTIONS

Drugs

3 *Probenecid:* Increased serum dyphylline concentrations

SPECIAL CONSIDERATIONS

• Though better tolerated, significantly less bronchodilating activity vs theophylline. Serious dosing errors possible if dyphylline monitored with theophylline serum assays

MONITORING PARAMETERS

• Minimal effective serum concentration 12 μg/ml

---

econazole

(e-kone'a-zole)

Rx: Spectazole

Chemical Class: Imidazole derivative

Therapeutic Class: Antifungal

CLINICAL PHARMACOLOGY

Mechanism of Action: Alteration of the fungal cell membrane, which allows leakage of essential intracellular components

Pharmacokinetics

TOP: Systemic absorption extremely low, inhibitory concentrations have been found as deep as the middle region of the dermis, <1% of applied dose recovered in urine and feces

INDICATIONS AND USES: Tinea pedis (athlete's foot), tinea cruris (jock itch), tinea corporis (ringworm), cutaneous candidiasis, tinea versicolor

Antifungal spectrum usually includes *Trichophyton rubrum, T. mentagrophytes, T. tonsurans, Microsporum canis, M. audouini, M. gypseum, Epidermophyton floccosum,* the yeasts, *Candida albicans, Pityrosporum orbiculare*

DOSAGE

Adult and Child

• TOP apply to affected area qd-bid depending on condition

$ **AVAILABLE FORMS/COST OF THERAPY**

• Cre—Top: 1%, 15, 30, 85, 100 g: **$27.36-$29.90**/30 g

PREGNANCY AND LACTATION: Pregnancy category C; excretion into breast milk unknown; limited systemic absorption would minimize possibility of exposure to nursing infant

---

*= non-FDA-approved use

SIDE EFFECTS/ADVERSE REACTIONS

SKIN: Burning, erythema, itching, pruritic rash, stinging

SPECIAL CONSIDERATIONS
PATIENT/FAMILY EDUCATION

• For external use only; avoid contact with eyes; cleanse skin with soap and water and dry thoroughly prior to application

• Use medication for full treatment time outlined by clinician, even though symptoms may have improved

• Notify clinician if no improvement after 2 wk (jock itch, ringworm) or 4 wk (athlete's foot)

---

edetate calcium disodium (calcium EDTA)

(ed'e-tate)

Rx: Calcium Disodium Versenate

Chemical Class: Chelating agent

Therapeutic Class: Lead antidote

CLINICAL PHARMACOLOGY

Mechanism of Action: The calcium in edetate calcium disodium is readily displaced by heavy metals, such as lead, to form stable complexes that are excreted in urine

Pharmacokinetics

IV/IM/SC: Not metabolized; distributed primarily in extracellular fluid; excreted in urine; $t_{1/2}$ 20-60 min

INDICATIONS AND USES: Acute and chronic lead poisoning, lead encephalopathy

DOSAGE
Adult

• *Acute lead encephalopathy:* IV 1.5 g/m²/day as either an 8-24 hr INF or divided into 2 doses q12h for 3-5 days, with dimercaprol; may be given again after 4 days off drug; IM (preferred route) 250 mg/m²/dose q4h for 3-5 days, with dimercaprol; may be given again after 4 days off drug

• *Lead poisoning:* IV 1 g/250-500 ml D_5W or 0.9% NaCl over 1-2 hr q12h for 3-5 days; may repeat after 2 days; do not exceed 50 mg/kg/day in mildly affected or asymptomatic individuals; IM 35 mg/kg bid, do not exceed 50 mg/kg/day in mildly affected or asymptomatic individuals

Child

• *Acute lead encephalopathy:* Same as adult

• *Lead poisoning:* IM 35 mg/kg/day in divided doses q8-12h for 3-5 days; off 4 days before next course

S **AVAILABLE FORMS/COST OF THERAPY**

• Inj, Sol—IV: 200 mg/ml, 5 ml: **$43.96**

CONTRAINDICATIONS: Anuria, active renal disease, hepatitis

PRECAUTIONS: Vomiting (may lead to dehydration and decreased urine flow), rapid IV INF (especially in lead encephalopathy)

PREGNANCY AND LACTATION: Pregnancy category B; excretion into breast milk unknown; use caution in nursing mothers

SIDE EFFECTS/ADVERSE REACTIONS

CNS: Chills, fever, *headache,* numbness, tingling, tremors

CV: Cardiac rhythm irregularities, hypotension

EENT: Lacrimation, nasal congestion, sneezing

GI: Anorexia, cheilosis, excessive thirst; *mild increases in AST, ALT;* nausea, vomiting

GU: ***Acute necrosis of proximal tubules,*** glycosuria, infrequent changes in distal tubules and glom-

---

eruli, microscopic hematuria and large epithelial cells in urinary sediment, proteinuria

HEME: Anemia, transient bone marrow suppression

METAB: Hypercalcemia, zinc deficiency

MS: Arthralgia, fatigue, myalgia

SKIN: Rash

MISC: Malaise, pain at inj site

SPECIAL CONSIDERATIONS

PATIENT/FAMILY EDUCATION

• Notify clinician immediately if no urine output in a 12 hr period

MONITORING PARAMETERS

• Urinalysis and urine sediment daily during therapy to detect signs of progressive renal tubular damage

• Renal function tests, liver function tests, and serum electrolytes before and periodically during therapy

• ECG during IV therapy

---

edetate disodium

(ed´e-tate)

Rx: Disotate, Endrate

Chemical Class: Chelating agent

Therapeutic Class: Antihypercalcemic; digitalis antidote

CLINICAL PHARMACOLOGY

Mechanism of Action: Forms chelates with many divalent and trivalent metals that are then excreted in urine

Pharmacokinetics

IV: Not metabolized; $t_{1/2}$ 20-60 min: following chelation 95% excreted in urine as chelates within 24-48 hr

INDICATIONS AND USES: Emergency treatment of hypercalcemia; ventricular dysrhythmias associated with digitalis toxicity

DOSAGE

Adult

• IV INF 50 mg/kg/day (not to exceed 3 g/day), diluted in 500 ml of D_5W or 0.9% NaCl and infused over 3-4 hr for 5 consecutive days followed by 2 days without medication

Child

• IV INF 15-50 mg/kg/day (not to exceed 3 g/day), diluted in 500 ml of D_5W or 0.9% NaCl and infused over 3-4 hr for 5 consecutive days followed by 5 days without medication

§ AVAILABLE FORMS/COST OF THERAPY

• Inj, Sol—IV: 150 mg/ml, 20 ml: **$3.48-$26.90**

CONTRAINDICATIONS: Anuria

PRECAUTIONS: Intracranial lesions, seizure disorder, CAD, peripheral vascular disease, tuberculosis, CHF, diabetes

PREGNANCY AND LACTATION: Pregnancy category C; excretion into breast milk unknown; use caution in nursing mothers

SIDE EFFECTS/ADVERSE REACTIONS

CNS: Febrile reactions, *headache,* numbness, *seizures,* transient circumoral paresthesia

CV: Dysrhythmias, thrombophlebitis, transient drop in blood pressure

GI: Diarrhea, nausea, vomiting

GU: Acute tubular necrosis, nephrotoxicity

HEME: Anemia

METAB: Hyperuricemia, hypocalcemia, hypokalemia, hypomagnesemia

MS: Back pain, muscle cramps

RESP: Respiratory arrest

SKIN: Exfoliative dermatitis, skin and mucous membrane reactions

SPECIAL CONSIDERATIONS

• Have patient remain supine for a short time after INF due to the possibility of orthostatic hypotension

---

MONITORING PARAMETERS
• ECG, blood pressure during INF
• Renal function before and during therapy
• Serum calcium, magnesium, potassium levels

---

edrophonium
(ed-roe-foe′nee-um)
Rx: Enlon, Reversol, Tensilon
Combinations
   Rx: with atropine (Enlon-Plus)
Chemical Class: Quaternary ammonium derivative
Therapeutic Class: Cholinergic; curare antidote

CLINICAL PHARMACOLOGY
Mechanism of Action: An acetylcholinesterase inhibitor, inhibits destruction of acetylcholine, facilitates transmission of impulses across myoneural junction
Pharmacokinetics
IM: Onset 2-10 min, duration 12-45 min
IV: Onset <1 min, duration 6-24 min
Hydrolyzed by cholinesterase and metabolized by microsomal enzymes of liver, excreted by kidneys; $t_{1/2}$ 1.8 hr

INDICATIONS AND USES: Diagnosis of myasthenia gravis; differentiation of myasthenic crisis from cholinergic crisis; evaluation of treatment requirements in myasthenia gravis; curare antagonist
DOSAGE
Adult
• *Diagnosis of myasthenia gravis:* IV 1-2 mg over 15-30 sec, then 8 mg if no response; IM 10 mg; if cholinergic reaction occurs, retest after ½ hr with 2 mg IM

• *Evaluation of treatment requirements in myasthenia gravis:* IV 1-2 mg 1 hr after PO dose of anticholinesterase; if strength improves, an increase in neostigmine or pyridostigmine dose is indicated
• *Differentiation of myasthenic crisis from cholinergic crisis:* IV 1 mg, if no response in 1 min, may repeat; *myasthenic crisis* clear improvement in respiration, *cholinergic crisis* increased oropharyngeal secretions and further weakening of respiratory muscles (intubation and controlled ventilation may be required)
• *Curare antagonist:* IV 10 mg over 30-45 sec; may repeat; not to exceed 40 mg
Child
• *Diagnosis of myasthenia gravis:* IV 0.04 mg/kg given over 1 min followed by 0.16 mg/kg given within 45 sec if no response; >34 kg IM 2 mg; <34 kg IM 1 mg; infant IV 0.1 mg, followed by 0.4 mg if no response, not to exceed 0.5 mg
• *Evaluation of treatment requirements in myasthenia gravis:* IV 0.04 mg/kg given 1 hr after PO intake of drug being used in treatment; if strength improves, an increase in neostigmine or pyridostigmine is indicated
$ **AVAILABLE FORMS/COST OF THERAPY**
• Inj, Sol—IM, IV: 10 mg/ml, 1, 10, 15 ml: **$4.68**/1 ml
CONTRAINDICATIONS: Mechanical, intestinal, and urinary obstructions
PRECAUTIONS: Seizure disorders, bronchial asthma, recent coronary occlusion, hyperthyroidism, dysrhythmias, peptic ulcer, megacolon, poor GI motility, bradycardia, hypotension

---

italic = common side effects   ***bold italic*** = life-threatening reactions

PREGNANCY AND LACTATION:
Pregnancy category C; because it is ionized at physiologic pH, would not be expected to cross placenta in significant amounts; may cause premature labor; because it is ionized at physiologic pH, would not be expected to be excreted into breast milk

SIDE EFFECTS/ADVERSE REACTIONS

CNS: Dizziness, drowsiness, headache, incoordination, loss of consciousness, paralysis, *seizures,* sweating, weakness

CV: AV block, bradycardia, *cardiac arrest, dysrhythmias,* ECG changes, hypotension, syncope, tachycardia

EENT: Blurred vision, lacrimation, miosis, visual changes

GI: Cramps, diarrhea, dysphagia, increased peristalsis, increased salivary and gastric secretions, nausea, vomiting

GU: Frequency, incontinence, urgency

MS: Arthralgia, fasciculations, muscle cramps and spasms, weakness

RESP: Bronchospasm, dyspnea, increased tracheobronchial secretions, *laryngospasm, respiratory arrest, respiratory depression*

SKIN: Rash, urticaria

INTERACTIONS

Drugs

3 *Procainamide:* Edrophonium tests in patients with myasthenia gravis may be unreliable in procainamide-treated patients

3 *Tacrine:* Increased cholinergic effects of edrophonium

SPECIAL CONSIDERATIONS
MONITORING PARAMETERS

• Preinjection and postinjection strength

• Heart rate, respiratory rate, blood pressure

---

efavirenz
(e-fahv'er-ins)
Rx: Sustiva
Chemical Class: Substituted benzoxazinone
Therapeutic Class: Nonnucleoside reverse transcriptase inhibitor

CLINICAL PHARMACOLOGY

Mechanism of Action: Noncompetitive inhibitor of reverse transcriptase of HIV-1

Pharmacokinetics

PO: Peak 5 hr; well absorbed PO, bioavailability increased by 50% with high-fat meal; 99% protein bound (mainly albumin); metabolized by hepatic P450 system, primarily CYP3A4 and CYP2B6; induces its own metabolism through the P450 system; excreted unchanged in stool (50%) and urine (1%) and as glucuronidated metabolites in urine (30%); $t_{1/2}$ single dose: 52-76 hr, multiple dose: 40-55 hr; crosses placenta; CSF level 1% of plasma level

INDICATIONS AND USES: Combination therapy for HIV-1

DOSAGE

Adult and Child >40 kg

• 600 mg qd

• For latest treatment guidelines, see www.hivatis.org

Child<40 kg

• 10-<15 kg: 200 mg qd; 15-<20 kg: 250 mg qd; 20-<25 kg: 300 mg qd; 25-<32.5 kg: 350 mg qd; 32.5<40 kg: 400 mg qd

• For latest treatment guidelines, see www.hivatis.org

$ **AVAILABLE FORMS/COST OF THERAPY**

• Cap—Oral: 50 mg, 30's: **$32.88**; 100 mg, 30's: **$74.94**; 200 mg, 90's: **$449.64**

---

* = non-FDA-approved use

PRECAUTIONS: Depression, liver disease, pregnancy (fetal malformations observed in monkeys)

PREGNANCY AND LACTATION: Pregnancy category C (fetal malformations observed in monkeys); breast feeding not recommended

SIDE EFFECTS/ADVERSE REACTIONS

CNS: CNS side effects seen in 52% of patients, abnormal dreams, amnesia, anxiety, confusion, depression, suicide ideation, *dizziness, impaired concentration, insomnia,* tremor

CV: Flushing, palpitations, tachycardia

EENT: Tinnitus

GI: Diarrhea, elevated transaminases, nausea

METAB: Hyperlipidemia

MS: Arthralgia, myalgia

*RESP: **Asthma***

SKIN: Rash (27%)

INTERACTIONS

Drugs

❷ *Amprenavir:* Efavirenz decreases amprenavir plasma level; amprenavir dose adjustment recommended

🔢 *Barbiturates:* Barbiturates decrease plasma efavirenz levels; dose adjustment not recommended

🔢 *Carbamazepine:* Carbamazepine decreases plasma efavirenz levels; dose adjustment not recommended

❷ *Cisapride:* Efavirenz increases cisapride plasma level; coadministration not recommended

🔢 *Clarithromycin:* Efavirenz decreases clarithromycin plasma levels; coadministration not recommended

❷ *Ergotamines:* Efavirenz increases ergotamine plasma level; coadministration not recommended

🔢 *Ethinyl estradiol:* Efavirenz increases ethinyl estradiol plasma levels; dose adjustment not recommended

🔢 *Indinavir:* Efavirenz reduces indinavir AUC by 31%; increase indinavir dose to 1000 mg q8h

🔢 *Lopinavir:* Decreased plasma lopinavir concentrations; consider increase dose of lopinavir/ritonavir combination to 533 mg lopinavir and 133 mg ritonavir

🔢 *Lovastatin:* Efavirenz increases lovastatin plasma level; dose adjustment not recommended

❷ *Midazolam:* Efavirenz increases midazolam plasma level; coadministration not recommended

🔢 *Nelfinavir:* Efavirenz increases nelfinavir AUC by 20%; dose adjustment not recommended

🔢 *Oral contraceptives:* Efavirenz increases ethinyl estradiol plasma levels; dose adjustment not recommended

🔢 *Phenobarbital:* Decreased plasma efavirenz concentrations

🔢 *Phenytoin:* Phenytoin decreases plasma efavirenz level; dose adjustment not recommended

🔢 *Psychoactive drugs:* Potential for additive CNS effects

❷ *Rifabutin:* Efavirenz decreases plasma rifabutin level by 35%; no change in plasma efavirenz level; increase rifabutin dose to 450 mg qd

🔢 *Rifampin:* Rifampin decreases plasma efavirenz level by 25%; dose adjustment not recommended

🔢 *Ritonavir:* Ritonavir increases efavirenz AUC by 21%; efavirenz increases ritonavir AUC by 18%; dose adjustment not recommended

🔢 *St. John's Wort (Hypericum perforatum):* Substantial decrease in plasma efavirenz concentrations

italic = common side effects   **bold italic** = life-threatening reactions

likely; coadministration not recommended

❷ *Saquinavir:* Saquinavir reduces efavirenz AUC by 12%; efavirenz reduces saquinavir AUC by 62%; coadministration not recommended

❸ *Simvastatin:* Efavirenz increases simvastatin plasma level; dose adjustment not recommended

❷ *Triazolam:* Efavirenz increases triazolam plasma level; coadministration not recommended

❸ *Warfarin:* Efavirenz potentially increases or decreases plasma warfarin concentrations

Labs

• *False positive:* Cannabinoid screening test by CEDIA DAU Multi-level THC assay

SPECIAL CONSIDERATIONS
PATIENT/FAMILY EDUCATION

• May be taken without regard for meals; absorption increased by a high-fat meal, which should be avoided

• Take at bedtime for first 2-4 wk of therapy; may continue at bedtime if desired

• Use caution in driving or other activities requiring alertness

• Avoid alcohol ingestion

MONITORING PARAMETERS

• ALT, AST, CBC, cholesterol, triglycerides

---

eflornithine
(eh-floor´ni-theen)
Rx: Ornidyl (Injection); Vaniqa (Topical)
Chemical Class: Ornithine decarboxylase inhibitor
Therapeutic Class: Antiprotozoal

CLINICAL PHARMACOLOGY
Mechanism of Action: Irreversibly inhibits ornithine decarboxylase; decarboxylation of ornithine by ornithine decarboxylase is an obligatory step in the biosynthesis of polyamines such as putrescine, spermidine, and spermine, which play important roles in cell division and differentiation in all mammalian and many non-mammalian cells; topical form retards hair growth, not a depilatory

Pharmacokinetics

IV: Not significantly bound to plasma proteins, crosses the blood-brain barrier; 80% excreted unchanged in urine within 24 hr; $t_{1/2}$ 3 hr

INDICATIONS AND USES: Treatment of meningoencephalitic stage of *Trypanosoma brucei gambiense* infection (sleeping sickness); reduction of unwanted facial hair in women (topical); *Pneumocystis carinii* pneumonia*

DOSAGE
Adult

• IV INF 100 mg/kg/dose infused over a minimum of 45 min q6h for 14 days

NOTE: Eflornithine for inj concentrate is hypertonic and must be diluted with sterile water for injection, USP, before inf

• TOP apply thin layer to affected areas bid, separate doses by at least 8 hr, do not wash treated area for at least 4 hr

---

* = non-FDA-approved use

$ AVAILABLE FORMS/COST OF THERAPY

• Inj, Sol—IV: 200 mg/ml, 100 ml: *Compassionate use through World Health Organization (WHO)*

• Cre—Topical: 13.9%, 30 g: **$43.71**

PRECAUTIONS: Seizure disorder, renal function impairment (reduced doses recommended)

PREGNANCY AND LACTATION: Pregnancy category C; excretion into breast milk unknown; use caution in nursing mothers

SIDE EFFECTS/ADVERSE REACTIONS

CNS: Asthenia, dizziness, headache, *seizures*

EENT: Hearing impairment

GI: Abdominal pain, anorexia, *diarrhea*

HEME: **Anemia (55%),** eosinophilia, **leukopenia (37%), myelosuppression, thrombocytopenia (14%)**

SKIN: Alopecia; Topical: stinging, erythema, tingling of skin, rash

MISC: Facial edema

SPECIAL CONSIDERATIONS

• The most frequent, serious, toxic effect of eflornithine is myelosuppression, which may be unavoidable if successful treatment is to be completed; decisions to modify dosage or to interrupt or cease treatment depend on the severity of the observed adverse event(s) and the availability of support facilities

MONITORING PARAMETERS

• Serial audiograms if feasible

• CBC with platelets before and twice weekly during therapy and qwk after completion of therapy until hematologic values return to baseline levels

• Follow-up for at least 24 mo is advised to ensure further therapy should relapses occur

enalapril
(en-al'a-pril)
Rx: Vasotec
Combinations
  Rx: with diltiazem (Teczem); with felodipine (Lexxel); with hydrochlorothiazide (Vaseretic)
Chemical Class: Nonsulfhydryl angiotensin-converting enzyme (ACE) inhibitor
Therapeutic Class: Antihypertensive

CLINICAL PHARMACOLOGY

Mechanism of Action: Antihypertensive, hypoproliferative, and cardioprotective effects attributable to competitive inhibition of angiotensin-converting enzyme (ACE) yielding decreased plasma concentrations of angiotensin II, plasma aldosterone concentrations, systemic vascular resistance, blood pressure, preload, and afterload, not accompanied by changes in heart rate, pressor sensitivity to exogenous norepinephrine, or baroreceptor sensitivity

Pharmacokinetics

PO: Peak ½-1½ hr (enalaprilat 3-4 hr), metabolized by liver to active metabolite (enalaprilat), excreted in urine and feces; $t_{1/2}$ 1½ hr (enalaprilat 11 hr)

IV: (enalaprilat): Onset 5-15 min

INDICATIONS AND USES: Hypertension, CHF, MI, erythrocytosis,* nephropathy,* retinopathy,* hyperaldosteronism,* rheumatoid arthritis*

DOSAGE

Adult and child >16 yr

• *Hypertension:* PO 2.5-5 mg qd, increase prn; usual dose range 10-40 mg/day divided qd-bid; IV 0.625 mg (with concomitant diuretic therapy)—1.25 mg (without concomitant diuretic therapy)/dose given over 5 min q6h

• *Congestive heart failure:* 2.5-10 mg qd-bid, generally given with digitalis and diuretics; maximum daily doses, 40 mg (or until systolic blood pressure 100 mm Hg) greater symptomatic benefits without differences in mortality or tolerability

• *Nephropathy:* 5 mg qd; increasing prn to 20 mg/day

Child

• Same as adult

§ AVAILABLE FORMS/COST OF THERAPY

• Inj, Sol—IV: 1.25 mg/ml, 1 ml: **$3.85-$15.90**

• Tab, Uncoated—Oral: 2.5 mg, 100's: **$76.86-$93.68**; 5 mg, 100's: **$88.00-$119.01**; 10 mg, 100's: **$103.10-$124.95**; 20 mg, 100's: **$146.70-$177.79**

PRECAUTIONS: History of anaphylaxis, renal insufficiency (<30 ml/min), hypotension (CHF, elderly, volume depletion—diuretics, dialysis, cirrhosis), aortic stenosis, hyperkalemia (potassium supplements, potassium—sparing diuretics, renal disease, diabetes), neutropenia (autoimmune diseases, collagen vascular, febrile illness, immunosuppressant drug therapy), proteinuria, renal artery stenosis, surgery/anesthesia (excessive hypotension, correctable with fluids)

PREGNANCY AND LACTATION: Pregnancy category C (1st trimester), category D (2nd and 3rd trimesters); ACE inhibitors can cause fetal and neonatal morbidity and death when administered to pregnant women; when pregnancy is detected, discontinue ACE inhibitors as soon as possible; detectable in breast milk in trace amounts; effect on nursing infant has not been determined; use with caution in nursing mothers

SIDE EFFECTS/ADVERSE REACTIONS

CNS: Anxiety, dizziness, fatigue, headache, insomnia, paresthesia

CV: Angina, hypotension, palpitations, postural hypotension, syncope (especially with 1st dose)

GI: Abdominal pain, constipation, melena, nausea, vomiting

GU: Decreased libido, impotence, increased BUN/creatinine, UTI

HEME: **Agranulocytosis, neutropenia**

METAB: Hyperkalemia, hyponatremia

MS: Arthralgia, arthritis, myalgia

RESP: Asthma, bronchitis, *cough,* dyspnea, sinusitis

SKIN: **Angioedema,** flushing, rash, sweating

INTERACTIONS

Drugs

❷ *Allopurinol:* Predisposition to hypersensitivity reactions to ACE inhibitors

❸ *Aspirin, NSAIDs:* Inhibition of the antihypertensive response to ACE inhibitors

❸ *Azathioprine:* Increased myelosuppression

❸ *Insulin:* Enhanced insulin sensitivity

❸ *Iron:* Increased risk of anaphylaxis with administration of parenteral (IV) iron

❸ *Lithium:* Increased risk of serious lithium toxicity

❸ *Loop diuretics:* Initiation of ACE inhibitor therapy in the presence of intensive diuretic therapy results in a precipitous fall in blood pressure in some patients; ACE inhibitors may induce renal insufficiency in the presence of diuretic-induced sodium depletion

E *Potassium:* Increased risk for hyperkalemia

E *Potassium-sparing diuretics:* Increased risk for hyperkalemia

E *Prazosin, terazosin, doxazosin:* Exaggerated first-dose hypotensive response to α-blockers

E *Trimethoprim:* Additive risk of hyperkalemia, especially in patient predisposed to renal insufficiency

Labs
• ACE inhibition can account for approximately 0.5mEq/L rise in serum potassium

SPECIAL CONSIDERATIONS
PATIENT/FAMILY EDUCATION
• Caution with salt substitutes containing potassium chloride
• Rise slowly to sitting/standing position to minimize orthostatic hypotension
• Dizziness, fainting, lightheadedness may occur during 1st few days of therapy
• May cause altered taste perception or cough; persistent dry cough usually does not subside unless medication is stopped; notify clinician if these symptoms persist

MONITORING PARAMETERS
• BUN, creatinine, potassium within 2 wk after initiation of therapy (increased levels may indicate acute renal failure)

---

enoxacin

(en-ox′a-sin)
Rx: Penetrex
Chemical Class: Fluoroquinolone derivative
Therapeutic Class: Antibiotic

CLINICAL PHARMACOLOGY
Mechanism of Action: Interferes with the enzyme DNA gyrase needed for the synthesis of bacterial DNA; bactericidal

Pharmacokinetics
PO: Peak 1-3 hr, excreted in urine as unchanged drug (80%) and metabolites (20%); $t_{1/2}$ 3-6 hr

INDICATIONS AND USES: Uncomplicated urethral or cervical gonorrhea; uncomplicated UTI; complicated UTI

Antibacterial spectrum usually includes: Gram-positive organisms: *Staphylococcus epidermidis, S. saprophyticus*

Gram-negative organisms: *Neisseria gonorrhoeae, E. Coli, Klebsiella pneumoniae, Proteus mirabilis, Pseudomonas, aeruginosa, Enterobacter cloacae*

DOSAGE
Adult
• *Uncomplicated UTI:* PO 200 mg q12h for 3-7 days
• *Complicated UTI:* PO 400 mg q12h for 14 days
• *Uncomplicated gonorrhea:* PO 400 mg as a single dose
• *Renal function impairment* (CrCl <30 ml/min/1.73 m^2): PO after a normal initial dose; use 50% recommended dose q12h

$ **AVAILABLE FORMS/COST OF THERAPY**
• Tab, Uncoated—Oral: 200 mg, 50's: **$170.34**; 400 mg, 50's: **$178.86**

PRECAUTIONS: Children <17 yr (potential for arthropathy and osteochondrosis), elderly, renal disease, seizure disorders

PREGNANCY AND LACTATION: Pregnancy category C; excretion into breast milk unknown; due to the potential for arthropathy and osteochondrosis use extreme caution in nursing mothers

SIDE EFFECTS/ADVERSE REACTIONS
CNS: Anxiety, depression, dizziness, fatigue, headache, insomnia, *seizures,* somnolence

---

italic = common side effects　　　**bold italic** = life-threatening reactions

EENT: Visual disturbances

GI: Abdominal pain, anorexia, diarrhea, dry mouth; flatulence, heartburn, increased AST, ALT; *nausea, pseudomembranous colitis,* vomiting

SKIN: Photosensitivity, pruritus, rash

INTERACTIONS

Drugs

3 *Aluminum:* Reduced absorption of enoxacin; do not take within 4 hr of dose

3 *Antacids:* Reduced absorption of enoxacin; do not take within 4 hr of dose

3 *Antipyrine:* Inhibits metabolism of antipyrine; increased plasma antipyrine level

3 *Caffeine:* Inhibits metabolism of caffeine; increased plasma caffeine level

3 *Calcium:* Reduced absorption of enoxacin; do not take within 4 hr of dose

3 *Cimetidine:* Reduced absorption of enoxacin

3 *Diazepam:* Inhibits metabolism of diazepam; increased plasma diazepam level

3 *Didanosine:* Markedly reduced absorption of enoxacin; take enoxacin 2 hr before didanosine

3 *Famotidine:* Reduced absorption of enoxacin

3 *Fenbufen:* Coadministration increases seizure risk

3 *Foscarnet:* Coadministration increases seizure risk

3 *Iron:* Reduced absorption of enoxacin; do not take within 4 hr of dose

3 *Lansoprazole:* Reduced absorption of enoxacin

3 *Magnesium:* Reduced absorption of enoxacin; do not take within 4 hr of dose

3 *Metoprolol:* Inhibits metabolism of metoprolol; increased plasma metoprolol level

3 *Nizatidine:* Reduced absorption of enoxacin

3 *Omeprazole:* Reduced absorption of enoxacin

3 *Pentoxifylline:* Inhibits metabolism of pentoxifylline; increased plasma pentoxifylline level

3 *Phenytoin:* Inhibits metabolism of phenytoin; increased plasma phenytoin level

3 *Propranolol:* Inhibits metabolism of propranolol; increased plasma propranolol level

3 *Ranitidine:* Reduced absorption of enoxacin

3 *Ropinirole:* Inhibits metabolism of ropinirole; increased plasma ropinirole level

3 *Sodium bicarbonate:* Reduced absorption of enoxacin; do not take within 4 hr of dose

3 *Sucralfate:* Reduced absorption of enoxacin; do not take within 4 hr of dose

3 *Tacrine:* Inhibits metabolism of tacrine; increased plasma tacrine level

2 *Theobromine:* Inhibits metabolism of theobromine; increased plasma theobromine level

2 *Theophylline:* Inhibits metabolism of theophylline; cut maintenance theophylline dose in half during therapy with enoxacin

3 *Warfarin:* Inhibits metabolism of warfarin; increases hypoprothrombinemic response to warfarin

3 *Zinc:* Reduced absorption of enoxacin; do not take within 4 hr of dose

SPECIAL CONSIDERATIONS

• No demonstrated advantage over other fluoroquinolones for UTI or gonorrhea; choice should be based on availability and cost

PATIENT/FAMILY EDUCATION
• Administer on an empty stomach (1 hr before or 2 hr after meals)
• Drink fluids liberally
• Do not take antacids containing magnesium or aluminum or products containing iron or zinc within 4 hr before or 2 hr after dosing

---

enoxaparin
(e-nox-ah-pair'in)
Rx: Lovenox
Chemical Class: Depolymerized heparin derivative (low-molecular-weight heparin)
Therapeutic Class: Anticoagulant

CLINICAL PHARMACOLOGY
Mechanism of Action: Enhances the inhibition of Factor Xa and thrombin by binding to and accelerating antithrombin activity; preferentially inhibits Factor Xa; activated partial thromboplastin time (aPTT) not affected
Pharmacokinetics
SC: Peak activity 3-5 hr; renal elimination $t_{1/2}$ 4½ hr
INDICATIONS AND USES: Prevention of deep vein thrombosis (DVT), which may lead to pulmonary embolism (PE) following hip or knee replacement surgery or abdominal surgery; in conjunction with warfarin-treatment of DVT with and without PE (inpatient) or treatment of acute DVT without PE (outpatient); unstable angina and non-Q-wave MI (in conjunction with aspirin); prevention of deep vein thrombosis (DVT) long term when other modalities inappropriate*

DOSAGE
Adult
• Prevention of DVT, hip or knee replacement surgery: SC 30 mg q12h; initial dose given 12-24 hr postoperatively provided hemostasis has been established; duration 7-14 days
• Prevention of DVT, abdominal surgery: SC 40 mg qd; initial dose given 2 hr prior to surgery; duration 7-12 days
• Treatment of DVT/PE: SC 1 mg/kg q12h or 1.5 mg/kg qd; initiate warfarin therapy concurrently and continue enoxaparin for a minimum of 5 days and until therapeutic oral anticoagulant effect has been achieved (INR 2-3)
• Unstable angina/non-Q-wave MI: SC 1 mg/kg q12h in conjunction with aspirin 100-325 mg PO qd; usual duration 2-8 days
🖪 **AVAILABLE FORMS/COST OF THERAPY**
• Inj, Sol—SC: 30 mg/0.3 ml: **$18.35**; 40 mg/0.4 ml: **$24.46**; 60 mg/0.6 ml: **$36.74**; 80 mg/0.8 ml: **$48.98**; 100 mg/1 ml: **$61.23**; 120 mg/0.8 ml: **$73.50**; 150 mg/1 ml: **$91.88**
CONTRAINDICATIONS: Active major bleeding; thrombocytopenia associated with positive *in vitro* tests for anti-platelet antibody in the presence of enoxaparin; hypersensitivity to heparin or pork products
PRECAUTIONS: Bacterial endocarditis, bleeding disorder, active ulceration, angiodysplastic GI disease, hemorrhagic stroke; recent brain, spinal, or ophthalmological surgery; history of heparin-induced thrombocytopenia; renal function impairment; elderly; children; neuraxial anesthesia; prosthetic heart valves
PREGNANCY AND LACTATION: Pregnancy category B; reports of

---

italic = common side effects   ***bold italic*** = life-threatening reactions

congenital anomalies and fetal death, cause and effect relationship has not been determined; excretion into breast milk unknown; use caution in nursing mothers

SIDE EFFECTS/ADVERSE REACTIONS

CNS: Confusion, fever

CV: Edema

GI: Increased ALT, AST; nausea

HEME: Hemorrhage, hypochromic anemia, ***thrombocytopenia***, epidural/spinal hematoma (with concurrent epidural/spinal anesthesia or spinal puncture)

SKIN: Ecchymosis, erythema at inj site, hematoma, local irritation, pain

INTERACTIONS

Drugs

❸ *Aspirin:* Increased risk of hemorrhage

❸ *Oral anticoagulants:* Additive anticoagulant effects

SPECIAL CONSIDERATIONS

• Cannot be used interchangeably with unfractionated heparin or other low molecular weight heparins

• 1.5 mg/kg qd dosing should not be used in patients with cancer or obese patients

• Recent labeling changes regarding use in patients with mechanical prosthetic heart valves based on study involving a small number of pregnant women with mechanical valves; other evidence exists to substantiate cautious use in non-pregnant patients with mechanical valves

PATIENT/FAMILY EDUCATION

• Administer by deep SC inj into abdominal wall; alternate inj sites

• Report any unusual bruising or bleeding to clinician

MONITORING PARAMETERS

• CBC with platelets, stool occult blood, urinalysis

• Monitoring aPTT is not required

---

entacapone
(en-tak′a-pone)
Rx: Comtan
Chemical Class: Catechol-O-methyl-tranferase (COMT) inhibitor
Therapeutic Class: Anti-Parkinson's agent

CLINICAL PHARMACOLOGY

Mechanism of Action: Alters the plasma pharmacokinetics of levodopa; when given in combination with levodopa/carbidopa, plasma levels of levodopa are more sustained and result in more constant dopaminergic stimulation in the brain, leading to greater effects on the signs and symptoms of Parkinson's disease; may allow decrease in levodopa dose requirements

Pharmacokinetics

PO: Peak 1 hr, bioavailability 35%; 98% bound to plasma proteins; 99.8% metabolized, main pathway is isomerization to the cis-isomer, followed by glucuronidation (inactive); 0.2% of a dose is found unchanged in the urine; $t_{1/2}$ 2.4 hr

INDICATIONS AND USES: As an adjunct to levodopa/carbidopa for the treatment of signs and symptoms of idiopathic Parkinson's disease in patients who experience "wearing off" symptoms at the end of a dosing interval

DOSAGE

Adult

• PO 200 mg dose, up to a max of 8 × /day; max daily dose 1600 mg/day; always administer with levodopa/carbidopa; to optimize therapy the levodopa/carbidopa dosage must be reduced, usually by 25%; this reduction is usually necessary when the patient is taking more than 800 mg of levodopa daily

$ AVAILABLE FORMS/COST OF THERAPY

• Tab—PO: 200 mg, 100's: **$175.00**

CONTRAINDICATIONS: Treatment with a nonselective MAO inhibitor (isocarboxide, phenelzine, or tranylcypromine)

PRECAUTIONS: May increase risk of orthostatic hypotension and syncope; may cause diarrhea, hallucinations; may cause or exacerbate dyskinesia; abrupt withdrawal; hepatic impairment, renal impairment

PREGNANCY AND LACTATION: Pregnancy category C; use caution in nursing mothers

SIDE EFFECTS/ADVERSE REACTIONS

CNS: Dyskinesia, dizziness, fatigue, hallucinations, anxiety, somnolence, agitation, hyperpyrexia, confusion

CV: Orthostatic hypotension, syncope

GI: Nausea, diarrhea, abdominal pain, constipation, vomiting, dry mouth, dyspepsia, flatulence, gastritis, taste perversion

GU: Brown-orange urine discoloration

MS: Hyperkinesia, hypokinesia, back pain, weakness

RESP: Dyspnea

SKIN: Purpura

MISC: Increased sweating, rhabdomyolysis, pulmonary fibrosis, retroperitoneal fibrosis

INTERACTIONS

Drugs

❷ *Nonselective MAO inhibitors (phenelzine, tranylcypromine):* Inhibition of the majority of the pathways responsible for normal catecholamine metabolism

❸ *Iron:* Decreased absorption of iron via chelation

❸ *Isoproterenol, epinephrine, norepinephrine, dopamine, dobutamine, alpha-methyldopa, apomorphine, isoetherine, and bitolterol:* Decreased metabolism of these drugs

---

ephedrine

(e-fed´rin)

OTC: Pretz-D, Kondon's Nasal

Combinations

Rx: with potassium iodide, phenobarbital, theophylline (Quadrinal), with hydroxyzine, theophylline (Hydrophed DF, Marax-DF); with guaifenesin (Broncholate, Ephex SR)

Chemical Class: Catecholamine

Therapeutic Class: Bronchodilator; vasopressor; decongestant

CLINICAL PHARMACOLOGY

Mechanism of Action: Stimulates α- and β-adrenergic receptors directly and via norepineperine release; produces bronchial smooth muscle relaxation, cardiac stimulation, and increased blood pressure; CNS effects similar to amphetamine

Pharmacokinetics

PO: Onset 15-60 min, duration 3-6 hr

IM: Onset 10-20 min

60%-77% of dose excreted as unchanged drug in urine; $t_{1/2}$ 2.5-3.6 hr

INDICATIONS AND USES: Bronchial asthma, nasal congestion (local treatment); vasopressor in shock, enuresis,* myasthenia gravis*

DOSAGE
Adult
• IM/SC 25-50 mg, not to exceed 150 mg/24 hr; IV 10-25 mg, not to exceed 150 mg/24 hr; PO 25-50 mg bid-tid
• *Nasal congestion:* TOP instill 3-4 gtt q4h or small amount of gel in each nostril q4h
Child
• PO/SC/IV 3 mg/kg/day in divided doses q4-6h
• *Nasal congestion:* TOP instill 3-4 gtt q4h or small amount of gel in each nostril q4h
💲 AVAILABLE FORMS/COST OF THERAPY
• Cap, Gel—Oral: 25 mg, 100's: **$4.50-$14.00**; 50 mg, 100's: **$3.86-$5.95**
• Inj, Sol—IM, IV, SC: 50 mg/ml, 1 ml: **$0.56-$1.86**
• Spray—Nasal: 0.25%, 50 ml: **$5.00**

CONTRAINDICATIONS: Narrow-angle glaucoma

PRECAUTIONS: Heart disease, coronary insufficiency, dysrhythmias, angina, hyperthyroidism, diabetes mellitus, prostatic hypertrophy, increased intracranial pressure, hypovolemia

PREGNANCY AND LACTATION: Pregnancy category C; routinely used to treat or prevent maternal hypotension following spinal anesthesia; may cause fetal heart rate changes; excretion into breast milk unknown; one case report of adverse effects (excessive crying, irritability, and disturbed sleeping patterns) in a 3-month-old nursing infant whose mother consumed disoephedrine

SIDE EFFECTS/ADVERSE REACTIONS
CNS: Anxiety, confusion, dizziness, hallucinations, headache, *insomnia, seizures, tremors*

CV: Chest pain, ***dysrhythmias,*** hypertension, palpitations, tachycardia

EENT: Burning, dryness, irritation, rebound congestion with prolonged use, sneezing, stinging

GI: Anorexia, nausea, vomiting

GU: Dysuria, urinary retention

METAB: Hyperglycemia

RESP: Respiratory difficulty

SKIN: Contact dermatitis, pallor

INTERACTIONS
Drugs
🛇 *Antacids:* Increased ephedrine serum concentrations

🛇 *Furazolidone:* Hypertensive response possible

🛇 *Guanadrel:* Inhibits antihypertensive response

🛇 *Guanethidine:* Inhibits antihypertensive response

❷ *MAOIs:* Substantially enhanced pressor response to ephedrine, severe hypertension

🛇 *Sodium bicarbonate:* Increased ephedrine serum concentrations

Labs
• *False increase:* Urine amino acids, urine 5-HIAA

SPECIAL CONSIDERATIONS
PATIENT/FAMILY EDUCATION
• May cause wakefulness or nervousness; take last dose 4-6 hr prior to bedtime
• Do not use nasal products for >3-5 days

MONITORING PARAMETERS
• Heart rate, ECG, blood pressure (when using for vasopressor effect)

epinephrine

(ep-i-nef′rin)

Rx: Vasopressor: Adrenalin, Sus-Phrine

Rx: Bronchodilator: Adrenaline, Ana-Guard, Sus-Phrine

OTC: Adrenalin, AsthmaHaler Mist, Asthma-Nefrin, microNefrin, Nephron, Primatene Mist, S-2,

OTC: Decongestant: Adrenalin

Rx: Antiglaucoma agent: Epifrin, Glaucon

Rx: Emergency Kit: Ana-Kit, EpiPen, EpiPen Jr.
Combinations

   Rx: with etidocaine (Duranest with Epinephrine); with prilocaine (Citanest Forte); with lidocaine (Xylocaine with Epinephrine); with pilocarpine (E-Pilo Ophthalmic)

Chemical Class: Catecholamine

Therapeutic Class: Vasopressor; antiglaucoma agent; bronchodilator; decongestant

CLINICAL PHARMACOLOGY

Mechanism of Action: Stimulates α-, β_1-, and β_2-adrenergic receptors resulting in bronchodilation, cardiac stimulation, nasal decongestion, and dilation of skeletal muscle vasculature; effects on vasculature are dose dependent, small doses produce vasodilation while large doses produce vasoconstriction; decreases production of aqueous humor and increases aqueous outflow; dilates the pupil by contracting the dilator muscle

Pharmacokinetics
SC: Onset 3-5 min
INH: Onset 1 min
OPHTH: Onset 1 hr
Taken up into the adrenergic neuron and metabolized by monoamine oxidase and catechol-o-methyltransferase; circulating drug metabolized by liver; inactive metabolites excreted in urine

INDICATIONS AND USES: Cardiac arrest, acute asthmatic attacks, nasal congestion, open-angle glaucoma, anaphylactic reactions

DOSAGE

Adult

• *Bronchodilator:* IM/SC (1:1000) 0.1-0.5 mg q12-15 min-4 hr; IV 0.1-0.25 mg (single dose max 1 mg); SC susp (1:200) 0.5-1.5 mg (0.1-0.3 ml); NEB instill 8-15 gtt into nebulizer reservoir, administer 1-3 inhalations 4-6 times/day; MDI 1-2 puffs at 1st sign of bronchospasm

• *Cardiac arrest:* IV/intracardiac 0.1-1 mg (1-10 ml of 1:10,000 dilution) q3-5 min prn; IV intermediate dose 2-5 mg q3-5 min; escalating dose 1 mg-3 mg-5 mg 3 min apart; high dose 0.1 mg/kg q3-5 min; intratracheal 1 mg q3-5 min (higher doses [e.g., 0.1 mg/kg] should be considered only after 1 mg doses have failed)

• *Hypotension:* IV INF 1-4 µg/min

• *Anaphylactic reaction:* IM/SC 0.2-0.5 mg q20 min-4 hr (single dose max 1 mg)

• *Glaucoma:* Ophth 1 gtt qd-bid

• *Nasal congestion:* Intranasal apply prn; do not use for >3-5 days

Child

• *Bronchodilator:* SC 10 µg/kg (0.01 ml/kg of 1:1000), max single dose 0.5 mg; susp (1:200) 0.005 ml/kg/dose (0.025 mg/kg/dose) q6h, max 0.15 ml (0.75 mg)/dose;

---

italic = common side effects   ***bold italic*** = life-threatening reactions

NEB 0.25-0.5 ml of 2.25% racemic epinephrine solution diluted in 3 ml NS q1-4h

• *Cardiac arrest:* IV/intratracheal 0.01 mg/kg (0.1 ml/kg) of 1:10,000 sol q3-5 min prn, max 5 ml

• *Refractory hypotension:* IV INF 0.1-4 µg/kg/min

• *Anaphylactic reaction:* SC 0.01 mg/kg q15 min for 2 doses then q4h prn, max 0.5 mg/dose

• *Nasal congestion* (>6 yr): Intranasal apply prn

Neonate

• *Cardiac arrest:* IV/intratracheal 0.01-0.03 mg/kg (0.1-0.3 ml/kg) of 1:10,000 sol q3-5 min prn

$ **AVAILABLE FORMS/COST OF THERAPY**

• Aer—INH: 0.22 mg/INH, 15 ml: **$7.88-$8.07**; 0.3 mg/INH, 15 ml: **$8.22-$9.35**

• Inj, Sol—IM: 0.15, 0.3 mg/0.3 ml, 1's: **$34.68-$47.88**

• Inj, Sol—IM, IV, SC: 0.1 mg/ml, 10 ml: **$13.75-$170.00**; 1 mg/ml, 1 ml: **$0.49-$22.15**

• Inj, Sus—SC: 5 mg/ml, 5 ml: **$38.50**

• Sol—INH: 1%, 7.5 ml: **$24.88**

• Sol—Nasal: 1 mg/ml, 30 ml: **$1.20-$20.06**

• Sol—Ophth: 0.5%, 15 ml: **$46.36**; 1%, 15 ml: **$49.69**; 2%, 15 ml: **$54.36**

CONTRAINDICATIONS: Cardiac dysrhythmias, angle-closure glaucoma, local anesthesia of fingers and toes, general anesthesia with halogenated hydrocarbons or cyclopropane, organic brain damage, labor, coronary insufficiency

PRECAUTIONS: Elderly, cardiovascular disease, hypertension, diabetes, hyperthyroidism, psychoneurotic individuals, thyrotoxicosis, parkinsonism

PREGNANCY AND LACTATION: Pregnancy category C; excreted into breast milk; use caution in nursing mothers

SIDE EFFECTS/ADVERSE REACTIONS

CNS: Anxiety, dizziness, fear, headache, hemiplegia, restlessness, **subarachnoid hemorrhage,** *tremor,* weakness

CV: Anginal pain, **dysrhythmias,** hypertension, palpitations

GI: Nausea, vomiting

GU: Urinary retention

RESP: Respiratory difficulty

SKIN: Hemorrhage at inj site, pallor, urticaria, wheal

INTERACTIONS

Drugs

🟥 *Antihistamines:* Effects of epinephrine may be potentiated by certain antihistamines; diphenhydramine, tripelennamine, d-chlorpheniramine

🟥 *β-blockers:* Noncardioselective β-blockers enhance pressor response to epinephrine resulting in hypertension and bradycardia

🟥 *Chlorpromazine, clozaril, thioridazine:* Reversal of epinephrine pressor response

❷ *Cyclic antidepressants:* Pressor response to IV epinephrine markedly enhanced

🟥 *Levothyroxine:* Effects of epinephrine may be potentiated

SPECIAL CONSIDERATIONS

PATIENT/FAMILY EDUCATION

• Do not exceed recommended doses

• Wait at least 3-5 min between inhalations with MDI

• Notify clinician of dizziness or chest pain

• Do not use nasal preparations for >3-5 days to prevent rebound congestion

- To avoid contamination of ophth preparations, do not touch tip of container to any surface
- Do not use ophth preparations while wearing soft contact lenses
- Transitory stinging may occur on instillation of ophth preparations
- Report any decrease in visual acuity immediately
- Use of OTC asthma preparations containing epinephrine should be discouraged

MONITORING PARAMETERS
- Blood pressure, heart rate
- Intraocular pressure

---

epoprostenol (prostacyclin)

(e-poe-pros'ten-ol)

Rx: Flolan

Chemical Class: Prostaglandin PGI_2

Therapeutic Class: Vasodilator; Pulmonary hypertension agent

CLINICAL PHARMACOLOGY

Mechanism of Action: Direct vasodilator of pulmonary and systemic arterial vascular beds; reduces right and left ventricular afterload, increases cardiac output and stroke volume, decreases pulmonary vascular resistance and mean systemic arterial pressure, inhibits platelet aggregation; may also induce bronchodilation, inhibit gastric acid secretion, and decrease gastric emptying

Pharmacokinetics

IV INF: Steady state reached in 15 min; extensively hydrolyzed in blood, some metabolites have pharmacological activity; excreted (82%) in urine; $t_{1/2}$ 6 min

INDICATIONS AND USES: Long-term IV treatment of primary pulmonary hypertension in New York Heart Association Class III and Class IV patients

DOSAGE

Adult

- IV INF, acute: 2 ng/kg/min, increase by 2 ng/kg/min q15 min until limited by adverse effects, mean maximum-tolerated dose in trials was 9.2-11.2 ng/kg/min
- IV INF, chronic: Initiate at 4 ng/kg/min less than maximum-tolerated rate or at ½ maximum-tolerated rate if maximum rate <5 ng/kg/min; increases in rate can be made by 1-2 ng/kg/min q 15 min, decreases by 2 ng/kg/min q 15 min

💲 AVAILABLE FORMS/COST OF THERAPY

- Inj, dry sol—IV: 0.5 mg/vial: **$189.36**; 1.5 mg/vial: **$36.55**

CONTRAINDICATIONS: CHF secondary to severe left ventricular systolic dysfunction, patients unable to commit to administration and care of indwelling central venous catheter

PRECAUTIONS: Elderly, concurrent vasodilator use

PREGNANCY AND LACTATION: Pregnancy category B; women with pulmonary hypertension should avoid pregnancy; unknown if excreted in breast milk

SIDE EFFECTS/ADVERSE REACTIONS

CNS: Agitation, anxiety, headache (49%), hyperesthesia, hypoesthesia, nervousness, paresthesia, tremor

CV: Bradycardia (5%), chest pain (11%), dizziness (8%), flushing (58%), hypotension (16%), syncope, *tachycardia*

GI: Abdominal pain, diarrhea, dyspepsia, *nausea/vomiting (32%)*

MS: Back pain, jaw pain, musculoskeletal pain, myalgia

RESP: Dyspnea

---

italic = common side effects **bold italic** = life-threatening reactions

MISC: Chills, fever, flu-like syndrome, sweating

INTERACTIONS

Drugs

❸ *Antihypertensives, diuretics, vasodilators:* Additive effects on blood pressure

❸ *Digoxin:* Possible elevations of plasma digoxin concentrations

SPECIAL CONSIDERATIONS

• Clinically shown to improve exercise capacity, dyspnea, and fatigue as early as 1st week of therapy

• Drug is administered chronically on an ambulatory basis with a portable infusion pump through a permanent central venous catheter; peripheral IV infusions may be used temporarily until central venous access obtained

• Patients must be taught sterile technique, drug reconstitution, and care of catheter

• Do not interrupt infusion or decrease rate abruptly, may cause rebound symptoms (dyspnea, dizziness, asthenia, death)

• Unless contraindicated, patients should be anticoagulated to reduce risk of pulmonary thromboembolism or systemic embolism through a patent foramen ovale

MONITORING PARAMETERS

• Postural BP and heart rate for several hr following dosage adjustments

---

eprosartan

(eh-pro-sar'tan)

Rx: Teveten

Chemical Class: Angiotensin II receptor antagonist

Therapeutic Class: Antihypertensive

CLINICAL PHARMACOLOGY

Mechanism of Action: Antihypertensive (inhibition of vasoconstrictor and aldosterone secretion), smooth muscle hypoproliferative, and cardioprotective effects are attributable to selective blockade of angiotensin II receptors found throughout the cardiovascular and renal systems; effects independent of angiotension II synthesis

Pharmacokinetics

PO: Peak 4 hr (range 2-6 hr)
PO bioavailability, 13%, possibly delayed or enhanced by concurrent food; 98% protein bound, 20% metabolized by liver (no active metabolites), 70% excreted in feces, 7% in urine; elimination $t_{\frac{1}{2}}$ 5-9 hr

INDICATIONS AND USES: Hypertension, congestive heart failure (left ventricular dysfunction),* chronic renal failure,* diabetic nephropathy*

DOSAGE

Adult and child >16 yr

• Initially, 400 mg qd or 200 mg bid, with titration to 800 mg per day (36%-50% response in reaching goal reductions in sitting diastolic blood pressure)

Dosage in Renal Failure

• Dose reduction necessary; peak plasma levels approximately 50% higher in moderate to severe renal failure

❺ **AVAILABLE FORMS/COST OF THERAPY**

• Tab—Oral: 400 mg, 100's: **$103.13**; 600 mg, 100's: **$137.14**

PRECAUTIONS: Angioedema (associated with aspirin and/or penicillin allergy), aortic or mitral valve stenosis, biliary cirrhosis or biliary obstruction, breast feeding period, coronary artery disease, elderly patients, hepatic dysfunction (adjust dose), hypertrophic cardiomyopathy, hypotension (sodium- or volume-depleted patients), pregnancy, renal artery stenosis, solitary kidney, or congestive heart failure

---

* = non-FDA-approved use

PREGNANCY AND LACTATION:
Pregnancy category C, first trimester—category D, second and third trimesters; drugs acting directly on the renin-angiotensin-aldosterone system are documented to cause fetal harm (hypotension, oligohydramnios, neonatal anemia, hyperkalemia, neonatal skull hypoplasia, anuria, and renal failure; neonatal limb contractures, craniofacial deformities, and hypoplastic lung development)

SIDE EFFECTS/ADVERSE REACTIONS

CNS: Dizziness (2.4%), fatigue (1.4%), headache (3.8%)

MS: Myalgia (1.9%)

RESP: Cough (1.8%-6.5%)

SKIN: Facial edema, angioedema, diaphoresis

MISC: Angioedema

SPECIAL CONSIDERATIONS

• Potentially as or more effective than angiotensin-converting enzyme inhibitors, without cough; no evidence for reduction in morbidity and mortality as first line agents in hypertension, yet; whether they provide the same cardiac and renal protection also still tentative; like ACE inhibitors, less effective in black patients

PATIENT/FAMILY EDUCATION

• Call your clinician immediately if note following side effects: wheezing, lip, throat, or face swelling; hives or rash

MONITORING PARAMETERS

• Baseline electrolytes, urinalysis, blood urea nitrogen and creatinine with recheck at 2-4 wk after initiation (sooner in volume-depleted patients); monitor sitting blood pressure; watch for symptomatic hypotension, particulary in volume-depleted patients

eptifibatide

(ep-tih-fib'ah-tide)

Rx: Integrilin

Chemical Class: Glycoprotein (GP) IIb/IIIa inhibitor

Therapeutic Class: Antiplatelet agent

CLINICAL PHARMACOLOGY

Mechanism of Action: Reversibly prevents fibrinogen, von Willebrand's factor, and other adhesion ligands from binding to platelet GP IIb/IIIa receptors, thereby inhibiting platelet aggregation

Pharmacokinetics

Steady state achieved within 4-6 hr; 25% bound in human plasma; 50% cleared by renal excretion; t½ 2.5 hr

INDICATIONS AND USES: Acute coronary syndromes (unstable angina and non Q-wave MI), including patients who are to be managed medically and those undergoing percutaneous coronary intervention (PCI)

DOSAGE

Adult

• Acute coronary syndrome: IV bolus 180 µg/kg as soon as possible following diagnosis, followed by continuous INF rate of 2 µg/kg/min until hospital discharge or initiation of CABG surgery, up to 72 hr; if patient to undergo PCI during INF, continue INF until hospital discharge or 18-24 hr after procedure, whichever comes first, allowing for up to 96 hr of therapy; patients >121 kg should receive max bolus of 22.6 mg followed by max INF rate of 15 mg/hr

• Nonemergent PCI: IV bolus 180 µg/kg immediately prior to procedure, followed by continuous INF of 2.0 µg/kg/min and a second 180 µg/kg bolus 10 min after the first bolus; continue infusion until hospital discharge or 18-24 hr, whichever comes first; minimum of 12 hr of infusion recommended; patients >121 kg should receive max bolus of 22.6 mg followed by max INF rate of 15 mg/hr

• Dosage in renal impairment: Serum creatinine 2.0-4.0 mg/dL, all IV bolus doses remain 180 µg/kg, reduce continuous INF rate to 1.0 µg/kg/min; patients weighing >121 kg and serum creatinine 2.0-4.0 mg/dL, all bolus doses remain 22.6 mg, reduce continuous INF rate to 7.5 mg/hr

⑤   AVAILABLE FORMS/COST OF THERAPY

• Inj, Sol—IV: 0.75 mg/ml, 100 ml: **$203.13**; 2 mg/ml, 10 ml: **$541.65**/100 ml

CONTRAINDICATIONS: Active internal bleeding or history of bleeding diathesis within previous 30 days; history of stroke within 30 days; history of hemorrhagic stroke; major surgical procedure or severe physical trauma within previous month; systolic blood pressure >200 mm Hg or diastolic blood pressure >110 mm Hg; history of intracranial hemorrhage, intracranial neoplasm, arteriovenous malformation or aneurysm; history, symptoms or findings of aortic dissection, acute pericarditis; serum creatinine >4 mg/dL, dependency on renal dialysis

PRECAUTIONS: Platelet count <100,000/mm³; serum creatinine 2-4 mg/dL; hemorrhagic retinopathy; IM injections, urinary catheters, nasotracheal intubation, nasogastric tubes; elderly

PREGNANCY AND LACTATION: Pregnancy category B; use caution in nursing mothers

SIDE EFFECTS/ADVERSE REACTIONS

CV: Hypotension

*HEME: **Bleeding*** (major bleeding 4.4%-10.8%, minor bleeding 10.5%-14.2%)

INTERACTIONS

Drugs

⑧ *Anticoagulants (heparin, warfarin), Antiplatelet agents (ticlopidine, clopidogrel, dipyridamole), Thrombolytics (alteplase, streptokinase), NSAIDs, aspirin:* Increased risk of bleeding

SPECIAL CONSIDERATIONS

• When bleeding cannot be controlled with pressure, discontinue INF

• Most major bleeding occurs at arterial access site for cardiac catheterization; prior to pulling femoral artery sheath, discontinue heparin for 3-4 hr and document activated clotting time (ACT) <150 sec or aPTT <45 sec; achieve sheath hemostasis 2-4 hr before discharge

• In patients who undergo CABG, discontinue eptifibatide INF prior to surgery

• Eptifibatide, tirofiban, and abciximab can all decrease the incidence of cardiac events associated with acute coronary syndromes; direct comparisons are needed to establish which, if any, is superior; for angioplasty, until more data become available, abciximab appears to be the drug of choice

MONITORING PARAMETERS

• Platelet count, hemoglobin, hematocrit, PT/aPTT (baseline, within 6 hr following bolus dose, then daily thereafter)

• In patients undergoing PCI, also measure ACT; maintain aPTT between 50 and 70 sec unless PCI is to be performed; during PCI, maintain ACT between 300 and 350 sec

ergocalciferol

(er-goe-kal-sif'e-role)

Rx: Calciferol, Drisdol, Deltalin

OTC: Calciferol Drops, Drisdol Drops

Chemical Class: Sterol derivative

Therapeutic Class: Vitamin D analog

CLINICAL PHARMACOLOGY

Mechanism of Action: Regulates calcium homeostasis; promotes active absorption of calcium and phosphorus by the small intestine; increases rate of accretion and resorption of bone minerals; promotes resorption of phosphate by renal tubules; also involved in magnesium metabolism

Pharmacokinetics

PO: Peak effect in approximately 1 mo following daily dosing, readily absorbed from GI tract, absorption requires intestinal presence of bile; inactive until hydroxylated in the liver and kidney to calcifediol and then to calcitriol (most active form)

INDICATIONS AND USES: Refractory rickets, osteoporosis, familial hypophosphatemia and hypoparathyroidism

DOSAGE

Adult

• *Dietary supplementation* (including prevention of osteoporosis): PO 400-800 IU qd

• *Hypoparathyroidism:* PO 25,000-200,000 IU qd (with calcium supplements)

• *Refractory rickets:* PO 12,000-500,000 IU qd (with phosphate supplements)

• *Familial hypophosphatemia:* PO 10,000-80,000 IU qd (with 1-2 g/day elemental phosphorus)

• IM therapy reserved for patients with GI, liver, or biliary disease associated with vitamin D malabsorption

Child

• *Dietary supplementation:* PO 400 IU qd

• *Hypoparathyroidism:* PO 50,000-200,000 IU qd (with calcium supplements)

• *Refractory rickets:* PO 400,000-800,000 IU qd (with phosphate supplements)

☒ AVAILABLE FORMS/COST OF THERAPY

• Cap, Elastic—Oral: 25,000 IU, 100's: **$8.00**; 50,000 IU, 100's: **$3.57-$36.00**

• Inj, Sol—IM: 50,000 IU/ml, 1 ml: **$32.45**

• Sol—Oral: 8,000 IU/ml, 60 ml: **$18.72-$88.86** (OTC)

• Tab, Plain Coated—Oral: 50,000 IU, 100's: **$5.99-$52.59**

CONTRAINDICATIONS: Hypercalcemia, malabsorption syndrome, hypervitaminosis D, decreased renal function

PRECAUTIONS: Renal stones, coronary disease, arteriosclerosis, elderly

PREGNANCY AND LACTATION: Pregnancy category A (category D if used in doses above the recommended daily allowance); excreted into breast milk in limited amounts; compatible with breast feeding, however, serum calcium levels of the infant should be monitored if mother is receiving pharmacologic doses

SIDE EFFECTS/ADVERSE REACTIONS

CNS: Anorexia, headache, hyperthermia, irritability, overt psychosis, somnolence

CV: **Dysrhythmia,** generalized vascular calcification, hypertension

---

italic = common side effects   ***bold italic*** = life-threatening reactions

EENT: Conjunctivitis (calcific), rhinorrhea

GI: Constipation, dry mouth, elevated AST and ALT, metallic taste, nausea, ***pancreatitis,*** polydipsia, vomiting

GU: Albuminuria, decreased libido, elevated BUN, nephrocalcinosis, nocturia, polyuria, reversible azotemia

METAB: Hypercholesterolemia, mild acidosis

MS: Bone pain, muscle pain, weakness

SKIN: Photophobia, pruritis

MISC: Weight loss

SPECIAL CONSIDERATIONS
MONITORING PARAMETERS

• The following monitoring suggestions are recommended for pharmacologic dosing, not dietary supplementation

• Serum and urinary calcium, phosphorus, and BUN

• X-ray bones monthly until condition is corrected and stabilized

• Ensure adequate calcium intake; maintain serum calcium concentration between 9-10 mg/dl

• Periodically determine magnesium and alk phosphatase

• 24 hr urinary calcium and phosphate (hypoparathyroid patients)

• Serum calcium times phosphorus should not exceed 70 mg/dl to avoid ectopic calcification

---

ergoloid mesylates
(er´goe-loid)

Rx: Gerimal, Hydergine
Chemical Class: Ergot alkaloid
Therapeutic Class: Cerebral metabolic enhancer

CLINICAL PHARMACOLOGY
Mechanism of Action: May increase brain metabolism, possibly increasing cerebral blood flow
Pharmacokinetics
PO: Rapidly absorbed, peak 0.6-3 hr; extensive 1st-pass metabolism by the liver; $t_{1/2}$ 2.6-5.1 hr

INDICATIONS AND USES: Age-related mental capacity decline

DOSAGE
Adult
• PO 1 mg tid initially, increase to 4.5-12 mg/day in divided doses

$ AVAILABLE FORMS/COST OF THERAPY
• Cap, Elastic—Oral: 1 mg, 100's: **$109.36**
• Liq—Oral: 1 mg/ml, 100 ml: **$72.72**
• Tab, Uncoated—Oral: 0.5 mg, 100's: **$8.75-$15.75**; 1 mg, 100's: **$11.10-$103.93**
• Tab—SL: 0.5 mg, 100's: **$8.85**; 1 mg, 100's: **$10.58**

CONTRAINDICATIONS: Acute or chronic psychosis

PRECAUTIONS: Acute intermittent porphyria

SIDE EFFECTS/ADVERSE REACTIONS
GI: Nausea, sublingual irritation, vomiting

SPECIAL CONSIDERATIONS
PATIENT/FAMILY EDUCATION
• Results may not be observed for 3-4 wk

• May cause transient GI disturbances; allow sublingual tablets to completely dissolve under tongue; do not chew or crush sublingual tablets

MONITORING PARAMETERS

• Before prescribing, exclude the possibility that the patient's signs and symptoms arise from a potentially reversible and treatable condition

• Periodically reassess the diagnosis and the benefit of current therapy to the patient; discontinue if no benefit

---

ergonovine

(er-gone-o´veen)

Rx: Ergotrate Maleate
Chemical Class: Ergot alkaloid
Therapeutic Class: Oxytocic

CLINICAL PHARMACOLOGY

Mechanism of Action: Partial agonist or antagonist at α-adrenergic, dopaminergic, and tryptaminergic receptors; increases the strength, duration, and frequency of uterine contractions and decreases uterine bleeding when used after placental delivery

Pharmacokinetics

IM: Onset 7-8 min, duration 45 min
IV: Onset 40 sec, duration 3 hr
Principally eliminated by nonrenal mechanisms (metabolism in liver, excretion in feces); $t_{1/2}$ ½-2 hr

INDICATIONS AND USES: Postpartum/postabortal hemorrhage due to uterine atony; adjunct to coronary arteriography to diagnose coronary artery spasm*; migraine headache*

DOSAGE

Adult

• IM/IV 0.2 mg, severe uterine bleeding may require repeated doses, but rarely more than 0.2 mg per 2-4 hr (confine IV route to emergencies)

AVAILABLE FORMS/COST OF THERAPY

• Inj, Sol—IV: 0.2 mg/ml, 1 ml: **$4.74-$4.94**

CONTRAINDICATIONS: Augmentation of labor; administration before delivery of placenta; threatened spontaneous abortion

PRECAUTIONS: Calcium deficiency, prolonged use, hypertension, heart disease, venoarterial shunts, mitral valve stenosis, obliterative vascular disease, sepsis, hepatic or renal impairment

PREGNANCY AND LACTATION: Not recommended for routine use prior to delivery of the placenta; may lower prolactin levels, which may decrease lactation

SIDE EFFECTS/ADVERSE REACTIONS

CNS: Dizziness, fainting, headache
CV: Chest pain, hypertension, *MI*
EENT: Tinnitus
GI: Nausea, vomiting
GU: Cramping
RESP: Dyspnea
SKIN: Sweating

INTERACTIONS

Drugs

3 *Dopamine:* Excessive vasoconstriction

SPECIAL CONSIDERATIONS

• Symptoms of ergotism occur with overdosage (nausea, vomiting, diarrhea, seizure, hallucinations delirium, numb/gangrenous extremities)

MONITORING PARAMETERS

• Blood pressure, pulse, and uterine response

---

italic = common side effects   ***bold italic*** = life-threatening reactions

ergotamine
(er-got'a-meen)
Rx: Ergomar
Combinations
  Rx: with caffeine (Cafergot, Ercaf, Wigraine); with belladonna alkaloids, phenobarbital (Bellergal-S)
Chemical Class: Ergot alkaloid
Therapeutic Class: Antimigraine agent

CLINICAL PHARMACOLOGY
Mechanism of Action: Partial agonist and/or antagonist activity against tryptaminergic, dopaminergic, and α-adrenergic receptors depending upon their site; uterine stimulant; causes constriction of peripheral and cranial blood vessels
Pharmacokinetics
PO: Peak 2 hr; metabolized in liver, excreted as metabolites in bile; plasma $t_{1/2}$ 2 hr
INDICATIONS AND USES: Abortive therapy for vascular headaches including migraine and cluster headaches
DOSAGE
Adult
• PO, SL 2 mg stat, then 1-2 mg q½h prn until relief, not to exceed 6 mg/day or 10 mg/wk; PR 1 supp stat, then ½ supp q1h prn until relief, not to exceed 2 mg per attack
Older Child and Adolescent
• PO or SL 1 mg stat, then 1 mg q½h prn until relief, not to exceed 3 mg/attack
💲 AVAILABLE FORMS/COST OF THERAPY
• Supp—PR (caffeine/ergotamine): 100 mg/2 mg, 12's: **$18.75-$82.72**
• Tab—Oral: 2 mg, 20's: **$113.49**
• Tab—Oral: (caffeine/ ergotamine) 100 mg/1 mg, 100's: **$66.26-$106.86**

CONTRAINDICATIONS: Pregnancy (or women at risk for pregnancy), peripheral vascular disease, hepatic or renal impairment, CAD, uncontrolled hypertension, sepsis
PRECAUTIONS: Prolonged administration, excessive dosage
PREGNANCY AND LACTATION: Pregnancy category X; excreted into breast milk; has caused symptoms of ergotism (e.g., vomiting, diarrhea) in the infant; excessive dosage or prolonged administration may inhibit lactation
SIDE EFFECTS/ADVERSE REACTIONS
CV: Chest pain, coronary vasoconstriction (large doses), increase or decrease in blood pressure, transient tachycardia or bradycardia
GI: Nausea, vomiting
MISC: Itching, localized edema, muscle pain in extremities, numbness and tingling of fingers and toes, weakness in legs
INTERACTIONS
Drugs
❷ *Azithromycin, dirithromycin, erythromycin:* Coadministration may result in ergotism
❷ *Nitroglycerin:* Decreased antianginal effects of nitroglycerin
SPECIAL CONSIDERATIONS
PATIENT/FAMILY EDUCATION
• Initiate therapy at 1st sign of attack
• DO NOT exceed recommended dosage
• Notify clinician of irregular heart beat, nausea, vomiting, numbness or tingling of fingers or toes, pain or weakness of extremities
• Regular use may lead to withdrawal headaches

* = non-FDA-approved use

erythromycin
(er-ith-roe-mye′sin)

Rx: *Systemic:* E-Mycin, Eryc, Ery-Tab, PCE Dispertab, Ilosone, E.E.S., Eryped, Ilotycin

Rx: *Topical:* A/T/S, Akne-Mycin, C-Solve 2, Emgel, Erycette, Eryderm, Erygel, Erymax, E-Solve 2, ETS-2%, Staticin, Theramycin Z, T-Stat

Rx: *Ophth:* AK-Mycin, Ilotycin

Combinations

> **Rx:** with sulfisoxazole (Pediazole); with benzoyl peroxide (Benzamycin)

Chemical Class: Macrolide derivative

Therapeutic Class: Antibiotic

CLINICAL PHARMACOLOGY

Mechanism of Action: Binds to 50S ribosomal subunits of susceptible bacteria and suppresses protein synthesis

Pharmacokinetics

PO: Peak 4 hr, duration 6 hr; 70% bound to plasma proteins; $t_{1/2}$ 1-3 hr; metabolized in liver, excreted in bile, feces

INDICATIONS AND USES: Systemic: treatment of infections caused by susceptible strains of the designated microorganisms; upper and lower respiratory tract infections caused by *Streptococcus pyogenes* and *Str. pneumoniae;* respiratory tract infections due to *Mycoplasma pneumoniae;* pertussis (whooping cough) caused by *Bordatella pertussis;* diphtheria, as an adjunct to antitoxin in infections due to *Corynebacterium diphtheriae;* erythrasma due to *Corynebacterium minutissimum;* intestinal amebiasis caused by *Entamoeba histolytica* (PO only); acute pelvic inflammatory disease caused by *Neisseria gonorrhoeae;* infections due to *Listeria monocytogenes;* skin and soft tissue infections caused by *Str. pyogenes* and *Staphylococcus aureus;* infections caused by *Chlamydia trachomatis* (conjunctivitis of the newborn, pneumonia of infancy, urogenital infections during pregnancy, uncomplicated urethral, endocervical, or rectal infections in adults); nongonococcal urethritis caused by *Ureaplasma urealyticum;* Legionnaires' disease caused by *Legionella pneumophila;* prevention of initial/recurrent attacks of rheumatic fever; prevention of bacterial endocarditis Topical: acne vulgaris

Ophthalmic: superficial ocular infections involving the conjunctiva or cornea; prophylaxis of ophthalmia neonatorum due to *Neisseria gonorrhoeae* or *Chlamydia trachomatis*

Systemic: diabetic gastroparesis*; as an alternative to penicillins in anthrax*; Vincent's gingivitis*; actinomycosis*; *Nocardia* infections (with a sulfonamide)*; *Eikenella corrodens* infections*; *Borrelia* infections (including early Lyme disease)*; campylobacter enteritis*; *Lymphogranuloma venereum*; chancroid*

DOSAGE

Adult

• PO base 333 mg q8h; estolate, stearate, or base 250-500 mg q6-12h; ethyl succinate 400-800 mg q6-12h; IV 15-20 mg/kg/day divided q6h; TOP apply to affected area bid; OPHTH apply ¼ in ribbon of ointment qd-qid as needed

• *Endocarditis prophylaxis:* PO ethyl succinate 800 mg 1 hr prior to procedure and 400 mg 6 hr after

---

italic = common side effects   **bold italic** = life-threatening reactions

Child

• PO base, ethyl succinate 30-50 mg/kg/day divided q6-8h; estolate: 30-50 mg/kg/day divided q8-12h; stearate 20-40 mg/kg/day divided q6h; IV lactobionate 20-40 mg/kg/day divided q6h, do not exceed 4 g/day; gluceptate: 20-50 mg/kg/day divided q6h; TOP apply to affected area bid; OPHTH apply ¼ in ribbon of ointment qd-qid as needed

§ AVAILABLE FORMS/COST OF THERAPY

Erythromycin Base

• Cap, Sus Action—Oral: 250 mg, 100's: **$24.23-$128.63**

• Gel—Top: 2%, 30, 50, 60 g: **$21.26-$36.71**/30 g

• Oint—Ophth: 0.5%, 3.5 g: **$1.89-$8.49**

• Oint—Top: 2%, 25 g: **$19.94-$36.13**

• Sol—Top: 1.5%, 60 ml: **$5.25-$29.54**; 2%, 60, 120 ml: **$3.95-$26.35**/60 ml

• Swab, Medicated—Top: 2%, 60's: **$18.05-$29.53**

• Tab, Plain Coated—Oral: 250 mg, 100's: **$15.56**; 500 mg, 100's: **$28.60**

• Tab, Sus Action—Oral: 250 mg, 100's: **$11.38-$39.90**; 333 mg, 100's: **$31.04-$50.85**; 500 mg, 100's: **$44.74**

Erythromycin Estolate

• Cap, Gel—Oral: 250 mg, 100's: **$27.75-$56.91**

• Susp—Oral: 125 mg/5 ml, 100, 120, 200, 480 ml: **$23.90-$47.01**/480 ml; 250 mg/5 ml, 100, 120, 200, 480 ml: **$35.00-$84.00**/480 ml

• Tab, Coated—Oral: 500 mg, 50's: **$49.56**

Erythromycin Ethyl Succinate

• Powder, Granules, Reconst—Oral: 200 mg/5 ml, 100, 200, 480 ml: **$14.02-$19.25**/200 ml; 400 mg/5 ml, 100, 200 ml: **$21.62-$25.03**/200 ml

• Powder, Reconst, Drops—Oral: 100 mg/2.5 ml, 50 ml: **$7.21**

• Susp—Oral: 200 mg/5 ml, 100, 480 ml: **$19.04-$23.50**/480 ml; 400 mg/5 ml, 100, 200, 480 ml: **$33.39-$42.50**/480 ml

• Plain Coated—Oral: 400 mg, 100's: **$20.75-$31.20**

• Tab, Chewable—Oral: 200 mg, 40's: **$22.79-$25.46**

Erythromycin Gluceptate

• Inj, Dry Sol—IV: 1 g/ampule, 50 ml: **$25.07**

Erythromycin Lactobionate

• Inj, Lyphl-Sol—IV: 500 mg/vial, 1's: **$3.55-$9.76**; 1 g/vial, 1's: **$11.59-$12.58**

Erythromycin Stearate

• Tab, Plain Coated—Oral: 250 mg, 100's: **$9.00-$18.16**; 500 mg, 100's: **$24.28-$56.00**

CONTRAINDICATIONS: Systemic: pre-existing liver disease (estolate); ophthalmic: epithelial herpes simplex keratitis; vaccinia, varicella, mycobacterial, fungal infections

PRECAUTIONS: Systemic: hepatic disease, prolonged or repeated therapy; ophthalmic: antibiotic hypersensitivity; topical: child <12 yr

PREGNANCY AND LACTATION: Pregnancy category B; excreted into breast milk; compatible with breast feeding

SIDE EFFECTS/ADVERSE REACTIONS

*CV: **Ventricular dysrhythmias*** (rare)

EENT: Hearing loss, overgrowth of nonsusceptible organisms (ophth), poor corneal wound healing, temporary visual haze, tinnitus

GI: Abdominal cramping and discomfort, anorexia, cholestatic hepatitis (most common with estolate), *diarrhea,* heartburn, *nausea,* pruritus ani, stomatitis, *vomiting*

GU: Moniliasis, vaginitis

SKIN: Pruritus, rash, thrombophlebitis, urticaria (IV site), burning; dry, scaly, oily skin; pruritus, rash, stinging; urticaria (top)

INTERACTIONS

Drugs

3 *Alfentanil:* Prolonged anesthesia and respiratory depression

3 *Alprazolam:* Increased plasma alprazolam concentration

3 *Amprenavir:* Plasma concentrations of erythromycin may be increased by amprenavir; plasma concentrations of amprenavir may be increased by erythromycin

⚠ *Astemizole:* QT prolongation and life-threatening dysrhythmia

3 *Atorvastatin:* Increased plasma atorvastatin concentration with risk of rhabdomyolysis

3 *Bromocriptine:* Increased bromocriptine concentration with toxicity

3 *Buspirone:* Increased plasma buspirone concentration

3 *Carbamazepine:* Markedly increased plasma carbamazepine concentrations

❷ *Cisapride:* QT prolongation and dysrhythmia

❷ *Clozapine:* Increased plasma clozapine concentrations

3 *Colchicine:* Potential colchicine toxicity

3 *Cyclosporine:* Increased plasma cyclosporine concentrations

3 *Diazepam:* Increased plasma concentration of diazepam

3 *Digoxin:* Reduced bacterial flora may increase plasma digoxin concentrations

3 *Disopyramide:* Increased plasma disopyramide concentrations

❷ *Ergotamine:* Potential for ergotism

3 *Ethanol:* Ethanol reduces plasma erythromycin concentration

3 *Felodipine:* Increased plasma felodipine concentrations

3 *Food:* Food may increase or decrease the bioavailability of erythromycin

3 *Indinavir:* Plasma concentrations of erythromycin may be increased by indinavir; plasma concentrations of indinavir may be increased by erythromycin

3 *Itraconazole:* Increased plasma itraconazole concentration

3 *Lovastatin:* Increased plasma lovastatin concentration with risk of rhabdomyolysis

3 *Methylprednisolone:* Increased plasma methylprednisolone concentrations

3 *Midazolam:* Increased plasma concentration of midazolam

3 *Nelfinavir:* Plasma concentrations of erythromycin may be increased by nelfinavir; plasma concentrations of nelfinavir may be increased by erythromycin

3 *Penicillin:* Decreased activity of penicillin

3 *Quinidine:* Increased plasma concentration of quinidine

3 *Ritonavir:* Plasma concentrations of erythromycin may be increased by ritonavir; plasma concentrations of ritonavir may be increased by erythromycin

3 *Saquinavir:* Plasma concentrations of erythromycin may be increased by saquinavir; plasma concentrations of saquinavir may be increased by erythromycin

3 *Sildenafil:* Increased plasma sildenafil concentration

italic = common side effects   ***bold italic*** = life-threatening reactions

❷ *Simvastatin:* Increased plasma simvastatin concentration with risk of rhabdomyolysis

❸ *Tacrolimus:* Increased plasma tacrolimus concentration

❸ *Theophylline:* Increased plasma theophylline concentration

❸ *Triazolam:* Increased plasma triazolam concentration

❸ *Valproic acid:* Increased plasma valproic acid concentration

❸ *Warfarin:* Markedly increased hypoprothrombinemic response to warfarin

❸ *Zafirlukast:* Reduced plasma zafirlukast concentration probably by reducing bioavailability

❸ *Zopiclone:* Increased plasma zopiclone concentration

Labs
• *False decrease:* Folate assay
• *False increase:* Urine 17-ketosteroids, AST, urine amino acids

SPECIAL CONSIDERATIONS
PATIENT/FAMILY EDUCATION
• Take with food to minimize GI discomfort
• Take each dose with 180-240 ml of water
• Wash, rinse, and dry affected area prior to top application
• Keep top preparations away from eyes, nose, and mouth
• Ophth ointments may cause temporary blurring of vision following administration

MONITORING PARAMETERS
• LFTs if hepatotoxicity suspected
• Check daily for vein irritation and phlebitis in patients receiving IV forms

---

erythropoietin (epoetin alfa)
(er-ith-row-poe´ee-tin)
Rx: Epogen, Procrit
Chemical Class: Amino acid glycoprotein
Therapeutic Class: Hematopoietic agent

CLINICAL PHARMACOLOGY
Mechanism of Action: Induces red blood cell production by stimulating the division and differentiation of committed erythroid progenitor cells; induces release of reticulocytes from bone marrow into the bloodstream, where they mature to erythrocytes

Pharmacokinetics
SC: Peak 5-24 hr, onset takes several days; elimination poorly understood; some metabolism in liver and bone marrow, 10% excreted unchanged in urine; $t_{1/2}$ 4-13 hr in patients with chronic renal failure (20% shorter in patients with normal renal function)

INDICATIONS AND USES: Anemia in patients with chronic renal failure; anemia related to zidovudine therapy in HIV-infected patients; anemia in cancer patients on chemotherapy and other patients requiring elective surgery (attempt to reduce the need for blood transfusions); anemia of prematurity*; pruritus associated with renal failure*

DOSAGE
Adult
• *Chronic renal failure:* IV (dialysis patients)/IV or SC (non-dialysis chronic renal failure patients) 50-100 U/kg 3 times/wk initially; increase dose if hct increases by <5-6 points after 8 wk and is below target range; decrease dose when target hct is reached or hct increases >4 points

---

* = non-FDA-approved use

in any 2 wk period; maintenance dose should be individualized, but is generally about 25 U/kg 3 times/wk

• *Zidovudine-treated HIV-infected patients:* IV/SC 100 U/kg 3 times/wk initially; after 8 wk adjust dose by 50-100 U/kg to a max of 300 U/kg 3 times/wk

• *Cancer patients on chemotherapy:* SC 150 U/kg 3 times/wk initially; after 8 wk adjust dose by 50-100 U/kg to a max of 300 U/kg 3 times/wk

• *Prior to elective surgery:* SC 300 U/kg/d for 10 days prior to surgery, the day of surgery and for 4 days after surgery

Neonate

• *Anemia of prematurity:* SC 150-250 U/kg 3 times/wk

💲 AVAILABLE FORMS/COST OF THERAPY

• Inj, Sol—IV, SC: 2000 U/ml, 1 ml: **$24.00-$27.83**; 3000 U/ml, 1 ml: **$36.00-$41.76**; 4000 U/ml, 1 ml: **$48.00-$55.65**; 10,000 U/ml, 1 ml: **$120.00-$139.12**; 20,000 U/ml, 1 ml: **$263.08-$284.73**

CONTRAINDICATIONS: Uncontrolled hypertension; hypersensitivity to mammalian cell-derived products or to human albumin; use to enhance athletic performance

PRECAUTIONS: Severe anemia, seizure disorder, vascular disease, history of thrombosis, children, porphyria

PREGNANCY AND LACTATION: Pregnancy category C; excretion into breast milk unknown; use caution in nursing mothers

SIDE EFFECTS/ADVERSE REACTIONS

CNS: Headache, **seizures**
CV: Hypertension, tachycardia
GI: Diarrhea, *nausea,* vomiting
HEME: Clotted vascular access
METAB: Hyperkalemia
MS: Arthralgia, myalgia

RESP: Shortness of breath
SKIN: Inj site stinging

SPECIAL CONSIDERATIONS

• Iron supplementation should be given during therapy to provide for increased requirements during expansion of red cell mass secondary to marrow stimulation by erythropoietin

• Use prior to elective surgery should be limited to patients with presurgery hemoglobin of >10 but ≤13 g/dl undergoing noncardiac, nonvascular procedures

PATIENT/FAMILY EDUCATION

• Do not shake vials as this may denature the glycoprotein rendering the drug inactive

• Notify clinician if severe headache develops

• Frequent blood tests required to determine optimal dose

MONITORING PARAMETERS

• Hct (target range 30%-33%, max 36%), serum iron, ferritin (keep >100 ng/dl)

• Baseline erythropoietin level (treatment of patients with erythropoietin levels >200 mU/ml is not recommended)

• Blood pressure

• BUN, uric acid, creatinine, phosphorus, potassium on a regular basis

---

esmolol

(ess'moe-lol)

Rx: Brevibloc
Chemical Class: β_1-selective (cardioselective) adrenoceptor blocker
Therapeutic Class: Antidysrhythmic (Class II)

CLINICAL PHARMACOLOGY

Mechanism of Action: Competitive β-adrenergic antagonist; produces negative inotropic and chronotropic

---

italic = common side effects   ***bold italic*** = life-threatening reactions

responses; slows AV nodal conduction; decreases heart rate; decreases myocardial oxygen consumption; antiarrhythmic effects (class II); reduction in platelet aggregation and blood viscosity; suppression of renin release; inhibition of central sympathetic outflow; decreases presynaptic receptor neurotransmitter release; no intrinsic sympathomimetic or membrane stabilizing activity; low lipid solubility

Pharmacokinetics

IV: Onset very rapid, duration short; 55% bound to plasma proteins; metabolized by hydrolysis of the ester linkage by esterases in the cytosol of red blood cells, excreted via kidneys; $t_{1/2}$ 9 min

INDICATIONS AND USES: Supraventricular arrhythmias (atrial fibrillation, atrial flutter, paroxysmal supraventricular tachycardia), aggressive behavior,* angina pectoris,* anxiety,* hyperthyroidism,* neuroleptic-induced akathisia,* aortic dissection,* cardiac surgery (myocardial protection),* electroconvulsive therapy,* pheochromocytoma,* tetanus,* neuroleptic-induced akathisia, angina pectoris,* anxiety,* postmyocardial infarction*

DOSAGE

Adult and child >16 yr

• *Acute myocardial ischemia:* IV loading INF 500 µg/kg, followed by 50-150 µg/kg/min INF

• *Arrhythmias:* IV 50-200 µg/kg/min

Child

• *Arrhythmias:* IV 300 µg/kg/min INF initially; titrate upward in 50-100 µg/kg/min increments every 10 minutes; mean effective doses much higher than adults

⑧ AVAILABLE FORMS/COST OF THERAPY

• Inj, Sol—IV: 10 mg/ml, 10, 250 ml: **$8.51**/10 ml; 250 mg/ml, 10 ml: **$100.74**

CONTRAINDICATIONS: Bronchial asthma, cardiogenic shock, overt cardiac failure, 2nd and 3rd degree AV block, severe sinus bradycardia

PRECAUTIONS: Anesthesia/surgery (myocardial depression), avoid abrupt withdrawal, bronchospastic airways, congestive heart failure, diabetes mellitus, hyperthyroidism/thyrotoxicosis, concurrent clonidine, peripheral vascular disease, renal disease

PREGNANCY AND LACTATION: Pregnancy category C; potential for hypotension and subsequent decreased uterine blood flow and fetal hypoxia should be considered; excretion into breast milk unknown; use caution in nursing mothers

SIDE EFFECTS/ADVERSE REACTIONS

CNS: Depression, *dizziness,* drowsiness, *fatigue,* hallucinations, insomnia, *lethargy,* memory loss, mental changes, strange dreams

CV: Bradycardia, **CHF,** cold extremities, *hypotension,* **2nd or 3rd degree heart block**

EENT: Dry, burning eyes; sore throat; visual disturbances

GI: Diarrhea, dry mouth, ***ischemic colitis, mesenteric arterial thrombosis,*** nausea, vomiting

GU: Impotence, sexual dysfunction

HEME: **Agranulocytosis, thrombocytopenia**

METAB: Masked hypoglycemic response to insulin (sweating excepted)

RESP: **Bronchospasm,** dyspnea, wheezing

---

* = non-FDA-approved use

SKIN: Alopecia, pruritis, rash

INTERACTIONS

Drugs

3 *Alpha-1 adrenergic blockers:* Potential enhanced first dose response (marked initial drop in blood pressure, particularly on standing (especially prazocin)

3 *Amiodarone:* Symptomatic bradycardia and sinus arrest; AV node refractory period is prolonged and sinus node automaticity is decreased by amiodarone. The sinus rate can be further slowed or AV block worsened in patients with bradycardia, sick sinus syndrome, or partial AV block

3 *Dihydropyridine calcium channel blockers:* Severe hypotension or impaired cardiac performance; most prevalent with impaired left ventricular function, cardiac arrhythmias, or aortic stenosis

3 *Digoxin:* Additive prolongation of atrioventricular (AV) conduction time

3 *Diltiazem:* Potentiates β-adrenergic effects; hypotension, left ventricular failure, and AV conduction disturbances problematic in elderly, patients with left ventricular dysfunction, aortic stenosis, or with large doses of either drug

3 *Hypoglycemic agents:* Masked hypoglycemia, hyperglycemia

3 *Verapamil:* Potentiates β-adrenergic effects; hypotension, left ventricular failure, and AV conduction disturbances problematic in elderly, patients with left ventricular dysfunction, aortic stenosis, or with large doses of either drug

SPECIAL CONSIDERATIONS

• Transfer to alternative agent (e.g., propranolol, digoxin, verapamil): ½ hr after 1st dose of alternative agent, reduce esmolol INF rate by 50%; following 2nd dose of alternative agent, monitor patient's response

and, if satisfactory control is maintained for the 1st hr, discontinue esmolol INF

• Do not discontinue abruptly; may require taper; rapid withdrawal may produce rebound hypertension or angina

MONITORING PARAMETERS

• Angina: Reduction in nitroglycerin usage; frequency, severity, onset, and duration of angina pain; heart rate

• Arrhythmias: Heart rate

• Hypertension: Blood pressure

• Postmyocardial infarction: Left ventricular function, lower resting heart rate

• Toxicity: Blood glucose, bronchospasm, hypotension, bradycardia, depression, confusion, hallucination, sexual dysfunction

---

esomeprazole

(es-om-eh-pray′zole)

Rx: Nexium

Chemical Class: Benzimidazole derivative

Therapeutic Class: Gastrointestinal antisecretory agent

CLINICAL PHARMACOLOGY

Mechanism of Action: Irreversibly inactivates proton pump in gastric parietal cells, which blocks the final step in secretion of hydrochloric acid; acid secretion is inhibited until additional enzyme is synthesized; inhibits basal and stimulated gastric acid secretion

Pharmacokinetics

PO: Peak 1.5 hr; systemic bioavailability 90% (following repeated dosing; decreased by administration with food); 97% bound to plasma proteins; extensively metabolized by hepatic cytochrome P450 enzymes (metabolites lack antisecretory activity); 80% of oral dose excreted in urine as inactive metabolites, the remainder is found as inactive metabolites in the feces; $t_{1/2}$ 1-1.5 hr

INDICATIONS AND USES: Short-term treatment (4-8 wk) in the healing and symptomatic resolution of diagnostically confirmed erosive esophagitis; maintenance of symptom resolution and healing of erosive esophagitis; treatment of heartburn and other symptoms associated with gastroesophageal reflux disease (GERD); eradication of *H. pylori* in patients with *H. pylori* infection and duodenal ulcer disease (active or history of within past 5 yr) in combination with amoxicillin and clarithromycin

DOSAGE

Adult

• *Healing of erosive esophagitis:* PO 20-40 mg qd for 4-8 wk; for patients who do not heal after 4-8 wk, and additional 4-8 wk of treatment may be considered

• *Maintenance of healing of erosive esophagitis:* PO 20 mg qd

• *GERD:* PO 20 mg qd for 4 wk; if symptoms do not resolve completely after 4 wk, an additional 4 wk of treatment my be considered

• *Eradication of H. pylori:* PO 40 mg qd in combination with amoxicillin 1 g bid and clarithromycin 500 mg bid for 10 days (triple therapy)

• *Dose adjustment in severe liver impairment:* PO a dose of 20 mg qd should not be exceeded

$ AVAILABLE FORMS/COST OF THERAPY

• Cap, Delayed-Release—Oral: 20 mg, 100's: **$399.66**; 40 mg, 100's: **$399.66**

PRECAUTIONS: Symptomatic response does not preclude gastric malignancy; children; hepatic function impairment

PREGNANCY AND LACTATION: Pregnancy category B; likely to be excreted into breast milk, use caution in nursing mothers (suppression of gastric acid secretion is potential effect in nursing infant, clinical significance unknown)

SIDE EFFECTS/ADVERSE REACTIONS

CNS: Asthenia, dizziness, headache
GI: Abdominal pain, constipation, diarrhea, flatulence, nausea, dry mouth
MS: Back pain
RESP: Cough
SKIN: Rash

INTERACTIONS

Drugs

3 *Ketoconazole, iron salts, digoxin:* Reduced gastric acidity may result in decreased absorption of these and other drugs where gastric pH is an important determinant of bioavailability

SPECIAL CONSIDERATIONS

• S-isomer of omeprazole (racemate)
• No advantage over other proton-pump inhibitors

PATIENT/FAMILY EDUCATION

• Take at least 1 hr before meals
• Capsules may be opened, mixed with cold applesauce and swallowed immediately without chewing for patients who cannot swallow capsules whole

---

* = non-FDA-approved use

estazolam

(ess-ta'zoe-lam)
Rx: ProSom
Chemical Class: Benzodiazepine
Therapeutic Class: Sedative-hypnotic
DEA Class: Schedule IV

E

CLINICAL PHARMACOLOGY

Mechanism of Action: CNS depressants via facilitation of inhibitory GABA at benzodiazepine receptor sites (BZ_1—associated with sleep; BZ_2—associated with memory, motor, sensory, and cognitive function); effects include muscle relaxation (spinal cord), anticonvulsant activity (brain stem), ataxia (cerebellum), emotional behavior (limbic and cortical areas), and anxiolytic effects (separate from general CNS depression); decreases sleep latency, the number of awakenings, and the time spent in stage 0 (awake) sleep; stage 2 (unequivocal sleep) is increased; in sum, sleep time increased

Pharmacokinetics

PO: Onset 15-45 min, peak 2 hr, duration 7-8 hr; 93% bound to plasma proteins; metabolized by liver, excreted by kidneys (inactive/active metabolites); $t_{1/2}$ 8-28 hr

INDICATIONS AND USES: Insomnia

DOSAGE

Adult

• PO 1-2 mg qhs; 0.5 mg in elderly or debilitated patients

💲 AVAILABLE FORMS/COST OF THERAPY

• Tab, Uncoated—Oral: 1 mg, 100's: **$88.70-$132.39**; 2 mg, 100's: **$98.92-$147.49**

PRECAUTIONS: Renal or hepatic function impairment, elderly, depression, history of drug abuse, abrupt withdrawal, respiratory depression, sleep apnea

PREGNANCY AND LACTATION: Pregnancy category X; may cause fetal damage when administered during pregnancy; excreted into breast milk; may accumulate in breast-fed infants and is therefore not recommended

SIDE EFFECTS/ADVERSE REACTIONS

CNS: Abnormal thinking, agitation, amnesia, anxiety, apathy, *asthenia,* ataxia, decreased libido, decreased reflexes, emotional lability, hangover, hostility, *hypokinesia,* neuritis, **seizures,** sleep disorder, *somnolence,* stupor, twitch

CV: **Dysrhythmia,** syncope

EENT: Ear pain; epistaxis, eye irritation, pain, pharyngitis, photophobia, rhinitis, sinusitis, swelling

GI: Abdominal pain, appetite changes; dyspepsia; enterocolitis, flatulence, gastritis, increased AST, melena, mouth ulceration

GU: Frequent urination, hematuria, menstrual cramps; nocturia, oliguria, penile discharge, urinary hesitancy, urgency; urinary incontinence, vaginal discharge, itching

HEME: **Agranulocytosis**

MS: Back pain, lower extremity pain

RESP: Asthma, cold symptoms, cough, dyspnea, hyperventilation

SKIN: Acne, dry skin, photosensitivity, urticaria

INTERACTIONS

Drugs

3 *Cimetidine:* Increased serum benzodiazepine concentrations

3 *Disulfiram:* May increase benzodiazepine serum concentrations

3 *Erythromycin:* Increased estazolam sedative effects

---

italic = common side effects   ***bold italic*** = life-threatening reactions

3 *Ethanol:* Enhanced adverse psychomotor effects of benzodiazepines

3 *Rifampin:* Reduced serum benzodiazepine concentrations

SPECIAL CONSIDERATIONS
PATIENT/FAMILY EDUCATION
• Do not discontinue abruptly after prolonged therapy
• May experience disturbed sleep for the 1st or 2nd night after discontinuing the drug

---

esterified estrogens
Rx: Estratab, Menest
Combinations
  Rx: with methyltestosterone
  (Estratest, Menogen)
Chemical Class: Estrogen derivative
Therapeutic Class: Estrogen; antineoplastic; antiosteoporotic

---

CLINICAL PHARMACOLOGY
Mechanism of Action: Necessary for adequate functioning of female reproductive system; affects release of pituitary gonadotropins, inhibits ovulation, inhibits bone resorption
Pharmacokinetics
PO: Well absorbed; metabolized and inactivated in the liver, excreted in urine

INDICATIONS AND USES: Symptoms associated with menopause (vasomotor symptoms, atrophic vaginitis, kraurosis vulvae), female hypogonadism, female castration, primary ovarian failure, breast cancer (palliation), prostatic carcinoma (palliation), postpartum breast engorgement,* osteoporosis*

DOSAGE
Adult
• *Menopause:* PO 0.3-1.25 mg qd or days 1-25 of mo (combined with progestin in women with intact uterus)
• *Female hypogonadism:* PO 2.5 to 7.5 mg/day in divided doses for 20 days, followed by 10 day rest period, repeat if bleeding does not occur by the end of this period; if bleeding occurs before the end of the 10 day period, begin 2.5-7.5 mg/day in divided doses days 1-20 of mo (administer oral progestin during last 5 days of estrogen cycle)
• *Female castration and primary ovarian failure:* PO 1.25 mg qd, 3 wk on, 1 wk off
• *Prostate cancer (inoperable, progressing):* 1.25-2.5 mg tid
• *Breast cancer (inoperable, progressing):* 10 mg tid for 3 mo or longer

§ **AVAILABLE FORMS/COST OF THERAPY**
• Tab, Sugar Coated—Oral: 0.3 mg, 100's: **$14.53-$45.88**; 0.625 mg, 100's: **$20.60-$61.72**; 1.25 mg, 100's: **$36.08-$58.15**; 2.5 mg, 100's: **$148.12**
• Tab—Oral: 0.625 mg/2.5 mg methyltestosterone, 100's: **$63.25-$130.57**; 1.25 mg/2.5 mg methyltestosterone, 100's: **$78.00-$159.86**

CONTRAINDICATIONS: Breast cancer (except in selected patients being treated for metastatic disease), active thromboembolic disorders, known or suspected estrogen-dependent neoplasia, undiagnosed abnormal genital bleeding
PRECAUTIONS: Hypertension, gallbladder disease, CHF, diabetes mellitus, depression, migraine headache, seizure disorders, hepatic disease, family history of breast or endometrial cancer, history of

---

* = non-FDA-approved use

thromboembolic disorders, uterine fibroids, hypertriglyceridemia, hypercalcemia

PREGNANCY AND LACTATION: Pregnancy category X; may decrease quantity and quality of breast milk

SIDE EFFECTS/ADVERSE REACTIONS

CNS: Depression, migraine headache, emotional lability

CV: **Arterial thromboembolism, pulmonary embolism, CVA, MI,** hypertension, venous thrombosis, edema

EENT: Contact lens intolerance, ***retinal thrombosis***

GI: Nausea and vomiting, gallbladder disease, bloating, benign hepatic tumors, ***mesenteric thrombosis***

GU: Breakthrough bleeding, spotting, amenorrhea, change in cervical secretions, breast enlargement, breast tenderness, ***testicular atrophy, endometrial cancer***

METAB: Hyperglycemia, hypertriglyceridemia, hypercalcemia

SKIN: Melasma

INTERACTIONS

Drugs

3 *P450 inducers (e.g., rifampin, barbiturates):* Decreased estrogen levels

3 *Corticosteroids:* Increased steroid effect

3 *Phenytoin:* Loss of seizure control, decreased estrogen levels

3 *Warfarin:* Theoretical increased risk thromboembolism

SPECIAL CONSIDERATIONS

• Progestins recommended in non-hysterectomized women

estradiol

(ess-tra-dye'ole)

Rx: *Oral:* Estrace, Vagifem

Rx: *Estradiol Cypionate Inj:* Depo-Estradiol, DepoGen, Estro-Cyp

Rx: *Estradiol Valerate Inj:* Delestrogen, Valergen

Rx: *Transdermal:* Estraderm, Climara, Vivelle, E_2 III

Rx: *Vaginal insert:* Estring
Combinations

   Rx: with medroxyprogesterone (Lunelle)

   Rx: with norgestimate (Ortho-Prefest)

   Rx: with testosterone cypionate (Depo-Testadiol)

   Rx: with testosterone enanthate (Deladumone)

   Rx: Transdermal with norethindrone (CombiPatch)

Chemical Class: Estrogen derivative

Therapeutic Class: Estrogen; antineoplastic; antiosteoporotic

CLINICAL PHARMACOLOGY

Mechanism of Action: Necessary for adequate functioning of female reproductive system; affects release of pituitary gonadotropins, inhibits bone resorption

Pharmacokinetics

PO/IM/TRANSDERM: Degraded in liver; excreted in urine; crosses placenta; excreted in breast milk

INDICATIONS AND USES: Symptoms associated with menopause (vasomotor symptoms, atrophic vaginitis, kraurosis vulvae), breast cancer, prostatic cancer, atrophic vaginitis, hypogonadism, castration, primary ovarian failure, prevention of osteoporosis

---

italic = common side effects   ***bold italic*** = life-threatening reactions

DOSAGE
Adult
• *Menopause/hypogonadism/castration/ovarian failure:* PO 1-2 mg qd 3wk on, 1 wk off or 5 days on, 2 days off; IM 1-5 mg q3-4wk (cypionate); 10-20 mg q4wk (valerate); TRANSDERM 0.05-0.1 mg worn continuously, change once (Climara, E$_2$III) or twice (Estraderm, Vivelle, CombiPatch) per week; VAG RING insert ring into vagina, change rings q3mo
• *Prostatic cancer:* IM 30 mg q1-2 wk (valerate); PO 1-2 mg tid (oral estradiol)
• *Breast cancer:* PO 10 mg tid for 3 mo or longer
• *Atrophic vaginitis:* Vag cre 2-4 g (marked on applicator) qd for 1-2 wk, then 1 g 1-3 times/wk

§ AVAILABLE FORMS/COST OF THERAPY
• Cre—Vag: 0.01%, 42.5 g: **$44.19-$52.02**
• Film, Cont Rel—Percutaneous: 0.025 mg/24 hr 4's: **$29.50** (Climara); 0.0375 mg/24 hr, 8's: **$25.13** (Vivelle); 0.05 mg/24 hr, 8's: **$24.60** (Vivelle); 0.05 mg/24 hr, 8's: **$18.35-$25.58** (Estraderm); 0.075 mg/24 hr, 8's: **$25.08-$25.65** (Vivelle); 0.1 mg/24 hr, 8's: **$25.56** (Vivelle); 0.1 mg/24 hr, 8's: **$20.04** (Estraderm)
• Film, Cont Rel-Percutaneous: 0.05 mg/0.14 mg norethindrone/24 hr (9 sq cm); 8's: **$33.60-$36.22**; .05 mg/0.25 mg norethindrone/24 hr (16 sq cm), 8's: **$34.40-$37.09**
• Inj (Cypionate)—IM: 5 mg/ml, 5, 10 ml: **$5.50-$17.92**/10 ml
• Inj (Valerate)—IM: 10 mg/ml, 5, 10 ml: **$6.25-$8.40**/10 ml; 20 mg/ml, 1, 5, 10 ml: **$6.47-$50.10**/10 ml; 40 mg/ml, 5, 10 ml: **$9.03-$80.43**/10 ml
• Insert, Ring, Cont Rel—Vag: 2 mg (0.0075 mg/24 hr), 1's: **$87.51**

• Tab, Uncoated—Oral: 0.5 mg, 100's: **$22.78-$42.94**; 1 mg, 100's: **$18.35-$57.22**; 1.5 mg, 100's: **$50.83**; 2 mg, 100's: **$25.41-$83.56**
• Tab—Oral: 1 mg/0.5 mg norethindrone, 28's: **$26.09** (Activella)

CONTRAINDICATIONS: Breast cancer (except in selected patients being treated for metastatic disease), active thromboembolic disorders, known or suspected estrogen-dependent neoplasia, undiagnosed abnormal genital bleeding

PRECAUTIONS: Hypertension, gallbladder disease, CHF, diabetes mellitus, depression, migraine headache, seizure disorders, hepatic disease, family history of breast or endometrial cancer, history of thromboembolic disorders, uterine fibroids, hypertriglyceridemia, hypercalcemia

PREGNANCY AND LACTATION: Pregnancy category X; may reduce quantity and quality of breast milk

SIDE EFFECTS/ADVERSE REACTIONS
CNS: Depression, migraine headache, emotional lability
CV: **Arterial thromboembolism, pulmonary embolism, CVA, MI,** hypertension, venous thrombosis, edema
EENT: Contact lens intolerance, **retinal thrombosis**
GI: Nausea and vomiting, gallbladder disease, bloating, benign hepatic tumors, **mesenteric thrombosis**
GU: Breakthrough bleeding, spotting, amenorrhea, change in cervical secretions, breast enlargement, breast tenderness, **testicular atrophy, endometrial cancer**
METAB: Hyperglycemia, hypertriglyceridemia, hypercalcemia
SKIN: Melasma

---

* = non-FDA-approved use

INTERACTIONS
Drugs
▣ *P450 inducers (e.g., rifampin, barbiturates):* Decreased estrogen levels

▣ *Corticosteroids:* Increased steroid effect

▣ *Phenytoin:* Loss of seizure control, decreased estrogen levels

▣ *Warfarin:* Theoretical increased risk thromboembolism

SPECIAL CONSIDERATIONS
• Progestins recommended in non-hysterectomized women. Estring may have minimal systemic absorption

---

estrogens, conjugated

Rx: Premarin, Cenestin
Combinations
  Rx: with medroxyprogesterone (Prempro daily product]), Premphase [cycled product]; with meprobamate (PMB); with methyltestosterone (Premarin with methyltestosterone)
Chemical Class: Estrogen derivative
Therapeutic Class: Estrogen; antineoplastic; antiosteoporotic

---

CLINICAL PHARMACOLOGY
Mechanism of Action: Necessary for adequate functioning of female reproductive system; affects release of pituitary gonadotropins, inhibits bone resorption

Pharmacokinetics
PO/IV/IM: Degraded in liver, excreted in urine, crosses placenta, excreted in breast milk

INDICATIONS AND USES: Menopause, breast cancer (inoperable, in postmenopausal women and men), prostatic cancer, dysfunctional uterine bleeding, hypogonadism, castration, primary ovarian failure, atrophic vaginitis, prevention of osteoporosis

DOSAGE
Adult
• *Menopause/atrophic vaginitis:* PO 0.3-1.25 mg qd cyclically or continuously, with medroxyprogesterone in women with an intact uterus

• *Atrophic vaginitis:* Vag cre 2-4 g qd cyclically, reduce dosage as tolerated (typically, 2-4 g once or twice weekly for maintenance)

• *Osteoporosis prevention:* PO 0.625 mg qd cyclically or continuously, with medroxyprogesterone in women with an intact uterus

• *Prostatic cancer:* PO 1.25-2.5 mg tid

• *Breast cancer:* PO 10 mg tid for 3 mo or longer

• *Dysfunctional uterine bleeding:* IV/IM 25 mg, repeat in 6-12 hr

• *Castration/primary ovarian failure:* PO 1.25 mg qd cyclically or continuously, with medroxyprogesterone in women with an intact uterus

• *Hypogonadism:* PO 2.5 mg qd-tid cyclically, with medroxyprogesterone in women with an intact uterus

▣ **AVAILABLE FORMS/COST OF THERAPY**
• Cre, Top—Vag: 0.625 mg/g, 42.5 g: **$52.89**

• Inj, Lyphl-Sol—IM, IV: 25 mg/5 ml, 5 ml: **$58.00**

• Tab, Sugar Coated—Oral: 0.3 mg, 100's: **$39.00-$56.50**; 0.625 mg, 100's: **$39.45-$75.54**; 0.9 mg, 100's: **$77.58-$90.93**; 1.25 mg, 100's: **$88.90-$104.83**; 2.5 mg, 100's: **$158.76-$179.83**

---

italic = common side effects   ***bold italic*** = life-threatening reactions

Combination Products

• Tab, Uncoated—Oral: 0.625 mg/2.5 mg medroxyprogesterone (both dosed qd), 28's: **$17.88-$33.08**; 0.625 mg/5.0 mg medroxyprogesterone (both dosed qd), 28's: **$21.60-$31.18**

• Tab, Uncoated—Oral: 0.625 mg/5 mg medroxyprogesterone (estrogen dosed qd day 1-28, medroxyprogesterone dosed day 15-28), 28's: **$18.38-$27.78**

CONTRAINDICATIONS: Breast cancer (except in selected patients being treated for metastatic disease), active thromboembolic disorders, known or suspected estrogen-dependent neoplasia, undiagnosed abnormal genital bleeding

PRECAUTIONS: Hypertension, gallbladder disease, CHF, diabetes mellitus, depression, migraine headache, seizure disorders, hepatic disease, family history of breast or endometrial cancer, history of thromboembolic disorders, uterine fibroids, hypertriglyceridemia, hypercalcemia

PREGNANCY AND LACTATION: Pregnancy category X; may decrease quantity and quality of breast milk

SIDE EFFECTS/ADVERSE REACTIONS

CNS: Depression, migraine headache, emotional lability

CV: **Arterial thromboembolism, pulmonary embolism, CVA, MI,** hypertension, venous thrombosis, edema

EENT: Contact lens intolerance, **retinal thrombosis**

GI: Nausea and vomiting, gallbladder disease, bloating, benign hepatic tumors, **mesenteric thrombosis**

GU: Breakthrough bleeding, spotting, amenorrhea, change in cervical secretions, breast enlargement, breast tenderness, **endometrial cancer**

METAB: Hyperglycemia, hypertriglyceridemia, hypercalcemia

SKIN: Melasma

INTERACTIONS

Drugs

3 *P450 inducers (e.g., rifampin, barbiturates):* Decreased estrogen levels

3 *Corticosteroids:* Increased steroid effect

3 *Phenytoin:* Loss of seizure control, decreased estrogen levels

3 *Warfarin:* Theoretical increased risk thromboembolism

SPECIAL CONSIDERATIONS

• Progestins recommended in non-hysterectomized women

• Premarin is derived from pregnant mare's urine; Cenestin from yams and soy. Although probably therapeutically equivalent, they are not substitutable by the pharmacist.

---

estrone

(ess'trone)

Rx: Estragyn-5, Estro-A, Kestrone-5, Primestrin
Chemical Class: Estrogen derivative
Therapeutic Class: Estrogen; antineoplastic

CLINICAL PHARMACOLOGY
Mechanism of Action: Necessary for adequate functioning of female reproductive system; affects release of pituitary gonadotropins, inhibits ovulation, inhibits bone resorption
Pharmacokinetics
IM: Degraded in liver, excreted in urine, crosses placenta, excreted in breast milk

---

INDICATIONS AND USES: Menopause, inoperable prostatic cancer, atrophic vaginitis, hypogonadism, primary ovarian failure, dysfunctional uterine bleeding

DOSAGE

Adult

• *Dysfunctional uterine bleeding:* IM 2-5 mg qd for several days

• *Menopause/atrophic vaginitis:* IM 0.1-0.5 mg 2-3 times/wk, cyclically or continuously

• *Female hypogonadism/primary ovarian failure:* IM 0.1-2 mg q wk in 1 dose or divided doses, cyclically or continuously

• *Prostatic cancer:* IM 2-4 mg 2-3 times/wk

$ **AVAILABLE FORMS/COST OF THERAPY**

• Inj, Susp—IM: 2 mg/ml, 10, 30 ml: **$5.00-$9.98**/10 ml; 5 mg/ml, 10, 30 ml: **$4.95-$18.50**/10 ml

CONTRAINDICATIONS: Breast cancer, active thromboembolic disorders, known or suspected estrogen-dependent neoplasia, undiagnosed abnormal genital bleeding

PRECAUTIONS: Hypertension, gallbladder disease, CHF, diabetes mellitus, migraine headache, hepatic disease, family history of breast or endometrial cancer, uterine fibroids, history of thromboembolic disorders, hypertriglyceridemia, hypercalcemia

PREGNANCY AND LACTATION: Pregnancy category X; may reduce quantity and quality of breast milk

SIDE EFFECTS/ADVERSE REACTIONS

CNS: Depression, migraine headache, emotional lability

CV: ***Arterial thromboembolism, pulmonary embolism, CVA, MI,*** hypertension, venous thrombosis, edema

EENT: Contact lens intolerance, ***retinal thrombosis***

GI: Nausea and vomiting, gallbladder disease, bloating, benign hepatic tumors, ***mesenteric thrombosis***

GU: Breakthrough bleeding, spotting, amenorrhea, change in cervical secretions, breast enlargement, breast tenderness, ***testicular atrophy, endometrial cancer***

METAB: Hyperglycemia, hypertriglyceridemia, hypercalcemia

SKIN: Melasma

INTERACTIONS

Drugs

3 *P450 inducers (e.g., rifampin, barbiturates):* Decreased estrogen levels

3 *Corticosteroids:* Increased steroid effect

3 *Phenytoin:* Loss of seizure control, decreased estrogen levels

3 *Warfarin:* Theoretical increased risk thromboembolism

SPECIAL CONSIDERATIONS

• Progestins recommended in non-hysterectomized women

---

estropipate

(es-tro-pip´ate)

Rx: Ogen, Ortho-Est

Chemical Class: Estrogen derivative

Therapeutic Class: Estrogen; antiosteoporotic

CLINICAL PHARMACOLOGY

Mechanism of Action: Necessary for adequate functioning of female reproductive system; affects release of pituitary gonadotropins, inhibits bone resorption

Pharmacokinetics

PO: Metabolized in liver (significant 1st-pass effect) primarily to estrone, excreted in urine

INDICATIONS AND USES: Vasomotor symptoms, atrophic vaginitis or kraurosis vulvae associated with

---

italic = common side effects   ***bold italic*** = life-threatening reactions

menopause; female hypogonadism, female castration, or primary ovarian failure; osteoporosis prevention; prevention of cardiovascular disease*

DOSAGE

Adult

• *Vasomotor symptoms:* PO 0.75-3 mg qd for 25-31 days monthly

• *Atrophic vaginitis:* PO 0.75-3 mg qd for 25-31 days monthly; vag 2-4 g qd initially, then weekly or twice weekly

• *Female hypogonadism, female castration, or primary ovarian failure:* PO 1.5-9 mg/day × 3 wk, followed by a rest period of 8-10 days, repeated cyclically

• *Osteoporosis prevention:* PO 0.75 mg qd for 25-31 days monthly

$ **AVAILABLE FORMS/COST OF THERAPY**

• Cre—Vag: 1.5 mg/g, 45 g: **$47.67**

• Tab, Uncoated—Oral: 0.75 mg, 100's: **$29.73-$80.89**; 1.5 mg, 100's: **$54.90-$112.99**; 3 mg, 100's: **$100.35-$196.68**

CONTRAINDICATIONS: Breast cancer (except in selected patients being treated for metastatic disease), active thromboembolic disorders, known or suspected estrogen-dependent neoplasia, undiagnosed abnormal genital bleeding

PRECAUTIONS: Hypertension, gallbladder disease, CHF, diabetes mellitus, depression, migraine headache, seizure disorders, hepatic disease, family history of breast or endometrial cancer, history of thromboembolic disorders, uterine fibroids, hypertriglyceridemia, hypercalcemia

PREGNANCY AND LACTATION: Pregnancy category X; may reduce quantity and quality of breast milk

SIDE EFFECTS/ADVERSE REACTIONS

CNS: Depression, migraine headache, emotional lability

CV: **Arterial thromboembolism, pulmonary embolism, CVA, MI,** hypertension, venous thrombosis, edema

EENT: Contact lens intolerance, **retinal thrombosis**

GI: Nausea and vomiting, gallbladder disease, bloating, benign hepatic tumors, **mesenteric thrombosis**

GU: Breakthrough bleeding, spotting, amenorrhea, change in cervical secretions, breast enlargement, breast tenderness, **endometrial cancer**

METAB: Hyperglycemia, hypertriglyceridemia, hypercalcemia

SKIN: Melasma

INTERACTIONS

Drugs

▣ *P450 inducers (e.g., rifampin, barbiturates):* Decreased estrogen levels

▣ *Corticosteroids:* Increased steroid effect

▣ *Phenytoin:* Loss of seizure control, decreased estrogen levels

▣ *Warfarin:* Theoretical increased risk thromboembolism

SPECIAL CONSIDERATIONS

• Unopposed estrogen increases risk of endometrial cancer; recommended administration of concurrent progestational agents for non-hysterectomized women

---

* = non-FDA-approved use

etanercept

(e-tan´er-cept)
Rx: Enbrel
Chemical Class: Recombinant human fusion protein
Therapeutic Class: Immunomodulatory agent; disease-modifying antirheumatic drug (DMARD)*

CLINICAL PHARMACOLOGY
Mechanism of Action: Tumor necrosis factor receptor p75 Fc fusion protein (TNFR:Fc); binds specifically with human TNF and blocks its interaction with cell surface TNF receptors, preventing TNF's contribution to the normal inflammatory and immune responses of rheumatoid arthritis
Pharmacokinetics
SQ: Cmax 72 hr; 2-5 fold increases in serum level with repeated dosing; 60% bioavailability; Vd 17 L; cleared via the reticuloendothelial system (liver, spleen); $t_{1/2}$ 115 hr
INDICATIONS AND USES: Rheumatoid arthritis, juvenile rheumatoid arthritis, psoriatic arthritis
DOSAGE
Adult and child >16 yr
• SQ 25 mg twice weekly (72-96 hr apart)
Children 4-17 yr
• SQ 0.4 mg/kg (max 25 mg) twice weekly (72-96 hr apart)
$ AVAILABLE FORMS/COST OF THERAPY
• Inj, Pow—SQ: 25 mg; 1's: **$155.70**
CONTRAINDICATIONS: Active infection (chronic or localized)
PRECAUTIONS: Immunogenicity, potential declines in host defenses against malignancies and infections; immunization-related infections; latex allergies

History of recurring infections, diabetes, CNS demyelinating disorders, history of hematologic abnormalities
PREGNANCY AND LACTATION: Pregnancy category B; information on breast milk excretion is unknown; breast feeding not advised
SIDE EFFECTS/ADVERSE REACTIONS
CNS: Headache, dizziness, asthenia, ***cerebral ischemia,*** *depression, dyspnea*
CV: Heart failure, ***MI,*** hypertension, hypotension
EENT: Rhinitis, pharyngitis, sinusitis
GI: Abdominal pain, dyspepsia, cholycystitis, ***pancreatitis, GI hemorrhage***
MS: Bursitis
RESP: Respiratory tract infections, cough
SKIN: Rash
MISC: Injection site reactions; infections (varicella), aseptic meningitis
SPECIAL CONSIDERATIONS
• Immunizations should be up to date, especially in children prior to starting therapy
PATIENT/FAMILY EDUCATION
• Review injection techniques to ensure safe self-administration
MONITORING PARAMETERS
• Efficacy: ESR, C-reactive protein, rheumatoid factor, improvement in tender/painful swollen joints, quality of life

---

italic = common side effects   ***bold italic*** = life-threatening reactions

ethacrynic acid
(eth-a-kri'nik)
Rx: Edecrin
Chemical Class: Ketone derivative of aryloxyacetic acid
Therapeutic Class: Loop diuretic

CLINICAL PHARMACOLOGY
Mechanism of Action: Inhibits absorption of sodium and chloride at proximal and distal tubule sites and in the loop of Henle
Pharmacokinetics
PO: Onset ½ hr, peak 2 hr, duration 6-8 hr
IV: Onset 5 min, peak 15-30 min, duration 2 hr
Hepatic metabolism; excreted in urine and feces, crosses placenta; $t_{1/2}$ 30-70 min

INDICATIONS AND USES: Pulmonary edema; edema (CHF, hepatic cirrhosis nephrotic syndrome, ascites); glaucoma*; hypertension (in combination with other agents),* hypercalcemia*

DOSAGE
Adult
• PO 50-200 mg/day; may give up to 200 mg bid, adjust dose in 25-50 mg increments; IV 50 mg or 0.5-1.0 mg/kg given over several min
Child
• PO 25 mg, increased by 25 mg/day until desired effect occurs; not established for infants or parenterally

$ **AVAILABLE FORMS/COST OF THERAPY**
• Inj, Sol—IV: 50 mg/vial: **$23.80**
• Tab, Uncoated—Oral: 25 mg, 100's: **$37.35**; 50 mg, 100's: **$53.24**

CONTRAINDICATIONS: Anuria, hypovolemia, electrolyte depletion, infants, hepatic coma

PRECAUTIONS: Fluid and electrolyte imbalance (including sodium, chloride, potassium, magnesium, calcium), renal disease, hepatic disease (may precipitate hepatic encephalopathy), gout, COPD, lupus erythematosus, diabetes mellitus, hyperparathyroidism, vomiting, diarrhea, elevated cholesterol/triglycerides

PREGNANCY AND LACTATION: Pregnancy category B; cardiovascular disorders such as pulmonary edema, severe hypertension, or CHF are probably the only valid indications for loop diuretics during pregnancy; no data on nursing; contraindicated per manufacturer

SIDE EFFECTS/ADVERSE REACTIONS
CNS: Encephalopathy in hepatic disease, fatigue, headache, vertigo, weakness
CV: Chest pain, *circulatory collapse,* ECG changes, hypotension
EENT: Blurred vision, ear pain, hearing loss, tinnitus
GI: Abdominal distension, abdominal pain, *acute pancreatitis,* anorexia, cramps, dry mouth, *GI bleeding,* jaundice, nausea, severe diarrhea, upset stomach, vomiting
GU: Glycosuria, polyuria, *renal failure,* sexual dysfunction
HEME: **Agranulocytosis, leukopenia, neutropenia, thrombocytopenia**
METAB: Decreased glucose tolerance, hyperglycemia, hyperuricemia, hypocalcemia, hypochloremic alkalosis, *hypokalemia,* hypomagnesemia, hyponatremia
MS: Arthritis, cramps, stiffness
SKIN: Photosensitivity, pruritis, purpura, rash, ***Stevens-Johnson syndrome,*** sweating

* = non-FDA-approved use

INTERACTIONS
Drugs
❷ *Aminoglycosides (gentamicin, kanamycin, neomycin, streptomycin):* Additive ototoxicity (ethacrynic acid > furosemide, torsemide, bumetanide)

3 *Angiotensin converting enzyme inhibitors:* Initiation of ACEI with intensive diuretic therapy may result in precipitous fall in blood pressure; ACEIs may induce renal insufficiency in the presence of diuretic-induced sodium depletion

3 *Barbiturates (phenobarbital):* Reduced diuretic response

3 *Bile acid-binding resins (cholestyramine, colestipol):* Resins markedly reduce the bioavailability and diuretic response

3 *Carbenoxolone:* Severe hypokalemia from coadministration

3 *Cephalosporins (cephaloridine, cephalothin):* Enhanced nephrotoxicity with coadministration

❷ *Cisplatin:* Additive ototoxicity (ethacrynic acid > furosemide, torsemide, bumetanide)

3 *Clofibrate:* Enhanced effects of both drugs, especially in hypoalbuminemic patients

3 *Corticosteroids:* Concomitant loop diuretic and corticosteroid therapy can result in excessive potassium loss

3 *Digitalis glycosides (digoxin, digitoxin):* Diuretic-induced hypokalemia may increase risk of digitalis toxicity

3 *Nonsteroidal antiinflammatory drugs (flurbiprofen, ibuprofen, indomethacin, naproxen, piroxicam, sulindac):* Reduced diuretic and antihypertensive effects

3 *Phenytoin:* Reduced diuretic response

3 *Serotonin-reuptake inhibitors (fluoxetine, paroxetine, sertraline):* Case reports of sudden death; enhanced hyponatremia proposed; causal relationships not established

3 *Tubocurarine:* Prolonged neuromuscular blockade

SPECIAL CONSIDERATIONS
• Inhibits reabsorption of filtered sodium more than other loop diuretics, therefore, may be effective in patients with significant degrees of renal insufficiency
• Reserve for patients not responding to or intolerant of furosemide or bumetanide

MONITORING PARAMETERS
• Urine volume, creatinine clearance, BUN, electolytes, reduction in edema, increased diuresis, decrease in body weight, reduction in blood pressure, glucose, uric acid, serum calcium (tetany), tinnitus, vertigo, hearing loss (especially in those at risk for ototoxicity—IV doses > 120 mg; concomitant ototoxic drugs; renal disease)

---

ethambutol
(e-tham'byoo-tole)
Rx: Myambutol
Chemical Class: Diisopropyl-ethylene diamide derivative
Therapeutic Class: Antituberculosis agent

CLINICAL PHARMACOLOGY
Mechanism of Action: Inhibits RNA synthesis, decreases tubercle bacilli replication
Pharmacokinetics
PO: Peak 2-4 hr, metabolized in liver; excreted in urine (unchanged drug/inactive metabolites), and feces, crosses placenta; $t_{1/2}$ 3-4 hr

INDICATIONS AND USES: Adjunct in treatment of pulmonary tuberculosis; mycobacterium avium complex (MAC) in AIDS (2nd line)*

DOSAGE

Adult and Child >13 yr

Tuberculosis

• *Initial treatment:* PO 15 mg/kg/day as a single daily dose
• *Retreatment:* PO 25 mg/kg/day as single dose for 2 mo with at least 1 other drug, then decrease to 15 mg/kg/day as single daily dose

Mycobacterium avium complex in AIDS

• PO: 15 mg/kg with 3 or 4 other antimycobacterial agents

$ AVAILABLE FORMS/COST OF THERAPY

• Tab, Uncoated—Oral: 100 mg, 100's: **$55.18-$59.33**; 400 mg, 100's: **$177.92-$198.50**

CONTRAINDICATIONS: Optic neuritis, child <13 yr

PRECAUTIONS: Renal disease, diabetic retinopathy, cataracts, ocular defects, hepatic and hematopoietic disorders, gout

PREGNANCY AND LACTATION: Pregnancy category B; compatible with breast feeding

SIDE EFFECTS/ADVERSE REACTIONS

CNS: Confusion, disorientation, dizziness, fever, hallucinations, headache, malaise
EENT: Bloody sputum, blurred vision, changes in color perception, decreased visual acuity, optic neuritis, photophobia
GI: Abdominal distress, anorexia, nausea, vomiting
HEME: **Thrombocytopenia**
METAB: Acute gout, elevated uric acid, liver function impairment
MS: Joint pain
SKIN: Dermatitis, pruritis

SPECIAL CONSIDERATIONS

• Initial therapy in tuberculosis should include 4 drugs: isoniazid, rifampin, pyrazinamide, and ethambutol, until drug susceptibility results available

PATIENT/FAMILY EDUCATION

• Administer with meals to decrease GI symptoms

MONITORING PARAMETERS

• Perform visual acuity testing before beginning therapy and periodically during drug administration (qmo if dose >15 mg/kg/day)

---

ethchlorvynol

(eth-klor-vi'nole)

Rx: Placidyl
Chemical Class: Tertiary acetylenic alcohol
Therapeutic Class: Sedative-hypnotic
DEA Class: Schedule IV

CLINICAL PHARMACOLOGY

Mechanism of Action: Produces cerebral depression; mechanism unknown

Pharmacokinetics

PO: Onset 15-60 min, peak 2 hr, duration 5 hr, extensive distribution to adipose tissue; metabolized by liver (90%), renal elimination; $t_{1/2}$ 10-20 hr

INDICATIONS AND USES: Insomnia (short-term therapy); sedation*

DOSAGE

Adult

• *Insomnia:* PO 500 mg-1 g ½ hr before hs, may repeat 200 mg if needed
• *Sedation:* PO 200 mg bid or tid

Child

• PO 25 mg/kg in 1 dose, not to exceed 1 g

---

* = non-FDA-approved use

💲 AVAILABLE FORMS/COST OF THERAPY

• Cap, Gel—Oral: 200 mg, 100's: **$130.64**; 500 mg, 100's: **$160.94**; 750 mg, 100's: **$213.58**

CONTRAINDICATIONS: Porphyria

PRECAUTIONS: Depression, hepatic disease, renal disease, suicidal tendencies, elderly, history of drug abuse, tartrazine sensitivity

PREGNANCY AND LACTATION: Pregnancy category C

SIDE EFFECTS/ADVERSE REACTIONS

CNS: Ataxia, dizziness, facial numbness, fatigue, giddiness, hangover, hysteria, nightmares, weakness

CV: Hypotension

EENT: Blurred vision

GI: Bitter aftertaste, cholestatic jaundice, nausea, vomiting

HEME: **Thrombocytopenia**

SKIN: Rash, urticaria

INTERACTIONS

Drugs

🔳 *Warfarin:* Decreased hypoprothrombinemic response to oral anticoagulents

SPECIAL CONSIDERATIONS

• Geriatric patients may be more sensitive to usual adult dose

• Do not prescribe for periods >1 wk

ethinyl estradiol

(eth-in´il ess-tra-dye´ole)

Rx: Estinyl

Combinations

See oral contraceptives monograph for combined oral contraceptives containing ethinyl estradiol

Chemical Class: Synthetic estrogen derivative

Therapeutic Class: Estrogen; contraceptive

E

CLINICAL PHARMACOLOGY

Mechanism of Action: Necessary for adequate functioning of female reproductive system; affects release of pituitary gonadotropins; inhibits bone resorption

Pharmacokinetics

PO: Peak 2-3 hr; addition of 17-α-ethinyl group to estradiol enhances potency and oral activity; degraded in liver; excreted in urine

INDICATIONS AND USES: Vasomotor symptoms associated with menopause; atrophic vaginitis, kraurosis vulvae*; breast engorgement*; female hypogonadism; osteoporosis*; contraceptive (combined with progestins, see oral contraceptives monograph); female breast cancer (inoperable, progressing); prostatic carcinoma (inoperable)

DOSAGE

Adult

• *Menopause:* PO 0.02-0.05 mg qd 3 wk on, 1 wk off (may add progestational agent during latter part of the cycle)

• *Prostatic cancer:* PO 0.15-2 mg qd

• *Hypogonadism:* PO 0.05 mg qd-tid × 2 wk/mo, then 2 wk progesterone; repeat cycle for 3-6 mo, then 2 mo off

• *Breast cancer:* PO 1 mg tid

---

italic = common side effects   ***bold italic*** = life-threatening reactions

• *Breast engorgement:* PO 0.5-1 mg qd × 3 days, then tapered off over 7 days

• *Combined oral contraceptive:* Combined with progestins, 20-80 μg qd cycled 21 days, off 7 days

💲 AVAILABLE FORMS/COST OF THERAPY

• Tab, Coated—Oral: 0.02 mg, 100's: **$40.96**; 0.05 mg, 100's: **$68.98**

CONTRAINDICATIONS: Breast cancer (except in selected patients being treated for metastatic disease), active thromboembolic disorders, known or suspected estrogen-dependent neoplasia, undiagnosed abnormal genital bleeding

PRECAUTIONS: Hypertension, gallbladder disease, CHF, diabetes mellitus, depression, migraine headache, seizure disorders, hepatic disease, family history of breast or endometrial cancer, history of thromboembolic disorders, uterine fibroids, hypertriglyceridemia, hypercalcemia

PREGNANCY AND LACTATION: Pregnancy category X; may reduce quantity and quality of breast milk

SIDE EFFECTS/ADVERSE REACTIONS

CNS: Depression, migraine headache, emotional lability

CV: **Arterial thromboembolism, pulmonary embolism, CVA, MI,** hypertension, venous thrombosis, edema

EENT: Contact lens intolerance, **retinal thrombosis**

GI: Nausea and vomiting, gallbladder disease, bloating, benign hepatic tumors, **mesenteric thrombosis**

GU: Breakthrough bleeding, spotting, amenorrhea, change in cervical secretions, breast enlargement, breast tenderness, **testicular atrophy, endometrial cancer**

METAB: Hyperglycemia, hypertriglyceridemia, hypercalcemia

SKIN: Melasma

MISC: Changes in libido, weight gain

INTERACTIONS

Drugs

🔳 *P450 inducers (e.g., rifampin, barbiturates):* Decreased estrogen levels

🔳 *Corticosteroids:* Increased steroid effect

🔳 *Phenytoin:* Loss of seizure control, decreased estrogen levels

🔳 *Warfarin:* Theoretical increased risk of thromboembolism

SPECIAL CONSIDERATIONS

• Unopposed estrogen increases risk of endometrial cancer; recommended administration of concurrent progestational agents for non-hysterectomized women

---

ethionamide
(e-thye-on'am-ide)
Rx: Trecator-SC
Chemical Class: Thiomine derivative
Therapeutic Class: Antituberculosis agent

CLINICAL PHARMACOLOGY

Mechanism of Action: Bacteriostatic against *Mycobacterium tuberculosis* via inhibition of peptide synthesis

Pharmacokinetics

PO: Peak 3 hr, metabolized in liver, renal excretion (primarily inactive metabolites); $t_{1/2}$ 3 hr

INDICATIONS AND USES: Pulmonary, extrapulmonary TB when other antitubercular drugs have failed

---

* = non-FDA-approved use

DOSAGE

Adult

• PO 500 mg-1 g qd in divided doses with another antitubercular drug and pyridoxine

Child

• PO 15-20 mg/kg/day in 3-4 doses, not to exceed 1 g; concomitant pyridoxine recommended

$ AVAILABLE FORMS/COST OF THERAPY

• Tab, Sugar Coated—Oral: 250 mg, 100's: **$247.90-$274.05**

CONTRAINDICATIONS: Severe hepatic disease

PRECAUTIONS: Renal disease, diabetes, hepatic impairment, children

PREGNANCY AND LACTATION: Pregnancy category D

SIDE EFFECTS/ADVERSE REACTIONS

CNS: Depression, dizziness, drowsiness, headache, peripheral neuritis, psychosis, *seizures,* tremors

CV: Postural hypotension

EENT: Blurred vision, olfactory disturbances, optic neuritis

GI: Anorexia, diarrhea (50% can't tolerate >500 mg), hepatitis (5%), jaundice, metallic taste, *nausea, vomiting*

GU: Impotence, menorrhagia

HEME: Purpura, ***thrombocytopenia***

METAB: Difficulty managing diabetes mellitus

SKIN: Acne, alopecia, dermatitis

MISC: Gynecomastia

INTERACTIONS

Labs

• *False decrease:* Urine alkaline phosphatase, urine lactate dehydrogenase

SPECIAL CONSIDERATIONS

• Use only with at least 1 other effective antituberculous agent

MONITORING PARAMETERS

• Serum transaminases (AST, ALT) biweekly during therapy

---

ethosuximide

(eth-oh-sux′i-mide)

Rx: Zarontin

Chemical Class: Succinimide derivative

Therapeutic Class: Anticonvulsant

E

CLINICAL PHARMACOLOGY

Mechanism of Action: Increases seizure threshold and inhibits spike-and-wave formation in absence (petit mal) seizures; decreases amplitude, frequency, duration, spread of discharge in minor motor seizures

Pharmacokinetics

PO: Peak 3-7 hr; steady state 4-7 days; rapid and complete absorption; freely distributed, except to fat; insignificant protein binding; metabolized by liver, excreted in urine (20% unchanged); $t_{1/2}$ 56-60 hr (adults), 26-30 hr (children)

INDICATIONS AND USES: Absence seizures, partial seizures*

DOSAGE

Adult and Child >6 yr

• PO 250 mg bid initially; may increase by 250 mg q4-7 days, not to exceed 1.5 g/day

Child 3-6 yr

• PO 250 mg/day or 125 mg bid initially; may increase by 250 mg q4-7 days, not to exceed 1 g/day (20 mg/kg/day)

$ AVAILABLE FORMS/COST OF THERAPY

• Cap, Gel—Oral: 250 mg, 100's: **$101.34**

• Syr—Oral: 250 mg/5 ml, 480 ml: **$78.00-$106.59**

PRECAUTIONS: Hepatic function impairment; renal dysfunction; acute intermittent porphyria; monotherapy with mixed types of epilepsy (may increase frequency of grand-mal seizures)

---

italic = common side effects   **bold italic** = life-threatening reactions

PREGNANCY AND LACTATION:
Pregnancy category C; freely enters breast milk; no adverse effects on infants reported; compatible with breast feeding

SIDE EFFECTS/ADVERSE REACTIONS

CNS: Aggressiveness, anxiety, depression, *dizziness, drowsiness, euphoria, fatigue,* headache, insomnia, irritability, *lethargy*

EENT: Blurred vision, myopia

GI: Abdominal pain, *anorexia,* constipation, cramps, diarrhea, gum hypertrophy, *heartburn,* hiccups, *nausea,* tongue swelling, *vomiting,* weight loss

GU: Hematuria, **renal damage,** vaginal bleeding

HEME: **Agranulocytosis, aplastic anemia,** eosinophilia, **leukocytosis, pancytopenia, thrombocytopenia**

SKIN: Hirsutism, pruritic erythema, **Stevens-Johnson syndrome,** urticaria

MISC: Systemic lupus erythematosis

SPECIAL CONSIDERATIONS

PATIENT/FAMILY EDUCATION

• Take doses at regularly spaced intervals

• OK with food or milk

MONITORING PARAMETERS

• Blood counts, renal function tests, liver function tests, urinalysis periodically

• Therapeutic serum concentrations 40-100 µg/ml

---

ethotoin
(eth-oh-to´in)
Rx: Peganone
Chemical Class: Hydantoin derivative
Therapeutic Class: Anticonvulsant

CLINICAL PHARMACOLOGY

Mechanism of Action: Stabilizes neuronal membranes decreasing seizure activity by increasing efflux or decreasing influx of sodium ions across cell membranes the motor cortex during generation of impulses

Pharmacokinetics

PO: Therapeutic serum concentration 15-50 µg/ml; rapid absorption; metabolized by liver (substantial nonlinear kinetics), excreted in urine; $t_{1/2}$ 3-9 hr

INDICATIONS AND USES: Generalized tonic-clonic or complex-partial seizures (2nd-line agent)

DOSAGE

Adult

• PO 250 mg qid initially; may increase over several days to 3 g/day in divided doses (<2 g/day ineffective in most adults)

Child

• PO initial dose should not exceed 750 mg/day in divided doses; usual maintenance dose 500 mg-1 g/day in 4-6 divided doses

$ **AVAILABLE FORMS/COST OF THERAPY**

• Tab, Uncoated—Oral: 250 mg, 100's: **$50.98**; 500 mg, 100's: **$83.30**

CONTRAINDICATIONS: Hematologic disease, hepatic disease

PRECAUTIONS: Geriatric patients metabolize hydantoins slowly

PREGNANCY AND LACTATION: Pregnancy category C (fetal hydantoin syndrome); excreted in breast milk

SIDE EFFECTS/ADVERSE REACTIONS

CNS: Ataxia, dizziness, *drowsiness,* fatigue, fever, headache, insomnia, numbness, slurred speech

CV: Chest pain

EENT: Diplopia, nystagmus

GI: Diarrhea, gingival hypertrophy, liver damage, nausea, toxic hepatitis, vomiting

HEME: **Agranulocytosis, leukopenia,** lymphadenopathy, **megaloblastic anemia, pancytopenia, thrombocytopenia**

SKIN: Rash

INTERACTIONS

Drugs

🔟 *Alcohol or CNS depression-producing drugs:* Enhanced CNS depression

🔟 *Amiodarone:* Increased plasma concentration of ethotoin

🔟 *Antacids:* Decrease bioavailability of ethotoin

🔟 *Chloramphenicol, Cimetidine, Disulfiram, Isoniazid, Phenylbutazone, Sulfonamides:* All inhibit metabolism and increase concentration of ethotoin

🔟 *Estrogen contraceptives, Corticosteroids, Corticotropin:* All may have effects decreased because of increased metabolism

🔟 *Fluconazole:* Decreases the metabolism of ethotoin

🔟 *Lidocaine:* Concurrent IV use may produce additive cardiac depressant effects

🔟 *Methadone:* Increased methadone metabolism, decreased activity

🔟 *Oral anticoagulants:* Increased serum concentration of ethotoin; increased anticoagulant effect initially, then decreased with continued use

🔟 *Oral diazoxide:* Decreased efficacy of both agents

🔟 *Rifampin:* Increased metabolism of ethotoin, decreased effect

🔟 *Streptozocin:* Ethotoin may protect pancreatic β-cells from the toxic effects of streptozocin

🔟 *Sucralfate:* Decreased ethotoin absorption

🔟 *Valproic acid:* Displaces ethotoin from binding sites, inhibits ethotoin metabolism, increased or additive liver toxicity

🔟 *Xanthines:* Increased hepatic xanthine metabolism, decreased serum concentration; xanthines inhibit ethotoin absorption with decreased serum ethotoin levels

SPECIAL CONSIDERATIONS

PATIENT/FAMILY EDUCATION

• Strictly enforced program of teeth cleaning and plaque control to prevent gingival hyperplasia is necessary

• Take doses at regularly spaced intervals

MONITORING PARAMETERS

• Therapeutic serum level: 40-100 µg/ml

---

etidronate

(ee-tid´roe-nate)

Rx: Didronel

Chemical Class: Synthetic analog of pyrophosphate

Therapeutic Class: Bisphosphonate

CLINICAL PHARMACOLOGY

Mechanism of Action: Binds to hydroxyapatite at sites of bone resorption, inhibiting normal and abnormal bone resorption ("crystal poison"); minimal secondary reduction in bone formation (resorption coupled to formation)

---

italic = common side effects   **bold italic** = life-threatening reactions

Pharmacokinetics

Therapeutic response, Paget's Disease, and osteoporosis 1-3 mo; hypercalcemia 24 hr; duration of effect, Paget's Disease 1 yr after discontinuing therapy; hypercalcemia 14 days of normocalcemia; poorly absorbed orally (1%-6%); chemically adsorbed to bone; not metabolized, excreted in urine/feces; $t_{1/2}$ 1-6 hr

INDICATIONS AND USES: Paget's disease, heterotropic ossification caused by spinal cord injury or complicating total hip replacement, hyperparathyroidism, bone pain in prostatic carcinoma and metastatic breast cancer, prevention of glucocorticoid-induced osteoporosis, hypercalcemia of malignancy (IV), osteoporosis*

DOSAGE

Adult

• *Paget's disease:* PO 5-10 mg/kg/day 2 hr ac with H_2O; not to exceed 20 mg/kg/day; max course 6 mo

• *Heterotropic ossification:* PO (due to spinal cord injury) 20 mg/kg qd × 2 wk, then 10 mg/kg/day for 10 wk, total 12 wk; (complicating total hip replacement) 20 mg/kg qd × 1 mo preoperatively, then 20 mg/kg qd for 3 mo postoperatively

• *Hypercalcemia:* IV 7.5 mg/kg/day for 3 successive days (diluted in at least 250 ml normal saline) over at least 2 hr; retreatment interval at least 7 days

• *Osteoporosis:* PO 400 mg qd 2 hr ac with H_2O × 2 wk, repeat every 3 mo

$ **AVAILABLE FORMS/COST OF THERAPY**

• Inj, Sol—IV: 300 mg/6 ml, 6 ml: **$67.00**

• Tab, Uncoated—Oral: 200 mg, 60's: **$177.39**; 400 mg, 60's: **$354.72**

CONTRAINDICATIONS: Severe renal disease, overt osteomalacia

PRECAUTIONS: Renal disease, restricted vitamin D and calcium intake, enterocolitis

PREGNANCY AND LACTATION: Pregnancy category B; breast milk excretion not known; problems in humans have not been documented

SIDE EFFECTS/ADVERSE REACTIONS

GI: Diarrhea, metallic taste, nausea

GU: Mild to moderate abnormalities in renal function

MS: Bone pain, decreased mineralization of nonaffected bones, hypocalcemia

SPECIAL CONSIDERATIONS

PATIENT/FAMILY EDUCATION

• Administer on empty stomach with H_2O, 2 hr ac

• Exceeding the 2 wk treatment periods for osteoporosis may lead to bone demineralization and osteomalacia

---

etodolac

(e-toe-doe'lak)

Rx: Lodine

Chemical Class: Acetic acid derivative

Therapeutic Class: NSAID with analgesic and antipyretic activity

---

CLINICAL PHARMACOLOGY

Mechanism of Action: Reversible cyclooxygenase (i.e., prostaglandin synthetase) inhibitor; non-selectively decreases the formation of both prostaglandins and thromboxane A_2; variable effects on lipoxygenase synthesis and subsequent leukotriene production; antiinflammatory, antipyretic, and analgesic activity; inhibits platelet aggregation

* = non-FDA-approved use

Pharmacokinetics

PO: Peak serum levels 1-2 hr; analgesic onset 30 min, analgesic duration 4-12 hr; rapidly and completely absorbed; serum protein binding >99%; metabolized by liver, metabolites excreted in urine and feces; $t_{1/2}$ 7.3 hr

INDICATIONS AND USES: Osteoarthritis; pain—mild to moderate; rheumatoid arthritis; soft tissue injuries*; prevention of cognitive decline*

DOSAGE

Adult

• *Osteoarthritis:* PO 800-1200 mg/day in divided doses initially, then adjust dose to 600-1200 mg/day in divided doses; do not exceed 1200 mg/day; patients <60 kg, not to exceed 20 mg/kg; Sus Action PO 400-1000 mg qd

• *Analgesia:* PO 200-400 mg q6-8h prn for acute pain, do not exceed 1200 mg/day; patients <60 kg, not to exceed 20 mg/kg

💲 AVAILABLE FORMS/COST OF THERAPY

• Cap, Gel—Oral: 200 mg, 100's: **$40.00-$145.20**; 300 mg, 100's: **$42.50-$164.44**
• Tab, Uncoated—Oral: 400 mg, 100's: **$45.00-$173.84**; 500 mg, 100's: **$139.00-$174.95**
• Tab, Sus Action—Oral: 400 mg, 100's: **$138.62-$159.49**; 500 mg 100's: **$146.48-$262.27**; 600 mg, 100's: **$144.86-$301.75**

CONTRAINDICATIONS: Bronchospasm, nasal polyps, angioedema precipitated by aspirin or other NSAIDs

PRECAUTIONS: History of GI ulceration, bleeding, or perforation; renal dysfunction, hypertension or cardiac conditions aggravated by fluid retention and edema, history of liver dysfunction

PREGNANCY AND LACTATION: Pregnancy category C (category D if used near term); breast milk excretion unknown; problems in humans have not been documented

SIDE EFFECTS/ADVERSE REACTIONS

CNS: Anxiety, confusion, depression, *dizziness,* drowsiness, fatigue, *headache,* insomnia, light-headedness, tremors, vertigo

CV: ***CHF, dysrhythmias,*** fluid retention, palpitations, peripheral edema, tachycardia

EENT: Blurred vision, hearing loss, tinnitus

GI: Anorexia, cholestatic hepatitis, constipation, cramps, diarrhea, dry mouth, dyspepsia, flatulence, ***GI bleeding,*** jaundice, *nausea,* peptic ulcer, vomiting

GU: Azotemia, cystitis, dysuria, hematuria, oliguria, UTI

HEME: ***Blood dyscrasias***

SKIN: Erythema, pruritus, purpura, rash, sweating, urticaria

INTERACTIONS

Drugs

🔳 *Aminoglycosides:* Reduced clearance with elevated aminoglycoside levels and potential for toxicity (especially indomethacin in premature infants; other NSAIDs probably)

🔳 *Antihypertensives (α-blockers, angiotensin-converting enzyme inhibitors, angiotensin II receptor blockers, β-blockers, diuretics):* Inhibition of antihypertensive and other favorable hemodynamic effects

🔳 *Corticosteroids:* Increased risk of GI ulceration

🔳 *Anticoagulants:* Excessive hypoprothrombinemia, decreased platelet aggregation with increased risk of GI bleeding; may be less likely to increase bleeding risk than other NSAIDs due to preferential effects on COX-2

---

italic = common side effects   ***bold italic*** = life-threatening reactions

3 *Cyclosporine:* Increased nephrotoxicity risk

3 *Lithium:* Decreased clearance of lithium (mediated via prostaglandins) resulting in elevated serum lithium levels and risk of toxicity

3 *Methotrexate:* Decreased renal secretion of methotrexate resulting in elevated methotrexate levels and risk of toxicity

3 *Phenylpropanolamine:* Possible acute hypertensive reaction

3 *Potassium-sparing diuretics:* Additive hyperkalemia potential

3 *Triamterene:* Acute renal failure reported with addition of indomethacin; caution with other NSAIDs

SPECIAL CONSIDERATIONS
MONITORING PARAMETERS

• Initial hemogram and fecal occult blood test within 3 mo of starting regular chronic therapy; repeat every 6-12 mo (more frequently in high-risk patients (>65 years, peptic ulcer disease, concurrent steroids or anticoagulants); electrolytes, creatinine, and BUN within 3 mo of starting regular chronic therapy; repeat every 6-12 mo

---

etretinate
(e-tret'in-ate)
Rx: Tegison
Chemical Class: Retinoic acid derivative
Therapeutic Class: Antipsoriatic

CLINICAL PHARMACOLOGY
Mechanism of Action: Unknown; might reduce cell proliferation by inhibiting ornithine decarboxylase, a rate-limiting enzyme in regulation of cell growth, proliferation, and differentiation

Pharmacokinetics
PO: Peak 2-6 hr during chronic therapy; absorbed in small intestine; accumulates in adipose tissue, especially the liver and subcutaneous fat; significant 1st-pass hepatic metabolism to active acid form; primarily biliary excretion; $t_{1/2}$ 120 days

INDICATIONS AND USES: Severe recalcitrant psoriasis, including erythrodermic and generalized pustular types; bronchial metaplasia,* mycosis fungoides,* actinic keratoses,* arsenical keratoses,* basal cell carcinomas,* genodermatosis,* pustular bacterids,* hyperkeratotic eczema of palms and soles,* cutaneous lupus erythematosus*

DOSAGE
Adult

• Psoriasis: PO 0.75-1 mg/kg/day in divided doses, not to exceed 1.5 mg/kg/day; maintenance dose 0.5-0.75 mg/kg/day generally beginning after 8-16 wk of therapy; terminate therapy in patients whose lesions have sufficiently resolved

$ **AVAILABLE FORMS/COST OF THERAPY**

• Cap, Gel—Oral: 10 mg, 30's: **$70.88**; 25 mg, 30's: **$110.84**

PRECAUTIONS: Children, hepatic disease, diabetes, obesity, increased alcohol intake, hypertriglyceridemia

PREGNANCY AND LACTATION: Pregnancy category X (effective contraception must be used at least 1 mo before, during, and following discontinuation of therapy for an indefinite period of time); excreted into milk of lactating rats; human breast milk data not available; not recommended during lactation

SIDE EFFECTS/ADVERSE REACTIONS

CNS: Amnesia, anxiety, depression, *dizziness, fatigue, fever, headache, pain,* pseudotumor cerebri

---

* = non-FDA-approved use

CV: Atrial fibrillation, chest pain, co-agulation disorders, CV obstruction, edema

EENT: Change in lacrimation, cheilitis, *double vision, dry nose, eyes; earache, eye irritation,* nosebleed, *otitis externa; pain,* sore tongue

GI: Abdominal pain, anorexia, constipation, diarrhea, flatulence, hepatitis, increased transaminases, *nausea,* weight loss

GU: Acetonuria, casts, dysuria, glycosuria; hematuria, hemoglobinuria, *increased BUN, creatinine;* proteinuria, *WBC in urine*

METAB: Decrease in HDL cholesterol; elevation of plasma triglycerides, total cholesterol; increased or decreased fasting blood sugar, increase or decrease K, Ca, P, Na, Cl

MS: Bone pain, cramps, gout, *hyperostosis,* hypertonia, *myalgia*

RESP: Cough, dyspnea

SKIN: Alopecia; bruising, dryness, itching, nail changes, onycholysis, paronychia, *peeling of palms, soles, fingertips; rash,* perspiration change, pyogenic granuloma, rash, red scaling face; sunburn

INTERACTIONS
Drugs
❷ *Methotrexate:* Increased potential for hepatotoxicity

❸ *Vitamin A:* Additive toxicity possible

SPECIAL CONSIDERATIONS
PATIENT/FAMILY EDUCATION
• Take with food or milk
• Contact lens intolerance is common
• Transient exacerbation of psoriasis common during initiation of therapy
• Do not take vitamin A supplements

MONITORING PARAMETERS
• Fasting lipid panels

famciclovir
(fam-si'klo-veer)
Rx: Famvir
Chemical Class: Acyclic purine nucleoside analog
Therapeutic Class: Antiviral

CLINICAL PHARMACOLOGY
Mechanism of Action: Converted to penciclovir in intestinal and hepatic tissue, then phosphorylated intracellularly to penciclovir triphosphate which inhibits viral DNA synthesis

Pharmacokinetics
PO: Onset 15 min, peak 45-55 min, duration 6 hr; bioavailability 80%; not affected by food; protein binding 20%; metabolized to penciclovir, which is excreted in urine (60%) and stool; $t_{1/2}$ 2 hr (longer in renal insufficiency), intracellular $t_{1/2}$ 10-20 hr

INDICATIONS AND USES: Acute herpes zoster infection, acute treatment of initial* and recurrent episodes of genital herpes simplex, suppression of recurrent genital herpes

DOSAGE
Adult
• *Herpes zoster:* 500 mg q8h for 7 days, initiated as soon as possible after diagnosis; if CrCl 40-59 ml/min, use 500 mg q12h for 7 days; if CrCl 20-39 ml/min, use 500 mg q24h for 7 days; if CrCl <20 ml/min, use 500 mg q48h

• *Genital herpes simplex:* 125 mg q12h for 5 days; if CrCl 20-39 ml/min, use 125 mg q24h for 5 days; if CrCl <20 ml/min, use 125 mg q48h for 5 days

• *Suppression of genital herpes:* 250 mg bid; if CrCl 20-39 ml/min, use 125 mg q12h; if CrCl <20 ml/min, use 125 mg q24h

§ AVAILABLE FORMS/COST OF THERAPY

• Tab—Oral: 125 mg, 30's: **$101.40**; 250 mg, 30's: **$110.25**; 500 mg, 30's: **$221.30**

PRECAUTIONS: Renal insufficiency, children

PREGNANCY AND LACTATION: Pregnancy category B; excreted in breast milk

SIDE EFFECTS/ADVERSE REACTIONS

CNS: Bradykinesia, confusion, dizziness, *headache,* somnolence

GI: Anorexia, constipation, *diarrhea (8%), nausea (13%)*

MS: Arthralgia

SKIN: Pruritus, purpura

SPECIAL CONSIDERATIONS

• Reserve chronic suppressive therapy for patients without prodromal symptoms who have frequent recurrences

---

famotidine

(fam-o'tah-deen)

Rx: Pepcid, Pepcid RPD

OTC: Mylanta AR, Pepcid AC

Chemical Class: Thiazole derivative

Therapeutic Class: Gastrointestinal antiulcer agent

CLINICAL PHARMACOLOGY

Mechanism of Action: Competitive, reversible inhibitor of histamine at gastric H_2-receptors; reduces gastric acid secretion

Pharmacokinetics

PO: Onset 30-60 min, duration 6-12 hr, peak 1-3 hr

IV: Onset immediate, peak 30-60 min, duration 6-12 hr

Oral absorption 50%; plasma protein binding 15%-20%; metabolized in liver 30%; 70% excreted by kidneys unchanged; $t_{1/2}$ 2½-3½ hr (>20 hr with CrCl <10 ml/min)

INDICATIONS AND USES: Short-term treatment of duodenal and benign gastric ulcers; maintenance therapy for duodenal ulcer; pathological hypersecretory conditions (e.g., Zollinger-Ellison syndrome, multiple endocrine adenomas); gastroesophageal reflux disease (GERD) and esophagitis due to GERD; heartburn, acid indigestion, and sour stomach (OTC), GI bleeding,* prophylaxis for aspiration pneumonitis*

DOSAGE

Adult

• *Duodenal ulcer:* PO 40 mg qd hs × 4-8 wk, then 20 mg qd hs if needed (maintenance); IV 20 mg q12h if unable to take PO

• *Gastric ulcer:* PO 40 mg qhs

• *GERD:* PO 20 mg bid for up to 6 wk; for esophagitis due to GERD, 20-40 mg bid for up to 12 wk

• *Hypersecretory conditions:* PO 20 mg q6h; may give 160 mg q6h if needed; IV 20 mg q12h if unable to take PO

• *Heartburn, acid indigestion, and sour stomach (OTC):* PO 10 mg bid prn; for prevention of heartburn, take 1 hr ac

• *Renal failure (CrCl <10 ml/min):* PO 20 mg qhs or increase dosing interval to 36-48 hr

§ AVAILABLE FORMS/COST OF THERAPY

• Granule, Reconst—Oral Susp: 40 mg/5 ml, 50 ml: **$107.71**

• Inj, Sol—IV: 10 mg/ml, 2, 4 ml: **$1.11-$45.10**/2 ml

• Tab, Chewable—Oral: 10 mg, 18's (OTC): **$6.15**

---

* = non-FDA-approved use

• Tab, Oral Disintegrating—Oral: 20 mg, 100's: **$202.79**; 40 mg, 100's: **$362.50**
• Tab, Plain Coated—Oral: 10 mg, 18's (OTC): **$3.08-$6.71**; 20 mg, 100's: **$170.00-$202.79**; 40 mg, 100's: **$297.78-$391.95**

PRECAUTIONS: Severe renal disease, severe hepatic function
PREGNANCY AND LACTATION: Pregnancy category B; concentrated in breast milk (less than cimetidine or ranitidine); no problems reported with other H_2-histamine receptor antagonists; compatible with breast feeding

SIDE EFFECTS/ADVERSE REACTIONS
CNS: Anxiety, depression, dizziness, fever, headache, insomnia, paresthesia, *seizures,* somnolence
EENT: Orbital edema, taste change, tinnitus
GI: Abnormal liver enzymes, anorexia, constipation, cramps, nausea, vomiting
HEME: **Thrombocytopenia**
MS: Arthralgia, myalgia
RESP: **Bronchospasm**
SKIN: Rash

INTERACTIONS
Drugs
3 *Cefpodoxime, cefuroxime, enoxacin, ketoconazole:* Reduction in gastric acidity reduces absorption, decreased plasma levels, potential for therapeutic failure
3 *Glipizide; glyburide; tolbutamide:* Increased absorption of these drugs, potential for hypoglycemia
3 *Nifedipine; nitrendipine; nisoldipine:* Increased concentrations of these drugs

SPECIAL CONSIDERATIONS
• No advantage over other agents in this class, base selection on cost
PATIENT/FAMILY EDUCATION
• Stagger doses of famotidine and antacids

felodipine
(fell-o´da-peen)
Rx: Plendil
Combinations
  Rx: with enalapril (Lexxel)
Chemical Class: Dihydropyridine
Therapeutic Class: Calcium channel blocker: antihypertensive; antianginal

F

CLINICAL PHARMACOLOGY
Mechanism of Action: Inhibits calcium ion influx across cell membrane in vascular smooth muscle and cardiac muscle; produces relaxation of coronary and peripheral vascular smooth muscle; hemodynamics: increases myocardial contractility and cardiac output; significantly decreases peripheral vascular resistance
Pharmacokinetics
PO: Onset 2-5 hr, peak 2.5-5 hr, rapid and complete absorption; extensive 1st pass metabolism; 15% systemic bioavailability; 99% protein bound; metabolized in liver, 0.5% excreted unchanged in urine; $t_{1/2}$ 11-16 hr

INDICATIONS AND USES: Hypertension, vasospastic angina,* effort-associated angina,* primary pulmonary hypertension,* Raynaud's disease,* CHF*
DOSAGE
Adult
• *Hypertension:* PO 5 mg qd initially (2.5 mg in elderly and impaired liver function), usual range 5-10 mg qd; do not exceed 20 mg qd; do not adjust dosage at intervals of <2 wk
$ **AVAILABLE FORMS/COST OF THERAPY**
• Tab, Uncoated, Sus Action—Oral: 2.5, 5 mg, 100's: **$100.50-$117.28**; 10 mg, 100's: **$180.59-$210.73**

---

italic = common side effects   ***bold italic*** = life-threatening reactions

PRECAUTIONS: Hypotension (<90 mm Hg systolic), hepatic injury, children, renal disease, elderly

PREGNANCY AND LACTATION: Pregnancy category C

SIDE EFFECTS/ADVERSE REACTIONS

CNS: Anxiety, depression, dizziness, fatigue, headache, insomnia, light headedness, tinnitus

CV: Edema, hypotension, *MI,* palpitations, pulmonary edema, tachycardia, syncope

EENT: Cough, epistaxis, nasal congestion

GI: Gastric upset, gingival hyperplasia

GU: Nocturia, polyuria

HEME: Anemia

RESP: Shortness of breath, wheezing

SKIN: Pruritus, rash

MISC: Flushing, sexual difficulties

INTERACTIONS

Drugs

▪ *Barbiturates:* Decreased felodipine bioavailability

▪ *Digitalis glycosides:* Increased digitalis levels; increased risk of toxicity

▪ *Erythromycin:* Increased felodipine concentrations

▪ *Fentanyl:* Severe hypotension or increased fluid volume requirements

▪ *Grapefruit juice:* Inhibits felodipine metabolism, 200% increase in AUC

▪ *Histamine H_2 antagonists:* Increased bioavailability of felodipine

▪ *Hydantoins:* Serum felodipine level may be decreased

▪ *Propranolol:* Enhanced hypotension, increased propranolol concentrations

SPECIAL CONSIDERATIONS

• Results of V-HeFT III indicate felodipine may be used safely in patients with left ventricular dysfunction

PATIENT/FAMILY EDUCATION

• Administer as whole tablet (do not crush or chew)

• Avoid grapefruit juice (see drug interactions)

---

fenofibrate

(fee-no-fye'brate)

Rx: Tricor

Chemical Class: Fibric acid derivative

Therapeutic Class: Lipid lowering agent

CLINICAL PHARMACOLOGY

Mechanism of Action: Activates the peroxisom proliferator activated receptor α (PPARα): 1) increases lipolysis and elimination of TG-rich particles from plasma by activating lipoprotein lipase and reducing production of apoprotein C-III (an inhibitor of lipoprotein lipase activity); resulting fall in TG produces an alteration in size and composition of LDL-cholesterol (from small, dense particles to large buoyant particles) which allows rapid catabolism; 2) increased synthesis of A-I, A-II, and HDL-cholesterol; 3) reduces serum uric acid via increase in renal excretion

Total cholesterol: 14% decrease; LDL-cholesterol: 10% decrease; HDL-cholesterol: 18% increase; Triglycerides: 43% decrease

Pharmacokinetics

PO: Peak plasma levels 6-8 hr post dose well absorbed, administration with food increases absorption by 35%; 99% plasma protein bound; completely metabolized by liver esterases (fenofibric acid, major metabolite), excreted in urine (60%)/feces (25%); $t_{1/2}$ 20 hr

INDICATIONS AND USES: Adjunctive therapy to diet to reduce elevated LDL-C, total cholesterol, TG, and Apo B and increase HDL-C in adults with primary hypercholesterolemia or mixed dyslipidemia (Fredrickson Types IIa and IIb).

DOSAGE

Adult

• *Primary hypercholesterolemia or mixed hyperlipidemia:* PO 134 mg qd; adjust dose in 4-8 wk intervals (max 200 mg qd)

• *Hypertriglyceridemia:* PO 67-200 mg qd

• *Severe renal impairment:* PO 67 mg qd

• *Elderly:* PO 67 mg qd

§ AVAILABLE FORMS/COST OF THERAPY

• Cap—Oral: 67 mg 90's: **$74.62**; 134 mg 90's: **$149.24**; 200 mg 90's: **$223.87**

• Tab—Oral: 54 mg 90's: **$77.54**; 160 mg 90's: **$232.60**

CONTRAINDICATIONS: Hypersensitivity, hepatic or severe renal dysfunction (including primary biliary cirrhosis), preexisting gallbladder disease

PREGNANCY AND LACTATION: Pregnancy category C; embryocidal and teratogenic in rats; no adequate and well-controlled studies in pregnant women; tumorigenicity seen in animal studies; avoid breast feeding

SIDE EFFECTS/ADVERSE REACTIONS

CNS: Headache

EENT: Rhinitis

GI: Cholelithiasis, constipation, increased LFTs (ALT, AST), nausea, pancreatitis

GU: Myoglobinuria, acute renal failure

HEME: Decreased hemoglobin, hematocrit, and WBC count

MS: Back pain, myopathy, elevated creatine kinase (CK), rhabdomyolysis

RESP: Respiratory disorder

MISC: Hypersensitivity reactions

INTERACTIONS

Drugs

3 *β-Blockers:* Antagonistic effects; exacerbate hypertriglyceridemia

3 *Estrogens:* Antagonistic effects; exacerbate hypertriglyderidemia

2 *HMG-CoA reductase inhibitors (statins):* Increased risk of markedly elevated creatine kinase (CK), rhabdomyolysis, myoglobinuria, acute renal failure

3 *Resins (bile acid sequestrants):* Decreased absorption if taken concomitantly; separate by 1 hr before or 4 hr after to avoid interaction

3 *Thiazide diuretics:* Antagonistic effects; exacerbate hypertriglyceridemia

3 *Warfarin:* Potentiation leading to prolonged PT/INR; all oral coumarin-type anticoagulants

Labs

• *Uric acid:* Decreased

SPECIAL CONSIDERATIONS

• Plasma concentrations of fenofibric acid after administration of 54 mg and 160 mg tablets are equivalent to 67 and 200 mg capsules

PATIENT/FAMILY EDUCATION

• Signs, symptoms, and resources for management of myositis

MONITORING PARAMETERS

• Serum cholesterol, triglycerides, LDL-cholesterol, HDL-cholesterol, LFTs (serum transaminases), periodic CBC

---

italic = common side effects   ***bold italic*** = life-threatening reactions

fenoldopam

(fhe-knowl'doh-pam)
Rx: Corlopam
Chemical Class: Benzazepine
derivative
Therapeutic Class: Vasodilator
(rapid acting)

CLINICAL PHARMACOLOGY

Mechanism of Action: Vasodilating effects in coronary, renal, mesenteric, and peripheral arteries via selective D_1-like dopamine receptor agonist activity; additional moderate affinity for α2-receptors

Pharmacokinetics

IV: Steady state concentrations attained in 20 minutes following constant infusion (approx. 3.5 g/ml following a 0.1 µg/kg/min infusion rate); metabolized primarily by conjugation (without CYP-450 participation - metabolites inactive); 90% excreted in urine; 10% feces (4% unchanged); $t_{1/2}$ 5 min; not influenced by age, gender, race, renal disease or hepatic failure

Pharmacodynamics

Average SBP/DBP drop over 1-24 hr on 0.4-0.8 µg/kg/min infusion: 23/20 mm Hg; heart rate, increase 20 BPM; most of effect seen after 15 minutes following initiation of dose change

INDICATIONS AND USES: Severe hypertension, when rapid (but quickly reversible) reduction of blood pressure is clinically indicated (i.e., malignant hypertension with deteriorating end-organ function); short-term, in-hospital treatment regimen (i.e., <48 hr), before changing to alternative long-term agents; oral antihypertensive can be administered concomitantly or following infusion (note hypotension could result)

DOSAGE
Adult and Child >16 yr

• IV infusion (calibrated, mechanical infusion pump): 0.1-0.6 µg/kg/min; no bolus dose; start at 0.1 µg/kg/min and up-titrate; dosage titrations no more frequently than q15 min in 0.05-0.1 µg/kg/min increments; after blood pressure control, fenoldopam infusions have been continued for up to 6 hours followed by gradual tapering (usually over hours)

$ **AVAILABLE FORMS/COST OF THERAPY**

• Inj—IV: 10 mg/ml single dose ampules: 1 ml: **$240.00-$264.00**; 2 ml: **$260.00-$462.00**; 5 ml: **$1,155.00**

CONTRAINDICATIONS: None known

PRECAUTIONS: Preparation contains metabisulfite, that can precipitate asthma symptoms in susceptible individuals

Glaucoma or intraocular hypertension: Caution, may raise intraocular pressure (approx. 6.5 mm Hg)

Hypokalemia

PREGNANCY AND LACTATION: Pregnancy category B; animal studies show no evidence of impaired fertility or fetal harm; no human data available; excreted into breast milk of rats; human information unknown

SIDE EFFECTS/ADVERSE REACTIONS

CNS: Anxiety, dizziness, headache, insomnia, nervousness

CV: Angina pectoris, extrasystoles, flushing, heart failure, hypotension, ischemic heart disease, myocardial infarction, palpitations, ST-T wave abnormalities (T-wave inversion), tachycardia

EENT: Blurred vision, nasal congestion, increased intraocular pressure

GU: Oliguria

MS: Back pain, limb cramp

RESP: Dyspnea, upper respiratory infection

SKIN: Sweating

INTERACTIONS

Drugs

🔳 *Acetaminophen:* May increase fenoldopam serum concentrations due to competition for sulfation (especially with oral fenoldopam)

Labs

• Hypokalemia, increased blood urea nitrogen and serum creatinine, elevated liver transaminases, elevated LDH

SPECIAL CONSIDERATIONS

• *Preparation of infusion solution:* Contents of ampules must be diluted prior to infusion: 1 ml of 10 mg/ml solution in 250 ml 0.9% sodium chloride or 5% dextrose yields a final concentration of 40 μg/ml

• *Potential advantage over sodium nitroprusside in hypertensive crisis:* Induction of naturesis, diuresis; ability to increase creatinine clearance, preserve renal function

MONITORING PARAMETERS

• Blood pressure, pulse, serum electrolytes, urine volume, urinary sodium, serum creatinine, blood urea nitrogen, electrocardiogram, hepatic function tests

---

fenoprofen

(fen-oh-proe′fen)

Rx: Nalfon

Chemical Class: Propionic acid derivative

Therapeutic Class: NSAID with analgesic and antipyretic activity

---

CLINICAL PHARMACOLOGY

Mechanism of Action: Reversible cyclooxygenase (i.e., prostaglandin synthetase) inhibitor; non-selectively decreases the formation of both prostaglandins and thromboxane A_2; variable effects on lipoxygenase synthesis and subsequent leukotriene production; antiinflammatory, antipyretic, and analgesic activity; inhibits platelet aggregation

Pharmacokinetics

PO: Rapid absorption, peak level 2 hr, metabolized in liver, metabolites excreted in urine; 99% protein binding to albumin; $t_{1/2}$ 3 hr

INDICATIONS AND USES: Osteoarthritis, rheumatoid arthritis, ankylosing spondylitis,* prevention of cognitive decline,* pain—mild to moderate, migraine headache,* tendonitis*

DOSAGE

Adult

• *Pain:* PO 200 mg q4-6h prn

• *Arthritis:* PO 300-600 mg tid-qid, not to exceed 3.2 g/day

💲 **AVAILABLE FORMS/COST OF THERAPY**

• Cap, Gel—Oral: 200 mg, 100's: **$23.60-$56.04**; 300 mg, 100's: **$27.37-$49.77**

• Tab, Uncoated—Oral: 600 mg, 100's: **$37.80-$70.66**

CONTRAINDICATIONS: Bronchospasm, nasal polyps, angioedema precipitated by aspirin or other NSAIDs

PRECAUTIONS: History of GI ulceration, bleeding, or perforation; renal dysfunction, hypertension or cardiac conditions aggravated by fluid retention and edema, history of liver dysfunction, history of coagulation deficits

PREGNANCY AND LACTATION: Pregnancy category B (category D, 3rd trimester); excreted in breast milk

SIDE EFFECTS/ADVERSE REACTIONS

CNS: Anxiety, confusion, depression, dizziness, drowsiness, fatigue, headache, insomnia, tremors

---

italic = common side effects   ***bold italic*** = life-threatening reactions

CV: **Dysrhythmias,** palpitations, peripheral edema, tachycardia

EENT: Blurred vision, hearing loss, tinnitus

GI: Anorexia, cholestatic hepatitis, *constipation,* cramps, diarrhea, dry mouth, *dyspepsia, nausea,* **peptic ulcer,** vomiting

GU: Azotemia, dysuria, hematuria, **interstitial nephritis**

HEME: **Agranulocytosis, aplastic anemia, hemolytic anemia, thrombocytopenia**

METAB: Hyperkalemia

SKIN: Pruritus, purpura, rash, sweating

INTERACTIONS

Drugs

⊠ *Aminoglycosides:* Reduced clearance with elevated aminoglycoside levels and potential for toxicity (especially indomethacin in premature infants; other NSAIDs probably)

⊠ *Antihypertensives (α-blockers, angiotensin-converting enzyme inhibitors, angiotensin II receptor blockers, β-blockers, diuretics):* Inhibition of antihypertensive and other favorable hemodynamic effects

⊠ *Corticosteroids:* Increased risk of GI ulceration

⊠ *Anticoagulants:* Excessive hypoprothrombinemia, decreased platelet aggregation with increased risk of GI bleeding

⊠ *Cyclosporine:* Increased nephrotoxicity risk

⊠ *Lithium:* Decreased clearance of lithium (mediated via prostaglandins) resulting in elevated serum lithium levels and risk of toxicity

⊠ *Methotrexate:* Decreased renal secretion of methotrexate resulting in elevated methotrexate levels and risk of toxicity

⊠ *Phenylpropranolamine:* Possible acute hypertensive reaction

⊠ *Potassium-sparing diuretics:* Additive hyperkalemia potential

⊠ *Triamterene:* Acute renal failure reported with addition of indomethacin; caution with other NSAIDs

Labs

• *False increase:* Free and total triiodothyronine levels, plasma cortisol

• *False positive:* Urine barbiturate, urine benzodiazepine

SPECIAL CONSIDERATIONS

• No significant advantage over other NSAIDs; cost should govern use

MONITORING PARAMETERS

• Initial hemogram and fecal occult blood test within 3 mo of starting regular chronic therapy; repeat every 6-12 mo (more frequently in high-risk patients (>65 years, peptic ulcer disease, concurrent steroids or anticoagulants); electrolytes, creatinine, and BUN within 3 mo of starting regular chronic therapy; repeat every 6-12 mo

---

fentanyl

(fen'ta-nill)

Rx: *Injection:* Sublimaze
Transdermal: Duragesic;
Lozenge: Fentanyl Oralet,
Actiq
Combinations
  Rx: with droperidol (Innovar)
Chemical Class: Synthetic opium alkaloid; phenylpiperidine derivative
Therapeutic Class: Narcotic analgesic
DEA Class: Schedule II

CLINICAL PHARMACOLOGY

Mechanism of Action: Narcotic agonist with activity at μ-receptors (supraspinal analgesia, euphoria, respiratory and physical depression, miosis, and reduced GI motility), Kappa receptors (pentazocine-like spinal analgesia, sedation, and miosis), and Delta receptors (dysphoria, psychotomimetic effects [e.g., hallucinations]); compared to morphine, equal analgesia, less respiratory depression and emesis

Pharmacokinetics

IM: Onset 7-15 min, peak 30 min, duration 1-2 hr

IV: Onset 1-2 min, peak 3-5 min, duration ½-1 hr

LOZ: Onset 5-15 min, peak 20-30 min; 50% bioavailability with rapid transmucosal and slower GI absorption

TRANS: Steady state plasma level 24 hr after application, 6 days after change of dose; plasma level $t_{1/2}$ 17 hr after patch removal due to some continued absorption

Metabolized by liver, excreted by kidneys, excretion $t_{1/2}$ 2½-4 hr; highly lipophilic, 80% bound to plasma proteins, crosses placenta, stored in fat and muscle (may lead to prolonged effect with repeated administration)

INDICATIONS AND USES: Perioperative analgesia; adjunct to general anesthesia (alone or combined with droperidol); general anesthesia; chronic pain (transdermal)

DOSAGE

Adult and Child >12 yr

• *Chronic pain:* Trans 25 µg/hr system initially; initial dose may be increased after 3 days, thereafter a minimum of 6 days should elapse between dosage increases; to convert patients already receiving other narcotics, refer to manufacturer product information; change system q72h

• *Sedation for minor procedure:* Buccal 5 µg/kg (max 400 µg) 20-40 min prior to procedure

• *Preoperatively:* IM 50-100 µg 30-60 min before surgery

• *Adjunct to general anesthesia:* IV 2-50 µg/kg

• *Adjunct to regional anesthesia:* IM/IV 50-100 µg when additional analgesia required

• *General anesthesia:* IV 50-100 µg/kg with oxygen and a muscle relaxant

• *Postoperatively:* IM 50-100 µg q1-2h prn

Child 2-12 yr

• *Sedation for minor procedure:* Buccal 5-10 µg/kg (max 400 µg) 20-40 min prior to procedure; children <40 kg may require doses of 10-15 µg/kg (max 400 µg); do not use in child <2 yr

• *Adjunct to anesthesia:* IV 2-3 µg/kg

Notes:

1. IV/IM dose of 0.1 mg fentanyl equianalgesic to 10 mg of morphine, 75 mg of meperidine

2. Transdermal fentanyl dose of 100 µg/hr equianalgesic to 60 mg morphine IM or 360 mg morphine PO per 24 hr

3. Buccal dose of 5 µg fentanyl equianalgesic to 1 µg IM fentanyl

💲 AVAILABLE FORMS/COST OF THERAPY

• Film, Cont Rel—Percutaneous: 25 µg/hr, 5's: **$66.74**; 50 µg/hr, 5's: **$111.28**; 75 µg/hr, 5's: **$176.59**; 100 µg/hr, 5's: **$222.11**

• Inj, Sol—IM, IV: 0.05 mg/ml, 2, 5, 10, 20, 30, 50 ml: **$0.64-$12.60**/2 ml

• Loz, Top—On a stick: 0.2 mg, 1's: **$7.43**; 0.4 mg, 1's: **$9.58**; 0.6 mg, 1's: **$11.72**; 0.8 mg, 1's: **$13.85**; 1.2 mg, 1's: **$18.27**; 1.6 mg, 1's: **$22.34**

• Loz, Top—Oral: 100, 200, 300, 400 µg, 1's: **$28.81-$30.86**

CONTRAINDICATIONS: Lozenge for child <15 kg, transdermal for child <12 yr

PRECAUTIONS: Elderly, respiratory depression, increased intracranial pressure, seizure disorders, severe respiratory disorders, cardiac dysrhythmias

PREGNANCY AND LACTATION: Pregnancy category C; excreted in breast milk

SIDE EFFECTS/ADVERSE REACTIONS

CNS: Asthenia, *confusion,* delirium, *dizziness,* euphoria, *somnolence*

CV: Bradycardia, hypotension or hypertension

EENT: Blurred vision, *dry mouth,* miosis

GI: Constipation, nausea, vomiting

GU: Urinary retention

MS: Muscle rigidity

RESP: Laryngospasm, ***respiratory depression***

SKIN: Pruritis, sweating

INTERACTIONS

Drugs

3 *Antihistamines, chloral hydrate, glutethimide, methocarbamol:* Enhanced depressant effects

3 *Barbiturates:* Additive respiratory and CNS-depressant effects

3 *Cimetidine:* Increased respiratory and CNS depression

3 *Diazepam:* Cardiovascular depression

3 *Ethanol:* Additive CNS effects

3 *Nitrous oxide:* Cardiovascular depression

Labs

• False elevations of serum amylase and lipase

SPECIAL CONSIDERATIONS

• Increased skin temperature increases absorption rate of transdermal preparation

• Lozenge should be used only in a monitored anesthesia care setting

• Following removal of transdermal system, 17 hr are required for 50% decrease in serum fentanyl concentrations

• Do not administer agonist/antagonist analgesics (i.e., pentazocine, nalbuphine, butorphanol, dezocine, buprenorphine) to patient who has received a prolonged course of fentanyl (a pure agonist). In opioid-dependent patients, mixed agonist/antagonist analgesics may precipitate withdrawal symptoms

---

* = non-FDA-approved use

ferrous salts

OTC: *Sulfate:* Feosol, Feratab, Fer-in-sol, Fer-Iron, Fero-Gradumet, Mol-Iron *Sulfate exsiccated:* Feosol, Fer-in-Sol, Ferra-TD, Slow Fe *Gluconate:* Fergon, Simron *Fumarate:* Femiron, Feostat, Hemocyte, Ircon, Nephro-Fer *Polysaccharide-Iron complex:* Hytinic, Niferex, Nu-Iron

Combinations

OTC: with magnesium and aluminum hydroxide (Fermalox); with docusate (Ferocyl, Ferro-Sequels, Ferro-Docusate, Ferro-dok TR, Ferro-DSS SR); with vitamin C (Mol-Iron with Vitamin C, Ferancee-HP, Vitron-C Plus, Cevi-Fer, Irospan, Fero-Grad, Hemaspan); with folate (Palafer CF); with multivitamins (Flintstones Plus Iron, Stresstabs with Iron)

Chemical Class: Iron preparation

Therapeutic Class: Hematinic

CLINICAL PHARMACOLOGY

Mechanism of Action: Replaces iron stores; hematologic response begins in 3 days

Pharmacokinetics

PO: Absorbed in duodenum and upper jejunum, absorption decreased by food and achlorhydria; bound to transferrin; crosses placenta; excreted in feces, urine

INDICATIONS AND USES: Prevention and treatment of iron deficiency anemia; adjunct to epoetin therapy*

DOSAGE (all expressed in elemental iron)

Adult

• *Iron deficiency:* PO 100-200 mg/day divided tid

• *Pregnancy:* PO 30 mg/day

Child

• *Iron deficiency:* (2-12 yr) PO 3 mg/kg/day divided tid-qid; (6 mo-2 yr) PO up to 6 mg/kg/day divided tid-qid; (infants) PO 10-25 mg/day divided tid-qid

• *Prophylaxis:* 1-2 mg/kg/day in 3 divided doses

NOTE: Ferrous fumarate is 33% elemental iron (325 mg has 106 mg); gluconate 12% elemental iron (325 mg has 38 mg); sulfate 20% elemental iron (325 mg has 65 mg)

§ AVAILABLE FORMS/COST OF THERAPY

Ferrous Fumarate

• Liq—Oral: 45 mg/0.6 ml, 60 ml: **$18.20**

• Susp—Oral: 100 mg/5 ml, 240 ml: **$23.16**

• Tab, Chewable—Oral: 100 mg, 100's: **$18.73**

• Tab—Oral: 63 mg, 40's: **$4.93-$5.87**; 200 mg, 100's: **$4.50**; 300 mg, 100's: **$3.00-$5.95**; 325 mg, 100's: **$0.77-$6.32**; 350 mg, 30's: **$13.10**

Ferrous Gluconate

• Cap, Soft Gel—Oral: 86 mg, 100's: **$35.65**

• Elixir—Oral: 300 mg/5 ml, 480 ml: **$17.50**

• Tab—Oral: 240 mg, 100's: **$3.79-$6.65**; 300 mg, 100's: **$1.69-$5.10**; 320 mg, 100's: **$4.02**; 325 mg, 100s: **$0.78-$4.43**

Ferrous Sulfate

• Cap, Sus Action—Oral: 159 mg, 100's: **$6.10**; 190 mg, 100's: **$9.70**; 250 mg, 100's: **$4.15-$5.77**

• Elixir—Oral: 220 mg/5 ml, 120, 480 ml: **$3.74-$14.59/480 ml**

• Liq—Oral: 75 mg/0.6 ml, 50 ml: **$3.25-$10.00**
• Syr—Oral: 90 mg/5 ml, 480 ml: **$14.75**
• Tab—Oral: 195 mg, 100's: **$5.42**; 200 mg, 100's: **$5.65-$7.71**; 300 mg, 100's: **$1.80-$3.96**; 325 mg, 100's: **$0.65-$20.25**
• Tab, Enteric Coated—Oral: 325 mg, 100's: **$3.09**
• Tab, Sus Action—Oral: 160 mg, 90's: **$18.02-$18.92**; 525 mg, 100's: **$27.65**

CONTRAINDICATIONS: Ulcerative colitis; regional enteritis, hemosiderosis; hemochromatosis, hemolytic anemia

PREGNANCY AND LACTATION: Pregnancy category A; excreted in breast milk

SIDE EFFECTS/ADVERSE REACTIONS

GI: Black stools, constipation, diarrhea, *epigastric pain, nausea,* vomiting

SKIN: Temporarily discolored tooth enamel (liq) and eyes

INTERACTIONS

Drugs

3 *Antacids:* Reduce iron absorption

3 *Ciprofloxacin, levodopa, levofloxacin, methyldopa, norfloxacin, penicillamine, tetracyclines, vitamin E:* Absorption reduced by iron

3 *Enalapril:* Three patients on enalapril developed systemic reactions following IV iron; causal relationship not established

Labs

• Urine discoloration black, brown, or dark color
• *Glucose:* Decreased with clinistix, diastix; no effect observed with testape
• *Occult blood:* 25-65% false positives

SPECIAL CONSIDERATIONS

PATIENT/FAMILY EDUCATION

• Best absorbed on empty stomach, may take with food if GI upset occurs
• Drink liquid iron preparations in water or juice and through a straw to prevent tooth stains
• 4-6 mo of therapy generally required
• Iron changes stools black or dark green

MONITORING PARAMETERS

• Hemoglobin, hematocrit

---

fexofenadine

(fex-oh-fen'eh-deen)
Rx: Allegra
Combinations
  Rx: with pseudoephedrine (Allegra-D)
Chemical Class: Piperidine derivative
Therapeutic Class: Antihistamine

CLINICAL PHARMACOLOGY

Mechanism of Action: Decreases allergic response by blocking histamine at H_1-receptors; no QT prolongation even at very high plasma concentrations

Pharmacokinetics

PO: Active metabolite of terfenadine; onset 1 hr, peak 2.6 hr, duration 12 hr; absorption 90%, protein binding 70%, minimal metabolism; $t_{1/2}$ 14.4 hr; excreted in stool (80%) and urine (11%)

INDICATIONS AND USES: Seasonal allergic rhinitis

DOSAGE

Adult and Child >12 yr

• *Seasonal allergic rhinitis:* PO 60 mg qd-bid or 180 mg qd
• *Chronic idiopathic urticaria:* PO 60 mg qd-bid

• *Renal function impairment:* PO 60 mg qd if CrCl <40 ml/min
Child 6-11 yr
• *Seasonal allergic rhinitis:* PO 30 mg qd-bid
• *Chronic idiopathic urticaria:* PO 30 mg qd-bid
• *Renal function impairment:* PO 30 mg qd in pediatric patients with CrCl <40 ml/min
$ AVAILABLE FORMS/COST OF THERAPY
• Cap—Oral: 60 mg, 100's: **$107.67-$123.29**
• Tab—Oral: 30 mg, 100's: **$67.86**; 60 mg, 100's: **$123.29**; 180 mg, 100's: **$235.15**
PRECAUTIONS: Concurrent use of macrolide antibiotics, azole antifungals, or agents that inhibit cytochrome P450 3A4 isozyme
PREGNANCY AND LACTATION: Pregnancy category C; breast milk excretion unknown
SIDE EFFECTS/ADVERSE REACTIONS
CNS: Drowsiness (1%), fatigue, headache
GI: Dyspepsia, nausea
GU: Dysmenorrhea
INTERACTIONS
Drugs
3 *Antacids:* Decreased plasma fexofenadine concentrations; avoid taking aluminum and magnesium containing antacids with fexofenadine
3 *Erythromycin:* Increased plasma fexofenadine concentrations
3 *Ketoconazole:* Increased plasma fexofenadine concentrations
SPECIAL CONSIDERATIONS
• Essentially the same as terfenadine without the potential for QT prolongation; relatively weak antihistamine with minimal sedation
• Consider alternating q hs chlorpeniramine with qam fexofenadine 60 mg to minimize cost

finasteride
(feen-as'ter-ide)
Rx: Proscar, Propecia
Chemical Class: 5α-reductase inhibitor
Therapeutic Class: Benign prostatic hypertrophy agent, hair growth stimulant

CLINICAL PHARMACOLOGY
Mechanism of Action: Inhibits the enzyme responsible for converting testosterone to 5α-dihydrotestosterone (DHT) reducing the levels of DHT available for development of the prostate gland and other DHT-dependent organs
Pharmacokinetics
PO: Bioavailability 63%, peak 1-2 hr, plasma protein binding 90%; metabolized in the liver, 39% excreted in urine (metabolites), 57% in feces; $t_{1/2}$ 6 hr; crosses blood-brain barrier
INDICATIONS AND USES: Symptomatic benign prostatic hypertrophy (<50% of patients experience an increase in urinary flow and improvement in symptoms), male pattern hair loss (vertex and anterior midscalp), prostate cancer*
DOSAGE
Adult
• *BPH:* PO 5 mg qd
• *Hair loss:* PO 1 mg qd; ≥3 mo necessary for benefit to be noted
$ AVAILABLE FORMS/COST OF THERAPY
• Tab, Plain Coated—Oral: 1 mg, 30's: **$49.35-$56.32**; 5 mg, 100's: **$252.94-$266.25**
CONTRAINDICATIONS: Children, women
PRECAUTIONS: Hepatic function impairment, obstructive uropathy

PREGNANCY AND LACTATION: Pregnancy category X; not indicated for use in women; pregnant women should not handle crushed tablets

SIDE EFFECTS/ADVERSE REACTIONS

GU: Decreased libido, decreased volume of ejaculate, impotence

SPECIAL CONSIDERATIONS

• Minimal benefit for benign prostatic hypertrophy if the prostate is not very large; response is not immediate

• Combination therapy with α-blocker may be optimal

• Whether long-term treatment can reduce prostate cancer risk is unknown; decreases prostate specific antigen (PSA)

PATIENT/FAMILY EDUCATION

• Condoms should be used if the female partner is at risk of pregnancy

• Withdrawal of drug for hair loss leads to reversal within 12 mo

MONITORING PARAMETERS

• 6-12 mo of therapy may be necessary in some patients to assess effectiveness (BPH), 3 or more mo for hair loss

---

flavoxate

(fla-vox′ate)

Rx: Urispas

Chemical Class: Flavone derivative

Therapeutic Class: Genitourinary muscle relaxant

CLINICAL PHARMACOLOGY

Mechanism of Action: Relaxes the detrusor and other smooth muscle by cholinergic blockade, also exerts a direct effect on the muscle

Pharmacokinetics

PO: Onset 55 min, peak 112 min; 57% excreted in urine within 24 hr

INDICATIONS AND USES: Relief of nocturia, incontinence, suprapubic pain, dysuria, frequency associated with urologic conditions (symptomatic only)

DOSAGE

Adult and Child >12 yr

• PO 100-200 mg tid-qid, reduce dose when symptoms improve

⑤ AVAILABLE FORMS/COST OF THERAPY

• Tab, Plain Coated—Oral: 100 mg, 100's: **$138.50-$142.81**

CONTRAINDICATIONS: Pyloric or duodenal obstruction, obstructive intestinal lesions or ileus, achalasia, GI hemorrhage, obstructive uropathies of the lower urinary tract

PRECAUTIONS: Glaucoma, children <12 yr

PREGNANCY AND LACTATION: Pregnancy category B; excretion into breast milk unknown; use caution in nursing mothers

SIDE EFFECTS/ADVERSE REACTIONS

CNS: Drowsiness, headache, mental confusion (especially in the elderly), nervousness, vertigo

CV: Tachycardia and palpitation

EENT: Blurred vision, disturbance in eye accommodation, increased ocular tension

GI: Dry mouth, *nausea,* vomiting

GU: Dysuria

HEME: Leukopenia (rare)

SKIN: Urticaria and other dermatoses

SPECIAL CONSIDERATIONS

• Urinary antispasmodic that is no more effective than propantheline or other similar agents

---

flecainide

(fle'kah-nide)

Rx: Tambocor

Chemical Class: Benzamide derivative

Therapeutic Class: Antidys-rhythmic (Class IC)

CLINICAL PHARMACOLOGY

Mechanism of Action: Produces a dose-related decrease in intracardiac conduction in all parts of the heart with the greatest effect on the His-Purkinje system; causes slight prolongation of refractory periods; decreases the rate of rise of the action potential without affecting its duration

Pharmacokinetics

PO: Peak 3 hr, 40%-50% bound to plasma proteins (α_1-glycoprotein), $t_{1/2}$ 12-27 hr; metabolized by liver, excreted by kidneys

INDICATIONS AND USES: Paroxysmal atrial fibrillation (PAF) and paroxysmal supraventricular tachycardias (PSVT) associated with disabling symptoms; documented life-threatening ventricular dysrhythmias

DOSAGE

Adult

• *PSVT and PAF:* PO 50 mg q12h; may increase q4d by 50 mg q12h to desired response; not to exceed 300 mg/day

• *Sustained ventricular tahcycardia:* PO 100 mg q12h; may increase q4d by 50 mg q12h to desired response; not to exceed 400 mg/day

Child

• PO 3 mg/kg/day divided tid; may increase up to 11 mg/kg/day for uncontrolled patients with subtherapeutic levels

$ **AVAILABLE FORMS/COST OF THERAPY**

• Tab, Uncoated—Oral: 50 mg, 100's: **$201.50**; 100 mg, 100's: **$316.06**; 150 mg, 100's: **$435.00**

CONTRAINDICATIONS: Severe heart block, cardiogenic shock, non-sustained ventricular dysrhythmias, frequent PVCs, non-life-threatening dysrhythmias (due to proarrhythmic effects), recent MI

PRECAUTIONS: Children, renal disease, liver disease, CHF, respiratory depression, myasthenia gravis, sick sinus syndrome, electrolyte disturbances

PREGNANCY AND LACTATION: Pregnancy category C; excreted into breast milk with milk-plasma ratios 1.6:3.7, but considered compatible with breast feeding

SIDE EFFECTS/ADVERSE REACTIONS

CNS: Amnesia, anxiety, ataxia, confusion, depression, *dizziness,* euphoria, *faintness, fatigue, headache,* hypoesthesia, insomnia, *lightheadedness,* malaise, neuropathy, paresis, paresthesia, **seizures,** somnolence, stupor, syncope, tremor, twitching, unsteadiness, vertigo, weakness

CV: Angina pectoris, **AV block, bradycardia,** chest pain, **CHF, dysrhythmia,** edema, hypertension, hypotension, palpitation, **sinus arrest, sinus pause,** tachycardia

EENT: Blurred vision, diplopia; eye pain, irritation; nystagmus, photophobia, visual disturbances

GI: Abdominal pain, anorexia, change in taste, *constipation,* dry mouth, dyspepsia, flatulence, *nausea,* vomiting

GU: Decreased libido, impotence, polyuria, urinary retention

HEME: **Leukopenia, thrombocytopenia**

MS: Arthralgia, myalgia

---

italic = common side effects   ***bold italic*** = life-threatening reactions

RESP: **Bronchospasm**

SKIN: Alopecia, **exfoliative derma-titis,** pruritus, rash, urticaria

INTERACTIONS

Drugs

3 *Acetazolamide, ammonium chloride, antacids, sodium bicarbonate:* Increases in urine pH decreases flecanide urinary clearance

3 *Amiodarone:* Reduced flecainide dosage requirements

3 *Cimetidine:* Inhibits metabolism of flecainide

3 *Propranolol:* Inhibitors of each other's metabolism; additive negative inotropic effects

3 *Sotolol:* Additive myocardial conduction depression; cardiac arrest reported

SPECIAL CONSIDERATIONS

• Not 1st line therapy

• Reserve for resistant arrhythmias due to proarrhythmic effects

• Initiate therapy in facilities capable of providing continuous ECG monitoring and managing life-threatening dysrhythmias

MONITORING PARAMETERS

• Monitor trough plasma levels periodically, especially in patients with moderate to severe chronic renal failure or severe hepatic disease and CHF; therapeutic range 0.2-1 µg/ml

---

fluconazole

(floo-con'a-zole)

Rx: Diflucan

Chemical Class: Triazole derivative

Therapeutic Class: Antifungal

CLINICAL PHARMACOLOGY

Mechanism of Action: Interferes with cytochrome P450 activity, decreasing ergosterol synthesis (principal sterol in fungal cell membrane) and inhibiting cell membrane formation

Pharmacokinetics

IV/PO: Peak 1-2 hr (PO), 11%-12% bound to plasma proteins, extensive distribution into all studied body fluids, $t_{1/2}$ 20-50 hr; cleared primarily by renal excretion

INDICATIONS AND USES: Oropharyngeal and esophageal candidiasis; candidal UTI, peritonitis and systemic candidal infections; vaginal candidiasis; prophylaxis of candidiasis in patients undergoing bone marrow transplant who receive cytotoxic chemotherapy or radiation therapy; cryptococcal meningitis

DOSAGE

Adult

• *Cryptococcal meningitis:* PO/IV 400 mg on 1st day, then 200 mg qd for 10-12 wk after CSF becomes culture negative; increase up to 400 mg/day based on response

• *Esophageal candidiasis:* PO/IV 200 mg on 1st day, then 100 mg qd for at least 3 wk and for 2 wk following resolution of symptoms; doses up to 400 mg/day may be used based on response

• *Oropharyngeal candidiasis:* PO/IV 200 mg on 1st day, then 100 mg qd for at least 2 wk

• *Other candidiasis:* PO/IV 50-200 mg/day, doses up to 400 mg/day may be used based on response

• *Prevention of candidiasis in bone marrow transplant:* PO/IV 400 mg qd, initiate several days before anticipated onset of neutropenia, continue 7 days after neutrophil count rises above 1000 cells/mm^3

• *Vaginal candidiasis:* PO 150 mg as a single dose

• *Renal function impairment:* PO/IV reduce dose by 50% in patients with CrCl <50 ml/min

* = non-FDA-approved use

Child

• Equivalent doses for children are 3 mg/kg for adult dose of 100 mg; 6 mg/kg for adult dose of 200 mg; 12 mg/kg for adult dose of 400 mg; do not exceed 600 mg dose

💲 AVAILABLE FORMS/COST OF THERAPY

• Inj, Sol—IV: 2 mg/ml, 100 ml: **$95.65**
• Powder—Oral: 50 mg/5 ml, 60 ml: **$33.09**; 200 mg/5 ml, 60 ml: **$120.23**
• Tab, Plain Coated—Oral: 50 mg, 30's: **$154.51**; 100 mg, 30's: **$224.06-$242.80**; 150 mg, 12's: **$154.59**; 200 mg, 30's: **$392.26-$397.30**

PRECAUTIONS: Hypersensitivity to other azoles, children, renal disease

PREGNANCY AND LACTATION: Pregnancy category C; excreted into breast milk in concentrations similar to plasma; not recommended in nursing mothers

SIDE EFFECTS/ADVERSE REACTIONS

CNS: Headache, *seizures*
GI: Cramping, diarrhea, flatus, *hepatic injury,* nausea, vomiting
HEME: **Leukopenia, thrombocytopenia**
METAB: Hypercholesterolemia, hypertriglyceridemia, hypokalemia
SKIN: **Exfoliative skin disorders**

INTERACTIONS

Drugs

🔳 *Alprazolam:* Increased plasma alprazolam concentration

🔳 *Atevirdine:* Increased plasma atevirdine concentration

🔳 *Atorvastatin:* Increased plasma atorvastatin concentration with risk of rhabdomyolysis

🔳 *Buspirone:* Increased plasma buspirone concentration

🔳 *Caffeine:* Increased plasma caffeine concentration

🔳 *Chlordiazepoxide:* Increased plasma chlordiazepoxide concentration

❷ *Cisapride:* QT prolongation and dysrhythmia

🔳 *Cyclosporine:* Increased plasma cyclosporine concentration

🔳 *Diazepam:* Increased plasma diazepam concentration

🔳 *Felodipine:* Increased plasma felodipine concentration

🔳 *Fluvastatin:* Increased plasma fluvastatin concentration with risk of rhabdomyolysis

🔳 *Losartan:* Reduced concentration of losartan's active metabolite may reduce efficacy of losartan

❷ *Lovastatin:* Increased plasma lovastatin concentration with risk of rhabdomyolysis

🔳 *Methadone:* Increased plasma methadone concentration

🔳 *Midazolam:* Increased plasma midazolam concentration

❷ *Phenytoin:* Markedly reduced plasma fluconazole concentration

🔳 *Pravastatin:* Increased plasma pravastatin concentration with risk of rhabdomyolysis

🔳 *Quinidine:* Increased plasma quinidine concentration

🔳 *Rifampin:* Decreased plasma fluconazole concentration; decreased plasma rifampin concentration

❷ *Simvastatin:* Increased plasma simvastatin concentration with risk of rhabdomyolysis

🔳 *Tacrolimus:* Increased plasma tacrolimus concentration

❷ *Triazolam:* Increased plasma triazolam concentration

---

3 *Tolbutamide:* Increased plasma tolbutamide concentration

3 *Warfarin:* Increased hypoprothrombinemic response

Labs

• *Benzoylecgonine:* False negative urine results

SPECIAL CONSIDERATIONS
MONITORING PARAMETERS

• Periodic liver function tests with prolonged therapy

---

flucytosine

(floo-sye'toe-seen)

Rx: Ancobon
Chemical Class: Fluorinated pyrimidine derivative
Therapeutic Class: Antifungal

CLINICAL PHARMACOLOGY

Mechanism of Action: Acts directly on fungal organisms by competitive inhibition of purine and pyrimidine uptake and indirectly by metabolism within the fungal organism to 5-fluorouracil, which inhibits synthesis of both DNA and RNA

Pharmacokinetics

PO: Peak 2 hr, $t_{1/2}$ 2-5 hr; excreted in urine (unchanged); well-distributed to peritoneal fluid, aqueous humor, joints, and other body fluids and tissues; CSF concentrations approximately 65%-90% of serum levels

INDICATIONS AND USES: Serious infections caused by susceptible strains of *Candida* (septicemia, endocarditis, UTIs) or *Cryptococcus* (meningitis, pulmonary, urinary tract infections, septicemia); treatment of chromomycosis*

DOSAGE

Adult and Child >50 kg

• PO 50-150 mg/kg/day divided q6h; initiate dose at the lower level if renal impairment is present

Adult and Child <50 kg

• PO 1.5-4.5 g/m²/day in 4 divided doses

$ **AVAILABLE FORMS/COST OF THERAPY**

• Cap, Gel—Oral: 250 mg, 100's: **$403.69**; 500 mg, 100's: **$698.30-$803.05**

PRECAUTIONS: Renal disease, impaired hepatic function, bone marrow depression, blood dyscrasias, radiation/chemotherapy

PREGNANCY AND LACTATION: Pregnancy category C; 4% of drug metabolized to 5-fluorouracil, an antineoplastic suspected of producing congenital defects in humans; excretion into breast milk unknown; use caution in nursing mothers

SIDE EFFECTS/ADVERSE REACTIONS

CNS: Ataxia, confusion, hallucinations, headache, hearing loss, paresthesia, parkinsonism, peripheral neuropathy, psychosis, pyrexia, sedation, vertigo

CV: **Cardiac arrest,** chest pain

GI: Abdominal pain, *anorexia,* bilirubin elevation, diarrhea, dry mouth, duodenal ulcer, elevation of hepatic enzymes, **GI hemorrhage,** hepatic dysfunction, jaundice, *nausea,* ulcerative colitis, *vomiting*

GU: Azotemia, creatinine and BUN elevation, crystalluria, **renal failure**

HEME: **Agranulocytosis,** anemia, **aplastic anemia,** eosinophilia, **leukopenia, pancytopenia, thrombocytopenia**

METAB: Hypoglycemia, hypokalemia

RESP: Dyspnea, **respiratory arrest**

SKIN: Photosensitivity, pruritus, rash, urticaria

INTERACTIONS

Drugs

3 *Cytosine arabinoside:* Inactivates antifungal activity by competitive inhibition

---

* = non-FDA-approved use

Labs
• *False increase:* Serum creatinine (when Ektachem analyzer is used)
SPECIAL CONSIDERATIONS
• Rarely used as monotherapy; generally used in combination with amphotericin B
PATIENT/FAMILY EDUCATION
• Reduce or avoid GI upset by taking caps a few at a time over a 15 min period
MONITORING PARAMETERS
• Creatinine, BUN, alk phosphatase, AST, ALT, CBC
• Serum flucytosine concentrations (therapeutic range 25-100 µg/ml)

---

fludrocortisone

(floo-droe-kor′ti-sone)
Rx: Florinef
Chemical Class: Synthetic mineralocorticoid
Therapeutic Class: Mineralocorticoid

CLINICAL PHARMACOLOGY
Mechanism of Action: Acts on the distal tubules of the kidney to enhance reabsorption of sodium from tubular fluid into the plasma; increases urinary excretion of both potassium and hydrogen
Pharmacokinetics
PO: Peak 1.7 hr, plasma $t_{1/2}$ 3½ hr, biological $t_{1/2}$ 18-36 hr; metabolized by liver, excreted in urine
INDICATIONS AND USES: Adrenocortical insufficiency in Addison's disease; salt-losing adrenogenital syndrome; severe orthostatic hypotension*
DOSAGE
Adult
• PO 0.05-0.2 mg qd
Child
• PO 0.05-0.1 mg qd

§ AVAILABLE FORMS/COST OF THERAPY
• Tab, Uncoated—Oral: 0.1 mg, 100's: **$83.26**
CONTRAINDICATIONS: Systemic fungal infections
PRECAUTIONS: Trauma, surgery, severe illness (supportive dosage may be required), abrupt discontinuation
PREGNANCY AND LACTATION: Pregnancy category C; observe newborn for signs and symptoms of adrenocortical insufficiency; corticosteroids are found in breast milk; use caution in nursing mothers
SIDE EFFECTS/ADVERSE REACTIONS
CNS: Headache
CV: ***CHF***, *edema,* enlargement of the heart, flushing, hypertension
METAB: Hypernatremia, hypokalemic alkalosis
MS: Fractures, osteoporosis, weakness
SKIN: Allergic rash, bruising, hives, increased sweating
INTERACTIONS
Drugs
3 *Amphotericin:* Excessive potassium depletion
3 *Diuretics, loop:* Opposite therapeutic effect; excessive potassium loss
3 *Diuretics, thiazide:* Opposite therapeutic effect; excessive potassium loss
3 *Digitalis:* Increased potential for digitalis toxicity associated with hypokalemia
SPECIAL CONSIDERATIONS
PATIENT/FAMILY EDUCATION
• Notify clinician of dizziness, severe headache, swelling of feet or lower legs, unusual weight gain
• Do not discontinue abruptly
MONITORING PARAMETERS
• Serum electrolytes, blood pressure, serum renin

---

italic = common side effects   ***bold italic*** = life-threatening reactions

flumazenil

(floo-maz´en-ill)

Rx: Romazicon

Chemical Class: Imidazoben-
zodiazepine derivative

Therapeutic Class: Benzodiazepine antagonist

CLINICAL PHARMACOLOGY

Mechanism of Action: Antagonizes
the actions of benzodiazepines in the
CNS; competitively inhibits activity
at the benzodiazepine recognition
site on the GABA/benzodiazepine
receptor

Pharmacokinetics

IV: 50% bound to plasma proteins,
metabolized in the liver, primarily
excreted in urine; terminal $t_{1/2}$ 41-79
min

INDICATIONS AND USES: Complete or partial reversal of sedative
effects of benzodiazepines

DOSAGE

Adult

• *Reversal of conscious sedation:* IV
0.2 mg (2 ml) initially over 15 sec,
repeat at 60 sec intervals prn to a
max total dose of 1 mg (10 ml)

• *Suspected benzodiazepine overdose:* IV 0.2 mg (2 ml) given over 30
sec; wait 30 sec, then give 0.3 mg (3
ml) over 30 sec if consciousness
does not occur; further doses of 0.5
mg (5 ml) can be given over 30 sec at
intervals of 1 min up to cumulative
dose of 3 mg; patients with a partial
response at 3 mg may require additional titration up to a total dose of 5
mg (administered slowly in the same
manner)

**§ AVAILABLE FORMS/COST
OF THERAPY**

• Inj, Sol—IV: 0.1 mg/ml, 5, 10 ml:
$10.40-$62.84/5 ml

* = non-FDA-approved use

CONTRAINDICATIONS: Serious
cyclic antidepressant overdose, patients given benzodiazepine for control of life-threatening condition

PRECAUTIONS: Children, elderly,
renal disease, seizure disorders,
head injury, labor and delivery, hepatic disease, hypoventilation,
panic disorder, drug and alcohol dependency, ambulatory patients (resedation may occur)

PREGNANCY AND LACTATION:
Pregnancy category C; excretion
into breast milk unknown; use caution in nursing mothers

**SIDE EFFECTS/ADVERSE REAC-
TIONS**

CNS: Agitation, confusion, *dizziness,* emotional lability, headache,
seizures, somnolence

CV: Bradycardia, *dysrhythmias,*
chest pain, cutaneous vasodilation,
hypertension, palpitations, tachycardia

EENT: Abnormal vision, blurred vision, tinnitus

GI: Hiccups, *nausea, vomiting*

SKIN: Increased sweating

MISC: Inj site pain, fatigue

SPECIAL CONSIDERATIONS

PATIENT/FAMILY EDUCATION

• Resedation may occur; do not engage in any activities requiring complete alertness or operate hazardous
machinery or a motor vehicle until at
least 18 to 24 hr after discharge

• Do not use any alcohol or non-prescription drugs for 18 to 24 hr after
flumazenil administration

MONITORING PARAMETERS

• Monitor for seizures, sedation, respiratory depression, or other residual benzodiazepine effects for an
appropriate period (up to 120 min)
based on dose and duration of effect
of the benzodiazepine employed;
pharmacokinetics of benzodiazepines are not altered in the presence
of flumazenil

flunisolide

(floo-niss´oh-lide)

Rx: *Aerosol INH:* AeroBid, *Nasal:* Nasalide, Nasarel

Chemical Class: Synthetic glucocorticoid

Therapeutic Class: Antiasthmatic; inhaled corticosteroid; nasal corticosteroid

CLINICAL PHARMACOLOGY

Mechanism of Action: Decreases inflammation by suppression of migration of polymorphonuclear leukocytes, fibroblasts, reversal of increased capillary permeability, and lysosomal stabilization

Pharmacokinetics

INH: Systemic availability 40%

NASAL: 50% absorption after nasal inhalation

Rapidly metabolized in liver to inactive metabolites; $t_{1/2}$ 1.8 hr; excreted in urine and feces

INDICATIONS AND USES: Seasonal or perennial rhinitis; (nasal sol); chronic asthma (oral inhaler)

DOSAGE

Adult

• NASAL SOL 2 sprays (50 µg) in each nostril bid-tid, max 8 sprays/nostril/day (400 µg/day); ORAL INHALER 2 inhalations (500 µg) bid, not to exceed 4 inhalations bid (2000 µg)

Child

• NASAL SOL 1 spray (25 µg) in each nostril tid or 2 sprays (50 µg) in each nostril bid, max 4 sprays/nostril/day (200 µg/day); ORAL INHALER (age 6-15 yr) 2 inhalations bid (1000 µg/day)

$ AVAILABLE FORMS/COST OF THERAPY

• Aer—Inhaler: 250 µg/inh, 100 doses: **$52.02-$79.43**

• Spray—Nasal: 25 µg/inh, 200 doses: **$31.22-$52.24**

CONTRAINDICATIONS: Fungal, bacterial infection of nose (nasal sol); status asthmaticus (oral inhaler)

PRECAUTIONS: Quiescent tuberculosis; nasal septal ulcers, recurrent epistaxis, nasal surgery or trauma; untreated fungal, bacterial, or viral infections

PREGNANCY AND LACTATION: Pregnancy category C; excretion into breast milk unknown, use caution in nursing mothers

SIDE EFFECTS/ADVERSE REACTIONS

CNS: Dizziness, headache, nervousness, restlessness

EENT: Candida infection of oral cavity, hoarseness/dysphonia, *sore throat* (oral sol); dryness, epistaxis, nasal irritation and stinging, rebound congestion, sneezing (nasal sol)

GI: Dry mouth, nausea, vomiting

SKIN: Urticaria

SPECIAL CONSIDERATIONS

PATIENT/FAMILY EDUCATION

• To be used on a regular basis, not for acute symptoms

• Use bronchodilators before oral inhaler (for patients using both)

• Nasal sol may cause drying and irritation of nasal mucosa

• Clear nasal passages prior to use of nasal sol

MONITORING PARAMETERS

• Monitor children for growth as well as for effects on the HPA axis during chronic therapy

• Monitor patients switched from chronic systemic corticosteroids to avoid acute adrenal insufficiency in response to stress

---

italic = common side effects   ***bold italic*** = life-threatening reactions

fluocinolone

(floo-oh-sin'oh-lone)

Rx: Derma-Smoothe/FS, FS Shampoo, Synalar, Synemol

Chemical Class: Synthetic glucocorticoid

Therapeutic Class: Topical corticosteroid, low potency (0.01% cream, solution, oil, shampoo), intermediate potency (0.025% cream, ointment)

CLINICAL PHARMACOLOGY

Mechanism of Action: Depresses formation, release, and activity of endogenous mediators of inflammation such as prostaglandins, kinins, histamine, liposomal enzymes, and the complement system resulting in decreased edema, erythema, and pruritus

Pharmacokinetics

Absorbed through the skin (increased by inflammation and occlusive dressings); metabolized primarily in the liver

INDICATIONS AND USES: Psoriasis, eczema, contact dermatitis, pruritus of corticosteroid responsive dermatoses; moderate to severe stable atopic dermatitis (0.01% oil) in patients ≥2 yr

DOSAGE

Adult

• *Atopic dermatitis:* TOP apply thin film to affected area tid, rub completely into skin

• *Scalp psoriasis:* TOP wet or dampen hair and scalp, apply thin film to scalp, massage well and cover scalp with shower cap; leave on overnight or minimum of 4 hr before washing off; wash hair with regular shampoo and rinse thoroughly

Child ≥ 2 yr

• *Atopic dermatitis:* TOP moisten skin, apply thin film to affected area bid for no longer than 4 wk, rub completely into skin

⑤ AVAILABLE FORMS/COST OF THERAPY

• Cre—Top: 0.01%, 15, 60, 100, 425 g: **$3.20-$4.95**/60 g; 0.025%, 15, 60, 100, 425 g: **$3.81-$52.09**/60 g

• Oil—Top: 0.01%, 120 ml: **$25.00**

• Oint—Top: 0.025%, 15, 30, 60 g: **$5.78-$52.09**/60 g

• Shampoo—Top: 0.01%, 120 ml: **$17.05-$30.44**

• Sol—Top: 0.01%, 20, 60 ml: **$8.64-$54.94**/60 ml

CONTRAINDICATIONS: Fungal infections; use on face, groin, or axilla

PRECAUTIONS: Viral infections, bacterial infections, children

PREGNANCY AND LACTATION: Pregnancy category C; unknown whether topical application could result in sufficient systemic absorption to produce detectable amounts in breast milk (systemic corticosteroids are secreted into breast milk in quantities not likely to have detrimental effects on infant)

SIDE EFFECTS/ADVERSE REACTIONS

SKIN: Acne, allergic contact dermatitis, atrophy, burning, dryness, folliculitis, hypertrichosis, hypopigmentation, irritation, itching, miliaria, perioral dermatitis, secondary infection, striae

MISC: Systemic absorption of topical corticosteroids has produced reversible HPA axis suppression (more likely with occlusive dressings, prolonged administration, application to large surface areas, liver failure, and in children)

SPECIAL CONSIDERATIONS

• Topical oil contains refined peanut oil

---

* = non-FDA-approved use

PATIENT/FAMILY EDUCATION
• Apply sparingly only to affected area
• Avoid contact with eyes
• Do not put bandages or dressings over treated area unless directed by clinician
• Do not use on weeping, denuded, or infected areas
• Discontinue drug, notify clinician if local irritation or fever develops

---

fluocinonide
(floo-oh-sin′oh-nide)

Rx: Lidex, Lidex-E
Chemical Class: Synthetic glucocorticoid
Therapeutic Class: Topical corticosteroid, high potency

CLINICAL PHARMACOLOGY
Mechanism of Action: Depresses formation, release, and activity of endogenous mediators of inflammation such as prostaglandins, kinins, histamine, liposomal enzymes, and the complement system resulting in decreased edema, erythema, and pruritus

Pharmacokinetics
Absorbed through the skin (increased by inflammation and occlusive dressings); metabolized primarily in the liver

INDICATIONS AND USES: Psoriasis, eczema, contact dermatitis, pruritus of corticosteroid responsive dermatoses

DOSAGE
Adult and Child
• TOP apply to affected area bid-tid, rub completely into skin

💲 AVAILABLE FORMS/COST OF THERAPY
• Cre—Top: 0.05%, 15, 30, 60, 120 g: **$7.30-$36.83**/30 g

• Gel—Top: 0.05%, 15, 30, 60, 120 g: **$27.40-$36.83**/60 g
• Oint—Top: 0.05%, 15, 30, 60, 120 g: **$21.00-$36.83**/30 g
• Sol—Top: 0.05%, 20, 60 ml: **$17.50-$59.86**/60 ml

CONTRAINDICATIONS: Fungal infections; use on face, groin, or axilla

PRECAUTIONS: Viral infections, bacterial infections, children

PREGNANCY AND LACTATION: Pregnancy category C; unknown whether topical application could result in sufficient systemic absorption to produce detectable amounts in breast milk (systemic corticosteroids are secreted into breast milk in quantities not likely to have detrimental effects on infant)

SIDE EFFECTS/ADVERSE REACTIONS
SKIN: Acne, allergic contact dermatitis, atrophy, burning, dryness, folliculitis, hypertrichosis, hypopigmentation, irritation, itching, miliaria, perioral dermatitis, secondary infection, striae
MISC: Systemic absorption of topical corticosteroids has produced reversible HPA axis suppression (more likely with occlusive dressings, prolonged administration, application to large surface areas, liver failure, and in children)

SPECIAL CONSIDERATIONS
PATIENT/FAMILY EDUCATION
• Apply sparingly only to affected area
• Avoid contact with eyes
• Do not put bandages or dressings over treated area unless directed by clinician
• Do not use on weeping, denuded, or infected areas
• Discontinue drug, notify clinician if local irritation or fever develops

fluorescein

(flure'e-seen)

Rx: AK-Fluor, Angioscein, Fluorescite, Fluorets, Fluor-I-Strip, Fluor-I-Strip-A.T., Ful-Glo, Ocu-Flur 10
Combinations
   Rx: with proparacaine (Fluoracaine)
Chemical Class: Xanthine dye
Therapeutic Class: Ophthalmic diagnostic agent

CLINICAL PHARMACOLOGY

Mechanism of Action: Breaks in corneal tissue absorb dye and appear bright green under cobalt blue light
INDICATIONS AND USES: Diagnostic aid in identifying foreign bodies, hard fitting contact lenses, fundus photography, tonometry, identifying corneal abrasions, retinal angiography

DOSAGE

Adult

• *Detection of foreign bodies/corneal abrasions:* Ophth 1 gtt 2% sol, allow a few sec for staining, wash out excess with sterile irrigating solution; strips moisten strip with sterile water, place moistened strip at the fornix in lower cul-de-sac close to the punctum, have patient close lid tightly over strip until desired amount of staining obtained

• *Retinal angiography:* IV 500-750 mg inj rapidly in antecubital vein

Child

• *Retinal angiography:* IV 7.5 mg/kg inj rapidly in antecubital vein

💲 AVAILABLE FORMS/COST OF THERAPY

• Inj, Sol—Intraocular: 10% 5 ml: **$3.90-$97.50**

• Inj, Sol—IV: 25%, 2 ml: **$5.52-$7.82**

• Sol—Ophth: 2%, 15 ml: **$14.19-$23.99**; 10%, 5 ml: **$0.25**

• Strip—Ophth: 0.6 mg, 300's: **$36.87**; 1 mg, 9 mg, 300's: **$67.20-$77.80**

CONTRAINDICATIONS: Soft contact lenses (lenses may become discolored)

PRECAUTIONS: History of allergies, asthma

PREGNANCY AND LACTATION: Pregnancy category C; avoid parenteral use, especially in 1st trimester; excreted into breast milk; use caution in nursing mothers

SIDE EFFECTS/ADVERSE REACTIONS

CNS: **Seizures,** dizziness, headache, paresthesia

CV: Bradycardia, ***cardiac arrest,*** hypotension, ***shock,*** syncope

EENT: Burning, conjunctival redness, pruritis, stinging, urticaria

GI: GI distress, nausea, strong taste, vomiting

GU: Bright yellow discoloration of urine

RESP: ***Acute pulmonary edema, bronchospasm, dyspnea***

SKIN: Severe local tissue damage with extravasation, yellowish discoloration of skin

SPECIAL CONSIDERATIONS

PATIENT/FAMILY EDUCATION

• May cause temporary yellowish discoloration of skin (fades in 6-12 hr)

• Urine will appear bright yellow (fades in 24-36 hr)

• Soft contact lenses may become stained, wait at least 1 hr after thorough rinsing of eye before replacing lenses

MONITORING PARAMETERS

• Luminescence appears in the retina and choroidal vessels 9-15 min following IV inj; can be observed by standard viewing equipment

fluoride, sodium

Rx: Fluorinse, Fluoritab, Flura, Gel-Kam, Karidium, Karigel, Listermint with Fluoride, Luride, Minute-Gel, Pediaflor, Pharmaflur, Phos-Flur, Prevident, Stop, Thera-Flur

OTC: Fluorigard, Gel-Tin
Chemical Class: Fluoride ion
Therapeutic Class: Antiosteoporotic; anti-dental caries agent

CLINICAL PHARMACOLOGY
Mechanism of Action: Needed for hard tooth enamel and for resistance to periodontal disease; reduces acid production by dental bacteria; potent stimulator of bone formation—increases bone mass in intermediate doses

Pharmacokinetics
PO: Absorption related to solubility; sodium fluoride almost completely absorbed; calcium or magnesium delays absorption; 50% deposited in bone and teeth; excreted in urine, feces, and breast milk; crosses placenta

INDICATIONS AND USES: Prevention of dental caries; osteoporosis*

DOSAGE
NOTE: 2.2 mg sodium fluoride equivalent to 1 mg of fluoride ion
Adult and Child >12 yr
• *Dental rinse:* Top apply 10 ml 0.2% sol qd after brushing teeth, rinse mouth for >1 min with sol then expectorate
Child
• *Brush-on gel:* After brushing with toothpaste, >6 yr apply thin ribbon of gel to teeth with toothbrush for at least 1 min hs, expectorate gel and rinse mouth thoroughly
• *Dental rinse:* Top 5 ml 0.2% sol qd after brushing teeth, rinse mouth for >1 min with sol then expectorate
• *Gel Drops >6 yr:* Use applicators supplied by dentist; apply 4-8 gtt to inner surface of applicator, spread evenly with tip of bottle; place applicator over upper and lower teeth and bite down gently for 6 min; remove and rinse mouth
• *Systemic protection from periodontal disease:* PO in areas where fluoride content of drinking water < 0.3 ppm, <2 yr 0.25 mg fluoride qd; 2-3 yr 0.5 mg qd; 3-12 yr 1 mg qd; in areas where fluoride content of drinking water is 0.3-0.7 ppm, <2 yr 0.125 mg fluoride qd; 2-3 yr 0.25 mg qd, 3-14 yr 0.25-0.75 mg qd

AVAILABLE FORMS/COST OF THERAPY
• Drops—Oral: 0.125 mg/gtt (0.275 mg sodium fluoride), 50 ml: **$5.10**; 0.25 mg/gtt (0.55 mg sodium fluoride), 23 ml: **$2.16**; 0.5 mg/ml (1.1 mg sodium fluoride), 50 ml: **$6.53-$15.18**
• Gel, Drops—Dental: 0.5% (1.1% sodium fluoride), 24 ml: **$5.62**
• Gel, Swab—Dental: 0.1% (0.4% sodium fluoride), 122 g, 12's: **$12.50**; 0.5% (1.1% sodium fluoride), 60 g: **$11.04**
• Rinse—Dental: 0.01% (0.02% sodium fluoride), 500 ml: **$7.55-$9.75**; 0.02% (0.05% sodium fluoride), 480 ml: **$2.71**; 0.09% (0.2% sodium fluoride); 480 ml: **$7.49**
• Tab, Chewable—Oral: 0.25 mg (0.55 mg sodium fluoride), 1000's: **$9.41-$14.99**; 0.5 mg (1.1 mg sodium fluoride), 1000's: **$7.19-$46.67**; 1 mg (2.2 mg sodium fluoride), 1000's: **$7.10-$55.44**

CONTRAINDICATIONS: Hypersensitivity

PRECAUTIONS: Drinking water with >0.7 ppm fluoride

PREGNANCY AND LACTATION: Administration from 3rd-9th mo of gestation safe (no information on teratogenicity); small amounts excreted into breast milk, inadequate therapeutically due to small amount of excretion and complexation with calcium

SIDE EFFECTS/ADVERSE REACTIONS

EENT: Watery eyes

GI: Black tarry stools, constipation, diarrhea, discoloration of teeth, *hematemesis,* increased salivation, loss of appetite, nausea, stomatitis, weight loss

METAB: Hypocalcemia

MS: Articular and juxta-articular pain, osteomalacia, stress fractures, tetany

RESP: Decreased respiration, *respiratory arrest*

SPECIAL CONSIDERATIONS

• Therapy begun prenatally and continued through age 16 is effective in reducing the number of decayed, missing, or filled surfaces and teeth; especially beneficial in areas where fluoride content of drinking water is below 0.7 ppm

• Treatment of osteoporosis, combined with 1 or more of the following—calcium, estrogen, or vitamin D—increases bone density, reduces rate of new vertebral fractures, if correct dose and in slow-release preparation; role in steroid-induced osteoporosis being investigated, reports to date indicate a poor response rate

PATIENT/FAMILY EDUCATION

• Avoid use with dairy products

---

fluoxetine

(floo-ox′e-teen)

Rx: Prozac, Prozac Weekly, Sarafem

Chemical Class: Trifluoro propylamine derivative

Therapeutic Class: Selective serotonin reuptake inhibitor (SSRI), antidepressant

---

CLINICAL PHARMACOLOGY

Mechanism of Action: Selective, potent inhibition of CNS neuronal uptake of serotonin (5HT); no significant affinity for histaminergic, α- or β-adrenergic, muscarinic, or dopaminergic receptors

Pharmacokinetics

PO: Peak 4-8 hr; 94.5% bound to plasma proteins; metabolized in liver (CYP2D6) to norfluoxetine (active); $t_{1/2}$ 48-216 hr (including active metabolite); excreted in urine

INDICATIONS AND USES: Depression, obsessive-compulsive disorder, bulimia nervosa, premenstrual dysphoric disorder, obesity*

DOSAGE

Adult

• *Depression, obsessive-compulsive disorder, premenstrual dysphoric disorder:* PO 20 mg qAM, increase after 4-6 wks prn, max 80 mg/day; doses >20 mg can be divided into morning and noon doses

• *Bulimia nervosa:* PO 60 mg qam; may be advisable to titrate to target dose over several days in some patients

• *Maintenace therapy in depression:* PO 20 mg qd or 90 mg qwk starting 7 days after last daily dose of 20 mg

---

* = non-FDA-approved use

§ AVAILABLE FORMS/COST OF THERAPY

• Cap, Gel—Oral: 10 mg, 100's: **$259.52-$316.11**; 20 mg, 100's: **$266.52-$324.25**; 40 mg, 100's: **$533.05-$533.56**
• Cap, Sus Action—Oral: 90 mg, 4's: **$78.75**
• Sol—Oral: 20 mg/5 ml, 120 ml: **$118.49-$144.00**
• Tab—Oral: 10 mg, 100's: **$273.10-$316.11**; 20 mg, 100's: **$280.06**

CONTRAINDICATIONS: Concurrent use with MAOI, or within 14 days of discontinuing MAOI; concurrent use with thioridazine or within 5 weeks after discontinuing fluoxetine

PRECAUTIONS: Renal or hepatic function impairment, elderly, children, bipolar affective disorder, seizure disorder, suicidal ideation, diabetes

PREGNANCY AND LACTATION: Pregnancy category B; excreted into breast milk; use caution in nursing mothers

SIDE EFFECTS/ADVERSE REACTIONS

CNS: Anxiety, apathy, decreased libido, delusions, *dizziness, drowsiness,* euphoria, *fatigue,* hallucinations, *headache, insomnia, nervousness,* psychosis, **seizures,** serotonergic syndrome (anxiety, hyperreflexia, confusion), *tremor*
CV: Hot flushes, palpitations
EENT: Blurred vision, visual disturbance
GI: Anorexia, constipation, *diarrhea,* dry mouth, *dyspepsia,* hyperbilirubinemia, *loose stools, nausea,* taste changes
GU: Painful menstruation, sexual dysfunction
METAB: Altered glycemic control, hypoglycemia
MS: Joint or muscle pain
SKIN: Pruritus, rash, sweating
MISC: Weight loss

INTERACTIONS
Drugs

§ *Benzodiazepines (alprazolam, diazepam):* Probable inhibition of metabolism (CYP3A4) leading to accumulation of diazepam and alprazolam

§ *Beta-blockers (metroprolol, propranolol, sotalol):* Inhibition of metabolism (CYP2D6) leads to increased plasma concentrations of selective beta blockers and potential cardiac toxicity; atenolol may be safer choice

§ *Buspirone:* Reduced therapeutic effect of both drugs; possible seizures

§ *Carbamazepine:* Inhibition of hepatic metabolism of carbamazepine, but the formation of carbamazepine epoxide is not inhibited, contributing to increased toxicity

§ *Clozapine:* Increased serum clozapine concentrations

§ *Cyproheptadine:* Serotonin antagonist may partially reverse antidepressant and other effects

§ *Dextromethorphan:* Inhibition of dextromethorphan's metabolism (CYP2D6) by fluoxetine and additive serotonergic effects

§ *Diuretics, loop (bumetanide, furosemide, torsemide):* Possible additive hyponatremia; 2 fatal case reports with furosemide and fluoxetine

❷ *Fenfluramine:* Duplicate effects on inhibition of serotonin reuptake; inhibition of dexfenfluramine metabolism (CYP2D6) exaggerates ef-

F

fect; both mechanisms increase risk of serotonin syndrome

3 *Haloperidol:* Inhibition of haloperidol's metabolism (CYP2D6) may increase risks of extrapyramidal symptoms

❷ *HMG-Co A reductase inhibitors (atorvastatin, lovastatin, simvastatin):* Inhibition of statin metabolism (CYP3A4), by fluoxetine, may lead to rhabdomyolysis

3 *Lithium:* Neurotoxicity (tremor, confusion, ataxia, dizziness, dysarthria, and abscence seizures) reported in patients receiving this combination; mechanism unknown

⚠ *MAOI's (isocarboxazid, phenelzine, tranylcypromine):* Increased CNS serotonergic effect has been associated with severe or fatal reactions with this combination

3 *Phenytoin:* Inhibition of metabolism and phenytoin toxicity

3 *Selegiline:* Sporadic cases of mania and hypertension

⚠ *Thioridazine:* Increased serum thioridazine concentrations resulting in an increased risk of QTc interval prolongation, serious ventricular arrhythmias, and death

3 *Tricyclic antidepressants (clomipramine, desipramine, doxepin, imipramine, nortriptylline, trazodone):* Marked increases in tricyclic antidepressant levels due to inhibition of metabolism (CYP2D6)

❷ *Tryptophan:* Additive serotonergic effects

3 *Warfarin:* Altered anti-coagulant effects, including increased bleeding

SPECIAL CONSIDERATIONS
PATIENT/FAMILY EDUCATION
• Therapeutic response may take 4-6 wk
• May cause insomnia, administer in AM; sedating antidepressants, in small doses (i.e. trazodone 50 mg), frequently administered H.S., concurrently

---

fluoxymesterone
(floo-ox-ee-mess'te-rone)
Rx: Halotestin
Chemical Class: Testosterone derivative
Therapeutic Class: Androgen; antineoplastic
DEA Class: Schedule III

CLINICAL PHARMACOLOGY
Mechanism of Action: Promotes weight gain via retention of nitrogen, potassium, and phosphorus, increased protein anabolism, and decreased catabolism; endogenous androgens are essential for normal growth and development of male sex organs and maintenance of secondary sex characteristics; androgenic activity is minor, effects are predominantly anabolic

Pharmacokinetics
PO: Metabolized in liver, excreted in urine; t$_{1/2}$ 9.2 hr

INDICATIONS AND USES: Males: primary hypogonadism (congenital or acquired), hypogonadotropic hypogonadism (congenital or acquired), delayed puberty; females: palliative therapy of metastatic breast cancer, postpartum breast pain/engorgement

DOSAGE
Adult Males
• *Hypogonadism:* PO 5-20 mg qd
• *Delayed puberty:* 2.5-20 mg qd for 4-6 mo
Adult Females
• *Breast cancer:* PO 10-40 mg/day in divided doses

• *Breast engorgement:* PO 2.5 mg after delivery, 5-10 mg/day in divided doses for 4-5 days

$ AVAILABLE FORMS/COST OF THERAPY

• Tab, Uncoated—Oral: 2 mg, 100's: **$264.60**; 5 mg, 100's: **$204.88**; 10 mg, 100's: **$51.00-$264.60**

CONTRAINDICATIONS: Serious cardiac, hepatic, or renal disease; carcinoma of breast or prostate (males); pregnancy, enhancement of athletic performance

PRECAUTIONS: Diabetes mellitus, cardiovascular disease, risk factors for atherosclerosis, hepatic disease, seizure disorder, renal disease, BPH (urethral obstruction), acute intermittent porphyria

PREGNANCY AND LACTATION: Pregnancy category X; causes virilization of external genitalia of female fetus; excretion into breast milk unknown; use extreme caution in nursing mothers

SIDE EFFECTS/ADVERSE REACTIONS

CNS: Anxiety, decreased or increased libido, dizziness, fatigue, flushing, headache, insomnia, lability, paresthesias, sweating, tremors
CV: Increased blood pressure, **CHF,** edema
EENT: Conjunctival edema, nasal congestion, deepening of voice
GI: **Cholestatic jaundice,** constipation, nausea, vomiting, weight gain, **hepatocellular neoplasm**
GU: Decreased breast size, gynecomastia, priapism, menstrual irregularities, oligospermia, testicular atrophy, vaginitis, virilization in females
HEME: Polycythemia, suppression of clotting factors

METAB: Hypercalcemia (in breast cancer), hypercholesterolemia, hyperglycemia, hyperkalemia
SKIN: Acneiform lesions, acne vulgaris, alopecia, flushing, hirsutism, oily hair, skin, rash, sweating

INTERACTIONS
Drugs
❷ *Cyclosporine, tacrolimus:* Increased cyclosporine and tacrolimus levels with potential toxicity
❷ *Oral anticoagulants:* Enhanced hypoprothrombinemic response to oral anticoagulants

SPECIAL CONSIDERATIONS
MONITORING PARAMETERS
• Frequent urine and serum calcium determinations (breast cancer)
• Periodic LFTs, Hct
• X-ray examinations of bone age q6mo during treatment of prepubertal males

---

fluphenazine
(floo-fen′a-zeen)
Rx: Permitil, Prolixin
Chemical Class: Piperazine; phenothiazine derivative
Therapeutic Class: Antipsychotic

CLINICAL PHARMACOLOGY
Mechanism of Action: Dopamine receptor antagonist, with higher affinity for D_2- over D_1-receptors, and variable selectivity among the cortical dopamine tracts; also activity on nondopaminergic sites, i.e., cholinergic, α_1-adrenergic, and histaminic receptors (explaining side effects); high risk extrapyramidal reactions; minimal orthostatic hypotension, sedation, and anticholinergic effects
Pharmacokinetics
PO: Peak 2-4 hr, onset 1 hr, duration 6-8 hr

---

italic = common side effects   ***bold italic*** = life-threatening reactions

IM/SC: (depends on salt): (HCl) peak 1.5-2 hr, onset 1 day; (enanthate) peak 2-3 days, onset 1-3 days, duration 1-3 wk; (decanoate) peak 1-2 days, onset 1-3 days, duration ≥4 wk

Widely distributed in tissues, 91%-99% bound to plasma proteins; metabolized in liver, excreted in urine and bile; $t_{1/2}$ 33 hr (salt delays absorption but does not alter $t_{1/2}$)

INDICATIONS AND USES: Management of psychotic disorders, Huntington's chorea,* control of acute agitation,* dementia*

DOSAGE

NOTE: 2 mg equivalent to chlorpromazine 100 mg

Adult and Child >16 yr

• PO 0.5-10 mg/day divided q6-8h initially, reduce dosage gradually to daily maintenance doses of 1-5 mg (may give as single daily dose); IM (HCl) 1.25-10 mg/day divided q6-8h; IM/SC (enanthate and decanoate) 12.5-25 mg q1-4 wk based on patient response, do not exceed 100 mg

Child <16 yr

• PO 0.25-3.5 mg/day in divided doses q 4-6 hr, max 10 mg/day

§ AVAILABLE FORMS/COST OF THERAPY

• Conc—Oral: 5 mg/ml, 120 ml: **$57.50-$160.44**
• Elixir—Oral: 2.5 mg/5 ml, 60 ml: **$16.10-$25.50**; 25 mg/ml, 480 ml: **$128.70-$203.33**
• Inj, Sol—IM, SC: 2.5 mg/ml, 10 ml: **$33.28-$68.82**
• Tab, Plain Coated—Oral: 1 mg, 100's: **$31.09-$125.24**; 2.5 mg, 100's: **$44.10-$155.40**; 5 mg, 100's: **$56.88-$229.06**; 10 mg 100's: **$74.03-$278.90**
• Inj, Sol (decanoate)—IM, SC: 25 mg/ml, 5 ml: **$14.29-$125.45**
• Inj, Sol (enanthate)—SC: 25 mg/ml, 5 ml: **$128.50**

CONTRAINDICATIONS: Liver damage, cerebral arteriosclerosis, CAD, severe hypertension/hypotension, blood dyscrasias, coma, subcortical brain damage, bone marrow depression

PRECAUTIONS: Depression, acute pulmonary infection, chronic respiratory disorders, cardiovascular disease, glaucoma, seizure disorder; impaired hepatic/renal function; elderly, children <12 yr, alcohol withdrawal, electroconvulsive therapy

PREGNANCY AND LACTATION: Pregnancy category C; EPS in the newborn have been attributed to *in utero* exposure; other reports have indicated that phenothiazines are relatively safe during pregnancy; excretion into breast milk unknown; use caution in nursing mothers

SIDE EFFECTS/ADVERSE REACTIONS

CNS: Drowsiness, *EPS: pseudoparkinsonism, akathisia, dystonia, **tardive dyskinesia;*** fatigue, headache, insomnia, **neuroleptic malignant syndrome, seizures,** vertigo

CV: **Cardiac arrest,** ECG changes, hypertension, *orthostatic hypotension,* tachycardia

EENT: Blurred vision, dry eyes, glaucoma

GI: Anorexia, constipation, diarrhea, *dry mouth,* **hepatitis,** jaundice, *nausea,* **paralytic ileus,** *vomiting,* weight gain

GU: Bladder paralysis, ejaculation inhibition, enuresis, male impotence, polyuria, priapism, urinary retention, frequency or incontinence

HEME: **Agranulocytosis,** anemia, **aplastic anemia, hemolytic anemia, leukocytosis, leukopenia, thrombocytopenia**

METAB: Amenorrhea, elevated prolactin levels, galactorrhea, hyperglycemia or hypoglycemia, hypona-

---

* = non-FDA-approved use

tremia, lactation, menstrual irregularities, moderate breast engorgement (females), SIADH

RESP: Bronchospasm, dyspnea, laryngospasm

SKIN: Dermatitis, photosensitivity, *rash*

MISC: Heat intolerance

INTERACTIONS

Drugs

❸ *Anticholinergics:* Inhibition of therapeutic response to neuroleptics, additive anticholinergic effects

❸ *Antimalarials (amodiaquine, chloroquine, sulfadoxine-pyrimethamine):* Increased neuroleptic concentrations

❸ *Barbiturates:* Reduced serum neuroleptic concentrations

❸ *Beta-blockers:* Potential increases in serum concentrations of both drugs

❸ *Bromocriptine:* Reduced effects of both drugs

❸ *Clonidine:* Acute organic brain syndrome

❸ *Cyclic antidepressants:* Increased serum concentrations of both drugs

❸ *Epinephrine:* Reversal of pressor response to epinephrine

❸ *Guanadrel:* Inhibits antihypertensive response

❷ *Levodopa:* Inhibition of the antiparkinsonian effect of levodopa

❸ *Lithium:* Rare cases of severe neurotoxicity have been reported in acute manic patients

❸ *Meperidine:* Hypotension, excessive CNS depression

❸ *Orphenadrine:* Reduced serum neuroleptic concentrations

Labs

• Urine pregnancy test: false positive

SPECIAL CONSIDERATIONS

• Concentrate must be diluted prior to administration; use only the following diluents: water, saline, 7-Up, homogenized milk, carbonated orange beverage, and pineapple, apricot, prune, orange, V-8, tomato, and grapefruit juices; do not mix with beverages containing caffeine, tannics (tea), or pectinates (apple juice), as physical incompatibility may result

PATIENT/FAMILY EDUCATION

• May cause drowsiness; use caution while driving or performing other tasks requiring alertness

• Avoid contact with skin when using concentrates

• Avoid prolonged exposure to sunlight

• May discolor urine pink or reddish-brown

• Use caution in hot weather, heatstroke may result

• Arise slowly from a reclining position

MONITORING PARAMETERS

• Monitor closely for the appearance of tardive dyskinesia

---

flurandrenolide

(flure-an-dren'oh-lide)

Rx: Cordran, Cordran SP, Cordran Tape

Chemical Class: Synthetic glucocorticoid

Therapeutic Class: Topical corticosteroid, intermediate potency

---

CLINICAL PHARMACOLOGY

Mechanism of Action: Depresses formation, release, and activity of endogenous mediators of inflammation such as prostaglandins, kinins, histamine, liposomal enzymes, and the complement system resulting in decreased edema, erythema, and pruritus of corticosteroid responsive dermatoses

---

italic = common side effects   ***bold italic*** = life-threatening reactions

Pharmacokinetics

Absorbed through the skin (increased by inflammation and occlusive dressings); metabolized primarily in the liver

INDICATIONS AND USES: Psoriasis, eczema, contact dermatitis, pruritus of corticosteroid responsive dermatoses

DOSAGE

Adult and Child

• TOP apply to affected area bid-tid; rub completely into skin; apply tape q12-24h

$ **AVAILABLE FORMS/COST OF THERAPY**

• Cre—Top: 0.025%, 30, 60 g: **$20.10**/30 g; 0.05%, 15, 30, 60 g: **$25.65**/30 g
• Lotion—Top: 0.05%, 15, 60 ml: **$37.20**/60 ml
• Oint—Top: 0.025%, 30, 60 g: **$20.10**/30 g; 0.05%, 15, 30, 60 g: **$25.65**/30 g
• Tape, Medicated—Top: 4 µg/cm², 24 × 3: **$18.84-$40.45**

CONTRAINDICATIONS: Fungal infections, use on face, groin, or axilla

PRECAUTIONS: Viral infections, bacterial infections, children

PREGNANCY AND LACTATION: Pregnancy category C; unknown whether topical application could result in sufficient systemic absorption to produce detectable amounts in breast milk (systemic corticosteroids are secreted into breast milk in quantities not likely to have detrimental effects on infant)

SIDE EFFECTS/ADVERSE REACTIONS

SKIN: Acne, allergic contact dermatitis, atrophy, burning, dryness, folliculitis, hypertrichosis, hypopigmentation, irritation, itching, miliaria, perioral dermatitis, secondary infection, striae

MISC: Systemic absorption of topical corticosteroids has produced reversible HPA axis suppression (more likely with occlusive dressings, prolonged administration, application to large surface areas, liver failure, and in children)

SPECIAL CONSIDERATIONS

PATIENT/FAMILY EDUCATION

• Apply sparingly only to affected area
• Avoid contact with the eyes
• Do not put bandages or dressings over treated area unless directed by clinician
• Do not use on weeping, denuded, or infected areas
• Discontinue drug, notify clinician if local irritation or fever develops

---

flurazepam

(flure-az′e-pam)
Rx: Dalmane
Chemical Class: Benzodiazepine
Therapeutic Class: Sedative-hypnotic
DEA Class: Schedule IV

CLINICAL PHARMACOLOGY

Mechanism of Action: CNS depressants via facilitation of inhibitory GABA at benzodiazepine receptor sites (BZ_1—associated with sleep; BZ_2—associated with memory, motor, sensory, and cognitive function); effects include muscle relaxation (spinal cord), anticonvulsant activity (brain stem), ataxia (cerebellum), emotional behavior (limbic and cortical areas), and anxiolytic effects (separate from general CNS depression; decreases sleep latency, the number of awakenings, and the time spent in stage 0 (awake) sleep; stage 2 (unequivocal sleep) is increased; in sum, sleep time increased

Pharmacokinetics

PO: Onset 15-45 min, peak ½-1 hr; 97% bound to plasma proteins; metabolized by liver to an active metabolite (N-desalkylflurazepam); $t_{1/2}$ of active metabolite 47-100 hr

INDICATIONS AND USES: Insomnia

DOSAGE

Adult

• PO 15-30 mg qhs

Elderly and Child >15 yr

• PO 15 mg qhs

§ AVAILABLE FORMS/COST OF THERAPY

• Cap, Gel—Oral: 15 mg, 100's: **$8.93-$167.18**; 30 mg, 100's: **$11.40-$154.65**

CONTRAINDICATIONS: Pregnancy

PRECAUTIONS: Renal or hepatic function impairment, elderly, depression, history of drug abuse, abrupt withdrawal, respiratory depression, sleep apnea

PREGNANCY AND LACTATION: Pregnancy category X; administration to nursing mothers is not recommended

SIDE EFFECTS/ADVERSE REACTIONS

CNS: Anxiety, confusion, *daytime sedation,* dizziness, *drowsiness,* headache, irritability, *lethargy,* light-headedness

CV: Chest pain, hypotension (rare), palpitations, pulse changes

GI: Abdominal pain, constipation, diarrhea, heartburn, increased liver function tests, nausea, vomiting

HEME: **Granulocytopenia** (rare), **leukopenia**

SKIN: Dermatitis or allergy, flushes, pruritus, rash, sweating

INTERACTIONS

Drugs

❷ *Azole antifungals (fulconazole, itraconazole, ketoconazole):* Increased serum concentrations of flurazepam via inhibition of oxidative metabolism (CYP3A4)

❸ *Beta blockers (labetaolol, metoprolol, propranolol):* Reduces the metabolism of benzodiazepines and may increase the pharmacodynamic effects

❸ *Cimetidine:* Increased plasma levels of flurazepam and metabolites via inhibition of hepatic oxidative metabolism

❸ *Clozapine:* Isolated cases of cardiorespiratory collapse, but a causal relationship not established

❸ *Disulfiram:* May increase serum concentrations of flurazepam via inhibition of oxidative metabolism (CYP3A4)

❸ *Isoniazid:* May increase flurazepam serum concentrations via inhibition of metabolism

❸ *Loxapine:* Isolated cases of respiratory depression, stupor, and hypotension reported; role of drug interaction not established

❸ *Macrolide antibiotics (clarithromycin, erythromycin, troleandomycin):* Macrolides increase flurazepam plasma concentrations via inhibition of metabolism (CYP3A4)

❸ *Omeprazole:* Increases plasma concentrations of flurazepam via inhibition of hepatic metabolism

❸ *Rifampin:* Reduced serum concentrations of flurazepam via enhanced hepatic metabolism (CYP3A4)

❸ *Serotonin reuptake inhibitors (fluoxetine, fluvoxamine):* May increase serum concentrations of flurazepam via inhibition of oxidative metabolism (CYP3A4)

---

italic = common side effects   ***bold italic*** = life-threatening reactions

SPECIAL CONSIDERATIONS
PATIENT/FAMILY EDUCATION
• Avoid alcohol and other CNS depressants
• Do not discontinue abruptly after prolonged therapy
• May experience disturbed sleep for the 1st or 2nd night after discontinuing the drug
• May cause drowsiness or dizziness; use caution while driving or performing other tasks requiring alertness; hangover daytime drowsiness possible secondary to long duration of action
• Inform clinician if you are planning to become pregnant, you are pregnant, or if you become pregnant while taking this medicine

---

flurbiprofen
(flure-bi'proe-fen)
Rx: Ansaid, Ocufen (ophthalmic)
Chemical Class: Propionic acid derivative
Therapeutic Class: NSAID with analgesic and antipyretic activity

---

CLINICAL PHARMACOLOGY
Mechanism of Action: Reversible cyclooxygenase (i.e., prostaglandin synthetase) inhibitor; non-selectively decreases the formation of both prostaglandins and thromboxane A_2; variable effects on lipoxygenase synthesis and subsequent leukotriene production; antiinflammatory, antipyretic, and analgesic activity; inhibits platelet aggregation; OPHTH: antiinflammatory and antimiotic

Pharmacokinetics
PO: Peak 1.5 hr, >99% bound to plasma proteins; extensively metabolized, excreted primarily in urine; $t_{1/2}$ 5.7 hr

INDICATIONS AND USES: Intraoperative miosis, ocular inflammation, ankylosing spondylitis,* prevention of cognitive decline,* prevention of colon cancer,* dysmenorrhea,* acute gout,* migraine headache, mild-moderate pain* (bursitis, dental, cancer, episiotomy, osteoarthritis, postoperative sickle cell disease), peridontal disease, rheumatoid arthritis, tendonitis, soft tissue injury,* sunburn

DOSAGE
Adult
• *Rheumatoid and osteoarthritis:* PO 200-300 mg/day divided bid-qid
• *Dysmenorrhea:* PO 50 mg qid
• *Inhibition of intraoperative miosis:* Ophth 1 gtt q30 min beginning 2 hr before surgery (total 4 gtt)

§ **AVAILABLE FORMS/COST OF THERAPY**
• Sol—Ophth: 0.03%, 2.5 ml: **$8.73-$20.48**
• Tab, Coated—Oral: 50 mg, 100's: **$68.02-$89.41**; 100 mg, 100's: **$106.38-$210.38**

CONTRAINDICATIONS: Bronchospasm, nasal polyps, angioedema precipitated by aspirin or other NSAIDs, dendritic keratitis (ophth)

PRECAUTIONS: History of GI ulceration, bleeding, or perforation; renal dysfunction, hypertension or cardiac conditions aggravated by fluid retention and edema, history of liver dysfunction, history of coagulation deficits

PREGNANCY AND LACTATION: Pregnancy category C; excreted into breast milk; use caution in nursing mothers

---

* = non-FDA-approved use

SIDE EFFECTS/ADVERSE REACTIONS

CNS: Dizziness, headache, lightheadedness

CV: Chest pain, **CHF,** dysrhythmias, edema, hypertension, hypotension, palpitation, tachycardia

EENT: Burning or stinging upon instillation, dry eyes, hearing disturbances, photophobia, tinnitus, visual disturbances

GI: Abdominal cramps, constipation, diarrhea, *dyspepsia,* flatulence, **gastric or duodenal ulcer with bleeding or perforation, hepatitis,** nausea, occult blood in stool, pancreatitis, vomiting

GU: **Acute renal failure**

HEME: **Agranulocytosis, eosinophilia, leukopenia, neutropenia, pancytopenia, thrombocytopenia**

METAB: Hyperglycemia, hyperkalemia, hypoglycemia, hyponatremia

RESP: Bronchospasm, dyspnea

SKIN: Photosensitivity, rash, urticaria

INTERACTIONS

Drugs

🔢 *Aminoglycosides:* Reduced clearance with elevated aminoglycoside levels and potential for toxicity (especially indomethacin in premature infants; other NSAIDs probably)

🔢 *Antihypertensives (α-blockers, angiotensin-converting enzyme inhibitors, angiotensin II receptor blockers, β-blockers, diuretics):* Inhibition of antihypertensive and other favorable hemodynamic effects

🔢 *Aspirin:* 50% decrease in plasma flurbiprofen concentrations, concurrent use not recommended

🔢 *Corticosteroids:* Increased risk of GI ulceration

🔢 *Anticoagulants:* Excessive hypoprothrombinemia, decreased platelet aggregation with increased risk of GI bleeding

🔢 *Cyclosporine:* Increased nephrotoxicity risk

🔢 *Lithium:* Decreased clearance of lithium (mediated via prostaglandins) resulting in elevated serum lithium levels and risk of toxicity

🔢 *Methotrexate:* Decreased renal secretion of methotrexate resulting in elevated methotrexate levels and risk of toxicity

🔢 *Phenylpropanolamine:* Possible acute hypertensive reaction

🔢 *Potassium-sparing diuretics:* Additive hyperkalemia potential

🔢 *Triamterene:* Acute renal failure reported with addition of indomethacin; caution with other NSAIDs

Labs

• *Cortisol:* Increased at high flurbiprofen levels

SPECIAL CONSIDERATIONS

PATIENT/FAMILY EDUCATION

• Avoid aspirin and alcoholic beverages

• Take with food, milk, or antacids to decrease GI upset

• Notify clinician if edema, black stools, or persistent headache occurs

MONITORING PARAMETERS

• Initial hemogram and fecal occult blood test within 3 mo of starting regular chronic therapy; repeat every 6-12 mo (more frequently in high-risk patients (>65 years, peptic ulcer disease, concurrent steroids or anticoagulants); electrolytes, creatinine, and BUN within 3 mo of starting regular chronic therapy; repeat every 6-12 mo

---

italic = common side effects   ***bold italic*** = life-threatening reactions

flutamide

(floo'ta-mide)
Rx: Eulexin
Chemical Class: Acetanilid
derivative
Therapeutic Class: Androgen
inhibitor; antineoplastic

CLINICAL PHARMACOLOGY
Mechanism of Action: Inhibits androgen uptake or inhibits nuclear binding of androgen in target tissues; arrests tumor growth in androgen-sensitive tissue, e.g., prostate gland
Pharmacokinetics
PO: Rapidly and completely absorbed, 94% bound to plasma proteins; excreted in urine and feces as metabolites; $t_{1/2}$ 6 hr, geriatric $t_{1/2}$ 8 hr
INDICATIONS AND USES: In combination with LHRH agonists (e.g., leuprolide) for management of locally confined stage B_2-C and Stage D_2 metastatic prostate carcinoma
DOSAGE
Adult
• PO 250 mg (125 mg × 2) q8h
💲 **AVAILABLE FORMS/COST OF THERAPY**
• Cap, Gel—Oral: 125 mg, 100's: **$209.22-$264.41**
PREGNANCY AND LACTATION: Pregnancy category D
SIDE EFFECTS/ADVERSE REACTIONS

CNS: Anxiety, confusion, depression, drowsiness, *hot flashes*
CV: Edema, hypertension
GI: Anorexia, *diarrhea,* **hepatitis,** increased liver function studies, *nausea, vomiting*
GU: Decreased libido, impotence
HEME: **Anemia, leukopenia, thrombocytopenia**
SKIN: Photosensitivity, rash
MISC: Galactorrhea, gynecomastia

INTERACTIONS
Drugs
3 *Warfarin:* Increased hypoprothrombinemic effect
SPECIAL CONSIDERATIONS
• Begin 8 wks before radiation therapy in Stage B_2-C carcinoma, continue during radiation
• In metastatic carcinoma continue until progression noted
PATIENT/FAMILY EDUCATION
• Feminization may occur during therapy
• Do not discontinue therapy without discussion with clinician
MONITORING PARAMETERS
• Periodic LFTs during long-term treatment

fluticasone

(flu-tic'a-zone)
Rx: Cutivate, Flonase, Flovent, Flovent Rotadisk
Combinations
   Rx: with salmeterol (Advair Diskus)
Chemical Class: Glucocorticoid
Therapeutic Class: Inhaled corticosteroid; nasal corticosteroid; topical corticosteroid, intermediate potency

CLINICAL PHARMACOLOGY
Mechanism of Action: Inhibits inflammatory cells and production or secretion of cell mediators of inflammation
Pharmacokinetics
INH: Peak (following 880 µg) 0.1-1 ng/ml, systemic bioavailability, 30% of dose delivered from the actuator; high total clearance due to efficient 1st-pass hepatic metabolism and minimally active metabolites

INDICATIONS AND USES: Asthma, chronic maintenance treatment; allergic rhinitis; corticosteroid-responsive dermatoses

DOSAGE

Adult

• *Asthma:* INH aerosol, previous therapy (bronchodilators alone or inhaled corticosteroids): 88-440 μg bid; (chronic oral corticosteroids): 880 μg bid; INH powder, previous therapy (bronchodilators alone or inhaled corticosteroids): 100-500 μg bid; (chronic oral corticosteroids): 1000 μg bid

• *Allergic rhinitis:* NASAL 1-2 sprays in each nostril qd or 1 spray in each nostril bid; do not exceed 2 sprays/nostril/day

• TOP apply to affected area qd-bid

Child

• Use not recommended in children <12 yr

Children ≥12 yr

• *Asthma:* INH aerosol, children ≥12 yr, previous therapy (bronchodilators alone or inhaled corticosteroids): 88-440 μg bid; (chronic oral corticosteroids): 880 μg bid; INH powder, children ≥4 yr, previous therapy (bronchodilators alone or inhaled corticosteroids): 50-100 μg bid

• *Allergic rhinitis:* NASAL, children ≥4 yr, 1 spray in each nostril qd; may increase to 2 sprays in each nostril qd

• TOP apply thin film to affected area qd-bid; may be used cautiously in pediatric patients ≥3 mo

💲 AVAILABLE FORMS/COST OF THERAPY

• Aer, metered—Inh: 44 μg/inh, 7.9 g (60 puffs): **$39.68**; 44 μg/inh, 13 g (120 puffs): **$46.94-$52.98**; 110 μg/inh, 13 g (120 puffs): **$51.06-$73.53**; 220 μg/inh, 13 g (120 puffs): **$80.81-$114.20**

• Aer, Metered—Nasal inh: 0.05 mg/inh, 16 g: **$53.35-$61.91**

• Cre—Top: 0.05%, 15, 30, 60 g: **$26.46**/30 g

• Disk—Inh: 50 μg/inh, 60's: **$35.05**; 100 μg/inh, 60's: **$55.53**; 250 μg/inh, 60's: **$77.23**

• Oint—Top: 0.005%, 15, 30, 60 g: **$26.46**/30 g

CONTRAINDICATIONS: Relief of acute bronchospasm

PREGNANCY AND LACTATION: Pregnancy category C; no information on excretion into human breast milk

SIDE EFFECTS/ADVERSE REACTIONS

CNS: Fatigue, headache

EENT: Dysphonia, nasal congestion or discharge, *oropharyngeal candidiasis,* sinusitis, upper respiratory tract infections

MS: Muscle soreness

*RESP: **Bronchospasm***

SKIN: Urticaria

MISC: Angioedema, ***hypersensitivity reactions*** (shortness of breath, tightness in chest, wheezing)

INTERACTIONS

Drugs

3 *Ketoconazole:* Possible increased plasma fluticasone concentrations

Labs

• Cholesterol: Increased

SPECIAL CONSIDERATIONS

• Improvement following inhalation, 24 hr to 1-2 wk

• Systemic corticosteroid effects from inhaled and nasal steroids inadequate to prevent adrenal insufficiency in most patients withdrawn abruptly from corticosteroids

• Observe for evidence of inadequate adrenal response following periods of stress; use caution with extended use in children and adolescents as reduction in growth velocity may occur

PATIENT/FAMILY EDUCATION
• Rinsing the mouth following INH and using a spacer device reduces common EENT adverse effects
• Review proper MDI administration technique regularly

---

fluvastatin
(floo´va-sta-tin)
Rx: Lescol, Lescol XL
Chemical Class: Substituted hexahydronaphthalene
Therapeutic Class: Antilipemic (HMG-CoA reductase inhibitor); "statin"

CLINICAL PHARMACOLOGY
Mechanism of Action: Competitively inhibits 3-hydroxy-3-methylglutaryl-coenzyme A (HMG-CoA) reductase, an early rate-limiting step in cholesterol biosynthesis; increases HDL cholesterol minimally [2.5%-7.8%], moderately decreases total and LDL cholesterol [15%-20%, 19%-35%, respectively, minimal lowering effect on triglycerides [3%-11%]
Pharmacokinetics
PO: Immed rel: onset 15 min, peak 30-60 min, $t_{1/2}$ 0.5-1 hr, duration 3-4 hr; Sus Action: peak 2.5-3 hr, $t_{1/2}$ 3 hr; fully absorbed if taken without food; high fat meal slows absorption and reduces peak by 50%; protein binding 98%; metabolized in liver (CYP2C9, CYP3A4), excreted in bile

INDICATIONS AND USES: Primary hypercholesterolemia (heterozygous familial and nonfamilial hypercholesterolemia), mixed dyslipidemia (Fredrickson Type IIa and IIb), secondary prevention of cardiovascular events, coronary atherosclerosis (slow the progression)

DOSAGE
Adult
• PO: 20-40 mg hs, increase to 40 mg bid if necessary or 80 mg extended release hs

🔢 AVAILABLE FORMS/COST OF THERAPY
• Cap—Oral: 20 mg, 40 mg, 100's: **$153.89**
• Tab, Coated, Sus Action—Oral: 80 mg, 100's: **$200.16**

CONTRAINDICATIONS: Pregnancy, lactation, active liver disease, unexplained transaminase elevations

PRECAUTIONS: History of liver disease, heavy ethanol use, patients at risk for rhabdomyolysis (acute infection, hypotension, major surgery, or trauma)

PREGNANCY AND LACTATION: Pregnancy category X; contraindicated in breast feeding—present in breast milk (2:1 milk: plasma ratio)

SIDE EFFECTS/ADVERSE REACTIONS
CNS: Headache, insomnia
GI: Diarrhea, dyspepsia, elevated transaminase levels (1%), *hepatotoxicity,* nausea
EENT: Posterior subcapsular abnormalities
MS: Myalgia, myopathy, *rhabdomyolysis*

INTERACTIONS
Drugs
🔳 *Alcohol:* 20 g of alcohol within 1 hr of dosing, increased fluvastatin AUC by 30%
❷ *Azole antifungals (fluconazole, itraconazole, ketoconazole, miconazole):* Increased fluvastatin levels via inhibition of metabolism with increased risk of rhabdomyolysis
🔳 *Cholestyramine, colestipol:* Reduced bioavailability of fluvastatin

---

3 *Cimetidine, ranitidine, omeprazole:* Coadministration increases fluvastatin Cmax 43%-70% with 18%-23% decrease in plasma clearance

3 *Cyclosporine:* Concomitant administration increases risk of severe myopathy or rhabdomyolysis

3 *Danazol:* Inhibition of metabolism (CYP3A4) thought to yield increased fluvastatin levels with increased risk of rhabdomyolysis

3 *Diclofenac:* Increased plasma diclofenac concentrations

3 *Fluoxetine:* Less likely to inhibit CYP3A4 hepatic metabolism (vs lovastatin) with less risk of rhabdomyolysis

2 *Gemfibrazil:* Small increased risk of myopathy with combination, especially at high doses of statin

3 *Glyburide:* Increased plasma concentrations of glyburide and fluvastatin

3 *Isradipine:* Isradipine probably decreases fluvastatin plasma concentrations minimally

3 *Macrolide antibiotics (clarithromycin, erythromycin, troleandomycin):* Increased fluvastatin levels via inhibition of metabolism with increased risk of rhabdomyolysis

3 *Niacin:* Concomitant administration increases risk of severe hepatotoxicity

3 *Nefazadone:* Less likely to inhibit CYP3A4 hepatic metabolism (vs lovastatin) with less risk of rhabdomyolysis

3 *Phenytoin:* Increased plasma concentrations of phenytoin and fluvastatin

3 *Rifampin:* Coadministration decreases fluvastatin Cmax and AUC

3 *Terbinafine:* Minimal effect on the metabolism of fluvastatin

3 *Warfarin:* Addition of fluvastatin may increase hypoprothrombinemic response to warfarin via inhibition of metabolism (CYP2C9)

SPECIAL CONSIDERATIONS
• Statin selection based on lipid-lowering prowess, cost, and availability

PATIENT/FAMILY EDUCATION
• Report symptoms of myalgia, muscle tenderness, or weakness
• Take daily doses in the evening for increased effect
• May take without regard to food

MONITORING PARAMETERS
• Cholesterol (max therapeutic response 4-6 wk)
• LFT's (AST, ALT) at baseline and at 12 wk of therapy; if no change, nor further monitoring necessary (discontinue if elevations persists at >3 times upper limit of normal)
• CPK in patients complaining of diffuse myalgia, muscle tenderness, or weakness

---

fluvoxamine

(floo-vox′a-meen)
Rx: Luvox
Chemical Class: Aralkylketone derivative
Therapeutic Class: Selective serotonin reuptake inhibitor (SSRI), antidepressant

CLINICAL PHARMACOLOGY
Mechanism of Action: Selectively inhibits CNS neuronal uptake of serotonin (5HT); no significant activity for histaminergic, α- or β- adrenergic, muscarinic, or dopaminergic receptors

Pharmacokinetics
PO: Peak 3-8 hr; 77%-80% bound to plasma proteins; primarily eliminated by kidneys; $t_{1/2}$ 13.6-15.6 hr

---

INDICATIONS AND USES: Obsessive-compulsive disorder (adults and children), depression

DOSAGE

Adult

• PO 50 mg qhs initially, increase in 50 mg increments q4-7d, as tolerated, until max therapeutic benefit is achieved; do not exceed 300 mg/day; doses >100 mg should be divided bid

Child

• PO 25 mg qhs initially, increase in 25 mg increments q4-6d, as tolerated, therapeutic benefit is achieved, or maximum daily dose of 200 mg; doses >100 mg should be divided bid

$ **AVAILABLE FORMS/COST OF THERAPY**

• Tab, Uncoated—Oral: 25 mg, 100's: **$229.18-$294.48**; 50 mg, 100's: **$257.35-$329.06**; 100 mg, 100's: **$262.67-$337.51**

CONTRAINDICATIONS: Combination with thioridazine or MAOIs. administration within 14 days of discontinuing MAOI therapy

PRECAUTIONS: History of mania, seizure disorder, liver dysfunction, suicidal ideation, children

PREGNANCY AND LACTATION: Pregnancy category C; excreted into breast milk; use caution in nursing mothers

SIDE EFFECTS/ADVERSE REACTIONS

CNS: Agitation, anxiety, decreased libido, depression, dizziness, *headache, insomnia,* nervousness, *somnolence,* tremor

CV: Hypertension, orthostatic hypotension, palpitations, syncope, tachycardia

EENT: Amblyopia, taste perversion/change

GI: Anorexia, constipation, *diarrhea, dry mouth, dyspepsia,* flatulence, *nausea,* vomiting

GU: Abnormal ejaculation, sexual dysfunction, urinary frequency

RESP: Dyspnea

SKIN: Sweating

INTERACTIONS

Drugs

⚠ *Antihistamines, nonsedating (astemizole, terfenadine):* Fluvoxamine inhibits metabolism (CYP3A4) for detoxifying these antihistamines; cardiac rhythm disturbances

3 *Benzodiazepines (alprazolam, midazolam, triazolam, diazepam):* Probable inhibition of metabolism (CYP3A4) leading to accumulation of benzodiazepines, avoid combination

3 *Beta-blockers (metoprolol, propranolol, sotalol):* Inhibition of metabolism (CYP2D6) leads to increased plasma concentrations of selective beta blockers and potential cardiac toxicity; atenolol may be safer choice

3 *Buspirone:* Reduced therapeutic effect of both drugs; possible seizures

3 *Carbamazepine:* Inhibition of hepatic metabolism of carbamazepine, but the formation of carbamazepine epoxide is not inhibited, contributing to increased toxicity

❷ *Clozapine:* Fluvoxamine markedly increases clozapine concentrations as a potent inhibitor of CYP1A2

3 *Cyclic antidepressants (clomipramine, desipramine, doxepin, imipramine, nortriptylline, trazadone):* Inhibition of metabolism (CYP1A2 and CYP3A4) leading to accumulation of cyclic antidepressants; dosage adjustments necessary

3 *Cyproheptadine:* Serotonin antagonist may partially reverse antidepressant and other effects

❷ *Dexfenfluramine:* Duplicate effects on inhibition of serotonin reuptake; inhibition of dexfenfluramine metabolism (CYP2D6) exaggerates effect; both mechanisms increase risk of serotonin syndrome

❷ *Fenfluramine:* Duplicate effects on inhibition of serotonin reuptake; inhibition of dexfenfluramine metabolism (CYP2D6) exaggerates effect; both mechanisms increase risk of serotonin syndrome

❷ *HMG-Co A reductase inhibitors (atorvastatin, lovastatin, simvastatin):* Inhibition of statin metabolism (CYP3A4), by fluoxetine, may lead to rhabdomyolysis

🅱 *Lithium:* Neurotoxicity (tremor, confusion, ataxia, dizziness, dysarthria, and abscence seizures) reported in patients receiving this combination; mechanism unknown

🅰 *MAOIs (isocarboxazid, phenelzine, tranylcypromine):* Increased CNS serotonergic effects have been associated with severe or fatal reactions with this combination

🅱 *Mexiletine:* Reduced clearance of mexiletine, monitor serum mexiletine levels if co-administered

🅱 *Methadone:* Significantly increased plasma methadone concentrations

🅱 *Phenytoin:* Inhibition of metabolism and phenytoin toxicity

❷ *Selegiline:* Sporadic cases of mania and hypertension

🅱 *Sumatriptan:* Reports of weakness, hyperreflexia and incoordination with SSRI and sumatriptan use, caution is advised

🅱 *Tacrine:* Increased plasma tacrine concentrations, cholinergic side effects possible

❷ *Theophylline:* Theophylline toxicity increased via accumulation due to inhibition of metabolism (CYP1A2) by fluvoxamine

🅰 *Thioridazine:* Dose related prolongation of the QTc interval, do not co-administer thioridazine and fluvoxamine

❷ *Tryptophan:* Additive serotonergic effects

🅱 *Warfarin:* Increased hypothrombinemic response

SPECIAL CONSIDERATIONS
PATIENT/FAMILY EDUCATION
• May cause dizziness or drowsiness; use caution driving or performing tasks requiring alertness

---

folic acid
(foe'lik)
Rx: Folic acid
OTC: Folic acid
Chemical Class: B complex vitamin
Therapeutic Class: Hematinic; vitamin

CLINICAL PHARMACOLOGY
Mechanism of Action: Required for nucleoprotein synthesis and maintenance of normal erythropoiesis; stimulates production of RBC, WBC, and platelets in certain megaloblastic anemias

Pharmacokinetics
PO: Peak 1 hr, metabolized in liver to 7,8-dihydrofolic acid and eventually to 5,6,7,8-tetrahydrofolic acid, excreted in urine (percentage dependent on dose)

INDICATIONS AND USES: Treatment of megaloblastic anemias due to folic acid deficiency; prophylaxis of fetal neural tube defects; hyperhomocysteinemia*

DOSAGE
Adult and Child >11 yr
• *Folic acid deficiency:* PO/IV/IM/SC 1 mg/day initially; maintenance dose 0.5 mg/day

---

• *Prophylaxis of fetal neural tube defects:* Low risk: PO at least 0.4 mg/day beginning at least 1 mo prior to conception and increasing to 0.8 mg/day during pregnancy; high risk: PO 4 mg/day at least 1 mo prior to conception and for 2 mo after conception

• Hyperhomocysteinemia: PO 0.4 mg qd

Child

• *Folic acid deficiency:* PO/IV/IM/SC 1 mg/day initially; maintenance dose 0.1-0.4 mg/day

Infants

• *Folic acid deficiency:* PO/IV/IM/SC 15 µg/kg/dose daily or 50 µg/day

$ **AVAILABLE FORMS/COST OF THERAPY**

• Inj, Sol—IM, IV, SC: 5 mg/ml, 10 ml: **$12.33-$14.33**

• Tab, Uncoated—Oral: 1 mg, 100's: **$0.66-$12.32**

• Tab—Oral: 0.4 mg, 100's (OTC): **$1.56-$2.15**; 0.8 mg, 100's (OTC): **$1.88-$3.94**

CONTRAINDICATIONS: Anemias other than megaloblastic/macrocytic anemia, vitamin B_{12} deficiency anemia

PREGNANCY AND LACTATION: Pregnancy category A; folic acid deficiency during pregnancy is a common problem in undernourished women and in women not receiving supplements; evidence has accumulated that folic acid deficiency, or abnormal folate metabolism, may be related to the occurrence of neural tube defects; actively excreted in human breast milk; compatible with breast feeding; recommended daily allowance during lactation is 0.5 mg/day

SIDE EFFECTS/ADVERSE REACTIONS

RESP: Bronchospasm (rare)

SKIN: Allergic reactions have been reported; itching, rash

INTERACTIONS

Drugs

3 *Phenytoin:* Decreased serum phenytoin concentrations; long-term phenytoin frequently leads to subnormal folate levels

2 *Pyrimethamine:* Inhibition of antimicrobial effect of pyrimethamine

SPECIAL CONSIDERATIONS

• Recent evidence supports the premise that lowering elevated plasma homocysteine levels may reduce the risk of coronary heart disease

PATIENT/FAMILY EDUCATION

• Take only under medical supervision

MONITORING PARAMETERS

• CBC; serum folate concentrations <0.005 µg/ml indicate folic acid deficiency and concentrations <0.002 µg/ml usually result in megaloblastic anemia

---

fomepizole

(foe-mep´i-zoll)

Rx: Antizol

Chemical Class: Pyrzole derivative

Therapeutic Class: Ethylene glycol (antifreeze) antidote

CLINICAL PHARMACOLOGY

Mechanism of Action: Competitively inhibits alcohol dehydrogenase; alcohol dehydrogenase catalyzes the oxidation of ethanol to acetaldehyde and the initial steps of ethylene glycol and methanol metabolism, which yields toxic metabolites

---

Pharmacokinetics

IV: Metabolized by the liver (autoinduction of metabolism occurs with multiple dosing); excreted primarily in urine; $t_{1/2}$ varies with dose and has not been calculated

INDICATIONS AND USES: Antidote for ethylene glycol (antifreeze) poisoning or for use in suspected ethylene glycol ingestion

DOSAGE

Adult

• *Treatment:* IV 15 mg/kg loading dose, followed by doses of 10 mg/kg q12h for 4 doses, then 15 mg/kg q12h thereafter until ethylene glycol levels have been reduced to <20 mg/dl; administer all doses as a slow IV infusion over 30 min

• *Dialysis:* Administer next scheduled dose at the beginning of dialysis if ≥6 hr since last dose; administer q4h during dialysis; at the end of dialysis, administer ½ of next scheduled dose if it has been 1-3 hr since last dose, or administer next scheduled dose if it has been >3 hr since last dose; for maintenance dosing of hemodialysis, administer next scheduled dose 12 hr from the last dose

⑤ AVAILABLE FORMS/COST OF THERAPY

• Conc—IV: 1 g/ml, 1.5 ml: **$1,150.00**

PRECAUTIONS: Elderly, children

PREGNANCY AND LACTATION: Pregnancy category C; use caution in nursing mothers

SIDE EFFECTS/ADVERSE REACTIONS

CNS: Headache, dizziness, **seizures,** vertigo, lightheadedness, nystagmus, feeling of drunkenness, strange feeling, slurred speech, decreased environmental awareness

CV: Bradycardia, tachycardia, hypotension, phlebosclerosis

GI: Nausea, vomiting, diarrhea, anorexia, heartburn

HEME: Lymphangitis, eosinophilia, anemia

RESP: Hiccups, pharyngitis

MISC: Abdominal pain, fever, somnolence, lumbalgia, hangover, rash, injection site reaction

INTERACTIONS

Drugs

❸ *Ethanol:* Reduced elimination rate of ethanol; reduced elimination rate of fomepizole

SPECIAL CONSIDERATIONS

MONITORING PARAMETERS

• Frequently monitor both ethylene glycol levels and acid-base balance, as determined by serum electrolyte (anion gap) or arterial blood gas analysis

• In patients with high ethylene glycol levels (≥50 mg/dl), significant metabolic acidosis or renal failure, consider hemodialysis to remove ethylene glycol and its toxic metabolites

• Treatment with fomepizole may be discontinued when ethylene glycol levels have been reduced to <20 mg/dl

---

fomvirsen

(fom-veer′-sen)

Rx: Vitravene

Chemical Class: Synthetic antisense oligonucleotide

Therapeutic Class: Antiviral

CLINICAL PHARMACOLOGY

Mechanism of Action: As an antisense oligonucleotide, fomvirsen is complementary to messenger RNA of the immediate-early transcriptional unit (IE2) of human CMV. Fomvirsen binding to this messenger

RNA results in selective inhibition of IE2 proteins necessary for CMV replication

Pharmacokinetics

INTRAVITREAL: No systemic absorption documented; metabolized intravitreally by exonucleases yielding shortened oligonucleotides and mononucleotides, which are further catabolized and excreted as low-molecular-weight metabolites

INDICATIONS AND USES: CMV retinitis in AIDS patients

DOSAGE

Adult

• *Intravitreal:* 330 µg day 1 and day 15, then 330 µg qmo

🛈 **AVAILABLE FORMS/COST OF THERAPY**

• Inj, Sol—Intravitreal: 330 µg/0.25 ml: **$1,000.00**

PRECAUTIONS: Ocular infection other than retinitis, ocular diseases/conditions (e.g., glaucoma), recent treatment with cidofovir (potential exacerbation of ocular inflammation)

PREGNANCY AND LACTATION: Pregnancy category C; breast milk excretion unlikely

SIDE EFFECTS/ADVERSE REACTIONS

EENT: Abnormal vision, cataract, eye pain, conjunctival hemorrhage, *increased intraocular pressure (19%), intaocular inflammation (e.g., iritis, vitreitis; 20%),* retinal hemorrhage

SPECIAL CONSIDERATIONS
PATIENT/FAMILY EDUCATION

• Does not treat systemic aspects of CMV infection

MONITORING PARAMETERS

• Ophthalmologic examination

---

formoterol

(for-moe′ter-ol)

Rx: Foradil

Chemical Class: Sympathomimetic amine; β₂-adrenergic agonist

Therapeutic Class: Antiasthmatic, bronchodilator

CLINICAL PHARMACOLOGY

Mechanism of Action: Causes bronchodilation by β₂-stimulation, resulting in relaxation of bronchial smooth muscle; inhibits mast cell degranulation; stimulates cilia to remove secretions

Pharmacokinetics

INH: Rapidly absorbed, peak plasma concentrations 5 min; some accumulation in plasma with repeated dosing; onset of effect 1-3 hr; majority of inhaled drug delivered is swallowed and absorbed from the GI tract; 61-64% bound to plasma proteins; metabolized primarily by glucuronidation; excreted in urine (59-62%) and feces (32-34%); $t_{1/2}$ 10 hr

INDICATIONS AND USES: Long-term maintenance treatment of asthma and prevention of bronchospasm in adults and children >5 yr with reversible obstructive airway disease; prevention of exercise-induced bronchospasm in adults and children >12 yr; long-term maintenance treatment of bronchoconstriction in patients with COPD

DOSAGE

Adult

• *Maintenance treatment of COPD:* INH one 12 µg capsule q12h using the Aerolizer Inhaler

Adult and Child >5 yr

• *Maintenance treatment of asthma:* INH one 12 µg capsule q12h using the Aerolizer Inhaler

---

Adult and Child >12 yr

• *Exercise-induced bronchospasm:*
INH one 12 μg capsule at least 15
min before exercise prn using the
Aerolizer Inhaler; additional doses
should not be used for 12 hr after administration of this drug; patients
using formoterol bid for maintenance treatment of asthma should
not use additional doses for prevention of exercise-induced bronchospasm

**$ AVAILABLE FORMS/COST
OF THERAPY**

• Cap, gelatin—Inh: 12 μg, 60's:
$73.00

PRECAUTIONS: Cardiovascular
disease (CAD, arrhythmias, hypertension); convulsive disorders; thyrotoxicosis; diabetes mellitus; children <5 yr

PREGNANCY AND LACTATION:
Pregnancy category C; β-agonists
may potentially interfere with uterine contractility during labor; excretion into breast milk unknown, use
caution in nursing mothers

**SIDE EFFECTS/ADVERSE REAC-
TIONS**

CNS: Nervousness, headache,
tremor, dizziness

CV: Angina, hypertension or hypotension, tachycardia, arrhythmias,
palpitation

EENT: Dysphonia, pharyngitis

GI: Dry mouth, nausea, abdominal
pain, dyspepsia

METAB: Hypokalemia, hyperglycemia, metabolic acidosis

MS: Muscle cramps

RESP: **Bronchospasm,** coughing

SKIN: Rash, pruritus

MISC: Fatigue, malaise, insomnia,
fever

INTERACTIONS

Drugs

3 *Non-potassium sparing diuretics, xanthine derivatives, steroids:*
Theoretical increase in the potential
for hypokalemia

2 *β-blockers:* Decreased action
of formoterol, cardioselective β-
blockers preferable if concurrent
use necessary (e.g., following myocardial infarction)

3 *MAO-inhibitors, tricyclic antidepressants:* Theoretical increase in
the potential for prolongation of
QTc interval

SPECIAL CONSIDERATIONS

• Not indicated for patients whose
asthma can be managed by occasional use of inhaled, short-acting,
β₂-agonists

• Can be used concomitantly with
short-acting β₂-agonists, inhaled or
systemic corticosteroids, and theophylline

• Does not eliminate the need for
treatment with an inhaled anti-inflammatory agent

• Do not initiate therapy in patients
with significantly worsening or
acutely deteriorating asthma

• For use only with the Aerolizer Inhaler

PATIENT/FAMILY EDUCATION

• Should never be used more frequently than twice daily (morning
and evening) at the recommended
dose; do not use to treat acute symptoms

• Discontinue the regular use of
short-acting β₂-agonists and use
them only for symptomatic relief of
acute asthma symptoms

• Seek medical advice immediately
if a previously effective asthma
medication regimen fails to provide
the usual response

• For inhalation only, do not take
orally

---

italic = common side effects   **bold italic** = life-threatening reactions

• Store in blister packaging, only remove immediately before use; handle capsules with dry hands
• Use the new Aerolizer Inhaler provided with each new prescription

MONITORING PARAMETERS
• Pulmonary function tests
• Serum potassium

---

foscarnet

(foss-car′net)
Rx: Foscavir
Chemical Class: Pyrophosphate analog
Therapeutic Class: Antiviral

CLINICAL PHARMACOLOGY
Mechanism of Action: Selective inhibition at the pyrophosphate binding site on virus-specific DNA polymerases and reverse transcriptases; does not require activation by thymidine kinase or other kinases

Pharmacokinetics
IV: 14%-17% bound to plasma proteins; 80%-90% excreted unchanged in urine; $t_{1/2}$ 2-8 hr in normal renal function

INDICATIONS AND USES: CMV retinitis in patients with AIDS; acyclovir-resistant HSV and herpes zoster infections; with ganciclovir for CMV retinitis after relapse with either agent alone

DOSAGE
Adult and Adolescent
• *Induction:* IV INF 60 mg/kg via infusion pump over 1 hr q8h for 2-3 wk depending on clinical response
• *Maintenance:* IV INF 90-120 mg/kg/day via infusion pump over 2 hr
• *Dose adjustment in renal impairment (based on CrCl ml/min/kg):* Induction for CrCl ≥1.6, 60 mg/kg/8 hr; CrCl 1.3, 50 mg/kg/8 hr; CrCl 1.0, 40 mg/kg/8 hr; CrCl 0.7, 30 mg/kg/8 hr; CrCl 0.4, 20 mg/kg/8 hr; maintenance for CrCl ≥1.4, 100 mg/kg/day; CrCl 0.7, 70 mg/kg/day; CrCl 0.5, 60 mg/kg/day

§ AVAILABLE FORMS/COST OF THERAPY
• Sol—IV: 24 mg/ml, 250 ml: **$79.80**; 24 mg/ml, 500 ml: **$158.97**

PRECAUTIONS: Renal function impairment, electrolyte disturbances, neurologic abnormalities, cardiac abnormalities, seizure disorder, elderly, children, severe anemia

PREGNANCY AND LACTATION: Pregnancy category C; excretion into breast milk unknown; use caution in nursing mothers

SIDE EFFECTS/ADVERSE REACTIONS
CNS: Fever, headache, *seizures*
CV: Bradycardia, *cardiac failure, arrest;* cardiomyopathy; dysrhythmias, ECG abnormalities (sinus tachycardia, 1st degree AV block, non-specific ST-T segment changes), extrasystole, flushing, hypertension, hypotension, palpitations, phlebitis
EENT: Conjunctivitis, eye abnormalities, eye pain, taste perversions, vision abnormalities
GI: Abdominal pain, anorexia, constipation, *diarrhea,* dry mouth, dyspepsia, dysphagia, flatulence, melena, *nausea, pancreatitis,* rectal hemorrhage, ulcerative stomatitis, *vomiting*
GU: **Abnormal renal function (acute renal failure, decreased CrCl and increased serum creatinine),** albuminuria, dysuria, nocturia, polyuria, urethral disorder, urinary retention, UTI
HEME: **Anemia, granulocytopenia, leukopenia,** lymphadenopathy, platelet abnormalities, ***thrombocytopenia,*** thrombosis, WBC abnormalities

---

METAB: Acidosis, cachexia, decreased weight, hypercalcemia, hypocalcemia, hypokalemia, hypomagnesemia, hyponatremia, hypophosphatemia or hyperphosphatemia, increased alkaline phosphatase, increased LDH and BUN, thirst

MS: Arthralgia, back pain, chest pain, myalgia

RESP: Bronchospasm, coughing, dyspnea, hemoptysis, pharyngitis, pneumonia, pneumothorax, pulmonary infiltration, respiratory disorders, rhinitis, sinusitis, stridor

SKIN: Erythematous rash, facial edema, maculopapular rash, pruritus, rash, seborrhea, skin discoloration, skin ulceration, sweating

INTERACTIONS
Drugs
3 *Quinolones: **Increased seizure risk (rare)***

SPECIAL CONSIDERATIONS
• Hydration to establish diuresis both prior to and during administration is recommended to minimize renal toxicity; the standard 24 mg/ml sol may be used undiluted via a central venous catheter, dilute to 12 mg/ml with D_5W or NS when a peripheral vein catheter is used

PATIENT/FAMILY EDUCATION
• Foscarnet is not a cure for CMV retinitis
• Notify clinician of perioral tingling, numbness in the extremities, or paresthesias (could signify electrolyte imbalances)

MONITORING PARAMETERS
• Serum creatinine, calcium, phosphorus, potassium, magnesium at baseline and 2-3 times/wk during induction and at least every 1-2 wk during maintenance
• Hemoglobin
• Regular ophthalmologic examinations

fosfomycin
(foss-fo-mye´sin)
Rx: Monurol
Chemical Class: Phosphoric acid derivative
Therapeutic Class: Antibiotic

CLINICAL PHARMACOLOGY
Mechanism of Action: Inactivates the enzyme enolpyruvul transferase; irreversibly blocks condensation of uridine diphosphate-N-acetylglucosamine with p-enolpyruvate which is one of the first steps in bacterial cell wall synthesis; bactericidal

Pharmacokinetics
PO: Peak 2 hr, absolute bioavailability 37% (reduced to 30% with food); not bound to plasma proteins, crosses the placenta; excreted unchanged in urine (38% of 3 g dose) and feces (18% of 3 g dose); $t_{1/2}$ 5.7 hr (11-50 hr in renal function impairment)

INDICATIONS AND USES: Uncomplicated acute cystitis in women
Antibacterial spectrum usually includes:
• Gram-positive organisms: *Enterococcus faecalis, E. faecalis*
• Gram-negative organisms: *Escherichia coli, Citrobacter diversus, C. freundii, Enterobacter aerogenes, Klebsiella oxytoca, K. pneumoniae, Proteus mirabilis, P. vulgaris, Serratia marcenscens*

DOSAGE
Adult ≥18 yr
• PO 3 g packet mixed with 90-120 ml of water as a single dose

$ **AVAILABLE FORMS/COST OF THERAPY**
• Granule—Oral: 3 g/packet, 3's: **$101.53**

PRECAUTIONS: Children

---

italic = common side effects   ***bold italic*** = life-threatening reactions

PREGNANCY AND LACTATION:
Pregnancy category B; excretion into breast milk unknown

SIDE EFFECTS/ADVERSE REACTIONS

CNS: Dizziness, headache

EENT: Pharyngitis, rhinitis

GI: Abdominal pain, *diarrhea,* dyspepsia, nausea

GU: Dysmenorrhea, vaginitis

HEME: **Aplastic anemia (rare)**

MS: Back pain

SKIN: Rash

MISC: Asthenia

INTERACTIONS

Drugs

3 *Metoclopramide:* Decreased serum concentration and urinary excretion of fosfomycin

SPECIAL CONSIDERATIONS

• Inferior 5-11 day posttherapy microbiologic eradication rates compared to ciprofloxacin and co-trimoxazole for acute cystitis; eradication rates comparable to nitrofurantoin

• Reserve for women unable to tolerate or unlikely to comply with 3-day courses of co-trimoxazole or trimethoprim

PATIENT/FAMILY EDUCATION

• Always mix with water before ingesting

---

fosinopril

(fo-sin′o-pril)

Rx: Monopril

Chemical Class: Nonsulfhydryl angiotensin-converting enzyme (ACE) inhibitor

Therapeutic Class: Antihypertensive

CLINICAL PHARMACOLOGY

Mechanism of Action: Antihypertensive, hypoproliferative, and cardioprotective effects attributable to competitive inhibition of angiotensin-converting enzyme (ACE) yielding decreased plasma concentrations of angiotensin II and plasma aldosterone concentrations, systemic vascular resistance, blood pressure, preload and afterload, not accompanied by changes in heart rate, pressor sensitivity to exogenous norepinephrine, or baroreceptor sensitivity

Pharmacokinetics

PO: Onset 1 hr, duration 24 hr, peak 3 hr; metabolized to active metabolite (fosinoprilat), $t_{1/2}$ (fosinoprilat) 12 hr; excreted in urine (50%) and feces (50%)

INDICATIONS AND USES: Hypertension, CHF (left ventricular dysfunction), MI, erythrocytosis,* nephropathy,* retinopathy*

DOSAGE

Adult and child >16 yr

• *Hypertension:* PO 10 mg qd; usual dose range, 20-40 mg qd; maximal dose 80 mg qd, though dose-response curve usually flat after 40 mg qd

• *Congestive heart failure:* PO 5 mg qd (for volume-depleted, moderate to severe renal failure) = 10 mg qd; usual dose range 20-40 mg qd or titrate to systolic blood pressure of 100 mm Hg

• *Myocardial infarction:* PO 5 mg initial dose, repeated in 24 hr, with progressive doubling to a maximum dose of 20 mg qd, if systolic blood pressure remains over 100 mm Hg (fosinopril in acute myocardial infarction study, FAMIS)

• *Dosage in renal failure:* PO ≤7.5 mg qd if CrCl <10 ml/min

$ AVAILABLE FORMS/COST OF THERAPY

• Tab, Uncoated—Oral: 10 mg, 100's: **$72.99-$110.41**; 20 mg, 100's: **$75.84-$109.82**; 40 mg, 90's: **$102.95**

---

* = non-FDA-approved use

PRECAUTIONS: History of anaphylaxis, renal insufficiency (<30 ml/min), hypotension (CHF, elderly, volume depletion—diuretics, dialysis, cirrhosis), aortic stenosis, hyperkalemia (potassium supplements, potassium-sparing diuretics, renal disease, diabetes), neutropenia (autoimmune and collagen vascular disease, febrile illness, immunosuppressant drug therapy), proteinuria, renal artery stenosis, surgery/anesthesia (excessive hypotension)

PREGNANCY AND LACTATION: Pregnancy category C (1st trimester), category D (2nd and 3rd trimesters); ACE inhibitors can cause fetal and neonatal morbidity and death when administered to pregnant women; when pregnancy is detected, discontinue ACE inhibitors as soon as possible; detectable in breast milk in trace amounts, a newborn would receive <0.1% of the mg/kg maternal dose; effect on nursing infant has not been determined; use with caution in nursing mothers

SIDE EFFECTS/ADVERSE REACTIONS

CNS: Anxiety, *dizziness, fatigue, headache,* insomnia, paresthesia

CV: Angina, hypotension, palpitations, postural hypotension, syncope (especially with 1st dose)

GI: Abdominal pain, constipation, melena, nausea, vomiting

GU: Decreased libido, impotence, increased BUN, creatinine, UTI

HEME: **Agranulocytosis, neutropenia**

METAB: Hyperkalemia, hyponatremia

MS: Arthralgia, arthritis, myalgia

RESP: Asthma, bronchitis, *cough,* dyspnea, sinusitis

SKIN: **Angioedema,** flushing, rash, sweating

INTERACTIONS
Drugs

❷ *Allopurinol:* Combination may predispose to hypersensitivity reactions

❸ *Alpha adrenergic blockers:* Exaggerated first dose hypotensive response when added to fosinopril

❸ *Aspirin:* May reduce hemodynamic effects of fosinopril; less likely at doses under 236 mg; less likely with nonacetylated salicylates

❸ *Azathioprine:* Increased myelosuppression

❸ *Cyclosporine:* Combination may cause renal insufficiency

❸ *Insulin:* Fosinopril may enhance insulin sensitivity

❸ *Iron:* Fosinopril may increase chance of systemic reaction to IV iron

❸ *Lithium:* Reduced lithium clearance

❸ *Loop diuretics:* Initiation of fosinopril may cause hypotension and renal insufficiency in patients taking loop diuretics

❸ *NSAIDs:* May reduce hemodynamic effects of fosinopril

❸ *Potassium-sparing diuretics:* Increased risk of hyperkalemia

❸ *Trimethoprim:* Additive risk of hyperkalemia, especially in patient predisposed to renal insufficiency

Labs

• ACE inhibition can account for approximately 0.5 mEq/L rise in serum potassium

SPECIAL CONSIDERATIONS
PATIENT/FAMILY EDUCATION

• Caution with salt substitutes containing potassium chloride

• Rise slowly to sitting/standing position to minimize orthostatic hypotension

• Dizziness, fainting, lightheadedness may occur during 1st few days of therapy

---

italic = common side effects   ***bold italic*** = life-threatening reactions

• May cause altered taste perception or cough; persistent dry cough usually does not subside unless medication is stopped; notify clinician if these symptoms persist

MONITORING PARAMETERS

• BUN, creatinine, potassium within 2 wk after initiation of therapy (increased levels may indicate acute renal failure)

---

furazolidone

(fyur-a-zoh´li-done)

Rx: Furoxone

Chemical Class: Synthetic nitrofuran derivative

Therapeutic Class: Antibiotic; antiprotozoal

CLINICAL PHARMACOLOGY

Mechanism of Action: Exerts bactericidal action via interference with several bacterial enzyme systems; MAOI

Pharmacokinetics

PO: Systemically absorbed; extensively metabolized (possibly in the intestine), colored metabolites excreted in urine

INDICATIONS AND USES: Bacterial or protozoal diarrhea and enteritis caused by susceptible organisms Antimicrobial spectrum usually includes:

• Gram-positive organisms: Staphylococci

• Gram-negative organisms: *E. coli, Salmonella, Shigella, Proteus, Enterobacter aerogenes, Vibrio cholerae;* protozoan organisms: *Giardia lamblia*

DOSAGE

Adult

• PO 100 mg qid

Child

• PO 25-50 mg qid (≥5 yr); 17-25 mg qid (1-4 yr); 8-17 mg qid (1 mo-1 yr)

💲 AVAILABLE FORMS/COST OF THERAPY

• Liq—Oral: 50 mg/15 ml, 60, 473 ml: **$16.06**/60 ml

• Tab, Coated—Oral: 100 mg, 100's: **$257.68**

CONTRAINDICATIONS: Infants <1 mo

PRECAUTIONS: Hypertension, diabetes, G-6-PD deficiency

PREGNANCY AND LACTATION: Pregnancy category C; could theoretically produce hemolytic anemia in a G-6-PD deficient newborn if given at term; excretion into breast milk unknown; use caution in nursing mothers

SIDE EFFECTS/ADVERSE REACTIONS

CNS: Fever, headache, malaise

*CV: **Hypertensive crisis,** orthostatic hypotension

GI: Anal pruritus, colitis, nausea, proctitis, staphylococcic enteritis, vomiting

HEME: Hemolysis in G-6-PD deficiency

METAB: Hypoglycemia

MS: Arthralgia

SKIN: Vesicular morbilliform rash

INTERACTIONS

Drugs

3 *Amphetamines:* Hypertensive crisis

3 *Ephedrine:* Hypertensive response

3 *Ethanol:* Disulfiram-like reaction

3 *Foods high in amine content:* Hypertensive crisis

3 *Phenylpropanolamine:* Hypertensive response

Labs

• *Urine discoloration:* Metabolites may produce brown color

• *Glucose:* Metabolites give false positive with Benedict's reagent

SPECIAL CONSIDERATIONS

PATIENT/FAMILY EDUCATION

• Avoid ingestion of alcohol during and within 4 days after furazolidone therapy

• Avoid foods containing tyramine, especially if therapy extends beyond 5 days

• Avoid OTC drugs containing sympathomimetic drugs

• May color the urine brown

---

furosemide

(fur-oh´se-mide)

Rx: Furocot, Fumide, Lasix, Lo-Aqua, Myrosemide, Terbolan

Chemical Class: Anthranilic acid

Therapeutic Class: Loop diuretic

CLINICAL PHARMACOLOGY

Mechanism of Action: Inhibits the absorption of sodium and chloride at proximal and distal tubule sites and in the loop of Henle

Pharmacokinetics

PO: Onset 1 hr, peak 1-2 hr, duration 6-8 hr, 60% bioavailability; oral absorption is slower and less complete in patients with decompensated CHF; IV administration or increased oral dosing overcomes this deficit

IV/IM: Onset 5 min (slightly delayed with IM), peak ½ hr (IM), duration 2 hr; 98% bound to plasma proteins; 50% of PO and 80% of IV dose excreted in the urine within 24 hr, remainder eliminated by non-renal pathways (liver metabolism, excreted unchanged in feces); $t_{1/2}$ 30 min (9 hr in renal failure)

INDICATIONS AND USES: Edema (CHF, hepatic cirrhosis, renal disease, nephrotic syndrome); hypertension, pulmonary edema, hypercalcemia*

DOSAGE

Adult

• PO 20-80 mg/day in AM; may give another dose in 6 hr; increase in increments of 20-40 mg up to 400 mg/day if response is not satisfactory

• IM/IV 20-40 mg, increased by 20 mg q2h until desired response (rule of thumb: IV dose = ½ PO dose)

• *Pulmonary edema:* IV 40 mg given over several min, repeated in 1 hr; increase to 80 mg if needed

Child

• PO/IM/IV 1-2 mg/kg/dose up to 6 mg/kg/day in divided doses q6-12h

⑤ AVAILABLE FORMS/COST OF THERAPY

• Inj, Sol—IM, IV: 10 mg/ml, 2, 4, 8, 10 ml: **$2.36-$38.75**/10 ml

• Sol—Oral: 10 mg/ml, 60, 120 ml: **$7.14-$12.00**/60 ml; 40 mg/5 ml, 500 ml: **$29.04**

• Tab, Uncoated—Oral: 20 mg, 100's: **$2.00-$22.00**; 40 mg, 100's: **$2.50-$47.60**; 80 mg, 100's: **$7.75-$43.70**

CONTRAINDICATIONS: Anuria, hepatic coma

PRECAUTIONS: Fluid and electrolyte imbalance (including sodium, chloride, potassium, magnesium, calcium), renal disease, hepatic disease (may precipitate hepatic encephalopathy), gout, COPD, lupus erythematosus, diabetes mellitus, hyperparathyroidism, vomiting, diarrhea, elevated cholesterol/triglycerides

PREGNANCY AND LACTATION: Pregnancy category C; cardiovascular disorders such as pulmonary edema, severe hypertension, or CHF are probably the only valid indica-

---

italic = common side effects   ***bold italic*** = life-threatening reactions

tions for this drug during pregnancy; furosemide has been used after the first trimester without causing fetal or newborn adverse effects; does not appear to significantly alter amniotic fluid volume; maternal use during pregnancy has not been associated with toxic or teratogenic effects, although metabolic complications have been observed (hyponatremia, hyperuricemia); reduces placental and/or maternal hepatic perfusion; excreted into breast milk; no reports of adverse effects in nursing infants

SIDE EFFECTS/ADVERSE REACTIONS

CNS: Dizziness, fever, headache, paresthesia, restlessness, vertigo

CV: Chest pain, **circulatory collapse,** ECG changes, orthostatic hypotension

EENT: Blurred vision, ototoxicity

GI: Anorexia, constipation, cramping, diarrhea, dry mouth, **ischemic hepatitis,** jaundice, *nausea,* oral and gastric irritation, pancreatitis, vomiting

GU: Glycosuria, hyperuricemia, urinary bladder spasm

HEME: **Agranulocytosis, anemia, aplastic anemia, leukopenia,** purpura, **thrombocytopenia**

METAB: Hyperglycemia

SKIN: Erythema multiforme, **exfoliative dermatitis,** interstitial nephritis, necrotizing angiitis, photosensitivity, pruritus, *rash,* urticaria

INTERACTIONS

Drugs

❷ *Aminoglycosides (gentamicin, kanamycin, neomycin, streptomycin):* Additive ototoxicity (ethacrynic acid > furosemide, torsemide, bumetanide)

❸ *Angiotensin converting enzyme inhibitors:* Initiation of ACEI with intensive diuretic therapy may result in precipitous fall in blood pressure;

ACEIs may induce renal insufficiency in the presence of diuretic-induced sodium depletion

❸ *Barbiturates (phenobarbital):* Reduced diuretic response

❸ *Bile acid-binding resins (cholestyramine, colestipol):* Resins markedly reduce the bioavailability and diuretic response of furosemide

❸ *Carbenoxolone:* Severe hypokalemia from coadministration

❸ *Cephalosporins (cephaloridine, cephalothin):* Enhanced nephrotoxicity with coadministration

❷ *Cisplatin:* Additive ototoxicity (ethacrynic acid > furosemide, torsemide, bumetanide)

❸ *Clofibrate:* Enhanced effects of both drugs, especially in hypoalbuminemic patients

❸ *Corticosteroids:* Concomitant loop diuretic and corticosteroid therapy can result in excessive potassium loss

❸ *Digitalis glycosides (digoxin, digitoxin):* Diuretic-induced hypokalemia may increase risk of digitalis toxicity

❸ *Nonsteroidal antiinflammatory drugs (flurbiprofen, ibuprofen, indomethacin, naproxen, piroxicam, aspirin, sulindac):* Reduced diuretic and antihypertensive effects

❸ *Phenytoin:* Reduced diuretic response

❸ *Serotonin-reuptake inhibitors (fluoxetine, paroxetine, sertraline):* Case reports of sudden death; enhanced hyponatremia proposed; causal relationships not established

❸ *Terbutaline:* Additive hypokalemia

❸ *Tubocurarine:* Prolonged neuromuscular blockade

Labs

• *Cortisol:* False increases

• *Glucose:* Falsely low urine tests with clinistix and diastix

- *Thyroxine:* Increased serum concentration
- *T_3 uptake:* Interference causes increased serum values

SPECIAL CONSIDERATIONS
PATIENT/FAMILY EDUCATION
- May cause GI upset, take with food or milk
- Take early in the day
- Avoid prolonged exposure to sunlight

MONITORING PARAMETERS
- Urine volume, creatinine clearance, BUN electrolytes, reduction in edema, increased diuresis, decrease in body weight, reduction in blood pressure, glucose, uric acid, serum calcium (tetany), tinnitus, vertigo, hearing loss (especially in those at risk for ototoxicity—IV doses >120 mg; concomitant ototoxic drugs; renal disease)

---

gabapentin
(ga′ba-pen-tin)
Rx: Neurontin
Chemical Class: Cyclohexan-acetic acid derivative
Therapeutic Class: Anticonvulsant; neuropathic pain, adjunct

CLINICAL PHARMACOLOGY
Mechanism of Action: Structurally related to gamma-aminobutyric acid (GABA) but does not interact with GABA receptors; binds to receptors in neocortex and hippocampus; identity and function remain to be elucidated
Pharmacokinetics
PO: Over dosage range of 300 to 600 mg tid, bioavailability drops 60%; not protein bound; not metabolized; elimination $t_{1/2}$ 5-7 hr if CrCl normal, 52 hr if CrCl <30 ml/min; removed by hemodialysis

INDICATIONS AND USES: Anticonvulsant adjunctive therapy for partial seizures with or without secondary generalization; adjunctive pain management*
DOSAGE
Adult and Child >12 yr
- PO 900 to 2400 mg/day given in 3 divided doses; start with 300 mg on day 1, 300 mg bid on day 2, and 300 mg tid on day 3
- *Adjustment for renal dysfunction:* CrCl >60 ml/min, daily dose 1200 mg; CrCl 30-60 ml/min, daily dose 600 mg; CrCl 15-30 ml/min, daily dose 300 mg; CrCl <15 ml/min, daily dose 150 mg; hemodialysis, 200-300 mg after dialysis
Child 3-12 yr
- PO Initial 10-15 mg/kg/day in 3 divided doses, titrate to effective dose over 3 days; effective dose in children 5 yr and older is 25-35 mg/kg/day in 3 divided doses; effective dose in children 3-4 yr is 40 mg/kg/day in 3 divided doses; doses up to 50 mg/kg/day have been well tolerated

💲 AVAILABLE FORMS/COST OF THERAPY
- Cap, Gel—Oral: 100 mg, 100's: **$49.66-$51.41**; 300 mg, 100's: **$124.54-$141.14**; 400 mg, 100's: **$149.48-$154.21**
- Sol—Oral: 250 mg/5 ml, 480 ml: **$100.68**
- Tab—Oral: 600 mg, 100's: **$212.00-$218.49**; 800 mg, 100's: **$254.29-$262.18**

PRECAUTIONS: Severe renal dysfunction, age <12 yr, tumorigenic in rats (pancreatic adenomas and carcinomas); significance to humans unknown

PREGNANCY AND LACTATION: Pregnancy category C; excretion into breast milk unknown

---

italic = common side effects   ***bold italic*** = life-threatening reactions

SIDE EFFECTS/ADVERSE REACTIONS

CNS: Abnormal thinking, amnesia, *ataxia (13%)*, depression, *dizziness (17%)*, dysarthria, *fatigue (11%)*, nervousness, *nystagmus (8%)*, somnolence (19%), tremor (7%)

EENT: Diplopia, rhinitis

GI: Dry mouth, dyspepsia

GU: Impotence

HEME: **Leukopenia (1%)**

MS: Myalgia, twitching

SKIN: Flushing, pruritus

INTERACTIONS

Drugs

3 *Antacids:* Reduce bioavailability of gabapentin by 20%

SPECIAL CONSIDERATIONS

PATIENT/FAMILY EDUCATION

• Do not stop abruptly; taper over 1 wk

MONITORING PARAMETERS

• Drug level monitoring not necessary

---

galantamine

(ga-lan´ta-mene)

Rx: Reminyl

Chemical Class: Benzazepine derivative

Therapeutic Class: Acetylcholinesterase inhibitor

CLINICAL PHARMACOLOGY

Mechanism of Action: Increases the concentration of available acetylcholine via reversible, competitive inhibition of cholinesterase, thus improving the neuronal function of the basal forebrain, cerebral cortex, and hippocampus, all of which are involved in memory, attention learning, and other cognitive processes; no evidence that the drug alters the course of the underlying dementing process

Pharmacokinetics

PO: Peak 1 hr, food decreases C_{max} 25%, T_{max} prolonged by 1.5 hr; Well absorbed (PO), bioavailability 90%; Vd 175 L, 18% protein bound; metabolized by liver (CYP2D6, CYP3A4, glucuronidation); 8 hr post dose, 39-77% of dose excreted (95% in urine; 5% feces); $t_{1/2}$ 7 hr

INDICATIONS AND USES: Mild to moderate dementia of the Alzheimer's type, anticholinergic syndrome*, mania*

DOSAGE

Adult

• 4 mg bid (with meals) initially; if tolerated, increase in 4 mg bid increments, every 4 weeks to 12 mg bid (max)

• Restart at lowest dose if interrupted for more than several days

§ **AVAILABLE FORMS/COST OF THERAPY**

• Sol—Oral: 4 mg/ml, 100 ml: **$150.00**

• Tab, Coated—Oral: 4 mg, 8 mg, 12 mg, 60's, all: **$135.00**

CONTRAINDICATIONS: Hypersensitivity

PRECAUTIONS: Cardiac conduction disorders (e.g., AV block), anesthesia, increased risk/history of GI ulceration, bladder outflow obstruction, asthma, COPD, seizures

PREGNANCY AND LACTATION: Pregnancy category B; breast milk excretion information not known

SIDE EFFECTS/ADVERSE REACTIONS

CNS: Syncope

CV: Bradycardia, AV block, palpitation, atrial fibrillation, QT prolongation, bundle branch block, supraventricular tachycardia

GI: Anorexia, diarrhea (12%), GI upset, nausea (24%), vomiting (10%)

---

* = non-FDA-approved use

GU: Incontinence, micturition, frequency, cystitis, urinary retention, nocturia, renal calculi

METAB: Weight loss (5%),

INTERACTIONS

Drugs

▪ *Anesthetics (inhaled):* Decreases neuromuscular blocking effects

▪ *Anesthetics (local, esters):* Increases effects (possible toxicity) of local anesthetic (pseudocholinesterase competition)

▪ *Anticholinergics:* Antagonistic effects; use to counteract undesirable muscarinic effects of cholinesterase inhibitors

❷ *Bethanechol, pilocarpine, dexpanthanol, echothiophate:* Galantamine potentiates cholinergic agonists

▪ *Cimetidine:* Increased bioavailability of galantamine (16%)

▪ *Ketoconazole:* Strong inhibitor of CYP3A4; increases AUC of galantamine by 30%

▪ *Erythromycin:* Moderate inhibitor of CYP3A4; increases AUC of galantamine 10%

▪ *Fluoxetine:* Inhibition of CYP2D6 may increase levels of galantamine

▪ *Fluvoxamine:* Inhibition of CYP2D6 may increase levels of galantamine

▪ *Paroxetine:* Strong inhibitor of CYP2D6; increases AUC of galantamine 40%

❷ *Succinylcholine:* Potentates neuromuscular blockade

SPECIAL CONSIDERATIONS

• Extracted from the bulbs of the daffodil, *Narcissus pseudonarcissus*

PATIENT/FAMILY EDUCATION

• Patient and caregiver should be advised of high incidence of gastrointestinal effects and directions for resource and resolution

MONITORING PARAMETERS

• Cognitive function (e.g., ADAS, Mini-Mental Status Exam [MMSE]), activities of daily living, global functioning, blood chemistry, complete blood counts, heart rate, blood pressure

---

gallium nitrate

(gal′ee-yum)

Rx: Ganite

Chemical Class: Hydrated nitrate salt of gallium

Therapeutic Class: Hypocalcemic agent

CLINICAL PHARMACOLOGY

Mechanism of Action: Inhibits calcium resorption from bone, reducing increased bone turnover

Pharmacokinetics

IV: Steady state achieved in 24-48 hr, not metabolized, excreted by the kidneys

INDICATIONS AND USES: Symptomatic cancer-related hypercalcemia unresponsive to adequate hydration

DOSAGE

Adult

• IV INF 200 mg/m^2/day for 5 consecutive days; dilute in 1 L NS or D$_5$W and infuse over 24 hr

💲 AVAILABLE FORMS/COST OF THERAPY

• Inj, Sol—IV: 25 mg/ml, 20, 200 ml: **$1,524.60**/200 ml

CONTRAINDICATIONS: Severe renal disease (serum creatinine >2.5 mg/dl)

PRECAUTIONS: Concurrent use of potentially nephrotoxic drugs, children, renal disease

PREGNANCY AND LACTATION: Pregnancy category C; excretion into breast milk unknown, use caution in nursing mothers

---

SIDE EFFECTS/ADVERSE REACTIONS

CNS: Confusion, fever, hypothermia, lethargy, paresthesia

CV: Edema, hypotension, tachycardia

EENT: Acute optic neuritis, decreased hearing, visual impairment

GI: Constipation, diarrhea, nausea, vomiting

GU: Acute renal failure, nephrotoxicity

HEME: Anemia (very high doses), *leukopenia*

METAB: Decreased serum bicarbonate, hypocalcemia, *transient hypophosphatemia*

RESP: Dyspnea, pleural effusion, pulmonary infiltrates, rales, rhonchi

SKIN: Rash

INTERACTIONS

Drugs

3 *Aminoglycosides:* Increased risk of nephrotoxicity

3 *Amphotericin B:* Increased risk of nephrotoxicity

SPECIAL CONSIDERATIONS

• Maintain adequate hydration throughout the treatment period; avoid overhydration in patients with compromised cardiovascular status

MONITORING PARAMETERS

• Serum creatinine daily (discontinue if exceeds 2.5 mg/dl)

• Urine output (≥2 L/day is recommended)

• Serum calcium and phosphorus

---

ganciclovir
(gan-sy'clo-ver)
Rx: Cytovene
Chemical Class: Synthetic nucleoside analog
Therapeutic Class: Antiviral

CLINICAL PHARMACOLOGY

Mechanism of Action: Preferentially phosphorylated in virus-infected cells to ganciclovir-triphosphate, which inhibits viral DNA synthesis

Pharmacokinetics

IV: $t_{1/2}$ 3.5 hr (prolonged in renal failure); excreted unchanged by the kidneys; crosses blood-brain barrier; 1%-2% bound to plasma proteins

PO: Bioavailability 5% fasting, 6-9% with food; elimination $t_{1/2}$ 4.8 hr

INDICATIONS AND USES: CMV retinitis in immunocompromised patients; prevention of CMV disease in transplant patients at risk; prevention of CMV in patients with advanced HIV infection; other CMV disease (e.g., pneumonitis, gastroenteritis, hepatitis)*

DOSAGE

Adult and Child >3 mo

• *CMV retinitis:* Induction IV 5 mg/kg q12h as a 1-2 hr INF for 14-21 days; maintenance IV 5 mg/kg/day as a single daily dose for 7 days/wk or 6 mg/kg/day for 5 days/wk; PO 1 g tid with food

• *CMV prevention in transplant recipients:* Induction IV 5 mg/kg q12h as a 1-2 hr INF for 7-14 days; maintenance IV 5 mg/kg/day as a single daily dose for 7 days/wk or 6 mg/kg/day for 5 days/wk

• *CMV prevention in AIDS patients:* PO 1 g tid with food

• *Renal function impairment (dosage for CrCl in ml/min)*

• CrCl 50-69 IV 2.5 mg/kg q12h (induction) and 2.5 mg/kg q24h (maintenance); PO 500 mg tid

• CrCl 25-49 IV 2.5 mg/kg q24h (induction) and 1.25 mg/kg q24h (maintenance); PO 500 mg bid

• CrCl 10-24 IV 1.25 mg/kg q24h (induction) and 0.625 mg/kg q24h (maintenance); PO 500 mg qd

• CrCl <10 IV 1.25 mg/kg 3 × /wk after hemodialysis (induction) and 0.625 mg/kg 3 × /wk after hemodialysis (maintenance); PO 500 mg 3 × /wk after hemodialysis

$ AVAILABLE FORMS/COST OF THERAPY

• Cap, Gel—Oral: 250 mg, 180's: **$780.90**; 500 mg, 180's: **$1,734.29**

• Inj, Lyphl-Sol—IV: 500 mg/vial: **$891.76-$966.08**

PRECAUTIONS: Pre-existing cytopenias, renal function impairment, children <6 mo, elderly, platelet count <25,000/mm^3

PREGNANCY AND LACTATION: Pregnancy category C; excretion into breast milk unknown, not recommended in nursing mothers due to potential for serious adverse reactions in the nursing infant; do not resume nursing for at least 72 hr after last dose of ganciclovir

SIDE EFFECTS/ADVERSE REACTIONS

CNS: Abnormal thoughts or dreams, ataxia, chills, *coma,* confusion, dizziness, fever, *headache,* malaise, nervousness, paresthesia, psychosis, somnolence, tremor

CV: Dysrhythmia, hypertension, hypotension

EENT: Retinal detachment in CMV retinitis

GI: Abdominal pain, abnormal LFTs, anorexia, diarrhea, *hemorrhage,* nausea, vomiting

GU: Hematuria; increased serum creatinine, BUN

HEME: **Anemia,** eosinophilia, ***granulocytopenia, thrombocytopenia***

METAB: Decrease in blood glucose

RESP: Dyspnea

SKIN: Alopecia, pruritus, rash, urticaria

MISC: Sepsis, infections

INTERACTIONS

Drugs

3 *Didanosine:* Increased hematological toxicity

▲ *Zidovudine:* Increased hematological toxicity

SPECIAL CONSIDERATIONS

PATIENT/FAMILY EDUCATION

• Compliance with laboratory monitoring is essential

MONITORING PARAMETERS

• CBC with differential and platelets q2 days during induction and weekly thereafter

• Serum creatinine q2 wk

---

gatifloxacin

(gah-tee-floks'a-sin)

Rx: Tequin

Chemical Class: Fluoroquinolone derivative

Therapeutic Class: Antibiotic

CLINICAL PHARMACOLOGY

Mechanism of Action: Inhibits DNA gyrase and topoisomerase 4, which are needed for the synthesis of bacterial DNA

Pharmacokinetics

IV: Peak 1-2 hr

PO: Bioavailability 96%, peak 1-2 hr; protein binding 20%; concentrated in respiratory tissue and bile; 1% metabolized by liver, remainder excreted in urine (75% unchanged after 48 hr); t$_{1/2}$ 7-9 hr (prolonged in patients with renal insufficiency)

INDICATIONS AND USES: Acute bacterial exacerbation of chronic bronchitis, acute sinusitis, and community-acquired pneumonia; cystitis, pyelonephritis, and complicated urinary tract infections caused by susceptible organisms; and, uncomplicated urethral or cervical gonorrhea, and acute, uncomplicated rectal gonorrhea in women

Antibacterial spectrum usually includes:

• Gram-positive organisms: *Staphylococcus aureus* (methicillin-susceptible strains only), *Staphylococcus epidermidis* (methicillin-susceptible strains only), *Staphylococcus saprophyticus, Streptococcus agalactiae, Streptococcus pneumoniae* (penicillin-susceptible and penicillin-resistant strains), *Streptococcus pyogenes, Streptococcus viridans* group

• Gram-negative organisms: *Acinetobacter lwoffi, Citrobacter freundii, Citrobacter koseri, Enterobacter aerogenes, Enterobacter cloacae, Escherichia coli, Haemophilus influenzae, Haemophilus parainfluenzae, Klebsiella oxytoca, Klebsiella pneumoniae, Legionella pneumophila, Moraxella catarrhalis, Morganella morganii, Neisseria gonorrhoeae, Proteus mirabilis*

• Anaerobes: *Fusobacterium* species, *Peptostreptococcus* species, *Prevotella* species

• Other organisms: *Chlamydia pneumoniae, Mycoplasma pneumoniae*

DOSAGE

Adult

• Acute bacterial exacerbation of chronic bronchitis PO 400 mg 7-10 days

• Acute sinusitis PO 400 mg 10 days

• Community-acquired pneumonia PO 400 mg 7-14 days

• Cystitis PO 400 mg single dose or PO 200 mg 3 days

• Complicated urinary tract infections PO 400 mg 7-10 days

• Acute pyelonephritis PO 400 mg 7-10 days

• *Gonorrhea:* uncomplicated urethral PO 400 mg single dose; endocervical or rectal in women PO 400 mg single dose

• *Dose adjustment for renal insufficiency:* CrCl <40 ml/min initial dose PO 400 mg, subsequent doses PO 200 mg every day; hemodialysis or peritoneal dialysis patients, initial dose PO 400 mg, subsequent doses PO 200 mg every day

$ AVAILABLE FORMS/COST OF THERAPY

• Inj, Sol—IV: 2 mg/ml, 100 ml: **$192.50**; 2 mg/ml, 200 ml: **$396.25**; 10 mg/ml, 20 ml: **$18.75**; 10 mg/ml, 40 ml: **$40.67**

• Tab—Oral: 200 mg 30's: **$255.85**; 400 mg 14's: **$114.41**; 400 mg 100's: **$777.92**

PRECAUTIONS: Children <18 yr; renal insufficiency (CrCl <40 ml/min); diabetes (may affect glucose control); may prolong the QT interval, avoid in patients with known prolongation of the QT interval, hypokalemia, and patients receiving class Ia (e.g., quinidine, procainamide) or class III (e.g., amiodarone, sotalol) antiarrhythmic agents, or cisapride, erythromycin, antipsychotics, and tricyclic antidepressants; bradycardia; acute myocardial infarction; known or suspected CNS disorders (e.g., severe cerebral arteriosclerosis, epilepsy) or in the presence of other risk factors that may predispose to seizures or lower the seizure threshold

PREGNANCY AND LACTATION: Pregnancy category C; breast milk excretion unknown

---

* = non-FDA-approved use

SIDE EFFECTS/ADVERSE REACTIONS

CNS: Anxiety, asthenia, confusion, dizziness (3%), depersonalization, headache (3%), incoordination, insomnia, somnolence, tremor, vertigo

CV: Bradycardia, edema, hypertension, hypotension, palpitation, tachycardia, vasodilatation

EENT: Taste perversion, tinnitus

GI: Abdominal pain (2%), diarrhea (4%), dyspepsia (1%), *nausea* (8%), vomiting (2%), abnormal liver function test (1%), increased amylase, **pseudomembranous colitis**

GU: Moniliasis, *vaginitis,* increase in BUN, creatinine

HEME: **Leukopenia,** prothrombin time decrease, prothrombin time increase, thrombocythemia *,* **thrombocytopenia**

METAB: Hyperglycemia, hypoglycemia (if taking hypoglycemic agents)

MS: Arthralgia, myalgia, tendon inflammation, tendon rupture

RESP: Asthma, cough increased, dyspnea

SKIN: Urticaria, rash, pruritus, sweating

INTERACTIONS

Drugs

🔟 *Aluminum:* Reduced absorption of gatifloxacin; do not take within 4 hr of dose

➋ *Amiodarone:* Additive cardiac toxicity

🔟 *Antacids (containing aluminum or magnesium):* Reduced absorption of gatifloxacin; do not take within 4 hr of dose

➋ *Antipsychotics:* Additive cardiac toxicity

🔟 *Didanosine (buffered formulation):* Markedly reduced absorption of gatifloxacin; take gatifloxacin 2 hr before didanosine

➋ *Erythromycin:* Coadministration may increase risk of cardiac toxicity due to gatifloxacin

🔟 *Foscarnet:* Coadministration increase seizure risk

🔟 *Iron:* Reduced absorption of gatifloxacin; do not take within 4 hr of dose

🔟 *Magnesium:* Reduced absorption of gatifloxacin; do not take within 4 hr of dose

🔟 *Probenecid:* Inhibits excretion of gatifloxacin

➋ *Procainamide:* Additive cardiac toxicity

➋ *Quinidine:* Additive cardiac toxicity

🔟 *Sodium bicarbonate:* Reduced absorption of gatifloxacin; do not take within 4 hr of dose

➋ *Sotalol:* Additive cardiac toxicity

🔟 *Sucralfate:* Reduced absorption of gatifloxacin; do not take within 4 hr of dose

➋ *Tricyclic antidepressants:* Additive cardiac toxicity

🔟 *Zinc:* Reduced absorption of gatifloxacin; do not take within 4 hr of dose

SPECIAL CONSIDERATIONS
PATIENT/FAMILY EDUCATION

• May be taken with or without meals

• Should be taken at least 4 hr before or 8 hr after multivitamins (containing iron or zinc), antacids (containing magnesium, calcium, or aluminum), sucralfate, or didanosine chewable/buffered tablets

• Discontinue treatment, rest and refrain from exercise, and inform prescriber if pain, inflammation, or rupture of a tendon occur

• Test reaction to this drug before operating an automobile or machinery or engaging in activities requiring mental alertness or coordination

---

italic = common side effects   ***bold italic*** = life-threatening reactions

gemfibrozil
(gem-fi'broe-zil)
Rx: Lopid
Chemical Class: Fibric acid derivative
Therapeutic Class: Antilipemic

CLINICAL PHARMACOLOGY
Mechanism of Action: Inhibits peripheral lipolysis and decreases hepatic extraction of free fatty acids, thus reducing hepatic triglyceride production; inhibits synthesis of VLDL carrier apolipoprotein B, leading to a decrease in VLDL production; in the process of decreasing triglyceride production, accelerates turnover and removal of cholesterol from the liver and increases excretion of cholesterol in the feces
Pharmacokinetics
PO: Peak 1-2 hr, >90% bound to plasma proteins, $t_{1/2}$ 1½ hr (biologic $t_{1/2}$ considerably longer due to enterohepatic recycling); metabolized in liver, excreted in urine (glucuronide conjugates)

INDICATIONS AND USES: Hypertriglyceridemia (Types IV and V hyperlipidemia); Type IIb hyperlipidemia; reduction of coronary heart disease risk in patients with low HDL cholesterol in addition to elevated LDL cholesterol and triglyceride levels that haven't responded to weight loss, dietary therapy, and other pharmacologic agents

DOSAGE
Adult
• PO 600 mg bid, 30 min before morning and evening meals

$ AVAILABLE FORMS/COST OF THERAPY
• Tab, Plain Coated—Oral: 600 mg, 100's: **$89.50-$138.66**

CONTRAINDICATIONS: Severe hepatic disease, pre-existing gallbladder disease, severe renal disease, primary biliary cirrhosis

PRECAUTIONS: Children, cholelithiasis

PREGNANCY AND LACTATION: Pregnancy category C; excretion into breast milk unknown; use caution in nursing mothers

SIDE EFFECTS/ADVERSE REACTIONS
CNS: Fatigue, headache, hypesthesia, paresthesia, vertigo
CV: Atrial fibrillation
EENT: Blurred vision, cataracts, retinal edema
GI: Abdominal pain, constipation, diarrhea, *dyspepsia,* nausea, taste perversion, vomiting, cholelithiasis
GU: Impotence
HEME: **Anemia, bone marrow hypoplasia,** eosinophilia, **leukopenia, thrombocytopenia**
METAB: Increased blood glucose
MS: Arthralgia, myalgia, myasthenia, myopathy, painful extremities, **rhabdomyolysis,** synovitis
SKIN: Alopecia, dermatitis, ***exfoliative dermatitis,*** pruritus
MISC: Weight loss, carcinogenesis

INTERACTIONS
Drugs
▌ *Binding resins:* Reduced bioavailability of gemfibrozil, separate doses by >2 hr
▌ *Glyburide:* Increased risk of hypoglycemia
❷ *HMG CoA reductase inhibitors (atorvastatin, fluvastatin, lovastatin, pravastatin, simvastatin):* Increased likelihood of drug-induced myopathy
❷ *Warfarin:* Increased hypoprothrombinemic, response to warfarin

* = non-FDA-approved use

SPECIAL CONSIDERATIONS
PATIENT/FAMILY EDUCATION
• May cause dizziness or blurred vision; use caution while driving or performing other tasks requiring alertness
• Notify clinician if GI side effects become pronounced

MONITORING PARAMETERS
• Serum CK level in patients complaining of muscle pain, tenderness, or weakness
• Periodic CBC during first 12 mo of therapy
• Periodic LFTs; discontinue therapy if abnormalities persist
• Blood glucose

---

gentamicin
(jen-ta-mye'sin)

Rx: *Cre/oint:* Ed-Mycin, G-Myticin, Garamycin
Ophth: Ed-Mycin, Garamycin, Genoptic, Gent-AK, Gentrasul, Infa-Gen, Spectro Genta
Systemic: G Mycin, Garamycin,
Combinations
   Rx: with prednisolone (Pred-G)
Chemical Class: Aminoglycoside
Therapeutic Class: Antibiotic

CLINICAL PHARMACOLOGY
Mechanism of Action: Interferes with protein synthesis in bacterial cell by binding to 30S ribosomal subunit, which causes misreading of genetic code; inaccurate peptide sequence forms in protein chain, causing bacterial death

Pharmacokinetics
IM: Onset rapid, peak 30-90 min
IV: Onset immediate, peak 30 min after a 30 min INF

<30% bound to plasma proteins, plasma $t_{1/2}$ 1-2 hr, duration 6-8 hr; not metabolized, eliminated unchanged in urine via glomerular filtration

INDICATIONS AND USES: Bacterial neonatal sepsis; bacterial septicemia; serious bacterial infections of the CNS (meningitis), urinary tract, respiratory tract, GI tract, skin, bone, and soft tissue; superficial ocular infections involving the conjunctiva or cornea; infection prophylaxis in minor cuts, wounds, burns, and skin abrasions; superficial infections of the skin; alternative regimen for PID (in combination with clindamycin)*

Antibacterial spectrum usually includes:
• Gram-positive organisms: *Staphylococcus* spp. (including penicillin- and methicillin-resistant strains), *Streptococcus faecalis* (in combination with cell wall synthesis inhibitor)
• Gram-negative organisms: *Escherichia coli, Proteus* spp. (indole-positive and indole-negative), *Pseudomonas aeruginosa, Klebsiella* spp., *Enterobacter* spp., *Serratia* spp., *Citrobacter* spp., *Providencia* spp., *Salmonella* spp. and *Shigella* spp., *Yersinia pestis*

DOSAGE
NOTE: Use ideal body weight for dosage calculations
Adult
• *Severe systemic infections:* IV INF 3-5 mg/kg/day diluted in 50-100 ml NS or D_5W and infused over 30-60 min in divided doses q8h, adjust dosage based on results of gentamicin peak and trough levels (once-daily dosage*: 7 mg/kg q24h; not for pediatrics, pregnant, burns, ascites, dialysis, enterococcal endocarditis); IM 3 mg/kg/day in divided doses

---

italic = common side effects   ***bold italic*** = life-threatening reactions

q8h, adjust dosage based on results of gentamicin peak and trough levels; intrathecal 4-8 mg/day

• *Conjunctivitis:* INSTILL 1 gtt q2-4h; OPHTH apply 1/4 in ribbon of ointment to conjunctival sac bid-tid

• TOP rub into affected area qd-qid, cover with sterile bandage if needed

Infants and Children <5 yr

• IV/IM 2.5 mg/kg/dose q8h, adjust dosage based on results of gentamicin peak and trough levels; INTRATHECAL (>3 mo) 1-2 mg/day

Child ≥5 yr

• IV/IM 1.5-2.5 mg/kg/dose q8h, adjust dosage based on results of gentamicin peak and trough levels

$ AVAILABLE FORMS/COST OF THERAPY

• Cre—Top: 0.1%, 15, 30 g: **$2.55-$25.14**/15 g

• Inj, Sol—IM; IV: 10 mg/ml, 2 ml: **$1.75-$2.25**; 40 mg/ml, 2 ml: **$2.15-$5.28**

• Oint—Ophth: 0.3%, 3.5 g: **$4.10-$23.82**

• Oint—Top: 0.1%, 15, 30, 45 g: **$2.10-$22.97**/15 g

• Sol—Ophth: 0.3%, 5, 15 ml: **$2.95-$22.03**/5 ml

PRECAUTIONS: Neonates, renal disease, myasthenia gravis, hearing deficits, Parkinson's disease, elderly, dehydration, hypokalemia, prolonged use

PREGNANCY AND LACTATION: Pregnancy category C; ototoxicity has not been reported as an effect of *in utero* exposure; 8th cranial nerve toxicity in the fetus is well known following exposure to other aminoglycosides and could potentially occur with gentamicin; potentiation of magnesium sulfate-induced neuromuscular weakness in neonates has been reported, use caution during the last 32 hr of pregnancy; data on excretion into breast milk are lacking

SIDE EFFECTS/ADVERSE REACTIONS

CNS: Confusion, **convulsions,** depression, dizziness, muscle twitching, myasthenia gravis-like syndrome, **neurotoxicity,** numbness, tremors, vertigo

CV: Hypertension, hypotension, palpitations

EENT: **Deafness, ototoxicity,** tinnitus, visual disturbances; Ophth, burning, conjunctival erythema, conjunctival paresthesia, inflammation, itching, lid itching, lid swelling, mydriasis, overgrowth of non-susceptible organisms, poor corneal wound healing, stinging, temporary visual haze (ointment), transient irritation

GI: *Anorexia,* hepatomegaly, increased ALT, AST, bilirubin; *nausea,* splenomegaly, *vomiting*

GU: **Azotemia, hematuria, nephrotoxicity, oliguria, renal damage, renal failure**

HEME: **Agranulocytosis,** anemia, **eosinophilia, leukopenia, thrombocytopenia**

METAB: Decreased serum calcium, sodium, potassium, magnesium

RESP: **Respiratory depression**

SKIN: Alopecia, burning, dermatitis, photosensitivity, pruritis, *rash,* urticaria

INTERACTIONS

Drugs

3 *Amphotericin B:* Synergistic nephrotoxicity

2 *Atracurium:* Gentamicin potentiates respiratory depression by atracurium

3 *Carbenicillin:* Potential for inactivation of gentamicin in patients with renal failure

3 *Carboplatin:* Additive nephrotoxicity or ototoxicity

3 *Cephalosporins:* Increased potential for nephrotoxicity in patients with preexisting renal disease

3 *Cisplatin:* Additive nephrotoxicity or ototoxicity

3 *Cyclosporine:* Additive nephrotoxicity

2 *Ethacrynic acid:* Additive ototoxicity

3 *Indomethacin:* Reduced renal clearance of gentamicin in premature infants

3 *Methoxyflurane:* Additive nephrotoxicity

2 *Neuromuscular blocking agents:* Gentamicin potentiates respiratory depression by neuromuscular blocking agents

3 *NSAIDs:* May reduce renal clearance of gentamicin

3 *Penicillins (extended spectrum):* Potential for inactivation of gentamicin in patients with renal failure

3 *Piperacillin:* Potential for inactivation of gentamicin in patients with renal failure

2 *Succinylcholine:* Gentamicin potentiates respiratory depression by succinylcholine

3 *Ticarcillin:* Potential for inactivation of gentamicin in patients with renal failure

3 *Vancomycin:* Additive nephrotoxicity or ototoxicity

2 *Vecuronium:* Gentamicin potentiates respiratory depression by vecuronium

Labs
• *Amino acids:* Increase in urine amino acids
• *AST:* False elevations
• *Protein:* False urine elevations

SPECIAL CONSIDERATIONS
PATIENT/FAMILY EDUCATION
• Report headache, dizziness, loss of hearing, ringing, roaring in ears, or feeling of fullness in head
• Tilt head back, place medication in conjunctival sac, and close eyes

• Apply light finger pressure on lacrimal sac for 1 min following instill (gtt)
• May cause temporary blurring of vision following administration
• Notify clinician if stinging, burning, or itching becomes pronounced or if redness, irritation, swelling, decreasing vision, or pain persists or worsens
• Do not touch tip of container to any surface
• For external use only
• Cleanse affected area of skin prior to application
• Notify clinician if condition worsens or if rash or irritation develops

MONITORING PARAMETERS
• Urinalysis for proteinuria, cells, casts
• Urine output
• Serum peak, drawn at 30-60 min after IV INF or 60 min after IM inj, trough level drawn just before next dose; adjust dosage per levels (usual therapeutic plasma levels, peak 4-8 µg/ml, trough ≤2 µg/ml)
• Serum creatinine for CrCl calculation
• Serum calcium, magnesium, sodium
• Audiometric testing, assess hearing before, during, after treatment

---

glatiramer
(gla-teer´a-mer)
Rx: Copaxone
Chemical Class: Synthetic polypeptide
Therapeutic Class: Multiple sclerosis agent

CLINICAL PHARMACOLOGY
Mechanism of Action: Inhibits the immune response to myelin basic protein and possibly other myelin

---

antigens that are thought to be involved in the pathogenesis of multiple sclerosis

Pharmacokinetics

SC: Substantial fraction hydrolyzed locally; some fraction enters lymphatic circulation; some may enter systemic circulation intact

INDICATIONS AND USES: Relapsing-remitting multiple sclerosis

DOSAGE

Adult

• SC 20 mg qd

§ **AVAILABLE FORMS/COST OF THERAPY**

• Inj—SC: 20 mg/vial, 32's: **$1,107.69**

PRECAUTIONS: Advanced relapsing-remitting multiple sclerosis, chronic-progressive multiple sclerosis

PREGNANCY AND LACTATION: Pregnancy category B; excretion into breast milk unknown, use caution in nursing mothers

SIDE EFFECTS/ADVERSE REACTIONS

CNS: Dizziness, faintness

CV: Transient chest pain

GI: Anorexia, constipation, nausea, vomiting

HEME: Transient eosinophilia

MS: Joint pain, muscle cramps

SKIN: Pain at injection site, rash, urticaria

MISC: Systemic reaction (combination of flushing, palpitations, chest tightness, diaphoresis, dyspnea, and/or anxiety)

SPECIAL CONSIDERATIONS

• May be useful for relapsing-remitting multiple sclerosis in patients who are not benefiting from, or are intolerant of, interferon β-1 a/b; less effective in patients with advanced disease or chronic-progressive multiple sclerosis; not a cure for multiple sclerosis and benefits achieved are relatively modest

• Sites for injection include arms, abdomen, hips, and thighs

---

glimepiride

(gly-mep´er-ide)

Rx: Amaryl

Chemical Class: Sulfonylurea (2nd generation)

Therapeutic Class: Oral hypoglycemic

CLINICAL PHARMACOLOGY

Mechanism of Action: Decreases blood sugar via stimulation of insulin secretion and increased tissue responsiveness to insulin; initial hypoglycemic effects due to stimulation of pancreatic islets (dependent upon functioning β-cells); extrapancreatic effect predominantly due to inhibition of hepatic glucose production, but may also facilitate improved insulin-insulin receptor binding

Pharmacokinetics

PO: Peak 2-3 hr, duration 24 hr; >99.5% bound to plasma proteins; completely metabolized by liver, metabolites excreted in urine (60%) and feces (40%)

INDICATIONS AND USES: Diabetes mellitus, type 2

DOSAGE

Adult

• PO 1-2 mg qd with breakfast or the 1st main meal; usual maintenance dose 1-4 mg qd; mfg. maximum dose 8 mg/day

(NOTE: Daily doses >4 mg provide little added benefit.)

§ **AVAILABLE FORMS/COST OF THERAPY**

• Tab—Oral: 1 mg, 100's: **$29.81**; 2 mg, 100's: **$48.30**; 4 mg, 100's: **$77.76-$91.11**

CONTRAINDICATIONS: Diabetes mellitus, type 1; ketoacidosis

---

* = non-FDA-approved use

PRECAUTIONS: Elderly, cardiac disease, severe renal disease, severe hepatic disease, thyroid disease, adrenal or pituitary insufficiency, debilitated or malnourished patients

PREGNANCY AND LACTATION: Pregnancy category C; inappropriate for use during pregnancy due to inadequacy for blood glucose control, potential for prolonged neonatal hypoglycemia, and risk of congenital abnormalities; insulin is the drug of choice for control of blood sugars during pregnancy; breast milk secretion, unknown; the potential for neonatal hypoglycemia dictates caution in nursing mothers

SIDE EFFECTS/ADVERSE REACTIONS

CNS: Dizziness, drowsiness, headache, paresthesia

EENT: Blurred vision, tinnitus, vertigo

GI: Cholestatic jaundice, constipation, diarrhea, elevated liver function tests, gastralgia, nausea

HEME: **Agranulocytosis, aplastic anemia, hemolytic anemia,** hepatic porphyria, **leukopenia, pancytopenia, thrombocytopenia**

METAB: Hypoglycemia, hyponatremia, SIADH

MS: Fatigue, weakness

SKIN: Eczema, erythema, morbilliform or maculopapular eruptions, pruritus, urticaria

INTERACTIONS

Drugs

�3 *Anabolic steroids:* Enhanced hypoglycemic response

�3 *Angiotensin converting enzyme inhibitors:* Increased risk of hypolycemia

�3 *Antacids:* Enhanced rate of absorption

�3 *Aspirin:* Enhanced hypoglycemic effect

�3 *β-Adrenergic blockers:* Altered response to hypoglycemia; prolonged recovery of normoglycemia, hypertension, blockade of tachycardia; may increase blood glucose concentration

�3 *Clofibrate:* Enhanced effects of oral hypoglycemic drugs

�3 *Corticosteroids:* Increased blood glucose in diabetic patients

�3 *Cyclosporine:* Increased cyclosporine levels

⚠ *Ethanol:* Excessive intake may lead to altered glycemic control; "Antabuse"-like reaction may occur

�3 *Gemfibrozil:* Increased risk of hypoglycemia

�3 *H2-receptor antagonists:* Enhanced rate of absorption

�3 *MAOIs:* Excessive hypoglycemia may occur in patients with diabetes

❷ *Phenylbutazole:* Increases serum concentrations of oral hypoglycemic drugs

�3 *Proton pump blockers:* Enhanced rate of absorption

�3 *Rifampin:* Reduced sulfonylurea concentrations

�3 *Sulfonamides:* Enhanced hypoglycemic effects of sulfonylureas

�3 *Thiazide diuretics:* Potential increased dosage requirement of antidiabetic drugs

SPECIAL CONSIDERATIONS

• No demonstrated advantage over existing 2nd generation sulfonylureas

PATIENT/FAMILY EDUCATION

• Multiple drug interactions, including alcohol and salicylates

• Symptoms of hypoglycemia: tingling lips/tongue, nausea, confusion, fatigue, sweating, hunger, visual changes (spots)

MONITORING PARAMETERS

• Self-monitored blood glucoses; glycosolated hemoglobin q 3-6 mo

---

italic = common side effects   **bold italic** = life-threatening reactions

glipizide

(glip'i-zide)

Rx: Glucotrol, Glucotrol XL
Chemical Class: Sulfonylurea
(2nd generation)
Therapeutic Class: Oral hypoglycemic

CLINICAL PHARMACOLOGY

Mechanism of Action: Decreases
blood sugar via stimulation of insulin secretion and increased tissue responsiveness to insulin; initial hypoglycemic effects due to stimulation of pancreatic islets (dependent
upon functioning β-cells); extrapancreatic effect predominantly due
to inhibition of hepatic glucose production, but may also facilitate improved insulin-insulin receptor
binding

Pharmacokinetics

PO: Completely absorbed by GI
route, onset 1-1½ hr, duration 10-24
hr, $t_{1/2}$ 2-4 hr; metabolized in liver to
inactive metabolites, excreted in
urine; 90%-95% bound to plasma
proteins

INDICATIONS AND USES: Type 2
diabetes mellitus

DOSAGE

Adult and child >16 yr

• PO 2.5-5 mg 30 min before breakfast; adjust dose in 2.5-5 mg increments; manufacturer recommended
max dose 40 mg/day; best to divide
dose if daily dose exceeds 10 mg
(i.e., 10 mg bid);
(NOTE: little if any benefit from
daily doses >20 mg)

💲 AVAILABLE FORMS/COST OF THERAPY

• Tab, Uncoated—Oral: 5 mg,
100's: **$27.30-$43.64**; 10 mg,
100's: **$50.12-$80.13**

• Tab, Coated, Sus Action—Oral: 5
mg, 100's: **$37.90**; 10 mg, 100's:
$75.00

CONTRAINDICATIONS: Diabetes
mellitus, type 1; ketoacidosis

PRECAUTIONS: Elderly, cardiac
disease, severe renal disease, severe
hepatic disease, thyroid disease, adrenal or pituitary insufficiency, debilitated or malnourished patients

PREGNANCY AND LACTATION:
Pregnancy category C; inappropriate for use during pregnancy due to
inadequate for blood glucose control, potential for prolonged neonatal hypoglycemia, and risk of congenital abnormalities; insulin is the
drug of choice for control of blood
sugars during pregnancy; breast
milk secretion unknown; the potential for neonatal hypoglycemia dictates caution in nursing mothers

SIDE EFFECTS/ADVERSE REACTIONS

CNS: Dizziness, drowsiness, headache, paresthesia

EENT: Tinnitus, vertigo

GI: Cholestatic jaundice, constipation, diarrhea, elevated liver function tests, gastralgia, nausea

GU: Mild to moderate elevations in
BUN and creatinine

HEME: **Agranulocytosis, aplastic
anemia, hemolytic anemia,** hepatic
porphyria, **leukopenia, pancytopenia, thrombocytopenia**

METAB: **Hypoglycemia,** SIADH

MS: Fatigue, weakness

SKIN: Eczema, erythema, morbilliform or maculopapular eruptions,
pruritus, urticaria

INTERACTIONS

Drugs

🔳 *Anabolic steroids:* Enhanced hypoglycemic response

🔳 *Angiotensin converting enzyme
inhibitor:* Increased risk of hypoglycemia

---

* = non-FDA-approved use

3 *Antacids:* Enhanced rate of absorption

3 *Aspirin:* Enhanced hypoglycemic effects

3 *β-Adrenergic blockers:* Altered response to hypoglycemia; prolonged recovery of normoglycemia, hypertension, blockade of tachycardia; may increase blood glucose concentration

3 *Clofibrate:* Enhanced effects of oral hypoglycemic drugs

3 *Corticosteroids:* Increased blood glucose in diabetic patients

A *Ethanol:* Excessive intake may lead to altered glycemic control; Antabuse-like reaction may occur

3 *Gemfibrozil:* Increased risk of hypoglycemia

3 *H₂-receptor antagonists (cimetidine, ranitidine, etc.):* Enhanced rate of absorption

3 *MAOIs:* Excessive hypoglycemia may occur in patient with diabetes

3 *Phenylbutazone:* Increases serum concentrations of oral hypoglycemics

3 *Rifampin:* Reduced sulfonylurea concentrations

3 *Sulfonamides:* Enhanced hypoglycemic effects of sulfonylureas

3 *Thiazide diuretics:* Potential increased dosage requirement of antidiabetic drugs

SPECIAL CONSIDERATIONS
PATIENT/FAMILY EDUCATION
• Administer 30 min ac
• Notify clinician of fever, sore throat, rash, unusual bruising, or bleeding
• Multiple drug interactions, including alcohol and salicylates
• Symptoms of hypoglycemia: tingling lips/tongue, nausea, confusion, fatigue, sweating, hunger, visual changes (spots)

• Notify clinician of fever, sore throat, rash, unusual bruising, or bleeding

MONITORING PARAMETERS
• Self-monitored blood glucose; glycosylated hemoglobin q 3-6 mo

glucagon
(gloo′ka-gon)
Rx: Glucagon
Chemical Class: Polypeptide hormone (pancreas)
Therapeutic Class: Antihypoglycemic agent

CLINICAL PHARMACOLOGY
Mechanism of Action: Accelerates liver glycogenolysis and inhibits glycogen synthetase resulting in blood glucose elevation; stimulates hepatic gluconeogenesis; relaxes smooth muscle of the GI tract

Pharmacokinetics

IV/IM/SC: Onset within 15 min; degraded in liver, kidney and plasma; t₁/₂ 3-6 min

INDICATIONS AND USES: Hypoglycemia; diagnostic aid in radiologic examination of GI tract when hypotonic state is advantageous

DOSAGE
Adult
• *Hypoglycemia:* IV/IM/SC 0.5-1 mg, may repeat in 20 min prn
• *Diagnostic aid:* IV/IM/SC 0.25-2.0 mg 10 min prior to procedure

Child
• *Hypoglycemia:* IV/IM/SC 30 μg/kg/dose, not to exceed 1 mg/dose, repeat in 20 min prn

Neonate
• *Hypoglycemia:* IV/IM/SC 30 μg/kg/dose, max 1 mg/dose

italic = common side effects   ***bold italic*** = life-threatening reactions

$ AVAILABLE FORMS/COST OF THERAPY
• Inj, Powder for Inj—IM, IV, SC: 1 mg: **$48.00-$57.60**
• Inj, Sol—IM, IV, SC: 1 mg/vial: (Glucagon emergency kit): **$77.34**
PRECAUTIONS: Insulinoma, pheochromocytoma
PREGNANCY AND LACTATION: Pregnancy category B; excretion into breast milk unknown; use caution in nursing mothers
SIDE EFFECTS/ADVERSE REACTIONS
CV: Hypotension
GI: Nausea, vomiting
RESP: Respiratory distress
SKIN: Urticaria
INTERACTIONS
Drugs
3 *Oral anticoagulants:* Enhanced hypoprothrombinemic response to warfarin and possibly other oral anticoagulants
SPECIAL CONSIDERATIONS
PATIENT/FAMILY EDUCATION
• Notify clinician when hypoglycemic reactions occur so that antidiabetic therapy can be adjusted
MONITORING PARAMETERS
• Blood sugar, level of consciousness

---

glyburide

(glye'byoor-ide)
Rx: DiaβEta, Glynase Prestab, Micronase
Chemical Class: Sulfonylurea (2nd generation)
Therapeutic Class: Oral hypoglycemic

CLINICAL PHARMACOLOGY
Mechanism of Action: Decreases blood sugar via stimulation of insulin secretion and increased tissue responsiveness to insulin; initial hypoglycemic effects due to stimulation of pancreatic islets (dependent upon functioning β cells); extrapancreatic effect predominantly due to inhibition of hepatic glucose production, but may also facilitate improved insulin-insulin receptor binding
Pharmacokinetics
PO: Completely absorbed by GI route, onset 2-4 hr, peak 2-8 hr, duration 24 hr, $t_{1/2}$ 10 hr (4 hr for micronized formulation); metabolized in liver to weakly active metabolites; excreted in urine, feces (metabolites); 90%-95% bound to plasma proteins
INDICATIONS AND USES: Diabetes mellitus, type 2
DOSAGE
Adult and child >16 yr
• PO 1.25-5 mg qd (0.75-3 mg for micronized formulation) with breakfast or 1st main meal; manufacturer max dose 20 mg/day (2 mg/day for micronized formulation); best to divide dose bid for doses >5 mg (i.e., 5 mg bid)
(NOTE: Daily doses >10 mg [6 mg for micronized] provide little added benefit)
$ AVAILABLE FORMS/COST OF THERAPY
• Tab, Uncoated—Oral: 1.25 mg, 100's: **$18.32-$34.49**; 2.5 mg, 100's: **$28.40-$57.45**; 5 mg, 100's: **$34.40-$100.90**
• Tab, Uncoated, Micronized—Oral: 1.5 mg, 100's: **$29.52-$48.96**; 3 mg, 100's: **$60.20-$82.76**; 6 mg, 100's: **$84.09-$121.96**
CONTRAINDICATIONS: Diabetes mellitus, type 1; ketoacidosis
PRECAUTIONS: Elderly, cardiac disease, severe renal disease, severe hepatic disease, thyroid disease, adrenal or pituitary insufficiency, debilitated or malnourished patients

PREGNANCY AND LACTATION:
Pregnancy category B; inappropriate for use during pregnancy due to inadequacy for blood glucose control, potential for prolonged neonatal hypoglycemia, and risk of congenital abnormalities; insulin is the drug of choice for control of blood sugars during pregnancy; breast milk secretion unknown; the potential for neonatal hypoglycemia dictates caution in nursing mothers

SIDE EFFECTS/ADVERSE REACTIONS

CNS: Dizziness, drowsiness, headache, paresthesia

EENT: Tinnitus, vertigo

GI: Cholestatic jaundice, constipation, diarrhea, elevated liver function tests, gastralgia, nausea

GU: Mild to moderate elevations in BUN and creatinine

HEME: **Agranulocytosis, aplastic anemia, hemolytic anemia,** hepatic porphyria, **leukopenia, pancytopenia, thrombocytopenia**

METAB: **Hypoglycemia,** SIADH

MS: Fatigue, weakness

SKIN: Eczema, erythema, morbilliform or maculopapular eruptions, pruritus, urticaria

INTERACTIONS

Drugs

🔢 *Anabolic steroids:* Enhanced hypoglycemic response

🔢 *Angiotensin converting enzyme inhibitor:* Increased risk of hypoglycemia

🔢 *Antacids:* Enhanced rate of absorption

🔢 *Aspirin:* Enhanced hypoglycemic effects

🔢 *β-Adrenergic blockers:* Altered response to hypoglycemia; prolonged recovery of normoglycemia, hypertension, blockade of tachycardia; may increase blood glucose concentration

🔢 *Clofibrate:* Enhanced effects of oral hypoglycemic drugs

🔢 *Corticosteroids:* Increased blood glucose in diabetic patients

⚠ *Ethanol:* Excessive intake may lead to altered glycemic control; Antabuse-like reaction may occur

🔢 *Gemfibrozil:* Increased risk of hypoglycemia

🔢 *H$_2$-receptor antagonists (cimetidine, ranitidine, etc.):* Enhanced rate of absorption

🔢 *MAOIs:* Excessive hypoglycemia may occur in patient with diabetes

🔢 *Phenylbutazone:* Increases serum concentrations of oral hypoglycemics

🔢 *Rifampin:* Reduced sulfonylurea concentrations

🔢 *Sulfonamides:* Enhanced hypoglycemic effects of sulfonylureas

🔢 *Thiazide diuretics:* Potential increased dosage requirement of antidiabetic drugs

Labs

• *Protein:* False-urine increases with Ponceaus dye method

SPECIAL CONSIDERATIONS

• Micronized formulations do not provide bioequivalent serum concentrations to non-micronized formulations; retitrate patients when transferring from any hypoglycemic to micronized glyburide

PATIENT/FAMILY EDUCATION

• Multiple drug interactions including alcohol and salicylates

• Notify clinician of fever, sore throat, rash, unusual bruising, or bleeding

MONITORING PARAMETERS

• Self-monitored blood glucose; glycosylated Hgb q3-6 mo

---

italic = common side effects   ***bold italic*** = life-threatening reactions

glycerin

(gli′ser-in)
OTC: *Laxative:* Fleets
Babylax, Glycerol, Sani-Supp
Rx: *Ophth:* Ophthalgan
Oral: Osmoglyn
Chemical Class: Trihydric alcohol
Therapeutic Class: Laxative;
antiglaucoma agent; osmotic
diuretic

CLINICAL PHARMACOLOGY
Mechanism of Action: (Laxative)
Osmotic shifts stimulate defecation;
(Ophth) Osmotic agent reduces intraocular pressure transiently
Pharmacokinetics
PO: Well absorbed, onset 10-60 min,
duration 5 hr
OPHTH: Onset 10 min, peak 20 min,
duration 4-8 hr
PR: Poorly absorbed, onset 15-30
min
Metabolized and eliminated by kidney
INDICATIONS AND USES: (Rect)
constipation; (Ophth) edematous
cornea; (Oral) interruption of acute
glaucoma attack, reduction of intraocular pressure preocular and
postocular surgery, lowering intracranial pressure*
DOSAGE
Adult
• *Constipation:* PR 1 adult supp 1-2
times/day prn or 5-15 ml as an enema
• *Reduction of corneal edema:*
OPHTH instill 1 gtt q3-4h
• *Reduction of intraocular pressure:*
PO 1-1.8 g/kg 1-1½ hr preoperatively; additional doses may be administered at 5 hr intervals
• *Reduction of intracranial pressure:* PO 1.5 g/kg/day divided q4h or
1 g/kg/dose q6h

* = non-FDA-approved use

Child
• *Constipation:* PR (<6 yr) 1 infant
supp 1-2 times/day prn or 2-5 ml as
an enema; (>6 yr) same as adult
• *Reduction of corneal edema:*
Same as adult
• *Reduction of intraocular pressure:*
Same as adult
• *Reduction of intracranial pressure:* Same as adult
Neonate
• *Constipation:* PR 0.5 ml/kg/dose
🟥 **AVAILABLE FORMS/COST
OF THERAPY**
• Sol—Ophth: 99.5%, 7.5 ml:
$26.98
• Sol—Oral: 50%, 220 ml: **$2.60**
• Supp—Rect: Adult 12's: **$0.69-
$4.82**; Pediatric 12's: **$0.69-$4.82**
CONTRAINDICATIONS: (Laxative) Symptoms of appendicitis,
acute surgical abdomen, fecal impaction, intestinal obstruction, undiagnosed abdominal pain; (Oral)
well-established anuria, severe dehydration, pulmonary edema, cardiac decompensation
PRECAUTIONS: (Laxative) fluid
and electrolyte imbalance, chronic
use, rectal bleeding; (Oral) hypervolemia, confused mental status,
CHF, diabetes, severe dehydration;
cardiac, renal, hepatic disease
PREGNANCY AND LACTATION:
Pregnancy category C; data regarding use in breast feeding are unavailable
SIDE EFFECTS/ADVERSE REACTIONS
CNS: Confusion, disorientation,
headache (oral); dizziness, fainting
(laxative)
CV: **Dysrhythmias** (oral); palpitations (laxative)
EENT: Pain or irritation upon instillation (ophth)

GI: Abdominal pain, bloating, excessive bowel activity, flatulence, perianal irritation (laxative); nausea, vomiting (oral)

METAB: **Hyperosmolar nonketotic coma**

INTERACTIONS
Labs
• *Increase:* Amniotic fluid phosphatidylglycerol, serum triglycerides
• *Decrease:* Serum ionized calcium

SPECIAL CONSIDERATIONS
PATIENT/FAMILY EDUCATION
• Do not use laxative in the presence of abdominal pain, nausea, or vomiting
• Do not use longer than 1 wk
• Prolonged or frequent use may result in dependency or electrolyte imbalance
• Notify clinician if unrelieved constipation, rectal bleeding, muscle cramps, weakness, or dizziness occurs

MONITORING PARAMETERS
• Blood glucose, intraocular pressure

---

glycopyrrolate
(glye-koe-pye′roe-late)
Rx: Robinul, Robinul Forte
Chemical Class: Quaternary ammonium derivative
Therapeutic Class: Anticholinergic; gastrointestinal antiulcer agent (adjunct)

CLINICAL PHARMACOLOGY
Mechanism of Action: Inhibits action of acetylcholine on structures innervated by postganglionic cholinergic nerves and on smooth muscles that respond to acetylcholine but lack cholinergic innervation; diminishes volume and free acidity of gastric secretions and controls excessive pharyngeal, tracheal, and bronchial secretions; antagonizes muscarinic symptoms (e.g., bronchorrhea, bronchospasm, bradycardia, and intestinal hypermotility) induced by cholinergic drugs such as the anticholinesterases

Pharmacokinetics
PO: Onset 1 hr, duration 6 hr
IM: Onset 15-30 min, duration 7 hr
IV: Onset 1-10 min, duration 7 hr
Does not penetrate CNS; excreted primarily unchanged via bile, feces

INDICATIONS AND USES: Peptic ulcer (adjunctive therapy); decreases secretions prior to induction of anesthesia, intubation, and surgery; interoperatively to counteract drug-induced or vagal traction reflexes with the associated dysrhythmias; protection against peripheral muscarinic effects of cholinergic agents such as neostigmine and pyridostigmine used to reverse neuromuscular blockade due to non-depolarizing muscle relaxants

DOSAGE
Adult
• *Preoperatively:* IM 0.004 mg/kg 0.5-1 hr before surgery
• *Intraoperative:* IV 0.1 mg repeat prn at 2-3 min intervals
• *Peptic ulcer:* PO 1-2 mg bid-tid; IM/IV 0.1-0.2 mg tid-qid
• *Reversal of neuromuscular blockade:* IV 0.2 mg for each 1 mg of neostigmine or 5 mg of pyridostigmine administered

Child
• *Preoperatively:* IM (<2 yr) 4.4-8.8 µg/kg 0.5-1 hr before surgery; (>2 yr) 4.4 µg/kg 0.5-1 hr before surgery
• *Intraoperative:* IV 4 µg/kg (max 0.1 mg), repeat prn at 2-3 min intervals
• *Reversal of neuromuscular blockade:* Same as adult

$ AVAILABLE FORMS/COST OF THERAPY
• Inj, Sol—IM, IV: 0.2 mg/ml, 1, 2, 5, 20 ml: **$0.88-$1.78**/2 ml
• Tab, Uncoated—Oral: 1 mg, 100's: **$21.16-$66.02**; 2 mg, 100's: **$33.70-$105.33**

CONTRAINDICATIONS: Narrow-angle glaucoma, obstructive uropathy, GI tract obstruction, paralytic ileus, intestinal atony, acute hemorrhage, severe ulcerative colitis, toxic megacolon, myasthenia gravis

PRECAUTIONS: Glaucoma, asthma, elderly, prostatic hypertrophy, renal disease, CHF, pulmonary disease, hyperthyroidism, CAD, hypertension

PREGNANCY AND LACTATION: Pregnancy category B; has been used prior to cesarean section to decrease gastric secretions; quaternary structure results in limited placental transfer; excretion into breast milk is unknown, but should be minimal due to quaternary structure

SIDE EFFECTS/ADVERSE REACTIONS
CNS: Anxiety, confusion, delusions, depression, dizziness, flushing, hallucinations, headache, incoherence, irritability, lethargy, restlessness, sedation, weakness
CV: Palpitations, paradoxical bradycardia, postural hypotension, tachycardia
EENT: Blurred vision, cycloplegia, difficulty swallowing, dilated pupils, increased intraocular pressure, mydriasis, nasal congestion, photophobia
GI: Abdominal distress, altered taste perception, *constipation, dry mouth,* nausea, paralytic ileus, vomiting
GU: Hesitancy, impotence, retention
SKIN: Allergic reactions, decreased sweating, urticaria

gonadorelin
(goe-nad-oh-rell'in)
Rx: Factrel
Chemical Class: Synthetic gonadotropin-releasing hormone (GnRH or LHRH)
Therapeutic Class: Diagnostic agent; ovulation stimulant

CLINICAL PHARMACOLOGY
Mechanism of Action: Stimulates release of lutenizing hormone (LH) from the anterior pituitary
Pharmacokinetics
IV: Rapidly metabolized to various biologically inactive peptide fragments, which are readily excreted in urine; $t_{1/2}$ 2-10 min (initial), 10-40 min (terminal)

INDICATIONS AND USES: Evaluating gonadotropic function of the anterior pituitary

DOSAGE
Adult
• *Evaluating functional capacity and response of gonadotropes of the anterior pituitary:* IV/SC: 100 µg; in females, perform the test in the early follicular phase (days 1-7) of menstrual cycle
Child
• *Evaluating functional capacity and response of gonadotropes of the anterior pituitary:* IV: 100 µg

$ AVAILABLE FORMS/COST OF THERAPY
• Inj, Sol—IV, SC: 100 µg/vial: **$212.61**; 250 µg/vial: **$206.90**

CONTRAINDICATIONS: Reproductive hormone-dependent tumor; ovarian cysts

PRECAUTIONS: Ovarian hyperstimulation is possible

PREGNANCY AND LACTATION: Pregnancy category B; possibility of fetal harm appears remote if used during pregnancy

* = non-FDA-approved use

SIDE EFFECTS/ADVERSE REACTIONS

CNS: Flushing, headache, lightheadedness

GI: Abdominal discomfort, nausea

GU: Multiple pregnancy, **ovarian hyperstimulation** (sudden ovarian enlargement, ascites, pleural effusion)

RESP: **Anaphylaxis**

INTERACTIONS

Drugs

3 *Androgen, Estrogen, Glucocorticoid, Progestin-containing preparations:* May reduce LH release from anterior pituitary

Labs

• Do not conduct diagnostic tests during administration of these agents

---

goserelin

(go'seh-rel-in)

Rx: Zoladex

Chemical Class: Synthetic gonadotropin-releasing hormone (GnRH or LHRH)

Therapeutic Class: Antineoplastic; antiendometriosis agent

CLINICAL PHARMACOLOGY

Mechanism of Action: Causes initial increase in serum luteinizing hormone (LH) and follicle stimulating hormone (FSH); chronic administration leads to sustained suppression of pituitary gonadotropins with subsequent reductions in serum testosterone (males) and estradiol (females)

Pharmacokinetics

SC: Peak 12-15 days; released from depot at slower rate for 1st 8 days, and then more rapidly during the remainder of the 28-day dosing period; $t_{1/2}$ 4.2 hr; cleared via a combination of hepatic metabolism and urinary excretion

INDICATIONS AND USES: Advanced prostate carcinoma, endometriosis, breast cancer,* endometrial thinning agent for dysfunctional uterine bleeding*

DOSAGE

Adult

• SC 3.6 mg into upper abdominal wall 4 wk; recommended duration in endometriosis is 6 mo

• Prostate carcinoma: SC 10.8 mg into upper abdominal wall q12 wk

$ **AVAILABLE FORMS/COST OF THERAPY**

• Implant, Cont Rel—SC: 3.6 mg: **$469.99**; 10.8 mg: **$1,409.98**

CONTRAINDICATIONS: Pregnancy

PRECAUTIONS: Patients at risk for osteoporosis (alcoholism, tobacco abuse, family history, chronic anticonvulsant therapy, chronic corticosteroid use)

PREGNANCY AND LACTATION: Pregnancy category X; excretion into breast milk unknown; use caution in nursing mothers

SIDE EFFECTS/ADVERSE REACTIONS

CNS: Anxiety, *depression, emotional lability, headaches,* insomnia, nervousness, **spinal cord compression**

CV: **Cerebrovascular accident,** chest pain, **dysrhythmia,** *hot flashes,* hypertension, **MI**

GI: Constipation, diarrhea, nausea, ulcer, vomiting

GU: Breakthrough bleeding, *decreased libido,* renal insufficiency, *spotting,* urinary obstruction, UTI, vaginal dryness

METAB: Gout, hyperglycemia

MS: Decreased bone mineral density, osteoneuralgia

---

italic = common side effects   ***bold italic*** = life-threatening reactions

SKIN: Alopecia, dry skin, pain on inj, rash, skin discoloration, *sweating*
MISC: Breast tenderness, *change in breast size*, gynecomastia

INTERACTIONS
Labs
• *Increase:* Alk phosphatase, estradiol, FSH, LH, testosterone levels (1st week)
• *Decrease:* Testosterone levels (after 1st week), progesterone

SPECIAL CONSIDERATIONS
PATIENT/FAMILY EDUCATION
• Notify clinician if regular menstruation persists (females)
• An initial flare in bone pain may occur (prostate cancer therapy)

MONITORING PARAMETERS
• Prostate-specific antigen, acid phosphatase, alk phosphatase
• Testosterone level (<25 ng/dl)
• Bone density if therapy prolonged

---

granisetron
(gra-ni′se-tron)
Rx: Kytril
Chemical Class: Carbazole derivative
Therapeutic Class: Antiemetic

CLINICAL PHARMACOLOGY
Mechanism of Action: Selectively blocks the action of serotonin at 5-HT$_3$ receptors; cytotoxic chemotherapy appears to be associated with release of serotonin from enterochromaffin cells of the small intestine, which may stimulate vagal afferents through 5-HT$_3$ receptors, initiating the vomiting reflex
Pharmacokinetics
PO: Onset 15-30 min
IV: Onset 1-3 min
Mean $t_{1/2}$ 9 hr in cancer patients (range 1-31 hr); mean 5 hr in normals (range 1-15 hr); 65% protein bound; metabolized by cytochrome P-450 3A, some metabolites active; 12% of drug excreted unchanged in urine; metabolites excreted in urine and feces

INDICATIONS AND USES: Prevention and treatment of emesis due to cancer chemotherapy; radiation; postsurgical nausea and vomiting*

DOSAGE
Adult
• IV 10 µg/kg infused over ½-5 min, beginning 30 min before initiation of chemotherapy, no adjustment for renal or hepatic disease
• PO 1 mg q12h, or 2 mg × 1, 1st dose given 1 hr before chemotherapy, only on the day(s) chemotherapy is given
Child 2-16 yr
• IV 10 µg/kg INF over 5 min, beginning 30 min before initiation of chemotherapy, no adjustment for renal or hepatic disease
• PO same as adult

☒ AVAILABLE FORMS/COST OF THERAPY
• Inj, Sol—IV: 1 mg/ml, 1, 4 ml: **$195.20**/1 ml
• Tab, Uncoated—Oral: 1 mg, 2's: **$94.10**

PRECAUTIONS: Child <2 yr
PREGNANCY AND LACTATION: Pregnancy category B; breast milk excretion unknown

SIDE EFFECTS/ADVERSE REACTIONS
CNS: Anxiety, *headache,* somnolence, weakness
CV: Atrioventricular block, hypertension, hypotension, ventricular ectopy
EENT: Dysgeusia
GI: Constipation, diarrhea, elevated transaminase
MISC: Fever

---

grepafloxacin

(gree-pah-floks´a-sin)

Rx: Raxar

Chemical Class: Fluoroquinolone derivative

Therapeutic Class: Antibiotic

NOTE: Removed from market October, 1999 due to ECG QT interval prolongation

CLINICAL PHARMACOLOGY

Mechanism of Action: Interferes with the enzyme DNA gyrase, needed for the synthesis of bacterial DNA

Pharmacokinetics

PO: Peak 2-3 hr; 70% bioavailable PO not affected by food; widely distributed, 50% protein bound; metabolized in liver by cytochrome P450 1A2 and 3A4 to inactive metabolites; $t_{1/2}$ 16 hr; 50% excreted in feces, 38% in urine as metabolites; clearance impaired in patients with hepatic insufficiency but not with renal insufficiency; clearance increased by 40% in cigarette smokers due to cytochrome P450 1A2 induction

INDICATIONS AND USES: Acute bacterial exacerbations of chronic bronchitis, community-acquired pneumonia, uncomplicated gonorrhea (urethral in males; endocervical and rectal in females), nongonococcal urethritis and cervicitis

Antibacterial spectrum usually includes:

• Gram-positive organisms: *Staphylococcus aureus* (methicillin-susceptible strains), *S. epidermidis*, *Streptococcus pneumoniae*, *S. pyogenes*

• Gram-negative organisms: *Citrobacter freundii*, *C. diversus*, *Enterobacter aerogenes*, *E. cloacae*, *Escherichia coli*, *H. influenza*, *H. parainfluenza*, *Klebsiella pneumoniae*, *Moraxella catarrhalis*, *Morganella morganii*, *N. gonorrhoeae*, *Proteus mirabilis*, *P. vulgaris*

• Other: *Chlamydia trachomatis*, *Mycoplasma pneumoniae;* not active against anaerobic bacteria

DOSAGE

Adult

• *Bronchitis:* PO 400-600 mg qd × 10 days

• *Community-acquired pneumonia:* PO 600 mg qd × 10 days

• *Non-gonococcal urethritis and cervicitis:* PO 400 mg qd × 7 days

• *Uncomplicated gonorrhea:* PO 400 mg as single dose (plus treatment for *chlamydia trachomatis*)

$ **AVAILABLE FORMS/COST OF THERAPY**

• Tab, Uncoated—Oral: 200 mg, 60's: **$148.10**; 400 mg, 10's: **$49.37**; 600 mg, 10's: **$67.63**

CONTRAINDICATIONS: Hepatic failure, patients with QT interval prolongation or taking other medications known to prolong the QT interval

PRECAUTIONS: Patients with hepatic insufficiency, seizure disorder, history of proarrhythmic conditions (e.g., hypokalemia, significant bradycardia, CHF, myocardial ischemia, atrial fibrillation), taking NSAIDs (increased risk of CNS side effects)

PREGNANCY AND LACTATION: Pregnancy category C; excreted in breast milk at levels similar to serum; do not breast feed within 48 hours after a dose

SIDE EFFECTS/ADVERSE REACTIONS

CNS: Anxiety, *dizziness,* headache, hyperkinesia, insomnia, somnolence, ***toxic psychosis***

CV: Arrhythmia, QT prolongation

EENT: Dry mouth, *dysgeusia (18%),* tinnitus

---

italic = common side effects   ***bold italic*** = life-threatening reactions

GI: Abdominal pain, anorexia, constipation, dyspepsia, *nausea (16%), vomiting*

GU: Vaginitis

MS: Arthralgia, tendon rupture

SKIN: Alopecia, photosensitivity, pruritus, rash, sweating

INTERACTIONS

Drugs

▪ *Antacids:* Reduced absorption of grepafloxacin; do not take within 4 hr of dose

▪ *Benzodiazepines:* May increase serum concentrations of benzodiazepines

▪ *β-Adrenergic blockers:* May increase serum concentrations of hepatically metabolized β-adrenergic blockers

▪ *Caffeine:* Inhibits metabolism of caffeine

▪ *Cyclosporine:* Inhibits metabolism of cyclosporine

▪ *Iron:* Reduced absorption of grepafloxacin; do not take within 4 hr of dose

▪ *Sucralfate:* Reduced absorption of grepafloxacin; do not take within 4 hr of dose

▪ *Theobromine:* Inhibits metabolism of theobromine

▪ *Theophylline:* Inhibits metabolism of theophylline; cut maintenance theophylline dose in half during therapy with grepafloxacin

▪ *Warfarin:* May increase hypoprothrombinemic response to warfarin

▪ *Zinc:* Reduced absorption of grepafloxacin; do not take within 4 hr of dose

Labs

• *Interference:* Urine coproporphyrin, urine uroporphyrin

SPECIAL CONSIDERATIONS
PATIENT/FAMILY EDUCATION

• Do not take antacids or iron within 4 hr of taking grepafloxacin

* = non-FDA-approved use

griseofulvin

(gri-see-oh-ful'vin)

Rx: Fulvicin P/G, Fulvicin-U/F, Grifulvin V, Grisactin, Grisactin 500, Grisactin-Ultra, Gris-PEG
Chemical Class: Penicillium *griseofulvum* derivative
Therapeutic Class: Antifungal

CLINICAL PHARMACOLOGY

Mechanism of Action: Deposited in the keratin precursor cells, which are gradually exfoliated and replaced by non-infected tissue; has a greater affinity for diseased tissue; tightly bound to the new keratin, which becomes highly resistant to fungal invasions

Pharmacokinetics

PO: GI absorption exhibits high interindividual variability; absorption increased by meals with high fat content; ultramicrosize absorbed 1.5 times more efficiently than conventional microsized formulation; peak 4 hr, $t_{1/2}$ 9-24 hr; metabolized in liver; excreted in urine (inactive metabolites), feces, perspiration

INDICATIONS AND USES: Fungal infections of the skin, hair, and nails (i.e., tinea corporis, tinea pedis, tinea cruris, tinea barbae, tinea capitis, and tinea unguium) caused by susceptible organisms

Antifungal spectrum usually includes: *Trichophyton rubrum, T. tonsurans, T. mentagrophytes, T. interdigitalis, T. verrucosum, T. megninii, T. gallinae, T. crateriform, T. sulphureum, T. schoenleinii, Microsporum audouinii, M. canis, M. gypseum, Epidermophyton floccosum*

DOSAGE
Adult
• PO (microsize) 500-1000 mg/day in single or divided doses; (ultramicrosize) 330-375 mg/day in single or divided doses, max 750 mg/day
Child ≥2 yr
• PO (microsize) 10-15 mg/kg/day in single or divided doses; (ultramicrosize) 5.5-7.3 mg/kg/day in single or divided doses
Duration
• *Tinea corporis:* 2-4 wk
• *Tinea capitis:* At least 4-6 wk
• *Tinea pedis:* 4-8 wk
• *Tinea unguium:* 3-6 mo
💲 AVAILABLE FORMS/COST OF THERAPY
Microsize
• Cap, Gel—Oral: 250 mg, 100's: **$87.68**
• Susp—Oral: 125 mg/5 ml, 120 ml: **$31.10-$33.99**
• Tab, Uncoated—Oral: 250 mg, 100's: **$59.25-$80.16**; 500 mg, 100's: **$162.88**
Ultramicrosize
• Tab, Uncoated—Oral: 125 mg, 100's: **$33.11-$63.30**; 165 mg, 100's: **$47.65-$85.19**; 250 mg, 100's: **$64.96-$125.00**; 330 mg, 100's: **$82.25-$157.73**
CONTRAINDICATIONS: Porphyria, hepatocellular failure
PRECAUTIONS: Penicillin allergy (possible cross-sensitivity), lupus erythematosus
PREGNANCY AND LACTATION: Pregnancy category C; since the use of an antifungal is seldom essential during pregnancy, avoid use during this time; excretion into breast milk unknown; use caution in nursing mothers
SIDE EFFECTS/ADVERSE REACTIONS
CNS: Dizziness, fatigue, headache, insomnia, mental confusion, paresthesias (chronic use)
GI: Diarrhea, epigastric distress, **GI bleeding, hepatic toxicity,** nausea, oral thrush, vomiting
GU: Menstrual irregularities, proteinuria
HEME: **Granulocytopenia, leukopenia**
SKIN: Angioneurotic edema, photosensitivity, *rash, urticaria*
INTERACTIONS
Drugs
⚅ *Aspirin:* Reduces plasma salicylate level
⚅ *Cyclosporine:* Reduces plasma cyclosporine level
⚅ *Oral contraceptives:* Menstrual irregularities, increased risk of pregnancy possible
⚅ *Phenobarbital:* Reduces plasma griseofulvin level
⚅ *Tacrolimus:* Reduces plasma tacrolimus level
⚅ *Warfarin:* Reduces anticoagulant response
SPECIAL CONSIDERATIONS
• Prior to therapy, the type of fungus responsible for the infection should be identified
PATIENT/FAMILY EDUCATION
• Response to therapy may not be apparent for some time; complete entire course of therapy
• Avoid prolonged exposure to sunlight or sunlamps
• Notify clinician if sore throat or skin rash occurs
• Store oral suspensions at room temp in light-resistant container
MONITORING PARAMETERS
• Periodic assessments of renal, hepatic, and hematopoietic function during prolonged therapy

---

italic = common side effects **bold italic** = life-threatening reactions

guaifenesin

(gwye-fen´e-sin)

Rx: Allfen, Amibid LA, Aquamist, Bidex, Duratuss G, Fenesin, GG-200 NR, Ganidin NR, Gua-SR, Guaibid-LA, Guaifenesin Expectorant, Guaifenesin LA, Guaifenesin-SR, Guaifenex G, Guaifenex LA, Humavent LA, Humibid LA, Humibid Pediatric, Iofen-NR, Iophen-NR, Liquibid, Monafed, Muco-Fen 800, Muco-Fen 1200, Muco-Fen LA, Orgadin, Organ-1 NEF, Organidin NR, Pneumomist, Q-Bid LA, Respa-GF, Simumist-SR, Touro EX

OTC: Anti-Tuss, Breonesin, Genatuss, Glytuss, Guiatuss, Hytuss, Hytuss 2X, Mytussin, Naldecon Senior EX, Robitussin

Combinations

    Rx: with codeine (Guiatussin AC); with dextromethorphan (Guaibid-DM); with hydrocodone (Hycotuss); with phenylpropanolamine (Entex LA)

Chemical Class: Glyceryl derivative

Therapeutic Class: Expectorant; mucolytic

CLINICAL PHARMACOLOGY

Mechanism of Action: Supposedly increases the output of respiratory tract fluid by reducing adhesiveness and surface tension; promotes ciliary action and facilitates removal of viscous mucus; lack of convincing studies to document efficacy

Pharmacokinetics

PO: Readily absorbed from GI tract; rapidly metabolized, excreted in urine; $t_{1/2}$ 1 hr

INDICATIONS AND USES: Dry, non-productive cough; sinusitis*

DOSAGE

Adult

• PO 100-400 mg q4-6h or 600 mg sustained release q12h, not to exceed 2.4 g/day

Child

• PO (6-12 yr) 100-200 mg q4h, not to exceed 1.2 g/day; (2-6 yr) 50-100 mg q4h, not to exceed 600 mg/day

$ **AVAILABLE FORMS/COST OF THERAPY**

• Cap—Oral: 200 mg, 100's: **$14.91-$18.79**

• Cap, Sus Action—Oral: 300 mg, 100's: **$55.73**

• Liq—Oral: 100 mg/5 ml, 480 ml: **$2.69-$125.17**; 200 mg/5 ml, 120 ml: **$5.96**

• Tab—Oral: 100 mg, 100's: **$9.21**; 200 mg, 100's: **$10.94-$48.98**

• Tab, Sus Action—Oral: 575 mg, 100's: **$43.00**; 600 mg 100's: **$12.80-$58.03**; 800 mg, 100's: **$26.29-$35.38**; 1000 mg, 100's: **$29.99-$60.70**; 1200 mg, 100's: **$32.25-$73.70**

PRECAUTIONS: Recurrent cough; cough associated with fever, rash, persistant headache, excessive secretions

PREGNANCY AND LACTATION: Pregnancy category C; excretion into breast milk unknown

SIDE EFFECTS/ADVERSE REACTIONS

CNS: Dizziness, drowsiness, headache

GI: Nausea, stomach pain, *vomiting*

SKIN: Rash

INTERACTIONS

Labs

• *Interference:* Urine 5-HIAA, VMA

SPECIAL CONSIDERATIONS
PATIENT/FAMILY EDUCATION

• Drink a full glass of water with each dose to help further loosen mucus

• Notify clinician if cough persists after medication has been used for 7 days or cough is associated with headache, high fever, skin rash, or sore throat

---

guanabenz
(gwan′a-benz)

Rx: Wytensin
Chemical Class: Dichlorobenzene derivative
Therapeutic Class: Antihypertensive, centrally acting sympathoplegic

CLINICAL PHARMACOLOGY

Mechanism of Action: Stimulates central α_2-adrenergic receptors resulting in reduced sympathetic outflow from the CNS to the heart, kidneys, and peripheral vasculature; decreases systolic and diastolic blood pressure, and pulse

Pharmacokinetics

PO: 75% bioavailable; onset 1 hr, duration 12 hr; 90% bound to plasma proteins; extensive metabolism excreted in urine (1% unchanged); $t_{1/2}$ approximately 7-10 hr

INDICATIONS AND USES: Hypertension

DOSAGE

Adult

• PO 4 mg bid initially, increase in 4-8 mg/day increments q1-2 wk prn, not to exceed 32 mg bid

⑤ AVAILABLE FORMS/COST OF THERAPY

• Tab, Uncoated—Oral: 4 mg, 100's: **$53.20-$98.55**; 8 mg, 100's: **$67.60-$135.75**

PRECAUTIONS: Severe coronary insufficiency, recent MI, cerebrovascular disease; severe renal, hepatic dysfunction; sudden discontinuation

PREGNANCY AND LACTATION: Pregnancy category C; excretion into breast milk unknown; use caution in nursing mothers

SIDE EFFECTS/ADVERSE REACTIONS

CNS: Anxiety, ataxia, depression, *dizziness, drowsiness, headache, sedation,* sleep disturbance, *weakness*
CV: Chest pain, dysrhythmias, edema, palpitations, ***rebound hypertension with abrupt cessation***
EENT: Blurred vision, nasal congestion
GI: Abdominal discomfort, constipation, diarrhea, *dry mouth,* epigastric pain, nausea, taste disorder, vomiting
GU: Disturbances of sexual function, urinary frequency
METAB: Gynecomastia
MS: Myalgias
RESP: Dyspnea
SKIN: Pruritis, rash

INTERACTIONS

Drugs

3 *β-blockers:* Rebound hypertension from guanabenz withdrawal exacerbated by noncardioselective β-blockers
3 *Tricyclic antidepressants:* Inhibit the antihypertensive response

SPECIAL CONSIDERATIONS
PATIENT/FAMILY EDUCATION

• Avoid hazardous activities, since drug may cause drowsiness
• Do not discontinue oral drug abruptly, or withdrawal symptoms may occur (anxiety, increased BP, headache, insomnia, increased pulse, tremors, nausea, sweating)
• Do not use OTC (cough, cold, or allergy) products unless directed by clinician

---

italic = common side effects   ***bold italic*** = life-threatening reactions

• Rise slowly to sitting or standing position to minimize orthostatic hypotension, especially elderly
• May cause dizziness, fainting, lightheadedness during 1st few days of therapy
• May cause dry mouth; use hard candy, saliva product, or frequent rinsing of mouth

MONITORING PARAMETERS

• Blood pressure (posturally), mental depression

---

guanadrel

(gwahn'a-drel)

Rx: Hylorel

Chemical Class: Guanidine derivative

Therapeutic Class: Antihypertensive, postganglionic adrenergic neuron inhibitor

---

CLINICAL PHARMACOLOGY

Mechanism of Action: Adrenergic neuron inhibitor: lowers arterial pressure secondary to decreased peripheral vascular resistance and cardiac output by depletion of catecholamines from adrenergic nerve endings, the myocardium, and vascular walls; hypotensive effects most pronounced in the erect position; approximately one-third as potent as guanethidine

Pharmacokinetics

PO: Peak levels 1½-2 hr, onset 2 hr, duration 4-14 hr; <20% bound to plasma proteins; metabolized in liver, excreted in urine (40% as unchanged drug); $t_{1/2}$ approximately 10 hr (high interindividual variation)

INDICATIONS AND USES: Hypertension (not 1st-line) thyrotoxicosis*

DOSAGE

Adult

• PO 10 mg/day as a single dose or divided bid; usual range 20-75 mg/day generally divided bid-qid
• *Renal function impairment:* CrCl 30-60 ml/min, 5 mg qd; CrCl <30 ml/min, 5 mg qod

§ AVAILABLE FORMS/COST OF THERAPY

• Tab, Uncoated—Oral: 10 mg, 100's: **$74.87-$181.58**; 25 mg, 100's: **$108.36**

CONTRAINDICATIONS: Pheochromocytoma, CHF, concurrent use with or within 1 wk of MAOI

PRECAUTIONS: Cerebral vascular disease, CAD, elective surgery, orthostatic hypotension, asthma, renal function impairment, children, peptic ulcer, elderly, diabetes (causes hypoglycemia unawareness)

PREGNANCY AND LACTATION: Pregnancy category B; excretion into breast milk unknown; use caution in nursing mothers

SIDE EFFECTS/ADVERSE REACTIONS

CNS: Confusion, depression, drowsiness, faintness, fatigue, headache, paresthesias, psychological problems, sleep disorder

CV: Bradycardia, chest pain, *CHF, orthostatic hypotension,* palpitations, *peripheral edema,* syncope

EENT: Double vision, dry burning eyes, *nasal stuffiness,* sore throat, *tinnitus,* visual changes

GI: Abdominal pain, anorexia, *constipation,* dry throat; glossitis, *increased bowel movements,* nausea, vomiting

GU: Ejaculation disturbances, impotence, hematuria; *nocturia; urinary frequency,* urgency

MS: Aching limbs, joint pain, leg cramps

RESP: Bronchospasm

---

* = non-FDA-approved use

SKIN: Alopecia, purpura, rash
MISC: Weight gain, loss

INTERACTIONS
Drugs
❷ *Amitriptyline:* Inhibits antihypertensive effect

❸ *Dextroamphetamine:* Inhibits antihypertensive effect

❸ *Ephedrine:* Inhibits antihypertensive effect

❸ *MAOIs:* Inhibits antihypertensive effect

❸ *Methylphenidate:* Inhibits antihypertensive effect

❸ *Norepinephrine:* Exaggerated pressor response to norepinephrine

❸ *Phenothiazines:* Inhibits antihypertensive effect

❸ *Tricyclic antidepressants:* Inhibit antihypertensive effect

Labs
• *Increase:* BUN
• *Decrease:* Urinary VMA excretion

SPECIAL CONSIDERATIONS
PATIENT/FAMILY EDUCATION
• Arise slowly from a reclining position, especially in the morning
• Avoid OTC medications except as directed by clinician
• Avoid driving, hazardous activities if drowsiness occurs
• Use alcohol with caution
• Use caution when standing for prolonged periods, exercising, and during hot weather (enhanced orthostatic hypotension)
• Do not discontinue abruptly

MONITORING PARAMETERS
• Sitting and standing blood pressure, pulse, weight, edema

guanethidine
(gwahn-eth'i-deen)
Rx: Ismelin
Chemical Class: Guanidine derivative
Therapeutic Class: Antihypertensive, postganglionic adrenergic neuron inhibitor

CLINICAL PHARMACOLOGY
Mechanism of Action: Adrenergic neuron inhibitor: lowers arterial pressure secondary to decreased peripheral vascular resistance and cardiac output by depletion of catecholamines from adrenergic nerve endings, the myocardium, and vascular walls; hypotensive effects most pronounced in the erect position

Pharmacokinetics
PO: Oral absorption highly variable (3%-50%), maximum hypotensive response in 14 days; metabolized in liver, excreted in urine (25%-50% as unchanged drug); $t_{1/2}$ 5-10 days

INDICATIONS AND USES: Hypertension (not 1st-line), angina (add on),* bladder instability,* exophthalmos,* glaucoma

DOSAGE
Adult
• *Ambulatory patients:* PO 10 mg qd, increase at 5-7 day intervals to a max of 25-50 mg/day
• *Hospitalized patients:* PO 25-50 mg qd; increase by 25-50 mg/day to desired therapeutic response

Child
• PO 0.2 mg/kg/day; increase by 0.2 mg/kg/day at 7-10 day intervals to a max of 3 mg/kg/day

💲 AVAILABLE FORMS/COST OF THERAPY
• Tab, Uncoated—Oral: 10 mg, 100's: **$62.82**; 25 mg, 100's: **$107.69**

---

italic = common side effects   ***bold italic*** = life-threatening reactions

CONTRAINDICATIONS: Pheochromocytoma, CHF, concurrent use with or within 1 wk of MAOI

PRECAUTIONS: Elective surgery (discontinue 2 wk prior to procedure), fever (reduced dosage requirements), asthma, recent MI, CAD, peptic ulcer, elderly, orthostatic hypotension, renal dysfunction, sexual dysfunction

PREGNANCY AND LACTATION: Pregnancy category C; breast milk excretion unknown

SIDE EFFECTS/ADVERSE REACTIONS

CNS: Dizziness, fatigue, *lassitude,* mental depression, tremor, *weakness*

CV: Angina, *bradycardia,* **CHF,** edema, fluid retention, *orthostatic hypotension,* syncope

EENT: Blurred vision, *nasal congestion,* ptosis, unpleasant taste

GI: Diarrhea, dry mouth, nausea, parotid tenderness, vomiting

GU: Impotence, *inhibition of ejaculation,* nocturia, priapism, rise in BUN, urinary incontinence, urinary retention

HEME: Anemia, *leukopenia, thrombocytopenia*

METAB: Weight gain, hyperglycemia

MS: Myalgia, myopathy

RESP: Asthma, dyspnea

SKIN: Alopecia, dermatitis

INTERACTIONS

Drugs

❷ *Amitriptyline:* Inhibits antihypertensive effect

❸ *Dextroamphetamine:* Inhibits antihypertensive effect

❸ *Ephedrine:* Inhibits antihypertensive effect

❸ *Haloperidol:* Inhibits antihypertensive effect

❸ *MAOIs:* Inhibits antihypertensive effect

❸ *Methylphenidate:* Inhibits antihypertensive effect

❸ *Norepinephrine:* Exaggerated pressor response to norepinephrine

❸ *Phenothiazines:* Inhibits antihypertensive effect

❸ *Phenylephrine:* Guanethidine enhances pupillary response to phenylephrine

❸ *Thiothixene:* Inhibits antihypertensive effect

❸ *Tricyclic antidepressants:* Inhibits antihypertensive effect

Labs

• *Increase:* BUN

• *Decrease:* Urinary VMA excretion

SPECIAL CONSIDERATIONS

PATIENT/FAMILY EDUCATION

• Arise slowly from a reclining position, especially in the morning

• Use alcohol with caution

• Use caution when standing for prolonged periods of time, exercising, and during hot weather (enhanced orthostatic hypotension)

• Avoid OTC medications unless discussed with clinician

• Avoid driving; hazardous activities if drowsiness occurs

• Do not discontinue abruptly

MONITORING PARAMETERS

• Sitting and standing blood pressure, pulse, weight, edema

guanfacine

(gwan'fa-seen)

Rx: Tenex

Chemical Class: Phenylacyl guanidine

Therapeutic Class: Antihypertensive, centrally acting sympathoplegic

CLINICAL PHARMACOLOGY

Mechanism of Action: Centrally acting antihypertensive stimulates central α_2-adrenergic receptors resulting in reduced sympathetic outflow from the CNS to the heart, kidneys, and peripheral vasculature; decreases systolic and diastolic blood pressure and pulse; considered more selective α-2 receptor agonist than clonidine; no dopamine inhibition; does not activate opiate receptors

Pharmacokinetics

PO: Bioavailability 80%; peak concentration 1-4 hr, onset (multiple doses) 1 wk, 70% bound to plasma proteins, 50% bound to erythrocytes; metabolized in liver, excreted in urine (40%-75% as unchanged drug); $t_{1/2}$ 17 hr

INDICATIONS AND USES: Hypertension, heroin withdrawal syndrome,* migraine headache*

DOSAGE

Adult

• PO 1 mg qd, increase to 2 mg qd after 3-4 wk prn

💲 AVAILABLE FORMS/COST OF THERAPY

• Tab, Uncoated—Oral: 1 mg, 100's: **$70.55-$120.60**; 2 mg, 100's: **$96.75-$165.33**

PRECAUTIONS: Chronic renal or hepatic failure, severe coronary insufficiency, recent MI, cerebrovascular disease

PREGNANCY AND LACTATION: Pregnancy category B; excretion into human breast milk unknown

SIDE EFFECTS/ADVERSE REACTIONS

CNS: Dizziness, fatigue, headache, somnolence, amnesia, depression

CV: Bradycardia, chest pain, palpitations, orthostatic hypotension/withdrawal symptoms—rebound phenomenon (hypertension and sympathetic overactivity)

EENT: Nasal congestion, rhinitis, taste change, tinnitus, vision change

GI: Constipation, cramps, diarrhea, *dry mouth,* nausea

GU: Impotence, urinary incontinence

MS: Leg cramps

RESP: Dyspnea

SKIN: Dermatitis, pruritus, purpura

INTERACTIONS

Drugs

🔼 *β-blockers:* Rebound hypertension from guanfacine withdrawal exacerbated by noncardioselective β-blockers

🔼 *Cyclosporine, tacrolimus:* Increased immunosuppressant plasma levels

🔼 *Insulin, sulfonylureas hypoglycemics:* Diminished symptoms of hypoglycemia

🔼 *Neuroleptics, nitroprusside:* Severe hypotension possible

🔼 *Tricyclic antidepressants:* Inhibit the antihypertensive response

SPECIAL CONSIDERATIONS

PATIENT/FAMILY EDUCATION

• Avoid hazardous activities, since drug may cause drowsiness

• Do not discontinue oral drug abruptly, or withdrawal symptoms may occur after 3-4 days (anxiety, increased BP, headache, insomnia, increased pulse, tremors, nausea, sweating)

• Do not use OTC (cough, cold, or allergy) products unless directed by clinician

• Rise slowly to sitting or standing position to minimize orthostatic hypotension, especially elderly

• Dizziness, fainting, lightheadedness may occur during 1st few days of therapy

• May cause dry mouth; use hard candy, saliva product, or frequent rinsing of mouth

MONITORING PARAMETERS

• Blood pressure (posturally), blood glucose in patients with diabetes mellitus; confusion, mental depression

---

halazepam
(hal-az′e-pam)
Rx: Paxipam
Chemical Class: Benzodiazepine
Therapeutic Class: Anxiolytic
DEA Class: Schedule IV

CLINICAL PHARMACOLOGY

Mechanism of Action: CNS depressants via facilitation of inhibitory GABA at benzodiazepine receptor sites (BZ_1—associated with sleep; BZ_2—associated with memory, motor, sensory, and cognitive function); effects include muscle relaxation (spinal cord), anticonvulsant activity (brain stem), ataxia (cerebellum), emotional behavior (limbic and cortical areas), and anxiolytic effects (separate from general CNS depression)

Pharmacokinetics

PO: Peak 1-3 hr; metabolized by the liver to active metabolites, eliminated in urine; $t_{1/2}$ 14 hr

INDICATIONS AND USES: Anxiety

DOSAGE

Adult

• PO 20-40 mg tid-qid

Geriatric

• PO 20 mg qd-bid

§ AVAILABLE FORMS/COST OF THERAPY

• Tab, Uncoated—Oral: 20 mg, 100's: **$58.14**; 40 mg, 100's: **$80.81**

CONTRAINDICATIONS: Narrow angle glaucoma, psychosis, pregnancy

PRECAUTIONS: Elderly, debilitated, hepatic disease, renal disease, history of drug abuse, abrupt withdrawal, respiratory depression

PREGNANCY AND LACTATION: Pregnancy category D; may cause fetal damage when administered during pregnancy; excreted into breast milk; may accumulate in breast-fed infants and is therefore not recommended

SIDE EFFECTS/ADVERSE REACTIONS

CNS: Abnormal thinking, agitation, amnesia, anxiety, apathy, *asthenia,* ataxia, decreased reflexes, decreased libido, emotional lability, hangover, hostility, *hypokinesia,* neuritis, seizures, sleep disorder, *somnolence,* stupor, twitch

CV: Dysrhythmia, syncope

EENT: Ear pain, epistaxis, eye irritation, pain, swelling; pharyngitis, photophobia, rhinitis, sinusitis

GI: Abdominal pain, decreased, increased appetite; dyspepsia, enterocolitis, flatulence, gastritis, increased serum transaminase levels, melena, mouth ulceration

GU: Frequent urination, hematuria, itching, menstrual cramps, nocturia, oliguria, penile discharge, urinary hesitancy, urgency; urinary incontinence, vaginal discharge

HEME: Agranulocytosis

MS: Back pain, lower extremity pain

RESP: Asthma, cold symptoms, cough, dyspnea, hyperventilation
SKIN: Acne, dry skin, photosensitivity, urticaria

INTERACTIONS
Drugs

⬛ *Carbamazepine:* Markedly reduces effect of halazepam

⬛ *Cimetidine:* Inhibits hepatic metabolism of halazepam

⬛ *Ciprofloxacin:* Inhibits hepatic metabolism of halazepam; may also competitively inhibit gamma amino butyric acid receptors

❷ *Clarithromycin:* Inhibits hepatic metabolism of halazepam

⬛ *Clozapine:* Additive respiratory and cardiovascular depression

⬛ *Delavirdine:* Inhibits hepatic metabolism of halazepam

⬛ *Disulfiram:* Inhibits hepatic metabolism of halazepam

⬛ *Erythromycin:* Inhibits hepatic metabolism of halazepam

⬛ *Ethanol:* Additive CNS effects

⬛ *Fluconazole:* Inhibits hepatic metabolism of halazepam

⬛ *Fluoxetine:* Inhibits hepatic metabolism of halazepam

⬛ *Fluvoxamine:* Inhibits hepatic metabolism of halazepam

⬛ *Isoniazid:* Inhibits hepatic metabolism of halazepam

⬛ *Itraconazole:* Inhibits hepatic metabolism of halazepam

⬛ *Ketoconazole:* Inhibits hepatic metabolism of halazepam

⬛ *Levodopa:* May reduce anti-Parkinsonian effect

⬛ *Metoprolol:* Inhibits hepatic metabolism of halazepam

⬛ *Omeprazole:* Inhibits hepatic metabolism of halazepam

⬛ *Phenytoin:* Markedly reduces effect of halazepam

⬛ *Quinolones:* Inhibits hepatic metabolism of halazepam; may also competitively inhibit gamma amino butyric acid receptors

⬛ *Rifampin:* Markedly reduces effect of halazepam

⬛ *Troleandomycin:* Inhibits hepatic metabolism of halazepam

SPECIAL CONSIDERATIONS
PATIENT/FAMILY EDUCATION

• Avoid alcohol and other CNS depressants

• Do not discontinue abruptly after prolonged therapy

• May cause drowsiness or dizziness, use caution while driving or performing other tasks requiring alertness

• Inform clinician if you are planning to become pregnant, you are pregnant, or if you become pregnant while taking this medicine

• May be habit forming

MONITORING PARAMETERS

• Periodic CBC, UA, blood chemistry analyses during prolonged therapy

---

halcinonide

(hal-sin′o-nide)
Rx: Halog, Halog-E
Chemical Class: Synthetic glucocorticoid
Therapeutic Class: Topical corticosteroid, high potency

CLINICAL PHARMACOLOGY
Mechanism of Action: Depresses formation, release, and activity of endogenous mediators of inflammation such as prostaglandins, kinins, histamine, liposomal enzymes, and the complement system resulting in decreased edema, erythema, and pruritus

Pharmacokinetics

Absorbed through the skin (increased by inflammation and occlusive dressings); metabolized primarily in the liver

---

italic = common side effects

bold italic = life-threatening reactions

INDICATIONS AND USES: Psoriasis, eczema, contact dermatitis, pruritus

DOSAGE

Adult and Child

• Top apply to affected area bid-tid, rub completely into skin

§ **AVAILABLE FORMS/COST OF THERAPY**

• Cre—Top: 0.1%, 15, 30, 60, 240 g: **$38.60**/30 g

• Oint—Top: 0.1%, 15, 30, 60, 240 g: **$38.60**/30 g

• Sol—Top: 0.1%, 20, 60 ml: **$28.44**/20 ml

CONTRAINDICATIONS: Fungal infections; use on face, groin, or axilla

PRECAUTIONS: Viral infections, bacterial infections, children

PREGNANCY AND LACTATION: Pregnancy category C; unknown whether top application could result in sufficient systemic absorption to produce detectable amounts in breast milk (systemic corticosteroids are secreted into breast milk in quantities not likely to have detrimental effects on infant)

SIDE EFFECTS/ADVERSE REACTIONS

SKIN: Acne, allergic contact dermatitis, atrophy, burning, dryness, folliculitis, hypertrichosis, hypopigmentation, irritation, itching, miliaria, perioral dermatitis, secondary infection, striae

MISC: Systemic absorption of topical corticosteroids has produced reversible HPA axis suppression (more likely with occlusive dressings, prolonged administration, application to large surface areas, liver failure, and in children)

SPECIAL CONSIDERATIONS

PATIENT/FAMILY EDUCATION

• Apply sparingly only to affected area

• Avoid contact with the eyes

• Do not put bandages or dressings over treated area unless directed by clinician

• Do not use on weeping, denuded, or infected areas

• Discontinue drug, notify clinician if local irritation or fever develops

---

halobetasol

(hal-oh-be′ta-sol)

Rx: Ultravate

Chemical Class: Synthetic glucocorticoid

Therapeutic Class: Topical corticosteroid, very high potency

CLINICAL PHARMACOLOGY

Mechanism of Action: Depresses formation, release, and activity of endogenous mediators of inflammation such as prostaglandins, kinins, histamine, liposomal enzymes, and the complement system resulting in decreased edema, erythema, and pruritus

Pharmacokinetics

Absorbed through the skin (increased by inflammation and occlusive dressings); metabolized primarily in the liver

INDICATIONS AND USES: Psoriasis, eczema, contact dermatitis, pruritus

DOSAGE

Adult and Child

• Top apply to affected area bid-tid, rub completely into skin; total dosage should not exceed 50 g/wk because of the drug's potential to suppress the hypothalamic-pituitary-adrenal (HPA) axis; treatment beyond 2 consecutive wk not recommended

AVAILABLE FORMS/COST OF THERAPY

• Cre—Top: 0.05%, 15, 50 g: **$27.25-$31.90**/15 g
• Oint—Top: 0.05%, 15, 50 g: **$31.90**/15 g

CONTRAINDICATIONS: Fungal infections; use on face, groin, or axilla; occlusive dressings

PRECAUTIONS: Viral infections, bacterial infections, children

PREGNANCY AND LACTATION: Pregnancy category C; unknown whether top application could result in sufficient systemic absorption to produce detectable amounts in breast milk (systemic corticosteroids are secreted into breast milk in quantities not likely to have detrimental effects on infant)

SIDE EFFECTS/ADVERSE REACTIONS

SKIN: Acne, allergic contact dermatitis, atrophy, burning, dryness, folliculitis, hypertrichosis, hypopigmentation, irritation, itching, miliaria, perioral dermatitis, secondary infection, striae

MISC: Systemic absorption of topical corticosteroids has produced reversible HPA axis suppression (more likely with occlusive dressings, prolonged administration, application to large surface areas, liver failure, and in children)

SPECIAL CONSIDERATIONS
PATIENT/FAMILY EDUCATION

• Apply sparingly only to affected area
• Avoid contact with the eyes
• Do not put bandages or dressings over treated area
• Do not use on weeping, denuded, or infected areas
• Discontinue drug, notify clinician if local irritation or fever develops
• Treatment should be limited to 2 wk, and amounts greater than 50 g/wk should not be used

---

haloperidol

(ha-loe-per'idole)
Rx: Haldol
Chemical Class: Butyrophenone derivative
Therapeutic Class: Antipsychotic

CLINICAL PHARMACOLOGY

Mechanism of Action: Dopamine receptor antagonist, with higher affinity for D_2- over D_1-receptors, and variable selectivity among the cortical dopamine tracts; also activity on nondopaminergic sites, i.e., cholinergic, α_1-adrenergic and histaminic receptors (explaining side effects); high risk extrapyramidal reactions; minimal orthostatic hypotension, sedation, and anticholinergic effects

Pharmacokinetics

PO: Peak 3-6 hr, $t_{1/2}$ 17 hr
IM: Peak 10-20 min, $t_{1/2}$ 17 hr
IM: (decanoate): Peak 3-9 days, $t_{1/2}$ approximately 3 wk
>90% bound to plasma proteins, metabolized by the liver, excreted in urine and feces

INDICATIONS AND USES: Psychosis, Gilles de la Tourette syndrome, severe behavioral problems, hyperactive children (short-term), prolonged parenteral neuroleptic therapy for chronic schizophrenia (decanoate), antiemetic* (small doses)

DOSAGE

NOTE: 2 mg equivalent to chlorpromazine 100 mg

Adult and child >16 yr

• *Psychosis/Tourette's syndrome:* PO 0.5-5 mg bid or tid initially depending on severity of condition, dose is increased to desired dose, max 100 mg/day; IM 2-5 mg q1-8h

---

italic = common side effects   ***bold italic*** = life-threatening reactions

• *Chronic schizophrenia:* IM 10-15 times the individual patient's stabilized PO dose q4 wk (decanoate)

Child 3-12 yr

• *Psychosis:* PO/IM 0.05-0.15 mg/kg/day in 2-3 divided doses

• *Tourette's syndrome:* PO 0.05-0.075 mg/kg/day in 2-3 divided doses

• *Hyperactivity:* PO 0.05-0.075 mg/kg/day in 2-3 divided doses

$ AVAILABLE FORMS/COST OF THERAPY

• Conc—Oral: 2 mg/ml, 15, 120 ml: **$15.00-$120.07**/120 ml

• Inj, Sol—IM: 5 mg/ml, 1, 10 ml: **$1.50-$8.91**/1 ml

• Inj, Sol—IM (decanoate): 50 mg/ml, 1, 5 ml: **$27.00-$37.50**; 100 mg/ml, 1, 5 ml: **$49.50-$68.94**/1 ml

• Tab, Uncoated—Oral: 0.5 mg, 100's: **$6.75-$46.70**; 1 mg, 100's: **$7.95-$69.12**; 2 mg, 100's: **$10.95-$95.34**; 5 mg, 100's: **$16.00-$155.83**; 10 mg, 100's: **$22.50-$199.91**; 20 mg, 100's: **$53.00-$387.36**

CONTRAINDICATIONS: Severe toxic CNS depression, comatose states from any cause, Parkinson's disease

PRECAUTIONS: Elderly, severe cardiac disorders, seizure disorder, hepatic dysfunction, child <3 yr, alcohol withdrawal, electroconvulsive therapy, abrupt withdrawal, glaucoma, COPD

PREGNANCY AND LACTATION: Pregnancy category C; has been used for hyperemesis gravidarum, chorea gravidarum, and manic-depressive illness during pregnancy; excreted into breast milk; effect on nursing infant unknown, but may be of concern

SIDE EFFECTS/ADVERSE REACTIONS

CNS: Agitation, anxiety, catatonic-like behavioral states, confusion, depression, *drowsiness, EPS (pseudoparkinsonism, akathisia, dystonia, tardive dyskinesia),* euphoria, exacerbation of psychotic symptoms including hallucinations, *headache,* insomnia, lethargy, **neuroleptic malignant syndrome,** restlessness, *seizures,* vertigo

CV: ECG changes, hypertension, hypotension, *tachycardia*

EENT: Blurred vision, cataracts, dry eyes, glaucoma, retinopathy

GI: Anorexia, constipation, diarrhea, *dry mouth,* dyspepsia, hypersalivation, *nausea,* vomiting

GU: Priapism, urinary retention

HEME: **Agranulocytosis,** anemia, leukocytosis, minimal decreases in red blood cell counts, transient leukopenia

METAB: Breast engorgement, gynecomastia, hyperglycemia, hyperprolactinemia, hypoglycemia, hyponatremia, impotence, increased libido, lactation, mastalgia, menstrual irregularities

RESP: Bronchospasm, increased depth of respiration, laryngospasm

SKIN: Diaphoresis, isolated cases of photosensitivity, loss of hair, maculopapular and acneiform skin reactions

INTERACTIONS

Drugs

3 *Anticholinergics:* Inhibition of therapeutic effect of neuroleptics

3 *Barbiturates:* Potential reduction of serum neuroleptic concentrations

3 *Bromocriptine:* Inhibition of bromocriptine's ability to lower serum prolactin concentrations in patients with pituitary adenoma; theoretical inhibition of antipsychotic effects of neuroleptics

---

* = non-FDA-approved use

▪ *Carbamazepine:* Decreased serum haloperidol concentrations
▪ *Guanethidine:* Inhibition of antihypertensive effect of guanethidine
❷ *Levodopa:* Inhibition of antiparkinsonian effects of levodopa
▪ *Lithium:* Rare reports of severe neurotoxicity in patients receiving lithium and neuroleptics
▪ *Quinidine:* Increases haldol concentrations; increased risk of toxicity

SPECIAL CONSIDERATIONS
PATIENT/FAMILY EDUCATION
• Do not mix liquid formulation with coffee or tea
• Use calibrated dropper
• Take with food or milk
• Arise slowly from reclining position
• Do not discontinue abruptly
• Use a sunscreen during sun exposure to prevent burns
• Take special precautions to stay cool in hot weather

MONITORING PARAMETERS
• Observe closely for signs of tardive dyskinesia

---

heparin
(hep′a-rin)
Rx: Heparin
Chemical Class: Sulfated glycosaminoglycan
Therapeutic Class: Anticoagulant

CLINICAL PHARMACOLOGY
Mechanism of Action: Potentiates inhibitory action of antithrombin III (heparin cofactor) on several activated coagulation factors, including thrombin (factor IIa) and factors IXa, Xa, XIa, and XIIa, by forming a complex with and inducing a conformational change in the antithrombin III molecule

Pharmacokinetics
IV: Onset immediate (if no loading dose is given, onset may depend on rate of INF)
SC: Onset 20-60 min
Highly bound to plasma proteins; primary route of removal from circulation via uptake by the reticuloendothelial system; also metabolized by liver, eliminated in urine usually as metabolites (50% of IV dose may be excreted unchanged); $t_{1/2}$ 90 min

INDICATIONS AND USES: Deep vein thrombosis (DVT), pulmonary embolism (PE), peripheral arterial embolism; coagulopathies (e.g., disseminated intravascular coagulation); DVT/PE prophylaxis; clotting prevention in arterial and heart surgery, blood transfusions, extracorporeal circulation, dialysis and blood samples; prophylaxis of LV thrombi and CVA after MI*; evolving stroke*; adjunctive therapy of coronary occlusion with acute MI*

DOSAGE
Adult
• *DVT/PE:* IV INF 80 U/kg bolus, then 18 U/kg/hr, adjust based on aPTT results; intermittent IV 10,000 U initially, then 75-125 U/kg q4-6h adjust based on aPTT results; SC 10,000-20,000 units initially, then 8000-10,000 U q8h, or 15,000-20,000 U q12h, adjust based on aPTT results drawn at mid-dosing interval
• *Prevention of DVT/PE:* SC 5000-7500 U q8-12h until patient is ambulatory
Child
• IV INF 50 U/kg initially, then 15-25 U/kg/hr, increase dose by 2-4 U/kg/hr q6-8h based on aPTT results; intermittent IV 50-100 U/kg initially, then 50-100 U/kg q4h adjust based on aPTT results

---

italic = common side effects   ***bold italic*** = life-threatening reactions

$ AVAILABLE FORMS/COST OF THERAPY

• Inj, Sol—IV, SC: 1000 U/ml, 1, 2, 10, 30 ml: **$0.54-$2.00**/ml; 2500 U/ml, 1 ml: **$0.95-$1.35**/ml; 5000 U/ml, 0.5, 1, 10, 20 ml: **$0.23-$1.61**/ml; 7500 U/ml, 1 ml: **$1.21-$2.15**/ml; 10,000 U/ml, 0.5, 1, 2, 4, 5, 10 ml: **$0.92-$4.75**/ml; 20,000 U/ml, 1, 2, 5 ml: **$2.76-$4.45**/ml; 40,000 U/ml, 1, 2, 5 ml: **$7.50**/ml

CONTRAINDICATIONS: Severe thrombocytopenia, uncontrolled bleeding (except when due to DIC), suspected intracranial hemorrhage, shock, severe hypotension

PRECAUTIONS: IM inj (avoid due to risk for hematoma), elderly, children, diabetes, renal insufficiency, severe hypertension, subacute bacterial endocarditis, acute nephritis, peptic ulcer disease, severe renal disease

PREGNANCY AND LACTATION: Pregnancy category C; does not cross the placenta, has major advantages over oral anticoagulants as the treatment of choice during pregnancy; is not excreted into breast milk due to its high molecular weight

SIDE EFFECTS/ADVERSE REACTIONS

CNS: Fever, headache

*CV: **Allergic vasospastic reactions, shock***

EENT: Lacrimation, rhinitis

GI: Nausea, vomiting

*GU: **Hematuria,** priapism*

*HEME: **Hemorrhage, heparin-induced thrombocytopenia (HIT), white clot syndrome (new thrombus formation associated with heparin administration)***

METAB: Rebound hyperlipidemia, suppressed aldosterone synthesis,

MS: Osteoporosis (after long-term, high doses)

*RESP: **Anaphylactoid reactions,** asthma*

SKIN: Chills, ***cutaneous necrosis,*** delayed transient alopecia, erythema, hematoma/ulceration, histamine-like reactions, local irritation, urticaria

INTERACTIONS

Drugs

$ *Aspirin:* Increased risk of hemorrhage

$ *Warfarin:* Warfarin may prolong the aPTT in patients receiving heparin; heparin may prolong the PT in patients receiving warfarin

SPECIAL CONSIDERATIONS

PATIENT/FAMILY EDUCATION

• Report any signs of bleeding: gums, under skin, urine, stools

MONITORING PARAMETERS

• aPTT (usual goal is to prolong aPTT to a value that corresponds to a plasma heparin level of 0.2 to 0.4 U/ml by protamine titration or to an antifactor Xa level of about 0.3 to 0.6 U/ml; this range must be determined for each individual laboratory), usually measure 6-8 hr after initiation of IV and 6-8 hr after INF rate changes; increase or decrease INF by 2-4 U/kg/hr dependent on aPTT

• For intermittent inj, measure aPTT 3.5-4 hr after IV inj

• Platelet counts, signs of bleeding, Hgb, hct

---

* = non-FDA-approved use

hydralazine

(hye-dral´a-zeen)

Rx: Apresoline
Combinations
Rx: with hydrochlorothiazide
(Apresazide); with hydro-
chlorothiazide, reserpine
(Ser-Ap-Es)
Chemical Class: Phthalazine
derivative
Therapeutic Class: Direct va-
sodilator antihypertensive;
congestive heart failure

CLINICAL PHARMACOLOGY

Mechanism of Action: Preferentially dilates arterioles with little effect on veins; interferes with calcium movement within vascular
smooth muscle responsible for initiating or maintaining the contractile
state; increases cardiac output, decreases systemic resistance, reduces
afterload

Pharmacokinetics

PO: Well absorbed; undergoes 1st-
pass metabolism; bioavailability
50% (slow acetylators) or 30% (fast
acetylators); peak 60 min, onset 45
min, duration 3-8 hr

IM: Onset 5-10 min, peak 1 hr, duration 2-4 hr

IV: Onset 10-20 min, duration 3-8 hr
Metabolized by liver (genetic variation among individuals in rate of
acetylation), excreted in urine; t₁/₂
0.44-0.47 hr (metabolite 2-4 hr)

INDICATIONS AND USES: Hyper-
tension, CHF,* afterload reduction
in severe aortic insufficiency and after valve replacement,* eclampsia*

DOSAGE

Adult

• PO 10 mg qid, increase by 10-25
mg/dose q2-5 days as needed to max
of 300 mg/day; IM/IV 10-20 mg q4-
6h, may increase to 40 mg/dose

Child

• PO 0.75-1 mg/kg/day divided bid-
qid, increase over 3-4 wk to 7.5
mg/kg/day divided bid-qid if necessary, do not exceed 200 mg/day;
IM/IV 0.1-0.2 mg/kg/dose q4-6h,
do not exceed 20 mg/dose

$ **AVAILABLE FORMS/COST
OF THERAPY**

• Inj, Sol—IM, IV: 20 mg/ml, 1 ml:
$8.75-$18.75
• Tab, Uncoated—Oral: 10 mg,
100's: **$2.63-$26.07**; 25 mg, 100's:
$1.02-$43.50; 50 mg, 100's: **$1.48-
$63.60**; 100 mg, 100's: **$5.95-
$81.96**

CONTRAINDICATIONS: CAD, mitral valvular rheumatic heart disease
PRECAUTIONS: Advanced renal
disease, children, pulmonary hypertension
PREGNANCY AND LACTATION:
Pregnancy category C; commonly
used in pregnant women; excreted
into breast milk; compatible with
breast feeding

SIDE EFFECTS/ADVERSE REAC-
TIONS

CNS: Anxiety, depression, *dizziness,
headache,* peripheral neuritis, psychotic reactions, *tremor*
CV: Angina, flushing, hypotension,
palpitations, reflex tachycardia
EENT: Nasal congestion
GI: Anorexia, constipation, *diarrhea,* hepatitis, *nausea,* paralytic ileus, *vomiting, pancreatitis*
GU: Frequency, glucosuria, polyuria, uremia incresed creatinine
BUN
HEME: **Agranulocytosis, aplastic
anemia,** hemolytic anemia, neutropenia, thrombocytopenia, eosinophilia, *leukopenia*
MS: Arthralgia, muscle cramps
RESP: Dyspnea
SKIN: Pruritus, rash, urticaria

---

italic = common side effects   ***bold italic*** = life-threatening reactions

MISC: Lupus-like syndrome (arthralgia, dermatoses, fever, splenomegaly, glomerulonephritis)

INTERACTIONS

Drugs

🔳 *Diazoxide:* Severe hypotension

🔳 *NSAIDs:* Inhibited antihypertensive response to hydralazine

Labs

• *False increase:* Ca^{++} (slight); urine 17-ketogenic steroids; glucose, uric acid

• *False decrease:* Glucose, uric acid

SPECIAL CONSIDERATIONS

• Lupus-like syndrome more common in "slow acetylators" and following higher doses for prolonged periods

PATIENT/FAMILY EDUCATION

• Take with meals

• Notify clinician of any unexplained prolonged general tiredness or fever, muscle or joint aching, or chest pain

• Stools may turn black

MONITORING PARAMETERS

• CBC and ANA titer before and during prolonged therapy

---

hydrochlorothiazide

(hye-droe-klor-oh-thye'a-zide)

Rx: Aquazide-H, Diaqua, Esidrix, Ezide, HydroDiuril, Hydro-Par, Lexor, Microzide, Oretic, Zide

Combinations

Rx: with angiotensin-converting inhibitors: quinapril (Accuretic); captopril (Acediur, Capozide); lisinopril (Prinzide, Zestoretic); benazepril (Lotensin HCT); moexipril (Uniretic); enalapril (Vaseretic); with spironolactone (Aldactazide, Spirozide) with methyldopa (Aldoril), with hydralazine (Apresazide) with reserpine (Aqwesine, Hydropres, Hydroserpine, Hydrotensin, Mallopres, Marpres, Unipres) with angiotensin II receptor blockers: irbesartan (Avalide), valsartan (Diovan HCT), losartan (Hyzaar), with hydralazine and reserpine (Cam-ap-es, H.H.R., Hyserp, Lo-Ten, Ser-A-Gen, Seralazide, Ser-Ap-Es, Serpex, Uni-Serp), with triamterene: (Dyazide, Maxzide) with potassium (Esidrix-K) with guanethidine (Esimil), with beta-blockers: propranolol: (Inderide); metoprolol: (Lopressor HCT); labetolol (Normazide, Trandate-HCT); timolol: (Timolide); bisoprolol (Ziac) with amiloride (Moduretic)

Chemical Class: Sulfonamide derivative

Therapeutic Class: Thiazide diuretic, antihypertensive

CLINICAL PHARMACOLOGY

Mechanism of Action: Inhibits reabsorption of sodium and chloride in cortical thick ascending limb of the loop of Henle and the early distal tubules, increasing the urinary excretion of sodium and chloride; sulfonamide moiety provides some carbonic anhydrase inhibition activity; other actions: increased potassium and bicarbonate excretion; decreased calcium excretion; uric acid retention; antihypertensive action dependent on sodium depletion, drop in peripheral vascular resistance, and reduction in extracellular volume

Pharmacokinetics

PO: Readily absorbed (60%-80% of dose) peak 4 hr, onset 2 hr, duration 6-12 hr; excreted unchanged in urine; $t_{1/2}$ 5.6-14.8 hr

INDICATIONS AND USES: Edema (CHF, hepatic cirrhosis, corticosteroid and estrogen therapy, nephrotic syndrome, acute glomerulonephritis); hypertension; calcium nephrolithiasis*; prevention of osteoporosis*; diabetes insipidus*

DOSAGE

Adult

• PO 12.5-50 mg qd, max 200 mg/day; doses >50 mg/day generally not recommended due to increased incidence of hypokalemia and other metabolic disturbances

Child

• PO (<6 mo) 1-3.3 mg/kg/day divided bid; (>6 mo) 2 mg/kg/day divided bid

$ AVAILABLE FORMS/COST OF THERAPY

• Sol—Oral: 50 mg/5 ml, 500 ml: **$16.91**

• Tab, Uncoated—Oral: 12.5 mg, 100's: **$42.45-$53.99**; 25 mg, 100's: **$0.69-$16.81**; 50 mg, 100's: **$0.74-$25.45**; 100 mg, 100's: **$1.04-$42.77**

CONTRAINDICATIONS: Anuria, renal decompensation

PRECAUTIONS: Fluid and electrolyte imbalance (including sodium, potassium, magnesium, calcium), renal disease, hepatic disease, gout, COPD, lupus erythematosus, diabetes mellitus, hyperparathyroidism, vomiting, diarrhea, elevated cholesterol/triglycerides

PREGNANCY AND LACTATION: Pregnancy category B; 1st trimester use may increase risk of congenital defects, use in later trimesters does not seem to carry this risk; therapy for preexisting hypertension can be continued throughout pregnancy with minimal risk; initiating for simple edema not recommended; few unequivocal indications for diuretic therapy in pregnancy except for pulmonary edema or congestive heart failure, excreted into breast milk in small amounts; considered compatible with breast feeding

SIDE EFFECTS/ADVERSE REACTIONS

CNS: Depression, *dizziness,* drowsiness, *fatigue,* headache, paresthesia, *weakness*

CV: **Arrhythmias,** irregular pulse, orthostatic hypotension, palpitations, volume depletion

EENT: Blurred vision

GI: *Anorexia,* constipation, cramps, diarrhea, *nausea,* pancreatitis, *vomiting*

GU: *Frequency,* decreased libido, impotence

HEME: **Agranulocytosis, aplastic anemia, hemolytic anemia, leukopenia, neutropenia, thrombocytopenia**

METAB: Hypercalcemia, *hyperglycemia, hyperuricemia,* hypochloremia, *hypokalemia,* hypomagnesemia, hyponatremia, increased crea-

---

tinine, BUN, lipid abnormalities (increased total triglycerides, LDL cholesterol)

SKIN: Fever, photosensitivity, purpura, *rash,* urticaria

INTERACTIONS

Drugs

❷ *Angiotensin-converting enzyme inhibitors:* Risk of postural hypotension when added to ongoing diuretic therapy; more common with loop diuretics; first dose hypotension possible in patients with sodium depletion or hypovolemia due to diuretics or sodium restriction; hypotensive response is usually transient; hold diuretic day of first dose

🔢 *Calcium (high doses):* Risk of milk-alkali syndrome; monitor for hypercalcemia

🔢 *Carbenoxolone:* Additive potassium wasting; severe hypokalemia

🔢 *Cholestyramine/colestipol:* Reduced serum concentrations of thiazide diuretics

🔢 *Corticosteroids:* Concomitant therapy may result in excessive potassium loss

🔢 *Diazoxide:* Hyperglycemia

🔢 *Digitalis glycosides:* Diuretic-induced hypokalemia may increase the risk of digitalis toxicity

🔢 *Hypoglycemic agents:* Thiazide diuretics tend to increase blood glucose, may increase dosage requirements of antidiabetic drugs

🔢 *Lithium:* Increased serum lithium concentrations, toxicity may occur

🔢 *Methotrexate:* Increased bone marrow suppression

🔢 *Nonsteroidal antiinflammatory drugs:* Concurrent use may reduce diuretic and antihypertensive effects

Labs

• *False decrease:* Urine estriol

SPECIAL CONSIDERATIONS

• May protect against osteoporotic hip fractures

• Loop diuretics or metolazone more effective if CrCl <40-50 ml/min

• Combinations with triamterene, lisinopril have potassium sparing effect

• Doses above 25 mg provide no further blood pressure reduction, but are more likely to induce metabolic disturbance (i.e., hypokalemia, hyperuricemia, etc.)

PATIENT/FAMILY EDUCATION

• Will increase urination temporarily (for about 3 wk); take early in the day

• May cause sensitivity to sunlight; avoid prolonged exposure to the sun and other ultraviolet light

• May cause gout attacks; notify clinician if sudden joint pain occurs

MONITORING PARAMETERS

• Weight, urine output, serum electrolytes, BUN, creatinine, CBC, uric acid, glucose, lipids

hydrocodone

(hye-droe-koe´done)

Rx: Hycodan

Combinations

Rx: with acetaminophen (Anexsia, Bancap-HC, Cetaplus, Co-gesic, Duocet, Hydrocet, Hydrogesic, Hy-Phen, Lorcet, Lortab, Margesic-H, Norco, Panacet, Stagesic, T-Gesic, Vidocin, Zydone); with aspirin (Alor, Azdone, Damason-P, Lortab); with ibuprofen (Vicoprofen); with pseudoephedrine, guaifenesin (Duratuss, Pizotuss-D, Deconamine CX, Entuss-D, Cophene XP, SRC Liquid, Tussafin), with pseudoephedrine, chlorpheniramine, guaifenesin (Ztuss); with phenylpropanolamine, pyrilamine, guaifenesin (Triaminic Expectorant DH, S-T Forte, Vetuss HC, Statuss); with phenindamine, guaifenesin (P-V-Tussin); with phenylpropanolamine, guaifenesin (Tussanil); with phenylephrine, chlorpheniramine (Atuss-HD); with phenylephrine, guaifenesin (Donatussin DC, Tussafed HC, Atuss-G)

Chemical Class: Semisynthetic opium alkaloid; phenanthrene derivative

Therapeutic Class: Narcotic analgesic; antitussive

DEA Class: Schedule III

CLINICAL PHARMACOLOGY

Mechanism of Action: Narcotic agonist with activity at Mu receptors (supraspinal analgesia, euphoria, respiratory and physical depression, miosis, and reduced GI motility), Kappa receptors (pentazocine-like spinal analgesia, sedation, and miosis), and Delta receptors (dysphoria, psychotomimetic effects [e.g., hallucinations], and respiratory and vasomotor stimulation caused by drugs with antagonist activity); compared to morphine, less analgesia, equal antitussive, less respiratory depression and less physical dependence

Pharmacokinetics

Peak 1.3 hr, duration 4.6 hr, $t_{1/2}$ 3.8 hr; metabolized in liver, excreted mainly in urine

INDICATIONS AND USES: Moderate to moderately severe pain, nonproductive cough

DOSAGE

NOTE: Only available commercially in combination (USA)

Adult

• PO 5-10 mg q4-6h prn

Child

• PO 0.6 mg/kg/day in 3-4 divided doses; do not exceed 1.25 mg/dose (<2 yr), 5 mg/dose (2-12 yr), 10 mg/dose (>12 yr)

💲 AVAILABLE FORMS/COST OF THERAPY

• Cap, Gel—Oral: 500 mg (acetaminophen)/5 mg, 100's: **$19.50-$343.88**

• Elixir—Oral: 500 mg (acetaminophen)/5 mg/15 ml, 480 ml: **$21.22-$89.44**; 100 mg (guiafenisen)/5 mg/15 ml, 480 ml: **$43.82-$58.12**

• Tab, Uncoated—Oral: 500 mg (acetaminophen)/2.5 mg, 100's: **$29.95-$81.07**; 500 mg (acetaminophen)/5 mg, 100's: **$8.70-$103.43**; 500 mg (acetaminophen)/7.5 mg, 100's: **$32.00-$89.79**; 500 mg (acetaminophen)/10 mg, 100's: **$53.27-$253.03**; 650 mg (acetaminophen)/7.5, 100's: **$34.25-$99.41**; 650 mg

---

italic = common side effects   ***bold italic*** = life-threatening reactions

(acetaminophen)/10 mg, 100's: **$50.72-$139.85**; 750 mg (acetaminophen)/7.5 mg, 100's: **$34.00-$65.05**; 200 mg (ibuprofen)/7.5 mg, 100's: **$109.38**

PRECAUTIONS: Head injury, increased intracranial pressure, acute abdominal conditions, elderly, severe impairment of hepatic or renal function, hypothyroidism, Addison's disease, prostatic hypertrophy, urethral stricture, history of drug abuse

PREGNANCY AND LACTATION: Pregnancy category B (category D if used for prolonged periods or in high doses at term); withdrawal could theoretically occur in infants exposed *in utero* to prolonged maternal ingestion; excretion into breast milk unknown; use caution in nursing mothers

SIDE EFFECTS/ADVERSE REACTIONS

CNS: Agitation, dependency, dizziness, *drowsiness,* lethargy, restlessness, *sedation*

CV: Bradycardia, orthostatic hypotension, palpitations, tachycardia

GI: Anorexia, constipation, nausea, vomiting

GU: Urinary retention

RESP: **Respiratory depression, respiratory paralysis**

SKIN: Flushing, rash, urticaria

INTERACTIONS

Drugs

3 *Antihistamines, chloral hydrate, glutethimide, methocarbamol:* Enhanced depressant effects

3 *Barbiturates:* Additive respiratory and CNS depressant effects

3 *Cimetidine:* Increased respiratory and CNS depression

3 *Ethanol:* Additive CNS effects

3 *Protease inhibitors:* Enhanced CNS and respiratory depression

Labs

• False elevations of amylase and lipase

SPECIAL CONSIDERATIONS

PATIENT/FAMILY EDUCATION

• Report any symptoms of CNS changes, allergic reactions

• Physical dependency may result when used for extended periods

• Change position slowly, orthostatic hypotension may occur

• Avoid hazardous activities if drowsiness or dizziness occurs

• Avoid alcohol, other CNS depressants

• Minimize nausea by administering with food and remain lying down following dose

• Do not administer agonist/antagonist analgesics (i.e., pentazocine, nalbuphine, butorphanol, dezocine, buprenorphine) to patient who has received a prolonged course of hydrocodone (a pure agonist). In opioid-dependent patients, mixed agonist/antagonist analgesics may precipitate withdrawal symptoms

hydrocortisone

(hye-dro-kor'ti-sone)

Rx: *Ano-Rectals:* Proctocort, Anusol-HC, Proctofoam-HC, Anucort-HC, Cortenema *Systemic:* Cortef, Hydrocortone, Hydrocortone Phosphate, Hydrocortone Acetate, Solu-Cortef *Topical:* Cetacort, Cort-Dome, Dermacort, Hytone, Locoid, Synacort, Westcort

OTC: Cortizone, Cortaid, Lanacort-5, Gynecort Female Creme, Dermolate, Tegrin-HC Combinations

Rx: with choloramphenicol (Chloromycetin/HC suspension—ophthalmic); with neomycin and polymyxin B (Cortisporin Otic, Drotic, Otocort—otic); with neomycin, polymyxin B, and bacitracin (Cortisporin Ointment, Neotricin HC—ophthalmic); with oxytetracycline (Terra-Cortril—ophthalmic); with urea (Carmol HC)

Chemical Class: Glucocorticoid

Therapeutic Class: Systemic and topical corticosteroid, low potency

---

CLINICAL PHARMACOLOGY

Mechanism of Action: Decreases inflammation by depressing migration of polymorphonuclear leukocytes and activity of endogenous mediators of inflammation, has many profound metabolic effects, possesses mineralocorticoid activity

Pharmacokinetics

PO: Onset 1-2 hr, peak 1 hr, duration 1-1½ days

PR: Onset 3-5 days

TOP: Absorbed through the skin (increased by inflammation and occlusive dressings); metabolized by liver, excreted in urine (17-OHCS, 17-KS)

INDICATIONS AND USES: Anti-inflammatory or immunosuppressant agent in the treatment of a variety of diseases of hematologic, allergic, inflammatory, neoplastic, and autoimmune origin; in replacement doses for primary or secondary adrenocortical insufficiency

DOSAGE

Adult and Child

• *Otitis externa:* With head tilted for 2 min instill 4 gtt 3-4 × /day
• *Inflammatory ocular conditions:* Instill 1 gtt or ointment q3-4h

Adult

• *Acute adrenal insufficiency:* PO 5-30 mg bid-qid; IM/IV/SC 15-240 mg q12h
• *Anti-inflammatory:* PO 5-30 mg bid-qid; IM/IV/SC 15-240 mg q12h
• *Shock:* IM/IV 500-2000 mg q2-6h
• *Rect:* Enema 100 mg nightly for 21 days; suppository 25 mg bid-qid prn
• *Intra-articular and soft tissue (acetate):* Large joints 25 mg; small joints 10-25 mg; bursae 25-37.5 mg; tendon sheaths 5-12.5 mg; soft tissue infiltration 25-50 mg; ganglia 12.5-25 mg

Child

• *Acute adrenal insufficiency:* IM/IV/SC 1-2 mg/kg bolus, then 25-150 mg/day in divided doses (infants and younger children); 1-2 mg/kg bolus, then 150-250 mg/day in divided doses (older children)

H

• *Physiologic replacement:* PO 0.5-0.75 mg/kg/day or 20-25 mg/m^2/day divided q8h; IM 0.25-0.35 mg/kg/day or 12-15 mg/m^2/day qd
• *Shock:* IM/IV 50 mg/kg initially, then repeated in 4 hr and/or q24h prn

Adult and Child

• TOP apply to affected area bid-qid, rub completely into skin

S **AVAILABLE FORMS/COST OF THERAPY**

• Aerosol, Foam (acetate)—Rect: 10%, 15 g: **$81.19**
• Aer—Top: 1%, 59 ml: **$4.33**
• Cre, Oint (butyrate)—Top: 0.1%, 15, 45 g: **$21.74-$26.94**/15 g
• Cre—Rect: 2.5%, 30 g: **$41.16**
• Cre—Top: 0.5%, 15, 30, 45, 60, 120, 454 g: **$1.32-$9.13**/30 g; 1%, 15, 30, 45, 60, 120, 454 g: **$1.05-$18.14**/30 g; 2.5%, 15, 30, 45, 60, 120, 454 g: **$5.25-$44.21**/30 g
• Enema—Rect: 100 mg/60 ml: **$5.42-$8.24**
• Inj, Susp (acetate)—Intra-Articular, IM: 25 mg/ml, 5, 10 ml: **$3.60-$26.19**/10 ml
• Inj, Lyph-Sol (sodium succinate)—IM, IV: 100 mg/vial: **$2.00-$3.75**; 250 mg/vial: **$3.51-$9.50**; 500 mg/vial: **$8.38-$15.00**; 1000 mg/vial: **$29.00**
• Inj, Sol (sodium phosphate)—IM, IV, SC: 50 mg/ml, 2, 10 ml: **$11.71**/2 ml
• Lotion—Top: 0.5%, 30, 60, 120 ml: **$3.37**/60 ml; 1%, 30, 60, 75, 120 ml: **$16.25-$30.03**/60 ml; 2.5%, 60, 120 ml: **$20.50-$54.10**/60 ml
• Oint—Top: 0.5%, 15, 30, 60, 120, 240 g: **$2.14-$3.49**/30 g; 1%, 20, 30, 60, 120, 454 g: **$1.92-$11.80**/30 g; 2.5%, 20, 30, 454 g: **$5.25-$20.66**/30 g
• Sol (butyrate)—Top: 0.1%, 20, 60 ml: **$31.43**/20 ml
• Sol—Top: 1%, 30, 60 ml: **$8.00**/30 ml; 2.5%, 30 ml: **$15.41-$21.61**

• Supp (acetate)—Rect: 25 mg, 12's: **$3.88**
• Susp (cypionate)—Oral: 10 mg/5 ml, 120 ml: **$28.26**
• Supp, Enema—Rect: 100 mg/60 ml: **$8.24-$10.45**
• Tab, Uncoated—Oral: 5 mg, 50's: **$10.26**; 10 mg, 100's: **$23.93-$36.33**; 20 mg, 100's: **$2.64-$68.88**

CONTRAINDICATIONS: Systemic fungal infections

PRECAUTIONS: Psychosis, diabetes mellitus, glaucoma, osteoporosis, seizure disorders, ulcerative colitis (intestinal perforation), CHF, hypertension, myesthenia gravis (if used with anticholinesterase agents), renal disease, esophagitis, peptic ulcer, latent tuberculosis or amebiasis (reactivation of disease). Topical: use on face, groin, or axilla, ocular herpes simplex

PREGNANCY AND LACTATION: Pregnancy category C; excreted in breast milk, could interfere with infant's growth and endogenous corticosteroid production

SIDE EFFECTS/ADVERSE REACTIONS

CNS: Depression, *mood changes, seizures*
CV: CHF, hypertension, tachycardia, *thromboembolism,* thrombophlebitis
EENT: Blurred vision, cataract, increased intraocular pressure
GI: Abdominal distension, diarrhea, GI hemorrhage, increased appetite, nausea, *pancreatitis*
GU: Menstrual irregularities
HEME: Increased neutrophils
METAB: Alkalosis, Cushingoid state, decreased glucose tolerance, growth suppression in children, HPA suppression
MS: Aseptic necrosis of femoral and humeral heads, fractures, muscle mass loss, osteoporosis, tendon rupture, weakness

SKIN: Acne, allergic contact dermatitis, atrophy, bruising, burning, dryness, ecchymosis, folliculitis, hypertrichosis, hypopigmentation, irritation, itching, miliaria, perioral dermatitis, petechiae, poor wound healing, secondary infection, striae, suppression of skin test reactions, thin fragile skin

INTERACTIONS

Drugs

▣ *Aminoglutethamide:* Enhanced elimination of hydrocortisone; reduction in corticosteroid response

▣ *Antidiabetics:* Increased blood glucose in patients with diabetes

▣ *Barbiturates:* Reduction in the serum concentrations of corticosteroids

▣ *Cholestyramine, colestipol:* Possible reduced absorption of corticosteroids

▣ *Cyclosporine:* Increased levels of both drugs increases the risk of seizures

▣ *Estrogens:* Enhanced effects of corticosteroids

▣ *Isoniazid (INH):* Reduced INH levels, enhanced corticosteroid effect

▣ *IUDs:* Inhibition of inflammation may decrease contraceptive effect

▣ *NSAIDs:* Increased risk GI ulceration

▣ *Phenytoin:* Reduced therapeutic effect of corticosteroids

▣ *Rifampin:* Reduced therapeutic effect of corticosteroids

▣ *Salicylates:* Enhanced elimination of salicylates; subtherapeutic salicylate concentrations possible

Labs

• *False negative:* Skin allergy tests

SPECIAL CONSIDERATIONS

PATIENT/FAMILY EDUCATION

• May cause GI upset; take with meals or snacks

• Take single daily doses in AM

• Increased dose of rapidly acting corticosteroids may be necessary in patients subjected to unusual stress

• Signs of adrenal insufficiency include fatigue, anorexia, nausea, vomiting, diarrhea, weight loss, weakness, dizziness, and low blood sugar

• Avoid abrupt withdrawal of therapy following high-dose or long-term therapy

• May mask infections

• Do not give live virus vaccines to patients on prolonged therapy

• Patients on chronic steroid therapy should wear medical alert bracelet

MONITORING PARAMETERS

• Serum K and glucose

• Edema, blood pressure, CHF, mental status, weight

• Growth in children on prolonged therapy

---

hydroflumethiazide

(hye-droe-flu-me-thye'a-zide)

Rx: Diucardin, Saluron

Combinations

  Rx: reserpine (Salutensin, Salutensin-Demi)

Chemical Class: Sulfonamide derivative

Therapeutic Class: Thiazide diuretic; antihypertensive

CLINICAL PHARMACOLOGY

Mechanism of Action: Inhibits reabsorption of sodium and chloride in cortical thick ascending limb of the loop of Henle and the early distal tubules, increasing the urinary excretion of sodium and chloride; sulfonamide moiety provides some carbonic anhydrase inhibition activity; other actions: increased potassium and bicarbonate excretion; decreased calcium excretion; uric acid retention; antihypertensive action

---

dependent on sodium depletion, drop in peripheral vascular resistance, and reduction in extracellular volume

Pharmacokinetics

PO: Onset 2 hr, peak 4 hr, duration 12-24 hr; metabolized and biphasic excreted in the urine; $t_{1/2}$ approximately 17 hr

INDICATIONS AND USES: Edema (CHF, hepatic cirrhosis, corticosteroid and estrogen therapy, nephrotic syndrome, acute glomerulonephritis); hypertension; calcium nephrolithiasis*; prevention of osteoporosis*; diabetes insipidus*

DOSAGE

NOTE: Equivalent hydrochlorothiazide dose: 50 mg-50 mg

Adult

• *Edema:* PO 50 mg qd-bid initially; maintenance 25-200 mg/day; administer in divided doses when dosage >100 mg/day

• *Hypertension:* PO 50 mg bid initially; maintenance 50-100 mg/day, do not exceed 200 mg/day

🛇 AVAILABLE FORMS/COST OF THERAPY

• Tab, Uncoated—Oral: 50 mg, 100's: **$59.05-$72.94**

CONTRAINDICATIONS: Anuria, renal decompensation

PRECAUTIONS: Fluid and electrolyte imbalance (including sodium, potassium, magnesium, calcium), renal disease, hepatic disease, gout, COPD, lupus erythematosus, diabetes mellitus, hyperparathyroidism, vomiting, diarrhea, elevated cholesterol/triglycerides, tartrazine sensitivity

PREGNANCY AND LACTATION: Pregnancy category C; therapy for preexisting hypertension can be continued throughout pregnancy with minimal risk; initiating for simple edema not recommended; few unequivocal indications for diuretic therapy in pregnancy except for pulmonary edema or congestive heart failure, excreted into breast milk in small amounts; considered compatible with breast feeding

SIDE EFFECTS/ADVERSE REACTIONS

CNS: Depression, *dizziness,* drowsiness, *fatigue,* headache, paresthesia

CV: **Arrhythmias** Orthostatic hypotension, palpitations, volume depletion

EENT: Blurred vision

GI: Anorexia, constipation, cramps, diarrhea, hepatitis, *nausea,* **pancreatitis,** *vomiting*

GU: Frequency, impotence, reduced libido, glucosuria, polyuria, increased creatinine, BUN

HEME: **Agranulocytosis, aplastic anemia, hemolytic anemia, leukopenia, neutropenia, thrombocytopenia**

METAB: Lipid abnormalities (incr total, LDL cholesterol, triglycerides); hypercalcemia, *hyperglycemia, hyperuricemia, hypokalemia,* hypomagnesemia, hyponatremia

SKIN: Photosensitivity, purpura, *rash,* urticaria

INTERACTIONS

Drugs

❷ *Angiotensin-converting enzyme inhibitors:* Risk of postural hypotension when added to ongoing diuretic therapy; more common with loop diuretics; first dose hypotension possible in patients with sodium depletion or hypovolemia due to diuretics or sodium restriction; hypotensive response is usually transient; hold diuretic day of first dose

❸ *Calcium (high dose):* Risk of milk-alkali syndrome. Monitor for hypoglycemia

❸ *Cholestyramine, Colestipol:* Reduced serum concentrations of thiazide diuretics

---

* = non-FDA-approved use

3 *Corticosteroids:* Concomitant therapy may result in excessive potassium loss

3 *Diazoxide:* Hyperglycemia

3 *Digitalis glycosides:* Diuretic-induced hypokalemia may increase the risk of digitalis toxicity

3 *Hypoglycemic agents:* Thiazide diuretics tend to increase blood glucose; may increase dosage requirements of hypoglycemic agents

3 *Lithium:* Increased serum lithium concentrations, toxicity may occur

3 *Methotrexate:* Increased bone marrow suppression

3 *Nonsteroidal antiinflammatory drugs:* Concurrent may reduce diuretic and antihypertensive effects

Labs
• *False decrease:* Urine estriol

SPECIAL CONSIDERATIONS
• Doses above 2.5 mg provide no further blood pressure reduction, but are more likely to induce metabolic disturbance (i.e., hypokalemia, hyperuricemia, etc.)
• May protect against osteoporotic hip fractures
• Loop diuretics or metolazone more effective if CrCl <40-50 ml/min

PATIENT/FAMILY EDUCATION
• Will increase urination temporarily (approximately 3 wk); take early in the day to prevent sleep disturbance
• May cause sensitivity to sunlight; avoid prolonged exposure to the sun and other ultraviolet light
• May cause gout attacks; notify clinician if sudden joint pain occurs

MONITORING PARAMETERS
• Weight, urine output, serum electrolytes, BUN, creatinine, CBC, uric acid, glucose, lipids

hydromorphone

(hye-droe-mor'fone)
Rx: Dilaudid
Chemical Class: Synthetic opium alkaloid; phenanthrene derivative
Therapeutic Class: Narcotic analgesic; antitussive
DEA Class: Schedule II

H

CLINICAL PHARMACOLOGY
Mechanism of Action: Narcotic agonist with activity at Mu receptors (supraspinal analgesia, euphoria, respiratory and physical depression, miosis, and reduced GI motility), Kappa receptors (pentazocine-like spinal analgesia, sedation, and miosis), and Delta receptors (dysphoria, psychotomimetic effects [e.g., hallucinations], and respiratory and vasomotor stimulation caused by drugs with antagonist activity); compared to morphine, equal analgesia, constipation, respiratory depression, and sedation; less emesis
Pharmacokinetics
PO: Peak 45 min
IM: Onset 15-30 min, peak 0.5-1½ hr, duration 4-5 hr
Metabolized by liver, excreted by kidneys

INDICATIONS AND USES: Moderate to severe pain, non-productive cough

DOSAGE
Adult
• *Pain:* PO/IM/IV/SC 1-4 mg q4-6h prn; PR 3 mg q6-8h
• *Antitussive:* PO 1 mg q3-4h prn
Child
• *Pain:* PO 0.03-0.08 mg/kg/dose q4-6h prn, max 5 mg/dose; IV 0.015 mg/kg/dose q4-6h prn
• *Antitussive:* (6-12 yr) 0.5 mg q3-4h prn

---

italic = common side effects   **bold italic** = life-threatening reactions

💲 AVAILABLE FORMS/COST OF THERAPY

• Inj, Sol—IM, IV, SC: 1 mg/ml, 1, 10 ml: **$0.97-$1.27**/1 ml; 2 mg/ml, 1, 10, 20 ml: **$1.05-$3.20**/1 ml; 4 mg/ml, 1, 10, 20 ml: **$1.01-$1.59**/1 ml; 10 mg/ml, 1, 5, 10 ml: **$3.50-$3.56**/1 ml

• Sol—Oral: 1 mg/ml, 120, 480 ml: **$108.18**/480 ml

• Supp—Rect: 3 mg, 6's: **$23.97**

• Tab, Uncoated—Oral: 2 mg, 100's: **$23.33-$49.34**; 4 mg, 100's: **$39.17-$80.54**; 8 mg, 100's: **$121.98-$146.59**

CONTRAINDICATIONS: Acute bronchial asthma, obstetrical anesthesia (parenteral)

PRECAUTIONS: Head injury, increased intracranial pressure, acute abdominal conditions, elderly, severe impairment of hepatic or renal function, hypothyroidism, Addison's disease, prostatic hypertrophy, urethral stricture, history of drug abuse, hypotension

PREGNANCY AND LACTATION: Pregnancy category C (category D if used for prolonged periods or in high doses at term); use during labor produces neonatal respiratory depression; excretion into breast milk unknown; use caution in nursing mothers

SIDE EFFECTS/ADVERSE REACTIONS

CNS: Agitation, dependency, dizziness, *drowsiness, sedation*

CV: Bradycardia, orthostatic hypotension, palpitations, tachycardia

GI: Anorexia, constipation, nausea, vomiting

GU: Urinary retention

RESP: **Respiratory depression**

SKIN: Flushing, rash, urticaria

METAB: Transient hyperglycemia

INTERACTIONS

Drugs

🔢 *Antihistamines, chloral hydrate, glutethimide, methocarbamol:* Enhanced depressant effects

🔢 *Barbiturates:* Additive respiratory and CNS depressant effects

🔢 *Cimetidine:* Increased respiratory and CNS depression

🔢 *Ethanol:* Additive CNS effects

Labs

• *False increase:* Amylase and lipase

SPECIAL CONSIDERATIONS

• Do not administer agonist/antagonist analgesics (i.e., pentazocine, nalbuphine, butorphanol, dezocine, buprenorphine) to patient who has received a prolonged course of hydromorphone (a pure agonist). In opioid-dependent patients, mixed agonist/antagonist analgesics may precipitate withdrawal symptoms.

PATIENT/FAMILY EDUCATION

• Physical dependency may result when used for extended periods

• Avoid hazardous activities if drowsiness or dizziness occurs

• Avoid alcohol, other CNS depressants unless directed by clinician

• Minimize nausea by administering with food and remain lying down following dose

hydroquinone

(hye-droe-kwin'own)

Rx: Alphaquin HP,
Eldopaque-Forte,
Eldoquin-Forte, Lustra,
Solaquin Forte, Melpaque
HP, Melquin HP, Melquin 3,
NuQuin HP, Melanex, Viquin
Forte

OTC: Esoterica Sensitive Skin
Formula, Eldopaque,
Solaquin

Chemical Class: Monobenzone
derivative

Therapeutic Class: Depigmenting agent

CLINICAL PHARMACOLOGY
Mechanism of Action: Depigments
hyperpigmented skin by inhibiting
the enzymatic oxidation of tyrosine
and suppressing other melanocyte
metabolic processes, thereby inhibiting melanin formation
INDICATIONS AND USES: Temporary bleaching of hyperpigmented
skin conditions (e.g., freckles, senile
lentigines, chloasma and melasma,
other forms of melanin hyperpigmentation)
DOSAGE
Adult and Child ≥12 yr
• *TOP:* apply to affected skin bid
**⑤ AVAILABLE FORMS/COST
   OF THERAPY**
• Cre—Top: 2%, 15, 30, 60, 90, 120
g: **$2.30**/30 g; 4%, 15, 30, 45, 60,
120 g: **$3.40-$71.25**/30 g
• Gel—Top: 4%, 15, 30, 60 g:
$29.00-$48.95/30 g
• Sol—Top: 3%, 30 ml: **$8.70-
$13.13**
PRECAUTIONS: Sulfite sensitivity
PREGNANCY AND LACTATION:
Pregnancy category C; degree of
systemic absorption unknown; ex-
cretion into breast milk unknown

**SIDE EFFECTS/ADVERSE REAC-
   TIONS**
SKIN: Contact dermatitis, dryness
and fissuring of paranasal and in-
fraorbital areas, erythema, irritation,
sensitization, stinging
INTERACTIONS
Labs
• *False decrease:* Urine glucose
SPECIAL CONSIDERATIONS
PATIENT/FAMILY EDUCATION
• Apply small amount to an unbro-
ken patch of skin and check in 24 hr;
if vesicle formation, itching, or excessive inflammation occurs, further treatment not advised
• Positive response may require 3
wk to 6 mo
• Protect the treated area from UV
light by using a sunscreen, sun
block, or protective clothing
• Avoid application to lips or near
eyes

hydroxocobalamin
(vitamin B₁₂)

(hye-drox'oh-co-bal'a-min)

Rx: Hydroxy-Cobal, LA-12
Chemical Class: B complex
vitamin
Therapeutic Class: Vitamin
supplement; blood modifier;
nitroprusside antidote

CLINICAL PHARMACOLOGY
Mechanism of Action: Physiologic
role is associated with methylation,
participating in nucleic acid and protein synthesis; participates in red
blood cell formation through activation of folic acid coenzymes
Pharmacokinetics
IM: Slowly absorbed from inj site;
distributed into liver, bone marrow,
and other tissue; available for urinary excretion when administered

parenterally in doses that exceed binding capacity of plasma, liver, and other tissues

INDICATIONS AND USES: Vitamin B_{12} deficiency (pernicious anemia, GI pathology, fish tapeworm infestation, malignancy of pancreas or bowel, gluten enteropathy, sprue, gastrectomy); increased vitamin B_{12} requirement (pregnancy, thyrotoxicosis, hemolytic anemia, hemorrhage, malignancy, hepatic or renal disease); Schilling test for vitamin B_{12} absorption; cyanide toxicity associated with sodium nitroprusside*

DOSAGE

Adult

• IM 30-100 µg/day for 5-10 days, followed by 100 µg q mo

Child

• IM 1-5 mg over 2 or more wk in doses of 100 µg, then 30-100 µg q mo for maintenance

§ AVAILABLE FORMS/COST OF THERAPY

• Inj, Sol—IM: 1000 µg/ml, 10, 30 ml: **$6.33-$38.26**/30 ml

CONTRAINDICATIONS: Hypersensitivity to cobalt

PRECAUTIONS: IV route, infection, uremia, concurrent iron or folic acid deficiency, severe megaloblastic anemia, hypokalemia

PREGNANCY AND LACTATION: Pregnancy category A (C if dose exceeds recommended daily allowance); vitamin B_{12} is an essential vitamin and needs are increased during pregnancy; excreted into breast milk; 2.6 µg/day should be consumed during pregnancy and lactation

SIDE EFFECTS/ADVERSE REACTIONS

CV: **CHF,** peripheral vascular thrombosis

GI: Diarrhea

METAB: Hypokalemia

SKIN: Pain at inj site

INTERACTIONS

Labs

• *False positive:* Intrinsic factor

• *Interference:* Methotrexate, pyrimethamine and most antibiotics interfere with vitamin B_{12} assay

SPECIAL CONSIDERATIONS

PATIENT/FAMILY EDUCATION

• Therapy may require life-long monthly injections

MONITORING PARAMETERS

• Serum potassium for 1st 48 hr during treatment of severe megaloblastic anemia

• Reticulocyte counts, Hct, vitamin B_{12}, iron, and folic acid plasma levels prior to treatment, between days 5 and 7 of treatment, then frequently until Hct is normal

---

hydroxychloroquine

(hye-drox-ee-klor′oh-kwin)

Rx: Plaquenil, Quineprox

Chemical Class: 4-aminoquinoline derivative

Therapeutic Class: Antimalarial; disease-modifying antirheumatic drug (DMARD)

CLINICAL PHARMACOLOGY

Mechanism of Action: Antimalarial: Inhibits DNA/RNA synthesis (mammalian and protozoal cells); within parasite: raises pH of organelles causing interference with utilization of host erythrocyte hemoglobin; interference with phospholipid metabolism

Inflammation: Suppress responsiveness of T cells to mitogens; decreases leukocyte chemotaxis; stabilizes lysosomal membranes; inhibits DNA/RNA synthesis; traps free radicals

---

* = non-FDA-approved use

Pharmacokinetics

PO: Rapidly and completely absorbed, peak 1-6 hr; protein-binding 55%; partially metabolized, slowly excreted by kidneys (parent drug and metabolites)

INDICATIONS AND USES: Prophylaxis and treatment of acute attacks of malaria due to *Plasmodium vivax, P. malariae, P. ovale,* and susceptible strains of *P. falciparum;* discoid and systemic lupus erythematosus; rheumatoid arthritis, juvenile rheumatoid arthritis,* sarcoid associated hypercalcemia,* polymorphous light eruption,* prophyria cutanea tarda,* urticaria solar,* chronic cutaneous vasculitis*

DOSAGE

NOTE: hydroxychloroquine sulfate 200 mg = 155 mg hydroxychloroquine base

Adult

• *Prophylaxis of malaria:* PO 400 mg q wk on same day each wk; begin 1-2 wk before exposure, continue 6-8 wk after leaving endemic area

• *Acute malaria attack:* PO 800 mg initial dose, followed by 400 mg in 6 hr on day 1, then 400 mg as single dose on days 2 and 3

• *Rheumatoid arthritis:* PO 400-600 mg qd initially, increase dose until optimal response achieved (usually 4-12 wk); maintenance dose 200-400 mg qd

• *Lupus erythematosus:* PO 400 mg qd-bid for several wk depending on response; maintenance 200-400 mg/day

Child

• *Prophylaxis of malaria:* PO 5 mg/kg (base) q wk on same day each wk; begin 1-2 wk before exposure, continue 6-8 wk after leaving endemic area; do not exceed recommended adult dose

• *Acute malaria attack:* PO 10 mg/kg (base) initial dose, followed by 5 mg/kg (base) in 6 hr on day 1, then 5 mg/kg (base) as a single dose on days 2 and 3

• *Juvenile rheumatoid arthritis/lupus erythematosus:* PO 3-5 mg/kg/day divided 1-2 times/day, max 400 mg/day

$ AVAILABLE FORMS/COST OF THERAPY

• Tab, Uncoated—Oral: 200 mg, 100's: **$100.00-$164.76**

CONTRAINDICATIONS: Retinal or visual field changes, children (long-term therapy)

PRECAUTIONS: Psoriasis, porphyria, children (NOTE: Children especially sensitive to the effects of the 4-aminoquinolones), hepatic function impairment, G-6-PD deficiency, alcoholism

PREGNANCY AND LACTATION: Pregnancy category C; excreted in breast milk; safe use during nursing has not been established

SIDE EFFECTS/ADVERSE REACTIONS

CNS: Headache, neuropathy, psychic stimulation, psychosis, *seizures*

CV: ECG changes (inversion or depression of T-wave, widening of QRS complex), hypotension

EENT: ***Irreversible retinal damage*** (prolonged high doses), nerve-type deafness (prolonged high doses), nyctalopia, reduced hearing, scotomatous vision, tinnitus, visual disturbances

GI: Abdominal cramps, *anorexia,* diarrhea, *nausea, vomiting*

HEME: ***Agranulocytosis, blood dyscrasias, hemolytic anemia***

MS: Muscular weakness

---

italic = common side effects   ***bold italic*** = life-threatening reactions

SKIN: Lichen planus-like eruptions, pleomorphic skin eruptions (prolonged therapy), pruritus, skin and mucosal pigmentary changes

INTERACTIONS

Drugs

3 *Digitalis glycosides:* Increased serum digoxin concentrations

3 *Praziquantel:* Reduced praziquantel concentration

SPECIAL CONSIDERATIONS

PATIENT/FAMILY EDUCATION

• Report any muscle weakness, visual disturbances, difficulty hearing, or ringing in ears to clinician

MONITORING PARAMETERS

• Baseline and periodic ophthalmologic examinations (visual acuity, slit lamp, funduscopic, and visual field tests); periodic tests of knee and ankle reflexes to detect muscular weakness

• Periodic CBCs during prolonged therapy

---

hydroxyprogesterone

(hye-drox-ee-proe-jess´te-rone)

Rx: Hylutin, Prodrox

Chemical Class: Progestin derivative

Therapeutic Class: Progestin; antineoplastic

CLINICAL PHARMACOLOGY

Mechanism of Action: Exerts a progestational effect on the endometrium, alters cervical mucus, suppresses evaluation in some patients

Pharmacokinetics

IM: Duration 9-17 days; metabolized primarily in the liver, excreted by the kidney

INDICATIONS AND USES: Amenorrhea (primary and secondary), dysfunctional uterine bleeding, metrorrhagia, metastatic endometrial carcinoma (palliative therapy)

DOSAGE

Adult

• *Amenorrhea and uterine bleeding:* IM 375 mg, repeated q4 wk prn

• *Endometrial carcinoma:* IM 1-7 g/wk

$ AVAILABLE FORMS/COST OF THERAPY

• Inj, Sol—IM: 250 mg/ml, 5 ml: **$9.95-$29.95**

CONTRAINDICATIONS: Active thromboembolic disorders or thrombophlebitis, cerebral hemorrhage, impaired liver function or disease, breast cancer, undiagnosed vaginal bleeding, missed abortion, use as a diagnostic test for pregnancy

PRECAUTIONS: Epilepsy, migraine, asthma, cardiac or renal dysfunction, depression, diabetes

PREGNANCY AND LACTATION: Pregnancy category D; an increased risk of hypospadias in the male fetus and mild virilization of the female fetus have been reported with progestin use; progestins compatible with breast feeding

SIDE EFFECTS/ADVERSE REACTIONS

CNS: Depression, dizziness, fatigue, headache

CV: Edema

GI: Anorexia, *cholestatic jaundice,* increased weight, *nausea,* vomiting

GU: Amenorrhea, breakthrough bleeding, breast changes, dysmenorrhea, *gynecomastia*

METAB: Hyperglycemia

SKIN: Acne, alopecia, hirsutism, melasma, rash

INTERACTIONS
Drugs
3 *Aminoglutethimide:* Decreases progestin concentration
SPECIAL CONSIDERATIONS
PATIENT/FAMILY EDUCATION
• Take protective measures against exposure to UV light or sunlight

---

hydroxyzine
(hye-drox'i-zeen)
Rx: Atarax, Vistaril, Vistazine
Chemical Class: Piperazine derivative
Therapeutic Class: Antihistamine; sedative/hypnotic; anxiolytic; antiemetic (parenteral)

CLINICAL PHARMACOLOGY
Mechanism of Action: Antianxiety: depresses subcortical levels of CNS; other: primary skeletal muscle relaxation, bronchodilator activity, antihistaminic and analgesic effects, antispasmodic and antiemetic effects
Pharmacokinetics
Onset 15-30 min, duration 4-6 hr, $t_{1/2}$ 3 hr
INDICATIONS AND USES: Anxiety, nausea, vomiting, to potentiate narcotic analgesics; sedation; pruritus
DOSAGE
Adult
• PO 10-100 mg q4-6h; IM 25-100 mg q4-6h
Child
• PO (>6 yr) 50-100 mg/day in divided doses; PO (<6 yr) 50 mg/day in divided doses; IM 1.1 mg/kg q4-6h

$ AVAILABLE FORMS/COST OF THERAPY
• Cap—Oral: 25 mg, 100's: **$7.95-$106.32**; 50 mg, 100's: **$11.25-$124.58**; 100 mg, 100's: **$18.95-$153.08**
• Inj—IM: 25 mg/ml, 10 ml: **$2.03-$12.90**; 50 mg/ml, 10 ml: **$2.63-$119.70**
• Sus—Oral: 25 mg/5 ml, 120, 480 ml: **$28.00-$38.98**/120 ml
• Syr—Oral: 10 mg/5 ml, 120 ml: **$3.85-$12.70**
• Tab—Oral: 10 mg, 100's: **$5.25-$69.68**; 25 mg, 100's: **$6.95-$102.19**; 50 mg, 100's: **$4.38-$153.08**; 100 mg, 100's: **$22.50-$153.08**
PRECAUTIONS: Elderly, debilitated, hepatic disease, renal disease, pregnancy, IM only (avoid IV, SC, or intraarterial administration)
PREGNANCY AND LACTATION: Pregnancy category C (but no excess in birth defects documented); safe during labor for relief of anxiety; no data on breast feeding
SIDE EFFECTS/ADVERSE REACTIONS
CNS: Confusion, depression, dizziness, *drowsiness,* fatigue, headache, *seizures,* tremor
GI: Dry mouth
GU: Urinary retention
INTERACTIONS
Labs
• *False increase:* Urine 17-hydroxycorticosteroids and 17-ketogenic steroids

H

---

hyoscyamine

(hye-oh-sye′a-meen)

Rx: A-Spas S/L, Anaspaz, Cystospaz, Cystospaz-M, Donnamar, ED-SPAZ, Gastrosed, Hyco Drops, Hyosol/SL, Hyospaz, Levbid, Levsin, Levsin/SL, Levsinex, Liqui-Sooth, Medispaz, Spacol, Spasdel, Symax-SL, Symax-SR
Combinations
   Rx: with phenobarbital (Levsin PB)
Chemical Class: Belladonna alkaloid
Therapeutic Class: Anticholinergic, gastrointestinal

CLINICAL PHARMACOLOGY

Mechanism of Action: Inhibits muscarinic actions of acetylcholine at postganglionic parasympathetic neuroeffector sites

Pharmacokinetics

PO: Duration 4-6 hr; metabolized by liver, excreted in urine; t₁/₂ 3.5 hr

$PO:$ Duration 4-6 hr; metabolized by liver, excreted in urine; $t_{1/2}$ 3.5 hr

INDICATIONS AND USES: Irritable bowel syndrome, biliary colic, hypermotility in cystitis, adjunctive treatment of peptic ulcer disease, renal colic, sinus bradycardia (parenteral), acute rhinitis; sialorrhea*; hyperhidrosis*

DOSAGE

Adult

• PO/SL 0.125-0.25 mg tid-qid ac, hs; Sus Action 0.375 mg q12h; IM/SC/IV 0.25-0.5 mg q6h

Child

• 2-12 yr ¼ − ½ adult dose; <2 yr ⅛ − ¼ adult dose

$ AVAILABLE FORMS/COST OF THERAPY

• Cap, Gel, Sus Action—Oral: 0.375 mg, 100's: **$39.95-$118.68**

• Elixir—Oral: 0.125 mg/5 ml, 480 ml: **$11.45-$38.10**

• Inj, Sol—IM, IV, SC: 0.5 mg/ml, 1 ml: **$16.65**

• Sol—Oral: 0.125 mg/ml, 15, 120 ml: **$8.40-$31.64**/15 ml

• Tab, Uncoated—SL: 0.125 mg, 100's: **$3.10-$62.39**

• Tab—Oral: 0.125 mg, 100's: **$3.10-$68.05**; 0.15 mg, 100's: **$21.25-$45.31**

• Tab, Sus Action—Oral: 0.375 mg, 100's: **$39.95-$105.51**

CONTRAINDICATIONS: Narrow-angle glaucoma, GI obstruction, myasthenia gravis, paralytic ileus, GI atony, toxic megacolon, prostatic hypertrophy

PRECAUTIONS: Hyperthyroidism, CAD, dysrhythmias, CHF, ulcerative colitis, hypertension, hiatal hernia, hepatic disease, renal disease, urinary retention

PREGNANCY AND LACTATION: Pregnancy category C; excreted in breast milk; infants sensitive to anticholinergics

SIDE EFFECTS/ADVERSE REACTIONS

CNS: Anxiety, *confusion,* dizziness, drowsiness, hallucination, headache, insomnia, *stimulation in elderly,* weakness

CV: Palpitations, tachycardia

EENT: Blurred vision, cycloplegia, increased intraocular pressure, mydriasis, photophobia

GI: Absence of taste, *constipation, dry mouth,* dysphagia, heartburn, ileus, nausea, vomiting

GU: Hesitancy, impotence, *retention*

SKIN: Anhidrosis, fever, pruritus, rash, urticaria

---

* = non-FDA-approved use

ibuprofen

(eye-byoo´pro-fen)

Rx: Motrin, Ibuprohm, IBU, Rufen, Saleto

OTC: Arthritis Foundation Pain Reliever, Advil, Ibuprin, Motrin IB, Nuprin

Combinations

  Rx: with Hydrocodone (Vicoprofen)

  OTC: With pseudoephedrine (Sine-Aid IB, Motrin IB Sinus)

Chemical Class: Propionic acid derivative

Therapeutic Class: NSAID with analgesic and antipyretic activity

CLINICAL PHARMACOLOGY

Mechanism of Action: Reversible cyclooxygenase (i.e., prostaglandin synthetase) inhibitor; nonselectively decreases the formation of both prostaglandins and thromboxane A2; variable effects on lipoxygenase synthesis and subsequent leukotriene production; antiinflammatory, antipyretic, and analgesic activity; inhibits platelet aggregation

Pharmacokinetics

PO: Onset ½ hour, peak 1-2 hr, $t_{1/2}$ 2-4 hr; metabolized in liver (inactive metabolites), excreted in urine (inactive metabolites) within 24 hr; does not enter breast milk; food decreases rate but not extent of absorption

INDICATIONS AND USES: Rheumatoid arthritis, osteoarthritis, primary dysmenorrhea, gout,* pain, fever, tocolysis in preterm labor*; prevention of cognitive decline,* colon cancer,* cystic fibrosis,* headache*

DOSAGE

Adult

• PO 200-800 mg qid, not to exceed 3200 mg/day

(NOTE: Doses <1600 mg/day analgesic only; >1600 mg/day needed for antiinflammatory activity)

Child

• PO 20-40 mg/kg/day divided tid or qid

🔢 AVAILABLE FORMS/COST OF THERAPY

• Cap—Oral: 200 mg, 40's: **$5.39**

• Susp—Oral: 40 mg/5 ml, 15 ml: **$4.50-$5.09**

• Tab, Chewable—Oral: 50 mg, 100's: **$11.05**; 100 mg, 100's: **$25.95**

• Tab—Oral: 200 mg, 100's: **$1.75-$23.42**; 300 mg, 100's: **$6.00-$8.30**; 400 mg, 100's: **$3.95-$41.00**; 600 mg, 100's: **$4.45-$45.90**; 800 mg, 100's: **$8.50-$49.71**

CONTRAINDICATIONS: Hypersensitivity to NSAIDs (including symptoms of asthma, nasal polyps, angioedema)

PRECAUTIONS: History of GI ulceration, bleeding, or perforation; renal dysfunction, hypertension or cardiac conditions aggravated by fluid retention and edema, history of liver dysfunction, history of coagulation

PREGNANCY AND LACTATION: Pregnancy category B; reduces amniotic fluid volume, constriction of the ductus arteriosus in 3rd trimester; compatible with breast feeding

SIDE EFFECTS/ADVERSE REACTIONS

CNS: Anxiety, confusion, depression, *dizziness,* drowsiness, fatigue, insomnia, tremors

CV: ***CHF,*** dysrhythmias, hypertension, palpitations, peripheral edema, tachycardia

EENT: Blurred vision, hearing loss, tinnitus

GI: Anorexia, cholestatic hepatitis, constipation, cramps, diarrhea, dry mouth, flatulence, **GI bleeding,** jaundice, nausea, peptic ulcer, vomiting

GU: Azotemia, hematuria, **nephrotoxicity,** oliguria

HEME: **Blood dyscrasias,** increased bleeding time

SKIN: Pruritus, purpura, rash, sweating

INTERACTIONS
Drugs
3 *Aminoglycosides:* Reduced clearance with elevated aminoglycoside levels and potential for toxicity (especially indomethacin in premature infants; other NSAIDs probably)

3 *Anticoagulants:* Excessive hypoprothrombinemia, decreased platelet aggregation with increased risk of GI bleeding

3 *Antihypertensives (α-blockers, angiotensin-converting enzyme inhibitors, angiotensin II receptor blockers, β-blockers, diuretics):* Inhibition of antihypertensive and other favorable hemodynamic effects

3 *Corticosteroids:* Increased risk of GI ulceration

3 *Cyclosporine:* Increased nephrotoxicity risk

3 *Lithium:* Decreased clearance of lithium (mediated via prostaglandins) resulting in elevated serum lithium levels and risk of toxicity

3 *Methotrexate:* Decreased renal secretion of methotrexate resulting in elevated methotrexate levels and risk of toxicity

3 *Phenylpropanolamine:* Possible acute hypertensive reaction

3 *Potassium-sparing diuretics:* Additive hyperkalemia potential

3 *Triamterene:* Acute renal failure reported with addition of indomethacin; caution with other NSAIDs

Labs
• *False decrease:* ALT, AST
SPECIAL CONSIDERATIONS
• Administer with food or antacids if GI symptoms occur
MONITORING PARAMETERS
• Initial hemogram and fecal occult blood test within 3 mo of starting regular chronic therapy; repeat every 6-12 mo (more frequently in high-risk patients, >65 years, peptic ulcer disease, concurrent steroids or anticoagulants); electrolytes, creatinine, and BUN within 3 mo of starting regular chronic therapy; repeat every 6-12 mo

---

ibutilide
(eye-byoo'ti-lide)
Rx: Corvert
Chemical Class: Methanesulfonamide derivative
Therapeutic Class: Antidysrhythmic (Class III)

CLINICAL PHARMACOLOGY
Mechanism of Action: Delays repolarization by activation of a slow, inward current (predominantly sodium); prolongs atrial and ventricular action potential duration and refractoriness; produces mild slowing of the sinus rate and AV conduction; produces dose-related prolongation of QT interval
Pharmacokinetics
IV: 40% bound to plasma proteins; metabolized to 8 metabolites (1 active), excreted in urine (80%) and feces (19%); t$_{1/2}$ 6 hr
INDICATIONS AND USES: Rapid conversion of atrial fibrillation or atrial flutter of recent onset to sinus rhythm (atrial arrhythmias of longer duration less likely to respond)

---

* = non-FDA-approved use

DOSAGE
Adult

• IV (≥60 kg) 1 mg (1 vial) infused over 10 min; (<60 kg) 0.01 mg/kg (0.1 ml/kg); if arrhythmia does not terminate within 10 min after end of initial infusion, a 2nd 10 min infusion of equal strength may be administered

$ **AVAILABLE FORMS/COST OF THERAPY**

• Sol—IV: 0.1 mg/ml, 10 ml: **$253.31**

PRECAUTIONS: Heart block; can worsen or induce ventricular dysrhythmias (including torsades de pointes)

PREGNANCY AND LACTATION: Pregnancy category C; excretion into breast milk unknown, breast feeding not recommended

SIDE EFFECTS/ADVERSE REACTIONS

CNS: Headache

CV: Bradycardia, bundle branch block, *CHF*, hypertension, hypotension, palpitation, postural hypotension, QT segment prolongation, syncope, tachycardia, ***ventricular dysrhythmias***

GI: Nausea

INTERACTIONS
Drugs

3 *Disopyramide, quninidine, procainamide, amiodarone, sotalol:* Potential to prolong refractoriness

2 *Phenothiazines, tricyclic antidepressants, terfenadine, astemizole:* Increased potential for prodysrhythmia due to prolongation of QT interval

SPECIAL CONSIDERATIONS
MONITORING PARAMETERS

• Continuous ECG monitoring for at least 4 hr following infusion or until QTc returns to baseline (longer monitoring if dysrhythmic activity noted). Defibrillator must be available

idoxuridine
(eye-dox-your'ih-deen)
Rx: Herplex
Chemical Class: Pyrimidine nucleoside
Therapeutic Class: Ophthalmic antiviral

CLINICAL PHARMACOLOGY

Mechanism of Action: Inhibits viral replication by interfering with viral DNA synthesis

Pharmacokinetics

Deactivated by deaminases and nucleotidases, penetrates cornea poorly

INDICATIONS AND USES: Herpes simplex keratitis, CMV, and varicella zoster keratitis*

DOSAGE
Adult and Child

• INSTILL 1 gtt q1h during day and q2h during night

$ **AVAILABLE FORMS/COST OF THERAPY**

• Sol, Ophth—Top: 0.1%, 10 ml: **$13.21**

PRECAUTIONS: Sensitivity to iodine

PREGNANCY AND LACTATION: Pregnancy category C; crosses placenta, teratogenic in rabbits and mice; no data available for breast feeding but shown to have tumorgenicity in animal studies

SIDE EFFECTS/ADVERSE REACTIONS

EENT: Overgrowth of non-susceptible organisms, photosensitivity, poor corneal wound healing, temporary visual haze

INTERACTIONS
Drugs

2 *Boric acid:* Precipitate formation

SPECIAL CONSIDERATIONS
PATIENT/FAMILY EDUCATION
• Wearing sunglasses decreases sensitivity to bright light. Notify clinician if no improvement in 14 days

---

imipenem-cilastin
(i-me-pen´em)
Rx: Primaxin
Chemical Class: Thienamycin antibiotic; renal dipeptidase inhibitor
Therapeutic Class: Antibiotic

CLINICAL PHARMACOLOGY
Mechanism of Action: Inhibits bacterial wall synthesis, results in cell lysis; formulated with cilastin, which prevents renal metabolism of imipenem; bactericidal
Pharmacokinetics
IV: Onset immediate, peak ½-1 hr, $t_{1/2}$ 1 hr
IM: Peak 2 hr, $t_{1/2}$ 6-8 hr
Excreted by kidney (75%) and unknown non-renal mechanism (25%); rapidly cleared by hemodialysis; $t_{1/2}$ longer in children (2 hr in neonates, 1.2 hr in older children)
INDICATIONS AND USES: Serious infections of the lower respiratory tract, urinary tract, skin; intra-abdominal infections, gynecologic infections, septicemia, endocarditis
Antibacterial spectrum usually includes:
• Gram-positive organisms: *Streptococcus pneumoniae,* group A β-hemolytic streptococci, *Staphylococcus aureus,* enterococci
• Gram-negative organisms: *Acinetobacter, Citrobacter, Enterobacter, E. Coli, Hemophilus, Klebsiella, Proteus, Pseudomonas aeruginosa, Salmonella, Serratia, Shigella*
• *Anaerobes: Bacteroides* including *B. fragilis, Peptococcus, Peptostreptococcus*
DOSAGE
Adult
• IV 250-500 mg q6h; severe infections may require 1 g q6h; max 50 mg/kg/day or 4 g/day (whichever is lower)
• IM 500 or 750 mg q12h to max 1500 mg qd
• *Dosage adjustment in impaired renal function:* CrCl 40-70 ml/sec, 250-500 mg q6-8h; CrCl 20-40 ml/sec, 250 mg q6-8h-500 mg q8h; CrCl 6-20 ml/sec, 250-500 mg q12h
• *Hemodialysis patients:* Supplemental dose after hemodialysis, unless scheduled dose within 4 hr
Child
• IV >40 kg, adult dose
• IV <40 kg, 60 mg/kg/day in divided doses
💲 AVAILABLE FORMS/COST OF THERAPY
• Inj, Dry-Sol—IM: 500 mg: **$31.43**; 750 mg: **$43.20**
• Inj, Dry-Sol—IV: 250 mg: **$16.70**; 500 mg: **$16.70-$17.34**
CONTRAINDICATIONS: IM: hypersensitivity to local anesthetics of the amide type (contains lidocaine)
PRECAUTIONS: Elderly, hypersensitivity to penicillins, seizure disorders, renal disease, children <12 yr
PREGNANCY AND LACTATION: Pregnancy category C; unknown if excreted in breast milk
SIDE EFFECTS/ADVERSE REACTIONS
CNS: Dizziness, fever, myoclonus, *seizures,* somnolence, weakness
CV: Hypotension, palpitations
GI: Diarrhea, glossitis, hepatitis, nausea, *pseudomembranous colitis,* vomiting
GU: Proteinuria, increased BUN/creatinine
HEME: Eosinophilia, *neutropenia*

RESP: Chest discomfort, dyspnea, hyperventilation

SKIN: Erythema at inj site, pain at inj site, phlebitis, pruritus, rash, urticaria

INTERACTIONS

Drugs

3 *Cyclosporine, tacrolimus:* Risk of CNS toxicity

3 *Theophylline:* Increased seizure risk without elevated theophylline levels

Labs

• *Interference:* Clindamycin, erythromycin, metronidazole, polymyxin, tetracycline, trimethoprim colistin levels

---

imipramine

(im-ip′ra-meen)

Rx: Tofranil, Tofranil PM

Chemical Class: Dibenzazepine derivative; tertiary amine, tertiary amine dibenzazepine derivative

Therapeutic Class: Tricyclic antidepressant; antiincontinence agent

---

CLINICAL PHARMACOLOGY

Mechanism of Action: Inhibits reuptake of norepinephrine and serotonin (blocking activity moderate and very high, respectively) at the presynaptic neuron, prolonging neuronal activity; inhibits histamine and acetylcholine activity; mild peripheral vasodilator effects and possible quinidine-like action on cardiac conduction; moderate anticholinergic and sedative, high orthostatic hypotensive side effects

Pharmacokinetics

PO: Steady state 2-5 days; metabolized by liver, excreted in urine, feces; crosses placenta; excreted in breast milk; $t_{1/2}$ 6-20 hr

INDICATIONS AND USES: Depression, enuresis in children, headache*

DOSAGE

Adult

• PO/IM 75-100 mg/day in divided doses, may increase by 25-50 mg to 200 mg, not to exceed 300 mg/day; may give daily dose hs

Child

• *Depression: PO:* 1.5 mg/kg/d, increasing by 1-1.5 mg/kg/d q 3-5 days to maximum 5 mg/kg/d

• *Enuresis:* (≥5 yr): *PO:* 25 mg qhs, increase to 50 mg in 1 wk Maximum dose 2.5 mg/kg/d or 75 mg

$ **AVAILABLE FORMS/COST OF THERAPY**

• Cap, Gel—Oral (pamoate): 75 mg, 100's: **$156.33**; 100 mg, 100's: **$205.59**; 125 mg, 100's: **$256.37**; 150 mg, 100's: **$292.17**

• Inj—IM: 25 mg/2 ml: **$2.42**

• Tab, Sugar Coated—Oral: 10 mg, 100's: **$3.00-$39.40**; 25 mg, 100's: **$3.42-$65.83**; 50 mg, 100's: **$4.50-$111.80**

CONTRAINDICATIONS: Hypersensitivity to tricyclic antidepressants, recovery phase of MI, convulsive disorders, prostatic hypertrophy

PRECAUTIONS: Suicidal patients, severe depression, increased intraocular pressure, narrow-angle glaucoma, urinary retention, cardiac disease, hepatic disease, hyperthyroidism, electroshock therapy, elective surgery, elderly

PREGNANCY AND LACTATION: Pregnancy category C

SIDE EFFECTS/ADVERSE REACTIONS

CNS: Anxiety, confusion, *dizziness, drowsiness,* EPS (elderly), headache, increased psychiatric symptoms, insomnia, nightmares, paresthesia, stimulation, tremors, weakness

---

italic = common side effects   ***bold italic*** = life-threatening reactions

CV: ECG changes, hypertension, *orthostatic hypotension,* palpitations, *tachycardia*

EENT: Blurred vision, mydriasis, tinnitus

GI: Cramps, *diarrhea, dry mouth,* epigastric distress, hepatitis, increased appetite, jaundice, nausea, paralytic ileus, stomatitis, vomiting

GU: Acute renal failure, impotence, *retention*

HEME: Bone marrow depression, eosinophilia

METAB: Hyperprolactinemia

SKIN: Photosensitivity, pruritus, rash, sweating, urticaria

INTERACTIONS

Drugs

❸ *Altretamine:* Orthostatic hypotension

❸ *Amphetamines:* Theoretical increase in amphetamine effect

❸ *Antidiabetics:* Possible enhanced hypoglycemic effects

❷ *Bethanidine, clonidine:* Inhibition of antihypertensive effect, possible hypertensive crisis

❸ *Carbamazepine, cholestyramine, colestipol, barbiturates:* Reduces imipramine levels

❷ *Epinephrine, norepinephrine:* Hypertension and dysrhythmias

❸ *Ethanol:* Enhanced motor skill impairment

❸ *Guanethidine, guanfacine:* Inhibition of antihypertensive effect

❸ *Isoproterenol and possibly other β-agonists:* Increased risk of arrhythmias

❸ *Lithium:* Possible increased CNS toxicity, especially in elderly

▲ *MAOIs:* Serotonin syndrome, some fatal

❷ *Moclobemide:* Risk serotonin syndrome

❸ *Phenothiazines, cimetidine (not with other H_2 blockers), calcium channel blockers, selective serotonin reuptake inhibitors, quinidine, ritonavir, indinavir:* Increased imipramine levels

❸ *Phenylephrine:* Enhanced pressor response

❸ *Propantheline:* Excessive anticholinergic effects

Labs

• *False increase:* Carbamazepine levels

• *False decrease:* Urine 5-HIAA, VMA

SPECIAL CONSIDERATIONS

PATIENT/FAMILY EDUCATION

• Withdrawal symptoms (headache, nausea, vomiting, muscle pain, weakness) may occur if drug discontinued abruptly

• At doses of 20 mg/kg ventricular arrhythmias occur

---

imiquimod

(im-ick′wih-mod)

Rx: Aldara

Chemical Class: Immune response modifier

Therapeutic Class: Antiviral

CLINICAL PHARMACOLOGY

Mechanism of Action: Unknown, but may involve the induction of cytokines, including interferon-α and others

Pharmacokinetics

TOP: Minimal systemic absorption; <0.9% of dose excreted in urine and feces

INDICATIONS AND USES: External genital and perianal warts (condyloma acuminata)

DOSAGE

Adult

• TOP apply to warts 3 times weekly prior to normal sleeping hours; leave on for 6-10 hr then wash off with mild soap and water; continue until warts are completely cleared or 16 wk, whichever comes first

💲 AVAILABLE FORMS/COST OF THERAPY

• Cre—Topical: 5%, 250 mg/single-use packet, 12's: **$124.80**

PRECAUTIONS: Urethral, intravaginal, cervical, rectal, or intra-anal warts; children <18 yr

PREGNANCY AND LACTATION: Pregnancy category B; excretion into breast milk unknown but would be expected to be small given minimal systemic absorption

SIDE EFFECTS/ADVERSE REACTIONS

CNS: Headache

MS: Myalgia

SKIN: Itching, erythema, erosion, burning, excoriation, flaking, edema, local pain, induration, ulceration, scabbing, vesicles, soreness

MISC: Flu-like symptoms

SPECIAL CONSIDERATIONS

• New option for treatment of genital and perianal warts which can be applied by patient at home and appears to have low toxicity compared to podofilox

• Response rates approximately 50% and relapses are common

PATIENT/FAMILY EDUCATION

• Apply thin layer to wart(s) and rub in until cream is no longer visible

• Do not occlude application site

• Should severe local reaction occur, remove cream by washing with soap and water; treatment may be resumed once skin reaction has subsided

indapamide

(in-dap'a-mide)

Rx: Lozol

Chemical Class: Indoline derivative

Therapeutic Class: Thiazide-like diuretic; antihypertensive

CLINICAL PHARMACOLOGY

Mechanism of Action: Structural and pharmacological similarities to thiazide diuretics; inhibits reabsorption of sodium and chloride in cortical thick ascending limb of the loop of Henle and the early distal tubules—minimal effect on glomerular filtration rate or renal plasma flow, unlike other thiazide diuretics; decreases peripheral resistance (perhaps via calcium channel blockade) with little or no effect on cardiac output, rate or rhythm. Antihypertensive effects decrease in patients with decreasing renal function; less effect on electrolyte excretion

Pharmacokinetics

PO: Onset 1-2 hr, peak 2 hr, duration up to 36 hr; excreted in urine, feces; $t_{1/2}$ 14-18 hr

INDICATIONS AND USES: Edema (CHF, cirrhosis, corticosteroid and estrogen therapy); hypercalciuria; hypertension, Raynaud's disease*

DOSAGE

Adult

• PO 2.5-5 mg qd in AM

NOTE: Equivalent hydrochlorothiazide dose: 2.5 mg-50 mg

💲 AVAILABLE FORMS/COST OF THERAPY

• Tab, Plain Coated—Oral: 1.25 mg, 100's: **$61.40-$99.16**; 2.5 mg, 100's: **$65.97-$122.65**

CONTRAINDICATIONS: Renal decompensation; anuria

---

italic = common side effects   ***bold italic*** = life-threatening reactions

PRECAUTIONS: Fluid and electrolyte imbalance (including sodium, potassium, chloride, magnesium, calcium), renal disease, hepatic disease, gout, COPD, lupus erythematosus, diabetes mellitus, hyperparathyroidism, vomiting, diarrhea

PREGNANCY AND LACTATION: Pregnancy category B; therapy for preexisting hypertension can be continued throughout pregnancy with minimal risk; initiating for edema not recommended; few unequivocal indications for diuretic therapy in pregnancy except for pulmonary edema or congestive heart failure; not known if excreted in breast milk

SIDE EFFECTS/ADVERSE REACTIONS

CNS: Vertigo, *dizziness,* fatigue, *headache,* paresthesias, *weakness*

CV: Dysrhythmias, orthostatic hypotension, palpitations

EENT: Blurred vision, increased intraocular pressure, loss of hearing, nasal congestion, tinnitus

GI: Abdominal pain, anorexia, constipation, cramps, diarrhea, dry mouth, hepatitis, jaundice, *nausea,* pancreatitis, vomiting

GU: Decreased libido, frequency, impotence, increased creatinine, BUN *HEME:* Inhibits platelet aggregation

METAB: Hypercalcemia, hyperglycemia, *hyperuricemia, hypochloremic alkalosis,* hypokalemia, *hypomagnesemia, hyponatremia*

MS: Cramps

SKIN: Photosensitivity, pruritus, rash, urticaria

INTERACTIONS

Drugs

❷ *Angiotensin-converting enzyme inhibitors:* Risk of postural hypotension when added to ongoing diuretic therapy; more common with loop diuretics; first dose hypotension possible in patients with sodium depletion or hypovolemia due to diuretics or sodium restriction; hypotensive response is usually transient; hold diuretic day of first dose

❸ *Corticosteroids:* Concomitant therapy may result in excessive potassium loss

❸ *Diazoxide:* Blunt insulin secretion; results in hyperglycemia

❸ *Lithium:* Concurrent use may result in elevated serum levels of lithium; monitor carefully

❸ *Nonsteroidal antiinflammatory drugs:* Concurrent may reduce diuretic and antihypertensive effects

SPECIAL CONSIDERATIONS

PATIENT/FAMILY EDUCATION

• May cause sensitivity to sunlight; avoid prolonged exposure to the sun and other ultraviolet light

• May cause gout attacks; notify clinician if sudden joint pain occurs

• May worsen control or increase requirements of hypoglycemic agents

MONITORING PARAMETERS

• Weight, urine output, serum electrolytes, BUN, creatinine, CBC, uric acid, glucose, lipids

---

indinavir

(in-din′ah-veer)

Rx: Crixivan

Chemical Class: HIV protease inhibitor

Therapeutic Class: HIV infection

CLINICAL PHARMACOLOGY

Mechanism of Action: Inhibits HIV protease preventing cleavage of viral polyproteins resulting in the formation of immature non-infectious viral particles

Pharmacokinetics

PO: Peak 0.8 hr; AUC decreased by high-calorie, fat and protein meals; 60% bound to plasma proteins; metabolized in liver to 7 metabolites, excreted in feces (83%) and urine; $t_{1/2}$ 1.8 hr

INDICATIONS AND USES: HIV infection when antiretroviral treatment is warranted

DOSAGE

Adult

• PO 800 mg (two 400 mg caps) q8h on an empty stomach; reduce dose to 600 mg q8h in mild-to-moderate hepatic insufficiency

• Adjust dose when used with ketoconazole, nelfinavir, rifabutin, ritonavir

• For latest treatment guidelines, see www.hivatis.org

🖫 AVAILABLE FORMS/COST OF THERAPY

• Cap—Oral: 200 mg, 270's: **$375.98**; 333 mg, 135's: **$326.76**; 400 mg, 180's: **$523.35**

CONTRAINDICATIONS: Concurrent use of rifampin

PRECAUTIONS: Renal and hepatic function impairment, dehydration, children

PREGNANCY AND LACTATION: Pregnancy category C; not recommended for breast-feeding mothers

SIDE EFFECTS/ADVERSE REACTIONS

CNS: Dizziness, headache, insomnia, somnolence

EENT: Taste perversion

GI: Acid regurgitation, anorexia, diarrhea, dry mouth, *hyperbilirubinemia, nausea,* vomiting

GU: Flank pain, hematuria, nephrolithiasis (4%)

METAB: Hyperbilirubinemia

MS: Back pain

INTERACTIONS

Drugs

▲ *Astemizole:* Increased plasma levels of astemizole

🖪 *Barbiturates:* Increased clearance of indinavir; reduced clearance of barbiturates

❷ *Carbamazepine:* Increased clearance of indinavir; reduced clearance of carbamazepine

▲ *Cisapride:* Increased plasma levels of cisapride

🖪 *Clarithromycin:* Indinavir reduces clearance of clarithromycin

🖪 *Delavirdine:* Decreased clearance of indinavir; reduce dose of indinavir to 600 mg q8h

❷ *Efavirenz:* Reduced indinavir level; increase indinavir dose to 1000 mg q8h

▲ *Ergot alkaloids:* Increased plasma levels of ergot alkaloids

🖪 *Erythromycin:* Reduced clearance of indinavir; indinavir reduces clearance of erythromycin

🖪 *Ketoconazole:* Decreased clearance of indinavir; decrease indinavir dose to 600 mg tid

▲ *Lovastatin:* Indinavir reduces clearance of lovastatin

▲ *Midazolam:* Increased plasma levels of midazolam and prolonged effect

🖪 *Nelfinavir:* Decreased clearance of indinavir; reduce dose of indinavir to 1200 mg bid

🖪 *Nevirapine:* Reduces plasma indinavir levels; no dose adjustment needed

🖪 *Oral contraceptives:* Indinavir may reduce efficacy

🖪 *Phenytoin:* Increased clearance of indinavir; reduced clearance of phenytoin

❷ *Rifabutin:* Increased clearance of indinavir; reduced clearance of rifabutin—reduce rifabutin dose to 150 mg qd and increase indinavir dose to 1000 mg tid

italic = common side effects   ***bold italic*** = life-threatening reactions

A *Rifampin:* Increased clearance of indinavir

R *Ritonavir:* Decreased clearance of indinavir; decrease indinavir dose to 400 mg bid

R *Saquinavir:* Decreased clearance of saquinavir; reduce dose of Fortovase (saquinavir soft gel capsule) to 800 mg tid

A *Simvastatin:* Indinavir reduces clearance of simvastatin

A *Terfenadine:* Increased plasma levels of terfenadine

A *Triazolam:* Increased plasma levels of triazolam and prolonged effect

R *Troleandomycin:* Reduced clearance of indinavir; indinavir reduces clearance of troleandomycin

SPECIAL CONSIDERATIONS
• Antiretroviral activity of indinavir may be increased when used in combination with reverse transcriptase inhibitors

PATIENT/FAMILY EDUCATION
• Drink plenty of water, at least 48 oz/day
• Take with water or light, low-fat meals (dry toast, apple juice, corn flakes, skim milk). High fat meals and grapefruit juice reduce absorption
• Capsules sensitive to moisture. Keep dessicant in bottle
• If dose is missed take next dose on schedule; do not double this dose
• Separate dosing with didanosine by 1 hour
• Take 1 hr before or 2 hr after meals; may take with skim milk or low-fat meal

indomethacin

(in-doe-meth′a-sin)
Rx: Indocin, Indocin IV, Indocin SR, Indochron, Indo-Lemmon
Chemical Class: Indole acetic acid derivative
Therapeutic Class: NSAID with analgesic and antipyretic activity

CLINICAL PHARMACOLOGY
Mechanism of Action: Reversible cyclooxygenase (i.e., prostaglandin synthetase) inhibitor; nonselectively decreases the formation of both prostaglandins and thromboxane A2; variable effects on lipoxygenase synthesis and subsequent leukotriene production; antiinflammatory, antipyretic, and analgesic activity; inhibits platelet aggregation
Pharmacokinetics
PO: Completely absorbed; onset 1-2 hr, peak 3 hr, duration 4-6 hr; metabolized in liver, kidneys; excreted in urine, bile, feces; 99% plasma protein binding
PR: 80%-90% absorbed
IV: $t_{1/2}$ 4½ in adults; in infants, inversely related to gestational age and wt (<7 days age, <1000 g, $t_{1/2}$ 20-21 hr; >7 days age, >1000 g, $t_{1/2}$ 12-15 hr)
INDICATIONS AND USES: Ankylosing spondylitis, apnea of prematurity,* cholecystitis,* cognitive decline—prevention,* colon cancer—prevention,* dysmenorrhea,* erythema nodosum,* fever,* gouty arthritis, headache,* heterotopic bone ossification—prevention,* hypotension,* interferon intrathecal toxicity,* male infertility,* muromonab (OKT3) toxicity,* neonatal intraventricular hemorrhage,* nephrotic syndrome,* neurogenic, osteoar-

thritis, pain,* patent ductus arteriosus (PDA), pericarditis,* polyhydramnios,* premature labor,* Reiter's syndrome,* renal tubular dysfunction,* rheumatoid arthritis,* shoulder—acute pain,* Sweet's syndrome,* systemic lupus erythematosus,* ureteral colic*

DOSAGE

Adult

• *Antirheumatic/anti - inflammatory:* PO 25-50 mg bid-qid, may increase by 25 mg/day q wk, not to exceed 200 mg/day; Sus Action 75 mg qd, may increase to 75 mg bid; PR 50 mg bid-qid

• *Gout:* PO 100 mg initially then 50 mg tid until pain relieved, then reduce dose; PR 50 mg bid-qid

Child

• *Antirheumatic / antiinflammatory:* PO/PR 1.5-2.5 mg/kg/day divided doses tid-qid to max 4 mg/kg/day or 150-200 mg qd

• *Patent ductus arteriosus:* IV (preferred)/PO/PR 200 µg/kg initial dose; may follow with 100 µg/kg (infants ≤48 hr age), 200 µg/kg (infants 2-7 days age), 250 µg/kg (infants >7 days age) q12-24 hr for 2 doses

$ AVAILABLE FORMS/COST OF THERAPY

• Cap, Gel—Oral: 25 mg, 100's: **$4.13-$67.46**; 50 mg, 100's: **$4.13-$110.14**

• Cap, Gel, Sus Action—Oral: 75 mg, 100's: **$57.60-$193.47**

• Inj, Lyphl-Sol—IV: 1 mg/vial: **$32.40**

• Supp—Rect: 50 mg, 30's: **$40.85-$55.39**

• Susp—Oral: 25 mg/5 ml, 237, 500 ml: **$50.65**/237 ml

CONTRAINDICATIONS: Bronchospasm, nasal polyps, angioedema precipitated by aspirin or other NSAIDs

PRECAUTIONS: History of GI ulceration, bleeding, or perforation; renal dysfunction, hypertension or cardiac conditions aggravated by fluid retention and edema, history of liver dysfunction, history of coagulation

PREGNANCY AND LACTATION: Pregnancy category B; crosses placenta; excreted in breast milk

SIDE EFFECTS/ADVERSE REACTIONS

CNS: Anxiety, confusion, depression, dizziness, drowsiness, fatigue, *headache,* insomnia, tremors

*CV: **CHF, dysrhythmias,** hypertension, palpitations, peripheral edema, tachycardia

EENT: Blurred vision, hearing loss, tinnitus

GI: Anorexia, cholestatic hepatitis, constipation, cramps, diarrhea, *dyspepsia,* flatulence, **GI bleeding,** green stools, jaundice, *nausea,* peptic ulcer

GU: Azotemia, hematuria, **nephrotoxicity,** oliguria

*HEME: **Blood dyscrasias***

RESP: Asthma

SKIN: Pruritus, purpura, rash, sweating

MISC: Fever

INTERACTIONS

Drugs

🔳 *Aminoglycosides:* Reduced clearance with elevated aminoglycoside levels and potential for toxicity (especially indomethacin in premature infants; other NSAIDs probably)

🔳 *Anticoagulants:* Excessive hypoprothrombinemia, decreased platelet aggregation with increased risk of GI bleeding

🔳 *Antihypertensives (alpha blockers, angiotensin-converting enzyme inhibitors, angiotensin II receptor blockers, beta blockers, diuretics:*

---

italic = common side effects   ***bold italic*** = life-threatening reactions

Inhibition of antihypertensive and other favorable hemodynamic effects

3 *Corticosteroids:* Increased risk of GI ulceration

3 *Cyclosporine:* Increased nephrotoxicity risk

3 *Lithium:* Decreased clearance of lithium (mediated via prostaglandins) resulting in elevated serum lithium levels and risk of toxicity

3 *Methotrexate:* Decreased renal secretion of methotrexate resulting in elevated methotrexate levels and risk of toxicity

3 *Phenylpropanolamine:* Possible acute hypertensive reaction

3 *Potassium-sparing diuretics:* Additive hyperkalemia potential

3 *Triamterene:* Acute renal failure reported with addition of indomethacin; caution with other NSAIDs

SPECIAL CONSIDERATIONS

PATIENT/FAMILY EDUCATION

• Take with food
• No significant advantage over other oral NSAIDs; cost and clinical situation should govern use

MONITORING PARAMETERS

• Renal and hepatic function with prolonged use: check after 3 months, then q6-12 months
• Initial CBC and fecal occult blood test within 3 months of starting regular chronic therapy; repeat q6-12 months (more frequently in high-risk patients)

infliximab

(in-flicks´ih-mab)

Rx: Remicade

Chemical Class: IgG1k chimeric monoclonal antibody
Therapeutic Class: Tumor necrosis factor alpha (TNFα) antibody

CLINICAL PHARMACOLOGY

Mechanism of Action: Binds and neutralizes the biological activity of TNFα, which includes: 1) induction of pro-inflammatory cytokines (interleukins), 2) enhancement of leukocyte migration, 3) activation of neutrophil and eosinophil functional activity, 4) induction of acute phase reactants and tissue degrading enzymes

Pharmacokinetics

IV: C_{max} 118 µg/ml following single 5 mg/kg dose; detectable in serum 12 weeks after infusion; Vd 3 L; $t_{1/2}$ 8.0-9.5 days

INDICATIONS AND USES: Rheumatoid arthritis, Crohn's disease, enterocutaneous fistulae, arthritis - Crohn's disease induced*, sarcoidosis*, ulcerative colitis*, Bechet's disease*, psoriasis/psoriatic arthritis*, pyoderma gangrenosum*

DOSAGE

Adult

• *Rheumatoid arthritis:* 3 mg/kg IV infusion (over not less than 2 hr) initially, then repeated at 2, 6, and q8wk thereafter; for patients with incomplete response, consider increasing dose to 10 mg/kg infusions (Note: given in conjunction with ongoing methotrexate therapy)
• *Crohn's disease:* 5 mg/kg IV infusion (over not less than 2 hr), followed by similar doses at 2 and 6 weeks

---

* = non-FDA-approved use

• Safety and efficacy not established in children

💲 AVAILABLE FORMS/COST OF THERAPY
• Inj, Sol—IV: 100 mg/20 ml vial: **$450.00-$665.01**

CONTRAINDICATIONS: Hypersensitivity to murine proteins; clinically important, active infection

PRECAUTIONS: History of allergic phenomena, multiple sclerosis (possible exacerbation), elderly (increased risk of infection), history of chronic or recurrent infection

PREGNANCY AND LACTATION: Pregnancy category B; breast milk excretion unknown, nursing not recommended

SIDE EFFECTS/ADVERSE REACTIONS
CNS: Headache
CV: Chest pain, hypotension, hypertension
GI: Cholecystitis, GI upset (nausea, vomiting, abdominal pain)
HEME: Anemia, ***splenic infarction, splenomegaly***
MS: Arthralgia, formation of autoantibodies (lupus-like syndrome), back pain, myalgia
RESP: Cough, pharyngitis, sinusitis
SKIN: Pruritus, rash
MISC: Fatigue, fever, infection (32%), infusion reactions (19%), ***malignancy,*** pain

INTERACTIONS
Drugs
• *Live virus vaccines:* No information on vaccine response or secondary transmission of infection

SPECIAL CONSIDERATIONS
• Evaluate for risk of TB (TB skin test) prior to initiating therapy

PATIENT/FAMILY EDUCATION
• More susceptible to infections; avoid crowds, people with URI, flu, etc

MONITORING PARAMETERS
• Decreased levels of serum IL-6, C-reactive protein, ESR, rheumatoid factor, signs and symptoms of disease, urinalysis, blood chemistry, human anti-cA2 titers, blood pressure (during and after infusion), temperature, body weight, signs and symptoms of infection (including TB)

---

italic = common side effects   ***bold italic*** = life-threatening reactions

insulin

(in′su-lin)

Rx: *RAPID-ACTING INSULIN ANALOG:* Humalog (Lispro), NovoLog (Aspart)
OTC: *RAPID ACTING: REGULAR INSULIN:* Humulin R, Regular Iletin II (Beef), Regular Iletin II (Pork), Regular Iletin I (Beef-Pork), Novolin R, Velosulin
PROMPT INSULIN-ZINC SUSPENSION: Semilente Iletin I/(Beef-Pork)
INTERMEDIATE ACTING: INSULIN-ZINC SUSPENSION: Humulin L, Lente Iletin I (Beef-Pork), Lente Iletin II (Pork), Iletin II (Pork), Novolin-L
ISOPHANE-INSULIN SUSPENSION (NPH): Humulin N, NPH Iletin III (Beef), NPH Iletin II (Pork), NPH Iletin I (Beef-Pork), Novolin N
LONG-ACTING INSULIN ANALOG: Lantus (Glargine)
EXTENDED INSULIN-ZINC SUSPENSION: Humulin-U, Ultralente Iletin I (Beef-Pork),
PROTAMINE ZINC-INSULIN SUSPENSION (PZI): PZI III (Beef), PZI II (Pork), PZI I (Beef-Pork)
INSULIN MIXTURES: ISOPHANE INSULIN AND REGULAR INSULIN: Humulin 50/50, Humulin 70/30, Novolin 70/30
CONCENTRATED INSULIN: REGULAR CONCENTRATED INSULIN: Humulin RU-500, Regular Iletin II U-500 (Pork)
Chemical Class: Exogenous insulin
Therapeutic Class: Antidiabetic

CLINICAL PHARMACOLOGY

Mechanism of Action: Stimulates carbohydrate metabolism; facilitates transfer of glucose into muscle and adipose tissue (lowers blood glucose); converts glucose to glycogen; stimulates both lipogenesis and protein synthesis; shifts potassium and magnesium intracellularly

Pharmacokinetics

See Insulins Table, p. 1123 SC and IM absorption not significantly different

Metabolized by liver, muscle, kidneys; excreted in urine; $T_{1/2}$ elimination: 5-15 minutes (IV administration); range: 1.6-5.2 hr (SC or IM administration) with $T_{1/2}$ increasing with increased dose

INDICATIONS AND USES: Diabetes mellitus types 1 and 2, ketoacidosis, hyperkalemia, nonketotic hyperosmolar syndrome; human insulin is insulin of choice in insulin allergy, insulin resistance, pregnancy

DOSAGE

Adult and Child

• *Ketoacidosis:* IV bolus or IM 0.1-0.25 U/kg regular insulin, then 0.1 U/kg/hr IV INF/IM q1h until blood glucose 250 mg/dl, then give SC replacement dose

• *Type I diabetes mellitus (DM) replacement:* SC dosage individualized by blood glucose levels; initial total daily dose based on presence of urine ketones; if ketones negative –moderate 0.5 U/kg; if ketones large 0.7 U/kg; give ⅔ total dose in AM, ⅓ in PM; use mixture regular/NPH insulin (ratio 1:2 for AM dose, 1:1 for PM dose)

• *Type II DM replacement:* SC dosage individualized by blood glucose levels; initial total daily dose 0.3 U/kg; give ⅔ total dose in AM, ⅓ in PM; use mixed insulin 70/30 or

50/50 or mixture of regular/NPH (ratio 1:2 for AM dose, 1:1 for PM dose)

• *Type II DM combination with oral agent* (unable to achieve targets on max dose oral agent, AM hyperglycemia): Decrease oral agent to ½ max dose, give as single AM dose; add insulin with evening snack SC 0.1 U/kg NPH

• *Nonketotic hyperosmolar syndrome:* IV 10-20 U regular insulin, then IV/IM 5-15 U/hr until glucose 250 mg/dl, then give SC replacement dose

• *Gestational DM:* SC dosage individualized by blood glucose levels; initial total daily dose 0.4 U/kg current wt given as mixture regular/NPH distributed as for Type I DM

• *Hyperkalemia:* Adult IV 5-10 U regular insulin with 25 g dextrose (1 ampule D_{50}); child: 0.5g/kg dextrose with 0.3 U regular insulin/g dextrose over 2 hr

💲 AVAILABLE FORMS/COST OF THERAPY

Rapid-Acting Insulin Analog
• Inj, Sol—SC: 100 U/ml, 1.5 ml, 5's: **$52.50**; 10 ml (Lispro): **$52.18**; 10 ml (Aspart): **$52.18**
Long-Acting Insulin Analog
• Inj, Sol—SC: 100 U/ml, 10 ml (Glargine): **$46.99**
Rapid-Acting Regular Insulin
• Inj, Sol—IM, IV, SC: 100 U/ml, (human) 1.5 ml, 5's: **$34.15-$42.60**; 10 ml: (human): **$27.66**; (beef/pork): **$17.68-$28.25**; (pork): **$46.13-$49.98**
Intermediate-Acting Insulin-Zinc Suspension
• Inj, Susp—SC: 100 U/ml, 10 ml (human): **$27.64**; (beef/pork): **$28.25**; (pork): **$46.13-$49.98**
Isophane Insulin Suspension (NPH)
• Inj, Susp—SC: 100 U/ml, (human) 1.5 ml, 5's: **$34.15-$44.74**; 10 ml: **$27.66**

Long-Acting Insulin-Zinc Suspension
• Inj, Vsp—SC: 100 U/ml, 10 ml: **$27.66**
Mixed Insulin 70/30 (NPH/Regular)
• Inj, Sol—SC: 100 U/ml, 1.5 ml, 5's: **$34.15-$44.74**; 10 ml: **$27.66**
Mixed Insulin 50/50 (NPH/Regular)
• Inj, Susp—SC: 50 U/ml, 10 ml: **$27.66**
Concentrated Regular Insulin
• Inj, Sol—SC: 500 U/ml, 20 ml: **$199.05**

PREGNANCY AND LACTATION: Pregnancy category B; insulin requirements of pregnant diabetic patients often decreased in 1st half and increased in the latter half of pregnancy; elevated blood glucose levels associated with congenital abnormalities; does not pass into breast milk

SIDE EFFECTS/ADVERSE REACTIONS

SKIN: Flushing, rash, urticaria, warmth, lipodystrophy, lipohypertrophy

METAB: **Hypoglycemia,** decreased K, Ca, PO_4, Mg

INTERACTIONS
Drugs

🔳 *Beta-blockers:* Increased glucose levels, hypoglycemia symptoms masked (except sweating)

🔳 *Cigarette smoking, marijuana, corticosteroids, thiazides:* Increased glucose levels

🔳 *Clonidine, Guanfacine, Guanabenz:* Hypoglycemia symptoms masked

⚠ *Ethanol (excessive):* Hypoglycemia

🔳 *Salicylates, ACE inhibitors, anabolic steroids, MAO inhibitors:* Enhanced hypoglycemic response

---

italic = common side effects   ***bold italic*** = life-threatening reactions

SPECIAL CONSIDERATIONS
PATIENT/FAMILY EDUCATION

• Symptoms of hypoglycemia include: fatigue, weakness, confusion, headache, convulsions, hunger, nausea, pallor, sweating, rapid breathing

• For hypoglycemia, give 1 mg glucagon, glucose 25 g IV (via dextrose 50% sol, 50 ml) or oral glucose if tolerated

• When mixing insulins, draw up short-acting first

• Dosage adjustment may be necessary when changing insulin products

• Human insulin considered insulin of choice secondary to antigenicity of animal insulins

---

interferon alfa-2a/2b

(in-ter-feer´on)

Rx: Roferon-A (alfa-2a), Intron-A (alfa-2b)
Combinations

> **Rx:** Interferon alfa 2b with ribavirin (Rebetron Combination Therapy)

Chemical Class: Recombinant interferon
Therapeutic Class: Antineoplastic, antiviral

CLINICAL PHARMACOLOGY

Mechanism of Action: Altered synthesis of RNA, DNA, cellular proteins

Pharmacokinetics

SC: Absorption >80%; $t_{1/2}$ (alfa-2a) 6-8 hr, peak 7.3 hr; $t_{1/2}$ (alfa-2b) 2-3 hr, peak 3-12 hr

IV: $t_{1/2}$ 4-8 hr

IM: Absorption >80%; $t_{1/2}$ (alfa-2a) 6-8 hr, peak 3.8 hr; $t_{1/2}$ (alfa-2b) 2-3 hr, peak 3-12 hr

INTRALESIONAL: Minimal systemic absorption

Excreted by kidney; unknown if excreted in human breast milk

INDICATIONS AND USES: Hairy cell leukemia, condylomata acuminata, chronic hepatitis C, chronic hepatitis B, malignant melanoma, AIDS-associated Kaposi's sarcoma, renal carcinoma,* chronic myelocytic leukemia, laryngeal papillomatosis,* non-Hodgkin's lymphoma,* multiple myeloma,* mycosis fungoides,* other cancers*

DOSAGE

A variety of dosage schedules have been used; consult medical literature prior to choosing specific dosage

INTERFERON ALFA-2A

Adult

• *Hairy cell leukemia:* IM/SC 3 million U qd for 16-24 wk then 3 million U 3 times/wk

• *Kaposi's sarcoma:* IM/SC 36 million U qd for 10-12 wk or 3 million U qd days 1-3 then 9 million U qd days 4-6, then 18 million U days 7-9, then 36 million U qd for remainder of 10-12 wk; maintenance with 36 million U 3 times/wk

• *Hepatitis C:* IM/SC 3 million U 3 times/wk × 12 months

• For relapse 3-6 million U 3 times/wk for 6-12 additional months

Child

• Not established; caution in adolescent females because interferes with serum estradiol and progesterone concentration

INTERFERON ALFA-2B

Adult

• *Hairy cell leukemia:* IM/SC 2 million U/m^2 body surface area 3 times/wk

• *Condylomata acuminata:* Intralesional 1 million U (0.1 ml) per wart (up to five warts) 3 times/wk for 3 wk; 2nd course may be given 12-16 wk after 1st course; treat more warts sequentially in groups of 5

---

* = non-FDA-approved use

• *Kaposi's sarcoma:* IM/SC 30 million U/m^2 body surface area 3 times/wk
• *Chronic active hepatitis:* IM/SC 3 million U 3 times/wk

Child
• Not established

💲 AVAILABLE FORMS/COST OF THERAPY

Interferon alfa-2a
• Inj, Dry-Sol—IM, SC: 3 million IU/vial: **$36.72**; 6 million IU/vial: **$73.42**; 9 million IU/vial: **$103.37**; 36 million IU/vial: **$419.26**

Interferon alfa-2b
• Inj, Dry-Sol,—IM, SC, ID: 3 million IU/vial: **$33.91**; 5 million IU/vial: **$52.51**; 10 million IU/vial: **$118.76**; 18 million IU/vial: **$245.93**; 25 million IU/vial: **$341.93**; 50 million IU/vial: **$551.83**

PRECAUTIONS: Severe hypotension, dysrhythmia, tachycardia, severe renal or hepatic disease, seizure disorder

PREGNANCY AND LACTATION: Pregnancy category C; abortifacient in animal models; avoid breast feeding

SIDE EFFECTS/ADVERSE REACTIONS

CNS: Amnesia, anxiety, **coma,** *confusion, dizziness,* hallucinations, mood changes, *numbness, paresthesias,* **seizures**
CV: Chest pain, **CHF,** dysrhythmias, hypertension, hypotension, palpitations
EENT: Blurred vision, *dry mouth*
GI: Anorexia, *diarrhea (15-45%), nausea (20-50%), taste changes, vomiting, weight loss*
GU: Impotence
HEME: **Anemia, leukopenia, thrombocytopenia**
SKIN: Alopecia, *dry skin,* flushing, *itching, rash*

MISC: Chills, *fatigue, fever (40-80%), flu-like syndrome, headache, myalgias*

INTERACTIONS

Drugs
3 *Theophylline:* Increased theophylline levels

SPECIAL CONSIDERATIONS
• Rebetron Combination Therapy (kit containing interferon alfa-2b inj plus ribavirin capsules) more effective than interferon alfa-2b monotherapy for chronic hepatitis C infection

PATIENT/FAMILY EDUCATION
• Drink plenty of fluids
• Flu-like symptoms decrease during treatment. Acetaminophen (do not exceed recommended dose) may alleviate fever and headache

---

interferon alfa-n3
(in-ter-feer'on)
Rx: Alferon N
Chemical Class: Human leukocyte interferon
Therapeutic Class: Antiviral

CLINICAL PHARMACOLOGY
Mechanism of Action: Altered synthesis of RNA, DNA, and cellular proteins

Pharmacokinetics
INJ: Unable to detect by assay although some systemic effects noted

INDICATIONS AND USES: Condylomata acuminata

DOSAGE

Adult ≥18 yr
• INTRALESIONAL (into base of wart): 0.05 ml (250,000 IU) per wart, given 2 times/wk for max 8 wk; max 0.5 ml/treatment session

💲 AVAILABLE FORMS/COST OF THERAPY
• Inj, Sol—ID, SC: 5 million U/ml: **$159.00-$159.11**

CONTRAINDICATIONS: Anaphylaxis to egg protein, neomycin, mouse IgG

PRECAUTIONS: CHF, angina (unstable), COPD, diabetes mellitus with ketoacidosis, hemophilia, pulmonary embolism, thrombophlebitis, bone marrow depression, seizure disorder

PREGNANCY AND LACTATION: Pregnancy category C: Abortifacient in animal models; unknown if excreted into breast milk

SIDE EFFECTS/ADVERSE REACTIONS

CNS: Dizziness, insomnia, sleepiness

GI: Diarrhea, heartburn, *nausea,* vomiting

SKIN: Pain at inj site, pruritis

MISC: Chills, fatigue, fever (40%), flu-like syndrome, myalgias

INTERACTIONS
Drugs

3 *Theophylline:* Increased theophylline levels

---

interferon alfacon-1

(in-ter-feer'on)

Rx: Infergen
Chemical Class: Recombinant interferon
Therapeutic Class: Antiviral

CLINICAL PHARMACOLOGY
Mechanism of Action: Binds to cell surfaces, has antiviral, immunoregulatory, antiproliferative effects
Pharmacokinetics
SC: Unable to detect serum levels; metabolism mainly by kidney
INDICATIONS AND USES: Chronic hepatitis C infection in adults with compensated liver disease

DOSAGE
Adult ≥18 yr
• No previous interferon therapy: SC 9 µg 3 times/wk for 24 wk
• Previous interferon therapy/relapse: SC 15 µg 3 times/wk for 6 months

§ AVAILABLE FORMS/COST OF THERAPY
• Inj, Sol—SC: 9 µg/0.3 cc vial: **$37.00-$38.80**; 15 µg/0.5 cc vial: **$61.66-$64.70**

CONTRAINDICATIONS: Hypersensitivity to *E. coli*-derived products

PRECAUTIONS: Cardiovascular disease, myelodepression or myelodepressive drugs, thyroid disorders, severe psychiatric disorders, transplant patients, immunosuppression

PREGNANCY AND LACTATION: Pregnancy category C; unknown if excreted in breast milk

SIDE EFFECTS/ADVERSE REACTIONS

CNS: Amnesia, confusion, *dizziness, insomnia, mild to moderate depression (26%), paresthesia,* somnolence, **suicide,** suicidal ideation (1%)

CV: Hypertension, palpitations, tachycardia

EENT: Cotton wool spots URI, retinal hemorrhages

GI: Abdominal pain, anorexia, constipation, diarrhea, dyspepsia, nausea, vomiting

GU: Dysmenorrhea

HEME: **Granulocytopenia** *(25%),* lymphadenopathy, **thrombocytopenia** *(18%)*

METAB: Abnormal thyroid test (5-9%), hypertriglyceridemia (6%)

MISC: Flu-like symptoms: arthralgia (45%), fatigue (65%), fever (50-60%), headache (80%), myalgia (55%); injection site erythema (20%)

INTERACTIONS
Drugs
3 *Theophylline:* Increased theophylline levels

SPECIAL CONSIDERATIONS
• Response rates (normal ALT, HCV RNA negative) of 9 μg dose approx 35%, about half those have sustained response 24 wk after treatment
• Withold dosage temporarily if severe adverse reaction occurs, consider decreasing dose to 7.5 μg

PATIENT/FAMILY EDUCATION
• Needs to be refrigerated (36-46° F), may allow to reach room temp before injection; call manufacturer for advice if left out

MONITORING PARAMETERS
• CBC, plts, TSH, triglycerides, LFTs initially, repeat after 2 wk treatment and periodically thereafter
• Withold for ANC $<0.5 \times 10^9$/L or platelets $<50 \times 10^9$/L

---

interferon beta

(in-ter-feer′on)

Rx: Betaseron
Chemical Class: Recombinant interferon
Therapeutic Class: Multiple sclerosis agent
See next monograph for updated information on interferon beta-1b (Betaseron)

CLINICAL PHARMACOLOGY
Mechanism of Action: Antiviral, immunoregulatory; action not clearly understood

Pharmacokinetics
SC: Serum levels very low or not detectable at recommended dose; at higher doses 50% bioavailable, peak 1-8 hr

INDICATIONS AND USES: Ambulatory patients with relapsing or remitting multiple sclerosis, treatment of AIDS,* AIDS-related Kaposi's sarcoma,* malignant melanoma,* metastatic renal cell carcinoma,* cutaneous T-cell lymphoma,* acute non-A, non-B hepatitis*

DOSAGE
Adult
• *Relapsing/remitting multiple sclerosis:* SC 0.25 mg (8 IU) qod
Child
• Not established

$ **AVAILABLE FORMS/COST OF THERAPY**
• Inj, Lyphl-Sol—SC: 0.3 mg/vial: **$72.00**

CONTRAINDICATIONS: Hypersensitivity to human albumin

PRECAUTIONS: Children under 18 yr, chronic progressive MS, depression, mental disorders, seizure disorder, heart disease

PREGNANCY AND LACTATION: Pregnancy category C; possible abortifacient; not known if excreted in breast milk; avoid in nursing mothers

SIDE EFFECTS/ADVERSE REACTIONS
CNS: Dizziness, mental changes
CV: Hypertension, palpitations, peripheral vascular disorders, tachycardia
EENT: Conjunctivitis
GI: Abdominal pain, constipation, diarrhea, vomiting
GU: Breast pain, cystitis, *dysmenorrhea, irregular menses, metrorrhagia*
HEME: Lymphadenopathy, lymphopenia, ***neutropenia***
RESP: Dyspnea, *sinusitis*
SKIN: Inj site reaction (85%), sweating
MISC: Flu-like syndrome (76%): chills, fever, headache, myalgias

---

italic = common side effects   ***bold italic*** = life-threatening reactions

INTERACTIONS
Drugs
• *Zidovudine, theophylline:* Increased levels

SPECIAL CONSIDERATIONS
• 31% reduction in annual exacerbation rate (1.31 in placebo group, 0.9 in treatment group)

PATIENT/FAMILY EDUCATION
• Use acetaminophen for relief of flu-like symptoms
• Avoid prolonged sun exposure (photosensitivity)

MONITORING PARAMETERS
• Follow CBC, platelets, LFTs q3mo
• D/C for ANC <750/mm³, ALT/AST >10 × upper limits normal, bilirubin >5 × upper limits normal; when labs return to these levels restart at 50% reduction dose

---

interferon beta-1 a/b
(in-ter-feer'on)
Rx: Avonex (beta-1a),
Betaseron (beta-1b)
Chemical Class: Purified protein product
Therapeutic Class: Multiple sclerosis agent

CLINICAL PHARMACOLOGY
Mechanism of Action: Binds to cell surfaces; has antiviral, immunoregulatory, antiproliferative effects
Pharmacokinetics
SC: Serum levels very low or not detectable at recommended dose; at higher doses 50% bioavailable; peak 1-8 hr
IM: Peak 9.8 hr; biologic response within 12 hr, maximal at 48 hr; duration at least 4 days, $t_{1/2}$ 10 hr

INDICATIONS AND USES: Relapsing forms of multiple sclerosis (slows the accumulation of physical disability and decreases frequency of clinical exacerbations); treatment of AIDS-related Kaposi's sarcoma,* metastatic renal cell carcinoma*; herpes of the lips, genitals*; malignant melanoma,* cutaneous T-cell lymphoma*; acute non-A, non-B hepatitis*

DOSAGE
Adult
• *Relapsing multiple sclerosis:* IM 30 µg IM q wk (Avonex); SC 0.25 mg (8 IU) qod (Betaseron)

💲 AVAILABLE FORMS/COST OF THERAPY
• Inj, Lyphl-Sol—SC: 0.3 mg/vial: **$72.00**
• Inj—IM: 33 µg/vial, 4's: **$985.20**

CONTRAINDICATIONS: Hypersensitivity to human albumin
PRECAUTIONS: Depression, seizure disorder, heart disease, children <18 yr, chronic progressive ms, mental disorders
PREGNANCY AND LACTATION: Pregnancy category C; possible abortifacient; not known if excreted into breast milk; avoid in nursing mothers

SIDE EFFECTS/ADVERSE REACTIONS
CNS: Dizziness, insomnia, **seizures,** mental changes
CV: Syncope, vasodilation, hypertension, palpitations, peripheral vascular disorders, tachycardia
EENT: Decreased hearing, conjunctivitis
GI: Abdominal pain, anorexia, diarrhea, dyspepsia, nausea
GU: Dysmenorrhea, irregular menses, metrorrhagia
HEME: Anemia, *eosinophilia,* **neutropenia**
RESP: Dyspnea, sinusitis, upper respiratory tract infection
SKIN: Alopecia, *inj site reaction,* urticaria, sweating

---

* = non-FDA-approved use

MISC: *Flu-like symptoms (61%-76%): chills, fever, headache, myalgias*

INTERACTIONS

Drugs

3 *Zidovudine, theophylline:* Increased levels of these drugs

SPECIAL CONSIDERATIONS

PATIENT/FAMILY EDUCATION

• Use acetaminophen for relief of flu-like symptoms
• Avoid prolonged sun exposure (photosensitivity)
• Benefit in chronic progressive multiple sclerosis has not been evaluated
• Patients treated × 2 yr had significantly longer time to progression of disability compared with placebo group

MONITORING PARAMETERS

• CBC, platelets, liver function tests, and blood chemistries q3 mo
• DC for ANC <750/m³, ALT/AST >10 × upper normal limits; when labs return to these levels, restart at 50% of dose

---

interferon gamma-1b

(in-ter-feer'on)
Rx: Actimmune
Chemical Class: Recombinant interferon
Therapeutic Class: Biologic response modifier

CLINICAL PHARMACOLOGY

Mechanism of Action: Interacts with other lymphokines (e.g., interleukin-2); activates macrophages, enhancing phagocytic function; enhances cellular cytotoxicity

Pharmacokinetics

SC: 89% dose absorbed, $t_{1/2}$ 5.9 hr, peak 7 hr

INDICATIONS AND USES: Reduction of frequency and severity of serious infections associated with chronic granulomatous disease

DOSAGE

Adult and Child

• SC 50 μg/m² (1.5 million U/m²) for patients with surface area of >0.5 m²; 1.5 μg/kg/dose for patient with a surface area of <0.5/m²; given 3 × /wk
• Reduce dose 50% for adverse reactions

$ **AVAILABLE FORMS/COST OF THERAPY**

• Inj, Sol—SC: 100 μg (3 million U)/0.5 ml: **$140.00-$200.45**

CONTRAINDICATIONS: Hypersensitivity to *E. coli*-derived products

PRECAUTIONS: Cardiac disease, seizure disorders, CNS disorders, myelosuppression, safety not established in children <1 yr

PREGNANCY AND LACTATION: Pregnancy category C; possible abortifacient; not known if excreted in breast milk; not recommended in breast feeding

SIDE EFFECTS/ADVERSE REACTIONS

CNS: *Chills, fatigue (14%), fever (52%), headache (33%)*
GI: Abdominal pain, *diarrhea, nausea (10%), vomiting, weight loss*
HEME: **Neutropenia, thrombocytopenia**
MS: *Myalgia*
SKIN: Pain at inj site, rash

INTERACTIONS

Drugs

3 *Theophylline, zidovudine:* Increased levels of these drugs

SPECIAL CONSIDERATIONS

• Optimal sites for inj are the right and left deltoid and anterior thigh

PATIENT/FAMILY EDUCATION

• Use acetaminophen to relieve fever, headache

---

italic = common side effects　　　**bold italic** = life-threatening reactions

iodinated glycerol
Rx: Iophen, Organidin, Par Glycerol, R-Gen
Combinations
Rx: with theophylline (Theo-Oridol, Theo-R-Gen); with codeine (Iophen-C Liquid, Tussi-Organidin Liquid)
Chemical Class: Iodopropylidene glycerol isomer
Therapeutic Class: Expectorant

CLINICAL PHARMACOLOGY
Mechanism of Action: Increases respiratory tract fluid by decreasing surface tension, increases removal of mucus
Pharmacokinetics
PO: Readily absorbed, concentrated in respiratory secretions; excreted by kidneys
INDICATIONS AND USES: Mucolytic expectorant in asthma, emphysema, bronchitis, cystic fibrosis, chronic sinusitis; **efficacy not proven**
DOSAGE
Adult
• PO tab 60 mg qid; ELI 5 ml qid; SOL 20 gtt qid
Child
• PO up to half adult dose depending on weight
$ **AVAILABLE FORMS/COST OF THERAPY**
• Eli—Oral: 60 mg/5 ml, 120 ml: **$1.25-$6.93**
• Sol—Oral: 50 mg/ml, 30 ml: **$5.50-$27.62**
• Tab, Uncoated—Oral: 30 mg, 100's: **$10.66-$18.07**
CONTRAINDICATIONS: Hypersensitivity to iodides, pulmonary TB, hyperthyroidism, hyperkalemia, newborns, lactation, acute bronchitis

PRECAUTIONS: Thyroid disease, cystic fibrosis (increased goitrogenic effect in children with cystic fibrosis)
PREGNANCY AND LACTATION: Contraindicated in pregnancy, category X; not recommended in nursing mothers (rash and thyroid suppression in infant)
SIDE EFFECTS/ADVERSE REACTIONS
CNS: CNS depression, fever, frontal headache, parkinsonism
EENT: Burning mouth, throat, eye irritation, swelling of eyelids
GI: Gastric irritation
METAB: Iodism, goiter, myxedema
RESP: Pulmonary edema
SKIN: **Angioedema,** rash
INTERACTIONS
Drugs
3 *Lithium, antithyroid drugs:* Increased hypothyroid effects

iodoquinol
(eye-oh-do-kwin'ole)
Rx: Yodoxin
Chemical Class: 8-hydroxyquinolone derivative
Therapeutic Class: Amebicide

CLINICAL PHARMACOLOGY
Mechanism of Action: Direct-acting amebicide; action occurs in intestinal lumen
Pharmacokinetics
PO: Poorly absorbed, excreted in feces
INDICATIONS AND USES: Intestinal amebiasis
DOSAGE
Adult
• PO 650 mg tid after meals for 20 days, not to exceed 2 g/day

Child

• PO 30-40 mg/kg/day in 3 divided doses for 20 days, not to exceed 1.95 g/24 hr for 20 days; do not repeat treatment before 2-3 wk

💲 AVAILABLE FORMS/COST OF THERAPY

• Tab, Uncoated—Oral: 210 mg, 100's: **$58.35**; 650 mg, 100's: **$19.50-$75.09**

CONTRAINDICATIONS: Hypersensitivity to iodine; renal disease, hepatic disease, severe thyroid disease, pre-existing optic neuropathy

PRECAUTIONS: Thyroid disease

PREGNANCY AND LACTATION: Pregnancy category C; excretion into breast milk unknown

SIDE EFFECTS/ADVERSE REACTIONS

CNS: Agitation, headache, malaise, peripheral neuropathy

EENT: Blurred vision, optic atrophy, optic neuritis, retinal edema, sore throat

GI: Abdominal cramps, anal itching, *anorexia,* constipation, diarrhea, epigastric distress, gastritis, *nausea,* rectal irritation, vomiting

HEME: **Agranulocytosis** (rare)

SKIN: Alopecia, discolored skin, hair, nails; pruritus; rash

MISC: Chills, fever, thyroid enlargement, vertigo

---

ipecac

(ip′e-kak)

OTC: Ipecac

Chemical Class: Cephaelis ipecacuanha derivative

Therapeutic Class: Emetic

CLINICAL PHARMACOLOGY

Mechanism of Action: Acts on chemoreceptor trigger zone to induce vomiting; irritates gastric mucosa

Pharmacokinetics

PO: Onset 15-30 min; minimal systemic absorption

INDICATIONS AND USES: In poisoning to induce vomiting

DOSAGE

Adult

• PO 15-30 ml, then 3-4 glasses water

Child 1-12 yr

• PO 15 ml, then 1-2 glasses water

Child <1 yr

• PO 5-10 ml, then ½-1 glass water, may repeat dose if needed

💲 AVAILABLE FORMS/COST OF THERAPY

• Liq—Oral (1.5-2.0% in ethanol): 30 ml: **$1.10-$23.11**

CONTRAINDICATIONS: Unconsciousness, semiconsciousness; depressed gag reflex, poisoning with petroleum products or caustic substances, seizures

PREGNANCY AND LACTATION: Pregnancy category C; not known if excreted in breast milk

SIDE EFFECTS/ADVERSE REACTIONS

CNS: **Coma, seizures**

CV: **Atrial fibrillation, dysrhythmias, fatal myocarditis, hypotension**

GI: Bloody diarrhea, nausea, vomiting

INTERACTIONS

Drugs

🔢 *Activated charcoal:* Decreased effect of ipecac; if both drugs used, give activated charcoal after emesis induced

SPECIAL CONSIDERATIONS

• May not work on empty stomach

• Do not confuse with ipecac fluid extract (14 times stronger)

---

italic = common side effects   ***bold italic*** = life-threatening reactions

ipratropium

(eye-pra-troep´ee-um)
Rx: Atrovent
Combinations
　Rx: with albuterol (Combiv-
　　ent)
Chemical Class: Quaternary
ammonium compound
Therapeutic Class: Bronchodi-
lator

CLINICAL PHARMACOLOGY

Mechanism of Action: Inhibits action of acetylcholine at receptor sites
on bronchial smooth muscle, resulting in bronchodilation; has antisecretory properties when applied
locally

Pharmacokinetics
INH: Onset 5-15 min; peak effect 1-2
hr, duration of action 3-6 hr; absorption minimal; does not cross blood-
brain barrier; 90% excreted in feces

INDICATIONS AND USES: Maintenance treatment of bronchospasm in
COPD; perennial rhinitis, rhinorrhea associated with the common
cold; bronchial asthma,* cough after respiratory infection* (not indicated for acute bronchospasm)

DOSAGE

Adult
• INH 1-2 puffs qid, not to exceed 12
puffs/24 hr
• SOL 500 µg via nebulizer q6-8 hr,
can be mixed with albuterol
• *Perennial rhinitis:* Nasal 2 sprays
of 0.03% sol bid-tid
• *Rhinitis associated with common
cold:* Nasal 2 sprays of 0.06% sol
tid-qid for 4 days

Child <12 yr
• *Perennial rhinitis:* Nasal 2 sprays
of 0.03% sol bid-tid
• *Rhinitis associated with common
cold:* Nasal 2 sprays of 0.06% sol
tid-qid for 4 days

💲 AVAILABLE FORMS/COST
OF THERAPY

• Aer—INH: 18 µg/inh, 14 g:
$38.87-$46.41
• Sol—INH: 0.2 mg/ml, 2.5 ml:
$0.74-$2.96
• Sol—Nasal: 21 µg/inh, 30 ml:
$42.46; 42 µg/inh 15 ml: **$36.38**

CONTRAINDICATIONS: Hypersensitivity to atropine

PRECAUTIONS: Angle-closure
glaucoma, prostatic hypertrophy,
bladder neck obstruction, urinary
retention

PREGNANCY AND LACTATION:
Pregnancy category B; not known if
excreted in breast milk, but little systemic absorption when administered by INH

SIDE EFFECTS/ADVERSE REAC-
TIONS

CNS: Anxiety, dizziness, headache,
nervousness
CV: Palpitations
EENT: Blurred vision, dry mouth,
metallic taste, stomatitis
GI: Cramps, *nausea,* vomiting
RESP: **Bronchospasm,** *cough, wors-
ening of symptoms*
SKIN: Rash

SPECIAL CONSIDERATIONS

• Bronchodilator of choice for
COPD

---

* = non-FDA-approved use

irbesartan

(erb'ba-sar-tan)

Rx: Avapro
Combinations
Rx: with hydrochlorothiazide
(Avalide)
Chemical Class: Angiotensin II
receptor antagonist
Therapeutic Class: Antihypertensive

CLINICAL PHARMACOLOGY

Mechanism of Action: Antihypertensive (inhibition of vasoconstriction and aldosterone secretion), smooth muscle hypoproliferative, and cardioprotective effects are attributable to selective blockade of angiotensin II (AT_1) receptors found throughout the cardiovascular and renal systems; effects independent of angiotensin II synthesis

Pharmacokinetics

PO: Peak, 1-2 hrs; peak response, 2 hrs (blood pressure reduction, increased plasma renin activity), 4-8 hrs (reductions in plasma aldosterone)

PO bioavailability, 60%-80%, no food effect; 90% protein bound; extensively metabolized by liver (CYP2C9) to inactive metabolite, 65% fecal, 20% renal excretion; elimination $t_{1/2}$, 11-15 hrs

INDICATIONS AND USES: Hypertension; congestive heart failure (left ventricular dysfunction),* myocardial infarction,* diabetic nephropathy*

DOSAGE

Adult

• PO 150-300 mg qd, no adjustment for hepatic or renal impairment (unless also volume depleted)

$ **AVAILABLE FORMS/COST OF THERAPY**
• Cap—Oral: 75 mg, 100's: **$123.80**; 150 mg, 100's: **$125.32**; 300 mg, 100's: **$210.88**

PRECAUTIONS: Angioedema (associated with aspirin and/or penicillin allergy), aortic or mitral valve stenosis, coronary artery disease, breast feeding, elderly patients, hypertrophic cardiomyopathy, hypotension (sodium or volume depleted patients), pregnancy, renal artery stenosis, solitary kidney, or CHF

PREGNANCY AND LACTATION: Pregnancy category C (first trimester—category D, second and third trimesters; drugs acting directly on the renin-angiotensin-aldosterone system are documented to cause fetal harm (hypotension, oligohydramnios, neonatal anemia, hyperkalemia, neonatal skull hypoplasia, anuria, and renal failure; neonatal limb contractures, craniofacial deformities, and hypoplastic lung development; breast milk excretion unknown

SIDE EFFECTS/ADVERSE REACTIONS

CNS: Dizziness, headache, weakness or tiredness
CV: First dose hypotension, fluid retention, orthostatic effects, syncope
GI: Diarrhea, dyspepsia/heartburn
MS: Trauma
RESP: Cough, upper respiratory infection
MISC: Angioedema

SPECIAL CONSIDERATIONS
• Potentially as or more effective than angiotensin-converting enzyme inhibitors, without cough; no evidence for reduction in morbidity and mortality as first line agents in hypertension, yet; whether they provide the same cardiac and renal pro-

tection also still tentative; Like ACE inhibitors, less effective in black patients

PATIENT/FAMILY EDUCATION

• Call your clinician immediately if note following side effects: wheezing; lip, throat or face swelling; hives or rash

MONITORING PARAMETERS

• Baseline electrolytes, urinalysis, blood urea nitrogen and creatinine with recheck at 2-4 weeks after initiation (sooner in volume depleted patients); monitor sitting blood pressure; watch for symptomatic hypotension, particularly in volume depleted patients

---

iron dextran

Rx: InFeD, Dexferrum
Chemical Class: Ferric hydroxide complexed with dextran
Therapeutic Class: Hematinic

CLINICAL PHARMACOLOGY

Mechanism of Action: Iron is carried by transferrin to bone marrow and incorporated into hemoglobin

Pharmacokinetics

IM: Excreted in feces, urine, bile, breast milk; crosses placenta; most absorbed through lymphatics; can be gradually absorbed over weeks/months from fixed locations

INDICATIONS AND USES: Iron deficiency anemia when oral administration not satisfactory; patients receiving epoetin therapy*

DOSAGE

To calculate total amount of iron (in mg) required to restore hemoglobin to normal levels and replenish iron stores in iron deficient anemia: $(0.3) \times (\text{weight in lb}) \times [100-(\text{Hgb in g/dl} \times 100/14.8)]$

Divide this result by 50 to obtain dose in ml

Adult

• IM 0.5 ml as a test dose by Z-track (pull skin laterally prior to injection); wait ≥1 hr before giving remainder of therapeutic dose; max dose 2 ml (100 μg) qd

• IV 0.5 ml as test dose; give slowly, ≤1 ml/min; follow same protocol and dose as for IM; alternatively the entire dose may be diluted in 500 ml of normal saline and infused over 4-6 hr if the test dose is tolerated

Child

• If <30 lb, total dose is 80% of dose as calculated by above formula

• IM/IV 0.5 ml as a test dose as above, then no more than the following per day: <10 lb 0.5 ml (25 mg); <20 lb 1 ml (50 mg)

$ **AVAILABLE FORMS/COST OF THERAPY**

• Inj, Sol—IM, IV: 50 mg/ml, 2 ml: **$37.70**

CONTRAINDICATIONS: Anemias other than iron deficiency anemia, hepatic disease

PRECAUTIONS: Acute renal disease, asthma, rheumatoid arthritis (IV), severe liver disease, infants <4 mo

PREGNANCY AND LACTATION: Pregnancy category C; excreted in breast milk

SIDE EFFECTS/ADVERSE REACTIONS

CNS: Dizziness, headache, paresthesia, *seizures,* shivering, weakness
CV: Chest pain, hypotension, *shock,* tachycardia
GI: Abdominal pain, dark stools, metallic taste, *nausea,* vomiting
HEME: Leukocytosis
RESP: Dyspnea
SKIN: Brown skin discoloration, chills, fever, necrosis, pain at inj site, phlebitis, pruritus, rash, sterile abscesses, sweating, urticaria

---

* = non-FDA-approved use

INTERACTIONS
Drugs
3 *Enalapril:* Three patients on enalapril receiving IV iron developed systemic reactions (GI symptoms, hypotension); causality not established

3 *Vitamin E:* Decreased reticulocyte response in anemic children
Labs
• *False increase:* Serum calcium, serum glucose, serum iron
• *False positive:* Stool guaiac
SPECIAL CONSIDERATIONS
• Discontinue oral iron before giving
• Delayed reaction (fever, myalgias, arthralgias, nausea) may occur 1-2 days after administration
• When giving IM, give only in gluteal muscle

---

isocarboxazid
(eye-soe-kar-box´a-zid)
Rx: Marplan
Chemical Class: Hydrazine derivative
Therapeutic Class: MAOI

CLINICAL PHARMACOLOGY
Mechanism of Action: Increases concentrations of endogenous epinephrine, norepinephrine, serotonin, dopamine in storage sites in CNS by inhibition of monoamine oxidase; increased concentrations reduce depression
Pharmacokinetics
PO: Duration up to 2 wk; metabolized by liver; excreted by kidneys
INDICATIONS AND USES: Depression uncontrolled by other means

DOSAGE
Adult
• PO 30 mg/day in single or divided doses; reduce dose to lowest effective dose (10-20 mg qd) when condition improves; full effect may take 3-4 wk
💲 AVAILABLE FORMS/COST OF THERAPY
• Tab, Uncoated—Oral: 10 mg, 100's: **$70.66**
CONTRAINDICATIONS: Elderly, hypertension, CHF, severe hepatic disease, pheochromocytoma, severe renal disease, severe cardiac disease
PRECAUTIONS: Suicidal patients, seizure disorders, severe depression, schizophrenia, hyperactivity, diabetes mellitus
PREGNANCY AND LACTATION: Pregnancy category C; breast feeding data not available
SIDE EFFECTS/ADVERSE REACTIONS
CNS: Anxiety, confusion, *dizziness, drowsiness,* fatigue, headache, hyperreflexia, insomnia, mania, stimulation, tremors, weakness
CV: **Dysrhythmias,** hypertension, **hypertensive crisis,** orthostatic hypotension
EENT: Blurred vision
GI: *Anorexia,* constipation, diarrhea, dry mouth, nausea, vomiting, weight gain
GU: Change in libido, frequency
HEME: Anemia
METAB: Hypoglycemia, syndrome of inappropriate antidiuretic hormone-like syndrome
SKIN: Flushing, increased perspiration, jaundice, rash
INTERACTIONS
Drugs
3 *Barbiturates:* Prolonged action of barbiturate

⚠ *Dextromethorphan:* Agitation, seizure, increased BP, hyperpyrexia

---

italic = common side effects   ***bold italic*** = life-threatening reactions

▲ *Ephedrine, amphetamines, phenylephrine, phenylpropanolamine, pseudoephedrine:* Hypertension, severe

▲ *Ethanol:* Alcoholic beverages containing tyramine may cause severe hypertensive reaction

3 *Guanethidine:* Decreased antihypertensive response to guanethidine

3 *Levodopa:* Hypertension, severe

2 *Lithium:* Hyperpyrexia possible

▲ *Meperidine:* Sweating, rigidity, hypertension

▲ *Methotrimeprazine:* Case report of fatality in patient taking these drugs, causality not established

3 *Norepinephrine:* Increased pressor response to norepinephrine

▲ *Reserpine:* Potential for hypertensive reaction, clinical evidence lacking

▲ *Sertraline, fluoxetine, fluvoxamine, paroxetine, venlafaxine:* Increased CNS effects (serotonergic)

▲ *Tricyclic antidepressants:* Excessive sympathetic response, mania, hyperpyrexia

SPECIAL CONSIDERATIONS
• Phentolamine for severe hypertension

PATIENT/FAMILY EDUCATION
• Avoid high-tyramine foods: cheese (aged), sour cream, beer, wine, pickled products, liver, raisins, bananas, figs, avocados, meat tenderizers, chocolate, yogurt; soy sauce, caffeine

• Do not discontinue medication quickly after long-term use

isoetharine
(eye-soe-eth′a-reen)
Rx: Isoetharine
Chemical Class: Sympathomimetic amine; B₂-adrenergic agonist
Therapeutic Class: Antiasthmatic, bronchodilator

CLINICAL PHARMACOLOGY
Mechanism of Action: Causes bronchodilation by β-₂ stimulation, resulting in relaxation of bronchial smooth muscle; inhibits mast cell degranulation; stimulates cilia to remove secretions

Pharmacokinetics
INH: Onset rapid, peak 5-15 min, duration 1-4 hr; metabolized in liver, GI tract, lungs; excreted in urine

INDICATIONS AND USES: Bronchial asthma; reversible bronchospasm that occurs with bronchitis and emphysema

DOSAGE
Adult
• NEB 1%, 0.25-0.5 ml, q4h prn

$ **AVAILABLE FORMS/COST OF THERAPY**
• Sol—INH: 1%, 30 ml: **$23.10-$96.11**

PRECAUTIONS: Ischemic heart disease, cardiac dysrhythmias, hyperthyroidism, diabetes mellitus, prostatic hypertrophy, hypertension

PREGNANCY AND LACTATION: Pregnancy category C; no breast feeding data available

SIDE EFFECTS/ADVERSE REACTIONS
CNS: Anxiety, dizziness, headache, insomnia, stimulation, *tremors*

CV: **Cardiac arrest, dysrhythmias,** hypertension, palpitations, tachycardia

GI: Nausea

METAB: Hyperglycemia

INTERACTIONS
Drugs
❷ *Beta-blockers:* Decreased action of isoetharine, cardioselective beta-blockers preferable if concurrent use necessary

❸ *Furosemide:* Potential for additive hypokalemia

SPECIAL CONSIDERATIONS
• Inhalation technique critical
• Re-educate routinely

---

isometheptene
(i-so-meh-thep´tene)
Only available in combination with dichloralphenazone and acetaminophen:
Rx: Amidrine Duradin, I.D.A., Iso-Acetazone, Midchlor, Midrin, Migrapap, Migratine, Migrazone, Migquin, Migrex, VA-Zone
Chemical Class: Sympathomimetic amine
Therapeutic Class: Vasoconstrictor (in combination with analgesic and sedative)

CLINICAL PHARMACOLOGY
Mechanism of Action: Indirect-acting sympathomimetic agent with vasoconstricting activity; vasoconstriction of cerebral blood vessels may reduce pulsation of cerebral arteries; dichloralphenazone is a mild sedative; acetaminophen an analgesic

INDICATIONS AND USES: Tension headache; possibly effective for relief of vascular headaches

DOSAGE
Adult
• *Tension headache:* PO 1-2 caps q4h prn to max 8 caps qd
• *Vascular headache:* PO 2 caps at once, then 1 cap qhr prn to max 5 caps/12 hr

💲 AVAILABLE FORMS/COST OF THERAPY
• Cap, Gel—Oral: acetaminophen 325 mg/dichloralphenazone 100 mg/isometheptene 65 mg, 100's: **$4.50-$55.65**

CONTRAINDICATIONS: Glaucoma, severe renal disease, severe hepatic disease (acetaminophen), organic heart disease, MAOI therapy

PRECAUTIONS: Hypertension, peripheral vascular disease, recent CVA

PREGNANCY AND LACTATION: Pregnancy category C; excretion into breast milk unknown

SIDE EFFECTS/ADVERSE REACTIONS
CNS: Dizziness
SKIN: Rash

INTERACTIONS
Drugs
⚠ *Bromocriptine:* Potential for hypertension and ventricular tachycardia
Labs
• *False positive:* Urine amphetamine

---

isoniazid (INH)
(eye-soe-nye´a-zid)
Rx: INH: Nydrazid
Combinations
  Rx: with rifampin (Rifamate); with rifampin, pyrazinamide (Rifater)
Chemical Class: Synthetic isonicotinic acid derivative
Therapeutic Class: Antituberculosis agent

CLINICAL PHARMACOLOGY
Mechanism of Action: Interferes with lipid and nucleic acid biosynthesis in growing tubercle bacilli;

active only against mycobacteria, primarily those that are actively dividing

Pharmacokinetics

PO: Peak 1-2 hr, duration 6-8 hr; Widely distributed to all fluids and tissues; low protein binding; metabolized in liver, primarily by acetylation; rate of metabolism genetically determined; eliminated in urine; $t_{1/2}$ 0.5-1.6 hr (fast acetylators), 2-5 hr (slow acetylators)

INDICATIONS AND USES: Treatment and prophylaxis of tuberculosis; severe tremor in patients with multiple sclerosis*

DOSAGE

Adult

• *Treatment:* PO or IM 5 mg/kg/day (up to 300 mg total) in a single dose; use in conjunction with other effective antituberculosis agents; duration of treatment 6 mo-2 yr

• *Disseminated disease:* PO 10 mg/kg/day in 1-2 divided doses

• *Prophylaxis:* PO or IM 300 mg qd

Child

• *Treatment:* PO or IM 10-20 mg/kg/day (up to 300 mg total) in 1-2 divided doses

• *Prophylaxis:* PO or IM 10 mg/kg/day qd, do not exceed 300 mg/day

💲 AVAILABLE FORMS/COST OF THERAPY

• Inj, Sol—IM: 100 mg/ml, 10 ml: **$20.26**

• Syr—Oral: 50 mg/ml, 480 ml: **$20.00-$22.50**

• Tab, Uncoated—Oral: 100 mg, 100's: **$0.68-$15.45**; 300 mg, 100's: **$5.48-$20.75**

CONTRAINDICATIONS: Previous isoniazid-associated hepatic injury, acute liver disease

PRECAUTIONS: Active chronic liver disease, severe renal dysfunction, malnutrition, slow acetylators, elderly, diabetes, alcoholics (increased risk of peripheral neuropathy)

PREGNANCY AND LACTATION: Pregnancy category C; the American Thoracic Society recommends use of isoniazid for tuberculosis during pregnancy; excreted in breast milk; women can safely breast feed their infants while taking isoniazid if the infant is periodically examined for signs and symptoms of peripheral neuritis or hepatitis

SIDE EFFECTS/ADVERSE REACTIONS

CNS: Fever, memory impairment, *peripheral neuropathy,* **seizures, toxic encephalopathy,** toxic psychosis

EENT: Optic neuritis and atrophy

GI: Epigastric distress, **hepatotoxicity** (mild and transient elevation of serum transaminases in 10%-20% does not require discontinuation; progressive liver damage rare in patients <20 yr, but is seen in as many as 2.3% of those >50 yr), nausea, vomiting

HEME: **Agranulocytosis;** eosinophilia, **hemolytic, sideroblastic, or aplastic anemia; thrombocytopenia**

METAB: Gynecomastia, hyperglycemia, hypocalcemia, hypophosphatemia, metabolic acidosis, pellagra, pyridoxine deficiency

SKIN: Skin eruptions, vasculitis

MISC: Rheumatic syndrome, systemic lupus erythematosis-like syndrome

INTERACTIONS

Drugs

3 *Acetaminophen:* Increased acetaminophen concentrations, potential for hepatotoxicity

3 *Antacids:* Reduced plasma isoniazid concentrations

---

* = non-FDA-approved use

❸ *Carbamazepine:* Increased serum carbamazepine concentrations, toxicity may occur

❸ *Corticosteroids:* Reduced plasma concentrations of isoniazid

❸ *Cycloserine:* Increased potential for CNS toxicity

❸ *Diazepam, triazolam:* Increased concentrations of these drugs

❷ *Disulfiram:* Adverse mental changes and coordination problems

❸ *Ethanol:* Higher incidence of isoniazid-induced hepatitis in alcoholics

❸ *Phenytoin:* Predictable increases in serum phenytoin concentrations, toxicity possible

❸ *Rifampin:* Increased hepatotoxicity of isoniazid in some patients; more common with slow acetylators of isoniazid, and/or pre-existing liver disease

❸ *Theophylline:* Increased theophylline concentrations, toxicity possible

❸ *Valproic acid:* Increased valproic acid concentration possible

❸ *Warfarin:* Potential for enhanced hypoprothrombinemic response to warfarin

Labs
• *False increase:* Serum AST, serum uric acid
• *False decrease:* Serum glucose
• *False positive:* Urine sugar

SPECIAL CONSIDERATIONS
PATIENT/FAMILY EDUCATION
• Take on empty stomach if possible; however, may be taken with food to decrease GI upset
• Minimize daily alcohol consumption to lessen the risk of hepatitis
• Notify clinician of weakness, fatigue, loss of appetite, nausea and vomiting, yellowing of skin or eyes, darkening of urine, numbness or tingling of hands and feet

MONITORING PARAMETERS
• Periodic ophthalmologic examinations even when visual symptoms do not occur
• Periodic liver function tests

---

isoproterenol
(eye-soe-proe-ter′e-nole)
Rx: Isuprel, Medihaler-Iso
Combinations
  Rx: with phenylephrine
  (Duo-Medihaler)
Chemical Class: Synthetic catecholamine
Therapeutic Class: β-adrenergic agonist: antiasthmatic, bronchodilator; vasopressor; sympathomimetic

---

CLINICAL PHARMACOLOGY
Mechanism of Action: Stimulates β_1- and β_2-adrenergic receptors resulting in relaxation of bronchial, GI, and uterine smooth muscle, increased heart rate and contractility, vasodilation of peripheral vasculature; increases renal perfusion, cardiac output, decreases total peripheral resistance, and increasing blood pressure in cardiogenic or septicemic shock

Pharmacokinetics
IV: Onset rapid, duration 10 min
INH: Onset immediate
SC: Onset 30 min, duration up to 2 hr
Metabolized by conjugation in many tissues including the liver and lungs; $t_{1/2}$ 2½-5 min; excreted in urine (principally as sulfate conjugates)

INDICATIONS AND USES: Mild or transient episodes of heart block; serious episodes of heart block and Stokes-Adams attacks (except when caused by ventricular tachycardia or fibrillation); cardiac arrest (until electric shock or pacemaker is avail-

---

able); bronchospasm occurring during anesthesia, asthma, chronic bronchitis, or emphysema; hypovolemic and septic shock, low cardiac output (hypoperfusion) states, congestive heart failure, cardiogenic shock

DOSAGE

Adult

• *Bronchospasm:* MDI 1-2 puffs 4-6 times/day; neb 0.25-0.5 ml of a 1% sol diluted in 2-3 ml normal saline or 0.25% and 0.5% undiluted, treatment may be repeated up to 5 times/day

• *Dysrhythmia/heart block:* IV 0.02-0.06 mg (1-3 ml of 1:50,000 dilution) bolus, followed by subsequent doses of 0.01-0.2 mg (0.5-10 ml of 1:50,000 dilution); IV INF 5 µg/min initially, titrate to desired response, usual range 2-20 µg/min; IM 0.2 mg (1 ml of 1:5,000 dilution) initially, subsequent doses of 0.02-1 mg (0.1-5 ml of 1:5,000 dilution); SC 0.2 mg (1 ml of 1:5,000 dilution) initially, subsequent doses of 0.15-0.2 mg (0.75-1 ml of 1:5,000 dilution); IC 0.02 mg (0.1 ml of 1:5,000 dilution)

• *Shock:* IV INF 0.5-5 µg/min (0.25-2.5 ml of 1:500,000 dilution), titrate to patient response

Child

• *Bronchospasm:* MDI 1-2 puffs up to 6 times/day; neb 0.01 ml/kg of 1% sol; min dose 0.1 ml, max dose 0.5 ml diluted in 2-3 ml normal saline

• *Shock:* IV INF 0.05-2 µg/kg/ min, rate (ml/hr) = dose (µg/kg/min) $\times$ weight (kg) $\times$ 60 min/hr divided by concentration (µg/ml)

$ AVAILABLE FORMS/COST OF THERAPY

• Inj, Sol—IV: 0.02 mg/ml, 10 ml: **$7.99**; 0.2 mg/ml, 1, 5, 10 ml: **$3.83-$19.57/5 ml**

• Sol—INH: 0.25%, 15 ml: **$12.50**

CONTRAINDICATIONS: Tachydysrhythmias, tachycardia or heart block caused by digitalis intoxication, ventricular dysrhythmias requiring inotropic therapy, angina pectoris

PRECAUTIONS: Hypovolemia, CAD, coronary insufficiency, diabetes, hyperthyroidism

PREGNANCY AND LACTATION: Pregnancy category C; no reports linking isoproterenol with congenital defects have been located; excretion into breast milk unknown; use caution in nursing mothers

SIDE EFFECTS/ADVERSE REACTIONS

CNS: Anxiety, dizziness, headache, *mild tremors,* nervousness, weakness

CV: Angina, hypertension, hypotension, palpitations, tachycardia, *tachydysrhythmias, ventricular dysrhythmias*

GI: Nausea, vomiting

RESP: Pulmonary edema

SKIN: Flushing of skin, sweating

INTERACTIONS

Drugs

3 *Amitriptyline:* Combined use may result in predisposition to cardiac arrhythmias

3 *Beta-blockers:* Reduced effectiveness of isoproterenol in the treatment of asthma

Labs

• *False increase:* Serum AST, serum bilirubin, serum glucose

isosorbide dinitrate/mononitrate

(eye-soe-sor'bide dye-nye'-trate/mon-oh-nye'trate)

Rx: Dinitrate (sublingual chewable): Isordil, Sorbitrate, Dilatrate-SR
Mononitrate (oral): Monoket, ISMO, Imdur, Isotrate ER
Chemical Class: Organic nitrate
Therapeutic Class: Antianginal

CLINICAL PHARMACOLOGY

Mechanism of Action: Stimulation of c-GMP production yields vascular smooth muscle relaxation; venous dilation predominates but dose-dependent dilation of arterial beds occurs; dilation of postcapillary vessels promotes venous pooling, decreases venous return to the heart, reducing left ventricular end-diastolic pressure (preload); arteriolar relaxation reduces systemic vascular resistance and arterial pressure (afterload); myocardial oxygen consumption/demand is decreased; blood pressure decreases with reflex

Pharmacokinetics

Dinitrate

PO: Onset 20-40 min, duration 4-6 hr

PO-SUS REL: Onset up to 4 hr, duration 6-8 hr

SL: Onset 2-5 min, duration 1-3 hr

Metabolized by liver, excreted in urine as metabolites

Mononitrate

PO: Onset 30-60 min

Not subject to 1st-pass metabolism; <4% bound to plasma proteins; metabolized to inactive metabolites; $t_{1/2}$ 5 hr

INDICATIONS AND USES: Prevention of angina pectoris; relief of acute anginal episodes and prophy-laxis prior to events likely to provoke an attack (SL dinitrate formulation only); CHF,* hypertension (acute)*

DOSAGE

Asymmetric dosing regimens provide a daily nitrate-free interval to minimize the development of tolerance

Adult

• *Dinitrate:* SL 2.5-5 mg initially, titrate upward until angina is relieved or side effects limit the dose; chewable tabs 5 mg initially, titrate upward until angina is relieved or side effects limit the dose; PO 5-20 mg bid-tid initially (last dose no later than 7 PM), maintenance 10-40 mg bid-tid (last dose no later than 7 PM); PO Sus Action 40 mg qd-bid initially (last dose no later than 2 PM), maintenance 40-80 mg qd-bid (last dose no later than 2 PM)

• *Mononitrate:* PO 5-20 mg bid (with the 2 doses 7 hr apart); PO Sus Action 30-60 mg qd initially, titrate to 120-240 mg qd if necessary

$ **AVAILABLE FORMS/COST OF THERAPY**

Dinitrate

• Cap, Gel, Sus Action—Oral: 40 mg, 100's: **$59.48-$77.03**

• Tab, Chewable—Oral: 5 mg, 100's: **$22.45**; 10 mg: **$23.88**

• Tab, Coated, Sus Action—Oral: 40 mg, 100's: **$5.83-$60.88**

• Tab, SL—Oral: 2.5 mg, 100's: **$4.35-$30.93**; 5 mg, 100's: **$2.50-$33.06**; 10 mg, 100's: **$36.14**

• Tab, Uncoated—Oral: 5 mg, 100's: **$2.60-$33.23**; 10 mg, 100's: **$1.88-$40.43**; 20 mg, 100's: **$3.23-$59.96**; 30 mg, 100's: **$5.25-$132.15**; 40 mg, 100's: **$4.95-$73.13**

Mononitrate

• Tab, Uncoated—Oral: 10 mg, 100's: **$91.04**; 20 mg, 100's: **$46.88-$91.46**

• Tab, Coated, Sus Action—Oral: 30 mg, 100's: **$111.56-$169.50**; 60 mg, 100's: **$117.40-$178.40**; 120 mg, 100's: **$189.05-$249.74**

CONTRAINDICATIONS: Hypersensitivity to nitrates, severe anemia, closed-angle glaucoma, postural hypotension, head trauma or cerebral hemorrhage (may increase intracranial pressure), acute MI or CHF (mononitrate)

PRECAUTIONS: Acute MI, hypertrophic cardiomyopathy, glaucoma, volume depletion, hypotension, abrupt withdrawal, continuous delivery without nitrate-free interval (tolerance will develop)

PREGNANCY AND LACTATION: Pregnancy category C; excretion into breast milk unknown; use caution in nursing mothers

SIDE EFFECTS/ADVERSE REACTIONS

CNS: Agitation, anxiety, apprehension, confusion, *dizziness,* dyscoordination, *headache,* hypoesthesia, hypokinesia, insomnia, nervousness, nightmares, restlessness, vertigo, weakness

CV: Atrial fibrillation, cardiovascular collapse, crescendo angina, dysrhythmias, edema, hypotension (sometimes with paradoxical bradycardia and increased angina), palpitations, *postural hypotension,* premature ventricular contractions, rebound hypertension, retrosternal discomfort, syncope, tachycardia

EENT: Blurred vision, diplopia

GI: Abdominal pain, diarrhea, dyspepsia, involuntary passing of feces, nausea, tenesmus, vomiting

GU: Dysuria, impotence, involuntary passing of urine, urinary frequency

HEME: Hemolytic anemia, methemoglobinemia

MS: Arthralgia, muscle twitching

SKIN: Cold sweat, crusty skin lesions, exfoliative dermatitis, *flushing,* pallor, perspiration, pruritis, rash

INTERACTIONS

Drugs

🔳 *Alcohol:* Exaggerated hypotension and cardiac collapse

🔳 *Calcium channel blockers:* Exaggerated symptomatic orthostatic hypotension

🔳 *Dihydroergotamine:* Increases the bioavailability of dihydroergotamine with resultant increase in mean standing systolic blood pressure; functional antagonism, decreasing effects

🔳 *Sildenafil:* Excessive hypotensive effects

SPECIAL CONSIDERATIONS

PATIENT/FAMILY EDUCATION

• Headache may be a marker for drug activity; do not try to avoid by altering treatment schedule; contact clinician if severe or persistent; aspirin or acetaminophen may be used for relief

• Dissolve SL tablets under tongue; do not crush, chew, or swallow

• Do not crush chewable tablets before administering

• Avoid alcohol

• Make changes in position slowly to prevent fainting

---

isotretinoin

(eye-soe-tret'i-noyn)

Rx: Accutane

Chemical Class: Vitamin A derivative

Therapeutic Class: Antiacne agent

CLINICAL PHARMACOLOGY

Mechanism of Action: Exact mechanism unknown; reduces sebaceous gland size and inhibits gland activity thereby decreasing sebum secretion; indirectly decreases the number of *Propionobacterium acnes* organisms within the follicle; exhibits antikeratinizing and anti-inflammatory actions

Pharmacokinetics

PO: Peak 3 hr; 99.9% bound to plasma proteins (almost exclusively to albumin); metabolized in liver and possibly in gut wall to 4-oxo-isotretinoin (active), eliminated via the bile and urine; t½ 10-20 hr

INDICATIONS AND USES: Severe recalcitrant cystic acne; keratinization disorders (keratosis follicularis, pityriasis rubra pilaris, lamellar ichthyosis, keratosis palmaris et plantaris, congenital ichthyosiform erythroderma, rosacea, lichen planus, psoriasis)*; cutaneous T-cell lymphoma (mycosis fungoides) and leukoplakia*; prevention of skin cancer in patients with xeroderma pigmentosum*; prevention of 2nd primary tumors in patients treated for squamous cell carcinoma of the head and neck*

DOSAGE

Adult

• PO 0.5-2 mg/kg/day divided bid for 15-20 wk or until total cyst count decreases by 70%; a 2nd course may be initiated after ≥2 mo off therapy if warranted by persistent or recurring severe cystic acne

$ AVAILABLE FORMS/COST OF THERAPY

• Cap, Elastic—Oral: 10 mg, 100's: **$782.83**; 20 mg, 100's: **$927.71**; 40 mg, 100's: **$458.78-$1,077.81**

CONTRAINDICATIONS: Pregnancy, hypersensitivity to parabens (preservative in gelatin capsule)

PRECAUTIONS: Diabetes, obesity, family history of hypertriglyceridemia, contact lens use, inflammatory bowel disease, liver disease, premature epiphyseal closure, hearing impairment, history of depression

PREGNANCY AND LACTATION: Pregnancy category X; isotretinoin is a potent human teratogen; excretion into breast milk unknown, but based on the close relationship to vitamin A, the presence of isotretinoin in breast milk should be expected; avoid use in nursing mothers

SIDE EFFECTS/ADVERSE REACTIONS

CNS: Depression, fatigue, headache, ***pseudotumor cerebri*** (headache, visual disturbances, papilledema)

CV: Edema, palpitations, tachycardia, transient chest pain, vasculitis

EENT: Cataracts, contact lens intolerance, *conjunctivitis,* corneal opacities, decreased night vision, *dry eyes, dry nose, epistaxis,* eyelid inflammation, optic neuritis, photophobia, visual disturbances

GI: Abdominal pain, anorexia, *dry mouth,* gingival bleeding and inflammation, ***hepatotoxicity,*** increased liver function tests, inflammatory bowel disease, *nausea, vomiting,* weight loss

GU: Abnormal menses, *hematuria, proteinuria,* pyuria

HEME: ***Anemia, thrombocytopenia,*** thrombocytosis

METAB: Glucose intolerance, *hypertriglyceridemia*

MS: Bone, joint, and muscle pain and stiffness

SKIN: Bruising, *cheilitis, drying of mucous membranes, dry skin,* erythema nodosum, exaggerated healing response, *facial skin desquamation,* hyperpigmentation, hypopigmentation, *nail brittleness,* paronychia, peeling of palms and soles, *petechiae,* photosensitivity, *pruritis,* pyogenic granuloma, *rash, skin fragility,* skin infections, thinning of hair, urticaria

---

italic = common side effects   ***bold italic*** = life-threatening reactions

INTERACTIONS

Drugs

3 *Carbamazepine:* Decreased concentrations of carbamazepine in one patient

3 *Vitamin A supplements:* Possible additive toxic effects

2 *Tetracyclines:* Concomitant use of isotretinoin and tetracyclines associated with pseudotumor cerebri

SPECIAL CONSIDERATIONS

• Have patient complete consent form included with package insert prior to initiating therapy

PATIENT/FAMILY EDUCATION

• Administer with meals
• Avoid alcohol
• Do not take vitamin supplements containing vitamin A
• **Women of childbearing potential should practice contraception during therapy and for 1 mo before and after therapy**
• Notify clinician immediately if pregnancy is suspected
• A transient exacerbation of acne may occur during the initiation of therapy
• Avoid prolonged exposure to sunlight or sunlamps
• Do not donate blood during and for 30 days after stopping therapy
• Use caution driving or operating any vehicle at night
• Discontinue drug if visual difficulties occur and have an ophthalmologic exam

MONITORING PARAMETERS

• Pregnancy test initially, during first 5 days of menstrual period then monthly
• CBC with differential, platelet count, baseline sedimentation rate, serum triglycerides (baseline and biweekly for 4 wk), liver enzymes

---

isoxsuprine

(eye-sox´syoo-preen)

Rx: Vasodilan, Voxsuprine
Chemical Class: Phenoxyiso-propdylnorsuprifen
Therapeutic Class: Peripheral vasodilator

CLINICAL PHARMACOLOGY

Mechanism of Action: Vasodilation by direct effect on vascular smooth muscle, primarily within skeletal muscle; little effect on cutaneous blood flow; α-adrenoreceptor antagonism and β-adrenoreceptor stimulation produce cardiac stimulation and uterine relaxation

Pharmacokinetics

PO: Onset 1 hr; partially conjugated in blood; eliminated primarily in urine; $t_{1/2}$ 1 ¼ hr

INDICATIONS AND USES: "Possibly effective" for cerebral vascular insufficiency, peripheral vascular disease or arteriosclerosis obliterans, thromboangiitis obliterans, and Raynaud's disease; dysmenorrhea*; threatened premature labor*

DOSAGE

Adult

• PO 10-20 mg tid-qid

$ AVAILABLE FORMS/COST OF THERAPY

• Tab, Uncoated—Oral: 10 mg, 100's: **$5.78-$46.18**; 20 mg, 100's: **$7.84-$54.00**

CONTRAINDICATIONS: Immediately postpartum, arterial bleeding

PREGNANCY AND LACTATION: Pregnancy category C; has been used to prevent premature labor; excretion into breast milk unknown; use caution in nursing mothers

SIDE EFFECTS/ADVERSE REACTIONS

CNS: Dizziness, weakness

CV: Chest pain, *hypotension,* tachycardia

GI: Abdominal distress, nausea, vomiting

SKIN: Flushing, *severe rash*

INTERACTIONS

Labs

• *False positive:* Urine amphetamine

SPECIAL CONSIDERATIONS

PATIENT/FAMILY EDUCATION

• Avoid sudden changes in posture to avoid dizziness (orthostatic hypotension)

---

isradipine

(is-rad'i-peen)

Rx: DynaCirc

Chemical Class: Dihydropyridine

Therapeutic Class: Calcium channel blocker: antihypertensive; antianginal

---

CLINICAL PHARMACOLOGY

Mechanism of Action: Inhibits calcium ion influx across cell membrane in vascular smooth muscle and cardiac muscle; produces relaxation of coronary and peripheral vascular smooth muscle; hemodynamics: decreases myocardial contractility; increases cardiac output; significantly decreases peripheral vascular resistance

Pharmacokinetics

PO: Peak serum concentration 1½ hr, onset 2 hr; significant first pass metabolism; oral bioavailability 17%, 95% bound to plasma proteins; metabolized in liver, excreted in urine and feces (metabolites); $t_{1/2}$ 5-11 hr

INDICATIONS AND USES: Hypertension, chronic stable angina*

DOSAGE

Adult

• PO 2.5 mg bid initially, increase in 2-4 wk intervals prn to max of 10 mg bid; Sus Action PO 5 mg qd, may increase by 5 mg increments at 2-4 wk intervals, max 20 mg/day

💲 AVAILABLE FORMS/COST OF THERAPY

• Cap, Gel—Oral: 2.5 mg, 100's: **$93.18-$107.16**; 5 mg, 100's: **$135.64-$155.98**

• Tab, Sus Action—Oral: 5 mg, 100's: **$127.60-$140.23**; 10 mg, 100's: **$203.32-$223.44**

PRECAUTIONS: CHF, hypotension, hepatic insufficiency, aortic stenosis, elderly, children

PREGNANCY AND LACTATION: Pregnancy category C; excretion into breast milk unknown; use caution in nursing mothers

SIDE EFFECTS/ADVERSE REACTIONS

CNS: Anxiety, asthenia, depression, dizziness, fatigue, headache, insomnia, malaise, nervousness, paresthesia, somnolence, tremor

CV: Bradycardia, *dysrhythmia,* hypotension, palpitations, *peripheral edema,* syncope, tachycardia

EENT: Epistaxis, nasal congestion, tinnitus

GI: Abdominal cramps, constipation, diarrhea, dry mouth, flatulence, gastric upset, nausea, vomiting

GU: Nocturia, polyuria, sexual dysfunction

SKIN: Hair loss, pruritus, rash, urticaria

MISC: Cough, flushing, muscle cramps, shortness of breath, sweating, weight gain

INTERACTIONS

Drugs

3 *Cimetidine:* Increased blood levels of nifedipine with cimetidine

---

italic = common side effects   ***bold italic*** = life-threatening reactions

3 *Digitalis glycosides:* Increased digitalis levels; increased risk of toxicity

3 *Fentanyl:* Severe hypotension or increased fluid volume requirements

3 *Lovastatin:* Decreased lovastatin concentrations

---

itraconazole

(it-ra-con´a-zol)
Rx: Sporanox
Chemical Class: Triazole derivative
Therapeutic Class: Antifungal

CLINICAL PHARMACOLOGY
Mechanism of Action: Inhibits the cytochrome P-450-dependent synthesis of ergosterol, which is a vital component of fungal cell membranes

Pharmacokinetics
PO: Peak 3-5 hr, requires acid pH for absorption, distributed poorly to CSF; 98% bound to plasma proteins; metabolized in liver to hydroxyitraconazole (active) and other metabolites; excreted in urine, bile, and feces; $t_{1/2}$ 60 hr

INDICATIONS AND USES: Blastomycosis, histoplasmosis, aspergillosis, oropharyngeal candidiasis (sol), esophageal candidiasis (sol), superficial mycoses (dermatophytoses, pityriasis versicolor, sebopsoriasis, candidiasis*), onychomycosis, systemic mycoses (candidiasis,* cryptococcal infections, paracoccidioidomycosis, coccidioidomycosis),* subcutaneous mycoses (sporotrichosis, chromomycosis),* cutaneous leishmaniasis,* fungal keratitis,* alternariosis,* zygomycosis*

DOSAGE
Adult
• *Oropharyngeal candidiasis:* PO 200 mg sol (20 ml) qd for 1-2 wk
• *Oropharyngeal candidiasis refractory to fluconazole:* PO 100 mg sol (10 ml) bid
• *Esophageal candidiasis:* PO 100 mg sol (10 ml) qd for 3 wk, treat for at least 2 wk past resolution of symptoms
• *Blastomycosis/histoplasmosis:* PO 200 mg qd; may increase if evidence of progressive disease to 300-400 mg/day in 2 divided doses
• *Aspergillosis:* PO 200-400 mg/day; doses >200 mg/day should be given in 2 divided doses
• *Life-threatening situations:* PO loading dose of 200 mg tid should be given for 1st 3 days
• *Onychomycosis:* PO 200 mg qd for at least 3 mo or 200 mg qd × 1 wk/mo

$ AVAILABLE FORMS/COST OF THERAPY
• Cap, Gel—Oral: 100 mg, 30's: **$216.56-$243.08**
• Susp—Oral: 10 mg/ml, 150 ml: **$127.39**

PRECAUTIONS: Hypersensitivity to other azole antifungals; pre-existing hepatic function abnormalities, children, hypochlorhydria (reduces drug absorption)

PREGNANCY AND LACTATION: Pregnancy category C; excreted into breast milk; do not administer to nursing mothers

SIDE EFFECTS/ADVERSE REACTIONS
CNS: Decreased libido, depression, dizziness, fatigue, fever, headache, insomnia, malaise, somnolence
CV: Edema, hypertension
GI: Abdominal pain, anorexia, diarrhea, hepatitis, liver function test abnormality, *nausea,* vomiting
GU: Albuminuria, impotence

---

* = non-FDA-approved use

METAB: Hypokalemia

SKIN: Pruritis, rash (more common in patients receiving immunosupressants)

INTERACTIONS

Drugs

🔢 *Alprazolam:* Increased plasma alprazolam concentration

🔢 *Aluminum:* Reduced itraconazole absorption

🔢 *Amprenavir:* Increased plasma amprenavir concentration

🔢 *Antacids:* Reduced itraconazole absorption

⚠️ *Astemizole:* QT prolongation and life-threatening dysrhythmia

🔢 *Atevirdine:* Increased plasma atevirdine concentration

🔢 *Atorvastatin:* Increased plasma atorvastatin concentration with risk of rhabdomyolysis

🔢 *Buspirone:* Increased plasma buspirone concentration

🔢 *Calcium:* Reduced itraconazole absorption

🔢 *Cerivastatin:* Increased plasma cerivastatin concentration with risk of rhabdomyolysis

🔢 *Chlordiazepoxide:* Increased plasma chlordiazepoxide concentration

🔢 *Cimetidine:* Reduced itraconazole absorption

⚠️ *Cisapride:* QT prolongation and life-threatening dysrhythmia

🔢 *Clarithromycin:* Increased plasma itraconazole concentration

🔢 *Cyclosporine:* Increased plasma cyclosporine concentration

🔢 *Diazepam:* Increased plasma diazepam concentration

🔢 *Digoxin:* Increased plasma digoxin concentration

🔢 *Didanosine:* Reduced itraconazole absorption

🔢 *Erythromycin:* Increased plasma itraconazole concentration

🔢 *Ethanol:* Disulfiram-like reaction possible

🔢 *Famotidine:* Reduced itraconazole absorption

🔢 *Felodipine:* Increased plasma felodipine concentration

🔢 *Fluvastatin:* Increased plasma fluvastatin concentration with risk of rhabdomyolysis

🔢 *Food:* Increased itraconazole absorption

🔢 *Indinavir:* Increased plasma indinavir concentration

🔢 *Lansoprazole:* Reduced itraconazole absorption

2️⃣ *Lovastatin:* Increased plasma lovastatin concentration with risk of rhabdomyolysis

🔢 *Magnesium:* Reduced itraconazole absorption

🔢 *Methadone:* Increased plasma methadone concentration

🔢 *Methylprednisolone:* Increased plasma methylprednisolone concentration

🔢 *Midazolam:* Increased plasma midazolam concentration

🔢 *Nelfinavir:* Increased plasma nelfinavir concentration

🔢 *Nizatidine:* Reduced itraconazole absorption

🔢 *Omeprazole:* Reduced itraconazole absorption

🔢 *Oral anticoagulants:* Increased hypoprothrombinemic response

2️⃣ *Phenytoin:* Markedly reduced plasma itraconazole concentration

⚠️ *Pimozide:* Increased plasma pimozide concentration, QT prolongation and life-threatening dysrhythmia

🔢 *Pravastatin:* Increased plasma pravastatin concentration with risk of rhabdomyolysis

⚠️ *Quinidine:* Increased plasma quinidine concentration, QT prolongation and life-threatening dysrhythmia

---

italic = common side effects   ***bold italic*** = life-threatening reactions

⬛ *Rifampin:* Decreased plasma itraconazole concentration; decreased plasma rifampin concentration

⬛ *Ritonavir:* Increased plasma ritonavir concentration

⬛ *Saquinavir:* Increased plasma saquinavir concentration

❷ *Simvastatin:* Increased plasma simvastatin concentration with risk of rhabdomyolysis

⬛ *Sodium bicarbonate:* Reduced itraconazole absorption

⬛ *Sucralfate:* Reduced intraconazole absorption

⬛ *Tacrolimus:* Increased plasma tacrolimus concentration

▲ *Terfenadine:* QT prolongation and life-threatening dysrhythmia

⬛ *Tolbutamide:* Increased plasma tolbutamide concentration

❷ *Triazolam:* Increased plasma triazolam concentration

⬛ *Warfarin:* Increased hypoprothrombinemic response

SPECIAL CONSIDERATIONS
PATIENT/FAMILY EDUCATION
• Take with food to ensure maximal absorption
• Avoid antacids within 2 hr of itraconazole administration

MONITORING PARAMETERS
• Liver function tests in patients with pre-existing abnormalities

---

ivermectin

(eye-vir-mek′tin)

Rx: Mectizan, Stromectol
Chemical Class: Avermectin derivative
Therapeutic Class: Anthelmintic

CLINICAL PHARMACOLOGY
Mechanism of Action: Acts as a glutamate and gamma amino butyric acid agonist causing hyperpolarization of invertebrate nerve and muscle cells and death of susceptible organisms

Pharmacokinetics
PO: Peak plasma level 4 hr; does not cross blood-brain barrier; metabolized by liver; excreted in feces; $t_{1/2}$ 18-38 hr

INDICATIONS AND USES: Oncocerciasis, intestinal strongyloidiasis, ascariasis,* bancroftian filariasis,* enterobiasis,* trichuriasis,* scabies,* pediculosis*

DOSAGE
Adult and Child >15 kg
• *Strongyloidiasis:* PO 3 mg (15-24 kg), 6 mg (25-35 kg), 9 mg (36-50 kg), 12 mg (51-65 kg), 15 mg (66-79 kg), 200 μg/kg (>80 kg)
• *Oncocerciasis:* PO 3 mg (15-24 kg), 6 mg (25-35 kg), 9 mg (36-50 kg), 12 mg (51-65 kg), 15 mg (66-79 kg), 150 μg/kg (>80 kg)
• *Ascariasis:* PO 50-200 μg/kg
• *Enterobiasis:* PO 50-200 μg/kg
• *Trichuriasis:* PO 200 μg/kg qd × 2 days
• *Scabies:* TOP 0.8% solution applied to entire body; PO 12 mg

💲 AVAILABLE FORMS/COST OF THERAPY
• Tab, Uncoated—Oral: 3 mg, 20's: **$108.80**; 6 mg, 10's: **$99.74**

PRECAUTIONS: Rapid killing of microfilariae may induce systemic or ocular inflammatory response (Mazzotti reaction)

PREGNANCY AND LACTATION: Pregnancy category C; excreted in breast milk in low concentrations

SIDE EFFECTS/ADVERSE REACTIONS
CNS: Dizziness, somnolence, tremor, vertigo

GI: Anorexia, constipation, diarrhea, increased transaminase levels, nausea

*HEME: **Leukopenia***

---

* = non-FDA-approved use

SKIN: Pruritus, rash, urticaria
MISC: Fatigue

SPECIAL CONSIDERATIONS
PATIENT/FAMILY EDUCATION
• Rapid killing of microfilariae may induce systemic or ocular inflammatory response (Mazzotti reaction, manifest by pruritus, rash, lymphadenopathy, and fever)

MONITORING PARAMETERS
• Stool for parasites; blood for microfilaria and eosinophils

---

kanamycin
(kan-a-mye′sin)
Rx: Kantrex
Chemical Class: Aminoglycoside
Therapeutic Class: Antibiotic

CLINICAL PHARMACOLOGY
Mechanism of Action: Interferes with protein synthesis in bacterial cell by binding to 30S ribosomal subunit, which causes misreading of genetic code; inaccurate peptide sequence forms in protein chain, causing bacterial death

Pharmacokinetics
IM: Onset rapid, peak 1-2 hr
IV: Onset immediate
Plasma $t_{1/2}$ 2-3 hr; not metabolized, excreted unchanged in urine

INDICATIONS AND USES: Severe systemic infections of CNS, respiratory, GI, urinary tract, bone, skin, soft tissues caused by susceptible organisms; *Mycobacterium avium* complex infections (as part of a multiple-drug regimen),* cystic fibrosis (inhaled),* suppression of intestinal bacteria (PO), hepatic coma (PO)
Antibacterial spectrum usually includes:
• Gram-positive organisms: penicillinase- and non-penicillinase-producing *Staphylococcus* spp. (in general, has a low order of activity against other Gram-positive organisms)
• Gram-negative organisms: *Escherichia coli, Proteus* spp. (indole-positive and indole-negative), *Providencia* spp., *Klebsiella-Enterobacter-Serratia* spp., *Acinetobacter* spp., *Citrobacter* spp., *Shigella* spp., *Yersinia pestis, Hemophilus influenzae, Neisseria* spp., *Salmonella* spp.

DOSAGE
Adult
• *Severe systemic infections:* IM/IV 15 mg/kg/day divided q8-12h; do not exceed 1.5 g/day
• *Suppression of intestinal bacteria:* PO 1g q1h for 4 hr, followed by 1 g q6h for 36-72 hr
• *Hepatic coma:* PO 8-12 g/day in divided doses
• *Aerosol treatment:* 250 mg bid-qid; withdraw 250 mg (1 ml) from 500 mg vial, dilute with 3 ml normal saline, and nebulize
• *Intraperitoneal:* 500 mg diluted in 20 ml sterile distilled water instilled through a polyethylene catheter into wound (absorption similar to IM use)

Child
• *Severe systemic infections:* IM/IV 15 mg/kg/day divided q8-12h; do not exceed 1.5 g/day

$ AVAILABLE FORMS/COST OF THERAPY
• Cap, Gel—Oral: 0.5 g, 100's: **$198.00**
• Inj, Sol—IM, IV: 75 mg/2 ml, 2 ml: **$3.25-$16.70**; 500 mg/2 ml, 2 ml: **$3.36-$33.60**; 1 g/3 ml, 3 ml: **$2.50-$66.50**

CONTRAINDICATIONS: Hypersensitivity to aminoglycosides
PRECAUTIONS: Neonates, renal disease, myasthenia gravis, hearing deficits, Parkinson's disease, elderly, dehydration

---

italic = common side effects   ***bold italic*** = life-threatening reactions

PREGNANCY AND LACTATION: Pregnancy category D; 8th cranial nerve toxicity in the fetus has been reported; excreted into breast milk in low concentrations; poor oral availability reduces potential for ototoxicity for the infant; compatible with breast feeding

SIDE EFFECTS/ADVERSE REACTIONS

CNS: Headache, **neuromuscular blockade,** paresthesia

EENT: Deafness, hearing loss, loss of balance, ototoxicity

GI: Diarrhea, nausea, vomiting

GU: Azotemia, hematuria, **nephrotoxicity, oliguria, renal failure**

MS: **Acute muscular paralysis**

RESP: Apnea

SKIN: Rash

INTERACTIONS

Drugs

3 *Amphotericin B:* Synergistic nephrotoxicity

2 *Atracurium:* Kanamycin potentiates respiratory depression by atracurium

3 *Carbenicillin:* Potential for inactivation of kanamycin in patients with renal failure

3 *Carboplatin:* Additive nephrotoxicity or ototoxicity

3 *Cephalosporins:* Increased potential for nephrotoxicity in patients with preexisting renal disease

3 *Cisplatin:* Additive nephrotoxicity or ototoxicity

3 *Cyclosporine:* Additive nephrotoxicity

2 *Ethacrynic acid:* Additive ototoxicity

3 *Indomethacin:* Reduced renal clearance of kanamycin in premature infants

3 *Methoxyflurane:* Additive nephrotoxicity

2 *Neuromuscular blocking agents:* Kanamycin potentiates respiratory depression by neuromuscular blocking agents

3 *NSAIDs:* May reduce renal clearance of kanamycin

3 *Penicillins (extended spectrum):* Potential for inactivation of kanamycin in patients with renal failure

3 *Piperacillin:* Potential for inactivation of kanamycin in patients with renal failure

2 *Succinylcholine:* Kanamycin potentiates respiratory depression by succinylcholine

3 *Ticarcillin:* Potential for inactivation of kanamycin in patients with renal failure

3 *Vancomycin:* Additive nephrotoxicity or ototoxicity

2 *Vecuronium:* Kanamycin potentiates respiratory depression by vecuronium

Labs

• *False increase:* Urine amino acids

SPECIAL CONSIDERATIONS

PATIENT/FAMILY EDUCATION

• Report headache, dizziness, loss of hearing, ringing, roaring in ears, or feeling of fullness in head

MONITORING PARAMETERS

• Urinalysis

• Urine output

• Serum peak drawn at 30-60 min after IV INF or 60 min after IM inj, trough level drawn just before next dose; adjust dosage per levels, especially in renal function impairment (usual therapeutic plasma levels; peak 15-30 mg/L, trough ≤10 mg/L)

• Serum creatinine for CrCl calculation

• Serum calcium, magnesium, sodium

• Audiometric testing; assess hearing before, during, after treatment

kaolin-pectin

(kay'o-lynn)

OTC: Kao-Spen, Kapectolin, Kaolinpec

Combinations

OTC: with bismuth subcarbonate (K-C); with bismuth subsalicylate (Kaodene nonnarcotic)

Chemical Class: Kaolin: hydrous magnesium aluminum silicate; pectin: purified carbohydrate product

Therapeutic Class: Antidiarrheal

CLINICAL PHARMACOLOGY
Mechanism of Action: May act as adsorbents and protectants; effects in the treatment of diarrhea remain to be clearly established

INDICATIONS AND USES: Diarrhea

DOSAGE

Adult
• PO 60-120 ml after each loose bowel movement

Child 6-12 yr
• PO 30-60 ml after each loose bowel movement

Child 3-6 yr
• PO 15-30 ml after each loose bowel movement

⑤ AVAILABLE FORMS/COST OF THERAPY
• Liq—Oral: 5.8 g (kaolin)/130 mg (pectin)/30 ml, 480 ml: **$3.74-$4.68**
• Susp—Oral: 5.2 g (kaolin)/260 mg (pectin)/30 ml, 480 ml: **$4.39**

PRECAUTIONS: Infants, debilitated elderly patients

PREGNANCY AND LACTATION: Pregnancy category C; neither agent is systemically absorbed; should have no effect on lactation or nursing infant

SIDE EFFECTS/ADVERSE REACTIONS
GI: Constipation

INTERACTIONS

Drugs
❷ *Clindamycin, lincomycin:* Reduced antibacterial efficacy of these drugs

❸ *Digoxin:* Reduced bioavailability of digoxin tablets, capsules not affected

❸ *Lovastatin:* Pectin inhibits cholesterol lowering effects of lovastatin

❸ *Quinidine:* Reduced plasma quinidine concentrations

SPECIAL CONSIDERATIONS

PATIENT/FAMILY EDUCATION
• Do not self-medicate diarrhea for >48 hr without consulting a provider

K

---

ketoconazole

(kee-toe-koe'na-zole)

Rx: Nizoral

Chemical Class: Imidazole derivative

Therapeutic Class: Antifungal

CLINICAL PHARMACOLOGY
Mechanism of Action: Inhibits biosynthesis of ergosterol or other sterols, damaging the fungal cell membrane and altering its permeability with resultant loss of essential intracellular elements; inhibits several fungal enzymes resulting in build-up of toxic concentrations of hydrogen peroxide; inhibits biosynthesis of triglycerides and phospholipids by fungi

Pharmacokinetics
PO: Bioavailability decreases as gastric pH increases, peak 1-4 hr; partially metabolized by liver to in-

---

italic = common side effects   ***bold italic*** = life-threatening reactions

active metabolites, excreted mainly in feces (57%) and urine (13%); $t_{1/2}$ 8 hr; CSF penetration poor

INDICATIONS AND USES: TAB: candidiasis, chronic mucocutaneous candidiasis, oral thrush, candiduria, blastomycosis, coccidioidomycosis, histoplasmosis, chromomycosis, paracoccidioidomycosis; severe recalcitrant dermatophyte infections, onychomycosis,* pityriasis versicolor*; tinea corporis, pedis, capitus, cruris*; vaginal candidiasis,* advanced prostate cancer (high doses)*; Cushing's syndrome (high doses)*; CRE: tinea corporis, cruris, pedis; pityriasis versicolor, cutaneous candidiasis, seborrheic dermatitis, SHAMPOO: seborrhea

DOSAGE

Adult

• PO 200 mg qd initially, increase to 400 mg qd for serious infections or if clinical response insufficient; duration 1-2 wk (candidiasis), 6 mo (other indicated systemic mycoses)

• CRE: apply qd to affected area for 2 wk (bid for 4 wk for seborrheic dermatitis)

• Shampoo twice weekly for 4 wk with at least 3 days between each shampooing, then intermittently prn

Child >2 yr

• PO 3.3-6.6 mg/kg/day as a single dose

§ AVAILABLE FORMS/COST OF THERAPY

• Cre—Top: 2%, 15, 30, 60 g: **$27.70-$35.11**/30 g

• Shampoo—Top: 2%, 120 ml: **$22.62-$33.22**

• Tab, Uncoated—Oral: 200 mg, 100's: **$303.83-$402.46**

CONTRAINDICATIONS: Fungal meningitis (poor CSF penetration)

PRECAUTIONS: Renal disease, hepatic disease, achlorhydria (drug-induced), children <2 yr, other hepatotoxic agents, sulfite sensitivity (CRE)

PREGNANCY AND LACTATION: Pregnancy category C; has been used, apparently without harm, for the treatment of vaginal candidiasis during pregnancy; not detected in plasma with chronic shampoo use; unknown if cre absorbed; oral ketoconazole probably excreted in breast milk; use in breast feeding not recommended

SIDE EFFECTS/ADVERSE REACTIONS

CNS: Dizziness, headache, somnolence

GI: Abdominal pain, anorexia, diarrhea, ***hepatotoxicity,*** nausea, vomiting

GU: Gynecomastia, impotence, oligospermia (high doses)

HEME: **Hemolytic anemia, leukopenia, thrombocytopenia**

SKIN: Dermatitis, pruritus, purpura, rash, urticaria

MISC: Chills, fever, photophobia

INTERACTIONS

Drugs

§ *Alprazolam:* Increased plasma alprazolam concentration

§ *Aluminum:* Reduced ketoconazole absorption

§ *Amprenavir:* Increased plasma amprenavir concentration

§ *Antacids:* Reduced ketoconazole absorption

▲ *Astemizole:* QT prolongation and life-threatening dysrhythmia

§ *Atevirdine:* Increased plasma atevirdine concentration

§ *Atorvastatin:* Increased plasma atorvastatin concentration with risk of rhabdomyolysis

§ *Buspirone:* Increased plasma buspirone concentration

---

* = non-FDA-approved use

3 *Calcium:* Reduced ketoconazole absorption

3 *Chlordiazepoxide:* Increased plasma chlordiazepoxide concentration

3 *Cimetidine:* Reduced ketoconazole absorption

2 *Cisapride:* QT prolongation and dysrhythmia

3 *Cyclosporine:* Increased plasma cyclosporine concentration

3 *Diazepam:* Increased plasma diazepam concentration

3 *Didanosine:* Reduced ketoconazole absorption

3 *Ethanol:* Disulfiram-like reaction possible

3 *Famotidine:* Reduced ketoconazole absorption

3 *Felodipine:* Increased plasma felodipine concentration

3 *Fluvastatin:* Increased plasma fluvastatin concentration with risk of rhabdomyolysis

3 *Indinavir:* Increased plasma indinavir concentration

3 *Lansoprazole:* Reduced ketoconazole absorption

2 *Lovastatin:* Increased plasma lovastatin concentration with risk of rhabdomyolysis

3 *Magnesium:* Reduced ketoconazole absorption

3 *Methadone:* Increased plasma methadone concentration

3 *Methylprednisolone:* Increased plasma methylprednisolone concentration

3 *Midazolam:* Increased plasma midazolam concentration

3 *Nelfinavir:* Increased plasma nelfinavir concentration

3 *Nizatidine:* Reduced ketoconazole absorption

3 *Omeprazole:* Reduced ketoconazole absorption

3 *Oral anticoagulants:* Increased hypoprothrombinemic response

3 *Pravastatin:* Increased plasma pravastatin concentration with risk of rhabdomyolysis

3 *Quinidine:* Increased plasma quinidine concentration

3 *Rifampin:* Decreased plasma ketoconazole concentration; decreased plasma rifampin concentration

3 *Ritonavir:* Increased plasma ritonavir concentration

3 *Saquinavir:* Increased plasma saquinavir concentration

2 *Simvastatin:* Increased plasma simvastatin concentration with risk of rhabdomyolysis

3 *Sodium bicarbonate:* Reduced ketoconazole absorption

3 *Sucralfate:* Reduced ketoconazole absorption

3 *Tacrolimus:* Increased plasma tacrolimus concentration

A *Terfenadine:* QT prolongation and life-threatening dysrhythmia

3 *Tolbutamide:* Increased plasma tolbutamide concentration

3 *Triazolam:* Increased plasma triazolam concentration

3 *Warfarin:* Increased hypoprothrombinemic response

SPECIAL CONSIDERATIONS
PATIENT/FAMILY EDUCATION

• For shampoo, moisten hair and scalp, apply shampoo, and gently massage over entire scalp for 1 min; rinse with warm water; repeat, leaving shampoo on scalp for additional 3 min

• Do not take tab with antacids or H₂-receptor antagonists; separate doses by at least 2 hr

• Take tablets with food

MONITORING PARAMETERS

• Liver function tests at baseline and periodically during treatment

---

italic = common side effects   ***bold italic*** = life-threatening reactions

ketoprofen

(kee-toe-proe'fen)

Rx: Orudis, Oruvail

OTC: Actron, Orudis KT

Chemical Class: Propionic acid derivative

Therapeutic Class: NSAID with analgesic and antipyretic activity

CLINICAL PHARMACOLOGY

Mechanism of Action: Reversible cyclooxygenase (i.e., prostaglandin synthetase) inhibitor; non-selectively decreases the formation of both prostaglandins and thromboxane A2; variable effects on lipoxygenase synthesis and subsequent leukotriene production; antiinflammatory, antipyretic, and analgesic activity; inhibits platelet aggregation

Pharmacokinetics

PO: Peak 0.5-2 hr, highly bound to plasma proteins; metabolized primarily in liver, excreted in urine (60%-75%) and feces; t$_{1/2}$ 1-4 hr

INDICATIONS AND USES: Biliary colic,* dysmenorrhea, fever, osteoarthritis, rheumatoid arthritis, renal colic,* soft tissue injuries,* ankylosing spondylitis,* prevention of cognitive decline,* pain—mild to moderate

DOSAGE

Adult

• PO 150-300 mg in divided doses tid-qid, not to exceed 300 mg/day; PO Sus 100-200 mg qd (not recommended for acute pain); PO (OTC) 12.5 mg q4-6h, if pain or fever persist for more than 1 hr, follow with additional 12.5 mg dose

$ **AVAILABLE FORMS/COST OF THERAPY**

• Cap, Gel—Oral: 25 mg, 100's: **$65.68-$99.99**; 50 mg, 100's: **$80.62-$122.75**; 75 mg, 100's: **$23.11-$136.53**

• Cap, Gel, Sus Action—Oral: 100 mg, 100's: **$181.48-$237.25**; 150 mg, 100's: **$220.58-$288.36**; 200 mg, 100's: **$219.85-$301.61**

• Tab—Oral: 12.5 mg, 100's (OTC): **$7.85**

CONTRAINDICATIONS: Bronchospasm, nasal polyps, angioedema precipitated by aspirin or other NSAIDs

PRECAUTIONS: History of GI ulceration, bleeding, or perforation; renal dysfunction, hypertension or cardiac conditions aggravated by fluid retention and edema, history of liver dysfunction, history of coagulation

PREGNANCY AND LACTATION: Pregnancy category B (category D if used in 3rd trimester); could cause constriction of the ductus arteriosus *in utero;* persistent pulmonary hypertension of the newborn or prolonged labor; unknown if excreted into human breast milk

SIDE EFFECTS/ADVERSE REACTIONS

CNS: Dizziness, headache, lightheadedness

CV: Chest pain, *CHF, dysrhythmias,* edema, hypertension, hypotension, palpitation, tachycardia

EENT: Dry eyes, hearing disturbances, photophobia, tinnitus, visual disturbances

GI: Abdominal cramps, constipation, diarrhea, *dyspepsia,* flatulence, *gastric or duodenal ulcer with bleeding or perforation,* hepatitis, *nausea,* occult blood in stool, *pancreatitis,* vomiting

GU: Acute renal failure

---

* = non-FDA-approved use

HEME: ***Agranulocytosis,*** eosinophilia, ***leukopenia, neutropenia, pancytopenia, thrombocytopenia***
METAB: Hyperglycemia, hyperkalemia, hypoglycemia, hyponatremia
RESP: Bronchospasm, dyspnea
SKIN: Photosensitivity, rash, urticaria

INTERACTIONS
Drugs
⬛ *Aminoglycosides:* Reduced clearance with elevated aminoglycoside levels and potential for toxicity (especially indomethacin in premature infants; other NSAIDs probably)

⬛ *Anticoagulants:* Excessive hypoprothrombinemia, decreased platelet aggregation with increased risk of GI bleeding

⬛ *Antihypertensives (α-blockers, angiotensin-converting enzyme inhibitors, angiotensin II receptor blockers, β-blockers, diuretics):* Inhibition of antihypertensive and other favorable hemodynamic effects

⬛ *Corticosteroids:* Increased risk of GI ulceration

⬛ *Cyclosporine:* Increased nephrotoxicity risk

⬛ *Lithium:* Decreased clearance of lithium (mediated via prostaglandins) resulting in elevated serum lithium levels and risk of toxicity

⬛ *Methotrexate:* Decreased renal secretion of methotrexate resulting in elevated methotrexate levels and risk of toxicity

⬛ *Phenylpropanolamine:* Possible acute hypertensive reaction

⬛ *Potassium-sparing diuretics:* Additive hyperkalemia potential

⬛ *Triamterene:* Acute renal failure reported with addition of indomethacin; caution with other NSAIDs

Labs
• *False decrease:* Serum ALT, AST; serum lactate dehydrogenase

SPECIAL CONSIDERATIONS
• No significant advantage over other NSAIDs; cost should govern use

PATIENT/FAMILY EDUCATION
• Avoid aspirin and alcoholic beverages
• Take with food, milk, or antacids to decrease GI upset

MONITORING PARAMETERS
• Initial hemogram and fecal occult blood test within 3 mo of starting regular chronic therapy; repeat every 6-12 mo (more frequently in high-risk patients (>65 years, peptic ulcer disease, concurrent steroids or anticoagulants); electrolytes, creatinine, and BUN within 3 mo of starting regular chronic therapy; repeat every 6-12 mo

K

---

ketorolac
(kee-toe′role-ak)
Rx: Systemic: Toradol
Ophthalmic: Acular, Acular PF
Chemical Class: Acetic acid derivative
Therapeutic Class: NSAID with analgesic and antipyretic activity

---

CLINICAL PHARMACOLOGY
Mechanism of Action: Reversible cyclooxygenase (i.e., prostaglandin synthetase) inhibitor; non-selectively decreases the formation of both prostaglandins and thromboxane A2; variable effects on lipoxygenase synthesis and subsequent leukotriene production; antiinflammatory, antipyretic, and analgesic activity; inhibits platelet aggregation

Pharmacokinetics
PO: Peak 0.5-1 hr
IM: Onset 10 min, duration up to 6 hr

99% bound to plasma proteins; metabolized in liver, excreted in urine (metabolites); t½ 2.4-8.6 hr (increased in elderly, renal impairment)

INDICATIONS AND USES: Cancer pain,* cataract extraction—inflammation, cholecystectomy pain,* conjunctivitis—seasonal allergic, corneal abrasion,* cystoid macular edema,* fracture reduction—pain,* gouty arthritis,* headache,* narcotic sparing effect,* ocular pain, pain control with regional anesthesia,* pain—moderately severe

DOSAGE

Adult

• IM (single-dose treatment) one 60 mg dose; (multiple-dose treatment) 30 mg q6h for no more than 5 days, max 120 mg/day; IV (single-dose treatment) one 30 mg dose; (multiple-dose treatment) 30 mg q6h for no more than 5 days, max 120 mg/day; PO (indicated only as continuation therapy for parenteral ketorolac) 20 mg as a 1st dose then 10 mg q4-6h for no longer than 5 days (including parenteral therapy), max 40 mg/day

• *Elderly (>65 yr), renal impairment, weight <50 kg:* IM (single-dose treatment) one 30 mg dose; (multiple-dose treatment) 15 mg q6h for no more than 5 days, max 60 mg/day; IV (single-dose treatment) one 15 mg dose; (multiple-dose treatment) 15 mg q6h for no more than 5 days, max 60 mg/day; PO 10 mg q4-6h for no more than 5 days (including parenteral therapy), max 40 mg/day

• OPHTH 1 gtt qid

$ **AVAILABLE FORMS/COST OF THERAPY**

• Inj, Sol—IV/IM: 15 mg/ml, 1 ml: **$3.62-$10.40**; 30 mg/ml, 1, 2, 10 ml: **$5.00-$11.01**/1 ml

• Sol—Ophth: 0.5%, 3, 5, 10 ml: **$27.36-$53.59**/5 ml

• Tab, Uncoated—Oral: 10 mg, 100's: **$92.97-$128.66**

CONTRAINDICATIONS: Bronchospasm, nasal polyps, angioedema precipitated by aspirin or other NSAIDs; active peptic ulcer disease, recent GI bleeding or perforation; advanced renal impairment, volume depletion; before any major surgery; suspected or confirmed cerebrovascular bleeding, hemorrhagic diathesis, incomplete hemostasis, and those at high risk of bleeding; concurrent ASA or NSAIDs; neuraxial (epidural or intrathecal) administration due to its alcohol content; concomitant use of probenecid; while wearing soft contact lenses (ophth)

PRECAUTIONS: History of GI ulceration, bleeding, or perforation; renal dysfunction, hypertension or cardiac conditions aggravated by fluid retention and edema, history of liver dysfunction, history of coagulation

PREGNANCY AND LACTATION: Pregnancy category C; excreted into breast milk; not recommended in lactation

SIDE EFFECTS/ADVERSE REACTIONS

CNS: Dizziness, headache, lightheadedness

CV: Chest pain, ***CHF, dysrhythmias,*** edema, hypertension, palpitation, tachycardia

EENT: Dry eyes, hearing disturbances, photophobia, tinnitus; visual disturbances; *burning, stinging upon instillation (ophth)*

GI: Abdominal cramps, constipation, diarrhea, *dyspepsia,* flatulence, ***gastric or duodenal ulcer with bleeding or perforation,*** hepatitis, *nausea,* occult blood in stool, ***pancreatitis,*** vomiting

---

* = non-FDA-approved use

*GU: **Acute renal failure***

*HEME: **Agranulocytosis,** eosino-philia, **leukopenia, neutropenia, pancytopenia, thrombocytopenia***

METAB: Hyperglycemia, hyperkale-mia, hypoglycemia, hyponatremia

*RESP: **Bronchospasm,** dyspnea*

SKIN: Photosensitivity, rash, urti-caria

INTERACTIONS

Drugs

▣ *Aminoglycosides:* Reduced clearance with elevated aminogly-coside levels and potential for toxic-ity (especially indomethacin in pre-mature infants; other NSAIDs prob-ably)

▣ *Anticoagulants:* Excessive hy-poprothrombinemia, decreased platelet aggregation with increased risk of GI bleeding

▣ *Antihypertensives (α-blockers, angiotensin-converting enzyme in-hibitors, angiotensin II receptor blockers, β-blockers, diuretics):* In-hibition of antihypertensive and other favorable hemodynamic ef-fects

▣ *Corticosteroids:* Increased risk of GI ulceration

▣ *Cyclosporine:* Increased nephro-toxicity risk

▣ *Lithium:* Decreased clearance of lithium (mediated via prostaglan-dins) resulting in elevated serum lithium levels and risk of toxicity

▣ *Methotrexate:* Decreased renal secretion of methotrexate resulting in elevated methotrexate levels and risk of toxicity

▣ *Phenylpropanolamine:* Possible acute hypertensive reaction

▣ *Potassium-sparing diuretics:* Additive hyperkalemia potential

▣ *Triamterene:* Acute renal failure reported with addition of indometh-acin; caution with other NSAIDs

SPECIAL CONSIDERATIONS
PATIENT/FAMILY EDUCATION

• Not for chronic use

• No significant advantage over other oral NSAIDs; cost and clinical situation should govern use; no rea-son to continue parenteral course of therapy with oral ketorolac (more expensive, more toxic)

• Combined use of ketorolac paren-teral and oral should not exceed 5 days

---

labelalol
(la-bet´a-lole)

Rx: Normodyne, Trandate
Combinations
  Rx: with hydrochlorothiazide
    (Normozide, Trandate
    HCT)
Chemical Class: Nonselective β-adrenergic blocker; periph-eral α-adrenergic blocker
Therapeutic Class: Antihyper-tensive

CLINICAL PHARMACOLOGY

Mechanism of Action: Combines both selective, competitive postsyn-aptic α_1-adrenergic blocking and nonselective, competitive β-adren-ergic blocking activity; produces re-duction in systemic arterial pressure and total peripheral resistance, with-out significant effects on resting heart rate or cardiac output; pro-duces negative inotropic and chro-notropic responses; slows AV nodal conduction; decreases heart rate; de-creases myocardial oxygen con-sumption; antiarrhythmic effects (class II); reduction in platelet ag-gregation and blood viscosity; sup-pression of renin release; inhibition of central sympathetic outflow; de-creases presynaptic receptor neu-rotransmitter release; weak intrinsic

---

italic = common side effects   ***bold italic*** = life-threatening reactions

sympathomimetic activity; no membrane stabilizing activity; moderate lipid solubility

Pharmacokinetics

PO: Onset 20 min-2 hr, peak 1-4 hr, duration 8-24 hr

IV: Onset 5 min, peak 5-15 min, duration 2-4 hr

50% bound to plasma proteins; metabolized in liver, excreted in urine and feces (metabolites); $t_{1/2}$ 5.5-8 hr

INDICATIONS AND USES: Hypertension, eclampsia, preeclampsia, postmyocardial infarction,* supraventricular arrhythmias (atrial fibrillation, atrial flutter, paroxysmal supraventricular tachycardia),* aggressive behavior,* angina pectoris,* anxiety,* congestive heart failure,* tremor,* aortic dissection,* drug withdrawal syndromes (clonidine, alcohol)* electroconvulsive therapy-induced adverse effects,* hypertensive urgencies and emergencies,* stimulant drug overdoses (cocaine, epinephrine, pseudoephedrine),* pheochromocytoma,* post- and intraoperative hypertension,* Raynaud's phenomenon, tetanus, tyramine-monoamine oxidase inhibitor interaction*

DOSAGE

Adult and child >16 yr

• *Angina pectoris:* PO 100-400 mg bid-tid

• *Hypertension:* PO 100 mg bid; increase q2-3 days in 100 mg bid increments; usually maintenance dose, 200-400 mg bid; max 1200-2400 mg bid dosing; IV bolus—1-2 mg/kg (may overshoot); alternate 20, 40, 80, 160 q1h or until satisfactory control; IV INF 2 mg/min allows for safe titration

• Reduce dose by 50% in patients with chronic liver disease

Child

• *Hypertension:* PO 0.2 to 1 mg/kg/day divided bid

🛡 **AVAILABLE FORMS/COST OF THERAPY**

• Inj, Sol—IV: 5 mg/ml, 4, 8, 20, 40 ml: **$5.28-$47.24**/20 ml

• Tab, Coated—Oral: 100 mg, 100's: **$48.01-$65.06**; 200 mg, 100's: **$68.10-$92.56**; 300 mg, 100's: **$90.59-$123.24**

CONTRAINDICATIONS: Bronchial asthma, cardiogenic shock, overt cardiac failure, second and third degree AV block, severe sinus bradycardia

PRECAUTIONS: Anesthesia/surgery (myocardial depression), avoid abrupt withdrawal, bronchospastic airways, congestive heart failure, diabetes mellitus, hyperthyroidism/thyrotoxicosis (labetolol, unlike propranolol, does not decrease T_3 levels), concurrent clonidine (discontinue labetolol several days prior to withdrawal of clonidine); peripheral vascular disease, renal disease

PREGNANCY AND LACTATION: Pregnancy category C; similar drug, atenolol, frequently used in the third trimester for treatment of hypertension (many studies of efficacy and safety of atenolol in pregnancy-induced hypertension); long-term use has been associated with intrauterine growth retardation; only a small amount of drug appears in milk (0.004% of dose); unlikely to be therapeutically significant

SIDE EFFECTS/ADVERSE REACTIONS

CNS: Anxiety, catatonia, depression, dizziness, drowsiness, fatigue, headache, lethargy, mental changes, nightmares, paresthesias (scalp tingling)

CV: AV block, bradycardia, chest pain, *CHF,* orthostatic hypotension, *ventricular dysrhythmias*

EENT: Double vision, dry burning eyes, sore throat, tinnitus, visual changes

GI: Diarrhea, nausea, vomiting

GU: Dysuria, ejaculatory failure, impotence, Peyronie's disease

HEME: **Agranulocytosis, thrombocytopenic purpura** (reported with other β-blockers only) (rare)

MS: Asthenia, muscle cramps, toxic myopathy

RESP: **Bronchospasm,** dyspnea, wheezing

SKIN: Alopecia, fever, pruritus, rash, urticaria

INTERACTIONS

Drugs

🔳 *α-1 adrenergic blockers:* Potential enhanced first dose response (marked initial drop in blood pressure, particularly on standing)

🔳 *Amiodarone:* Symptomatic bradycardia and sinus arrest; AV node refractory period prolonged and sinus node automaticity decreased, especially patients with bradycardia, sick sinus syndrome, or partial AV

🔳 *Cimetidine:* Increased plasma labetolol concentrations

🔳 *Clonidine:* Withdrawal of clonidine abruptly may exaggerate the hypertension due to unopposed alpha stimulation; safer than other β-blockers, however

🔳 *Digoxin:* Additive prolongation of atrioventricular (AV) conduction time

🔳 *Dihydropyridine calcium channel blockers:* Severe hypotension or impaired cardiac performance; most prevalent with impaired left ventricular function, cardiac arrhythmias, or aortic stenosis

🔳 *Diltiazem:* Potentiates β-adrenergic effects; hypotension, left ventricular failure, and AV conduction disturbances problematic in elderly, patients with left ventricular dysfunction, aortic stenosis, or with large doses of either drug

🔳 *Epinephrine:* Increased diastolic pressure and bradycardia during epinephrine infusions

🔳 *Hypoglycemic agents:* Masked hypoglycemia, hyperglycemia

🔳 *NSAIDs:* Reduced hypotensive effects of β-blockers

❷ *Theophylline:* Antagonistic pharmacodynamic effects

🔳 *Verapamil:* Potentiates β-adrenergic effects; hypotension, left ventricular failure, and AV conduction disturbances problematic in elderly, patients with ventricular dysfunction, aortic stenosis, or with large doses of either drug

Labs

• *False positive:* Urine amphetamine

• *False increase:* Urinary catecholamines, plasma epinephrine

SPECIAL CONSIDERATIONS
PATIENT/FAMILY EDUCATION

• Do not discontinue abruptly; may require taper; rapid withdrawal may produce rebound hypertension or angina

• Transient scalp tingling may occur, especially when treatment is initiated

• May mask the symptoms of hypoglycemia, except for sweating, in diabetic patients

MONITORING PARAMETERS

• Angina: Reduction in nitroglycerin usage; frequency, severity, onset, and duration of angina pain; heart rate

• Arrhythmias: Heart rate

• Congestive heart failure: Functional status, cough, dyspnea on exertion, paroxysmal nocturnal dyspnea, exercise tolerance, and ventricular function

• Hypertension: Blood pressure

• Postmyocardial infarction: Left ventricular function, lower resting heart rate

---

italic = common side effects   ***bold italic*** = life-threatening reactions

• Toxicity: Blood glucose, broncho-spasm, hypotension, bradycardia, depression, confusion, hallucination, sexual dysfunction

---

lactulose

(lak´tyoo-lose)
Rx: Cephulac, Cholac, Chronulac, Constilac, Constulose, Duphalac, Enulose, Generlac, Kristalose
Chemical Class: Synthetic disaccharide analog of lactose
Therapeutic Class: Ammonia detoxicant; laxative

CLINICAL PHARMACOLOGY

Mechanism of Action: Hydrolyzed by colonic bacteria to low molecular weight acids, which convert ammonia (NH_3) to ammonium ion (NH_4+), trapping it and preventing its absorption; laxative action due to increased osmotic pressure of colonic contents and increased stool water content

Pharmacokinetics

PO: Poorly absorbed, does not produce effect until reaching colon, 24-48 hr may be required to produce normal bowel movement

INDICATIONS AND USES: Constipation; portal-systemic encephalopathy

DOSAGE

Adult

• *Constipation:* PO 15-30 ml qd; increase to 60 ml qd if necessary

• *Portal-systemic encephalopathy:* PO 30-45 ml tid-qid, adjust dose to produce 2-3 soft stools/day; PR mix 300 ml lactulose with 700 ml water, instill 180 ml via rectal balloon catheter and retain for 30-60 min, repeat q4-6h

Child

• *Constipation:* PO 7.5 ml qd after breakfast

• *Portal-systemic encephalopathy:* PO 40-90 ml/day divided tid-qid; adjust dose to produce 2-3 soft stools/day

Infant

• *Portal-systemic encephalopathy:* PO 2.5-10 ml/day divided tid-qid; adjust dose to produce 2-3 soft stools/day

$ AVAILABLE FORMS/COST OF THERAPY

• Powder, Packet—Oral: 10 g/packet, 30's: **$30.25**; 20 g/packet 30's: **$46.92**

• Syr—Oral: 10 g/15 ml, 480 ml: **$23.95-$34.75**

CONTRAINDICATIONS: Patients requiring a low galactose diet

PRECAUTIONS: Electrocautery procedures (may spark explosion), diabetes

PREGNANCY AND LACTATION: Pregnancy category B; breast feeding risk to fetus and the newborn negligible

SIDE EFFECTS/ADVERSE REACTIONS

GI: Abdominal discomfort, belching, diarrhea, *flatulence, gaseous distension, nausea,* vomiting

INTERACTIONS

Labs

• *False increase:* Serum creatinine

SPECIAL CONSIDERATIONS

PATIENT/FAMILY EDUCATION

• May be mixed with fruit juice, water, or milk to increase palatability

• Do not take other laxatives while on lactulose therapy

MONITORING PARAMETERS

• Serum electrolytes, carbon dioxide periodically during chronic treatment

lamivudine (3TC)

(la-miv'yoo-deen)

Rx: Epivir, Epivir-HBV
Combinations
  Rx: with zidovudine: (Combivir)
Chemical Class: Nucleoside analog
Therapeutic Class: Antiretroviral

CLINICAL PHARMACOLOGY

Mechanism of Action: Phosphorylated to active 5'-triphosphate metabolite, which inhibits HIV reverse transcription via viral DNA chain termination; also inhibits the RNA- and DNA-dependent DNA polymerase activities of reverse transcriptase

Pharmacokinetics

PO: Rapidly absorbed, bioavailability 86%; <36% bound to plasma proteins, 54%-57% bound to erythrocytes; majority eliminated unchanged in urine; $t_{1/2}$ 5-7 hr (prolonged in renal failure)

INDICATIONS AND USES: HIV infection in combination with zidovudine, chronic hepatitis B*

DOSAGE

Adult and Child ≥12 yr

• *HIV:* PO 150 mg bid in combination with zidovudine; in renal failure adjust dose as follows: CrCl 30-49 ml/min 150 mg qd; CrCl 15-29 ml/min 150 mg × 1, then 100 mg qd; CrCl 5-14 ml/min 150 mg × 1, then 50 mg qd; CrCl <5 ml/min 50 mg × 1, then 25 mg qd

• For latest treatment guidelines, see www.hivatis.org

• *Chronic hepatitis B:* PO 100 mg qd

Child 3 mo-11 yr

• *HIV:* PO 4 mg/kg bid (up to maximum of 150 mg bid) in combination with zidovudine; adjust dose in renal failure (see adult dose)

• For latest treatment guidelines, see www.hivatis.org

$ **AVAILABLE FORMS/COST OF THERAPY**

• Sol—Oral: 5 mg/ml, 240 ml: **$51.97**; 10 mg/ml, 240 ml: **$84.28**

• Tab, Film Coated—Oral: 100 mg, 60's: **$316.04**; 150 mg, 60's: **$208.35-$316.04**

PRECAUTIONS: Impaired renal function; patients at risk for pancreatitis (especially in children)

PREGNANCY AND LACTATION: Pregnancy category C; not recommended in nursing mothers

SIDE EFFECTS/ADVERSE REACTIONS

CNS: Depression, dizziness, fatigue, *headache,* insomnia, neuropathy

EENT: Nasal signs and symptoms

GI: Abdominal cramps, abdominal pain, anorexia, *diarrhea,* dyspepsia, increased ALT/AST, *nausea, **pancreatitis (incidence ~15% in children),*** vomiting

HEME: **Anemia, neutropenia, thrombocytopenia**

MS: Arthralgia, musculoskeletal pain, myalgia

RESP: Cough

SKIN: Rash

L

lamotrigine

(la-moe-trih'jeen)

Rx: Lamictal, Lamictal CD
Chemical Class: Phenyltriazine derivative
Therapeutic Class: Anticonvulsant

CLINICAL PHARMACOLOGY
Mechanism of Action: Inhibits voltage-sensitive sodium channels thereby stabilizing neuronal membranes and consequently modulating presynaptic transmitter release of excitatory amino acids (e.g., glutamate and aspartate)

Pharmacokinetics

PO: Peak 1.4-4.8 hr; 55% bound to plasma proteins; metabolized by glucuronic acid conjugation, eliminated in urine as unchanged drug (10%) and inactive glucuronides (86%); induces its own metabolism; $t_{1/2}$ 25.4-32.8 hr

INDICATIONS AND USES: Adjunctive therapy of partial seizures; generalized tonic-clonic,* absence,* atypical absence,* myoclonic seizures*; Lennox-Gastaut syndrome*

DOSAGE
Adult

• *Patients receiving enzyme-inducing antiepileptic drugs (AEDs) and no valproic acid:* PO 50 mg qd for 2 wk, followed by 50 mg bid for 2 wk, then 300-500 mg/day divided bid (escalate dose by 100 mg/day qwk)

• *Patients receiving enzyme-inducing AEDs plus valproic acid:* PO 25 mg qod for 2 wk, followed by 25 mg qd for 2 wk, then 100-150 mg/day divided bid (escalate dose by 25-50 mg/day q1-2 wk)

💲 AVAILABLE FORMS/COST OF THERAPY
• Tab, Uncoated—Oral: 25 mg, 100's: **$180.72-$259.66**; 100 mg, 100's: **$175.54-$278.51**; 150 mg, 60's: **$110.66-$175.61**; 200 mg, 60's: **$116.00-$184.07**
• Tab, Chewable—Oral: 5 mg, 100's: **$247.94**; 25 mg, 100's: **$259.66**

CONTRAINDICATIONS: Children <16 yr (high incidence of severe, potentially life-threatening rashes)

PRECAUTIONS: Abrupt discontinuation (reduce by 50% qwk over at least 2 wk), renal/hepatic function impairment, children, cardiac function impairment

PREGNANCY AND LACTATION: Pregnancy category C; passes into breast milk, effects on infants exposed by this route are unknown

SIDE EFFECTS/ADVERSE REACTIONS
CNS: Anxiety, *ataxia,* chills, confusion, decreased memory, depression, *dizziness,* emotional lability, fever, *headache,* insomnia, irritability, *seizure exacerbation,* sleep disorder, *somnolence,* speech disorder, tremor, vertigo

CV: Hot flushes, palpitations

EENT: Blurred vision, diplopia, ear pain, tinnitus

GI: Abdominal pain, *nausea, vomiting*

GU: Amenorrhea, dysmenorrhea, vaginitis

MS: Arthralgia, joint disorder, myasthenia, neck pain

RESP: Dyspnea, increased cough, pharyngitis, rhinitis

SKIN: Acne, alopecia, angioedema, photosensitivity, pruritus, *rash,* **Stevens-Johnson syndrome, toxic epidermal necrolysis**

---

* = non-FDA-approved use

INTERACTIONS
Drugs
3 *Carbamazepine:* Increased carbamazepine epoxide levels; decreased lamotrigine levels

3 *Phenobarbital,   primidone, phenytoin:* Decreased lamotrigine concentrations

3 *Valproic acid:* Increased lamotrigine concentration; decreased valproic acid concentration

SPECIAL CONSIDERATIONS
PATIENT/FAMILY EDUCATION
• Notify clinician immediately if a skin rash develops
• Avoid prolonged exposure to direct sunlight

---

lansoprazole
(lan-soe′pray-zole)
Rx: Prevacid
Chemical Class: Substituted benzimidazole derivative
Therapeutic Class: Gastrointestinal antisecretory agent

CLINICAL PHARMACOLOGY
Mechanism of Action: Irreversibly inactivates proton pump in gastric parietal cells, which blocks the final step in secretion of hydrochloric acid; acid secretion is inhibited until additional enzyme is synthesized; inhibits basal and stimulated gastric acid secretion

Pharmacokinetics
PO: Peak 1.7 hr, duration >24 hr; 97% bound to plasma proteins; extensively metabolized in the liver, eliminated as metabolites in urine (33%) and feces (66%); $t_{1/2}$ <2 hr (does not reflect duration of acid suppression)

INDICATIONS AND USES: Short-term treatment of duodenal ulcer; maintenance of healed duodenal ulcers (for up to 1 yr); in combination with clarithromycin and/or amoxicillin for the eradication of *H. pylori* infection in patients with active or recurrent duodenal ulcers; short-term treatment of benign gastric ulcer; short-term treatment of erosive esophagitis; maintenance of healed erosive esophagitis (for up to 1 yr); pathologic hypersecretory conditions (Zollinger-Ellison syndrome, multiple endocrine adenomas, systemic mastocytosis); treatment of GERD; treatment of NSAID-associated gratric ulcers, risk reduction of NSAID-associated gastric ulcer

DOSAGE
Adult and Child >16 yr
• *Duodenal ulcer:* PO 15 mg qd before eating for 4 wk; maintenance 15 mg qd
• *H. pylori:* PO 30 mg plus 500 mg clarithromycin and 1 g amoxicillin all given bid for 14 days; or 30 mg plus 1 g amoxicillin given tid for 14 days (intolerance to clarithromycin)
• *Benign gastric ulcer:* PO 30 mg qd before eating for 8 wk
• *NSAID-associated gastric ulcer:* Treatment PO 30 mg qd before eating for 8 wk; Prevention PO 15 mg qd before eating for 12 wk
• *GERD:* PO 15 mg qd before eating for 8 wk
• *Erosive esophagitis:* PO 30 mg qd before eating for 8 wk; may treat an additional 8 wk if complete healing not present; maintenance 15 mg qd
• *Zollinger-Ellison syndrome:* PO 60 mg qd initially; increase as needed up to 180 mg/day; doses >120 mg/day should be divided bid

S **AVAILABLE FORMS/COST OF THERAPY**
• Cap, Gel, Sus Action—Oral: 15 mg, 30's: **$102.24-$131.16**; 30 mg, 100's: **$445.53**
• Susp—Oral: 15 mg packets, 30's: **$131.16**; 30 mg packets, 30's: **$133.66**

PRECAUTIONS: Children, maintenance therapy in duodenal ulcer; symptomatic response does not preclude gastric cancer

PREGNANCY AND LACTATION: Pregnancy category B; excretion into breast milk unknown

SIDE EFFECTS/ADVERSE REACTIONS

CNS: Headache

GI: Abdominal pain, diarrhea, increased ALT and AST, nausea

INTERACTIONS

Drugs

3 *Cefpodoxime, cefuroxime, ketoconazole, enoxacin:* Reduced concentrations of these drugs

3 *Digoxin, nifedipine:* Increased serum concentrations of these drugs

3 *Food:* 50% decrease in absorption if given 30 min after food compared to the fasting condition

3 *Glipizide, glyburide, tolbutamide:* Increased concentrations of these drugs, potential for hypoglycemia

3 *Sucralfate:* Delayed absorption of lansoprazole and reduced bioavailability, administer lansoprazole at least 30 min prior to sucralfate

SPECIAL CONSIDERATIONS

• For patients with a nasogastric tube, capsules may be opened and the intact granules mixed with 40 ml of apple juice and injected through tube into stomach

• For patients unable to swallow capsules, capsule can be opened and the intact granules sprinkled on 1 tablespoon of applesauce and swallowed immediately; do not crush or chew granules

• For oral suspension, empty contents of packet into 30 ml of water only, don't use other liquids, do not crush or chew granules, if material remains add more water, stir, and drink immediately

---

leflunomide
(le-flu′na-mide)

Rx: Arava

Chemical Class: Isoxazole derivative

Therapeutic Class: Immunomodulatory agent; disease-modifying antirheumatic drug (DMARD)*

CLINICAL PHARMACOLOGY

Mechanism of Action: T-cell pyrimidine biosynthesis inhibitor—antiproliferative and antiinflammatory effects; disease-modifying antirheumatic effects not completely evaluated

Pharmacokinetics

PO: 80% bioavailable; no food effect on absorption; metabolized to active metabolite (which is responsibe for immunomodulating activity); peak metabolite levels at 6 to 12 hr with low Vd and extensive albumin binding (>93%); renal elimination following further hepatic metabolism (renal elimination predominates over the first 96 hr, after which fecal elimination becomes more prominent); elimination half-life of major metabolite, approximately 14 days (4-28 days)—long half-life mandates loading dose to facilitate rapid attainment of steady-state blood levels and clinical effects

INDICATIONS AND USES: Rheumatoid arthritis, organ transplantation*

DOSAGE

Adult and Child <18 yr

• *Rheumatoid arthritis: Loading dose* 100 mg qd for 3 days; *Maintenance dose* 20 mg daily (10 mg qd if side effects intolerable); *Drug elimination procedure:* cholestyramine 8 g tid × 11 days (consecutive days not necessary); without these extra

---

* = non-FDA-approved use

measures, nondetectable plasma levels would take ≤2 years, after drug discontinuation

$ AVAILABLE FORMS/COST OF THERAPY

• Tab, Coated—Oral: 10 mg, 20 mg, 30's: **$283.81**; 100 mg, 3's: **$135.15**

CONTRAINDICATIONS: Preexisting liver impairment

PRECAUTIONS: Hepatotoxicity, renal insufficiency, immunodeficiency, bone-marrow dysplasia, severe infections (potential for immunosuppression)

PREGNANCY AND LACTATION: Pregnancy category X; amount of excretion into breast milk unknown; use of leflunomide by nursing mothers is not recommended since the potential risk to nursing infants is considered serious

SIDE EFFECTS/ADVERSE REACTIONS

CNS: Headache, dizziness, paresthesia
CV: Hypertension
GI: Diarrhea, nausea, abdominal pain, hepatitis, abnormal liver enzymes
GU: Polyuria, dysuria
METAB: Weight loss
RESP: Respiratory infection, bronchitis
SKIN: Alopecia, rash, pruritis

INTERACTIONS

Drugs

3 *Cholestyramine, charcoal:* Coadministration results in rapid and significant decrease in active metabolite

3 *Nonsteroidal antiinflammatory drugs:* Inhibition of CYP 2C9, decreases the metabolism of many NSAIDS

3 *Rifampin:* Leflunomide levels increased 40%

SPECIAL CONSIDERATIONS

• Discuss potential risks of pregnancy and recommend appropriate contraception

MONITORING PARAMETERS

• *Efficacy:* ESR, C-reactive protein, platelet count, hemoglobin, improvement of RA; *toxicity:* LFTs (baseline, then monthly until stable)

---

lepirudin

(leh-peer'u-din)
Rx: Refludan
Chemical Class: Polypeptide
Therapeutic Class: Anticoagulant

CLINICAL PHARMACOLOGY

Mechanism of Action: Binds to and directly inhibits the thrombogenic activity of thrombin; a recombinant hirudin (natural hirudin is produced in trace amounts by the leech *Hirudo medicinalis*)

Pharmacokinetics

IV: Likely metabolized by catabolic hydrolysis; approximately 48% excreted in urine (35% as unchanged drug); terminal $t_{1/2}$ 1.3 hr (prolonged in patients with marked renal insufficiency)

INDICATIONS AND USES: Anticoagulation in patients with heparin-induced thrombocytopenia (HIT) and associated thromboembolic disease in order to prevent further thromboembolic complications

DOSAGE

Adult

• *Initial dose:* IV 0.4 mg/kg (max 44 mg) injected over 15-20 sec, followed by 0.15 mg/kg/hr (max 16.5 mg/hr) as continuous INF for 2-10 days or longer if clinically needed

• *Dose modifications:* If aPTT ratio is above target range (1.5-2.5), stop INF for 2 hr; at restart, decrease INF

---

italic = common side effects   ***bold italic*** = life-threatening reactions

rate by 50% (no additional IV bolus should be administered); determine aPTT ratio again in 4 hr; if aPTT ratio is below target range, increase INF rate in steps of 20%, determine aPTT again in 4 hr

• *Renal function impairment:* IV 0.2 mg/kg injected over 15-20 sec, followed by continuous INF based on creatinine clearance, 0.075 mg/kg/hr (creatine clearance 45-60 ml/min), 0.045 mg/kg/hr (30-44 mg/min), 0.0225 mg/kg/hr (15-29 ml/min); avoid if creatinine clearance <15 ml/min; additional aPTT monitoring is highly recommended

• *Concomitant use with thrombolytic therapy:* IV 0.2 mg/kg bolus, followed by 0.1 mg/kg/hr as continuous INF

• *Patients scheduled to switch to oral anticoagulation:* Gradually reduce lepirudin dose in order to reach an aPTT ratio just above 1.5 before initiating oral anticoagulation; stop lepirudin as soon as international normalized ratio (INR) of 2.0 is reached

$ AVAILABLE FORMS/COST OF THERAPY

• Inj, powder—IV: 50 mg, 1 vial: **$1,446.90**

PRECAUTIONS: Recent puncture of large vessels or organ biopsy; anomaly of vessels or organs; recent cerebrovascular accident, stroke, intracerebral surgery or other neuraxial procedures; severe uncontrolled hypertension; bacterial endocarditis; advanced renal impairment; hemorrhagic diathesis; recent major surgery; recent major bleeding; children; severe liver dysfunction; prolonged therapy

PREGNANCY AND LACTATION: Pregnancy category B; use caution in nursing mothers

SIDE EFFECTS/ADVERSE REACTIONS

CV: **Heart failure**
GI: Abnormal liver function
GU: Abnormal kidney function
HEME: **Bleeding**
SKIN: Allergic skin reactions
MISC: Fever, **multiorgan failure**, allergic reactions

INTERACTIONS
Drugs

❸ *Thrombolytics (tPA, streptokinase, urokinase, reteplase):* Increased risk of bleeding complications; enhanced effect of lepirudin on aPTT prolongation

❸ *Antithrombotic agents (warfarin, aspirin, ticlopidine, clopidogrel, dipyridamole):* Inceased risk of bleeding

SPECIAL CONSIDERATIONS

• Untreated, HIT can lead to thrombosis, venous thromboembolism, acute MI, peripheral artery occlusion, and stroke; mortality rate approaches 20% to 30%

• All sources of heparin must be discontinued as soon as HIT is detected

• In clinical trials the cumulative risk of death 35 days after starting treatment was 9% in the lepirudin-treated patients, compared with 18% in historical controls; cumulative risk of new thromboembolic complications was 6% with lepirudin and 22% in historical controls

MONITORING PARAMETERS

• aPTT ratio (patient aPTT over median of laboratory normal range for aPTT); target range 1.5-2.5; do not start in patients with baseline aPTT ratio ≥2.5; determine aPTT ratio 4 hr following start of INF and at least daily thereafter

• CBC with platelet count (to detect bleeding complications and monitor recovery of platelets)

leucovorin

(loo-koe-vor'in)
Rx: Leucovorin
Chemical Class: Folic acid
derivative
Therapeutic Class: Dihydrofolate reductase inhibitor
antidote; hematinic

CLINICAL PHARMACOLOGY
Mechanism of Action: Reduced
form of folic acid that does not require reduction by dihydrofolate reductase and, therefore, is not affected by blockage of this enzyme
by dihydrofolate reductase inhibitors (e.g., methotrexate)
Pharmacokinetics
PO: Peak 1.72 hr, onset 20-30 min,
duration 3-6 hr
IM: Peak 0.71 hr, onset 10-20 min,
duration 3-6 hr
IV: Onset <5 min, duration 3-6 hr
Metabolized by liver and intestinal
mucosa to active metabolite, eliminated in the urine (80%-90%) and
feces (5%-8%); $t_{1/2}$ 6.2 hr
INDICATIONS AND USES: Rescue
therapy following high-dose methotrexate therapy in osteosarcoma
and inadvertent overdoses of dihydrofolate reductase inhibitors
(methotrexate, pyrimethamine, tri-
metrexate, trimethoprim); megaloblastic anemias due to folic acid deficiency (parenteral); palliative
therapy of advanced colorectal cancer in combination with 5-fluoro-
uracil (parenteral)
DOSAGE
Adult and Child
• Give parenterally when individual
doses are >25 mg
• *Folate deficient megaloblastic
anemia:* IM 1 mg/day

• *Megaloblastic anemia secondary
to congenital deficiency of dihydrofolate reductase:* IM 3-6 mg/day
• *Rescue dose:* PO/IV/IM 15 mg
(approximately 10 mg/m^2) every 6
hr for 10 doses starting 24 h after the
beginning of the methotrexate INF
(administer parenterally in the presence of GI toxicity, nausea, or vomiting); if serum creatinine is elevated
>50% 24 hr after methotrexate **or**
the 24 hr serum methotrexate level is
>5 × 10^{-6}M, increase dose to 100
mg/m^2/dose q3h until serum methotrexate level is <5 × 10^{-8}M
• *Advanced colorectal cancer:* Consult current protocols
**AVAILABLE FORMS/COST
OF THERAPY**
• Inj, Sol—IV/IM: 50 mg/vial:
$21.53-$56.25; 100 mg/vial: **$36.69-
$56.25**; 200 mg/vial: **$10.19-$350.00**;
350 mg/vial: **$81.46-$137.95**
• Tab, Uncoated—Oral: 5 mg, 100's:
$202.68-$551.87; 10 mg, 100's:
$138.33; 15 mg, 24's: **$195.62-
$200.96**; 25 mg, 25's: **$453.00-
$680.34**
CONTRAINDICATIONS: Pernicious anemia and other megaloblastic anemias secondary to vitamin
B$_{12}$ deficiency
PRECAUTIONS: Third-space fluid
accumulation (i.e., ascites, pleural
effusion), renal insufficiency, or inadequate hydration (may increase
leucovorin requirement to prevent
methotrexate toxicity)
PREGNANCY AND LACTATION:
Pregnancy category C; has been
used in the treatment of megaloblastic anemia during pregnancy; compatible with breast feeding
**SIDE EFFECTS/ADVERSE REAC-
TIONS**
RESP: ***Anaphylactoid reactions,***
wheezing
SKIN: Urticaria

SPECIAL CONSIDERATIONS
• Administer as soon as possible following overdoses of dihydrofolate reductase inhibitors

MONITORING PARAMETERS
• CBC with differential and platelets, electrolytes, and liver function tests prior to each treatment with leucovorin/5-fluorouracil combination
• Plasma methotrexate concentrations as a therapeutic guide to high-dose methotrexate therapy with leucovorin rescue; continue leucovorin until plasma methotrexate concentrations are $<5 \times 10^{-8}$M (see dosage)
• Serum creatinine

---

leuprolide
(loo´proe-lide)
Rx: Lupron, Oaklide, Lupron Depot, Lupron Depot-Ped, Viadur
Chemical Class: Synthetic gonadotropin-releasing hormone (GnRH)
Therapeutic Class: Antineoplastic; antiendometriosis agent

CLINICAL PHARMACOLOGY
Mechanism of Action: GnRH agoist; inhibits gonadotropin secretion when given continuously in therapeutic doses; after initial stimulation, chronic leuprolide results in suppression of ovarian and testicular steroidogenesis, which is reversible upon discontinuation

Pharmacokinetics
SC: Peak 3 hr
IM: (depot): Peak 4 hr, duration >4 wk

7%-15% bound to plasma proteins; $t_{1/2}$ 3 hr

INDICATIONS AND USES: Advanced prostate cancer, endometriosis, central precocious puberty; breast, ovarian, and endometrial cancer*; leiomyoma uteri,* infertility,* prostatic hypertrophy*

DOSAGE
Adult
• *Advanced prostate cancer:* SC 1 mg qd; IM (depot) 7.5 mg/dose given qmo, or 22.5 mg/dose given q3mo, or 30 mg/dose given q4mo; implant SC 65 mg (1 implant), remove old implant and replace q12mo
• *Endometriosis/uterine leiomyomata:* IM (depot) 3.75 mg/dose given once qmo or 11.25 mg/dose given q3mo for 6 consecutive mo (3-6 mo for fibroids); repeated courses not recommended

Child
• *Precocious puberty:* SC 50 μg/kg/day, titrate upward by 10 μg/kg qd if total suppression of ovarian or testicular steroidogenesis is not achieved; IM/SC (depot) 7.5 mg q4wk (children <25 kg), 11.25 mg q4wk (children 25-37.5 kg), 15 mg q4wk (children >37.5 kg); titrate upward in 3.75 mg/dose increments q4wk until clinical or laboratory tests indicate no progression of disease

$ AVAILABLE FORMS/COST OF THERAPY
• Inj, Sol—SC: 5 mg/ml, 2.8 ml: **$254.90-$2,219.47**
• Inj, Susp (Depot)—IM: 3.75 mg/vial, 1's: **$440.63-$518.64**; 7.5 mg/vial, 1's: **$594.65-$643.75**
• Inj, Susp (Depot-3)—IM: 11.25 mg/vial, 1's: **$1,455.48-$1,555.92**; 22.5 mg/vial, 1's: **$1,783.95-$1,931.25**
• Inj, Susp (Depot-4)—IM: 30 mg/vial, 1's: **$2,378.60-$2,575.00**

---

* = non-FDA-approved use

• Kit (Depot-Ped)—IM: 7.5 mg/vial, 1's: **$540.63-$643.75**; 11.25 mg/vial, 1's: **$931.88**; 15 mg/vial, 1's: **$1,081.25-$1,287.50**

CONTRAINDICATIONS: Undiagnosed vaginal bleeding

PRECAUTIONS: Edema, hepatic disease, CVA, MI, seizures, hypertension, diabetes mellitus, thromboembolic disease

PREGNANCY AND LACTATION: Pregnancy category X; spontaneous abortions or intrauterine growth retardation are possible; not recommended during lactation

SIDE EFFECTS/ADVERSE REACTIONS

CNS: Dizziness, headache, insomnia, pain, *hot flashes* (50%-80%)

CV: Cardiac murmurs, **CHF,** ECG changes, *edema, hypertension, ischemia,* thrombosis

GI: Anorexia, constipation, nausea, vomiting

GU: Amenorrhea, anovulation, urinary frequency, vaginal bleeding, vaginal discharge, vaginitis, *gynecomastia/breast tenderness*

METAB: Androgen-like effects, decreased libido, decreased testicular size, impotence

MS: Bone pain (with initiation in prostate cancer), myalgia

RESP: Dyspnea, sinus congestion

SPECIAL CONSIDERATIONS

PATIENT/FAMILY EDUCATION

• May cause increase in bone pain and difficulty urinating during 1st few wk of treatment for prostate cancer, may also cause hot flashes

• Gonadotropin and sex steroids rise above baseline initially; side effects greatest in 1st weeks

• Continuous therapy vital for treatment of central precocious puberty

• Females may experience menses or spotting during 1st 2 mo of therapy for central precocious puberty; notify provider if continues into 2nd treatment mo; non-hormonal contraception should be used

MONITORING PARAMETERS

• Monitor response to therapy for prostate cancer by measuring prostate specific antigen (PSA) levels

• GnRH stimulation test and sex steroid levels 1-2 mo after starting therapy for central precocious puberty, measurement of bone age for advancement q6-12mo

---

levetiracetam
(leva-tir-ass´eh-tam)

Rx: Keppra
Chemical Class: Pyrrolidone derivative
Therapeutic Class: Antiepileptic agent

CLINICAL PHARMACOLOGY

Mechanism of Action: S-enantiomer binds to the synaptic plasma membrane in the central nervous system and stimulates several neurochemical systems, including dopaminergic, cholinergic, and glutamanergic neurotransmission

Pharmacokinetics

PO: Onset 1 hr; duration 6-30 hr; peak plasma concentration 20-120 min; 100% bioavailability, not affected by food; minimal metabolism (no CYP systems), metabolites inactive; renal excretion of unchanged drug; $t_{1/2}$ 7 hr

INDICATIONS AND USES: Adjunctive therapy of partial seizures

DOSAGE

Adult and Child >16 yr

• *Adjunctive therapy of partial onset seizures:* PO 1 g-4 g qd, given in 2 equally divided doses; initiate with 500 mg bid with dosing increments increased by 1000 mg/day at 2 wk intervals

---

italic = common side effects   ***bold italic*** = life-threatening reactions

• *Renal impairment:* CrCl 50-80 ml/min: 500-1000 mg bid; for CrCl 30-50 ml/min: 250-750 mg bid; for CrCl <30 ml/min 250-500 mg bid; hemodialysis 500-1000 mg qd, 250-500 mg supplemental dose following hemodialysis recommended

$ AVAILABLE FORMS/COST OF THERAPY

• Tabs—Oral: 250 mg, 120's: **$188.74**; 500 mg, 120's: **$230.69**; 750 mg, 120's: **$329.17**

PRECAUTIONS: Neuropsychiatric conditions (somnolence and fatigue, coordination difficulties, behavioral abnormalities); withdrawal seizures (withdraw slowly to minimize potential); hematologic abnormalities; hepatic abnormalities

PREGNANCY AND LACTATION: Pregnancy category C; developmental toxicity in animals; excretion into breast milk unknown

SIDE EFFECTS/ADVERSE REACTIONS

CNS: Asthenia, amnesia, anxiety, ataxia, depression, *dizziness, emotional lability,* hostility, *nervousness,* paresthesia, *somnolence,* vertigo, confusion, insomnia, tremor
CV: Chest pain
EENT: Diplopia, ambylopia, otitis media
GI: Abdominal pain, constipation, diarrhea, dyspepsia, gastroenteritis, gingivitis, nausea, vomiting, weight gain
HEME: Ecchymosis
MS: Arthralgia, back pain
RESP: Cough, *pharyngitis,* rhinitis, sinusitis, bronchitis
SKIN: Rash
MISC: Infection, fever, flu syndrome

SPECIAL CONSIDERATIONS

• Reserve as an alternative treatment for patients with partial onset seizures not responding to first-line agents

* = non-FDA-approved use

PATIENT/FAMILY EDUCATION

• Notify clinician if female patients intend to or become pregnant
• Caution about common adverse effects, i.e., dizziness and somnolence

MONITORING PARAMETERS

• Therapeutic plasma concentrations not established; base dosing on therapeutic response (reduction in severity and frequency of seizures)

---

levodopa

(lee-voe-doe′pa)
Rx: Larodopa
Combinations
  Rx: with Carbidopa (Sinemet, Sinemet CR)
Chemical Class: Catecholamine precursor
Therapeutic Class: Anti-Parkinson's agent; antidyskinetic

CLINICAL PHARMACOLOGY

Mechanism of Action: Decarboxylated to dopamine, which stimulates dopaminergic receptors in the basal ganglia, improving the balance between cholinergic and dopaminergic activity; improves modulation of voluntary nerve impulses transmitted to the motor cortex; carbidopa in combination product inhibits peripheral decarboxylation of levodopa making more levodopa available for transport to brain and conversion to dopamine

Pharmacokinetics

PO: Peak 1-3 hr, 0.7 hr (Sinemet), 2.4 hr (Sinemet CR); onset 2-3 wk, duration up to 5 hr/dose; 95% converted to dopamine by L-aromatic amino acid decarboxylase enzyme in the lumen of the stomach and intestines and on 1st pass through the liver (reduced by carbidopa); <1% reaches CNS due to extensive metabolism in the periphery and liver (improved by carbidopa); excreted by the kidneys as metabolites; $t_{1/2}$ 1-3 hr

INDICATIONS AND USES: Idiopathic Parkinson's disease, postencephalitic parkinsonism, symptomatic parkinsonism following injury to the nervous system by carbon monoxide or manganese intoxication, parkinsonism associated with cerebral arteriosclerosis; herpes zoster,* restless legs syndrome*

DOSAGE

Adult

• Parkinson's disease (L-dopa): PO 0.5-1 g qd divided bid-qid with meals; may increase gradually by up to 0.75 g/day q3-7 days as tolerated, do not exceed 8 g/day unless closely supervised; (Sinemet) PO 1 tab of 25 mg carbidopa/100 mg levodopa tid or 10 mg/100 mg tid-qid; increase by 1 tab qd-qod prn until dosage of 8 tabs/day is reached; provide at least 70-100 mg of carbidopa/day; (Sinemet CR) PO 1 tab bid at intervals of not <6 hr; usual dose is 2-8 tabs/day in divided doses at intervals of 4-8 hr while awake; allow at least 3 days between dosage adjustments

• Restless legs: PO 1 tab 25 mg/100 mg qhs

§ AVAILABLE FORMS/COST OF THERAPY

• Cap—Oral: 100 mg, 100's: **$28.00**; 250 mg, 100's: **$54.80**; 500 mg, 100's: **$74.70**

• Tab, Uncoated—Oral: 100 mg, 100's: **$23.40**; 250 mg, 100's: **$37.37**; 500 mg, 100's: **$64.18**

• (Sinemet) Tab, uncoated—Oral: 10 mg/100 mg, 100's: **$52.10-$82.69**; 25 mg/100 mg, 100's: **$26.05-$93.36**; 25 mg/250 mg, 100's: **$71.30-$118.96**

• (Sinemet CR) Tab, Sus Action—Oral: 25 mg/100 mg, 100's: **$89.60-$104.59**; 50 mg/200 mg, 100's: **$170.70-$201.16**

CONTRAINDICATIONS: Narrow-angle glaucoma, concurrent MAOI therapy, history of melanoma or suspicious undiagnosed skin lesions (can activate malignant melanoma)

PRECAUTIONS: Severe cardiovascular or pulmonary disease, bronchial asthma, occlusive cerebrovascular disease; renal, hepatic, endocrine disease; affective disorders, major psychoses, cardiac dysrhythmias, history of peptic ulcer, wide-angle glaucoma

PREGNANCY AND LACTATION: Pregnancy category C; do not use in nursing mothers

SIDE EFFECTS/ADVERSE REACTIONS

CNS: Anxiety, ataxia, *choreiform or dystonic movements,* confusion, delusions, depression, dizziness, euphoria, hallucinations, headache, increased hand tremor, insomnia, mental changes, nightmares, "on-off" phenomenon

CV: Edema, hypertension, orthostatic hypotension, palpitations, phlebitis

EENT: Blepharospasm, blurred vision, dilated pupils, diplopia, hoarseness, oculogyric crisis

GI: Abdominal pain, anorexia, burning sensation of tongue, constipation, diarrhea, *dry mouth, dysgeusia, dysphagia,* flatulence, ***GI bleeding, nausea,*** sialorrhea, *vomiting*

GU: Dark urine, priapism, urinary incontinence, urinary retention

HEME: ***Agranulocytosis, hemolytic anemia, leukopenia***

RESP: Bizarre breathing patterns, hiccups

SKIN: Dark sweat, flushing, hot flushes, increased sweating, loss of hair, rash

---

italic = common side effects   ***bold italic*** = life-threatening reactions

MISC: Weight gain
INTERACTIONS
Drugs
3 *Benzodiazepines:* Diazepam and chlordiazepoxide have exacerbated parkinsonism in a few patients receiving levodopa, effect of other benzodiazepines not clinically established
3 *Food:* High-protein diets may inhibit the efficacy of levodopa
3 *Iron:* Reduced levodopa bioavailability possible
3 *Methionine, phenytoin, pyridoxine, spiramycin, tacrine:* Inhibited clinical response to levodopa
3 *Moclobemide:* Increased risk of adverse effects from levodopa
3 *MAOIs:* Hypertensive response
2 *Neuroleptics:* Inhibited clinical response to levodopa
Labs
• *False positive:* Urine ferric chloride test, urine ketones, urine glucose, Coombs test
• *False negative:* Urine glucose (glucose oxidase), urine guaiacols spot test
• *False increase:* Serum acid phosphatase, urine amino acids, serum AST, serum bilirubin, plasma catecholamines, serum cholinesterase, serum creatinine, urine creatinine, creatinine clearance, serum glucose, urine hydroxy-methoxymandelic acid, urine ketones, serum lithium, urine protein, urine sugar, serum uric acid, urine uric acid
• *False decrease:* Serum bilirubin (conjugated and unconjugated), serum glucose, urine glucose, serum triglycerides, serum urea nitrogen, serum uric acid, VMA
SPECIAL CONSIDERATIONS
• Combination with carbidopa is preferred preparation
PATIENT/FAMILY EDUCATION
• Full benefit may require up to 6 mo

• Take with food to minimize GI upset
• Avoid sudden changes in posture
• May cause darkening of the urine or sweat
MONITORING PARAMETERS
• CBC, renal function, liver function, ECG, intraocular pressure

---

levofloxacin

(levo-flox′a-sin)
Rx: *Oral:*Levaquin
*Ophthalmic:*Quixin
Chemical Class: Fluoroquinolone derivative
Therapeutic Class: Antibiotic

CLINICAL PHARMACOLOGY
Mechanism of Action: Interferes with the enzyme DNA gyrase needed for the synthesis of bacterial DNA; bactericidal
Pharmacokinetics
PO: Rapidly and completely absorbed, peak 1-2 hr; can be administered without regard to food
IV: Interchangeable with PO route; Widespread distribution into body tissues; 24%-38% bound to plasma proteins; primarily excreted unchanged in the urine; $t_{1/2}$ 6-8 hr (prolonged in renal failure)
INDICATIONS AND USES: Acute maxillary sinusitis, acute bacterial exacerbation of chronic bronchitis, community acquired pneumonia, uncomplicated and complicated skin and skin structure infections, uncomplicated and complicated urinary tract infection, acute pyelonephritis, bacterial conjunctivitis (ophthalmic)

Antibacterial spectrum usually includes:

• Gram-positive organisms: *Enterococcus faecalis, Staphylococcus aureus, Streptococcus pneumoniae, S. pyogenes*

• Gram-negative organisms: *Enterobacter cloacae, Escherichia coli, Haemophilus influenzae, H. parainfluenzae, Klebsiella pneumoniae, Legionella pneumophila, Moraxella catarrhalis, Proteus mirabilis, Pseudomonas aeruginosa*

• Other organisms: *Chlamydia pneumoniae, Mycoplasma pneumoniae*

DOSAGE
Adult

• *Bronchitis:* PO/IV 500 mg q24h × 7 days

• *Pneumonia:* PO/IV 500 mg q24h × 7-14 days

• *Sinusitis:* PO/IV 500 mg q24h × 10-14 days

• *Uncomplicated skin and skin structure infections:* PO/IV 500 mg q24h × 7-10 days

• *Complicated skin and skin structure infections:* PO/IV 750 mg q24h × 7-14 days

• *Uncomplicated UTI:* PO/IV 250 mg q24h × 3 days

• *Complicated UTI, pyelonephritis:* PO/IV 250 mg q24h × 10 days

• *Bacterial conjunctivitis:* Ophth 1-2 gtt q2h while awake up to 8 times per day for 1st 2 days, then qid for additional 5 days

Dosage in renal failure

• *Bronchitis, pneumonia, sinusitis, uncomplicated skin and skin structure infections:* PO/IV CrCl 20-49 ml/min, 500 mg × 1, then 250 mg q24h; CrCl 10-19 ml/min, 500 mg × 1, then 250 mg q48h; Hemodialysis/CAPD, 500 mg × 1, then 250 mg q48h

• *Complicated skin and skin structure infections:* PO/IV CrCl 20-49 ml/min, 750 mg × 1, then 750 mg q48h; CrCl 10-19 ml/min, 750 mg × 1, then 500 mg q48h; Hemodialysis/CAPD, 750 mg × 1, then 500 mg q48h

• *Complicated UTI, pyelonephritis:* PO/IV CrCl 10-19 ml/min 250 mg × 1, then 250 mg q48h, no dosages adjustment required in uncomplicated UTI

$ AVAILABLE FORMS/COST OF THERAPY

• Sol—IV: 500 mg/20 ml, 1's: **$34.40**

• Sol—Ophth: 0.5%, 5 ml: **$34.40**

• Tab, Film Coated—Oral: 250 mg, 50's: **$395.78**; 500 mg, 50's: **$462.25**; 750 mg, 50's: **$563.55**

PRECAUTIONS: Children (potential for arthropathy and osteochondrosis), renal disease, seizure disorders, diabetes mellitus, rare post-marketing reports of torsades de pointes, infuse IV slowly over 60 min (250-500 mg) to 90 min (750 mg) to avoid hypotension

PREGNANCY AND LACTATION: Pregnancy category C; excretion into breast milk unknown; due to the potential for arthropathy and osteochondrosis, use extreme caution in nursing mothers

SIDE EFFECTS/ADVERSE REACTIONS

CNS: Anxiety, depression, dizziness, fatigue, headache, insomnia, *seizures,* somnolence

EENT: Dizziness, visual disturbances, transient ocular burning and discomfort, photophobia

GI: Abdominal pain, anorexia, diarrhea, dry mouth, flatulence, heartburn, increased AST, ALT; nausea, ***pseudomembranous colitis,*** vomiting

SKIN: Photosensitivity, pruritus, rash

---

italic = common side effects   ***bold italic*** = life-threatening reactions

INTERACTIONS
Drugs

3 *Aluminum:* Reduced absorption of levofloxacin; do not take within 4 hr of dose

3 *Antacids:* Reduced absorption of levofloxacin; do not take within 4 hr of dose

3 *Calcium:* Reduced absorption of levofloxacin; do not take within 4 hr of dose

3 *Cimetidine:* Reduced absorption of levofloxacin

3 *Didanosine:* Markedly reduced absorption of levofloxacin; take levofloxacin 2 hr before didanosine

3 *Famotidine:* Reduced absorption of levofloxacin

3 *Iron:* Reduced absorption of levofloxacin; do not take within 4 hr of dose

3 *Lansoprazole:* Reduced absorption of levofloxacin

3 *Magnesium:* Reduced absorption of levofloxacin; do not take within 4 hr of dose

3 *Nizatidine:* Reduced absorption of levofloxacin

3 *Omeprazole:* Reduced absorption of levofloxacin

3 *Ranitidine:* Reduced absorption of levofloxacin

3 *Sodium bicarbonate:* Reduced absorption of levofloxacin; do not take within 4 hr of dose

3 *Sucralfate:* Reduced absorption of levofloxacin; do not take within 4 hr of dose

3 *Warfarin:* May increase hypoprothrombinemic response to warfarin

3 *Zinc:* Reduced absorption of levofloxacin; do not take within 4 hr of dose

SPECIAL CONSIDERATIONS
• L-isomer of the racemate, ofloxacin (a commercially available quinolone antibiotic)

PATIENT/FAMILY EDUCATION
• Avoid direct exposure to sunlight (even when using sunscreen)
• Drink fluids liberally

---

levonorgestrel
(lee-voe-nor-jess'trel)
Rx: Norplant System, Mirena, Plan B
Combinations
> **Rx:** See oral contraceptives monograph for combined oral contraceptives containing levonorgestrel

Chemical Class: 19-Nortestosterone derivative; progestin
Therapeutic Class: Contraceptive; progestin

CLINICAL PHARMACOLOGY
Mechanism of Action: Exerts a progestational effect on the endometrium, alters cervical mucus, suppresses ovulation in some patients, renders the endometrium hostile to implantation

Pharmacokinetics
IMPLANT: Max concentrations within 24 hr; duration 5 yr; concentrations show considerable interindividual variation depending on individual clearance rates, body weight, and possibly other factors; metabolized by reduction followed by conjugation

PO: Peak 0.5-2 hr, $t_{1/2}$ 11-45 hr, highly bound to albumin and sex hormone binding globulin

INDICATIONS AND USES: Prevention of pregnancy (Norplant, Mirena), emergency contraception (Plan B)

DOSAGE
Adult
• IMPLANT 216 mg (6 × 36 mg caps) subdermally in the upper arm during 1st 7 days after onset of

---

menses; implantation should be fan-like, 15 degrees apart, 8 cm (3 in) above the crease of the elbow

• *Emergency contraception:* PO 0.75 mg within 72 hr of unprotected intercourse, followed by 0.75 mg 12 h later

• INTRAUTERINE 52 mg inserted into uterine cavity during 1st 7 days after onset of menses or immediately after first trimester abortion

§ **AVAILABLE FORMS/COST OF THERAPY**

• Device—Intrauteral: 52 mg, 1 device: **$395.00**

• Kit: 216 mg, 1 kit (36 mg/implant, 6's): **$491.25**

• Tab—Oral: 0.75 mg package of 2: **$21.86**

• Tab—Oral: 0.05 mg ethinyl estradiol/0.25 mg levonorgestrel, 4's: **$12.50**

CONTRAINDICATIONS: Active thrombophlebitis or thromboembolic disorders, undiagnosed abnormal genital bleeding, pregnancy, acute liver disease, liver tumors, breast cancer, hypersensitivity, Intrauterine Device: congenital or acquired uterine anomaly including fibroids, acute pelvic inflammatory disease or history unless subsequent intrauterine pregnancy, postpartum endometritis or infected abortion in past 3 mo, uterine or cervical neoplasia or unresolved, abnormal Pap smear, untreated lower genital tract infections, genital actinomycosis, history of ectopic pregnancy

PRECAUTIONS: Diabetes mellitus, impaired liver function, conditions aggravated by fluid retention, history of depression, contact lens wearers

PREGNANCY AND LACTATION: Pregnancy category X; compatible with breast feeding

SIDE EFFECTS/ADVERSE REACTIONS

CNS: Dizziness, headache, nervousness

CV: Edema

EENT: Contact lens intolerance

GI: Weight gain, change of appetite, nausea

GU: Ovarian cysts, amenorrhea, cervicitis, *irregular bleeding, many bleeding days, prolonged bleeding, spotting,* vaginitis, galactorrhea, mastalgia

METAB: Altered glucose tolerance

MS: Musculoskeletal pain

SKIN: Acne, dermatitis, hirsutism, hypertrichosis, infection at inj site; pain, itching at inj site, scalp hair loss

INTERACTIONS

Drugs

§ *Carbamazepine, phenobarbital, phenytoin:* Decreased efficacy of levonorgestrel, pregnancy has occurred

SPECIAL CONSIDERATIONS

PATIENT/FAMILY EDUCATION

• Most women can expect some variation in menstrual bleeding; these irregularities should diminish with continued use

• Capsules can be removed at any time for any reason or at the end of 5 yr. Removal is more difficult than insertion.

• Failure rate 0.2-1.0%, increases to 5% in patients ≥70 kg (Norplant)

• Efficacy of emergency contraception is better as soon as possible after unprotected intercourse. Causes less nausea and vomiting than other products for emergency contraception. Decreases risk of pregnancy from 8% to 19%

• Based on WHO study, levonorgesterel (norgestrel) only pills preferred emergency contraception; equal efficacy and 50% less nausea, vomiting compared to combined regimen

• About 80% of women wishing to become pregnant conceived within 12 mo after removal of intrauterine device

levorphanol

(lee-vor´fa-nole)
Rx: Levo-Dromoran
Chemical Class: Synthetic opium alkaloid; phenanthrene derivative
Therapeutic Class: Narcotic analgesic
DEA Class: Schedule II

CLINICAL PHARMACOLOGY

Mechanism of Action: Narcotic agonist with activity at Mu receptors (supraspinal analgesia, euphoria, respiratory and physical depression, miosis, and reduced GI motility), Kappa receptors (pentazocine-like spinal analgesia, sedation, and miosis), and Delta receptors (dysphoria, psychotomimetic effects [e.g., hallucinations], and respiratory and vasomotor stimulation caused by drugs with antagonist activity); compared to morphine, equal analgesia, constipation, respiratory depression, and sedation; less emesis

Pharmacokinetics

PO/SC: Peak analgesia 1-1½ hr, duration 6-8 hr

IV: Peak analgesia 20 min, duration 6-8 hr

Metabolized by liver, excreted in urine as glucuronide conjugate; $t_{1/2}$ 11 hr

INDICATIONS AND USES: Moderate to severe pain, preoperative sedation (parenteral)

DOSAGE

Adult

• PO/SC/IV 2-3 mg q6-8h prn

* = non-FDA-approved use

💲 AVAILABLE FORMS/COST OF THERAPY

• Inj, Sol—SC: 2 mg/ml, 1 ml: **$3.96**
• Tab, Uncoated—Oral: 2 mg, 100's: **$56.23-$75.44**

CONTRAINDICATIONS: Acute bronchial asthma, upper airway obstruction

PRECAUTIONS: Head injury, increased intracranial pressure, acute abdominal conditions, elderly, severe impairment of hepatic or renal function, hypothyroidism, Addison's disease, prostatic hypertrophy, urethral stricture, history of drug abuse

PREGNANCY AND LACTATION: Pregnancy category B (category D if used for prolonged periods or in high doses at term); use during labor produces neonatal depression

SIDE EFFECTS/ADVERSE REACTIONS

CNS: Agitation, dependency, dizziness, *drowsiness,* lethargy, restlessness, *sedation*

CV: Bradycardia, orthostatic hypotension, palpitations, tachycardia

GI: Anorexia, constipation, nausea, vomiting

GU: Urinary retention

*RESP: **Respiratory depression, respiratory paralysis***

SKIN: Flushing, rash, urticaria

INTERACTIONS

Drugs

🔢 *Antihistamines, chloral hydrate, glutethimide, methocarbamol:* Enhanced depressant effects

🔢 *Barbiturates:* Additive respiratory and CNS depressant effects

🔢 *Cimetidine:* Increased respiratory and CNS depression

🔢 *Ethanol:* Additive CNS effects

Labs

• *False increase:* Amylase and lipase

SPECIAL CONSIDERATIONS

• Do not administer agonist/antagonist analgesics (i.e., pentazocine, nalbuphine, butorphanol, dezocine, buprenorphine) to patient who has received a prolonged course of levorphanol (a pure agonist). In opioid-dependent patients, mixed agonist/antagonist analgesics may precipitate withdrawal symptoms

PATIENT/FAMILY EDUCATION

• Physical dependency may result when used for extended periods
• Change position slowly; orthostatic hypotension may occur
• Minimize nausea by administering with food and remain lying down following dose

---

levothyroxine

(lee-voe-thye-rox'een)

Rx: Levo-T, Levothroid, Levoxine, Synthroid, Levoxyl
Combinations
   Rx: with liothyronine (Euthroid, Thyrolar)
Chemical Class: Synthetic *levo* isomer of thyroxine (T_4)
Therapeutic Class: Thyroid hormone

CLINICAL PHARMACOLOGY

Mechanism of Action: Increases metabolic rate, increases cardiac output, O_2 consumption, body temperature, blood volume, growth, development at cellular level, metabolism of carbohydrates, lipids, and proteins; exerts profound effects on every organ system, especially CNS

Pharmacokinetics
IV: Onset 6-8 hr
PO: Extent of absorption increased by the fasting state, peak 12-48 hr;

>99% bound to plasma proteins; 35% of T_4 is converted in the periphery to T_3; $t_{1/2}$ 6-7 days (3-4 days in hyperthyroidism, 9-10 days in myxedema)

INDICATIONS AND USES: Hypothyroidism (including cretinism, myxedema, non-toxic goiter), pituitary TSH suppression (thyroid nodules, Hashimoto's disease, multinodular goiter, thyroid cancer), thyrotoxicosis (with antithyroid drugs)

DOSAGE
Adult
• *Hypothyroidism:* PO 50 µg qd to start, increase by 25-50 µg/day at intervals of 2-4 wk, usual dose 100-200 µg/day; use ≤25 µg/day in patients with long-standing hypothyroidism if cardiovascular impairment present; IM/IV 50% of oral dose
• *Myxedema:* IV 200-500 µg 1 time, then 100-300 µg the next day prn; resume oral therapy as soon as clinical situation stabilized
• *TSH suppression:* PO larger amounts than needed for replacement are required; optimal dose determined by laboratory findings and clinical response
Child
• PO 8-10 µg/kg or 25-50 µg qd (0-6 mo); 6-8 µg/kg or 50-75 µg qd (6-12 mo); 5-6 µg/kg or 75-100 µg qd (1-5 yr); 4-5 µg/kg or 100-150 µg qd (6-12 yr); 2-3 µg/kg or ≥150 µg qd (>12 yr); IM/IV 50%-75% of oral dose

$ AVAILABLE FORMS/COST OF THERAPY
• Inj, Lyphl-Sol—IM, IV: 0.2 mg/vial: **$4.38-$62.56**; 0.5 mg/vial: **$4.38-$89.50**
• Tab, Uncoated—Oral: 0.025 mg, 100's: **$4.95-$31.64**; 0.05 mg, 100's: **$4.64-$120.88**; 0.075 mg, 100's: **$4.74-$39.70**; 0.088 mg, 100's: **$14.48-$40.41**; 0.1 mg, 100's: **$3.05-**

$142.56; 0.112 mg, 100's: **$14.48-$47.00**; 0.125 mg, 100's: **$5.40-$47.65**; 0.137 mg, 100's: **$14.48-$36.68**; 0.15 mg, 100's: **$3.15-$49.06**; 0.175 mg, 100's: **$14.48-$69.21**; 0.2 mg, 100's: **$3.30-$7.28**; 0.3 mg, 100's: **$7.47-$79.60**

CONTRAINDICATIONS: Adrenal insufficiency, MI, thyrotoxicosis

PRECAUTIONS: Cardiovascular disease, diabetes mellitus or insipidus, elderly, decreased bone mineral density (long-term therapy in women)

PREGNANCY AND LACTATION: Pregnancy category A; little or no transplacental passage at physiologic serum concentrations; excreted into breast milk in low concentrations (inadequate to protect a hypothyroid infant; too low to interfere with neonatal thyroid screening programs)

SIDE EFFECTS/ADVERSE REACTIONS

CNS: Headache, *insomnia,* nervousness, *tremors*

CV: Angina pectoris, **cardiac arrest, cardiac dysrhythmias,** *palpitations, tachycardia*

GI: Diarrhea, gastric intolerance, nausea

GU: Menstrual irregularities

METAB: Bone demineralization (osteoporosis)

MISC: Fever, heat intolerance, sweating, weight loss

INTERACTIONS

Drugs

🔳 *Aluminum and magnesium antacids, bile acid sequestrants, calcium carbonate, ferrous sulfate, kayexalate, simethicone, sucralfate:* Reduced serum thyroid concentrations through binding and delaying or preventing absorption of levothyroxine, administer these agents at least 4 hr apart

🔳 *Antidepressants (tricyclics, tetracyclics, selective serotonin reuptake inhibitors):* Potential increase in therapeutic and toxic effects of levothyroxine and tri/tetracyclics; increased levothyroxine requirements with sertraline

🔳 *Carbamazepine, phenobarbital, phenytoin, rifampin:* Increased elimination of thyroid hormones; possible increased requirement for thyroid hormones in hypothyroid patients

🔳 *Digoxin:* Levothyroxin may reduce therapeutic effects of digitalis glycosides

❷ *Ketamine:* Concurrent use with thyroid hormones may cause hypertension and tachycardia

🔳 *Oral anticoagulants:* Thyroid hormones increase catabolism of vitamin K-dependent clotting factors; an increase or decrease in clinical thyroid status will increase or decrease the hypoprothrombinemic response to oral anticoagulants

🔳 *Sympathomimetics:* Concurrent use may increase the effects of thyroid hormones or sympathomimetics

🔳 *Theophylline:* Reduced serum theophylline concentrations with initiation of thyroid therapy

Labs

• *False increase:* Serum triiodothyronine

SPECIAL CONSIDERATIONS

• Bioequivalence problems have been documented in the past for products marketed by different manufacturers; however, studies in patients have shown comparable clinical efficacy between brands based on the results of thyroid function tests; brand interchange should be limited to products with demonstrated therapeutic equivalence

---

* = non-FDA-approved use

PATIENT/FAMILY EDUCATION
• Transient, partial hair loss may be experienced by children in the 1st few mo of therapy
• Take as a single daily dose, preferably before breakfast
MONITORING PARAMETERS
• TSH

lidocaine (local, topical)

(lye'doe-kane)

Rx: *Local:* Dilocaine, Duo-Trach Kit, Lidoject, Nervocaine, Octocaine, Xylocaine
Topical: Anestacon, Xylocaine
OTC: *Topical:* DermaFlex, Solarcaine, Zilactin-L
Combinations
  Rx: with epinephrine (Xylocaine with Epinephrine); Prilocaine (EMLA)
Chemical Class: Aminoacyl amide
Therapeutic Class: Local anesthetic

CLINICAL PHARMACOLOGY
Mechanism of Action: Prevents the generation and conduction of nerve impulses by reducing sodium permeability, increasing electrical excitation threshold, slowing nerve impulse propagation, and reducing rate of rise of the action potential
Pharmacokinetics
TOP: Peak 2-5 min, duration 30-60 min
LOCAL: Onset 0.5-1 min (5-15 min for epidural), duration 0.5-1 hr (1-3 hr for epidural)
55%-65% bound to plasma proteins; metabolized primarily in the liver, excreted in urine and bile as metabolites

INDICATIONS AND USES: LOCAL: infiltration anesthesia, nerve block techniques (peripheral, sympathetic, epidural [including caudal], spinal), intraperitoneal anesthesia*; TOP (spray, oint, sol): anesthesia of skin and accessible mucous membranes
TOP (jelly): anesthesia of urethra, anesthetic lubricant for endotracheal intubation
DOSAGE
Adult and Child
• LOCAL varies with procedure, degree of anesthesia desired, vascularity of tissue, duration of anesthesia required, and physical condition of patient; max 4.5 mg/kg/dose, do not repeat within 2 hr
• TOP apply to affected area prn, max 3 mg/kg/dose, do not repeat within 2 hr

AVAILABLE FORMS/COST OF THERAPY
Top
• Aer, Spray—Oral; Top: 10%, 30 ml: **$51.36**
• Cream—Top: 0.5%, 120 g: **$3.00**; 5%, 30 g: **$37.45**
• Gel—Top; Oral: 2%, 30 g: **$15.52-$23.75**
• Oint—Top: 5%, 3, 35, 50, 454 g: **$2.10-$17.34**/35 g
• Sol—Top: 2.5%, 60, 105, 120, 240, 450 ml: **$3.55**/120 ml
Local
• Inj, Sol: 0.5%, 50 ml: **$3.98-$24.13**; 1%, 50 ml: **$1.35-$4.20**; 1.5%, 20 ml: **$7.24**; 2%, 50 ml: **$0.96-$4.20**; 4%, 25 ml: **$1.16-$2.41**; 10%, 10 ml: **$9.07**; 20%, 10 ml: **$5.78-$9.56**
CONTRAINDICATIONS: Hypersensitivity to amide anesthetics, heart block (large doses), septicemia (spinal anesthesia), ophth use (top preparations), spinal anesthesia (preparations containing preservatives)

PRECAUTIONS: Inflammation, sepsis, shock, elderly, children, severe liver disease

PREGNANCY AND LACTATION: Pregnancy category C; has been used as a local anesthetic during labor and delivery; may produce CNS depression and bradycardia in the newborn with high serum levels; compatible with breast feeding

SIDE EFFECTS/ADVERSE REACTIONS

CNS: Anxiety, disorientation, drowsiness, loss of consciousness, restlessness, *seizures,* shivering, tremors

CV: Bradycardia, *cardiac arrest, dysrhythmias,* hypertension, hypotension, *myocardial depression*

EENT: Blurred vision, pupil constriction, tinnitus

GI: Nausea, vomiting

RESP: **Respiratory arrest, status asthmaticus**

SKIN: Allergic reactions, burning, edema, irritation, rash, sensitization (top), skin discoloration at inj site, tissue necrosis, urticaria

INTERACTIONS

Drugs

3 *Disopyramide:* Induction of dysrhythmia or heart failure in predisposed patients

3 *Metoprolol, nadolol, propranolol, cimetidine:* Increased serum lidocaine concentrations

Labs

• *False increase:* Serum creatinine, CSF protein

SPECIAL CONSIDERATIONS

PATIENT/FAMILY EDUCATION

• Do not ingest food for 60 min following oral use (impairs swallowing)

---

lidocaine (systemic)
(lye´doe-kane)
Rx: Xylocaine
Chemical Class: Aminoacyl amide
Therapeutic Class: Antidysrhythmic (Class IB)

CLINICAL PHARMACOLOGY

Mechanism of Action: Decreases depolarization, automaticity, and excitability in the ventricles during the diastolic phase by a direct action on the tissues, especially the Purkinje network, without involvement of the autonomic system; contractility, systolic arterial blood pressure, atrioventricular (AV) conduction velocity, absolute refractory period are not altered by usual therapeutic doses

Pharmacokinetics

IV: Onset immediate, duration 10-20 min

IM: Onset 5-15 min, duration 60-90 min

60%-80% bound to plasma proteins; metabolized by liver to active metabolites, eliminated in urine (10% as unchanged drug); $t_{1/2}$ 1-2 hr

INDICATIONS AND USES: Acute ventricular dysrhythmias

DOSAGE

Adult

• IV bolus 50-100 mg over 2-3 min, repeat q3-5 min, not to exceed 300 mg in 1 hr, begin IV INF; IV INF 20-50 µg/kg/min (1-4 mg/min); decrease the dose in patients with CHF, acute MI, shock, or hepatic disease; IM 200-300 mg in deltoid muscle, additional doses may be given after 60-90 min if necessary; ET 2-2.5 times the IV dose

---

Child

• IV/ET/IO 1 mg/kg loading dose, repeat if needed in 10-15 min × 2 doses, begin IV INF; IV INF 20-50 µg/kg/min

💲 AVAILABLE FORMS/COST OF THERAPY

For Direct IV Administration

• Inj, Sol—IV: 0.5%, 50 ml: **$3.92-$10.62**; 1%, 5 ml: **$0.65-$12.82**; 1.5%, 20 ml: **$4.54-$11.64**; 2%, 5 ml: **$1.93-$12.10**

For IV Admixture

• Inj, Sol: 4%, 5 ml: **$6.38-$7.17**; 10%, 10 ml: **$10.50**; 20%, 10 ml: **$5.78-$9.56**

CONTRAINDICATIONS: Hypersensitivity to amide anesthetics, Stokes-Adams syndrome, Wolff-Parkinson-White syndrome, severe heart block (in absence of a pacemaker)

PRECAUTIONS: Children, renal disease, liver disease, CHF, reduced cardiac output, digitalis toxicity accompanied by AV block, respiratory depression, genetic predisposition to malignant hyperthermia, atrial fibrillation or flutter

PREGNANCY AND LACTATION: Pregnancy category C; compatible with breast feeding

SIDE EFFECTS/ADVERSE REACTIONS

CNS: Apprehension, confusion, *dizziness,* drowsiness, euphoria, hallucinations, lightheadedness, mood changes, nervousness, **seizures,** tremors, twitching, unconsciousness

CV: Bradycardia, **cardiovascular collapse,** edema, **heart block,** hypotension

EENT: Blurred or double vision, tinnitus

GI: Vomiting

RESP: **Respiratory depression and arrest**

SKIN: Rash, swelling, urticaria

MISC: Febrile response, **malignant hyperthermia,** phlebitis at inj site

INTERACTIONS

Drugs

🛑 *Disopyramide:* Induction of dysrhythmia or heart failure in predisposed patients

🛑 *Metoprolol, nadolol, propranolol, cimetidine:* Increased serum lidocaine concentrations

Labs

• *False increase:* Serum creatinine, CSF protein

SPECIAL CONSIDERATIONS

MONITORING PARAMETERS

• Constant ECG monitoring, blood pressure

• Therapeutic serum concentrations are 1.5-6 µg/ml (concentrations >6-10 µg/ml are usually associated with toxicity)

---

lindane (gamma benzene hexa-chloride)

(lin′dane)

Rx: Lindane

Chemical Class: Cyclic chlorinated hydrocarbon

Therapeutic Class: Scabicide/pediculicide

CLINICAL PHARMACOLOGY

Mechanism of Action: Absorbed through the exoskeleton of arthropods, stimulates the nervous system resulting in seizures and death

Pharmacokinetics

TOP: Slowly and incompletely absorbed through intact skin; stored in body fat; metabolized by the liver, excreted in urine and feces

INDICATIONS AND USES: *Pediculus capitis* (head lice), *Pediculus pubis* (crab lice) and their ova; *Sarcoptes scabiei* (scabies)

---

italic = common side effects   **bold italic** = life-threatening reactions

DOSAGE

Adult and Child

• *Lotion:* (Crab lice) apply sufficient quantity only to cover the hair and skin of the pubic area and adjacent infested areas, leave in place for 12 hr then wash thoroughly, may repeat in 7 days if necessary, treat sexual contacts concurrently; (head lice) apply a sufficient quantity to cover only the affected area, rub into scalp, and leave in place for 12 hr then wash thoroughly, may repeat in 7 days if necessary; (scabies) make total body application from neck down, leave on 8-12 hr (adults), 6-8 hr (children), 6 hr (infants), remove by thorough washing, 60 ml usually sufficient for adults

• *Shampoo:* (Head lice and crab lice) apply a sufficient quantity to dry hair, work thoroughly into hair and allow to remain in place for 4 min, add small quantities of water until a good lather forms, rinse hair thoroughly and towel briskly; comb with a fine-toothed comb or use tweezers to remove any remaining nits or nit shells, retreatment not usually necessary; short hair requires approximately 30 ml, long hair 60 ml

💲 **AVAILABLE FORMS/COST OF THERAPY**

• Lotion—Top: 1%, 60, 100, 480, 3840 ml: **$2.10-$15.18**/60 ml
• Shampoo—Top: 1%, 60, 100, 480, 3840 ml: **$2.30-$16.40**/60 ml

CONTRAINDICATIONS: Premature neonates, seizure disorder

PRECAUTIONS: Children, infants, avoid contact with eyes; inflammation of skin, abrasions, or breaks in skin

PREGNANCY AND LACTATION: Pregnancy category B; use no more than twice during a pregnancy; amounts excreted in breast milk probably clinically insignificant

SIDE EFFECTS/ADVERSE REACTIONS

CNS: Dizziness, *seizures,* stimulation

SKIN: Eczematous eruptions due to irritation

SPECIAL CONSIDERATIONS

PATIENT/FAMILY EDUCATION

• Do not exceed prescribed dosage
• Do not apply to face
• Avoid getting in eyes
• Wear rubber gloves for application
• Do not use oil-based hair products (e.g., conditioners) after using product
• Treat sexual and household contacts concurrently

---

linezolid

(li-nee′zoh-lid)

Rx: Zyvox

Chemical Class: Oxazolidinone derivative

Therapeutic Class: Antibiotic

CLINICAL PHARMACOLOGY

Mechanism of Action: Inhibits bacterial protein synthesis through a mechanism of action different from that of other antibacterial agents; by binding to a site on the bacterial 23S ribosomal RNA of the 50S subunit and preventing the formation of a functional 70S initiation complex; bacteriostatic against enterococci and staphylococci, bactericidal against streptococci

Pharmacokinetics

PO: Well absorbed, bioavailability 100%; peak 1-2 hr; 30% protein bound; 65% oxidatively metabolized by liver (does not affect cytochrome P450 system), renally excreted (30% unchanged, 50% metabolites, remainder in stool (75% unchanged after 24 hr); $t_{1/2}$ 4-8 hr (10% shorter in children); no dose adjustment in renal or hepatic insufficiency; give dose after hemodialysis

INDICATIONS AND USES: Vancomycin-resistant *Enterococcus faecium* infections including bacteremia, nosocomial or community acquired pneumonia, complicated skin and skin structure infections caused susceptible organisms

Antibacterial spectrum usually includes:

• Gram-positive organisms: *Enterococcus faecalis* (including vancomycin-resistant strains), *Enterococcus faecium* (vancomycin-susceptible and vancomycin-resistant strains), *Staphylococcus aureus* (including methicillin-resistant strains), *Staphylococcus epidermidis* (including methicillin-resistant strains), *Staphylococcus haemolyticus,* *Streptococcus agalactiae,* *Streptococcus pneumoniae* (penicillin-susceptible and penicillin-resistant strains only), *Streptococcus pyogenes,* Viridans group streptococci

• Gram-negative organisms: *Pasteurella multocida*

DOSAGE

Adult

• *Vancomycin-resistant Enterococcus faecium infections including bacteremia:* PO or IV 600 mg q12h for 14-28 days

• *Nosocomial pneumonia:* PO or IV 600 mg q12h for 10-14 days

• *Community-acquired pneumonia:* PO or IV 600 mg q12h for 10-14 days

• *Complicated skin and skin structure infections:* PO or IV 600 mg q12h for 10-14 days

• *Uncomplicated skin and skin structure infections:* PO 400 mg q12h for 10-14 days

Child

• *Vancomycin-resistant Enterococcus faecium infections including bacteremia:* PO or IV 10 mg/kg q12h for 14-28 days

§ AVAILABLE FORMS/COST OF THERAPY

• Inj, Sol—IV: 2 mg/ml, 100 ml: **$38.10**; 2 mg/ml, 300 ml: **$76.19**

• Pow—Oral: 100 mg/5 ml when reconstituted, 150 ml: **$281.56**

• Tab, Coated—Oral: 400 mg; 600 mg, 20's: **$1,126.25**

PRECAUTIONS: Monoamine oxidase inhibition, uncontrolled hypertension, pheochromocytoma, carcinoid syndrome, or untreated hyperthyroidism, myelosuppression (including anemia, leukopenia, pancytopenia, and thrombocytopenia)

PREGNANCY AND LACTATION: Pregnancy category C; breast milk excretion unknown

SIDE EFFECTS/ADVERSE REACTIONS

CNS: Dizziness, *headache* (7%), insomnia

EENT: Altered taste, thrush

GI: Constipation, *diarrhea* (8%), *increased transaminase levels* (7%), *nausea,* **pseudomembranous colitis,** *vomiting*

GU: Vaginal candidiasis

HEME: **Agranulocytosis, anemia** (7%), **aplastic anemia, leukopenia** (2%), **thrombocytopenia** (5%)

SKIN: Rash

INTERACTIONS

Drugs

❷ *Amphetamines, alcoholic beverages containing tyramine, metaraminol, phenylephrine, phenylpropanolamine, pseudoephedrine, tyramine:* Severe hypertensive reaction

❷ *Antidepressants, cyclic:* Excessive sympathetic response

❷ *Dextromethorphan:* Severe hypertensive reaction

---

italic = common side effects   ***bold italic*** = life-threatening reactions

❷ *Dopamine:* Severe hypertensive reaction

❷ *Epinephrine:* Severe hypertensive reaction

❸ *Levodopa:* Hypertension

❷ *Meperidine:* Severe hypertensive reaction

❷ *Selective serotonin reuptake inhibitors (SSRIs):* Serotonin syndrome (hyperpyrexia, cognitive dysfunction)

❷ *Sibutramine:* Serotonin syndrome (hyperpyrexia, cognitive dysfunction)

❷ *Trazodone:* Serotonin syndrome (hyperpyrexia, cognitive dysfunction)

❷ *Venlafaxine:* Serotonin syndrome (hyperpyrexia, cognitive dysfunction)

SPECIAL CONSIDERATIONS
• Most appropriate use is when Vancomycin-resistant *Enterococcus faecium* infection is documented or strongly suspected, or for oral therapy of methicillin resistant *Staphylococcus aureus* infection

PATIENT/FAMILY EDUCATION
• Avoid high tyramine foods (consume less than 100 mg per meal)

MONITORING PARAMETERS
• CBC weekly if treatment longer than 2 weeks, ALT, AST, renal function

---

liothyronine (T3)
(lye-oh-thye′roe-neen)
Rx: Cytomel, Triostat
Combinations
   Rx: with levothyroxine (Euthroid, Thyrolar)
Chemical Class: Synthetic triiodothyronine (T$_3$)
Therapeutic Class: Thyroid hormone

CLINICAL PHARMACOLOGY
Mechanism of Action: Increases metabolic rate, increases cardiac output, O$_2$ consumption, body temperature, blood volume, growth, development at cellular level, metabolism of carbohydrates, lipids and proteins; exerts profound effects on every organ system, especially CNS
Pharmacokinetics
PO: Peak 48-72 hr, duration following withdrawal of chronic therapy up to 72 hr; >99% bound to plasma proteins; t$_{1/2}$ 0.6-1.4 hr

INDICATIONS AND USES: Hypothyroidism (including cretinism, myxedema, non-toxic goiter), pituitary TSH suppression (thyroid nodules, Hashimoto's disease, multinodular goiter, thyroid cancer), T$_3$ suppression test

DOSAGE
Adult
• *Hypothyroidism:* PO 25 µg/day; increase by 12.5-25 µg q1-2 wk to max of 100 µg/day
• *T$_3$ suppression test:* PO 75-100 µg/day for 7 days
• *Myxedema coma:* IV 25-50 µg; repeat prn at 4-12 hr intervals
Elderly
• *Hypothyroidism:* PO 5 µg/day; increase by 5 µg/day q1-2wk; usual maintenance dose 25-75 µg/day

---

Child
• *Congenital hypothyroidism:* PO 5 µg/day, increase by 5 µg q3d to 20 µg/day (infants), 50 µg/day (child 1-3 yr), adult dose (child >3 yr)

$ **AVAILABLE FORMS/COST OF THERAPY**
• Inj, Sol—IV: 10 µg/ml, 1 ml, 1's: **$399.58-$452.99**
• Tab, Uncoated—Oral: 5 µg, 100's: **$20.18-$52.33**; 25 µg, 100's: **$24.33-$63.04**; 50 µg, 100's: **$37.14-$96.29**

CONTRAINDICATIONS: Adrenal insufficiency, MI, thyrotoxicosis
PRECAUTIONS: Cardiovascular disease, diabetes mellitus or insipidus, elderly

PREGNANCY AND LACTATION: Pregnancy category A; little or no transplacental passage at physiologic serum concentrations; excreted into breast milk in low concentrations; (inadequate to protect a hypothyroid infant; too low to interfere with neonatal screening programs)

SIDE EFFECTS/ADVERSE REACTIONS
CNS: Headache, *insomnia,* nervousness, *tremors*
CV: Angina pectoris, ***cardiac arrest, cardiac arrhythmias,*** *palpitations, tachycardia*
GI: Diarrhea, gastric intolerance, vomiting
GU: Menstrual irregularities
METAB: Bone demineralization (osteoporosis)
MISC: Fever, heat intolerance, sweating, weight loss

INTERACTIONS
Drugs
3 *Bile acid sequestrants:* Reduced serum thyroid hormone concentrations

3 *Carbamazepine, phenytoin, rifampin:* Increased elimination of thyroid hormones; possible increased requirement for thyroid hormones in hypothyroid patients
3 *Oral anticoagulants:* Thyroid hormones increase catabolism of vitamin K-dependent clotting factors; an increase or decrease in clinical thyroid status will increase or decrease the hypoprothrombinemic response to oral anticoagulants
3 *Theophylline:* Reduced serum theophylline concentrations with initiation of thyroid therapy

SPECIAL CONSIDERATIONS
PATIENT/FAMILY EDUCATION
• Transient, partial hair loss may be experienced by children in the 1st few mo of therapy
• Other thyroid products have longer half-lives. Take this into consideration when switching from them to liothyronine.
• Take as single daily dose, preferably before breakfast

MONITORING PARAMETERS
• TSH

---

lisinopril
(ly-sin'oh-pril)
Rx: Prinivil, Zestril
Combinations
Rx: with hydrochlorothiazide (Prinzide, Zestoretic)
Chemical Class: Nonsulfhydryl angiotensin-converting enzyme (ACE) inhibitor
Therapeutic Class: Antihypertensive

CLINICAL PHARMACOLOGY
Mechanism of Action: Antihypertensive, hypoproliferative, and cardioprotective effects attributable to competitive inhibition of angiotensin-converting enzyme (ACE)

yielding decreased plasma concentrations of angiotensin II, plasma aldosterone concentrations, systemic vascular resistance, blood pressure, preload and afterload; not accompanied by changes in heart rate, pressor sensitivity to exogenous norepinephrine, or baroreceptor sensitivity

Pharmacokinetics

PO: Peak 7 hr, onset 1 hr, duration 24 hr; excreted unchanged in urine; t$_{1/2}$ 12 hr (prolonged in renal dysfunction)

INDICATIONS AND USES: Hypertension, CHF, MI, erythrocytosis,* nephropathy,* retinopathy*

DOSAGE

Adult and child >16 yr

• *Hypertension:* PO 10 mg qd; usual dosage range 20-40 mg/day

• *CHF:* PO 5 mg qd; usual dosage range 5-20 mg/day

• *Acute MI:* PO in hemodynamically stable patients within 24 hr of acute MI, 5 mg followed by 5 mg after 24 hr, 10 mg after 48 hr, then 10 mg qd; continue for 6 wk (or longer if concurrent hypertension or CHF)

• *Nephropathy (proteinuria):* PO 5 to 20 mg qd; (dose titration maximal response is required)

• *Renal impairment:* PO initial dose 5 mg qd (serum creatinine ≥3 mg/dl); initial dose 2.5 mg qd (dialysis patients)

$ **AVAILABLE FORMS/COST OF THERAPY**

• Tab, Uncoated—Oral: 2.5 mg, 100's: **$68.05-$71.39**; 5 mg, 100's: **$25.51-$107.04**; 10 mg, 100's: **$84.54-$114.04**; 20 mg, 100's: **$80.95-$118.33**; 30 mg: **$167.51**; 40 mg, 100's: **$132.17-$173.04**

CONTRAINDICATIONS: Hereditary or idiopathic angioedema, history of angioedema related to previous ACE inhibitor therapy

PRECAUTIONS: Renal insufficiency (<30 ml/min), hypotension (CHF, elderly, volume depletion—diuretics, dialysis, cirrhosis), aortic stenosis, hyperkalemia (potassium supplements, potassium-sparing diuretics, renal disease, diabetes), neutropenia (autoimmune diseases, collagen vascular, febrile illness, immunosuppressant drug therapy), proteinuria, renal artery stenosis, surgery/anesthesia (excessive hypotension, correctable with fluids)

PREGNANCY AND LACTATION: Pregnancy category C (1st trimester), category D (2nd and 3rd trimesters); ACE inhibitors can cause fetal and neonatal morbidity and death when administered to pregnant women; when pregnancy is detected, discontinue ACE inhibitors as soon as possible; detectable in breast milk in trace amounts; a newborn would receive <0.1% of the mg/kg maternal dose; effect on nursing infant has not been determined

SIDE EFFECTS/ADVERSE REACTIONS

CNS: Anxiety, *dizziness, fatigue, headache,* insomnia, paresthesia

CV: Angina, hypotension, palpitations, postural hypotension, syncope (especially with 1st dose)

GI: Abdominal pain, constipation, melena, nausea, vomiting

GU: **Acute renal failure,** decreased libido, impotence, increased BUN, creatinine

HEME: **Agranulocytosis, neutropenia**

METAB: Hyperkalemia, hyponatremia

MS: Arthralgia, arthritis, myalgia

RESP: Asthma, bronchitis, *cough,* dyspnea, sinusitis

SKIN: **Angioedema,** flushing, rash, sweating

---

* = non-FDA-approved use

INTERACTIONS
Drugs
❷ *Allopurinol:* Predisposition to hypersensitivity reactions to ACE inhibitors

❸ *Aspirin, NSAIDs:* Inhibition of the antihypertensive response to ACE inhibitors

❸ *Azathioprine:* Increased myelosuppression

❸ *Insulin:* Enhanced insulin sensitivity

❸ *Lithium:* Increased risk of serious lithium toxicity

❸ *Loop diuretics:* Initiation of ACE inhibitor therapy in the presence of intensive diuretic therapy results in a precipitous fall in blood pressure in some patients; ACE inhibitors may induce renal insufficiency in the presence of diuretic-induced sodium depletion

❸ *Potassium-sparing diuretics:* Increased risk for hyperkalemia

❸ *Prazosin, terazosin, doxazosin:* Exaggerated first-dose hypotensive response to α-blockers

❸ *Trimethoprim:* Additive risk of hyperkalemia, especially in patient predisposed to renal insufficiency

Labs
• ACE inhibition can account for approximately 0.5mEq/L rise in serum potassium

SPECIAL CONSIDERATIONS
PATIENT/FAMILY EDUCATION
• Caution with salt substitutes containing potassium chloride
• Rise slowly to sitting/standing position to minimize orthostatic hypotension
• Dizziness, fainting, lightheadedness may occur during 1st few days of therapy
• May cause altered taste perception or cough; persistent dry cough usually does not subside unless medication is stopped; notify clinician if these symptoms persist

MONITORING PARAMETERS
• BUN, creatinine, potassium within 2 wk after initiation of therapy (increased levels may indicate acute renal failure)

---

lithium
(li'thee-um)
Rx: *Tablets:* Eskalith, Lithane, Lithotabs, Lithobid
Capsules: Eskalith, Lithonate
Syrup: Cibalith-S
Chemical Class: Monovalent cation
Therapeutic Class: Antimanic; psychotherapeutic agent

CLINICAL PHARMACOLOGY
Mechanism of Action: Alters sodium transport in nerve and muscle cells; effects a shift toward intraneuronal metabolism of catecholamines; affects the synthesis, storage, release and reuptake of central monoamine neurotransmitters (norepinephrine, serotonin, dopamine, acetylcholine, and GABA); antimanic effects as a result of increases in norepinephrine uptake and increased serotonin receptor sensitivity

Pharmacokinetics
PO: Peak ½ hr (syr), 1-3 hr (cap or tabs), 3-4 hr (Sus Action formulations); onset 1-3 wk; not bound to plasma proteins; excreted unchanged in urine (95%); $t_{1/2}$ 18-36 hr

INDICATIONS AND USES: Manic episodes of bipolar affective disorder; prophylaxis of cluster headache,* premenstrual syndrome,* bulimia,* alcoholism,* SIADH,* tardive dyskinesia,* hyperthyroidism,* postpartum affective psychosis*

---

italic = common side effects   ***bold italic*** = life-threatening reactions

DOSAGE

Adult

• *Acute mania:* PO 600 mg tid or 900 mg bid (Sus Action formulations); determine serum lithium concentrations twice weekly until stabilized

• *Maintenance:* PO 300 mg tid-qid; adjust to maintain therapeutic serum lithium concentration

Child

• PO 15-60 mg/kg/day in 3-4 divided doses; adjust to maintain therapeutic serum lithium concentration; do not exceed usual adult dose

§ AVAILABLE FORMS/COST OF THERAPY

Lithium Carbonate

• Cap, Gel—Oral: 150 mg, 100's: **$13.97**; 300 mg, 100's: **$3.33-$29.75**; 600 mg, 100's: **$34.92-$41.90**

• Tab, Uncoated—Oral: 300 mg, 100's: **$9.11-$19.21**

• Tab, Coated, Sus Action—Oral: 300 mg, 100's: **$38.76**; 450 mg, 100's: **$51.94**

Lithium Citrate

• Syr—Oral: 300 mg/5 ml, 480 ml: **$15.50-$19.29**

CONTRAINDICATIONS: Severe cardiovascular or renal disease

PRECAUTIONS: Toxicity closely related to serum levels (facilities for serum lithium determinations required to monitor therapy); dehydration, sodium depletion, elderly, children <12 yr, concomitant infection, thyroid disease, tartrazine sensitivity, diabetes mellitus

PREGNANCY AND LACTATION: Pregnancy category D; avoid use in pregnancy if possible, especially during the 1st trimester; contraindicated in nursing mothers

SIDE EFFECTS/ADVERSE REACTIONS

CNS: Ataxia, clonic movements, confusion, *dizziness, drowsiness, fine hand tremor, headache,* memory loss, ***pseudotumor cerebri,*** restlessness, **seizures,** slurred speech, stupor, twitching

CV: Bradycardia, ***circulatory collapse, dysrhythmias,*** ECG changes, edema, *hypotension*

EENT: Blurred vision, tinnitus

GI: Abdominal pain, *anorexia, diarrhea, dry mouth,* excessive salivation, flatulence, gastritis, metallic taste, *nausea, vomiting*

GU: Albuminuria, decreased creatinine clearance, glycosuria, polydipsia, *polyuria,* proteinuria, sexual dysfunction, symptoms of nephrogenic diabetes, urinary incontinence

METAB: Euthyroid goiter, hyperthyroidism (rare), hyponatremia, hypothyroidism, transient hyperglycemia

MS: Arthralgia

SKIN: Acne, anesthesia of skin, ***angioedema,*** chronic folliculitis, drying and thinning of hair, exacerbation of psoriasis, generalized pruritis

MISC: Excessive weight gain, thirst

INTERACTIONS

Drugs

§ *ACE inhibitors, methyldopa:* Increased risk of lithium toxicity

§ *Diltiazem, verapamil, amitriptyline, carbamazepine, fluoxetine, fluvoxamine:* Neurotoxicity, including seizures

❷ *MAOIs:* Malignant hyperpyrexia

§ *Neuroleptics:* Reduced neuroleptic response; severe neurotoxicity possible in acute manic patients receiving lithium and neuroleptics

§ *NSAIDs:* Increased lithium concentrations

---

8 *Phenytoin:* Development of lithium toxicity has been reported

8 *Potassium iodide:* Increased risk for hypothyroidism

8 *Sodium bicarbonate:* Decreased plasma lithium concentrations

8 *Sodium chloride:* High sodium intake may reduce serum lithium concentrations; sodium restriction may increase serum lithium

8 *Theophylline:* Increased lithium renal clearance, decreased lithium efficacy

8 *Thiazide diuretics:* Increased lithium concentrations

Labs
• *False increase:* Serum creatinine

SPECIAL CONSIDERATIONS
PATIENT/FAMILY EDUCATION
• Take with meals to avoid stomach upset
• Discontinue medication and contact clinician for diarrhea, vomiting, unsteady walking, coarse hand tremor, severe drowsiness, muscle weakness
• Drink 8-12 glasses of water or other liquid every day
• Do not restrict sodium in diet

MONITORING PARAMETERS
• Serum lithium concentrations drawn immediately prior to next dose (8-12 hr after previous dose), monitor biweekly until stable then q2-3mo; therapeutic range 0.8-1.2 mEq/L (acute), 0.5-1.0 mEq/L (maintenance)
• Serum creatinine, CBC, urinalysis, serum electrolytes, fasting glucose, ECG, TSH

lomefloxacin
(lome-flock'sa-sin)
Rx: Maxaquin
Chemical Class: Fluoroquinolone
Therapeutic Class: Antibiotic

CLINICAL PHARMACOLOGY
Mechanism of Action: Interferes with the enzyme DNA gyrase needed for synthesis of bacterial DNA; bactericidal
Pharmacokinetics
PO: Peak 1-2 hr, absorption decreased by coadministration with food; excreted in urine as active drug, metabolites; $t_{1/2}$ 6-8 hr

INDICATIONS AND USES: Infections of the lower respiratory tract, urinary tract; prevention of UTI in patients undergoing transurethral procedures; gonorrhea*
Antibacterial spectrum usually includes:
• Gram-positive organisms: *Staphylococcus saprophyticus*
• Gram-negative organisms: *Citrobacter diversus, Enterobacter cloacae, Escherichia coli, Haemophilus influenzae, Klebsiella pneumoniae, Moraxella catarrhalis, Proteus mirabilis, Pseudomonas aeruginosa* (urinary tract only)

DOSAGE
Adult
• *Lower respiratory tract:* PO 400 mg qd for 10 days
• *Urinary tract:* PO 400 mg qd for 3-14 days
• *Prophylaxis:* PO 400 mg as a single dose 2-6 hr prior to surgery
• *Gonorrhea:* PO 400 mg as a single dose
• *Renal function impairment:* PO 400 mg loading dose, then 200 mg qd for duration of treatment (CrCl <40 ml/min/1.73 m²)

L

§ AVAILABLE FORMS/COST OF THERAPY

• Tab, Coated—Oral: 400 mg, 20's: **$132.08-$138.68**

CONTRAINDICATIONS: Hypersensitivity to quinolones

PRECAUTIONS: Children (potential for arthropathy and osteochondrosis), elderly, renal disease, seizure disorders, phototoxicity

PREGNANCY AND LACTATION: Pregnancy category C; excretion into breast milk unknown; due to the potential for arthropathy and osteochondrosis, use extreme caution in nursing mothers

SIDE EFFECTS/ADVERSE REACTIONS

CNS: Anxiety, depression, dizziness, fatigue, headache, insomnia, seizures, somnolence

EENT: Dizziness, visual disturbances

GI: Abdominal pain, anorexia, diarrhea, dry mouth, flatulence, heartburn, increased AST, ALT; *nausea,* **pseudomembranous colitis,** vomiting

SKIN: Photosensitivity, pruritus, rash

INTERACTIONS

Drugs

▪ *Aluminum:* Reduced absorption of lomefloxacin; do not take within 4 hr of dose

▪ *Antacids:* Reduced absorption of lomefloxacin; do not take within 4 hr of dose

▪ *Calcium:* Reduced absorption of lomefloxacin; do not take within 4 hr of dose

▪ *Cimetidine:* Interference with the elimination of other quinolones

▪ *Cyclosporine:* Increased plasma cyclosporine concentrations with other quinolones

▪ *Didanosine:* Markedly reduced absorption of lomefloxacin; take lomefloxacin 2 hr before didanosine

▪ *Iron:* Reduced absorption of lomefloxacin; do not take within 4 hr of dose

▪ *Magnesium:* Reduced absorption of lomefloxacin; do not take within 4 hr of dose

▪ *Probenecid:* Probenecid slows the renal elimination of lomefloxacin resulting in increased plasma lomefloxacin concentrations

▪ *Sodium bicarbonate:* Reduced absorption of lomefloxacin; do not take within 4 hr of dose

▪ *Sucralfate:* Reduced absorption of lomefloxacin; do not take within 4 hr of dose

▪ *Warfarin:* May increase hypoprothrombinemic response to warfarin

▪ *Zinc:* Reduced absorption of lomefloxacin; do not take within 4 hr of dose

SPECIAL CONSIDERATIONS

PATIENT/FAMILY EDUCATION

• Avoid direct exposure to sunlight (even when using sunscreen)
• Drink fluids liberally
• Do not take antacids containing magnesium or aluminum or products containing iron or zinc within 4 hr before or 2 hr after dosing

---

* = non-FDA-approved use

loperamide

(loe-per'a-mide)

Rx: Imodium

OTC: Imodium A-D, Maalox Anti-Diarrheal Combinations

OTC: with simethicone (Imodium Advanced)

Chemical Class: Piperidine derivative

Therapeutic Class: Antidiarrheal

CLINICAL PHARMACOLOGY

Mechanism of Action: Direct action on intestinal muscles to decrease GI peristalsis

Pharmacokinetics

PO: 40% absorbed, onset 30-60 min, peak 5 hr (capsule) and 2½ hr (liquid); metabolized in liver; excreted in feces as unchanged drug, small amount in urine; $t_{1/2}$ 7-14 hr

INDICATIONS AND USES: Diarrhea (acute non-specific); chronic diarrhea (inflammatory bowel disease); reduction of volume from ileostomy; traveler's diarrhea

DOSAGE

Adult

• PO 4 mg, then 2 mg after each loose stool, max 16 mg/day; maintenance for chronic diarrhea usually 4-8 mg/day

Child

• <2 yr, use not recommended

• 13-20 kg PO 1 mg tid on day 1, then 0.1 mg/kg after each loose stool

• 20-30 kg PO 2 mg bid on day 1, then 0.1 mg/kg after each loose stool

• >30 kg PO 2 mg tid on day 1, then 0.1 mg/kg after each loose stool

⑤ AVAILABLE FORMS/COST OF THERAPY

• Cap, Gel—Oral: 2 mg, 100's: **$14.00-$87.35**

• Liq—Oral: 1 mg/5 ml, 60, 120 ml (OTC): **$1.87-$6.47**/120 ml

• Tab—Oral: 2 mg, 12's (OTC): **$1.50-$17.76**

CONTRAINDICATIONS: Acute diarrhea due to invasive organisms (enteroinvasive *E. coli, Salmonella, Shigella*) or pseudomembranous colitis

PRECAUTIONS: Liver disease, dehydration, severe ulcerative colitis (toxic megacolon), children (greater variability in response)

PREGNANCY AND LACTATION: Pregnancy category B; unknown if excreted in breast milk; compatible with breast feeding

SIDE EFFECTS/ADVERSE REACTIONS

CNS: Fatigue, fever, dizziness, drowsiness

GI: Abdominal pain, anorexia, *constipation, dry mouth, nausea,* **toxic megacolon,** vomiting

RESP: Respiratory depression

SKIN: Rash

SPECIAL CONSIDERATIONS
PATIENT/FAMILY EDUCATION

• Do not self-medicate diarrhea for >48 hr without consulting provider

lopinavir/ritonavir

(lop-in'a-veer/rit-on'a-veer)

Rx: Kaletra

Chemical Class: HIV protease inhibitor

Therapeutic Class: Antiviral

CLINICAL PHARMACOLOGY

Mechanism of Action: Lopinavir inhibits HIV protease, preventing cleavage of the Gag-Pol polyprotein, resulting in the production of immature, non-infectious viral particles; Kaletra is a co-formulation of lopinavir and ritonavir; as co-formulated in Kaletra, ritonavir inhibits the CYP3A-mediated metabolism of lopinavir, thereby providing increased plasma levels of lopinavir

Pharmacokinetics

PO: Peak 2-4 hr; absolute bioavailability unknown, AUC increased by 48% (capsule) and 80% (liquid) when taken with food; 98% protein bound; 100% metabolized by liver (almost exclusively by CYP3A, which is inhibited by ritonavir); excreted in stool as unchanged drug (20%), and metabolites (80%); $t_{1/2}$ 5-6 hr

INDICATIONS AND USES: HIV infection, as part of combination therapy

DOSAGE

Adult and child >12 yr

• PO 400/100 mg (3 capsules) bid with food

Child 6 mo - 12 yr

• PO 12/3 mg/kg (for those 7 to <15 kg) or 10/2.5 mg/kg (for those 15 to 40 kg) taken bid with food, up to a maximum dose of 400/100 mg bid

$ AVAILABLE FORMS/COST OF THERAPY

• Cap—Oral: 133.3 mg lopinavir with 33.3 mg ritonavir, 180's: **$703.50**

• Liquid—Oral: 400 mg lopinavir with 100 mg ritonavir/5 ml, 160 ml: **$351.75**

CONTRAINDICATIONS: Co-administration with drugs highly metabolized by CYP3A or CYP2D6, including antiarrhythmics: flecainide, propafenone; antihistamines: astemizole, terfenadine; ergot derivatives: dihydroergotamine, ergonovine, ergotamine, methylergonovine; GI motility agent: cisapride; neuroleptic: pimozide; sedative/hypnotics: midazolam, triazolam

PRECAUTIONS: Co-administration with drugs primarily metabolized by CYP3A or CYP2D6, diabetes, hepatic disease, hyperlipidemia

PREGNANCY AND LACTATION: Pregnancy category C; breast milk excretion unknown; the CDC recommends that HIV-infected mothers not breast-feed their infants to avoid risking postnatal transmission of HIV

SIDE EFFECTS/ADVERSE REACTIONS

CNS: Insomnia

GI: Abdominal pain (3%), *diarrhea* (14%), *nausea* (6%), vomiting

METAB: Hyperglycemia, hyperlipidemia

SKIN: Rash

INTERACTIONS

Drugs

❷ *Amiodarone:* Increased plasma levels of amiodarone

❸ *Amprenavir:* Increased plasma level of amprenavir; consider dose adjustment of amprenavir to 750 mg bid

⚠ *Astemizole:* Increased plasma levels of astemizole

❸ *Atorvastatin:* Increased plasma level of atorvastatin

❸ *Atovaquone:* Decreased level of atovaquone

❸ *Barbiturates:* Increased clearance of lopinavir/ritonavir; reduced clearance of barbiturates

❷ *Bepredil:* Increased plasma levels of bepredil

❷ *Carbamazepine:* Increased clearance of lopinavir/ritonavir; reduced clearance of carbamazepine

❸ *Cerivastatin:* Increased plasma level of cerivastatin

⚠ *Cisapride:* Increased plasma levels of cisapride

❷ *Clarithromycin:* Reduced clearance of lopinavir/ritonavir; lopinavir/ritonavir reduces clearance of clarithromycin; reduce clarithromycin dose for renal insufficiency if co-administered

🔳 *Cyclosporine:* Increased plasma level of cyclosporine

🔳 *Dexamethasone:* Decreased plasma level of lopinavir/ritonavir

🔳 *Didanosine (buffered formulation):* Reduces absorption of lopinavir/ritonavir, take didanosine 1 hr before or 2 hr after dose of lopinavir/ritonavir

🔳 *Dihydropyridine calcium channel blockers (amlodipine, felodipine, nifedipine, nicardipine):* Increased plasma level of these drugs

🔳 *Efavirenz:* Increased clearance of lopinavir/ritonavir, increase dose to 533/133 mg bid

❷ *Encainide:* Increased plasma levels of encainide

🔺 *Ergot alkaloids:* Increased plasma levels of ergot alkaloids

🔳 *Erythromycin:* Reduced clearance of lopinavir/ritonavir; lopinavir/ritonavir reduces clearance of erythromycin

🔺 *Flecainide:* Increased plasma levels of flecainide

🔺 *Flurazepam:* Increased plasma levels of flurazepam

🔳 *Indinavir:* Increased plasma level of indinavir; consider dose reduction to 600 mg bid

🔳 *Itraconazole:* Lopinavir/ritonavir reduces clearance of itraconazole; reduce itraconazole dose

🔳 *Ketoconazole:* Lopinavir/ritonavir reduces clearance of ketoconazole; reduce ketoconazole dose

❷ *Lidocaine:* Increased plasma levels of lidocaine

❷ *Lovastatin:* Lopinavir/ritonavir reduces clearance of lovastatin

❷ *Meperidine:* Increased plasma levels of meperidine

🔳 *Methadone:* Lopinavir/ritonavir reduces methadone plasma concentration by 50%

🔺 *Midazolam:* Increased plasma levels of midazolam and prolonged effect

🔳 *Nevirapine:* Increased clearance of lopinavir/ritonavir, increase dose to 533/133 mg bid

🔳 *Oral contraceptives:* Lopinavir/ritonavir may reduce efficacy

🔳 *Phenytoin:* Increased clearance of lopinavir/ritonavir; reduced clearance of phenytoin

🔺 *Pimozide:* Increased plasma levels of pimozide

🔺 *Propafenone:* Increased plasma levels of propafenone

❷ *Propoxyphene:* Increased plasma levels of propoxyphene

❷ *Quinidine:* Increased plasma levels of quinidine

🔳 *Rapamycin:* Increased plasma level of rapamycin

❷ *Rifabutin:* Increased clearance of lopinavir/ritonavir; reduced clearance of rifabutin; reduce rifabutin dose to 150 mg qod

❷ *Rifampin:* Increased clearance of lopinavir/ritonavir

🔳 *Saquinavir:* Decreased clearance of saquinavir; reduce dose of Fortovase (saquinavir soft gel capsule) to 800 mg bid

❷ *Sildenafil:* Increased plasma level of sildenafil, reduce dose to 25 mg q48h

❷ *Simvastatin:* Lopinavir/ritonavir reduces clearance of simvastatin

❷ *St. John's Wort (hypericum perforatum):* Increased clearance of lopinavir/ritonavir

🔳 *Tacrolimus:* Increased plasma level of tacrolimus

🔺 *Terfenadine:* Increased plasma levels of terfenadine

🔳 *Tenofovir:* Lopinavir/ritonavir increases tenofovir AUC by 34%; tenofovir decreases AUC of lopinavir/ritonavir by 24% (when co-administered with lopinavir/ritonavir, tenofovir should be administered 2 hours before or one hour after administration of lopinavir/ritonavir)

▲ *Triazolam:* Increased plasma levels of triazolam and prolonged effect

❸ *Troleandomycin:* Reduced clearance of lopinavir/ritonavir; lopinavir/ritonavir reduces clearance of troleandomycin

❸ *Warfarin:* May reduce warfarin effect

❷ *Zolpidem:* Increased plasma levels of zolpidem

SPECIAL CONSIDERATIONS
PATIENT/FAMILY EDUCATION
• Take with food to improve bioavailability
• Be aware of many potential drug interactions

MONITORING PARAMETERS
• Plasma glucose, lipid levels, hepatic function tests

---

loracarbef
(lor-a-kar´bef)
Rx: Lorabid
Chemical Class: Carbacephem derivative (structurally related to cephalosporins, 2nd generation)
Therapeutic Class: Antibiotic

CLINICAL PHARMACOLOGY
Mechanism of Action: Inhibits bacterial cell wall synthesis
Pharmacokinetics
PO: Well absorbed from GI tract, slower with food; peak 1 hr (cap), ½ hr (susp); 25% bound to plasma proteins; excreted in urine as unchanged drug; $t_{1/2}$ 1 hr

INDICATIONS AND USES: Infections of the upper and lower respiratory tract (including pharyngitis and tonsillitis); urinary tract (cystitis, pyelonephritis), skin infections; otitis media, sinusitis

Antibacterial spectrum usually includes:
• Gram-positive organisms: *Streptococcus pneumoniae, Str. pyogenes, Staphylococcus aureus, S. saprophyticus*
• Gram-negative organisms: *Haemophilus influenzae, E. coli, Proteus mirabilis, Klebsiella* spp., *Moraxella catarrhalis*

DOSAGE
Adult
• *UTI:* PO 200 mg q24h for 7 days
• *Pyelonephritis:* PO 400 mg q12h for 14 days
• *Upper and lower respiratory tract:* PO 200-400 mg q12h
• *Skin:* PO 200 mg q12h
Child 6 mo-12 yr
• *Acute otitis media, sinusitis:* PO 15 mg/kg/day divided q12h for 10 days
• *Pharyngitis, skin infections:* PO 7.5 mg/kg q12h
• *Renal function impairment:* CrCl ≥50 ml/min, use regular dose; CrCl 10-49 ml/min, use half regular dose at regular interval; CrCl <10 ml/min, use regular dose q3-5d; repeat after hemodialysis

💲 AVAILABLE FORMS/COST OF THERAPY
• Cap, Gel—Oral: 200 mg, 100's: **$453.15**; 400 mg, 100's: **$637.88**
• Susp—Oral: 100 mg/5 ml, 100 ml: **$37.44-$44.00**; 200 mg/5 ml, 100 ml: **$61.69-$71.85**

CONTRAINDICATIONS: Hypersensitivity to cephalosporins
PRECAUTIONS: Children <6 mo, renal disease, hypersensitivity to penicillins (10% cross reactivity)
PREGNANCY AND LACTATION: Pregnancy category B; unknown if excreted into breast milk

SIDE EFFECTS/ADVERSE REACTIONS

CNS: Chills, confusion, dizziness, fatigue, fever, headache, paresthesia
GI: Abdominal pain, anorexia, **bleeding,** colitis, diarrhea, dysgeusia, flatulence, glossitis, heartburn, increased LFTs, jaundice, nausea, stomach cramps, vomiting, diarrhea
GU: Candidiasis, **nephrotoxicity,** pruritus, pyuria, reversible interstitial nephritis, vaginitis
HEME: **Bone marrow suppression,** eosinophilia, **hemolytic anemia,** leukocytosis, lymphocytosis
RESP: Dyspnea
SKIN: Dermatitis, rash, urticaria

SPECIAL CONSIDERATIONS

• Essentially same spectrum and utility as cefaclor
• Take 1h before eating or 2h after eating

---

loratadine

(loer-at′ah-deen)
Rx: Claritin, Claritin Reditabs
Combinations
  Rx: with pseudoephedrine
  (Claritin-D)
Chemical Class: Piperidine derivative
Therapeutic Class: Antihistamine

CLINICAL PHARMACOLOGY

Mechanism of Action: Decreases allergic response by blocking histamine at H_1-receptors; provides antihistamine action without sedation

Pharmacokinetics
PO: Absorption limited by food, peak 1-2 hr metabolized in liver to active metabolite (descarboethoxyloratadine), excreted in urine and feces; elimination $t_{1/2}$ 8.4 hr

INDICATIONS AND USES: Seasonal allergic rhinitis; idiopathic chronic urticaria

DOSAGE

Adult
• PO 10 mg qd; give qod in hepatic impairment or renal insufficiency (CrCl <30 ml/min)

💲 AVAILABLE FORMS/COST OF THERAPY

• Syr—Oral: 5 mg/5 ml, 480 ml: **$122.40-$155.36**
• Tab, Uncoated—Oral: 10 mg, 100's: **$237.85-$277.83**
• Tab, Rapidly Disintegrating—Oral: 10 mg, 30's: **$246.65-$312.95**

PRECAUTIONS: Increased intraocular pressure, hepatic disease, renal insufficiency

PREGNANCY AND LACTATION: Pregnancy category B; excreted into breast milk at levels equivalent to serum levels

SIDE EFFECTS/ADVERSE REACTIONS

CNS: Insomnia, sedation (more common with increased doses)
GI: Dry mouth

INTERACTIONS

Drugs
3 *Itraconazole, ketoconazole, miconazole:* Increased loratadine levels but no increase in toxicity reported

SPECIAL CONSIDERATIONS

• Effective, but expensive nonsedating antihistamine; reserve for patients unable to tolerate sedating antihistamines like chlorpheniramine

L

---

italic = common side effects   ***bold italic*** = life-threatening reactions

lorazepam

(lor-a'ze-pam)
Rx: Ativan
Chemical Class: Benzodiazepine
Therapeutic Class: Anxiolytic; sedative/hypnotic; anticonvulsant
DEA Class: Schedule IV

CLINICAL PHARMACOLOGY

Mechanism of Action: CNS depressants via facilitation of inhibitory GABA at benzodiazepine receptor sites (BZ_1—associated with sleep; BZ_2— associated with memory, motor, sensory, and cognitive function); effects include muscle relaxation (spinal cord), anticonvulsant activity (brain stem), ataxia (cerebellum), emotional behavior (limbic and cortical areas), and anxiolytic effects (separate from general CNS depression); other effects include sedative, appetite-stimulating and weak analgesic actions

Pharmacokinetics
PO: Peak 1-6 hr, duration 3-6 hr
IM: Peak 60-90 min
Metabolized by liver to inactive metabolites; excreted by kidneys; crosses placenta, breast milk; $t_{1/2}$ 10-20 hr

INDICATIONS AND USES: Anxiety disorders, preoperative sedation (inj); insomnia,* acute alcohol withdrawal symptoms,* initial treatment of status epilepticus (inj), adjunct in endoscopic procedures,* chemotherapy-induced nausea and vomiting*

DOSAGE
Adult
• *Anxiety:* PO 2-6 mg/day in divided doses bid-tid; largest dose at hs; not to exceed 10 mg/day

• *Insomnia:* PO 2-4 mg hs; only minimally effective after 2 wk continuous therapy
• *Elderly:* 1-2 mg/day in divided doses
• *Preoperatively:* IM 0.05 mg/kg to max 4 mg given ≥2 hr before procedure; IV 0.044-0.05 mg/kg, max 4 mg, 15-20 min before procedure
Child
• Not recommended IM/IV <18 yr, PO <12 yr

💲 AVAILABLE FORMS/COST OF THERAPY
• Inj, Sol—IM, IV: 2 mg/ml, 0.5, 1, 2, 10 ml: **$1.03-$16.37**/1 ml; 4 mg/ml, 1, 2, 10 ml: **$1.04-$16.97**/1 ml
• Sol—Oral: 2 mg/ml, 30 ml: **$40.22**
• Tab, Uncoated—Oral: 0.5 mg, 100's: **$3.38-$86.95**; 1 mg, 100's: **$4.13-$113.24**; 2 mg, 100's: **$4.50-$165.08**

CONTRAINDICATIONS: Acute narrow-angle glaucoma, psychosis
PRECAUTIONS: Elderly, debilitated, hepatic disease, renal disease, suicidal patients, COPD, history of drug abuse

PREGNANCY AND LACTATION: Pregnancy category D (other benzodiazepines associated with cleft lip, cleft palate, microcephaly, pyloric stenosis); neonatal withdrawal, hypotonia; excreted into breast milk in low quantities; effect on infant unknown

SIDE EFFECTS/ADVERSE REACTIONS

CNS: Anxiety, confusion, depression, *dizziness, drowsiness,* fatigue, hallucinations, headache, insomnia, stimulation, tremors, unsteadiness
CV: ECG changes, *orthostatic hypotension,* tachycardia
EENT: Blurred vision, mydriasis, tinnitus
GI: Anorexia, constipation, diarrhea, dry mouth, nausea, vomiting

* = non-FDA-approved use

SKIN: Dermatitis, itching, rash
INTERACTIONS
Drugs
3 *Ethanol:* Increased adverse psychomotor effects of lorazepam
2 *Fluconazole:* Potential for increased lorazepam concentrations
3 *Itraconazole:* Potential for increased lorazepam concentrations
SPECIAL CONSIDERATIONS
• A good choice for elderly or patients with liver dysfunction who need benzodiazepines due to phase II metabolism to inactive metabolites (less likely to accumulate)
PATIENT/FAMILY EDUCATION
• Do not discontinue abruptly after long-term use, withdrawal syndrome (seizures, anxiety, insomnia, nausea, vomiting, flu-like illness, confusion, hallucinations, memory impairment) can occur

---

losartan
(lo-sar'tan)
Rx: Cozaar
Combinations
  Rx: with hydrochlorothiazide
  (Hyzaar)
Chemical Class: Angiotension II receptor antagonist
Therapeutic Class: Antihypertensive

CLINICAL PHARMACOLOGY
Mechanism of Action: Antihypertensive (inhibition of vasoconstriction and aldosterone secretion), smooth muscle hypoproliferative, and cardioprotective effects are attributable to selective blockade of angiotensin II (AT1) receptors found throughout the cardiovascular and renal systems; effects independent of angiotensin II synthesis

Pharmacokinetics
PO: Peak, 1-1.5 hrs; peak response, 6 hrs PO bioavailability, 25-35%, <10% food effect; 98+% protein bound (parent and active metabolite), extensively metabolized by liver (CYP2C9, 3A4) to active metabolite, minimal excretion via urine (13%); elimination $t_{1/2}$, 1.5-2 hrs (metabolite, 4-9 hrs)
INDICATIONS AND USES: Hypertension, CHF (left ventricular dysfunction),* myocardial infarction,* diabetic nephropathy*
DOSAGE
Adult >18 yr
• PO 25-50 mg qd; range 25-100 mg qd; divide bid if effect at trough inadequate
• *Hepatic impairment:* PO 25 mg qd initially
§ **AVAILABLE FORMS/COST OF THERAPY**
Cozaar
• Tab, Uncoated—Oral: 25, 50 mg; 100's: **$143.03**; 100 mg, 100's: **$194.81**
Hyzaar
• Tab, Uncoated—Oral: 12.5-50 mg, 100's: **$143.03**; 25-100 mg, 100's: **$194.81**
PRECAUTIONS: Angioedema (associated with aspirin and/or penicillin allergy), aortic or mitral valve stenosis, biliary cirrhosis or biliary obstruction, breast feeding period, coronary artery disease, elderly patients, hepatic dysfunction (adjust dose), hypertrophic cardiomyopathy, hypotension (sodium or volume depleted patients), pregnancy, renal artery stenosis, solitary kidney, or congestive heart failure
PREGNANCY AND LACTATION: Pregnancy category C, first trimester—Category D, second and third trimesters; drugs acting directly on the renin-angiotensin-aldosterone system are documented to cause fe-

---

italic = common side effects   ***bold italic*** = life-threatening reactions

tal harm (hypotension, oligohydramnios, neonatal anemia, hyperkalemia, neonatal skull hypoplasia, anuria, and renal failure; neonatal limb contractures, craniofacial deformities, and hypoplastic lung development)

SIDE EFFECTS/ADVERSE REACTIONS

CNS: Dizziness, insomnia

CV: Orthostatic effects, syncope

EENT: Nasal congestion, sinus disorder

GI: Diarrhea, dyspepsia, elevated liver enzymes

GU: Increased BUN, creatinine

HEME: Decreased hct, purpura

METAB: Hyperkalemia

MS: Back pain, leg pain, muscle cramps, myalgia

RESP: Cough

MISC: Angioedema

INTERACTIONS

Drugs

3 *Fluconazole:* Decreased conversion to active metabolite (CYP2C9 inhibition), loss of antihypertensive effects

2 *Lithium:* Increased renal lithium reabsorption at the proximal tubular site due to the natriuresis associated with the inhibition of aldosterone secretion; increased risk of lithium toxicity

3 *Rifampin:* Induced metabolism of losartan and metabolite, resulting in a decrease in the area under the concentration-time curve (AUC) and half-life of both compounds and reduced losartan efficacy

SPECIAL CONSIDERATIONS

• Potentially as or more effective than angiotensin-converting enzyme inhibitors, without cough; no evidence for reduction in morbidity and mortality as first line agents in hypertension, yet; whether they provide the same cardiac and renal pro-

tection also still tentative; like ACE inhibitors, less effective in black patients

PATIENT/FAMILY EDUCATION

• Call your clinician immediately if note following side effects: wheezing; lip, throat or face swelling; hives or rash

MONITORING PARAMETERS

• Baseline electrolytes, urinalysis, blood urea nitrogen and creatinine with recheck at 2-4 weeks after initiation (sooner in volume depleted patients); monitor sitting blood pressure; watch for symptomatic hypotension, particularly in volume-depleted patients

---

lovastatin

(lo´va-sta-tin)

Rx: Mevacor

Combinations

  Rx: With niacin extended release (Advicor)

Chemical Class: Substituted hexahydronaphthlene

Therapeutic Class: Antilipemic (HMG-CoA reductase inhibitor); "statin"

CLINICAL PHARMACOLOGY

Mechanism of Action: Competitively inhibits 3-hydroxy-3-methylglutaryl-coenzyme A (HMG-CoA) reductase, an early rate-limiting step in cholesterol biosynthesis; increases HDL cholesterol mildly [2%-10%], significantly decreases total and LDL cholesterol [16%-29%, 21%-40% respectively], minimal lowering effect on triglycerides [6%-10%]

Pharmacokinetics

PO: Peak 2-4 hr; metabolized in liver (metabolites); highly protein bound (>95%); excreted in urine (10%), feces (83%); crosses placenta; excreted in breast milk; max effect on lipid levels in 4-6 wk

INDICATIONS AND USES: Primary hypercholesterolemia (heterozygous familial and nonfamilial hypercholesterolemia), mixed dyslipidemia (Fredrickson types IIa and IIb), and secondary prevention of cardiovascular events

DOSAGE

Adult

• PO 10-20 mg qd with evening meal; may increase to 20-80 mg/day in single or divided doses, not to exceed 80 mg/d; dosage adjustments should be made qmo; for cholesterol levels >300 mg/dl initiate at 40 mg/day

$ AVAILABLE FORMS/COST OF THERAPY

• Tab, Uncoated—Oral: 10 mg, 60's: **$80.64-$89.70**; 20 mg, 60's: **$137.41-$158.19**; 40 mg, 60's: **$242.98-$284.76**

CONTRAINDICATIONS: Active liver disease

PRECAUTIONS: Past liver disease, alcoholics, severe acute infections, trauma, hypotension, uncontrolled seizure disorders, severe metabolic disorders, electrolyte imbalances

PREGNANCY AND LACTATION: Pregnancy category X (may produce skeletal malformations); not recommended in nursing mothers

SIDE EFFECTS/ADVERSE REACTIONS

CNS: Dizziness, headache, insomnia
EENT: Blurred vision, dysgeusia, lens opacities
GI: Abdominal pain, constipation, diarrhea, dyspepsia, flatus, heartburn, hepatotoxicity, increased transaminases, nausea
MS: Muscle cramps, myalgia, myositis, ***rhabdomyolysis***
SKIN: Pruritus, rash

INTERACTIONS

Drugs

❸ *Cholestyramine, colestipol:* Decreased bioavailability of lovastatin possible, effect likely overcome by additive lipid-lowering effects of concurrent therapy

❸ *Clarithromycin, cyclosporine, danazol, erythromycin, niacin:* Severe myopathy or rhabdomyolysis

❷ *Clofibrate, gemfibrozil, nefazodone:* Severe myopathy or rhabdomyolysis with combination, especially at high doses

❸ *Cyclosporine:* Concomitant administration increases risk of severe myopathy or rhabdomyolysis

❷ *Fluconazole, itraconazole:* Large increases in lovastatin concentration, myopathy or rhabdomyolysis possible

❸ *Isradipine:* Reduction in lovastatin concentration

❸ *Niacin:* Concomitant administration increases risk of severe myopathy or rhabdomyolysis

❸ *Pectin:* Reduced cholesterol-lowering effect of lovastatin

❸ *Warfarin:* Increased prothrombin times and bleeding reported with concomitant use

SPECIAL CONSIDERATIONS

• Less effective in homozygous familial hypercholesterolemia (lack of functional LDL receptors); these patients also more likely to have adverse reaction of elevated transaminases

• Statin selection based on lipid-lowering prowess, cost, and availability

PATIENT/FAMILY EDUCATION

• Report symptoms of myalgia, muscle tenderness, or weakness

• Take daily doses in the evening for increased effect

MONITORING PARAMETERS

• Cholesterol (max therapeutic response 4-6 wk)

italic = common side effects   ***bold italic*** = life-threatening reactions

• LFTs (AST, ALT) at baseline and at 12 wk of therapy; if no change, no further monitoring necessary (discontinue if elevations persist >3 × upper limit of normal)

• CPK in patients complaining of diffuse myalgia, muscle tenderness, or weakness

loxapine
(lox'a-peen)
Rx: Loxitane
Chemical Class: Dibenzox-azepine derivative
Therapeutic Class: Antipsy-chotic

CLINICAL PHARMACOLOGY
Mechanism of Action: Dopamine receptor antagonist, with higher affinity for D_2- over D_1-receptors, and variable selectivity among the cortical dopamine tracts; also activity on nondopaminergic sites, i.e., cholinergic, alpha$_1$-adrenergic and histaminic receptors (explaining side effects); moderate risk extrapyramidal reactions; minimal sedation, orthostatic hypotension and anticholinergic effects
Pharmacokinetics
PO: Onset 20-30 min, peak 1-2 hr, duration 12 hr
IM: Onset 15-30 min, peak 5 hr, duration 12 hr
Metabolized by liver to active and inactive metabolites, excreted in urine (30%-40%) and feces (50%); crosses placenta; enters breast milk; terminal $t_{1/2}$ 19 hr
INDICATIONS AND USES: Psychotic disorders
DOSAGE
NOTE: 15 mg equivalent to chlorpromazine 100 mg

Adult and child>16yr
• PO 10 mg bid-qid initially, may be rapidly increased depending on severity of condition, range 60-100 mg/day divided bid-qid, reduce to maintenance 20-60 mg/day in divided doses; IM 12.5-50 mg q4-6 hr until desired response, then start PO form

⑤ AVAILABLE FORMS/COST OF THERAPY
• Cap, Gel—Oral: 5 mg, 100's: **$47.25-$113.93**; 10 mg, 100's: **$69.45-$147.21**; 25 mg, 100's: **$108.68-$222.43**; 50 mg, 100's: **$139.95-$296.78**
• Inj, Sol—IM: 50 mg/ml, 10 ml: **$116.58-$128.24**
• Liq—Oral: 25 mg/ml, 120 ml: **$270.86-$297.95**
CONTRAINDICATIONS: Coma, severe drug-induced depressed states
PRECAUTIONS: Seizure disorders, hepatic disease, cardiac disease, prostatic hypertrophy, child <16 yr, glaucoma, COPD
PREGNANCY AND LACTATION: Pregnancy category C; no data in lactating women
SIDE EFFECTS/ADVERSE REACTIONS

CNS: Akathisia, confusion, *drowsiness,* dystonia, headache, pseudo-parkinsonism, *seizures,* tardive dyskinesia

CV: Cardiac arrest, ECG changes, hypertension, *orthostatic hypotension,* tachycardia

EENT: Blurred vision, glaucoma

GI: Anorexia, *constipation,* diarrhea, *dry mouth,* jaundice, nausea, vomiting, weight gain

GU: Amenorrhea, enuresis, gynecomastia, impotence, urinary frequency, urinary retention

HEME: Agranulocytosis, anemia, leukocytosis, *leukopenia, thrombocytopenia*

---

* = non-FDA-approved use

RESP: Dyspnea, laryngospasm, *respiratory depression*

SKIN: Dermatitis, photosensitivity, rash

INTERACTIONS

Drugs

3 *Anticholinergics:* Decreased neuroleptic effect

3 *Bromocriptine:* Decreased lowering of prolactin by bromocriptine in patients with pituitary adenoma

3 *Lithium:* Increased neurotoxicity

3 *Lorazepam:* Isolated cases of respiratory depression, stupor and hypotension have been observed

---

mafenide

(ma'fe-nide)

Rx: Sulfamylon

Chemical Class: Sulfonamide derivative

Therapeutic Class: Topical antibiotic

CLINICAL PHARMACOLOGY

Mechanism of Action: Reduces bacterial population present in avascular tissue of 2nd and 3rd degree burns; permits spontaneous healing of deep partial-thickness burns; inhibits carbonic anhydrase

Pharmacokinetics

TOP: Absorbed through devascularized areas, peak concentration 24 hr after initial dose; rapidly metabolized to inactive metabolite, excreted in urine

INDICATIONS AND USES: Adjunctive treatment in burns (2nd, 3rd degree); bacteriostatic against many Gram-positive and Gram-negative organisms, including *Pseudomonas* and some anaerobes

DOSAGE

Adult and Child >2 mo

• TOP apply thin layer ($\frac{1}{16}$ in) to clean and debrided affected area qd-bid, reapply if washed off

[§] AVAILABLE FORMS/COST OF THERAPY

• Cre—Top: 85 mg/g, 60, 120, 454 g: **$23.60**/60 g

• Pow—Top: 50 g/packet: **$122.50**

PRECAUTIONS: Impaired pulmonary function, impaired renal function, G-6-PD deficiency, blood dyscrasias, inhalation injury

PREGNANCY AND LACTATION: Pregnancy category C; compatible with breast feeding except in G-6-PD deficiency and ill, jaundiced, or premature infants

SIDE EFFECTS/ADVERSE REACTIONS

HEME: **Bone marrow suppression,** eosinophilia, **fatal hemolytic anemia**

METAB: Metabolic acidosis

RESP: Tachypnea

SKIN: Bleeding, blisters, *burning,* erythema, excoriation of new skin, facial edema, hives, pruritus, rash, *stinging,* superinfections, urticaria

INTERACTIONS

Labs

• *False increase:* Urine amino acids

M

---

magaldrate

(mag'al-drate)
OTC: Riopan
Combinations
   OTC: with simethicone (Riopan Plus)
Chemical Class: Mixture of aluminum and magnesium hydroxide and sulfate
Therapeutic Class: Antacid

CLINICAL PHARMACOLOGY
Mechanism of Action: Neutralizes gastric acidity
Pharmacokinetics
PO: Duration 20-60 min (fasting), 1-3 hr (if given 1 hr after meals)
INDICATIONS AND USES: Hyperacidity; peptic ulcer disease,* GERD,* prevention of stress ulcer bleeding*
DOSAGE
Adult and Child
• *Peptic ulcer disease:* 5-10 ml 1 and 3 hr after meals and at hs for 4-6 wk
• *Gastroesophageal reflux:* 5-10 ml q30-60 min for severe symptoms, or as for peptic ulcer disease
• *GI bleeding:* Administer q hr to keep nasogastric aspirate pH >3.5
• *Before anesthesia:* 5-10 ml 30 min before anesthesia
§ AVAILABLE FORMS/COST OF THERAPY
• Liq/Susp—Oral: 540 mg/5 ml, 360 ml: **$2.27-$5.49**
PRECAUTIONS: Elderly, fluid restriction, decreased GI motility, GI obstruction, dehydration, renal disease, Na-restricted diets, CHF, edema, cirrhosis
PREGNANCY AND LACTATION: Pregnancy category C
SIDE EFFECTS/ADVERSE REACTIONS
GI: Constipation, diarrhea
METAB: Hypermagnesemia

INTERACTIONS
Drugs
3 *Allopurinol, cefpodoxime, ciprofloxacin, isoniazid, ketoconazole, quinolones, tetracyclines, digoxin, iron salts, indomethacin:* Decreased GI absorption of these drugs
3 *Pseudoephedrine, enteric coated aspirin, diazepam:* Increased GI absorption of these drugs
3 *Quinidine:* Increased quinidine levels
3 *Salicylates:* Increased urinary excretion of salicylates

magnesium

OTC: *Magnesium oxide:* Mag-Ox 400, Maox, Uro-Mag
OTC: *Magnesium hydroxide:* Milk of Magnesia, Phillips' Chewable
OTC: *Magnesium citrate:* Evac-Q-Mag, Citro-Nesia, Citroma
OTC: *Magnesium sulfate:* Epsom Salts
OTC: *Magnesium gluconate:* Almora, Magonate, Magtrate
OTC: *Magnesium chloride:* Slow-Mag
Chemical Class: Divalent cation
Therapeutic Class: Antacid; laxative; antiarrhythmic, uterine relaxant, electrolyte supplement

CLINICAL PHARMACOLOGY
Mechanism of Action: Antacid products: neutralize gastric acidity magnesium citrate: causes osmotic retention of fluid in GI tract, increases peristalsis

* = non-FDA-approved use

Magnesium sulfate: decreases acetylcholine release at neuromuscular junction; slows rate of SA node impulse formation, prolongs conduction time

Pharmacokinetics

Magnesium citrate: renal excretion

Magnesium hydroxide/oxide: onset of laxative action 4-8 hr; renal excretion (30%), unabsorbed drug excreted in feces

Magnesium sulfate: PO onset of laxative action 1-2 hr; IM onset 1 hr, duration 3-4 hr; IV onset immediate, duration 30 min; excreted by kidneys and in stool

Magnesium gluconate: PO 15%-30% absorbed; renal excretion

INDICATIONS AND USES: Magnesium citrate: bowel evacuation prior to procedures

Magnesium oxide/hydroxide/sulfate (PO): laxative

Magnesium hydroxide/oxide: antacid; hypomagnesemia (oxide)

Magnesium gluconate: hypomagnesemia

Magnesium sulfate (parenteral): hypomagnesemia, eclampsia prophylaxis, preterm labor,* cardiac dysrhythmias,* acute MI,* acute exacerbations of asthma*

DOSAGE

Adult

• Magnesium citrate: PO ½-1 full bottle

• Magnesium hydroxide: PO 30-60 ml qd (laxative); 5-15 ml or 622-1244 mg (tabs) up to qid (antacid)

• Magnesium oxide: PO 2-4 g hs with water (laxative); 140 mg (caps) tid-qid or 400-840 mg/day (tabs) (antacid)

• Magnesium gluconate: PO 1-2 tabs bid-tid

• Magnesium sulfate: IM 4-5 g of 50% Sol q4h prn; IV 4 g of a 10%-20% Sol initially then 4-5 g in 250 ml of D₅W or NS at a rate not exceeding 3 ml/min by infusion (preeclampsia); IM/IV 1 g q6h for 4 doses; for severe deficiency, 8-12 g/day in divided doses (hypomagnesemia); PO 10-15 g in a glass of water (laxative)

Child

• Magnesium citrate: PO (<6 yr) 0.5 ml/kg to max 200 ml repeated q 4-6 hr until clear; (6-12 yr) ⅓-½ bottle

• Magnesium hydroxide: Laxative PO (<2 yr) 0.5 ml/kg/dose, (2-5 yr) 5-15 ml/day or divided, (6-12 yr) 15-30 ml/day or divided; antacid PO 2.5-5 ml qd-qid as needed

• Magnesium gluconate: PO 3-6 mg/kg/d divided tid-qid, max 400 mg/day

• Magnesium sulfate: Neonate IV 25-50 mg/kg/dose q 8-12 hr for 2-3 doses; Child IM/IV 25-50 mg/kg/dose q 4-6 hr for 3-4 doses, max single dose 2000 mg (hypomagnesemia); PO 5-10 g in a glass of water (laxative)

$ AVAILABLE FORMS/COST OF THERAPY

Magnesium Citrate

• Liq—Oral: 8.85%, 300 ml: **$0.81-$4.86**

Magnesium Chloride

• Inj, Sol—IV: 200 mg/ml, 50 ml: **$3.20-$12.50**

Magnesium Gluconate

• Tab—Oral: 500 mg, 100's: **$2.51-$29.10**

Magnesium Hydroxide

• Liq—Oral: 16%, 240 ml: **$4.34**; 16%, 480 ml: **$1.20-$4.56**

• Tab—Oral: 100's: **$8.00**

• Tab, Chewable—Oral: 325 mg, 100's: **$4.34-$4.56**

Magnesium Oxide

• Tab—Oral: 250 mg, 100's: **$1.50-$3.09**; 400 mg, 100's: **$8.53-$9.99**

Magnesium Sulfate

• Inj, Conc-Sol—IV; IM: 500 mg/ml, 10 ml: **$0.79-$14.72**

---

italic = common side effects   ***bold italic*** = life-threatening reactions

• Inj, Sol—IV: 2 meq/ml, 150 ml: **$11.15**
• Inj, Sol—IV; IM: 100 mg/ml, 20 ml: **$1.24-$5.75**
• Sol—IV: 1%, 100 ml: **$3.19**; 2%, 500 ml: **$3.60**; 4%, 100 ml: **$7.15**; 8%, 50 ml: **$7.15**

CONTRAINDICATIONS: Renal failure (Mg toxicity), hypermagnesemia; do not use cathartics in patients with appendicitis, impaction, intestinal obstruction, or perforation; do not use parenterally in patients with heart block, myocardial damage

PRECAUTIONS: Diarrhea, digitalized patients, impaired renal function (monitor Mg levels)

PREGNANCY AND LACTATION: Pregnancy category B; compatible with breast feeding

SIDE EFFECTS/ADVERSE REACTIONS

CNS: **Coma,** *depressed deep tendon reflexes, depression, lethargy, weakness*

CV: Decreased BP, **heart block,** *increased pulse*

GI: Belching, cramps, (PO) diarrhea, flatulence, impaction, nausea, obstruction, pain, vomiting

METAB: Hypermagnesemia

RESP: **Respiratory depression**

INTERACTIONS

Drugs

🛛 *Allopurinol, cefpodoxime, ciprofloxacin, atenolol, tetracyclines, iron salts, isoniazid, ketoconazole, lomefloxacin, norfloxacin, ofloxacin, pefloxacin, penicillamine, trovafloxacin:* Decreased PO effectiveness of these drugs with PO magnesium products

🛛 *Aspirin:* Decreased salicylate concentrations due to alkinization of urine with oral magnesium hydroxide

🛛 *Glipizide, glyburide:* Increased absorption of these drugs with oral magnesium hydroxide

🛛 *Nifedipine:* Decreased effect of nifedipine with parenteral magnesium sulfate

🛛 *Quinidine:* Increased quinidine concentrations with oral magnesium products

🛛 *Sodium polystyrene sulfonate:* Systemic alkalosis with oral magnesium products

🛛 *Succinylcholine:* Increased toxicity of these drugs with parenteral magnesium sulfate

Labs

• *False increase:* Serum alkaline phosphatase

SPECIAL CONSIDERATIONS
MONITORING PARAMETERS

• Parenteral magnesium: knee jerk reflexes prior to each dose (do not administer if absent), respiration rate (do not administer if <16/min), urine output (do not administer if <100 ml during 4 hr preceding each dose), serum magnesium concentrations (normal 1.5-3 mEq/L; therapeutic concentrations for preeclampsia, eclampsia, convulsions 4-7 mEq/L)

---

magnesium salicylate
Rx: Mobidin
OTC: Doan's pills
Chemical Class: Salicylic acid derivative
Therapeutic Class: Nonnarcotic analgesic; NSAID

CLINICAL PHARMACOLOGY
Mechanism of Action: Inhibits prostaglandin synthesis; analgesic, antiinflammatory, antipyretic actions

Pharmacokinetics

PO: Onset 15-30 min, peak 1-2 hr, duration 4-6 hr; 50%-90% bound to plasma proteins; metabolized in liver, eliminated in urine; $t_{1/2}$ 2 hr

INDICATIONS AND USES: Mild to moderate pain, rheumatoid arthritis, osteoarthritis, related rheumatic disorders

DOSAGE

Adult

• PO 650 mg q4h or 1090 mg tid, may increase to 3.6-4.8 g/day in 3-4 divided doses

$ AVAILABLE FORMS/COST OF THERAPY

• Tab, Uncoated—Oral: 325 mg, 24's (OTC): **$3.84-$4.39**; 500 mg, 100's: **$25.00-$96.85**; 545 mg, 100's: **$56.86**; 600 mg, 100's: **$23.22**; 750 mg, 100's: **$30.00-$120.23**; 1000 mg, 100's: **$38.00-$155.02**

CONTRAINDICATIONS: Hypersensitivity to NSAIDs, hemophilia, bleeding ulcers, hemorrhagic states, advanced chronic renal insufficiency

PRECAUTIONS: Children; teenagers with chickenpox or influenza (association with Reye's syndrome); impaired hepatic function, history of peptic ulcer disease, diabetes mellitus, gout

PREGNANCY AND LACTATION: Pregnancy category C; excreted into breast milk; use caution in nursing mothers due to potential adverse effects in nursing infant

SIDE EFFECTS/ADVERSE REACTIONS

CNS: Confusion, dizziness, drowsiness, headache

EENT: Dimness of vision, reversible hearing loss, tinnitus

GI: Anorexia, diarrhea, *dyspepsia,* epigastric discomfort, *GI bleeding,* heartburn, hepatotoxicity, *nausea*

HEME: Decreased plasma iron concentration, *leukopenia,* prolonged bleeding time, shortened erythrocyte survival time, *thrombocytopenia*

METAB: Hypermagnesemia, hypoglycemia, hypokalemia, hyponatremia

RESP: Hyperpnea, wheezing

SKIN: Angioedema, bruising, hives, rash, urticaria

MISC: Fever, thirst

INTERACTIONS

Labs

• *False increase:* Serum bicarbonate, CSF protein, serum theophylline

• *False decrease:* Urine cocaine, urine estrogen, serum glucose, urine 17-hydroxycorticosteroids, urine opiates

• *False positive:* Urine ferric chloride test

SPECIAL CONSIDERATIONS

• Consider for patients with GI intolerance to aspirin or patients in whom interference with normal platelet function by aspirin or other NSAIDs is undesirable

MONITORING PARAMETERS

• AST, ALT, bilirubin, creatinine, CBC, hct if patient is on long-term therapy

M

---

mannitol

(man´i-tall)

Rx: Osmitrol, Resectisol
Chemical Class: Hexahydric alcohol
Therapeutic Class: Osmotic diuretic; genitourinary irrigant; antiglaucoma agent

---

CLINICAL PHARMACOLOGY

Mechanism of Action: Induces diuresis by elevating the osmolarity of the glomerular filtrate, thereby hindering the tubular reabsorption of water; excretion of sodium and chloride is increased

Pharmacokinetics

IV: Onset 30-60 min, peak 1 hr, duration 6-8 hr; mainly excreted unchanged in the urine; $t_{1/2}$ 15-100 min

INDICATIONS AND USES: Reduction of intracranial pressure associated with cerebral edema; reduction of intraocular pressure; improvement of renal function in oliguric phase of acute renal failure; irrigation in transurethral prostatic resection or other transurethral surgical procedures (2.5% only); promotion of urinary excretion of toxic substances

DOSAGE

Adult

• *Oliguria (prevention):* IV 50-100 g of 5%-25% sol

• *Oliguria (treatment):* IV 50-100 g of 15%-20% sol

• *Intraocular pressure, intracranial pressure:* IV 1.5-2 g/kg of 15%-25% sol over 30-60 min

• *Diuresis in drug intoxication:* IV 5%-10% sol continuously up to 200 g while maintaining urine output of 100-500 ml/hr

• *Urologic irrigation:* Add contents of two 50 ml vials of 25% mannitol to 900 ml sterile water for inj and use as irrigation

Child

• IV 0.5-1 g/kg initially, then 0.25-0.5 g/kg q4-6hr for maintenance

$ AVAILABLE FORMS/COST OF THERAPY

• Inj, Sol—IV: 5%, 1000 ml: **$6.47-$54.09**; 10%, 1000 ml: **$6.47-$76.99**; 15%, 500 ml: **$3.20-$69.95**; 20%, 500 ml: **$18.28-$58.40**; 25%, 50 ml: **$1.85-$5.50**

CONTRAINDICATIONS: Active intracranial bleeding, anuria, severe pulmonary congestion or edema, severe dehydration

PRECAUTIONS: Fluid and electrolyte imbalances, renal function impairment (consider use of 0.2 g/kg test dose followed by monitoring for increased urine flow), hepatic function impairment

PREGNANCY AND LACTATION: Pregnancy category C

SIDE EFFECTS/ADVERSE REACTIONS

CNS: Confusion, dizziness, headache, rebound increased intracranial pressure, *seizures*

CV: Angina-like chest pains, **CHF,** edema, hypertension, hypotension, tachycardia, thrombophlebitis

EENT: Blurred vision, loss of hearing, nasal congestion

GI: Diarrhea, dry mouth, *nausea, vomiting*

GU: Osmotic nephrosis, urinary retention

METAB: Acidosis, dehydration, electrolyte loss, fluid and electrolyte imbalances

SKIN: Skin necrosis, urticaria

MISC: Chills, fever

INTERACTIONS

Labs

• *False increase:* Serum osmolality, serum phosphate, CSF protein

• *False decrease:* Serum phosphate

SPECIAL CONSIDERATIONS

MONITORING PARAMETERS

• Serum electrolytes, urine output

---

* = non-FDA-approved use

maprotiline

(ma-proe'ti-leen)
Rx: Ludiomil
Chemical Class: Dibenzo-bicy-clo-octadiene derivative
Therapeutic Class: Tetracyclic antidepressant

CLINICAL PHARMACOLOGY

Mechanism of Action: Blocks reuptake of norepinephrine presynaptically, prolonging neuronal activity; moderate-anticholinergic and sedative; slight orthostatic hypotensive activity

Pharmacokinetics

PO: Peak 9-16 hr, onset of therapeutic effect 2-3 wk; 88% bound to plasma proteins; metabolized in the liver, excreted in bile (30%) and urine (65%); $t_{1/2}$ 27-58 hr (active metabolite 60-90 hr)

INDICATIONS AND USES: Major depression, dysthymic disorder, anxiety associated with depression, depressive phase of bipolar disorder

DOSAGE

Adult

• PO 75 mg/day initially, increase by 25 mg q2 wk up to 150-225 mg/day divided qd-tid; elderly may require smaller doses

💲 AVAILABLE FORMS/COST OF THERAPY

• Tab, Coated—Oral: 25 mg, 100's: **$27.95-$62.29**; 50 mg, 100's: **$39.49-$92.22**; 75 mg, 100's: **$54.75-$131.84**

CONTRAINDICATIONS: Acute recovery phase of MI, concurrent use of MAOIs, seizure disorder

PRECAUTIONS: Suicidal patients, prostatic hypertrophy, psychiatric disease, severe depression, increased intraocular pressure, narrow-angle glaucoma, urinary retention, cardiac disease; hepatic/renal disease; hyperthyroidism, electroshock therapy, elective surgery, elderly, abrupt discontinuation

PREGNANCY AND LACTATION: Pregnancy category B; excreted into breast milk, milk; plasma ratios of 1.5 and 1.3 have been reported, significance to the nursing infant unknown

SIDE EFFECTS/ADVERSE REACTIONS

CNS: Anxiety, confusion (especially in elderly), *dizziness, drowsiness,* EPS (elderly), fatigue, headache, increased psychiatric symptoms, insomnia, memory impairment, nervousness, nightmares, panic, *seizures* (dose related), stimulation, tremors, weakness

CV: ***Dysrhythmias,*** hypertension, *orthostatic hypotension,* palpitations, syncope, tachycardia

EENT: Blurred vision, increased intraocular pressure, mydriasis, nasal congestion, ophthalmoplegia, tinnitus

GI: Constipation, cramps, diarrhea, *dry mouth,* epigastric distress, hepatitis, increased appetite, jaundice, nausea, ***paralytic ileus,*** stomatitis, vomiting

GU: Urinary retention

HEME: ***Agranulocytosis,*** eosinophilia, ***leukopenia, thrombocytopenia***

SKIN: Photosensitivity, pruritus, rash, sweating, urticaria

INTERACTIONS

Drugs

3 *Barbiturates:* Reduced serum concentrations of cyclic antidepressants

2 *Bethanidine:* Reduced antihypertensive effect of bethanidine

3 *Carbamazepine:* Reduced cyclic antidepressant serum concentrations

3 *Cimetidine:* Increased maprotiline concentrations

---

italic = common side effects   ***bold italic*** = life-threatening reactions

❷ *Clonidine:* Reduced antihypertensive response to clonidine; enhanced hypertensive response with abrupt clonidine withdrawal

❸ *Debrisoquin:* Inhibited antihypertensive response of debrisoquin

❷ *Epinephrine:* Markedly enhanced pressor response to IV epinephrine

❸ *Ethanol:* Additive impairment of motor skills; abstinent alcoholics may eliminate cyclic antidepressants more rapidly than non-alcoholics

❸ *Fluoxetine, fluvoxamine, grapefruit juice:* Marked increases in cyclic antidepressant plasma concentrations

❸ *Guanethidine:* Inhibited antihypertensive response to guanethidine

❷ *Moclobemide:* Potential association with fatal or non-fatal serotonin syndrome

⚠ *MAOIs:* Excessive sympathetic response, mania, or hyperpyrexia possible

❸ *Neuroleptics:* Increased therapeutic and toxic effects of both drugs

❷ *Norepinephrine:* Markedly enhanced pressor response to norepinephrine

❷ *Phenylephrine:* Enhanced pressor response to IV phenylephrine

❸ *Propantheline:* Excessive anticholinergic effects

❸ *Propoxyphene:* Enhanced effect of cyclic antidepressants

❸ *Quinidine:* Increased cyclic antidepressant serum concentrations

❸ *Tolazemide:* Enhanced hypoglycemic effects of tolazemide

Labs
• *False negative:* Serum tricyclic antidepressants screen

SPECIAL CONSIDERATIONS
• Not first-line agent due to risk of seizures

PATIENT/FAMILY EDUCATION
• Use caution in driving or other activities requiring alertness
• Do not discontinue abruptly after long-term use

MONITORING PARAMETERS
• CBC
• Weight
• Mental status: mood, sensorium, affect, suicidal tendencies
• Determination of maprotiline plasma concentrations is not routinely recommended, but may be useful in identifying toxicity, drug interactions, or noncompliance (adjustments in dosage should be made according to clinical response not plasma concentrations); therapeutic plasma levels 200-300 ng/ml (including active metabolite)

---

mazindol
(may´zin-dole)
Rx: Mazanor, Sanorex
Chemical Class: Imadazoline derivative
Therapeutic Class: Anorexiant
DEA Class: Schedule IV

CLINICAL PHARMACOLOGY
Mechanism of Action: Acts on adrenergic and dopaminergic pathways, directly stimulating the satiety center in the hypothalamic and limbic regions; produces CNS stimulation and blood pressure elevation; tolerance phenomenon demonstrated

Pharmacokinetics
PO: Onset 30-60 min, duration 8-15 hr; excreted primarily in urine as unchanged drug and conjugated metabolites

INDICATIONS AND USES: Exogenous obesity (as a short-term adjunct to caloric restriction)

DOSAGE
Adult
• PO 1 mg tid 1 hr ac, or 2 mg qd 1 hr before lunch

💲 AVAILABLE FORMS/COST OF THERAPY
• Tab, Uncoated—Oral: 1 mg, 100's: **$154.25**; 2 mg, 100's: **$244.75**

CONTRAINDICATIONS: Hypersensitivity to sympathomimetic amines, glaucoma, history of drug abuse, cardiovascular disease, moderate to severe hypertension, advanced arteriosclerosis, agitated states, hyperthyroidism, within 14 days of MAOI administration

PRECAUTIONS: Diabetes mellitus, seizure disorders, mild hypertension, children

PREGNANCY AND LACTATION: Pregnancy category C

SIDE EFFECTS/ADVERSE REACTIONS
CNS: Dizziness, dysphoria, exacerbation of schizophrenia, headache, *insomnia,* mental depression, *nervousness, overstimulation, restlessness,* shivering, tremor

CV: Chest pain, palpitation, *tachycardia*

GI: Constipation, diarrhea, *dry mouth,* nausea, unpleasant taste

GU: Dysuria, impotence, pollakiuria

SKIN: Clamminess, excessive sweating, pallor, rash

INTERACTIONS
Drugs
3 *Furazolidone:* Hypertensive crisis

3 *Guanethidine:* Decreased antihypertensive effects

2 *MAOIs:* Hypertensive crisis

3 *Tricyclic antidepressants:* Decreased anorexiant effects

Labs
• *False positive:* Chlordiazepoxide, flurazepam, methadone, methapyrilene, methylphenidate, phendimetrazine

SPECIAL CONSIDERATIONS
PATIENT/FAMILY EDUCATION
• May cause insomnia; avoid taking late in the day
• Use caution while driving or performing other tasks requiring alertness; may cause dizziness or blurred vision
• Take with food if stomach upset occurs
• Do not discontinue abruptly

---

mebendazole
(me-ben´da-zole)
Rx: Vermox
Chemical Class: Benzimidazole derivative
Therapeutic Class: Anthelmintic

CLINICAL PHARMACOLOGY
Mechanism of Action: Causes degeneration of parasite's cytoplasmic microtubules and thereby selectively and irreversibly blocks glucose uptake in susceptible adult intestine-dwelling helminths and their tissue-dwelling larvae

Pharmacokinetics
PO: Poorly absorbed (5%-10%), peak 2-5 hr; 90%-95% bound to plasma proteins; metabolized by liver to inactive metabolites, eliminated primarily in feces (95%); $t_{1/2}$ 2.5-5.5 hr (35 hr in liver dysfunction)

INDICATIONS AND USES: Single or mixed infections due to *Trichuris trichiura* (whipworm), *Enterobius vermicularis* (pinworm), *Ascaris lumbricoides* (roundworm), *Ancy-*

---

lostoma duodenale (common hookworm), *Necator americanus* (American hookworm)

DOSAGE

Adult and Child

• *Pinworms:* PO 100 mg as a single dose; may need to repeat after 3 wk

• *Whipworms, roundworms, hookworms:* PO 100 mg bid for 3 consecutive days; repeat course in 3-4 wk if necessary

$ AVAILABLE FORMS/COST OF THERAPY

• Tab, Chewable—Oral: 100 mg, 12's: **$61.39-$80.76**

PRECAUTIONS: Child <2 yr

PREGNANCY AND LACTATION: Pregnancy category C; consider treatment if the parasite is causing clinical disease or may cause public health problems; it is doubtful that enough mebendazole is absorbed to be excreted into breast milk in significant quantities

SIDE EFFECTS/ADVERSE REACTIONS

CNS: Dizziness, fever

GI: Diarrhea, transient abdominal pain

INTERACTIONS

Drugs

3 *Carbamazepine:* Decreased mebendazole concentrations and effect via induction of metabolism

2 *Phenytoin:* Decreased mebendazole concentrations; possible impairment of therapeutic effect

SPECIAL CONSIDERATIONS

PATIENT/FAMILY EDUCATION

• Chew or crush tablets and administer with food

• Parasite death and removal from digestive tract may take up to 3 days after treatment

• Consult clinician if not cured in 3 wk

• For pinworms, all household contacts of patient should be treated

• Strict hygiene essential to prevent reinfection; disinfect toilet facilities, change and launder undergarments, bed linens, towels, and nightclothes

---

mecamylamine

(mek-a-mill´a-meen)

Rx: Inversine

Chemical Class: Ganglionic blocker

Therapeutic Class: Ganglionic blocker: antihypertensive

CLINICAL PHARMACOLOGY

Mechanism of Action: Blocks transmission of impulses at both sympathetic and parasympathetic ganglia; hypotensive effect is due to reduction in sympathetic tone, vasodilation, reduced cardiac output; predominantly orthostatic

Pharmacokinetics

PO: Onset 0.5-2 hr, duration 6-12 hr; mostly excreted unchanged in urine

INDICATIONS AND USES: Moderate to severe hypertension (not 1st line)

DOSAGE

Adult

• PO 2.5 mg bid initially, may increase in increments of 2.5 mg q2 days until desired response, usual maintenance dose 25 mg/day divided bid-qid

$ AVAILABLE FORMS/COST OF THERAPY

• Tab, Uncoated—Oral: 2.5 mg, 100's: **$13.50-$255.31**

CONTRAINDICATIONS: Mild, labile hypertension; coronary insufficiency, recent MI; uremia; glaucoma; organic pyloric stenosis; patients receiving sulfonamides or antibiotics

PRECAUTIONS: Cerebral arteriosclerosis, recent CVA, renal insufficiency, abrupt discontinuation, prostatic hypertrophy, bladder neck obstruction, urethral stricture

PREGNANCY AND LACTATION: Pregnancy category C; not recommended in nursing mothers

SIDE EFFECTS/ADVERSE REACTIONS

CNS: Choreiform movements, *fatigue,* mental aberrations, paresthesia, *sedation,* **seizures,** tremor, weakness

CV: Orthostatic dizziness, syncope

EENT: Blurred vision, dilated pupils

GI: Anorexia, constipation, dry mouth, glossitis, nausea, ***paralytic ileus,*** vomiting

GU: Decreased libido, impotence, urinary retention

SPECIAL CONSIDERATIONS

PATIENT/FAMILY EDUCATION

• Take after meals

• Arise slowly from reclining position

• Orthostatic changes are exacerbated by alcohol, exercise, hot weather

MONITORING PARAMETERS

• Maintenance doses should be limited to dose that causes slight faintness or dizziness in the standing position

meclizine

(mek'li-zeen)

Rx: Antivert, Medivert, Meclicot

OTC: Bonine

Chemical Class: Piperazine derivative

Therapeutic Class: Antihistamine; antivertigo agent

CLINICAL PHARMACOLOGY

Mechanism of Action: Central anticholinergic actions; diminishes vestibular stimulation, depresses labyrinthine function; an action on medullary chemoreceptive trigger zone may also be involved in antiemetic effect; also has antihistaminic, CNS depressant, and local anesthetic effects

Pharmacokinetics

PO: Onset 1 hr, duration 8-24 hr, $t_{1/2}$ 6 hr

INDICATIONS AND USES: Motion sickness; "possibly effective" in vertigo associated with diseases affecting vestibular system

DOSAGE

Adult and Child >12 yr

• *Motion sickness:* PO 25-50 mg 1 hr prior to travel; may repeat qd for duration of journey

• *Vertigo:* PO 25-100 mg/day in divided doses, usually tid

💲 AVAILABLE FORMS/COST OF THERAPY

• Tab, Chewable—Oral: 25 mg, 100's: **$1.01-$29.17**

• Tab, Uncoated—Oral: 12.5 mg, 100's: **$0.77-$43.89**; 25 mg, 100's: **$3.25-$69.39**; 30 mg, 100's: **$24.65**; 50 mg, 100's: **$114.18-$128.03**

PRECAUTIONS: Children <12 yr, glaucoma; obstructive GI, GU disease; prostatic hypertrophy

---

italic = common side effects   ***bold italic*** = life-threatening reactions

PREGNANCY AND LACTATION: Pregnancy category B; used for treatment of nausea and vomiting during pregnancy; excretion into breast milk unknown

SIDE EFFECTS/ADVERSE REACTIONS

CNS: Drowsiness, excitation (paradoxical reaction in children), restlessness

CV: Hypotension, palpitations, tachycardia

EENT: Blurred vision, diplopia, dry nose, dry throat

GI: Anorexia, constipation, diarrhea, *dry mouth,* nausea, vomiting

GU: Difficult urination, urinary frequency, urinary retention

SKIN: Rash, urticaria

---

meclofenamate

(me′kloe-fen′a-mate)

Rx: Meclomen, Meclodium
Chemical Class: Anthranilic acid derivative
Therapeutic Class: NSAID with analgesic and antipyretic activity

---

CLINICAL PHARMACOLOGY

Mechanism of Action: Reversible cyclooxygenase (i.e., prostaglandin synthetase) inhibitor; nonselectively decreases the formation of both prostaglandins and thromboxane A2; variable effects on lipoxygenase synthesis and subsequent leukotriene production; antiinflammatory, antipyretic, and analgesic activity; inhibits platelet aggregation

Pharmacokinetics

PO: Peak 0.5-2 hr (completely bioavailable); >90% bound to plasma proteins; metabolized by liver, excreted in urine (metabolites); $t_{1/2}$ 2-3.3 hr

INDICATIONS AND USES: Acute gouty arthritis,* menorrhagia, nephrotic syndrome,* dysmenorrhea, osteoarthritis, rheumatoid arthritis, ankylosing spondylitis,* pain— mild to moderate, psoriatic arthritis*

DOSAGE

Adult

• *Mild to moderate pain:* PO 50 mg q4-6h; max 400 mg/day

• *Primary dysmenorrhea:* PO 100 mg tid for up to 6 days; start at onset of menstrual flow

• *Arthritis:* PO 200-400 mg/day in 3-4 divided doses

§ AVAILABLE FORMS/COST OF THERAPY

• Cap, Gel—Oral: 50 mg, 100's: **$24.38-$183.00**; 100 mg, 100's: **$36.90-$339.75**

CONTRAINDICATIONS: Bronchospasm, nasal polyps, angioedema precipitated by aspirin or other NSAIDs

PRECAUTIONS: History of GI ulceration, bleeding, or perforation; renal dysfunction, hypertension or cardiac conditions aggravated by fluid retention and edema, history of liver dysfunction, history of coagulation

PREGNANCY AND LACTATION: Pregnancy category B (category D if used in 3rd trimester); may inhibit labor and prolong pregnancy, cause constriction of the ductus arteriosus *in utero,* or cause persistent pulmonary hypertension of the newborn

SIDE EFFECTS/ADVERSE REACTIONS

CNS: Dizziness, headache, lightheadedness

CV: Chest pain, *CHF, dysrhythmias,* edema, hypertension, hypotension, palpitation, tachycardia

EENT: Dry eyes, hearing disturbances, photophobia, tinnitus, visual disturbances

---

* = non-FDA-approved use

GI: Abdominal cramps, constipation, *diarrhea, dyspepsia,* flatulence, ***gastric or duodenal ulcer with bleeding or perforation,*** hepatitis, *nausea,* occult blood in stool, ***pancreatitis,*** vomiting

GU: ***Acute renal failure***

HEME: ***Agranulocytosis,*** eosinophilia, ***leukopenia, neutropenia, pancytopenia, thrombocytopenia***

METAB: Hyperglycemia, hyperkalemia, hypoglycemia, hyponatremia

RESP: Bronchospasm, dyspnea

SKIN: Photosensitivity, rash, urticaria

INTERACTIONS

Drugs

🔳 *Aminoglycosides:* Reduced clearance with elevated aminoglycoside levels and potential for toxicity (especially indomethacin in premature infants; other NSAIDs probably)

🔳 *Anticoagulants:* Excessive hypoprothrombinemia, decreased platelet aggregation with increased risk of GI bleeding

🔳 *Antihypertensives (α-blockers, angiotensin-converting enzyme inhibitors, angiotensin II receptor blockers, β-blockers, diuretics):* Inhibition of antihypertensive and other favorable hemodynamic effects

🔳 *Corticosteroids:* Increased risk of GI ulceration

🔳 *Cyclosporine:* Increased nephrotoxicity risk

🔳 *Lithium:* Decreased clearance of lithium (mediated via prostaglandins) resulting in elevated serum lithium levels and risk of toxicity

🔳 *Methotrexate:* Decreased renal secretion of methotrexate resulting in elevated methotrexate levels and risk of toxicity

🔳 *Phenylpropanolamine:* Possible acute hypertensive reaction

🔳 *Potassium-sparing diuretics:* Additive hyperkalemia potential

🔳 *Triamterene:* Acute renal failure reported with addition of indomethacin; caution with other NSAIDs

SPECIAL CONSIDERATIONS
• No significant advantage over other NSAIDs; cost should govern use

MONITORING PARAMETERS
• Initial hemogram and fecal occult blood test within 3 mo of starting regular chronic therapy; repeat every 6-12 mo (more frequently in high-risk patients (>65 years, peptic ulcer disease, concurrent steroids or anticoagulants); electrolytes, creatinine, and BUN within 3 mo of starting regular chronic therapy; repeat every 6-12 mo

---

medroxyprogesterone
(me-drox´ee-proe-jess´te-rone)
Rx: Amen, Curretab, Cycrin, Depo-Provera, Provera
Combinations
  Rx: with estradiol (Lunelle)
Chemical Class: 17 α-hydroxyprogesterone derivative
Therapeutic Class: Progestin; contraceptive; antineoplastic

CLINICAL PHARMACOLOGY
Mechanism of Action: Exerts a progestational effect on the endometrium, alters cervical mucus, suppresses ovulation in some patients, renders the endometrium hostile to implantation

Pharmacokinetics
Metabolized in the liver
IM: Peak levels 3 wk, $t_{1/2}$-50 days

INDICATIONS AND USES: Dysfunctional uterine bleeding, secondary amenorrhea, endometrial cancer, renal cancer, contraception, menopause,* obesity-hypoventilation syndrome (Pickwickian syndrome),* obstructive sleep apnea,* hirsutism,* homozygous sickle-cell disease*

DOSAGE

Adult

• *Secondary amenorrhea:* PO 5-10 mg qd for 5-10 days; withdrawal bleeding usually occurs 3-7 days after therapy ends

• *Endometrial/renal cancer:* IM 400-1000 mg/wk; maintenance of improvement may require as little as 400 mg/mo

• *Uterine bleeding:* PO 5-10 mg qd for 5-10 days; withdrawal bleeding usually occurs 3-7 days after therapy ends

• *Contraceptive:* Depot IM 150 mg q3 mo; medroxyprogesterone/estradiol (Lunelle) IM 0.5 ml q28-30 days not to exceed 33 days

• *Menopause:* PO 10 mg qd days 16-25 of month; or 2.5-5 mg qd (in combination with estrogen)

🅂 AVAILABLE FORMS/COST OF THERAPY

• Inj, Susp—IM: 125 mg/ml, 1 ml: **$41.29**; 150 mg/ml, 1 ml: **$48.10**; 400 mg/ml, 2, 2.5, 10 ml: **$110.39**/2.5 ml

• Tab, Uncoated—Oral: 2.5 mg, 100's: **$21.17-$61.09**; 5 mg, 100's: **$16.45-$92.21**; 10 mg, 100's: **$13.08-$124.68**

CONTRAINDICATIONS: Impaired liver function or disease, breast cancer, undiagnosed vaginal bleeding, missed abortion, use as a diagnostic test for pregnancy

PRECAUTIONS: Epilepsy, migraine, asthma, cardiac or renal dysfunction, depression, diabetes

PREGNANCY AND LACTATION: Pregnancy category X; compatible with breast feeding

SIDE EFFECTS/ADVERSE REACTIONS

CNS: Depression, *dizziness, headache, insomnia, fatigue*

CV: Edema

GI: **Cholestatic jaundice;** *increased weight (approx 4 lbs/yr), nausea, appetite changes*

GU: Amenorrhea, breakthrough bleeding, breast changes, decreased libido, delayed return to fertilty, hot flashes, leukorrhea

METAB: Decreased bone density

SKIN: Acne, alopecia, hirsutism, melasma, oily skin, photosensitivity, rash, melasma

INTERACTIONS

Drugs

🔳 *Aminoglutethimide:* Reduced plasma medroxyprogesterone concentrations

Labs

• *Feces:* Green color

SPECIAL CONSIDERATIONS

PATIENT/FAMILY EDUCATION

• Take protective measures against exposure to ultraviolet light

• Diabetic patients must monitor blood glucose carefully during therapy

• Take with food if GI upset occurs

• When used as contraceptive, menstrual cycle may be disrupted and irregular and unpredictable bleeding or spotting results; usually decreases to the point of amenorrhea as treatment continues (55% at 1 yr)

• After stopping injections, 50% of women who become pregnant will do so in about 10 mo after the last injection, 93% within 18 mo; not related to length of time drug used; women with lower body weights conceive sooner

• Failure rate 0.3% in first year of constant use

mefenamic acid

(me-fe-nam´ik)

Rx: Ponstel

Chemical Class: Anthranilic acid derivative

Therapeutic Class: NSAID with analgesic and antipyretic activity

CLINICAL PHARMACOLOGY

Mechanism of Action: Reversible cyclooxygenase (i.e., prostaglandin synthetase) inhibitor; nonselectively decreases the formation of both prostaglandins and thromboxane A2; variable effects on lipoxygenase synthesis and subsequent leukotriene production; antiinflammatory, antipyretic, and analgesic activity; inhibits platelet aggregation

Pharmacokinetics

PO: Peak 2-4 hr; >90% bound to plasma proteins; metabolized by liver, excreted in urine (metabolites); $t_{1/2}$ 2-4 hr

INDICATIONS AND USES: Dysmenorrhea, fever,* menorrhagia,* osteoarthritis,* pain, low back pain, premenstrual syndrome,* rheumatoid arthritis*

DOSAGE

Adult and Child >14 yr

• *Acute pain:* PO 500 mg, then 250 mg q6h prn; not to exceed 1 wk of therapy

• *Primary dysmenorrhea:* PO 500 mg, then 250 mg q6h; start with onset of bleeding and associated symptoms

💲 AVAILABLE FORMS/COST OF THERAPY

• Cap, Gel—Oral: 250 mg, 100's: **$133.80**

CONTRAINDICATIONS: Bronchospasm, nasal polyps, angioedema precipitated by aspirin or other NSAIDs

PRECAUTIONS: History of GI ulceration, bleeding, or perforation; renal dysfunction, hypertension or cardiac conditions aggravated by fluid retention and edema, history of liver dysfunction, history of coagulation

PREGNANCY AND LACTATION: Pregnancy category C (category D if used in 3rd trimester)

SIDE EFFECTS/ADVERSE REACTIONS

CNS: Dizziness, headache, lightheadedness

CV: Chest pain, CHF, *dysrhythmias,* edema, hypertension, hypotension, palpitation, tachycardia

EENT: Dry eyes, hearing disturbances, photophobia, tinnitus, visual disturbances

GI: Abdominal cramps, constipation, *diarrhea, dyspepsia,* flatulence, *gastric or duodenal ulcer with bleeding or perforation, hepatitis, nausea,* occult blood in stool, pancreatitis, vomiting

GU: **Acute renal failure**

HEME: **Agranulocytosis,** eosinophilia, **leukopenia, neutropenia, pancytopenia, thrombocytopenia**

METAB: Hyperglycemia, hyperkalemia, hypoglycemia, hyponatremia

RESP: Bronchospasm, dyspnea

SKIN: Photosensitivity, rash, urticaria

INTERACTIONS

Drugs

3 *Aminoglycosides:* Reduced clearance with elevated aminoglycoside levels and potential for toxicity (especially indomethacin in premature infants; other NSAIDs probably)

3 *Anticoagulants:* Excessive hypoprothrombinemia, decreased platelet aggregation with increased risk of GI bleeding

M

---

italic = common side effects   ***bold italic*** = life-threatening reactions

3 *Antihypertensives (α-blockers, angiotensin-converting enzyme inhibitors, angiotensin II receptor blockers, β-blockers, diuretics):* Inhibition of antihypertensive and other favorable hemodynamic effects

3 *Corticosteroids:* Increased risk of GI ulceration

3 *Cyclosporine:* Increased nephrotoxicity risk

3 *Lithium:* Decreased clearance of lithium (mediated via prostaglandins) resulting in elevated serum lithium levels and risk of toxicity

2 *Methotrexate:* Decreased renal secretion of methotrexate resulting in elevated methotrexate levels and risk of toxicity

3 *Phenylpropanolamine:* Possible acute hypertensive reaction

3 *Potassium-sparing diuretics:* Additive hyperkalemia potential

3 *Triamterene:* Acute renal failure reported with addition of indomethacin; caution with other NSAIDs

SPECIAL CONSIDERATIONS

• No significant advantage over other NSAIDs; cost should govern use
• Use beyond 1 wk is not recommended

MONITORING PARAMETERS

• Initial hemogram and fecal occult blood test within 3 mo of starting regular chronic therapy; repeat 6-12 mo (more frequently in high-risk patients (>65 years, peptic ulcer disease, concurrent steroids or anticoagulants); electrolytes, creatinine, and BUN within 3 mo of starting regular chronic therapy; repeat every 6-12 mo

---

mefloquine
(me'flow-quine)
Rx: Lariam
Chemical Class: Quinolinemethanol derivative
Therapeutic Class: Antimalarial

CLINICAL PHARMACOLOGY
Mechanism of Action: Blood schizonticide
Pharmacokinetics
PO: 98% bound to plasma proteins, concentrated in blood erythrocytes; metabolized in liver; $t_{1/2}$ 15-33 days

INDICATIONS AND USES: Treatment and prevention of *Plasmodium falciparum* and *P. vivax* malaria infections

DOSAGE
Adult
• *Treatment:* PO 1250 mg (5 tabs) as a single dose
• *Prevention:* PO 250 mg qwk for 4 wk, then 250 mg q2wk; CDC recommends 250 mg qwk starting 1 wk prior to travel, continued weekly during travel and for 4 wk after leaving endemic area
Child
• PO: CDC recommends following doses to be taken weekly starting 1 wk prior to travel, continued weekly during travel, and for 4 wk after leaving endemic area: 15-19 kg, ¼ tab; 20-30 kg, ½ tab; 31-45 kg, ¾ tab; >45 kg, 1 tab

$ **AVAILABLE FORMS/COST OF THERAPY**
• Tab, Uncoated—Oral: 250 mg, 25's: **$198.98-$280.15**

PRECAUTIONS: Children, cardiac dysrhythmias, neurologic disease

PREGNANCY AND LACTATION: Pregnancy category C; use caution during the 1st 12-14 wk of pregnancy; excreted in breast milk in amounts not thought to be harmful to the nursing infant and insufficient to provide adequate protection against malaria

SIDE EFFECTS/ADVERSE REACTIONS

CNS: Anxiety, ***coma,*** confusion, disorientation, dizziness, hallucinations, headache, ***seizures,*** syncope
CV: Bradycardia, extrasystole
EENT: Retinal, lens, corneal abnormalities (rats only), tinnitus
GI: Abdominal pain, diarrhea, loss of appetite, nausea, transiently increased transaminases, vomiting
HEME: Leukopenia, thrombocytopenia
MS: Myalgia
SKIN: Itching, rash

SPECIAL CONSIDERATIONS
PATIENT/FAMILY EDUCATION
• Do not take on an empty stomach
• Take medication with at least 8 oz water
• Caution, initially, when driving, operating machinery, where concentration necessary

MONITORING PARAMETERS
• Liver function tests and ophthalmic examinations during prolonged therapy

---

megestrol
(me-jess'trole)
Rx: Megace
Chemical Class: Progesterone derivative (methylpregnadienedione)
Therapeutic Class: Antineoplastic; appetite stimulant

CLINICAL PHARMACOLOGY
Mechanism of Action: Antineoplastic effect may result from suppression of luteinizing hormone by inhibition of pituitary function or a local effect on cancerous cells; effects on weight gain may be related to appetite-stimulation or metabolic effects

Pharmacokinetics
PO: Peak 1-5 hr; metabolized in liver, eliminated in urine and feces; $t_{1/2}$ 60 min

INDICATIONS AND USES: Anorexia, cachexia, or unexplained weight loss in patients with AIDS (suspension); advanced breast or endometrial cancer

DOSAGE
Adult
• *Breast cancer:* PO 40 mg qid for at least 2 mo
• *Endometrial cancer:* PO 40-320 mg/day in divided doses for at least 2 mo
• *Anorexia, cachexia:* PO 800 mg/day (20 ml susp/day) initially; daily doses of 400-800 mg have been shown to be effective

$ AVAILABLE FORMS/COST OF THERAPY
• Susp—Oral: 40 mg/ml, 236 ml: **$166.59**
• Tab, Uncoated—Oral: 20 mg, 100's: **$52.50-$75.88**; 40 mg, 100's: **$87.40-$134.96**

CONTRAINDICATIONS: As a diagnostic test for pregnancy, known or suspected pregnancy, prophylactic use to avoid weight loss

PRECAUTIONS: Children, HIV-infected women

PREGNANCY AND LACTATION: Pregnancy category X; not recommended during the 1st 4 mo of pregnancy

SIDE EFFECTS/ADVERSE REACTIONS
CNS: Headache, confusion, depression, hypesthesia, neuropathy, paresthesia
CV: Edema, palpitation
GI: Abdominal pain, nausea, vomiting, weight gain, flatulence

GU: Gynecomastia, breast tenderness, impotence, breakthrough bleeding

HEME: Thrombophlebitis, ***pulmonary embolism***

RESP: Dyspnea

SPECIAL CONSIDERATIONS

• Average weight gain in AIDS patients 11 lbs in 12 wk. Begin therapy only after treatable causes of weight loss are sought and addressed

---

meloxicam

(mel-oks'i-kam)

Rx: Mobic

Chemical Class: Oxicam derivative

Therapeutic Class: Nonsteroidal antiinflammatory drug (NSAID)

CLINICAL PHARMACOLOGY

Mechanism of Action: Nonsteroidal antiinflammatory drug with antiinflammatory, analgesic, and antipyretic activity related to prostaglandin synthetase (cyclooxygenase) inhibition; some selectivity for inducible isoform of cyclooxygenase (cyclooxygenase-2)

Pharmacokinetics

PO: Peak 5 hr, prolonged drug absorption (PO), absolute bioavailability 89%, no food effect; 99.4% bound to plasma proteins; synovial fluid concentrations 40-50% of serum concentration; completely metabolized to 4 pharmacologically inactive metabolites by liver (major metabolite, 5´-carboxy meloxicam) via CYP2C9 and CYP3A4; metabolites excreted equally in feces (significant biliary and/or enteral secretion) and urine; $t_{1/2}$ 15-20 hr; crosses the placenta

INDICATIONS AND USES: Osteoarthritis, rheumatoid arthritis*, sciatica*

DOSAGE

Adult and Child >16 yr

• 7.5 mg qd; max 15 mg qd

• No dosage alterations necessary for mild-moderate hepatic or renal (CrCl >15 ml/min) impairment

🟥 AVAILABLE FORMS/COST OF THERAPY

• Tab, Coated—Oral: 7.5 mg, 100's: **$225.00-$227.38**; 15 mg, 100's: **$250.35**

CONTRAINDICATIONS: Hypersensitivty, aspirin allergy (asthma, urticaria, or allergic-type reactions)

PRECAUTIONS: Renal disease (CrCl <15 ml/min), history of GI ulcer/bleed (increased risk of GI adverse reactions: extended course of high dose NSAID or corticosteroid therapy), smoker, alcoholics, bleeding disorders, hepatic dysfunction, dehydration, fluid retention, heart failure, hypertension, asthma, elderly, 3rd trimester pregnancy

PREGNANCY AND LACTATION: Pregnancy category C; animal studies document both teratogenic and nonteratongenic (premature PDA closure) in animals; no studies in humans; no human studies on breast milk excretion; in rats, milk concentrations are twice that of plasma

SIDE EFFECTS/ADVERSE REACTIONS

CNS: Headache, dizziness, insomnia

CV: Edema

GI: (25%) Abdominal pain, diarrhea, dyspepsia, flatulence, nausea, ulceration/bleed, elevated transaminases (evidence exists documenting less GI toxicity than other NSAIDs without COX-2 selectivity)

HEME: Anemia

SKIN: Rash, pruritus

---

* = non-FDA-approved use

INTERACTIONS
Drugs
❷ *Anticoagulants (heparin, low molecular weight heparin, warfarin, etc.):* Increased risk of hematoma and major and minor bleeding

❷ *Aspirin:* Increased risk of GI ulceration, especially with high dose aspirin; potential negation of protective cardiac effects

❸ *ACE inhibitors, angiotensin II receptor blockers:* Diminished antihypertensive effect

❸ *β-blockers:* Diminished antihypertensive effect

❸ *Cholestyramine:* Increases clearance of meloxicam (50%), with reduction in $t_{1/2}$ and AUC

❸ *Corticosteroids:* Additive effects; increased risk of GI bleeding, sodium/water retention

❸ *Cyclosporine:* Additive nephrotoxicity

❸ *Diuretics:* Reduced natriuretic effects

❷ *Lithium:* Addition of meloxicam may result in increased lithium blood levels (21%)

❷ *Warfarin:* Additive effects on coagulation; prothrombin times as INR have increased with the addition of meloxicam

Labs
• *Guaiac (Hemoccult) assay:* False positives

SPECIAL CONSIDERATIONS
• Partial, not pure, COX-2 selective inhibitor; most studies have compared it with non-selective agents, making final assessment of place in therapy difficult

PATIENT/FAMILY EDUCATION
• Take with food or milk; report gastrointestinal adverse effects

MONITORING PARAMETERS
• Acute phase reactants for efficacy in rheumatoid arthritis; pain, stiffness, number of swollen joints, range of motion, functional capacity, structural damage, fecal occult blood, hemogram, renal and hepatic function

---

menotropins
(men-oh-troe'pins)
Rx: Humegon, Pergonal, Repronex
Chemical Class: Purified preparation of human pituitary gonadotropins, (FSH and LH)
Therapeutic Class: Ovarian stimulant; fertility agent

CLINICAL PHARMACOLOGY
Mechanism of Action: Women: produces ovarian follicular growth in the absence of primary ovarian failure; does not induce ovulation; Men: with human chorionic gonadotropin (HCG), induces spermatogenesis in the presence of primary or secondary pituitary hypofunction

Pharmacokinetics
IM: $t_{1/2}$ of FSH and LH 70 hr and 4 hr, respectively; 8% of dose excreted unchanged in urine

INDICATIONS AND USES: Stimulation of ovarian follicular growth prior to induction of ovulation by HCG; induction of multiple follicles in ovulatory patients participating in an *in vitro* fertilization program; stimulation of spermatogenesis in men with primary or secondary hypogonadotropic hypogonadism (in conjunction with HCG)

DOSAGE
Adult
• Women: IM 75 IU FSH/LH qd for 7-12 days, followed by 10,000 IU HCG 1 day after last dose of menotropins; repeat for at least 2 more cycles if evidence of ovulation, but no pregnancy, then increase to 150 IU FSH/LH qd for 7-12 days,

---

followed by 10,000 IU HCG 1 day after last dose of menotropins, repeat as above

• Men: IM 75 IU FSH/LH 3 times/wk with HCG 2000 IU 2 times/wk for 4 mo (following pretreatment with HCG alone 5000 IU 3 times/wk for 4-6 mo)

$ AVAILABLE FORMS/COST OF THERAPY

• Inj, Sol—IM: 75 U, 1's: **$57.00-$84.72**; 150 U, 1's: **$113.12-$129.66**

CONTRAINDICATIONS: Women: Primary ovarian failure, abnormal bleeding; thyroid, adrenal dysfunction; organic intracranial lesion, ovarian cysts, pregnancy; men: primary testicular failure, normal pituitary function, infertility disorder other than hyopgonadotropic hypogonadism

PREGNANCY AND LACTATION: Pregancy category X

SIDE EFFECTS/ADVERSE REACTIONS

CNS: Chills, dizziness, febrile reactions, headache, malaise, *stroke*

CV: Tachycardia, *venous, arterial thromboembolism*

GI: Abdominal pain, bloating, cramps, diarrhea, *nausea,* vomiting

GU: Adnexal torsion, *ectopic pregnancy, hemoperitoneum, hyperstimulation syndrome* (sudden ovarian enlargement and ascites, with or without pain or pleural effusion), ovarian cysts, *ovarian enlargement* (20%)

MS: Joint pains, musculoskeletal aches

RESP: **Acute respiratory distress syndrome,** atelectasis, dyspnea, tachypnea

SKIN: Body rashes, pain, rash, irritation at inj site

MISC: Gynecomastia (men)

SPECIAL CONSIDERATIONS

PATIENT/FAMILY EDUCATION

• Multiple births occur in approximately 20% of women treated with menotropins and HCG

• Couple should engage in intercourse daily, beginning on the day prior to HCG administration, until ovulation occurs

• Ovarian enlargement regresses without treatment in 2-3 wk

MONITORING PARAMETERS

• Urinary estrogen; do not administer HCG if >150 µg/24 hr (increased risk of hyperstimulation of ovaries syndrome)

• Sonographic visualization of ovaries; estradiol levels

---

mepenzolate

(me-pen′zoe-late)

Rx: Cantil

Chemical Class: Quaternary ammonium compound

Therapeutic Class: Gastrointestinal antispasmodic agent; gastrointestinal antiulcer agent (adjunct)

CLINICAL PHARMACOLOGY

Mechanism of Action: Inhibits GI motility and diminishes gastric acid secretion

Pharmacokinetics

PO: Onset 1 hr, duration 3-4 hr, poor lipid solubility; 3%-22% of dose excreted in urine, remainder excreted in feces (probably as unabsorbed drug)

INDICATIONS AND USES: Peptic ulcer disease (in combination with other drugs); functional GI disorders (diarrhea, pylorospasm, hypermotility, neurogenic colon)*; irritable bowel syndrome (spastic colon, mucous colitis)*; acute entero-

---

* = non-FDA-approved use

colitis,* ulcerative colitis,* diverticulitis,* mild dysenteries,* pancreatitis,* splenic flexure syndrome*

DOSAGE

Adult

• PO 25-50 mg qid with meals, hs

$ AVAILABLE FORMS/COST OF THERAPY

• Tab, Uncoated—Oral: 25 mg, 100's: **$108.05**

CONTRAINDICATIONS: Hypersensitivity to anticholinergic drugs, narrow-angle glaucoma, obstructive uropathy, obstructive disease of the GI tract, paralytic ileus, intestinal atony, unstable cardiovascular status in acute hemorrhage, severe ulcerative colitis, toxic megacolon complicating ulcerative colitis, myasthenia gravis

PRECAUTIONS: Hyperthyroidism, CAD, dysrhythmias, CHF, ulcerative colitis, hypertension, hiatal hernia, hepatic disease, renal disease, urinary retention, prostatic hypertrophy, elderly, children, glaucoma

PREGNANCY AND LACTATION: Pregnancy category C; excretion into breast milk unknown, although would be expected to be minimal due to quaternary structure

SIDE EFFECTS/ADVERSE REACTIONS

CNS: Anxiety, confusion, dizziness, drowsiness, hallucination, headache, insomnia, stimulation (especially in elderly), weakness

CV: Palpitations, tachycardia

EENT: Blurred vision, cycloplegia, increased ocular tension, mydriasis, photophobia

GI: Absence of taste, *constipation, dry mouth,* dysphagia, heartburn, nausea, ***paralytic ileus,*** vomiting

GU: Hesitancy, impotence, *retention*

SKIN: Allergic reactions, anhidrosis, fever, pruritis, rash, urticaria

SPECIAL CONSIDERATIONS

PATIENT/FAMILY EDUCATION

• Take drug 30-60 min before a meal

• Drug may cause drowsiness, dizziness, or blurred vision; use caution while driving or performing other tasks requiring alertness

• Notify clinician if eye pain occurs

---

meperidine

(me-per′i-deen)
Rx: Demerol
Combinations
   Rx: with promethazine (Mepergan)
Chemical Class: Synthetic opium alkaloid; phenylpiperidine derivative
Therapeutic Class: Narcotic analgesic
DEA Class: Schedule II

M

CLINICAL PHARMACOLOGY

Mechanism of Action: Narcotic agonist with activity at Mu receptors (supraspinal analgesia, euphoria, respiratory and physical depression, miosis, and reduced GI motility), Kappa receptors (pentazocine-like spinal analgesia, sedation, and miosis), and Delta receptors (dysphoria, psychotmimetic effects [e.g., hallucinations], and respiratory and vasomotor stimulation caused by drugs with antagonist activity); compared to morphine, equal analgesia, respiratory depression, and physical dependence, less antitussive, constipation, sedation

Pharmacokinetics

PO: Peak analgesia within 1 hr, duration 2-4 hr

IM: Peak analgesia 30-50 min, duration 2-4 hr

SC: Peak analgesia 40-60 min, duration 2-4 hr

---

italic = common side effects   ***bold italic*** = life-threatening reactions

IV: Peak analgesia 5-30 min, duration 2-4 hr

60%-80% bound to plasma proteins; metabolized by liver (normeperidine is an active metabolite with half the analgesic potency but twice the CNS stimulant potency of the parent drug), eliminated in urine; $t_{1/2}$ 3-5 hr (normeperidine $t_{1/2}$ 8-21 hr; may be prolonged in renal impairment)

INDICATIONS AND USES: Moderate to severe pain, preoperative sedation (parenteral)

DOSAGE

Oral doses are about half as effective as parenteral doses

Adult

• *Analgesia:* PO/IM/IV/SC 50-150 mg q3-4h prn

• *Preoperative sedation:* IM/SC 50-100 mg 30-90 min before beginning anesthesia

Child

• *Analgesia:* PO/IM/IV/SC 1-1.5 mg/kg/dose q3-4h prn; max 100 mg/dose

• *Preoperative sedation:* IM/SC 1-2 mg/kg 30-90 min before beginning anesthesia

$ AVAILABLE FORMS/COST OF THERAPY

• Inj, Sol—IM, IV, SC: 10 mg/ml, 30 ml: **$11.80-$170.40**; 25 mg/ml, 1 ml: **$0.54-$1.18**; 50 mg/ml, 1 ml: **$0.59-$1.75**; 75 mg/ml, 1 ml: **$0.93-$1.21**; 100 mg/ml, 1 ml: **$0.82-$1.33**

• Syr—Oral: 50 mg/5 ml, 480 ml: **$105.85**

• Tab, Uncoated—Oral: 50 mg, 100's: **$24.70-$94.32**; 100 mg, 100's: **$38.70-$179.40**

CONTRAINDICATIONS: Concurrent use and within 14 days of MAOI therapy

PRECAUTIONS: Head injury, increased intracranial pressure, acute abdominal conditions, asthma and respiratory conditions, elderly, renal function impairment (normeperidine may accumulate, resulting in increased CNS adverse reactions), hepatic impairment, hypothyroidism, Addison's disease, prostatic hypertrophy, urethral stricture, history of drug abuse

PREGNANCY AND LACTATION: Pregnancy category B (category D if used for prolonged periods or in high doses at term); use during labor may produce neonatal respiratory depression; compatible with breast feeding

SIDE EFFECTS/ADVERSE REACTIONS

CNS: Agitation, dependency, dizziness, *drowsiness,* lethargy, myoclonus, restlessness, *sedation,* **seizures,** tremors, twitches

CV: Bradycardia, orthostatic hypotension, palpitations, tachycardia

GI: Anorexia, constipation, increased amylase, lipase; *nausea, vomiting*

GU: Urinary retention

RESP: **Respiratory depression, respiratory paralysis**

SKIN: Flushing, rash, urticaria

INTERACTIONS

Drugs

3 *Antihistamines, chloral hydrate, glutethimide, methocarbamol:* Enhanced depressant effects

3 *Barbiturates:* Additive respiratory and CNS depressant effects

3 *Cimetidine:* Increased respiratory and CNS depression

3 *Ethanol:* Additive CNS effects

⚠ *MAOIs:* Accumulation of CNS serotonin leading to agitation, blood pressure changes, hyperpyrexia, seizures

3 *Neuroleptics:* Hypotension, excessive CNS depression

3 *Phenytoin:* Enhanced metabolism; reduced meperidine concentrations

---

* = non-FDA-approved use

❷ *Selegiline:* Though primarily MAO-B inhibitor, residual MAO-A activity; see MAOI description

Labs

• *False increase:* Amylase and lipase

SPECIAL CONSIDERATIONS
PATIENT/FAMILY EDUCATION

• Physical dependency may result when used for extended periods

• Do not administer agonist/antagonist analgesics (i.e., pentazocine, nalbuphine, butorphanol, dezocine, buprenorphine) to patient who has received a prolonged course of meperidine (a pure agonist). In opioid-dependent patients, mixed agonist/antagonist analgesics may precipitate withdrawal symptoms.

• Change position slowly; orthostatic hypotension may occur

• Avoid hazardous activities if drowsiness or dizziness occurs

• Avoid alcohol, other CNS depressants unless directed by clinician

• Minimize nausea by administering with food and remain lying down following dose

---

mephentermine
(me-fen´ter-meen)
Rx: Wyamine
Chemical Class: Amphetamine derivative
Therapeutic Class: Antihypotensive

CLINICAL PHARMACOLOGY
Mechanism of Action: Primarily an indirect sympathomimetic that releases norepinephrine from its storage sites; increases blood pressure by increasing cardiac output (positive inotropic effect) and, to a lesser degree, by increasing peripheral resistance due to vasoconstriction

Pharmacokinetics
IM: Onset 5-15 min, duration 1-4 hr
IV: Onset almost immediate, duration 15-30 min
Metabolized by liver, eliminated in urine

INDICATIONS AND USES: Hypotension during spinal anesthesia

DOSAGE

Adult

• *Prevention of hypotension during spinal anesthesia:* IM 30-45 mg 10-20 min prior to anesthesia

• *Hypotension following spinal anesthesia:* IV 30-45 mg, repeat doses of 30 mg prn to maintain blood pressure; IV INF use 0.1% sol in D_5W (1 mg/ml), titrate to patient response

💲 **AVAILABLE FORMS/COST OF THERAPY**

• Inj, Sol—IM, IV: 15 mg/ml, 2 ml: **$6.33**

CONTRAINDICATIONS: Hypotension induced by chlorpromazine, concurrent use with any MAOI

PRECAUTIONS: Cardiovascular disease, chronically ill patients, hemorrhagic shock, hyperthyroidism, hypertension

PREGNANCY AND LACTATION: Pregnancy category C

SIDE EFFECTS/ADVERSE REACTIONS

CNS: Anxiety, confusion, drowsiness, incoherence, tremors
CV: Hypertension, palpitations, tachycardia

INTERACTIONS

Drugs

❸ *Halogenated hydrocarbon anesthetics:* Sensitization of myocardium to effects of catecholamines; serious dysrhythmia may result
❸ *MAOIs:* Hypertensive crisis

Labs

• *Amphetamines:* False positive for amphetamine, methamphetamine in urine

mephenytoin
(me-fen'i-toyn)
Rx: Mesantoin
Chemical Class: Hydantoin derivative
Therapeutic Class: Anticonvulsive

CLINICAL PHARMACOLOGY
Mechanism of Action: Stabilizes neuronal membranes decreasing seizure activity by increasing efflux or decreasing influx of sodium ions across cell membranes in the motor cortex during generation of nerve impulses
Pharmacokinetics
PO: Onset 30 min, duration 24-48 hr; metabolized by liver to active metabolite, excreted in urine; $t_{1/2}$ 144 hr
INDICATIONS AND USES: Tonic-clonic, partial, Jacksonian, and psychomotor seizures in patients refractory to less toxic anticonvulsants
DOSAGE
Adult
• PO 50-100 mg/day initially, increase by 50-100 mg at weekly intervals; usual maintenance dose 200-600 mg/day divided tid; max 800 mg/day
Child
• PO 3-15 mg/kg/day divided tid; usual maintenance dose 100-400 mg/day divided tid
$ AVAILABLE FORMS/COST OF THERAPY
• Tab, Uncoated—Oral: 100 mg, 100's: **$34.69**
PRECAUTIONS: Abrupt withdrawal, elderly, impaired liver function, hyperglycemia, acute intermittent porphyria
PREGNANCY AND LACTATION: Pregnancy category C

SIDE EFFECTS/ADVERSE REACTIONS
CNS: Ataxia, choreiform movements, depression, dizziness, *drowsiness,* dysarthria, fatigue, insomnia, irritability, mental confusion, nervousness, psychotic disturbances, tremor
CV: Edema
EENT: Diplopia, nystagmus, photophobia
GI: Hepatitis, jaundice, nausea, vomiting
GU: Nephrosis
HEME: **Agranulocytosis,** anemia, **aplastic anemia, hemolytic anemia, leukopenia,** lymphadenopathy, **megaloblastic anemia, neutropenia, pancytopenia, thrombocytopenia**
METAB: Hyperglycemia
MS: Osteomalacia, polyarthropathy
RESP: **Pulmonary fibrosis**
SKIN: Alopecia, erythema multiforme, **exfoliative dermatitis,** maculopapular, morbilliform, scarlantiniform, urticarial, purpuric, and non-specific skin rashes; **toxic epidermal necrosis**
MISC: Lupus erythematosus syndrome, weight gain
INTERACTIONS
Drugs
3 *Acetaminophen:* Enhanced hepatotoxic potential of overdose
3 *Acetazolamide:* Increased risk of osteomalacia
3 *Antidepressants:* Increased mephenytoin concentrations; reduced cyclic antidepressant concentrations
3 *Antineoplastics (cisplatin), diazoxide, folic acid, rifampin:* Reduced plasma mephenytoin concentrations

3 *Carbamazepine:* Combined use may decrease serum concentrations of both drugs; mephenytoin may either increase or decrease when carbamazepine is added

3 *Chloramphenicol, cimetidine, disulfiram, felbamate, fluconazole, flouroquinolones, fluoxetine, isoniazid, omeprazole, sulfonamides, sulthiame:* Increased serum mephenytoin concentrations

3 *Cyclosporine:* Reduced cyclosporine concentrations

3 *Loop diuretics:* Reduced diuretic response

3 *Mebendazole:* Reduced plasma mebendazole concentrations

3 *Methadone:* Reduced serum methadone concentrations

3 *Metyrapone:* Invalidated metyrapone test

3 *Mexiletine:* Reduced mexiletine concentrations

2 *Oral anticoagulants:* Transient increase followed by inhibition of hypoprothrombinemic response to oral anticoagulants

3 *Oral contraceptives:* Inhibited effect of oral contraceptives

3 *Primidone:* Enhanced conversion of primidone to phenobarbital

3 *Quinidine:* Decreased serum quinidine concentrations

3 *Theophylline:* Reduced serum theophylline concentrations

3 *Thyroid hormones:* Increased thyroid replacement dose requirements

3 *Valproic acid:* Increased, decreased, or unaltered plasma mephenytoin concentrations

Labs

• *Phenytoin:* Decreased serum level of phenytoin

SPECIAL CONSIDERATIONS
PATIENT/FAMILY EDUCATION
• Take with food
• Drug may cause drowsiness, dizziness, or blurred vision
• Avoid alcohol
• Notify clinician of skin rash, severe nausea or vomiting, swollen glands, bleeding, swollen or tender gums, yellowish discoloration of skin or eyes, joint pain, unexplained fever, sore throat, persistent headache, pregnancy

MONITORING PARAMETERS
• CBC with differential and platelet count at baseline, 2 wk after dosage changes, q1 mo for 1 yr, then q3 mo thereafter
• Therapeutic serum concentrations 25-40 µg/ml (mephenytoin plus active metabolite)

mephobarbital
(me'foe-bar'bi-tal)
Rx: Mebaral
Chemical Class: Barbituric acid derivative
Therapeutic Class: Sedative/hypnotic; anticonvulsant
DEA Class: Schedule IV

CLINICAL PHARMACOLOGY
Mechanism of Action: CNS depressant: depresses the sensory cortex, decreases motor activity, alters cerebellar function, produce drowsiness, sedation, and hypnosis; little analgesic action at subanesthetic doses (may increase reaction to painful stimuli); anticonvulsant activity in subhypnotic doses; dose-dependent respiratory depression (hypnotic doses produce respiratory depression similar to physiologic sleep)

Pharmacokinetics
PO: Onset 20-60 min, duration 10-16 hr; metabolized by the liver to phenobarbital, excreted in urine; $t_{1/2}$ 11-67 hr

---

italic = common side effects   ***bold italic*** = life-threatening reactions

INDICATIONS AND USES: Sedative (relief of anxiety, tension), partial and generalized tonic-clonic and cortical focal seizures

DOSAGE

Adult
- *Sedative:* PO 32-100 mg tid-qid
- *Epilepsy:* PO 400-600 mg/day in 2-4 divided doses

Child
- *Sedative:* PO 16-32 mg tid-qid
- *Epilepsy:* PO 4-10 mg/kg/day in 2-4 divided doses

$ AVAILABLE FORMS/COST OF THERAPY
- Tab, Uncoated—Oral: 32 mg, 250's: **$43.15-$59.68**; 50 mg, 250's: **$62.01-$85.44**; 100 mg, 250's: **$84.47-$114.52**

CONTRAINDICATIONS: Respiratory depression, severe liver impairment, porphyria

PRECAUTIONS: Myasthenia gravis, myxedema, anemia, hepatic disease, renal disease, elderly, mental depression, history of drug abuse, abrupt discontinuation, children, hyperthyroidism, fever, diabetes

PREGNANCY AND LACTATION: Pregnancy category D; has caused major adverse effects in some nursing infants; should be given with caution to nursing women

SIDE EFFECTS/ADVERSE REACTIONS

CNS: CNS depression, dizziness, *drowsiness,* headache, *lethargy,* lightheadedness, mental depression, physical dependence, slurred speech, stimulation in the elderly and children, vertigo

CV: Bradycardia, hypotension

GI: Constipation, diarrhea, nausea, vomiting

HEME: **Agranulocytosis,** megaloblastic anemia (long-term treatment), ***thrombocytopenia***

RESP: **Apnea, bronchospasm, depression, laryngospasm**

SKIN: **Angioedema,** erythema multiforme, pain, *rash,* **Stevens-Johnson syndrome,** thrombophlebitis, urticaria

MISC: Rickets, osteomalacia (prolonged use)

INTERACTIONS

Drugs

3 *Acetaminophen:* Enhanced hepatotoxic potential of acetaminophen overdoses

3 *Antidepressants:* Reduced serum concentration of cyclic antidepressants

3 *Beta-adrenergic blockers:* Reduced serum concentrations of beta-blockers which are extensively metabolized

3 *Calcium channel blockers:* Reduced serum concentrations of verapamil and dihydropyridines

3 *Chloramphenicol:* Increased barbiturate concentrations; reduced serum chloramphenicol concentrations

3 *Corticosteroids:* Reduced serum concentrations of corticosteroids; may impair therapeutic effect

3 *Cyclosporine:* Reduced serum concentration of cyclosporine

3 *Digitoxin:* Reduced serum concentration of digitoxin

3 *Disopyramide:* Reduced serum concentration of disopyramide

3 *Doxycycline:* Reduced serum doxycycline concentrations

3 *Estrogen:* Reduced serum concentration of estrogen

3 *Ethanol:* Excessive CNS depression

3 *Griseofulvin:* Reduced griseofulvin absorption

3 *Methoxyflurane:* Enhanced nephrotoxic effect

3 *MAOIs:* Prolonged effect of barbiturates

---

* = non-FDA-approved use

3 *Narcotic analgesics:* Increased toxicity of meperidine; reduced effect of methadone; additive CNS depression

3 *Neuroleptics:* Reduced effect of either drug

2 *Oral anticoagulants:* Decrease hypoprothrombinemic response to oral anticoagulants

3 *Oral contraceptives:* Reduced efficacy of oral contraceptives

3 *Phenytoin:* Unpredictable effect on serum phenytoin levels

3 *Propafenone:* Reduced serum concentration of propafenone

3 *Quinidine:* Reduced quinidine plasma concentrations

3 *Tacrolimus:* Reduced serum concentration of tacrolimus

3 *Theophylline:* Reduced serum theophylline concentrations

3 *Valproic acid:* Increased serum concentrations of amobarbital

2 *Warfarin:* See oral anticoagulants

Labs

• *Phenobarbital:* Falsely increased result

SPECIAL CONSIDERATIONS
PATIENT/FAMILY EDUCATION

• Avoid driving or other activities requiring alertness

• Avoid alcohol ingestion or CNS depressants

• Do not discontinue medication abruptly after long-term use

• Notify clinician of fever, sore throat, mouth sores, easy bruising or bleeding, broken blood vessels under skin

MONITORING PARAMETERS

• Periodic CBC, liver and renal function tests, serum folate, vitamin D during prolonged therapy

---

meprobamate
(me-proe'ba-mate)
Rx: Equanil, Miltown, Neuramate
Chemical Class: Carbamate derivative
Therapeutic Class: Anxiolytic; sedative/hypnotic
DEA Class: Schedule IV

CLINICAL PHARMACOLOGY
Mechanism of Action: CNS depressant activity at multiple sites in CNS including hypothalamus, thalamus, limbic system, and spinal cord; mildly tranquilizing; some anticonvulsant and muscle relaxant properties

Pharmacokinetics
PO: Onset 1 hr, peak concentration 1-3 hr; metabolized in liver, excreted in urine (metabolites); $t_{1/2}$ 6-17 hr

INDICATIONS AND USES: Anxiety disorders

DOSAGE
Adult
• PO 1.2-1.6 g/day divided tid-qid, do not exceed 2.4 g/day; sustained release 400-800 mg bid

Child 6-12 yr
• PO 100-200 mg bid-tid; SR 200 mg bid

§ AVAILABLE FORMS/COST OF THERAPY
• Tab, Uncoated—Oral: 200 mg, 100's: **$1.08-$202.18**; 400 mg, 100's: **$1.44-$246.50**; 600 mg, 100's: **$234.86**

CONTRAINDICATIONS: Acute intermittent porphyria

PRECAUTIONS: History of drug abuse, renal and hepatic function impairment, elderly, children <6 yr, epilepsy

M

PREGNANCY AND LACTATION:
Pregnancy category D; excreted into breast milk in concentrations 2-4 times that of maternal plasma; effect on nursing infant unknown

SIDE EFFECTS/ADVERSE REACTIONS

CNS: Ataxia, *dizziness, drowsiness,* euphoria, fast EEG activity, headache, overstimulation, paradoxical excitement, **seizures,** slurred speech, vertigo, weakness

CV: Hypotensive crises, palpitations, peripheral edema, syncope, tachycardia, transient ECG changes, **various dysrhythmias**

EENT: Impairment of visual accommodation

GI: Diarrhea, nausea, proctitis, stomatitis, vomiting

GU: **Anuria, oliguria**

HEME: **Agranulocytosis, aplastic anemia, eosinophilia, leukopenia,** thrombocytopenic purpura

RESP: **Bronchospasm**

SKIN: Ecchymoses, **erythema multiforme, exfoliative dermatitis,** fixed drug eruption, petechiae, rash, **Stevens-Johnson syndrome**

MISC: Angioneurotic edema, exacerbation of porphyric symptoms

INTERACTIONS

Drugs

3 *Ethanol:* Enhanced CNS depression

Labs

• *17-Hydroxycorticosteroids:* Urine, increased

• *17-Ketogenic Steroids:* Urine, increased

SPECIAL CONSIDERATIONS

PATIENT/FAMILY EDUCATION

• Avoid alcohol

• Do not discontinue abruptly following long-term use

MONITORING PARAMETERS

• Periodic CBC with differential and platelets during prolonged therapy

---

meropenem
(mear-ro-pen′em)
Rx: Merrem
Chemical Class: Carbapenem
Therapeutic Class: Antibiotic

CLINICAL PHARMACOLOGY
Mechanism of Action: Inhibits bacterial cell wall synthesis; bactericidal

Pharmacokinetics
IV: $t_{1/2}$ 1.5 hr, excreted by kidney

INDICATIONS AND USES: As monotherapy for intra-abdominal infections and bacterial meningitis caused by susceptible organisms, respiratory infections (including in cystic fibrosis patients), skin infections, urinary-tract infections, infections in immunocompromised patients

Antibacterial spectrum usually includes:

Gram-positive organisms: *Streptococcus pneumonia* (not penicillin-resistant strains), *Staphylococcus aureus* (not MRSA), *Staphylococcus epidermidis,* Viridans group streptococci

Gram-negative organisms: *E. coli, Haemophilus influenzae, Klebsiella pneumoniae, Neisseria meningitidis, Pseudomonas aeruginosa*

Anaerobes: *Bacteroides fragilis, Peptostreptococcus* species

DOSAGE

Adult

• IV 0.5-1 g q8h by INF over 15-30 min or via bolus over 3-5 min

• *Meningitis:* IV 2 g q8h

• *Dosage adjustment in impaired renal function:* CrCl 26-50 ml/min usual dose q12h; CrCl 10-25 ml/min one-half usual dose q12h; CrCl <10 ml/min one-half usual dose q24h

---

Child >3 mo and <50 kg
- IV 10-20 mg/kg q8h (max 2 g q8h)
- *Meningitis:* IV 40 mg/kg q8h
- *Cystic fibrosis:* IV 25-40 mg/kg q8h

💲 AVAILABLE FORMS/COST OF THERAPY
- Inj, Dry-Sol—IV: 500 mg: **$227.10-$263.10**; 1 g: **$525.60-$541.20**

CONTRAINDICATIONS: Hypersensitivity to penicillin, beta-lactam antibiotics

PRECAUTIONS: Seizure disorder, CNS lesions, impaired renal function

PREGNANCY AND LACTATION: Pregnancy category B; unknown if excreted into human milk

SIDE EFFECTS/ADVERSE REACTIONS

CNS: **Seizures,** headache

CV: **Shock**

GI: Diarrhea, **Pseudomembranous colitis,** nausea, vomiting, constipation, elevated LFTs

HEME: **Thrombocytopenia,** anemia, **neutropenia**

SKIN: Injection site reaction, rash, pruritus, **Stevens-Johnson syndrome,** erythema multiforme

INTERACTIONS
Drugs

3 *Probenecid:* Inhibits renal excretion of meropenem

3 *Valproic acid:* Two reports of decreased valproate concentrations

SPECIAL CONSIDERATIONS
- Less likely to induce seizures than imipenem-cilastin

MONITORING PARAMETERS
- Renal, hepatic and hematopoietic function during prolonged therapy

mesalamine

(mez-al′a-meen)

Rx: Asacol, Pentasa, Rowasa
Chemical Class: 5-amino derivative of salicylic acid
Therapeutic Class: GI anti-inflammatory

CLINICAL PHARMACOLOGY
Mechanism of Action: May act by blocking cyclooxygenase and inhibiting prostaglandin production in the colon; appears to produce a local inhibitory effect on the mucosal production of arachidonic acid metabolites, which are increased in patients with chronic inflammatory bowel disease

Pharmacokinetics

PR: Poorly absorbed; excreted principally in feces

PO: (TABS): Designed to release drug in terminal ileum and beyond; 28% absorbed; peak 4-12 hr

PO: (CAPS): Designed to release drug throughout the GI tract; 20%-30% absorbed; peak 3 hr

Unabsorbed drug eliminated in feces; absorbed drug metabolized and eliminated in urine (metabolite); $t_{1/2}$ 42 min (following IV administration)

INDICATIONS AND USES: Remission and treatment of ulcerative colitis (oral); treatment of distal ulcerative colitis, proctosigmoiditis or proctitis (rectal)

DOSAGE
Adult
- PO (tabs) 800 mg tid for 6 wk; PO (caps) 1 g qid for up to 8 wk; PR (supp) 1 supp (500 mg) bid for 3-6 wk, retain supp in rectum for 1-3 hr if possible; PR (enema) 60 ml (4 g) instilled qd, preferably hs, and retained for 8 hr, treat for 3-6 wk

---

italic = common side effects   ***bold italic*** = life-threatening reactions

☒ AVAILABLE FORMS/COST OF THERAPY

• Cap, Gel, Sus Action—Oral: 250 mg, 240's: **$94.50-$135.48**
• Enema—Rect: 4 g/60 ml, 60 ml; 7's: **$103.07**
• Supp—Rect: 500 mg, 12's: **$46.85**
• Tab, Enteric Coated—Oral: 400 mg, 100's: **$77.29-$90.54**

PRECAUTIONS: Hypersensitivity to sulfasalazine, renal function impairment, sulfite sensitivity (enema), children

PREGNANCY AND LACTATION: Pregnancy category B; has produced adverse effects in a nursing infant and should be used with caution during breast feeding; observe nursing infant closely for changes in stool consistency

SIDE EFFECTS/ADVERSE REACTIONS

CNS: Asthenia, fatigue, *headache,* insomnia, malaise, mental depression, weakness
CV: **Pericarditis,** peripheral edema
GI: Abdominal pain, colitis, constipation, *cramps,* difficulty retaining enema, *discomfort;* extension of inflammation to entire colon (rectal), flatulence, hemorrhoids, nausea, pain on enema insertion, **pancreatitis,** rectal pain, worsening diarrhea
GU: Urinary burning
MS: Back pain, leg or joint pain
SKIN: Acne, alopecia, pruritis, rash, **Stevens-Johnson syndrome**
MISC: Acute intolerance syndrome (cramping, abdominal pain, bloody diarrhea, fever, headache, rash)

SPECIAL CONSIDERATIONS
PATIENT/FAMILY EDUCATION

• Swallow tabs whole, do not break the outer coating
• Intact or partially intact tabs may be found in stool; notify clinician if this occurs repeatedly
• Avoid excess handling of suppositories
• Lie on left side during enema administration (to facilitate migration into the sigmoid colon)

---

mesna
(mess´na)
Rx: Mesnex, Mesnex VHA Plus
Chemical Class: Thiol derivative
Therapeutic Class: Ifosfamide antidote

CLINICAL PHARMACOLOGY
Mechanism of Action: Binds with and detoxifies acrolein and other urotoxic metabolites of ifosfamide and cyclophosphamide
Pharmacokinetics
IV: Rapidly oxidized to mesna disulfide (dimesna); dimesna rapidly eliminated by kidneys; dimesna reduced to free thiol compound (mesna) in the kidney; $t_{1/2}$ 0.36 hr (dimesna 1.17 hr)

INDICATIONS AND USES: Prevention of ifosfamide-induced and (cyclophosphamide-induced)* hemorrhagic cystitis

DOSAGE
Adult and Child

• IV give 20% of ifosfamide dosage (by weight) at the time of ifosfamide administration and 4 and 8 hr after each dose of ifosfamide

☒ AVAILABLE FORMS/COST OF THERAPY

• Inj, Sol—IV: 100 mg/ml, 10 ml: **$148.14-$1,850.00**

PRECAUTIONS: Children

PREGNANCY AND LACTATION: Pregnancy category B; use caution in nursing mothers

SIDE EFFECTS/ADVERSE REACTIONS

CNS: Fatigue, headache
CV: Hypotension

---

* = non-FDA-approved use

GI: Bad taste in mouth, diarrhea, nausea, soft stools, vomiting
MS: Limb pain

INTERACTIONS

Labs
• *False positive:* Urinary ketones, β-hydroxybutyrate

SPECIAL CONSIDERATIONS
MONITORING PARAMETERS
• Urinalysis each day prior to ifosfamide administration
• Reduction or discontinuation of ifosfamide may be initiated in patients developing hematuria (>50 RBC/hpf)

---

mesoridazine

(mez-oh-rid'a-zeen)

Rx: Serentil

Chemical Class: Piperidine phenothiazine derivative
Therapeutic Class: Antipsychotic

CLINICAL PHARMACOLOGY

Mechanism of Action: Dopamine receptor antagonist, with higher affinity for D_2- over D_1-receptors, and variable selectivity among the cortical dopamine tracts; also activity on nondopaminergic sites, i.e., cholinergic, α_1-adrenergic and histaminic receptors (explaining side effects); high rates of sedation and anticholinergic effects; moderate orthostatic hypotension; minimal risk of extrapyramidal reaction

Pharmacokinetics

PO: Peak 2-4 hr, onset 0.5-1 hr, duration 4-6 hr; 91%-99% bound to plasma proteins; metabolized in liver, eliminated mostly in urine; $t_{1/2}$ 24-48 hr

INDICATIONS AND USES: Schizophrenia; behavioral problems associated with mental deficiency and chronic brain syndrome; adjunctive treatment of alcoholism; personality disorders; anxiety and tension associated with neuroses

DOSAGE

NOTE: 50 mg equivalent to chlorpromazine 100 mg

Adult and Child>16yr

• *Schizophrenia:* PO 50 mg tid initially; usual range 100-400 mg/day
• *Mental deficiency, chronic brain syndrome:* PO 25 mg tid initially; usual range 75-300 mg/day
• *Alcoholism:* PO 25 mg bid initially; usual range 50-200 mg/day
• *Neuroses:* PO 10 mg tid initially; usual range 30-150 mg/day
• IM 25 mg as a single dose, may repeat in 30-60 min prn; do not exceed 200 mg/day

$ **AVAILABLE FORMS/COST OF THERAPY**

• Inj, Sol—IM: 25 mg/ml, 1 ml: **$6.60**
• Liq—Oral: 25 mg/ml, 120 ml: **$71.66**
• Tab, Plain Coated—Oral: 10 mg, 100's: **$82.85**; 25 mg, 100's: **$111.08**; 50 mg, 100's: **$113.35**; 100 mg, 100's: **$153.45**

CONTRAINDICATIONS: Severe CNS depression, coma

PRECAUTIONS: Children <12 yr, elderly, prolonged use, severe cardiovascular disorders, epilepsy, hepatic or renal disease, glaucoma, prostatic hypertrophy, hypocalcemia (increased susceptibility to dystonic reactions), COPD

PREGNANCY AND LACTATION: Pregnancy category C; bulk of evidence indicates that phenothiazines are safe for mother and fetus; effect on nursing infant is unknown, but may be of concern

SIDE EFFECTS/ADVERSE REACTIONS

CNS: Agitation, anxiety, confusion, depression, *drowsiness;* EPS (akathisia, dystonia, pseudoparkinsonism, tardive dyskinesia); euphoria, exacerbation of psychotic symptoms including catatonic-like behavioral states, hallucinations; heat or cold intolerance, *headache,* insomnia, lethargy, ***neuroleptic malignant syndrome,*** restlessness, ***seizures***

CV: ECG changes, hypertension, hypotension, tachycardia

EENT: Blurred vision, cataracts, dry eyes, glaucoma, pigmentation of retina or cornea, retinopathy, vertigo

GI: Anorexia, *constipation,* diarrhea, *dry mouth,* dyspepsia, hypersalivation, increased LFTs, *nausea,* vomiting

GU: Priapism, sexual dysfunction, urinary retention

HEME: **Agranulocytosis,** anemia, **aplastic anemia, hemolytic anemia,** minimal decreases in red blood cell counts; transient leukopenia, leukocytosis

METAB: Breast engorgement, gynecomastia, hypercholestreolemia, hyperglycemia, hypoglycemia, hyponatremia, impotence, increased libido, lactation, mastalgia, menstrual irregularities

RESP: **Bronchospasm,** increased depth of respiration, laryngospasm

SKIN: Diaphoresis, loss of hair, maculopapular and acneiform skin reactions, photosensitivity

INTERACTIONS

Drugs

3 *Anticholinergics:* Inhibited therapeutic response to antipsychotic; enhanced anticholinergic side effects

3 *Antidepressants:* Increased serum concentrations of some cyclic antidepressants

3 *Antimalarials:* Mesoridazine serum levels increased

3 *Attapulgite:* Reduced mesoridazine via decreased absorption

3 *Barbiturates:* Reduced effect of antipsychotic

3 *Beta-blockers:* Enhanced effects of both drugs

3 *Bromocriptine, lithium:* Reduced effects of both drugs

3 *Clonidine:* Hypotension

3 *Epinephrine:* Reversed pressor response to epinephrine

3 *Guanadrel:* Mesoridazine inhibits antihypertensive response

3 *Guanethidine:* Inhibited antihypertensive response to guanethidine

2 *Levodopa:* Inhibited effect of levodopa on Parkinson's disease

3 *Narcotic analgesics:* Excessive CNS depression, hypotension, respiratory depression

3 *Orphenadrine:* Reduced serum neuroleptic concentrations; excessive anticholinergic effects

3 *Phenylpropanolamine:* Case report of patient death on combination of these two drugs

SPECIAL CONSIDERATIONS
PATIENT/FAMILY EDUCATION

• Do not discontinue abruptly

• Concentrate may be diluted just prior to administration with distilled water, acidified tap water, orange or grape juice

MONITORING PARAMETERS

• Observe closely for signs of tardive dyskinesia

• Periodic CBC with platelets during prolonged therapy

metaproterenol

(met-a-proe-ter'e-nole)

Rx: Alupent

Chemical Class: Sympathomimetic amine; β_2-adrenergic agonist

Therapeutic Class: Antiasthmatic, bronchodilator

CLINICAL PHARMACOLOGY

Mechanism of Action: Causes bronchodilation by β_2-stimulation, resulting in relaxation of bronchial smooth muscle; inhibits mast cell degranulation; stimulates cilia to remove secretions

Pharmacokinetics

PO: Onset 15 min, peak 1 hr, duration 4 hr

INH: Onset 1 min (MDI), 5-30 min (neb), peak 1 hr, duration 4 hr

Metabolized in the liver, eliminated in urine (40% as unchanged drug)

INDICATIONS AND USES: Bronchial asthma, reversible bronchospasm associated with bronchitis and emphysema

DOSAGE

Adult

• PO 20 mg tid-qid; MDI 2-3 puffs q3-4h prn; NEB 5-15 inhalations of undiluted 5% sol or 0.2-0.3 ml of 5% sol diluted in 2.5-3 ml normal saline q4-6h (can be given more frequently according to need)

Child

• PO (<2 yr) 0.4 mg/kg/dose tid-qid, in infants the dose can be given q8-12h; (2-6 yr) 1-2.6 mg/kg/day divided q6-8h; (6-9 yr) 10 mg tid-qid; NEB 0.01-0.12 ml/kg of 5% sol (min dose 0.1 ml, max dose 0.3 ml) diluted in 2-3 ml normal saline q4-6h (may be given more frequently according to need)

$ **AVAILABLE FORMS/COST OF THERAPY**

• MDI—INH: 0.65 mg/puff, 200 puffs: **$26.00-$29.25**

• Sol—INH: 0.4%, 2 ml: **$0.48-$1.38**; 0.6%, 2 ml: **$0.71-$1.38**; 5%, 30 ml: **$29.25-$57.37**

• Syr—Oral: 10 mg/5 ml, 480 ml: **$7.52-$31.87**

• Tab, Uncoated—Oral: 10 mg, 100's: **$12.51-$36.47**; 20 mg, 100's: **$17.75-$51.80**

CONTRAINDICATIONS: Pre-existing cardiac dysrhythmias associated with tachycardia

PRECAUTIONS: Ischemic heart disease, cardiac dysrhythmias, hypertension, hyperthyroidism, diabetes mellitus

PREGNANCY AND LACTATION: Pregnancy category C; has been used to prevent premature labor; long-term evaluation of infants exposed *in utero* to β-agonists has been reported, but not specifically for metaproterenol, no harmful effects were observed

SIDE EFFECTS/ADVERSE REACTIONS

CNS: Anxiety, dizziness, headache, insomnia, nervousness, stimulation, tremors

*CV: **Cardiac arrest, dysrhythmias,** hypertension, palpitations, tachycardia*

EENT: Throat irritation

GI: Bad taste, GI distress, nausea, vomiting

METAB: Hypokalemia

MS: Muscle cramps in extremities

RESP: Cough, dyspnea

INTERACTIONS

Drugs

3 *Furosemide:* Potential for additive hypokalemia

2 *β-blockers:* Decreased action of metaproterenol, cardio selective beta-blockers preferable if concurrent use necessary

M

Labs
• *Glucose:* Urine, increase via Benedict's reagent
SPECIAL CONSIDERATIONS
PATIENT/FAMILY EDUCATION
• Proper inhalation technique is vital for MDIs
• Excessive use may lead to adverse effects
• Notify clinician if no response to usual doses

---

metaraminol

(met-ar-am′e-nol)
Rx: Aramine
Chemical Class: Synthetic catecholamine
Therapeutic Class: α-Adrenergic sympathomimetic amine; vasopressor

---

CLINICAL PHARMACOLOGY
Mechanism of Action: Increases both systolic and diastolic blood pressure, primarily by vasoconstriction, which is usually accompanied by marked reflex bradycardia; acts predominantly by a direct effect on α-adrenergic receptors; also has an indirect effect by releasing norepinephrine from its storage sites
Pharmacokinetics
IV: Onset 1-2 min, duration 20-60 min
IM: Onset 10 min, duration 20-60 min
SC: Onset 5-20 min, duration 20-60 min
Pharmacologic effect terminated principally by uptake into tissues and urinary excretion
INDICATIONS AND USES: Acute hypotensive states associated with spinal anesthesia, hemorrhage, reactions to medications, surgical complications; shock associated with brain damage resulting from

trauma or tumor; "probably effective" in hypotension due to cardiogenic shock or septicemia
DOSAGE
Adult
• SC/IM 2-10 mg; IV INF dilute 15-500 mg in 500 ml of D_5W or normal saline, administer at a rate adjusted to maintain desired blood pressure; IV 0.5-5 mg as a single dose in severe shock, follow with IV INF
Child
• SC/IM 0.1 mg/kg or 3 mg/m²; IV INF 0.4 mg/kg or 12 mg/m², diluted and administered at a rate adjusted to maintain desired blood pressure; IV 0.01 mg/kg or 0.3 mg/m² as a single dose in severe shock, follow with IV INF
$ **AVAILABLE FORMS/COST OF THERAPY**
• Inj, Sol—IM, IV, SC: 10 mg/ml, 10 ml: **$13.36-$14.00**
CONTRAINDICATIONS: Use with cyclopropane or halothane anesthesia
PRECAUTIONS: Prolonged administration, heart disease, thyroid disease, hypertension, diabetes, cirrhosis, extravasation (phentolamine is antidote), history of malaria (may provoke relapse), sulfite sensitivity
PREGNANCY AND LACTATION: Pregnancy category D; use could cause reduced uterine blood flow and fetal hypoxia
SIDE EFFECTS/ADVERSE REACTIONS
CNS: Apprehension, dizziness, headache, tremors
CV: ***Cardiac arrest;*** flushing, hypertension, hypotension (following cessation); palpitation; sinus tachycardia, ***ventricular tachycardia, other dysrhythmias***
GI: Nausea
SKIN: Extravasation (abscess, tissue necrosis, sloughing at inj site), sweating

---

* = non-FDA-approved use

INTERACTIONS
Drugs

3 *Guanethidine:* Reversed antihypertensive effects

2 *Halogenated hydrocarbon anesthetics:* Sensitized myocardium to the effects of catecholamines, arrhythmias possible

A *MAOIs:* Severe hypertensive response

3 *Oxytocic drugs:* Concomitant use may cause severe persistent hypertension

3 *Tricyclic antidepressant:* Vasopressor response decreased; higher sympathomimetic may be necessary

SPECIAL CONSIDERATIONS
MONITORING PARAMETERS

• Maximum effect is not immediately apparent; allow at least 10 min to elapse before increasing the dose
• BP and pulse

---

metaxalone

(me-tax′a-lone)
Rx: Skelaxin
Chemical Class: Oxazolidinone derivative
Therapeutic Class: Skeletal muscle relaxant

CLINICAL PHARMACOLOGY

Mechanism of Action: General CNS depressant; has no direct action on contractile mechanism of striated muscle, the motor endplate, or nerve fiber

Pharmacokinetics

PO: Peak 2 hr, onset 1 hr, duration 4-6 hr; metabolites excreted in urine; $t_{1/2}$ 2-3 hr

INDICATIONS AND USES: Adjunctive therapy to rest and physical therapy for acute, painful musculoskeletal conditions

DOSAGE
Adult and Child >12 yr

• PO 800 mg tid-qid

S **AVAILABLE FORMS/COST OF THERAPY**

• Tab, Uncoated—Oral: 400 mg, 100's: **$49.90-$89.11**

CONTRAINDICATIONS: Tendency to drug-induced hemolytic or other anemia; significantly impaired renal or hepatic function

PRECAUTIONS: Liver function impairment, children

SIDE EFFECTS/ADVERSE REACTIONS

CNS: Dizziness, *drowsiness,* headache, irritability, nervousness

GI: GI upset, jaundice, nausea, vomiting

HEME: **Hemolytic anemia, leukopenia**

SKIN: Hypersensitivity reaction (light rash with or without pruritus)

INTERACTIONS
Labs

• *False positive:* Glucose, urine via Benedict's reagent

---

metformin

(met-for′min)
Rx: Glucophage
Chemical Class: Biguanide
Therapeutic Class: Antidiabetic

CLINICAL PHARMACOLOGY

Mechanism of Action: Potentiates the effect of insulin; decreases hepatic glucose production, decreases intestinal glucose absorption, and improves insulin sensitivity by increasing peripheral glucose uptake and utilization; does not stimulate pancreatic β-cells to increase secretion of insulin; does not produce hypoglycemia by itself

M

Pharmacokinetics

PO: Peak 1-3 hr; 50%-60% bioavailable; food decreases the extent and delays the time to achieve maximum absorption; peak serum concentrations may be 40% lower; 90% excreted unchanged in urine; $t_{1/2}$ 6.2 hr; crosses placenta

INDICATIONS AND USES: Diabetes mellitus, type 2; polycystic ovary syndrome[*]

DOSAGE

Adult

• PO 250-500 mg qd-bid with meals; increase by 250-500 mg at 3-5 day-weekly intervals to 1000 mg bid
• Combination therapy: If after 4 wk and a 2 g daily dose of metformin, there is an inadequate response, sulfonylurea should be added; if at maximum doses of a sulfonylurea and metformin the patient still has an inadequate response, both agents should be stopped, and insulin should be started
• Adding metformin to insulin therapy: Continue current insulin dose; initial recommended dosage of metformin is 250-500 mg daily; increase by 250-500 mg/day at intervals of 1 wk or more; max dose is 2,000 mg/day; fasting plasma glucose concentrations below 120 mg/dL call for decreasing insulin dose by 10%-25% and closer monitoring
• Transferring sulfonylurea to metformin: (except chlorpropamide to metformin), no transition period is necessary; if transferring from chlorpropamide, careful monitoring for 2 wk due to an increased risk of hypoglycemia
• Geriatric dosing: Conservative initial and maintenance doses due to decreased renal function; make dosage adjustments carefully and conservatively; maximal doses should not be used

NOTE: Lower initiation doses (i.e., 250 mg qd) with gradual titration (i.e., 250 mg q3-5 days) may attenuate GI adverse effect

$ AVAILABLE FORMS/COST OF THERAPY

• Tab, Uncoated—Oral: 500 mg, 100's: **$59.24-$81.19**; 850 mg, 100's: **$100.27-$138.01**; 1000 mg, 100's: **$144.25-$167.24**

CONTRAINDICATIONS: Congestive heart failure requiring drug therapy, acute or chronic metabolic acidosis, including ketoacidosis, renal impairment (e.g., serum creatinine > 1.5 mg/dL in males; 1.4 mg/dL in females); during (temporarily) radiology studies using iodinated contrast media

PRECAUTIONS: Hypoxemia, dehydration, hepatic disease, severe congestive failure, fever, trauma, infection, megaloblastic anemia, thyroid disease, excessive alcohol intake; during and after surgical procedures

PREGNANCY AND LACTATION: Pregnancy category B; breast milk excretion unknown

SIDE EFFECTS/ADVERSE REACTIONS

CNS: Headache
GI: Abdominal bloating, anorexia, diarrhea, flatulence, metallic taste, *nausea, vomiting*
HEME: Megaloblastic anemia (impaired vitamin B_{12} absorption)
METAB: Hypoglycemia (rare); ***lactic acidosis (diarrhea; severe muscle pain, cramping; shallow and fast breathing, unusual tiredness and weakness, unusual sleepiness)***
SKIN: Dermatitis, rash

---

* = non-FDA-approved use

INTERACTIONS
Drugs
▪ *Cimetidine:* Increased metformin AUC 50%, peak concentrations 81%, and decreased renal clearance 27%, increasing the risk of lactic acidosis

▪ *Monoamine oxidase (MAO) inhibitors:* Stimulate insulin secretion via β-adrenergic stimulation; excessive and prolonged hypoglycemia may occur in some individuals

SPECIAL CONSIDERATIONS
• May also lower triglycerides
• May decrease insulin requirement in insulin-requiring diabetics

PATIENT/FAMILY EDUCATION
• Administer with food
• Avoid excessive alcohol
• Notify clinician of diarrhea, severe muscle pain or cramping, shallow and fast breathing, unusual tiredness and weakness, unusual sleepiness (signs of lactic acidosis)

MONITORING PARAMETERS
• Glycosylated hemoglobin q 3-6 mo (<7.0%); self-monitored preprandial blood sugars <150 mg/dL; absence of hyperglycemia (e.g., polyuria, polyphagia, polydipsia, blurred vision)
• Renal and hepatic function tests before and annually during therapy
• Serum vitamin B_{12} annually during chronic therapy

methacholine
(meth-a-ko'leen)
Rx: Provocholine
Chemical Class: Acetylcholine derivative
Therapeutic Class: Diagnostic agent

CLINICAL PHARMACOLOGY
Mechanism of Action: Causes bronchoconstriction; when inhaled in a sodium chloride solution, patients with asthma are significantly more sensitive to methacholine-induced bronchoconstriction than are healthy individuals

INDICATIONS AND USES: Diagnosis of bronchial airway hyperreactivity in subjects who do not have clinically apparent asthma (methacholine challenge test)

DOSAGE
Adult and Child >5 yr
• INH 5 inhalations at each of 5 concentrations in ascending order as follows: 0.025 mg/ml, 0.25 mg/ml, 2.5 mg/ml, 10 mg/ml, and 25 mg/ml (see monitoring parameters); administer via nebulizer that permits intermittent delivery time of 0.6 sec by either a Y-tube or a breath-actuated timing device; following the procedure, a β-agonist inhalation may be administered to help return FEV_1 to baseline and relieve patient discomfort

▪ **AVAILABLE FORMS/COST OF THERAPY**
• Powder—INH: 100 mg, 1's: **$299.63**

CONTRAINDICATIONS: Repeated challenge tests on the same day; use in patients receiving any β-adrenergic blocking agent

PRECAUTIONS: Epilepsy; cardiovascular disease accompanied by bradycardia; vagotonia; peptic ulcer

---

italic = common side effects   ***bold italic*** = life-threatening reactions

disease; thyroid disease; urinary tract obstruction; child <5 yr; **for diagnostic purposes only**

PREGNANCY AND LACTATION: Pregnancy category C

SIDE EFFECTS/ADVERSE REACTIONS

CNS: Headache, lightheadedness
EENT: Throat irritation
SKIN: Itching

INTERACTIONS

Drugs

3 *Beta-blockers:* Exaggerated response to methacholine challenge, prolonged recovery, poor response to treatment

SPECIAL CONSIDERATIONS
MONITORING PARAMETERS

• FEV_1 3-5 min after administration of each serial concentration; procedure is complete when there is a ≥20% reduction in FEV_1 compared to baseline (positive response) or when 5 inhalations have been administered at each concentration and FEV_1 has been reduced by ≤14% (negative response)

---

methadone

(meth′a-done)
Rx: Dolophine
Chemical Class: Synthetic opium alkaloid; diphenylheptane derivative
Therapeutic Class: Narcotic analgesic
DEA Class: Schedule II

CLINICAL PHARMACOLOGY

Mechanism of Action: Narcotic agonist with activity at Mu receptors (supraspinal analgesia, euphoria, respiratory and physical depression, miosis, and reduced GI motility), Kappa receptors (pentazocine-like spinal analgesia, sedation, and miosis), and Delta receptors (dysphoria, psychotomimetic effects [e.g., hallucinations], and respiratory and vasomotor stimulation caused by drugs with antagonist activity); compared to morphine, equal analgesia, antitussive, constipation, respiratory depression; less sedation, emesis, and physical dependence

Pharmacokinetics

PO: Onset 30-60 min, prolonged duration compared to parenteral therapy

IM: Onset 10-20 min, peak 30-60 min, duration 4-6 hr (22-48 hr after repeated administration)

SC: Onset 10-20 min, peak 50-90 min, duration 4-6 hr (22-48 hr after repeated administration)

Highly bound to tissue protein; metabolized by liver, eliminated in urine and feces; $t_{1/2}$ 13-47 hr

INDICATIONS AND USES: Severe pain; detoxification and maintenance of opiate dependence

DOSAGE

Adult

• *Pain:* SC/IM 2.5-10 mg q3-4h prn; PO 2.5-10 mg q6h prn; adjust dose according to severity of pain and response, tolerance of patient

• *Detoxification:* PO 15-40 mg/day should suppress withdrawal symptoms; reductions of 10%-20% qod usually tolerated; treatment should not exceed 21 days and may not be repeated earlier than 4 wk after completion of preceding course

• *Maintenance of opiate dependence:* PO 20-120 mg/day

Child

• *Pain:* PO/SC/IM 0.7 mg/kg/day divided q4-6h prn or 0.1-0.2 mg/kg q4-12h prn; max 10 mg/dose

💲 AVAILABLE FORMS/COST OF THERAPY

• Conc—Oral: 10 mg/ml, 946 ml: **$79.87-$103.99**

• Inj, Sol—IM, SC: 10 mg/ml, 20 ml: **$12.26-$15.89**

• Sol—Oral: 1 mg/ml, 500 ml: **$30.85**; 10 mg/5 ml, 500 ml: **$53.43**
• Tab, Uncoated—Oral: 5 mg, 100's: **$8.68-$34.16**; 10 mg, 100's: **$14.10-$38.86**; 40 mg, 100's: **$31.55-$37.75**

PRECAUTIONS: Head injury, increased intracranial pressure, acute abdominal conditions, elderly, severe impairment of hepatic or renal function, hypothyroidism, Addison's disease, prostatic hypertrophy, urethral stricture, history of drug abuse, acute asthma, upper airway obstruction

PREGNANCY AND LACTATION: Pregnancy category B (category D if used for prolonged periods or in high doses at term); compatible with breast feeding if mother consumes ≤20 mg/24 hr

SIDE EFFECTS/ADVERSE REACTIONS

CNS: Agitation, dependency, dizziness, *drowsiness,* lethargy, restlessness, *sedation*

CV: Bradycardia, orthostatic hypotension, palpitations, tachycardia

GI: Anorexia, constipation, increased amylase, *nausea, vomiting*

GU: Urinary retention

RESP: **Respiratory depression, respiratory paralysis**

SKIN: Excessive sweating, flushing, rash, urticaria

INTERACTIONS

Drugs

3 *Anticoagulants:* Potentiation of warfarin's anticoagulant effect

3 *Antihistamines, chloral hydrate, glutethimide, methocarbamol:* Enhanced depressant effects

3 *Barbiturates:* Additive respiratory and CNS depressant effects

3 *Carbamazepine, phenobarbital, primidone, rifampin:* Reduced serum methadone concentrations; increased symptoms associated with narcotic withdrawal

3 *Cimetidine:* Increased effect of narcotic analgesics

3 *Ethanol:* Additive CNS effects

3 *Neuroleptics:* Hypotension and excessive CNS depression

❷ *Phenytoin:* As with carbamazepine above

3 *Protease inhibitors:* Increased respiratory and CNS depression

Labs

• *Morphine:* Urine, increased

• *Pregnancy tests:* Urine, false positive (Gravindex)

• *False increase:* Amylase and lipase

SPECIAL CONSIDERATIONS

• **When used for the treatment of narcotic addiction in detoxification or maintenance programs, can only be dispensed by approved hospital pharmacies, approved community pharmacies, and maintenance programs approved by the Food and Drug Administration and the designated state authority**

• Do not administer agonist/antagonist analgesics (i.e., pentazocine, nalbuphine, butorphanol, dezocine, buprenorphine) to patient who has received a prolonged course of methadone (a pure agonist). In opioid-dependent patients, mixed agonist/antagonist analgesics may precipitate withdrawal symptoms.

PATIENT/FAMILY EDUCATION

• Change position slowly; orthostatic hypotension may occur

• Minimize nausea by administering with food and remain lying down following dose

M

---

methamphetamine

(meth-am-fet'a-meen)

Rx: Desoxyn

Chemical Class: Amphetamine derivative

Therapeutic Class: Anorexiant; CNS stimulant

DEA Class: Schedule II

CLINICAL PHARMACOLOGY

Mechanism of Action: Sympatho-mimetic amines with CNS stimulant activity increases release of norepi-nephrine from central noradrenergic neurons; at higher doses, dopamine may be released in the mesolimbic system; peripheral α- and β-activity includes elevation of systolic and di-astolic blood pressures and weak bronchodilator and respiratory stimulation action; heart rate re-flexly slowed at standard doses, ar-rhythmias with overdose

Pharmacokinetics

PO: Duration 8-24 hr; metabolized in liver to amphetamine (4%-7%) and other metabolites; eliminated in urine; biologic $t_{1/2}$ 4-5 hr (increased by alkaline urine)

INDICATIONS AND USES: Short-term adjunct to caloric restriction in exogenous obesity **(high potential for abuse, use only when alterna-tive therapies have failed);** atten-tion deficit disorder with hyperac-tivity

DOSAGE

Adult

• *Obesity:* PO 5 mg 30 min before each meal; sustained release PO 10-15 mg q AM; treatment duration should not exceed a few weeks

Child

• *Attention deficit disorder with hy-peractivity:* PO 5 mg qd-bid ini-tially; increase in increments of 5 mg/day at weekly intervals until an optimum response is achieved; usual effective dose 20-25 mg/day (divided bid with conventional tab-lets or qd with sustained release for-mulations)

$ AVAILABLE FORMS/COST OF THERAPY

• Tab, Uncoated—Oral: 5 mg, 100's: **$89.11**; 10 mg, 100's: **$300.00**

• Tab, Uncoated, Sus Action—Oral: 5 mg, 100's: **$208.27**; 10 mg, 100's: **$270.41**; 15 mg, 100's: **$344.95**

CONTRAINDICATIONS: Hyper-thyroidism, moderate to severe hy-pertension, glaucoma, severe arte-riosclerosis, history of drug abuse, symptomatic cardiovascular dis-ease, agitated states, within 14 days of MAOI administration

PRECAUTIONS: Mild hyperten-sion, child <3 yr, Tourette's disor-der, motor and phonic tics, tartrazine sensitivity (15 mg sustained release preparation)

PREGNANCY AND LACTATION: Pregnancy category C; use of am-phetamine for medical indications does not pose a significant risk to the fetus for congenital anomalies; mild withdrawal symptoms may be ob-served in the newborn; illicit mater-nal use presents significant risks to the fetus and newborn including in-trauterine growth retardation, pre-mature delivery, and the potential for increased maternal, fetal, and neonatal morbidity; concentrated in breast milk; contraindicated during breast feeding

SIDE EFFECTS/ADVERSE REAC-TIONS

CNS: Addiction, aggressiveness, changes in libido, chills, depen-dence, dizziness, dyskinesia, dys-phoria, euphoria, headache, *hyper-activity, insomnia,* irritability, over-stimulation, psychotic episodes, *restlessness,* talkativeness, tremor

CV: ***Arrhythmias*** (at larger doses), dysrhythmias, hypertension, *palpitations,* reflex decrease in heart rate, *tachycardia*

GI: Anorexia, constipation, cramps, diarrhea, dry mouth, metallic taste, nausea, vomiting, weight loss

GU: Impotence

METAB: Reversible elevations in serum thyroxine (T_4) with heavy use

SKIN: Urticaria

INTERACTIONS
Drugs

3 *Acetazolamide:* Increased serum amphetamine concentrations and prolonged amphetamine effects

3 *Antidepressants:* Increased effect of amphetamines, clinical evidence lacking

3 *Furazolidone:* Hypertensive reactions

3 *Guanadrel, guanethidine:* Inhibition of the antihypertensive response

▲ *MAOIs:* Severe hypertensive reactions possible

3 *Selegiline:* Potential for enhanced pressor effect if used in combination

3 *Sodium bicarbonate:* Large doses of sodium bicarbonate inhibit the elimination and increase the effect of amphetamines

Labs

• *Amino acids:* Urine, increased

• *Amphetamine:* Urine, positive at 1.0 µg/ml

SPECIAL CONSIDERATIONS
PATIENT/FAMILY EDUCATION

• Take early in the day

• Do not discontinue abruptly

• Avoid hazardous activities until stabilized on medication

• Avoid OTC preparations unless approved by clinician

---

methazolamide
(meth-ah-zole′ah-mide)
Rx: Neptazane
Chemical Class: Carbonic anhydrase inhibitor; sulfonamide derivative
Therapeutic Class: Antiglaucoma agent

CLINICAL PHARMACOLOGY
Mechanism of Action: Kidney: Increased excretion of sodium, potassium, bicarbonate, and water—alkaline diuresis; *CNS:* reduction in rate of aqueous humor formation—decreased intraocular pressure (IOP)

Pharmacokinetics

PO: Onset 2-4 hr, peak 6-8 hr, duration 10-18 hr; 55% bound to plasma proteins; partially metabolized in liver, excreted in urine; $t_{1/2}$ 14 hr

INDICATIONS AND USES: Adjunctive treatment of open-angle glaucoma; preoperatively in acute angle-closure glaucoma when delay of surgery is desired to lower intraocular pressure; acute mountain sickness

DOSAGE
Adult

• PO 50-100 mg bid-tid

$ **AVAILABLE FORMS/COST OF THERAPY**

• Tab, Uncoated—Oral: 25 mg, 100's: **$27.13-$71.68**; 50 mg, 100's: **$65.44-$106.98**

CONTRAINDICATIONS: Renal disease, severe hepatic disease, electrolyte imbalance (hyponatremia, hypokalemia, hyperchloremic acidosis), adrenalcortical insufficiency, cirrhosis, long-term use in angle-closure glaucoma

PRECAUTIONS: Children, severe loss of respiratory capacity, diabetes mellitus, hypercalciuria, gout

---

PREGNANCY AND LACTATION:
Pregnancy category C

SIDE EFFECTS/ADVERSE REACTIONS

CNS: Ataxia, confusion, depression, dizziness, drowsiness, excitement, fatigue, flaccid paralysis, headache, irritability, lassitude, malaise, nervousness, *paresthesia,* sedation, *seizures,* tremor, vertigo

EENT: Altered smell, myopia, tinnitus

GI: Abdominal distention, altered taste, *anorexia,* constipation, diarrhea, dry mouth, excessive thirst, *nausea, vomiting,* weight loss

GU: Crystalluria, dysuria, glycosuria, hematuria, phosphaturia, polyuria, renal calculi, renal colic, sulfonamide-like renal lesions, *urinary frequency*

HEME: **Agranulocytosis, aplastic anemia, hemolytic anemia, leukopenia, thrombocytopenia**

METAB: Hyperglycemia, hypokalemia, increased serum uric acid

MS: Muscular weakness

SKIN: **Exfoliative dermatitis,** photosensitivity, pruritus, rash, skin eruptions, urticaria

INTERACTIONS

Drugs

3 *Amphetamines:* Increased amphetamine serum concentrations and prolonged effects

3 *Antiarrhythmics (flecainide, mexiletine):* Alkalinization of urine increases concentrations of these drugs

3 *Cyclosporine:* Increased trough cyclosporine levels with potential for neurotoxicity and nephropathy

3 *Ephedrine:* Increased ephedrine concentrations

3 *Methenamine compounds:* Interference with antibacterial activity

3 *Phenytoin:* Increased risk of osteomalacia with prolonged use of both agents

3 *Quinidine:* Alkalinization of urine increases quinidine concentrations

2 *Salicylates:* Increased concentrations of methazolamide leading to CNS toxicity; also see furosemide for other general diuretic interactions

Labs

• *Increase:* Blood glucose levels, bilirubin, blood ammonia, calcium, chloride

• *Decrease:* Urine citrate, serum potassium

• *False positive:* Urinary protein

SPECIAL CONSIDERATIONS

PATIENT/FAMILY EDUCATION

• Take with food if GI upset occurs

MONITORING PARAMETERS

• Intraocular pressure, reduction in AMS symptoms, serum electrolytes, creatinine, CO_2

---

methenamine

(meth-en´a-meen)

Rx: *Hippurate:* Hiprex, Urex
Mandelate: Mandelamine
Chemical Class: Formaldehyde precursors
Therapeutic Class: Urinary anti-infectives

CLINICAL PHARMACOLOGY

Mechanism of Action: Hydrolyzed by acids to form formaldehyde and ammonia; formaldehyde is a nonspecific antibacterial agent that is bactericidal in action; acid portions of methenamine salts (hippuric acid, mandelic acid) have some non-specific bacteriostatic activity and may enhance liberation of formaldehyde by maintaining urinary acidity

---

* = non-FDA-approved use

Pharmacokinetics

PO: Peak formaldehyde concentrations in acid urine in 2-8 hr; some hepatic metabolism (10%-25%), 70%-90% excreted unchanged in urine; $t_{1/2}$ 3-6 hr

INDICATIONS AND USES: Prophylaxis or suppression of recurrent UTI **(should not be used alone for acute infections)**

DOSAGE

Adult

• *Hippurate:* PO 1 g bid
• *Mandelate:* PO 1 g qid ac and hs

Child 6-12 yr

• *Hippurate:* PO 25-50 mg/kg/day divided q12h
• *Mandelate:* PO 50-75 mg/kg/day divided q6h

§ AVAILABLE FORMS/COST OF THERAPY

Methenamine Hippurate
• Tab, Uncoated—Oral: 1 g, 100's: **$43.83-$144.76**
Methenamine Mandelate
• Susp—Oral: 500 mg/5 ml, 480 ml: **$38.80-$55.05**
• Tab, Enteric Coated—Oral: 500 mg, 100's: **$1.59-$43.35**; 1 g 100's: **$6.95-$69.33**

CONTRAINDICATIONS: Renal insufficiency, severe hepatic impairment (hippurate), severe dehydration (hippurate)

PRECAUTIONS: Tartrazine sensitivity (Hiprex tablets), patients susceptible to lipoid pneumonitis (mandelate susp)

PREGNANCY AND LACTATION: Pregnancy category C; excreted into breast milk; no adverse effects on nursing infants have been reported

SIDE EFFECTS/ADVERSE REACTIONS

CNS: Headache
CV: Edema
EENT: Tinnitus
GI: Abdominal cramps, anorexia, diarrhea, nausea, stomatitis; transient elevations in serum AST and ALT (hippurate), *vomiting*
GU: Dysuria, hematuria
MS: Muscle cramps
SKIN: Pruritus, rash, urticaria

INTERACTIONS

Drugs

3 *Acetazolamide:* Acetazolamide interferes with the urinary antibacterial activity of methenamine

3 *Antacids (magnesium, aluminum, sodium bicarbonate):* Interfere with urinary antibacterial activity of methenamine

3 *Sulfadiazine (sulfamethizole, sulfathiazole):* Combination may yield crystalluria

Labs

• *Catecholamines:* Plasma, increased
• *Estriol:* Urine, decreased
• *Estrogens:* Urine, decreased
• *PSP Excretion:* Urine, increased
• *Sugar:* Urine, increased via Benedict's reagent
• *Urobilinogen:* Urine, increased

SPECIAL CONSIDERATIONS

PATIENT/FAMILY EDUCATION

• Keep urine acidic (pH <5.5) by eating food that acidifies urine (meats, eggs, fish, gelatin products, prunes, plums, cranberries); may need to add ascorbic acid
• Fluids must be increased to 3 L/day to avoid crystallization in kidneys
• Take at evenly spaced intervals around clock for best results

MONITORING PARAMETERS

• Periodic liver function tests (hippurate); urine pH

M

---

italic = common side effects   ***bold italic*** = life-threatening reactions

methicillin

(meth-i-sill'in)
Rx: Staphcillin
Chemical Class: Semisynthetic
penicillinase-resistant penicillin
Therapeutic Class: Antibiotic

CLINICAL PHARMACOLOGY
Mechanism of Action: Inhibits biosynthesis of cell wall mucopeptide in susceptible organisms; the cell wall, rendered osmotically unstable, swells and bursts from osmotic pressure; bactericidal when adequate concentrations are reached; resistant to inactivation by most staphylococcal penicillinases

Pharmacokinetics
IM: Peak 30-60 min, duration 4 hr
IV: Peak 15 min, duration 2 hr
30%-50% bound to plasma proteins; not metabolized to any appreciable extent, excreted in urine; $t_{1/2}$ 0.4-0.5 hr (normal renal function)

INDICATIONS AND USES: Infections of the upper and lower respiratory tract, skin and skin structures, bones and joints, urinary tract; meningitis, septicemia and endocarditis caused by penicillinase-producing staphylococci; perioperative prophylaxis*

Antibacterial spectrum usually includes:

• Gram positive organisms: Penicillinase-producing and non-penicillinase-producing strains of *Staphylococcus aureus, S. epidermis, S. saprophyticus:* groups A, B, C, and G streptococci, *Streptococcus pneumoniae,* some viridans streptococci, *Bacillus anthracis*

DOSAGE
Adult
• IM 1 g q4-6h; IV 1 g q6h
• *Endocarditis, acute or chronic osteomyelitis:* IV 1.5-2 g q4h

• *Dose adjustment in renal impairment:* Administer q8-12h for CrCl <10 ml/min

Child
• IM/IV 150-200 mg/kg/day divided q6h, 200-400 mg/kg/day divided q4-6h has been used for severe infections, max 12 g/day

$ AVAILABLE FORMS/COST OF THERAPY
• Inj, Dry-Sol—IM, IV: 1 g/vial, 10's: **$61.44**; 4 g/vial, 10's: **$533.28**; 10 g/vial, 10's: **$223.80**

PRECAUTIONS: Hypersensitivity to cephalosporins, renal insufficiency, prolonged or repeated therapy, neonates

PREGNANCY AND LACTATION: Pregnancy category B; potential exists for modification of bowel flora in nursing infant; allergy/sensitization and interference with interpretation of culture results if fever workup required

SIDE EFFECTS/ADVERSE REACTIONS
CNS: Chills, fever, headache
CV: Phlebitis, thrombophlebitis
GI: Increased AST, ALT
GU: Hemorrhagic cystitis, interstitial nephritis, nephropathy
*HEME: **Eosinophilia, granulocytopenia, hemolytic anemia, leukopenia, neutropenia,** positive Coombs test, **thrombocytopenia***
MS: Myalgia
SKIN: Pain at inj site, pruritis, rash, sterile abscess at inj site
MISC: Serum sickness-like reactions

INTERACTIONS
Drugs
3 *Chloramphenicol:* Inhibited antibacterial activity of methicillin; ensure adequate amounts of both agents are given and administer methicillin a few hours before chloramphenicol

3 *Macrolides (clarithromycin, erythromycin, azithromycin, dirithromycin):* Inhibit bacterial activity of methicillin

3 *Methotrexate:* Increased serum methotrexate concentrations

3 *Oral contraceptives:* Occasional impairment of oral contraceptive efficacy; consider use of supplementary contraception during cycles in which methicillin is used

3 *Probenecid:* Increased methicillin concentrations

3 *Tetracyclines:* Inhibited antibacterial activity of methicillin; ensure adequate amounts of both agents are given and administer methicillin a few hours before tetracycline

3 *Warfarin:* Inhibition of hypoprothrombinemic response via metabolism enhancement

Labs
• *Phosphate:* Serum, increased
• *Protein:* CSF, increased
• *Triglycerides:* Serum, increased

SPECIAL CONSIDERATIONS
• Because acute interstitial nephritis has been reported more frequently with methicillin, nafcillin or oxacillin may be preferable
• Should not be used for organisms susceptible to penicillin G

MONITORING PARAMETERS
• Urinalysis, BUN, serum creatinine, CBC with differential, periodic liver function tests

---

methimazole
(meth-im′a-zole)
Rx: Tapazole
Chemical Class: Thioimidazole derivative
Therapeutic Class: Antithyroid agent

CLINICAL PHARMACOLOGY
Mechanism of Action: Inhibits synthesis of thyroid hormones by interfering with the incorporation of iodine into tyrosyl residues of thyroglobulin; does not inhibit action of already-formed or exogenously administered thyroid hormones; partially inhibits peripheral conversion of T_4 to T_3

Pharmacokinetics
PO: Peak 1 hr; onset 30-40 min; excreted in urine; $t_{1/2}$ 6-13 hr

INDICATIONS AND USES: Hyperthyroidism; preparation for thyroidectomy or radioactive iodine therapy

DOSAGE
Adult
• PO 15-60 mg/day divided q8h initially, 5-15 mg/day maintenance × 18-24 months; single daily doses (30-40 mg) are as effective as divided doses

Child
• PO 0.4 mg/kg/day in 3 divided doses initially, 0.2 mg/kg/day in 3 divided doses maintenance × 18-24 months; single daily doses (30-40 mg) are as effective as divided doses

$ **AVAILABLE FORMS/COST OF THERAPY**
• Tab, Uncoated—Oral: 5 mg, 100's: **$18.38-$53.33**; 10 mg, 100's: **$68.54-$92.13**

PRECAUTIONS: Thyroid storm, infection, bone marrow depression, hepatic disease

M

PREGNANCY AND LACTATION:
Pregnancy category D; use smallest possible dose to control maternal disease (propylthiouracil preferable, less likely to cross the placenta); excreted into breast milk

SIDE EFFECTS/ADVERSE REACTIONS

CNS: CNS stimulation, depression, drowsiness, headache, neuritis, neuropathies, paresthesias, vertigo

CV: Edema

GI: Epigastric distress, hepatitis, jaundice, loss of taste, *nausea,* sialadenopathy, *vomiting*

GU: Nephritis

HEME: **Agranulocytosis, aplastic anemia, granulocytopenia, hypoprothrombinemia, leukopenia, thrombocytopenia,** lymphadenopathy

METAB: Insulin autoimmune syndrome (may result in **hypoglycemic coma**)

MS: Arthralgia, myalgia

RESP: Interstitial pneumonitis

SKIN: Abnormal hair loss, erythema nodosum, **exfoliative dermatitis,** lupus-like syndrome, pruritis, skin pigmentation, rash, urticaria

INTERACTIONS

Drugs

3 *Oral anticoagulants:* Reduced hypoprothrombinemic response to oral anticoagulants

3 *Theophylline:* Physiologic response to antithyroid drug will increase theophylline concentrations via decreased clearance

Labs

• *False increase:* Glucose

SPECIAL CONSIDERATIONS

• Methimazole is the thioamide of choice based on improved patient adherence and outcomes

PATIENT/FAMILY EDUCATION

• Notify clinician of fever, sore throat, unusual bleeding or bruising, rash, yellowing of skin, vomiting

MONITORING PARAMETERS

• CBC periodically during therapy (especially during initial 3 mo), TSH

---

methocarbamol

(meth-oh-kar′ba-mole)

Rx: Robaxin, Robaxin-750
Combinations

  Rx: with aspirin (Robaxisal)

Chemical Class: Carbamate derivative

Therapeutic Class: Skeletal muscle relaxant

CLINICAL PHARMACOLOGY

Mechanism of Action: General CNS depressant; no direct action on contractile mechanism of striated muscle, motor endplate, or nerve fiber

Pharmacokinetics

PO: Peak 2 hr, onset 30 min; extensively metabolized by liver, excreted in urine and small amounts in feces; $t_{1/2}$ 1-2 hr

INDICATIONS AND USES: Adjunctive therapy to rest and physical therapy for acute painful musculoskeletal conditions; tetanus

DOSAGE

Adult

• *Musculoskeletal conditions:* PO 1.5 g qid for 2-3 days, then decrease to 4-4.5 g/day in 3-6 divided doses; IM/IV 1 g q8h, max 3 g/day for 3 consecutive days (unless treating tetanus), may be reinstituted after 2 drug-free days

---

* = non-FDA-approved use

• *Tetanus:* IV 1-2 g, followed by additional 1-2 g (max 3 g total); repeat with 1-2 g q6h until nasogastric tube or PO therapy possible; total daily dose of up to 24 g may be needed

Child

• *Tetanus:* IV 15 mg/kg/dose or 500 mg/m²/dose; may repeat q6h prn; max 1.8 g/m²/day for 3 days only

§ AVAILABLE FORMS/COST OF THERAPY

• Inj, Sol—IM, IV: 100 mg/ml, 10 ml: **$2.50-$15.77**
• Tab, Plain Coated—Oral: 500 mg, 100's: **$2.64-$71.58**; 750 mg, 100's: **$3.70-$102.30**

CONTRAINDICATIONS: Known or suspected renal pathology (parenteral)

PRECAUTIONS: Child <12 yr, extravasation, seizure disorder (inj)

PREGNANCY AND LACTATION: Pregnancy category C; compatible with breast feeding

SIDE EFFECTS/ADVERSE REACTIONS

CNS: Dizziness, drowsiness, fever, headache, *lightheadedness,* ***seizures*** (IV administration), vertigo

CV: Bradycardia, flushing, hypotension, syncope

EENT: Blurred vision, conjunctivitis, diplopia, nasal congestion, nystagmus

GI: Anorexia, GI upset, metallic taste, nausea

HEME: **Leukopenia** (rare), small amount of hemolysis (IV administration)

SKIN: Extravasation (thrombophlebitis, sloughing, pain at injection site), pruritus, rash, skin eruptions, urticaria

MISC: Muscular incoordination

INTERACTIONS

Labs

• *Color:* Urine brown, green, blue or black on standing

• *5-hydroxyindole acetic acid:* Urine, increased
• *Vanillylmandelic acid (VMA):* Urine, increased

---

methotrexate

(meth-oh-trex′ate)
Rx: Folex, Mexate, Rheumatrex, Trexall
Chemical Class: Dihydrofolate reductase inhibitor
Therapeutic Class: Antineoplastic; antipsoriatic; disease-modifying antirheumatic drug (DMARD)

CLINICAL PHARMACOLOGY

Mechanism of Action: Reversibly inhibits dihydrofolate reductase, the enzyme that reduces folic acid to tetrahydrofolic acid; limits the availability of one-carbon fragments necessary for synthesis of purines and the conversion of deoxyuridylate to thymidylate in the synthesis of DNA and cell reproduction; also has immunosuppressive activity

Pharmacokinetics

IM/IV: Peak 0.5-2 hr

PO: Peak 1-4 hr

Widely distributed into body tissues; 50% bound to plasma proteins; does not appear to be appreciably metabolized; excreted primarily by kidneys and small amounts in feces; t½ 3-10 hr

INDICATIONS AND USES: Abortion—therapeutic,* arthritis-rheumatoid, asthma,* bladder carcinoma,* brain cancer,* breast cancer, bullous phemphigoid,* Burkitt's lymphoma, cardinomatous meningitis,* cerebral vasculitis,* cervical carcinoma,* choriocarcinoma,* cochleovestibular disorders,* Crohn's disease,* cutaneous lupus erythematosus,* dermatomyositis,* diffuse large cell lymphoma, ectopic pregnancy,* esophageal cancer,* Felty's syndrome,* gestational trophoblastic neoplasms, graft vs. host disease,* head and neck cancer, hepatitis—idiopathic granulomatous,* inflammatory bowel disease,* leukemia - acute lymphocytic,* acute myelogenous,* chronic myelogenous,* meningeal*; lymphona—Hodgkin's,* mantle cell,* meningeal,* non-Hodgkin's, intraocular*; lymphomatoid papulosis,* mesothelioma,* multiple sclerosis,* osteogenic sarcoma, polymyalgia rheumatica,* primary biliary cirrhosis,* primary sclerosing cholangitis,* psoriasis,* pyoderma gangrenosum,* rejection cardiac transplant,* Reiter's syndrome,* reticulohistiocytosis—multicentric,* retinoblastoma,* sarcoidosis,* S Aaezary syndrome,* Still's disease,* Takayasu's disease,* toxoplasmosis chorioretinitis,* vasculitis,* Wegener's granuloma*

DOSAGE

NOTE: Administration and dosage vary significantly depending on the diagnosis and indication for drug use; check carefully

Adult

• *Abortion—therapeutic:* IM/PO 50 mg/m^2, followed by PV misoprostol 800 mg 7 days later; misoprostol may not be necessary

• *Trophoblastic neoplasms:* PO/IM 15-30 mg qd for 5 days; repeat 3-5 times as required, with rest periods of 1 or more wk interposed between courses

• *Acute lymphoblastic leukemias:* PO 3.3 mg/m^2 in combination with 60 mg/m^2 of prednisone qd for 4-6 wk to induce remission (not drug of choice for induction); IM/PO 20-30 mg/m^2/wk divided twice weekly or IV 2.5 mg/kg q14 days for maintenance therapy

• *Meningeal leukemia:* Intrathecal 12 mg/m^2; max 15 mg at 2-5 day intervals until the cell count of the CSF returns to normal, then 1 additional dose (use preservative-free preparation only)

• *Burkitt's lymphoma:* PO 10-25 mg/day for 4-8 days; usually given as several courses interposed with 7-10 day rest periods

• *Mycosis fungoides:* PO 2.5-10 mg/day for weeks to months; IM 50 mg qwk or 25 mg twice weekly

• *Psoriasis:* PO/IM/IV 10-25 mg qwk or PO 2.5 mg q12h for 3 doses each wk; adjust gradually to achieve optimal clinical response; max 30 mg/wk; once response achieved reduce to lowest possible effective dose

• *Rheumatoid arthritis:* PO 7.5 mg qwk or 2.5 mg q12h for 3 doses each wk; adjust gradually to achieve an optimal response; max 20 mg/wk; once response achieved reduce to lowest possible effective dose

Child

• *Acute lymphoblastic leukemias:* Same as adult

• *Meningeal leukemia:* Intrathecal (≤3 mo) 3 mg, (4-11 mo) 6 mg, (1 yr) 8 mg, (2 yr) 10 mg at 2-5 day intervals until the cell count of the CSF returns to normal, then 1 additional dose (use preservative-free preparation only)

• *Rheumatoid arthritis:* PO/IM 5-15 mg/m^2/wk as a single dose or in 3 divided doses given 12 hr apart

§ **AVAILABLE FORMS/COST OF THERAPY**

• Inj, Lyphl-Sol—Intrathecal: 25 mg/vial, 2 ml: **$4.38-$15.20**

---

* = non-FDA-approved use

• Inj, Sol—IM, IV: 25 mg/ml, 2 ml: **$4.38-$15.20**; 4 ml: **$5.13-$30.18**; 8 ml: **$7.44-$59.10**; 10 ml: **$9.38-$70.19**

• Tab, Uncoated—Oral: 2.5 mg, 100's: **$269.45-$525.41**; 5 mg, 30's: **$228.80**; 7.5 mg, 30's: **$343.20**; 10 mg, 30's: **$457.60**; 15 mg, 30's: **$686.40**

CONTRAINDICATIONS: Severe renal or hepatic impairment, pre-existing profound bone marrow depression

PRECAUTIONS: Infection, peptic ulcer, ulcerative colitis, elderly, pre-existing bone marrow suppression, renal or hepatic impairment, ascites, pleural effusion, dehydration

PREGNANCY AND LACTATION: Pregnancy category D; contraindicated in breast feeding

SIDE EFFECTS/ADVERSE REACTIONS

CNS: Dizziness, drowsiness, headache, malaise, *seizures*

EENT: Blurred vision, eye discomfort, tinnitus

GI: Abdominal distress, *anorexia,* diarrhea, enteritis, gingivitis, glossitis, hematemesis, *hepatotoxicity,* melena, *nausea,* pharyngitis, *stomatitis,* ulcerations and bleeding of the mucous membranes of the mouth or other portion of the GI tract, *vomiting*

GU: Azotemia, defective spermatogenesis, hematuria, menstrual irregularities, *renal failure,* uric acid nephropathy, urinary retention

HEME: **Anemia, hemorrhage, leukopenia, pancytopenia, thrombocytopenia**

METAB: Increased serum uric acid

MS: Arthralgia, myalgia, osteoporosis

RESP: Pneumonitis, *pulmonary fibrosis*

SKIN: Acne, *alopecia,* depigmentation, dermatitis, ecchymoses, *erythematous rashes,* folliculitis, furunculosis, hyperpigmentation, petechiae, photosensitivity, pruritus, telangiectasia, urticaria, vasculitis

MISC: Effects following intrathecal administration (headache, back pain, nuchal rigidity, fever, paresis, leukoencephalopathy)

INTERACTIONS

Drugs

3 *Aminoglycosides, oral (neomycin, vancomycin):* Reduction of 30-50% in methotrexate absorption in patient receiving concurrent oral aminoglycosides

3 *Antimalarials (chloroquine, hydroxychloroquine):* Methotrexate concentrations reduced by concurrent antimalarial administration

3 *Binding resins:* Reduced methotrexate concentrations

3 *Co-trimoxazole, omeprazole, penicillins:* Increased methotrexate concentrations, possible toxicity

3 *Cyclosporine:* Increased toxicity of both agents

3 *Ethanol:* Increased risk of methotrexate-induced liver injury

3 *Etretinate:* Increased risk of hepatotoxicity

❷ *NSAIDs, probenecid, salicylates, sulfinpyrazone, trimethoprim/sulfamethoxazole:* Increased methotrexate concentrations, possible toxicity

⚠ *Vaccines:* Increased risk of infection following use of live vaccines; reduced seroconversion rate to vaccine

Labs

• *Alanine aminotransferase:* Serum, decreased

• *Alkaline phosphatase:* Serum, increased

• *Bilirubin:* Serum, increased

• *Cholesterol:* Serum, increased

• *Color:* Feces, black

---

italic = common side effects   ***bold italic*** = life-threatening reactions

• *Ethanol:* Serum, increased
• *Lactate dehydrogenase:* Serum, decreased
• *Phosphate:* Serum, increased
• *Protein:* CSF, increased
• *Triglycerides:* Serum, decreased
• *Uric acid:* Serum, decreased

SPECIAL CONSIDERATIONS
PATIENT/FAMILY EDUCATION
• Notify clinician of black, tarry stools, chills, fever, sore throat, bleeding, bruising, cough, shortness of breath, dark or bloody urine
• Hair may be lost during treatment
• Drink 10-12 glasses of fluid/day
• Avoid alcohol, salicylates

MONITORING PARAMETERS
• Tumor response: Objective remissions are usually associated with a 50% decrease in the size of solid tumor as measured by physical measurement or test parameter (e.g., chest X-ray). After intrathecal administration, clearing of malignant cells in the cerebrospinal fluid indicates a positive response
• Rheumatoid arthritis: Tender, swollen joints, visual analogue scale for pain; acute phase reactants (ESR, C-reactive protein), duration of early morning stiffness, preservation of function
• CBC and platelets at 7, 10, and 14 days postdrug administration/injection; due to the possibility of early-onset pancytopenia, a lower initial dose for rheumatoid arthritis treatment along with intensified monitoring during early therapy is recommended—CBC's at 1, 2, and 4 wk of treatment; if stable dose may be increased and subsequent CBC's should be performed at monthly intervals
• BUN, serum uric acid, urine ClCr, electrolytes before, during therapy
• Liver function tests before and during therapy

---

methotrimeprazine

(meth-oh-trye-mep′ra-zeen)
Rx: Levoprome
Chemical Class: Phenothiazine derivative
Therapeutic Class: Nonnarcotic analgesic; anxiolytic; sedative

CLINICAL PHARMACOLOGY
Mechanism of Action: Depresses subcortical area of the brain at the levels of the thalamus, hypothalamus, and reticular and limbic systems; suppresses sensory impulses, reduces motor activity, alters temperature regulation, causes sedation and tranquilization; appears to have some analgesic effects possibly by raising pain threshold

Pharmacokinetics
IM: Maximum analgesia 20-40 min, duration 4 hr; metabolized in liver, excreted primarily in urine (metabolites); $t_{1/2}$ 15-30 hr

INDICATIONS AND USES: Moderate to severe pain in nonambulatory patients; preoperative sedation; analgesia and sedation during labor

DOSAGE
Adult
• *Analgesia:* IM 10-20 mg q4-6h; max 40 mg/dose
• *Preoperative sedation:* IM 2-20 mg 0.75-3 hr prior to surgery
• *Labor:* IM 15-20 mg

$ **AVAILABLE FORMS/COST OF THERAPY**
• Inj, Sol—IM: 20 mg/ml, 10 ml: **$191.06**

CONTRAINDICATIONS: Severe renal, cardiac, or hepatic disease; seizure disorders; coma; during overdoses of CNS depressants; child <12 yr; clinically significant hypotension

---

* = non-FDA-approved use

PRECAUTIONS: Ambulatory patients (can cause substantial orthostatic hypotension), elderly, use for >30 days, sulfite sensitivity

PREGNANCY AND LACTATION: Pregnancy category C; does not affect force, duration, and frequency of uterine contractions during labor

SIDE EFFECTS/ADVERSE REACTIONS

CNS: Amnesia, disorientation, drowsiness, euphoria, excessive sedation, extrapyramidal reactions, headache, *seizures,* slurred speech, weakness

CV: Bradycardia, *orthostatic hypotension* (fainting, weakness, dizziness), palpitation, tachycardia

EENT: Blurred vision, nasal congestion

GI: Abdominal discomfort, anorexia, dry mouth, *hepatotoxicity,* jaundice, nausea, vomiting

GU: Dysuria, hematuria, hesitancy, retention, uterine inertia (rare)

HEME: Agranulocytosis, hemolytic anemia (long-term, high dose), *leukopenia, neutropenia, thrombocytopenia*

RESP: Respiratory depression

SKIN: Pain at inj site

INTERACTIONS

Drugs

⚠ *MAOIs:* Coadministration with pargyline associated with fatality in 1 reported case

Labs

• *Ferric chloride test:* Urine, positive

• *Phenylketones:* Urine, positive

SPECIAL CONSIDERATIONS
MONITORING PARAMETERS

• CBC with differential and platelets; liver function tests during prolonged therapy

methoxamine
(meth-ox′a-meen)
Rx: Vasoxyl
Chemical Class: Synthetic catecholamine
Therapeutic Class: Sympathomimetic amine, vasopressor

CLINICAL PHARMACOLOGY
Mechanism of Action: α-adrenergic receptor stimulant that produces prompt and prolonged rise in blood pressure; no β-adrenergic effects; minimal arrhythmogenic potential

Pharmacokinetics
IV: Onset immediate, peak 0.5-2 min, duration 5-15 min
IM: Peak 15-20 min, duration 60-90 min
Metabolic fate and route of excretion unknown

INDICATIONS AND USES: Hypotension during anesthesia; supraventricular paroxysmal tachycardia; hypotension and shock*; diagnosis of heart murmurs*

DOSAGE
Adult
• *During spinal anesthesia:* IM 10-20 mg shortly before or with spinal anesthesia; repeat prn
• *Emergencies:* IV 3-5 mg injected slowly
• *Supraventricular tachycardia:* IV 10 mg injected slowly

$ AVAILABLE FORMS/COST OF THERAPY
• Inj, Sol—IM, IV: 20 mg/ml, 1 ml ampul: **$24.42**

CONTRAINDICATIONS: Severe hypertension

PRECAUTIONS: Children, hypovolemia, extravasation (phentolamine can be used as antidote), hyperthyroidism, bradycardia, partial heart block, myocardial disease, severe arteriosclerosis, sulfite sensitivity

PREGNANCY AND LACTATION:
Pregnancy category C; could reduce uterine blood flow, thereby producing fetal hypoxia and bradycardia; may also interact with oxytocics or ergot derivatives to produce severe persistent maternal hypertension; ephedrine may be a more suitable pressor agent

SIDE EFFECTS/ADVERSE REACTIONS

CNS: Anxiety, headache (often severe)

CV: Excessive blood pressure elevation, ventricular ectopic beats

GI: Nausea, vomiting (often projectile)

GU: Fetal bradycardia, urinary urgency, uterine hypertonus

SKIN: Pilomotor response, sweating

INTERACTIONS

Drugs

🔳 *β-blockers (nadolol, pindolol, practolol, propranolol, timolol):* Non-cardioselective β-blockers enhance the pressor response to alpha stimulation, resulting in hypertension and bradycardia

▲ *Bromocriptine:* Case report of hypertension and ventricular tachycardia with combination of a related sympathomimetic

🔳 *Furazolidone:* Enhanced hypertensive response when sympathomimetics used concurrently

🔳 *Guanadrel, guanethidine:* Reversal of antihypertensive effects

🔳 *Indomethacin:* Hypertensive reactions

❷ *Moclobemide:* Enhanced pressor response to methoxamine (headache, palpitations, and lightheadedness)

▲ *Monamine oxidase inhibitors (MAOI) (isocarboxazid, phenelzine, procarbazine, tranylcypromine):* Hypertensive reactions

🔳 *Oxytocic drugs:* May cause severe persistent hypertension

❷ *Tricyclic antidepressants (imipramine, protriptyline):* Predisposition to cardiac arrhythmias; enhanced pressor response

SPECIAL CONSIDERATIONS

MONITORING PARAMETERS
• Blood pressure and pulse

---

methoxsalen

(meth-ox´a-len)

Rx: 8-Mop, Oxsoralen, Oxsoralen-Ultra
Chemical Class: Psoralen or Furocoumarin compound
Therapeutic Class: Pigmenting agent; antipsoriatic

CLINICAL PHARMACOLOGY

Mechanism of Action: Increases tyrosinase activity in melanin-producing cells, as well as inhibits DNA synthesis, cell division, and epidermal turnover; successful pigmentation requires the presence of functioning melanocytes

Pharmacokinetics

PO: Peak serum concentration 1.5-6 hr (hard gelatin capsule), 0.5-4 hr (soft gelatin capsule); peak photosensitivity 3.9-4.25 hr (hard capsule), 1.5-2.1 hr (soft capsule); duration approximately 8 hr; highly protein bound; activated by long-wavelength ultraviolet light (UVA), further metabolized by liver; eliminated mainly in urine as metabolites; $t_{1/2}$ 1.1 hr (hard capsule), 2 hr (soft capsule)

INDICATIONS AND USES: Severe, refractory, disabling psoriasis, in conjunction with UVA—treatment known as PUVA (psoralen plus ultraviolet light A); repigmentation in the treatment of vitiligo (PUVA); cutaneous T-cell lymphoma (in conjunction with photopheresis)

DOSAGE

Adult

• *Psoriasis:* PO (hard caps) administer with food or milk 2 hr before UVA exposure, separate doses by at least 48 hr, (<30 kg) 10 mg, (30-50 kg) 20 mg, (51-65 kg) 30 mg, (66-80 kg) 40 mg, (81-90 kg) 50 mg, (91-115 kg) 60 mg, (>115 kg) 70 mg; (soft caps) administer with low-fat food or milk 1.5-2 hr before UVA exposure, separate doses by at least 48 hr, (<30 kg) 10 mg, (30-50 kg) 10-20 mg, (51-65 kg) 20-30 mg, (66-80 kg) 20-40 mg, (81-90 kg) 30-50 mg, (91-115 kg) 30-60 mg, (>115 kg) 40-70 mg

• *Vitiligo:* PO 20 mg 2-4 hr before measured periods of UVA exposure, 2-3 times/wk (at least 48 hr apart); TOP apply to small, well-defined lesion, then expose to UVA light once/wk or less depending on results

• *Cutaneous T-cell lymphoma:* PO (hard capsules) 0.6 mg/kg administered 2 hr before obtaining blood for extracorporeal exposure of extracted leukocytes to high-intensity UVA light

💲 AVAILABLE FORMS/COST OF THERAPY

• Cap, Gel—Oral: 10 mg, 50's: **$338.58** (soft caps) **$338.58** (hard caps)

• Lotion—Top: 1%, 30 ml: **$113.03** (do not dispense to patient)

CONTRAINDICATIONS: Hypersensitivity to psoralens, diseases associated with photosensitivity, melanoma, invasive squamous cell carcinoma, aphakia (oral)

PRECAUTIONS: Cardiac disease, hepatic disease, children <12 yr, contains tartrazine (hard caps), photosensitizing agents

PREGNANCY AND LACTATION: Pregnancy category C; excretion into breast milk unknown

SIDE EFFECTS/ADVERSE REACTIONS

CNS: Dizziness, headache, insomnia, malaise, nervousness, psychological depression

CV: Edema, hypotension

EENT: Cataract formation

GI: Nausea

MS: Leg cramps

SKIN: Basal cell epitheliomas, cutaneous tenderness, *erythema,* extension of psoriasis, folliculitis, herpes simplex, hypopigmentation, nonspecific rash, *pruritus,* severe burns, urticaria, vesication and bullae formation

SPECIAL CONSIDERATIONS

• Hard and soft caps are not equivalent

PATIENT/FAMILY EDUCATION

• Do not sunbathe during 24 hr prior to methoxsalen ingestion and UVA exposure

• Wear UVA-absorbing sunglasses for 24 hr following treatment to prevent cataract

• Avoid sun exposure for at least 8 hr after methoxsalen ingestion

• Avoid concurrent photosensitizing drugs

• Avoid furocoumarin-containing foods (e.g., limes, figs, parsley, parsnips, mustard, carrots, celery)

• Repigmentation of vitiligo may require 6-9 mo

M

---

italic = common side effects   **bold italic** = life-threatening reactions

methscopolamine

(meth-skoe-pol′a-meen)
Rx: Pamine
Chemical Class: Quaternary ammonium derivative
Therapeutic Class: Gastrointestinal antiulcer agent (adjunctive)

CLINICAL PHARMACOLOGY

Mechanism of Action: Inhibits GI motility and diminishes gastric acid secretion

Pharmacokinetics

PO: Onset 1 hr, duration 4-6 hr; incompletely absorbed from GI tract, excreted mainly in urine as unchanged drug and metabolites, remainder excreted in feces (probably as unabsorbed drug)

INDICATIONS AND USES: Adjunctive treatment of peptic ulcer

DOSAGE

Adult

• PO 2.5-5 mg qid (½ hr ac, hs)

Child

• PO 0.2 mg/kg or 6 mg/m^2 daily, given in 4 equally divided doses

$ AVAILABLE FORMS/COST OF THERAPY

• Tab, Uncoated—Oral: 2.5 mg, 100's: **$61.71**

CONTRAINDICATIONS: Narrow-angle glaucoma, obstructive uropathy, obstructive disease of the GI tract, paralytic ileus, intestinal atony, unstable cardiovascular status in acute hemorrhage, severe ulcerative colitis, toxic megacolon complicating ulcerative colitis, myasthenia gravis

PRECAUTIONS: Hyperthyroidism, CAD, dysrhythmias, CHF, ulcerative colitis, hypertension, hiatal hernia, hepatic disease, renal disease, urinary retention, prostatic hypertrophy, elderly, children, glaucoma

PREGNANCY AND LACTATION: Pregnancy category C; excretion into breast milk unknown, although would be expected to be minimal due to quaternary structure (see also atropine)

SIDE EFFECTS/ADVERSE REACTIONS

CNS: Anxiety, confusion, dizziness, drowsiness, hallucination, headache, insomnia, stimulation (especially in elderly), weakness

CV: Palpitations, tachycardia

EENT: Blurred vision, cycloplegia, increased ocular tension, mydriasis, photophobia

GI: Absence of taste, *constipation, dry mouth,* dysphagia, heartburn, nausea, *paralytic ileus,* vomiting

GU: Hesitancy, impotence, *retention*

SKIN: Allergic reactions, anhidrosis, fever, pruritus, rash, urticaria

INTERACTIONS

Drugs

🔳 *Amantadine, rimantadine:* Methscopolamine potentiates the CNS side effects of antivirals; antivirals potentiate the anticholinergic side effects of other anticholinergics

🔳 *Antidepressants (amitriptylline, doxepin, imipramine, maprotiline, nortriptyline, protriptyline, trimipramine):* Excessive anticholinergic effects

🔳 *Neuroleptics (chlorpromazine, haloperidol):* Methscopolamine may inhibit the therapeutic response to neuroleptics; excessive anticholinergic effects with combination

🔳 *Tacrine:* Tacrine may inhibit the therapeutic effects of anticholinergic agents; centrally acting anticholinergics may inhibit the therapeutic effects of tacrine

SPECIAL CONSIDERATIONS

• Has not been shown to be effective in contributing to the healing of peptic ulcer, decreasing the rate of recurrence, or preventing complications

---

methsuximide

(meth-sux´i-mide)

Rx: Celontin
Chemical Class: Succinimide derivative
Therapeutic Class: Anticonvulsant

CLINICAL PHARMACOLOGY

Mechanism of Action: Increases the seizure threshold and suppresses paroxysmal spike-and-wave pattern in absence seizures; depresses nerve transmission in the motor cortex

Pharmacokinetics

PO: Peak 1-3 hr; rapidly demethylated in liver to *N*-desmethylmethsuximide (active), excreted in urine (metabolites); $t_{1/2}$ 2-4 hr (*N*-desmethylmethsuximide 26-80 hr)

INDICATIONS AND USES: Refractory absence (petit mal) seizures

DOSAGE

Adult

• PO 300 mg/day for 1st wk; may increase by 300 mg/day at weekly intervals up to 1.2 g/day divided bid-qid

Child

• PO 10-15 mg/kg/day divided tid-qid initially; increase weekly up to max of 30 mg/kg/day

$ AVAILABLE FORMS/COST OF THERAPY

• Cap, Gel—Oral: 150 mg, 100's: **$60.68**; 300 mg, 100's: **$99.49**

PRECAUTIONS: Hepatic, renal function impairment; abrupt withdrawal; monotherapy with mixed types of epilepsy (may increase frequency of grand-mal seizures)

PREGNANCY AND LACTATION: Pregnancy category C

SIDE EFFECTS/ADVERSE REACTIONS

CNS: Aggressiveness, *ataxia,* confusion, depression, *dizziness,* dreamlike state, *drowsiness,* euphoria, fatigue, headache, hyperactivity, hypochondriacal behavior, inability to concentrate, insomnia, instability, irritability, lethargy, mental slowness, nervousness, night terrors

EENT: Blurred vision, myopia, periorbital edema, photophobia

GI: *Anorexia,* constipation, cramps, diarrhea, epigastric and abdominal pain, *nausea,* swelling of tongue, *vague gastric upset, vomiting,* weight loss

GU: Microscopic hematuria, renal damage, urinary frequency, vaginal bleeding

HEME: **Agranulocytosis, eosinophilia, granulocytopenia, leukopenia, monocytosis, pancytopenia**

MS: Muscle weakness

SKIN: Alopecia, **erythema multiforme,** hirsutism, pruritic erythematous rashes, pruritus, skin eruptions, **Stevens-Johnson syndrome,** urticaria

MISC: Systemic lupus erythematosus

INTERACTIONS

Labs

• *Ethosuximide:* False positive metabolite cross-reacts

SPECIAL CONSIDERATIONS
PATIENT/FAMILY EDUCATION

• Take with food or milk
• Do not discontinue abruptly

MONITORING PARAMETERS

• CBC with differential; liver enzymes

M

• Serum *N*-desmethylmethsuximide concentrations at trough for efficacy (range 10-40 μg/ml) and 3 hr post-dose for toxicity (>40 μg/ml)

---

methyclothiazide
(meth-ee-cloh-thye′a-zide)
Rx: *Aquatensen, Enduron*
Combinations
  Rx: with reserpine (Di-utensen-R)
Chemical Class: Sulfonamide derivative
Therapeutic Class: Thiazide diuretic; antihypertensive

CLINICAL PHARMACOLOGY
Mechanism of Action: Inhibits reabsorption of sodium and chloride in cortical thick ascencing limb of the loop of Henle and the early distal tubules—increasing the urinary excretion of sodium and chloride; sulfonamide moiety provides some carbonic anhydrase inhibition activity; other actions—increased potassium and bicarbonate excretion; decreased calcium excretion; uric acid retention; antihypertensive action dependent on sodium depletion, drop in peripheral vascular resistance, and reduction in extracellular volume.
Pharmacokinetics
PO: Onset 2 hr, peak effect 6 hr, duration 24 hr; excreted in urine (inactive metabolite and unchanged drug)
INDICATIONS AND USES: Edema (CHF, hepatic cirrhosis, corticosteroid and estrogen therapy, nephrotic syndrome, acute glomerulonephritis); hypertension; calcium nephrolithiasis,* prevention of osteoporosis*; diabetes insipidus*

* = non-FDA-approved use

DOSAGE
NOTE: Equivalent hydrochlorothiazide dose: 5 mg = 50 mg
Adult
• *Edema:* PO 2.5-10 mg qd
• *Hypertension:* PO 2.5-5 mg qd
 💲 **AVAILABLE FORMS/COST OF THERAPY**
• Tab, Uncoated—Oral: 2.5 mg, 100's: **$6.60-$60.38**; 5 mg, 100's: **$7.43-$177.43**
CONTRAINDICATIONS: Anuria, renal decompensation
PRECAUTIONS: Fluid and electrolyte imbalance (including sodium, potassium, magnesium, calcium), renal disease, hepatic disease, gout, COPD, lupus erythematosus, diabetes mellitus, hyperparathyroidism, vomiting, diarrhea, elevated cholesterol/triglycerides, tartrazine sensitivity
PREGNANCY AND LACTATION: Pregnancy category B; therapy for preexisting hypertension can be continued throughout pregnancy with minimal risk; initiating for simple edema not recommended; few unequivocal indications for diuretic therapy in pregnancy except for pulmonary edema or congestive heart failure; excreted into breast milk in small amounts; considered compatible with breast feeding
SIDE EFFECTS/ADVERSE REACTIONS
CNS: Anxiety, depression, *dizziness,* drowsiness, *fatigue,* headache, paresthesia, *weakness*
CV: Arrhythmias, irregular pulse, orthostatic hypotension, palpitations, volume depletion, angina
EENT: Blurred vision, nasal congestion
GI: Anorexia, constipation, cramps, diarrhea, GI irritation, hepatitis, *nausea,* pancreatitis, *vomiting*

GU: Frequency, glucosuria, poly-uria, uremia, increased creatinine, BUN

*HEME: **Agranulocytosis, aplastic anemia, hemolytic anemia, leuko-penia, neutropenia, thrombocyto-penia***

METAB: Hypercalcemia, *hypergly-cemia, hyperuricemia,* hypochlore-mia, *hypokalemia,* hypomagnese-mia, hyponatremia, lipid abnormali-ties (increased total LDL-choles-terol, triglycerides)

SKIN: Fever, photosensitivity, pur-pura, *rash,* urticaria

INTERACTIONS

Drugs

❷ *Angiotensin converting enzyme inhibitors:* Risk of postural hypo-tension when added to ongoing di-uretic therapy; more common with loop diuretics; first dose hypoten-sion possible in patients with so-dium depletion or hypovolemia due to diuretics or sodium restriction; hypotensive response is usually transient; hold diuretic day of first dose

❸ *Calcium:* Large doses can lead to milk-alkali syndrome

❸ *Carbenoxolone:* Severe hypoka-lemia

❸ *Binding resins (cholestyramine, colestipol):* Reduces thiazide serum levels and lessened diuretic effects

❸ *Corticosteroids:* Concomitant therapy may result in excessive po-tassium loss

❸ *Diazoxide:* Hyperglycemia

❸ *Digitalis glycosides:* Diuretic-induced hypokalemia may potenti-ate the risk of digitalis toxicity

❸ *Hypoglycemic agents:* Thiazide diuretics tend to increase blood glu-cose; may increase dosage require-ments of hypoglycemic agents.

❸ *Insulin:* Increased blood glu-cose, increased dosage requirement of antidiabetic drugs

❸ *Lithium:* Increased lithium con-centrations

❸ *Methotrexate:* Increased meth-otrexate effects; potentiates bone marrow toxicity

❸ *Nonsteroidal antiinflammatory drugs:* Concurrent use may reduce diuretic and antihypertensive ef-fects.

SPECIAL CONSIDERATIONS

• Doses above 2.5 mg provide no further blood pressure reduction, but are more likely to induce meta-bolic disturbance (i.e., hypokale-mia, hyperuricemia, etc.)

• May protect against osteoporotic hip fractures

• Loop diuretics or metolazone more effective if CrCl <40-50 ml/min

PATIENT/FAMILY EDUCATION

• Will increase urination tempo-rarily (approx. 3 weeks); take early in the day to prevent sleep distur-bance

• May cause sensitivity to sunlight; avoid prolonged exposure to the sun and other ultraviolet light

• May cause gout attacks; notify cli-nician if sudden joint pain occurs

MONITORING PARAMETERS

• Weight, urine output, serum elec-trolytes, BUN, creatinine, CBC, uric acid, glucose, lipids

italic = common side effects   ***bold italic*** = life-threatening reactions

methylcellulose
(meth-ill-sell'yoo-lose)
OTC: Citrucel
Chemical Class: Hydrophilic semisynthetic cellulose derivative
Therapeutic Class: Bulk laxative

CLINICAL PHARMACOLOGY
Mechanism of Action: Attracts water, expands in intestine to increase peristalsis; also absorbs excess water in stool; decreases diarrhea
Pharmacokinetics
PO: Not absorbed, onset 12-24 hr, full effect may not be apparent for 2-3 days
INDICATIONS AND USES: Constipation
DOSAGE
Adult and Child >12 yr
• PO 1 heaping tablespoon in 8 oz cold water, 1-3 times daily
Child
• PO 1 level tablespoon in 4 oz cold water, 1-3 times daily
$ AVAILABLE FORMS/COST OF THERAPY
• Powder—Oral: 2 g/heaping tablespoon, 480 g: **$7.63**; packet, 120's: **$8.03**
CONTRAINDICATIONS: Nausea, vomiting, or other symptom of appendicitis; acute surgical abdomen; fecal impaction; intestinal obstruction; undiagnosed abdominal pain
PRECAUTIONS: Rectal bleeding; esophageal stricture; intestinal ulcerations, stenosis, or disabling adhesions
PREGNANCY AND LACTATION: Bulk forming laxatives are the laxative of choice during pregnancy; compatible with breast feeding

SIDE EFFECTS/ADVERSE REACTIONS
GI: Abdominal distension, obstruction
SPECIAL CONSIDERATIONS
PATIENT/FAMILY EDUCATION
• Notify clinician of unrelieved constipation, rectal bleeding
• Ensure adequate fluids, proper dietary fiber intake and regular exercise

methyldopa
(meth-ill-doe'pa)
Rx: Aldomet
Combinations
Rx: with HCTZ (Aldoril); with chlorothiazide (Aldoclor)
Chemical Class: Catecholamine derivative
Therapeutic Class: Antihypertensive, centrally acting sympathoplegic

CLINICAL PHARMACOLOGY
Mechanism of Action: Stimulates inhibitory central α_2-adrenergic receptors by false transmitter, α-methylnorepinephrine, resulting in reduced sympathetic outflow from the CNS to the heart, kidneys, and peripheral vasculature; reduced peripheral resistance and plasma renin activity levels may also contribute to its effect
Pharmacokinetics
PO: Peak effect 3-6 hr
IV: (methyldopate): Onset 4-6 hr, duration 10-16 hr
50% of PO dose absorbed; weakly bound to plasma proteins; extensively metabolized in GI tract and liver, eliminated in urine; $t_{1/2}$ 7-16 hr (24% unchanged) and feces (50%)
INDICATIONS AND USES: Moderate to severe hypertension

DOSAGE

Adult

• PO 250 mg bid-tid, increase q2d prn, usual dose 1-1.5 g/day in 2-4 divided doses, max 3 g/day; IV (methyldopate) 250-1000 mg q68h, max 4 g/day

• *Dosing interval in renal impairment:* CrCl >50 ml/min q8h; CrCl 10-50 ml/min q8-12h; CrCl <10 ml/min q12-24h

Child

• PO 10 mg/kg/day in 2-4 divided doses, increase q2d prn to max dose of 65 mg/kg/day, do not exceed 3 g/day; IV 2-4 mg/kg/dose; if response not seen within 4-6 hr, may increase to 5-10 mg/kg/dose; administer doses q6-8h; max daily dose 65 mg/kg or 3 g, whichever is less

• *Dosing interval in renal impairment:* CrCl >50 ml/min q8h; CrCl 10-50 ml/min q8-12h; CrCl <10 ml/min q12-24h

⑤ AVAILABLE FORMS/COST OF THERAPY

• Inj, Sol—IV: 50 mg/ml, 5, 10 ml: **$1.69-$13.50**/5 ml (methyldopate)
• Susp—Oral: 250 mg/5 ml, 480 ml: **$65.27**
• Tab, Plain Coated—Oral: 125 mg, 100's: **$9.75-$30.83**; 250 mg, 100's: **$12.50-$44.92**; 500 mg, 100's: **$14.72-$71.73**

CONTRAINDICATIONS: Active hepatic disease

PRECAUTIONS: History of liver disease, pheochromocytoma, sulfite sensitivity, renal failure, autonomic dysfunction

PREGNANCY AND LACTATION: Pregnancy category B (oral); C (IV); no adverse reactions have been reported despite rather wide use during pregnancy; compatible with breast feeding

SIDE EFFECTS/ADVERSE REACTIONS

CNS: Asthenia, Bell's palsy, decreased mental acuity, depression, *dizziness, headache,* involuntary choreoathetotic movements, lightheadedness, paresthesias, parkinsonism, psychic disturbances, *sedation,* symptoms of cerebrovascular insufficiency

CV: Aggravation of angina pectoris, bradycardia, edema, myocarditis, orthostatic hypotension, paradoxical pressor response, pericarditis, prolonged carotid sinus hypersensitivity

EENT: Dry mouth, nasal stuffiness

GI: Abnormal liver function tests, colitis, constipation, diarrhea, distension, flatus, hepatitis, jaundice, nausea, **pancreatitis,** sialadenitis, vomiting

GU: Decreased libido, failure to ejaculate, impotence

HEME: **Bone marrow depression,** eosinophilia, **granulocytopenia, hemolytic anemia,** *positive Coombs test (10-20%),* positive tests for antinuclear antibody, LE cells, and rheumatoid factor

METAB: Amenorrhea, breast enlargement, galactorrhea, hyperprolactinemia

MS: Arthralgia, myalgia

SKIN: Rash, **toxic epidermal necrolysis**

MISC: Fever, lupus-like syndrome

INTERACTIONS

Drugs

3 *β-blockers:* Rebound hypertension from methyldopa withdrawal exacerbated by noncardioselective β-blockers

3 *Iron:* Inhibited antihypertensive response to methyldopa

3 *Lithium:* Lithium toxicity not necessarily associated with excessive lithium concentrations

M

3 *Tricyclic antidepressants:* Inhibit the antihypertensive response
Labs
• *Interference:* Plasma and urine catecholamines, serum creatinine, glucose, serum, urine uric acid, and acetaminophen, AST
• *False increase:* Urine amino acids, serum bilirubin, urine ferric chloride test, urine ketones, metanephrines, VMA
• *False decrease:* Serum cholesterol, triglycerides
• *False positive:* Guaiacols spot test, urine melanogen, urine Thormahlen test

SPECIAL CONSIDERATIONS
• Perform both direct and indirect Coombs test if blood transfusion needed. If indirect Coombs test positive, interference may occur with cross match. Positive direct Coombs test will not interfere

PATIENT/FAMILY EDUCATION
• Urine exposed to air after voiding may darken
• Do not discontinue abruptly
• Initial sedation usually improves

MONITORING PARAMETERS
• CBC, liver function tests periodically during therapy
• Direct Coombs test before therapy and after 6-12 mo. If positive rule out hemolytic anemia

methylene blue

(meth´i-leen)
Rx: Urolene Blue
Chemical Class: Thiazine dye
Therapeutic Class: Antidote, cyanide; antidote, drug-induced methemoglobinemia; diagnostic agent

CLINICAL PHARMACOLOGY
Mechanism of Action: Combines with cyanide to form cyanmethemoglobin, preventing interference of cyanide with the cytochrome system (high concentrations only); directly inhibits calcium binding by oxalate; possesses weak antiseptic and tissue-staining properties
Pharmacokinetics
PO/IV: Rapidly reduced in tissues to leukomethylene blue, excreted in urine and bile

INDICATIONS AND USES: Methemoglobinemia; cyanide poisoning; urolithiasis (ineffective in dissolving previously formed stones); genitourinary antiseptic (use is obsolete); cutaneous viral infections (in conjunction with polychromatic light)*; diagnosis of gastroesophageal reflux in infants and children*; delineation of body structures and fistulas through dye effect*; diagnosis of premature rupture of membrane*

DOSAGE
Adult
• IV 1-2 mg/kg (0.1-0.2 ml/kg) or 25-50 mg/m^2 over several min, may be repeated after 1 hr if necessary; PO 65-130 mg tid with a full glass of water
Child
• IV 1-2 mg/kg (0.1-0.2 ml/kg) or 25-50 mg/m^2 over several min, may be repeated after 1 hr if necessary

$\boxed{\text{S}}$ AVAILABLE FORMS/COST OF THERAPY

• Inj, Sol—IV: 1%, 1 ml: **$4.50-$9.80**

• Tab, Uncoated—Oral: 65 mg, 100's: **$30.15**

CONTRAINDICATIONS: Renal insufficiency, instraspinal inj

PRECAUTIONS: G6PD deficiency, prolonged administration, analine-induced methemoglobinemia (may precipitate Heinz body formation and hemolytic anemia)

PREGNANCY AND LACTATION: Pregnancy category C (category D if inj intra-amniotically); deep blue staining of the newborn, hemolytic anemia, hyperbilirubinemia, and methemoglobinemia in the newborn may occur after inj into the amniotic fluid

SIDE EFFECTS/ADVERSE REACTIONS

CNS: Dizziness, fever, *headache,* mental confusion

GI: Abdominal pain, blue-green stool, diarrhea, *nausea, vomiting*

GU: Bladder irritation, blue-green urine

HEME: Hemolytic anemia, methemoglobinemia (large doses)

SKIN: Profuse sweating, stains skin blue (may be removed by hypochlorite solution)

SPECIAL CONSIDERATIONS
PATIENT/FAMILY EDUCATION

• Photosensitivity may occur

MONITORING PARAMETERS

• Hct

---

methylergonovine
(meth-ill-er-goe-noe′veen)
Rx: Methergine
Chemical Class: Ergot alkaloid
Therapeutic Class: Oxytocic

CLINICAL PHARMACOLOGY

Mechanism of Action: Partial agonist or antagonist at α-adrenergic, dopaminergic, and tryptaminergic receptors; increases the strength, duration, and frequency of uterine contractions and decreases uterine bleeding when used after placental delivery

Pharmacokinetics

IV: Onset immediate, duration 3 hr

IM: Onset 2-5 min, duration 3 hr

PO: Onset 5-10 min, duration 3 hr

Excretion partially renal and partially hepatic; $t_{1/2}$ 20-30 min

INDICATIONS AND USES: Postpartum, postabortal hemorrhage due to uterine atony; subinvolution; routine management after delivery of the placenta

DOSAGE
Adult

• IM/IV 0.2 mg after delivery of the placenta, after delivery of the anterior shoulder, or during the puerperium; repeat q2-4h prn; PO 0.2 mg tid-qid in the puerperium for a max of 1 wk

$\boxed{\text{S}}$ AVAILABLE FORMS/COST OF THERAPY

• Inj, Sol—IM, IV: 0.2 mg/ml, 1's: **$3.74-$4.25**

• Tab, Coated—Oral: 0.2 mg, 100's: **$73.91-$77.06**

CONTRAINDICATIONS: Hypertension, toxemia, hypersensitivity to ergots

PRECAUTIONS: Rapid IV INF (may induce sudden hypertension

---

italic = common side effects   ***bold italic*** = life-threatening reactions

and CVAs), sepsis, obliterative vascular disease; hepatic/renal impairment

PREGNANCY AND LACTATION: Pregnancy category C; small quantity appears in breast milk; adverse effects have not been described

SIDE EFFECTS/ADVERSE REACTIONS

CNS: Dizziness, hallucinations, *headache,* paresthesias, ***seizure***

CV: Hypertension, palpitations, temporary chest pain, thrombophlebitis

EENT: Tinnitus

GI: Diarrhea, foul taste, nausea, vomiting

MS: Leg cramps

RESP: Dyspnea

SKIN: Diaphoresis

SPECIAL CONSIDERATIONS

PATIENT/FAMILY EDUCATION

• Report increased blood loss, severe abdominal cramps, increased temperature, or foul-smelling lochia.

• Symptoms of ergotism occur with overdosage (nausea, vomiting, diarrhea, seizure, hallucinations, delirium, numb/gangrenous extremities)

MONITORING PARAMETERS

• Blood pressure, pulse, and uterine response

---

methylphenidate

(meth-ill-fen´i-date)

Rx: Concerta, Ritalin, Ritalin-SR

Chemical Class: Piperidine derivative of amphetamine

Therapeutic Class: Cerebral stimulant

DEA Class: Schedule II

CLINICAL PHARMACOLOGY

Mechanism of Action: Sympathomimetic amine with CNS stimulant activity; like amphetamines, increases release of norepinephrine from central noradrenergic neurons; at higher doses, dopamine released in mesolimbic system; peripheral α- and β-activity includes elevation of systolic and diastolic blood pressures and weak bronchodilator and respiratory stimulation action; heart rate reflexly slowed at standard doses, arrhythmias with overdose

Pharmacokinetics

PO: Peak 1-3 hr (sustained release 4-7 hr), duration 3-6 hr (sustained-release 8 hr, Concerta 12 hr); 80% metabolized to ritalinic acid, excreted in urine

INDICATIONS AND USES: Attention deficit disorders; narcolepsy; depression in elderly, cancer, and poststroke patients*

DOSAGE

Adult

• *Narcolepsy:* PO 10 mg bid-tid; 30-45 min ac; may increase up to 40-60 mg/day

Child ≥6 yr

• *Attention deficit disorder:* PO 0.3 mg/kg/dose or 2.5-5 mg/dose given before breakfast and lunch; increase by 0.1 mg/kg/dose or 5-10 mg/day at weekly intervals; usual dose 0.5-1 mg/kg/day; max 2 mg/kg/day or 60 mg/day; sustained release may be used when the 8 hr dosage of sustained release corresponds to the titrated 8 hr dose of immediate-release tabs

• *Concerta:* If not on other methylphenidate products begin at 18 mg QAM, increase weekly by 18 mg/day to maximum 54 mg QAM

If switching from other methylphenidate products to Concerta: Methylphenidate daily dose of 5 mg bid/tid: 18 mg QAM; 10 mg bid/tid: 36 mg QAM; 15 mg big/tid: 54 mg QAM

Methylphenidate-SR daily dose of 20 mg: 18 mg QAM; 40 mg: 36 mg QAM; 60 mg: 54 mg QAM

$ AVAILABLE FORMS/COST OF THERAPY

• Tab, Plain Coated, Sus Action—Oral: 10 mg, 100's: **$93.09-$102.06**; 20 mg, 100's: **$78.92-$144.19**

• Tab, Sus Action—Oral (Concerta): 18 mg, 100's: **$243.75**; 36 mg, 100's: **$256.25**; 54 mg, 100's: **$275.00**

• Tab, Uncoated—Oral: 5 mg, 100's: **$25.12-$45.29**; 10 mg, 100's: **$35.76-$64.56**; 20 mg, 100's: **$54.95-$118.57**

CONTRAINDICATIONS: Marked anxiety, tension, and agitation; glaucoma; history of Tourette's syndrome or motor tics, prevention of normal fatigue

PRECAUTIONS: Severe depression, seizure disorders, hypertension, history of drug abuse, children <6 yr, symptoms associated with acute stress reactions

PREGNANCY AND LACTATION: Pregnancy category C

SIDE EFFECTS/ADVERSE REACTIONS

CNS: Akathisia, dizziness, dyskinesia, fever, headache, *hyperactivity, insomnia, restlessness,* talkativeness, Tourette's syndrome (rare)

CV: Angina, blood pressure changes, ***dysrhythmias,*** *palpitations, tachycardia*

GI: Abdominal pain, anorexia, dry mouth, nausea, weight loss

GU: Uremia

HEME: Anemia, ***leukopenia***

METAB: Growth retardation

MS: Arthralgia

SKIN: ***Erythema-multiforme, exfoliative dermatitis,*** rash, scalp hair loss, urticaria

INTERACTIONS
Drugs
3 *Guanethidine:* Inhibition of guanethidine antihypertensive effect

2 *MAOIs:* Hypertensive reactions

3 *Phenytoin:* Increased phenytoin levels with risk of toxicity

3 *Tricyclic antidepressants:* Increased serum concentrations of tricyclic antidepressants

Labs
• *False positive:* Urine amphetamine

SPECIAL CONSIDERATIONS
• Overdosage may cause vomiting, agitation, tremor, muscle twitching, seizures, confusion, tachycardia, hypertension, arrhythmias

PATIENT/FAMILY EDUCATION
• Take last daily dose prior to 6 PM to avoid insomnia
• Do not discontinue abruptly
• Avoid OTC preparations unless approved by clinician
• Do not crush or chew sustained release formulation

MONITORING PARAMETERS
• Periodic CBC with differential and platelet count

---

methylprednisolone
(meth-il-pred-niss'oh-lone)
Rx: *Methylprednisolone:* Medrol
Acetate: Depo-Medrol, depMedalone, Depoject, Depopred, D-Med, Duralone, Medralone, M-Prednisol, Rep-Pred
Sodium Succinate: A-MethaPred, Solu-Medrol
Chemical Class: Synthetic glucocorticoid
Therapeutic Class: Systemic corticosteroid

CLINICAL PHARMACOLOGY
Mechanism of Action: Decreases inflammation by depressing migra-

tion of polymorphonuclear leukocytes and activity of endogenous mediators of inflammation. Has many profound metabolic effects, does not possess mineralocorticoid activity

Pharmacokinetics

PO: Peak effect 1-2 hr, duration 30-36 hr

IM: (acetate): Peak effect 4-8 days, duration 1-4 wk

INTRA-ARTICULAR: Peak effect 1 wk, duration 1-5 wk

Metabolized in liver, excreted in urine and bile; biologic $t_{1/2}$ 18-36 hr

INDICATIONS AND USES: *Systemic:* Antiinflammatory or immunosuppressant agent in the treatment of a variety of diseases of hematologic, allergic, inflammatory, neoplastic, and autoimmune origin

Intra-articular: Synovitis, osteoarthritis

Intradermal: Keloids, alopecia areata, inflammatory skin lesions

DOSAGE

Adult

• PO 4-48 mg/day initially, adjust until satisfactory response is noted, taper gradually if used continuously for >10 days

• *Sodium succinate:* IM/IV 10-40 mg initially, may repeat q6h prn; for acute spinal cord injury, give 30 mg/kg IV over 15 min followed in 45 min by a continuous INF of 5.4 mg/kg/hr for 23 hr

• *Acetate:* IM 40-120 mg q1-2 wk; intra-articular/intralesional 4-40 mg, up to 80 mg for large joints q1-5 wk

Child

• PO/IM/IV 0.12-1.7 mg/kg/day or 5-25 mg/m^2/day in divided doses q6-12h

• *Status asthmaticus:* IV 2 mg/kg loading dose, then 0.5-1 mg/kg/dose q6h

§ AVAILABLE FORMS/COST OF THERAPY

• Tab, Uncoated—Oral: 2 mg, 100's: **$48.09**; 4 mg, 100's (dosepack): **$14.29-$97.51**; 4 mg, 21's: **$6.25-$19.72**; 8 mg, 25's: **$31.93**; 16 mg, 50's: **$98.66**; 24 mg, 25's: **$55.36**; 32 mg, 25's: **$73.46**

Methylprednisolone Acetate

• Inj, Sol—IM, intraarticular, intralesional: 20 mg/ml, 10 ml: **$7.50**; 40 mg/ml, 10 ml: **$12.95-$45.31**; 80 mg/ml, 5 ml: **$9.50-$45.31**

Methylprednisolone Sodium Succinate

• Inj, Lyphl-Sol—IM,IV: 40 mg/vial, 1's: **$2.05-$3.09**; 125 mg/vial, 1's: **$3.41-$12.50**; 500 mg/vial, 1's: **$6.08-$37.50**; 1 g/vial, 1's: **$9.71-$65.00**

• Inj, Sol—IM, IV: 2 g/vial, 1's: **$36.09**

CONTRAINDICATIONS: Systemic fungal infections, idiopathic thrombocytopenic purpura (IM), premature infants (sodium succinate, acetate, secondary to gasping syndrome from benzyl alcohol), intrathecal administration

PRECAUTIONS: Psychosis, diabetes mellitus, glaucoma, osteoporosis, seizure disorders, ulcerative colitis (intestinal perforation), CHF, hypertension, myesthenia gravis (if used with anticholinesterase agents), renal disease, esophagitis, peptic ulcer, latent tuberculosis or amebiasis (reactivation of disease). Topical: use on face, groin, or axilla, ocular herpes simplex

PREGNANCY AND LACTATION: Pregnancy category C; excreted in breast milk, could suppress infant's growth and interfere with endogenous corticosteroid production

SIDE EFFECTS/ADVERSE REACTIONS

CNS: Depression, headache, *mood changes, **seizures,** vertigo*

CV: ***CHF,*** hypertension, tachycardia, thromboembolism, thrombophlebitis

EENT: Blurred vision, cataract, increased intraocular pressure

GI: Abdominal distension, diarrhea, ***GI hemorrhage,*** *increased appetite, nausea,* ***pancreatitis***

METAB: Cushingoid state, decreased glucose tolerance, growth suppression in children, HPA suppression

MS: Aseptic necrosis of femoral and humeral heads, fractures, muscle mass loss, osteoporosis, weakness

SKIN: Acne, bruising, ecchymosis, petechiae, poor wound healing, striae, thin fragile skin

INTERACTIONS

Drugs

3 *Aminoglutethamide:* Enhanced elimination of corticosteroids; marked reduction in corticosteroid response; increased clearance of methylprednisolone; doubling of dose may be necessary

3 *Antidiabetics:* Increased blood glucose

3 *Barbiturates, carbamazepine:* Reduced serum concentrations of corticosteroids; increased clearance of methylprednisolone

3 *Cholestyramine, colestipol:* Possible reduced absorption of corticosteroids

3 *Cyclosporine:* Possible increased concentration of both drugs, seizures

3 *Erythromycin, troleandomycin, clarithromycin, ketoconazole:* Possible enhanced steroid effect

3 *Estrogens, oral contraceptives:* Enhanced effects of corticosteroids

3 *Isoniazid:* Reduced plasma concentrations of isoniazid

3 *IUDs:* Inhibition of inflammation may decrease contraceptive effect

3 *NSAIDs:* Increased risk GI ulceration

3 *Rifampin:* Reduced therapeutic effect of corticosteroids; may reduce hepatic clearance of methylprednisolone

3 *Salicylates:* Subtherapeutic salicylate concentrations possible

Labs

• *False increase:* Cortisol, digoxin, theophylline level

• *False decrease:* Urine glucose (Clinistix, Diastix only, Testape no effect)

• *False negative:* Skin allergy tests

SPECIAL CONSIDERATIONS

PATIENT/FAMILY EDUCATION

• Take single daily doses in AM

• May mask infections

• Increased dose of rapidly acting corticosteroids may be necessary in patients subjected to unusual stresses

• Signs of adrenal insufficiency include fatigue, anorexia, nausea, vomiting, diarrhea, weight loss, weakness, dizziness, and low blood sugar

• Avoid abrupt withdrawal of therapy following high dose or long-term therapy. Relative insufficiency may exist for up to 1 yr after discontinuation

• Patients on chronic steroid therapy should wear Medic Alert bracelet

• Do not give live virus vaccines to patients on prolonged therapy

MONITORING PARAMETERS

• Serum K and glucose

• Growth of children on prolonged therapy

methyltestosterone

(meth-ill-tess-toss'teh-rone)
Rx: Android, Methitest,
Testred, Virilon
Chemical Class: Testosterone
derivative
Therapeutic Class: Androgen;
antineoplastic
DEA Class: Schedule III

CLINICAL PHARMACOLOGY
Mechanism of Action: Promotes
weight gain via retention of nitrogen, potassium, and phosphorus, increased protein anabolism and decreased catabolism; endogenous androgens essential for normal growth
and development of male sex organs
and maintenance of secondary sex
characteristics

Pharmacokinetics
PO: Half as potent as buccally administered tablets; metabolized in
liver, excreted in urine

INDICATIONS AND USES: Males:
primary hypogonadism (congenital
or acquired), hypogonadotropic hypogonadism (congenital or acquired), delayed puberty; females:
palliative therapy of metastatic
breast cancer, postpartum breast
pain, engorgement,* moderate to severe vasomotor symptoms of menopause (in conjunction with estrogens)

DOSAGE
Adult
• *Male hypogonadism:* PO 10-50
mg qd; buccal 5-25 mg qd
• *Delayed puberty:* PO 10 mg qd for
4-6 mo; buccal 5 mg qd for 4-6 mo
• *Breast cancer:* PO 50-200 mg qd;
buccal 25-100 mg qd
• *Postpartum breast pain and engorgement:* PO 80 mg qd for 3-5
days after parturition; buccal 40 mg
qd for 3-5 days after parturition

• *Menopause:* PO 1.25-10 mg qd
(with estrogen)

🛇 AVAILABLE FORMS/COST OF THERAPY
• Cap, Gel—Oral: 10 mg, 100's:
$43.00-$220.46
• Tab—Uncoated—Oral: 10 mg,
100's: **$3.52-$201.11**; 25 mg, 100's:
$10.30-$343.32

CONTRAINDICATIONS: Severe
cardiac, hepatic, or renal disease;
carcinoma of breast or prostate
(males); pregnancy; enhancement
of athletic performance

PRECAUTIONS: Epilepsy, migraine headaches, children, benign
prostatic hypertrophy, acute intermittent porphyria, risk factors for
atherosclerosis, coronary artery disease

PREGNANCY AND LACTATION:
Pregnancy category X; causes virilization of female fetuses; excretion
into breast milk unknown; use extreme caution in nursing mothers

SIDE EFFECTS/ADVERSE REACTIONS
CNS: Anxiety, decreased or increased libido, dizziness, emotional
lability, fatigue, flushing, headache,
insomnia, paresthesias, sweating,
tremors

CV: Increased blood pressure, ***CHF,***
edema

EENT: Conjunctival edema, deepening of voice (women), nasal congestion

GI: Cholestatic jaundice, constipation, nausea, ***peliosis hepatis,*** stomatitis (buccal), vomiting, weight
gain

GU: Amenorrhea, *clitoral hypertrophy,* excessive frequency and duration of erection, hematuria, libido
changes, oligospermia, testicular atrophy, vaginitis, menstrual changes

HEME: Polycythemia, suppression
of clotting factors II, V, VII, and X

METAB: Abnormal GTT; decreased TBG (causes decreased total T_4, increased T_3 resin uptake, but normal free T_4), hypercalcemia; increased serum cholesterol, retention of sodium, chloride, water, potassium, and inorganic phosphate

MS: Cramps, spasms

SKIN: Acneiform lesions, acne vulgaris, hirsutism, male pattern baldness, oily hair, skin, rash, sweating

MISC: Decreased breast size, gynecomastia, *virilization (females)*

INTERACTIONS

Drugs

3 *Cyclosporine:* Increased cyclosporine concentrations

❷ *Warfarin:* Enhanced hypoprothrombinemic response to oral anticoagulants

SPECIAL CONSIDERATIONS

PATIENT/FAMILY EDUCATION

• Do not swallow buccal tablets, allow to dissolve between cheek and gum

• Avoid eating, drinking, or smoking while buccal tablet in place

MONITORING PARAMETERS

• LFTs, lipids, Hct

• Growth rate in children (Xrays for bone age q6 mo)

---

methysergide
(meth-i-ser′jide)
Rx: Sansert
Chemical Class: Semisynthetic ergot alkaloid
Therapeutic Class: Antimigraine agent

CLINICAL PHARMACOLOGY

Mechanism of Action: Exact mechanism of action in preventing migraine unknown; may be related to antiserotonin effect

Pharmacokinetics

PO: Onset of action 1-2 days, duration 1-2 days; metabolized in liver, excreted in urine (unchanged drug and metabolites); $t_{1/2}$ 10 hr

INDICATIONS AND USES: Prevention of vascular headache (not 1st-line); diarrhea in patients with carcinoid disease*

DOSAGE

Adult

• PO 4-8 mg/day in divided doses with meals; **a drug-free interval of 3-4 wk must follow each 6 mo course. Reduce dose gradually during last 2-3 wk to avoid "headache rebound"**

⑤ AVAILABLE FORMS/COST OF THERAPY

• Tab, Coated—Oral: 2 mg, 100's: **$265.60**

CONTRAINDICATIONS: Peripheral vascular disease; severe arteriosclerosis; severe hypertension; CAD; phlebitis or cellulitis of lower limbs; pulmonary disease; collagen diseases or fibrotic processes; impaired liver or renal function; valvular heart disease; peptic ulcer; debilitated states; serious infections

PRECAUTIONS: Tartrazine sensitivity, uninterrupted administration (increases risk of fibrotic complications)

PREGNANCY AND LACTATION: Contraindicated in pregnancy due to oxytocic properties; ergot derivatives in the milk of nursing mothers have caused symptoms of ergotism (e.g., vomiting, diarrhea) in the infant

SIDE EFFECTS/ADVERSE REACTIONS

CNS: Ataxia, dizziness, drowsiness, hyperesthesia, insomnia, lightheadedness, mild euphoria, unworldly feelings, weakness

---

italic = common side effects   ***bold italic*** = life-threatening reactions

*CV: **Cardiac fibrosis,*** edema, vaso-constriction of small and large arteries (chest pain, abdominal pain, cold, numb, painful extremities, diminished or absent pulses)

GI: Abdominal pain, constipation, diarrhea, heartburn, nausea, vomiting

*GU: **Retroperitoneal fibrosis***

HEME: Eosinophilia, ***neutropenia***

MS: Arthralgia, myalgia

*RESP: **Pleuropulmonary fibrosis***

SKIN: Facial flush, increased hair loss, non-specific rashes, telangiectasia

MISC: Weight gain

SPECIAL CONSIDERATIONS
• Reserve for patients who have failed to respond to safer agents (e.g., β-blockers, TCAs, and calcium channel blockers)

PATIENT/FAMILY EDUCATION
• Continuous administration should not exceed 6 mo
• Notify clinician of cold, numb, or painful extremities; leg cramps when walking; girdle, flank, or chest pain; painful urination; or shortness of breath (i.e. fibrotic symptoms)

MONITORING PARAMETERS
• Consider baseline urography, repeated q6-12 mo during therapy
• Monitor for new cardiac murmurs

---

metoclopramide
(met´oh-kloe-pra´mide)
Rx: Reglan
Chemical Class: Paraminobenzoic acid derivative
Therapeutic Class: Gastrointestinal prokinetic agent; antiemetic

---

CLINICAL PHARMACOLOGY
Mechanism of Action: Inhibits gastric smooth muscle relaxation produced by dopamine, thus enhancing cholinergic responses of GI smooth muscle; increases resting pressure of the lower esophageal sphincter, increases amplitude of esophageal peristaltic contractions; dopamine antagonist action raises the threshold of activity in the chemoreceptor trigger zone and decreases input from afferent visceral nerves; stimulates prolactin secretion

Pharmacokinetics

PO: Onset 30-60 min, duration 1-2 hr

IM: Onset 10-15 min, duration 1-2 hr

IV: Onset 1-3 min, duration 1-2 hr

13%-22% bound to plasma proteins; partially metabolized in liver, eliminated in urine; $t_{1/2}$ 4-6 hr

INDICATIONS AND USES: Gastroesophageal reflux disease (GERD); diabetic gastroparesis; chemotherapy-induced nausea and vomiting (parenteral); facilitation of small bowel intubation; postoperative nausea and vomiting; prevention of aspiration pneumonitis presurgery*; slow gastric emptying*; gastic stasis in preterm infants*; vascular headache*; lactation deficiency*; diabetic cystoparesis*; esophageal variceal bleeding*

DOSAGE

Adult

• *GERD/gastroparesis:* PO/IM/IV 10-15 mg 30 min ac and hs; PR 25 mg (5 oral tabs compounded in polyethylene glycol) 30 min ac and hs

• *Intubation of small bowel:* IV 10 mg.

• *Postoperative nausea and vomiting:* IM 10-20 mg near the end of surgery

• *Chemotherapy-induced nausea and vomiting:* IV 1-2 mg/kg/dose 30 min before chemotherapy then q2h for 2 doses, then q3h for 3 doses; dilute in 50 ml of parenteral sol and infused over at least 15 min; initial 2

---

doses 2 mg/kg for highly emetogenic regimens, 1 mg/kg/dose may be used for less emetogenic regimens

• *Esophageal erosions and ulcerations:* PO/IM/IV 15 mg qid as tolerated, healing documented in one controlled trial

• *Dosing adjustment in renal failure:* CrCl 10-50 ml/min administer 75% of recommended dose; CrCl <10 ml/min, administer 25-50% of recommended dose

Child

• *GERD:* PO/IM/IV 0.4-0.8 mg/kg/day divided qid

• *Intubation of small bowel:* IV (<6 yr) 0.1 mg/kg; (6-14 yr) 2.5-5 mg

• *Chemotherapy-induced nausea and vomiting:* IV 1-2 mg/kg/dose q2-4 hr

💲 AVAILABLE FORMS/COST OF THERAPY

• Conc—Oral: 10 mg/ml, 30 ml: **$19.49**

• Inj, Sol—IM, IV: 5 mg/ml, 2 ml: **$0.93-$3.95**

• Syr—Oral: 5 mg/5 ml, 480 ml: **$6.25-$62.04**

• Tab, Uncoated—Oral: 5 mg, 100's: **$24.80-$58.25**; 10 mg, 100's: **$3.55-$94.32**

CONTRAINDICATIONS: GI hemorrhage, mechanical obstruction or perforation of the GI tract, pheochromocytoma, seizure disorder

PRECAUTIONS: History of depression, Parkinson's disease, hypertension, anastomosis or closure of the gut, CHF and cirrhosis (risk of fluid retention)

PREGNANCY AND LACTATION: Pregnancy category B; has been used during pregnancy as an antiemetic and to decrease gastric emptying time; excreted into milk; use during lactation a concern because of the potent CNS effects the drug is capable of producing

SIDE EFFECTS/ADVERSE REACTIONS

CNS: Dizziness, *drowsiness, EPS* (dystonia, parkinson-like symptoms, akathisia, tardive dyskinesia 1-9%), *fatigue,* hallucinations, *headache, restlessness, sedation, seizures, sleeplessness*

CV: Bradycardia, hypertension, hypotension, supraventricular tachycardia

EENT: Visual disturbances

GI: Bowel disturbances, *diarrhea,* nausea

GU: Incontinence, urinary frequency

HEME: **Agranulocytosis, leukopenia, methemoglobinemia** (especially overdoses in neonates), **neutropenia,** porphyria

METAB: Amenorrhea, elevated aldosterone, galactorrhea, gynecomastia, impotence (hyperprolactinemia)

SKIN: Rash, urticaria

MISC: **Neuroleptic malignant syndrome**

INTERACTIONS

Drugs

🔢 *Cyclosporine:* Increased bioavailability and serum concentrations of cyclosporine

🔢 *Digitalis glycosides:* Reduced serum digoxin concentration when coadministered with generic formulations

🔢 *Ethanol:* Increased sedative effects of ethanol

🔢 *MAOIs:* Metoclopramide releases catecholamines, use cautiously with MAOIs

🔢 *Insulin:* Dosage and timing of insulin may need to be adjusted

SPECIAL CONSIDERATIONS

• Dystonic reactions can be managed with 50 mg diphenhydramine or 1-2 mg benztropine IM

M

---

italic = common side effects   ***bold italic*** = life-threatening reactions

PATIENT/FAMILY EDUCATION
• Use caution while diving or during other activities requiring alertness; may cause drowsiness

---

metolazone
(met-tole´a-zone)
Rx: Mykrox (rapid acting),
Zaroxolyn (slow acting)
Chemical Class: Quinazoline
derivative
Therapeutic Class: Thiazide-
like diuretic; antihypertensive

CLINICAL PHARMACOLOGY
Mechanism of Action: Structural and pharmacological similarities to thiazide diuretics; inhibits reabsorption of sodium and chloride in cortical thick ascending limb of the loop of Henle and the early distal tubules—increasing the urinary excretion of sodium and chloride; retains some proximal tubule activity via carbonic anhydrase inhibition activity; other actions—increased potassium and bicarbonate excretion; decreased calcium excretion; uric acid retention; antihypertensive action dependent on sodium depletion, drop in peripheral vascular resistance, and reduction in extracellular volume; more effective than thiazides in patients with impaired renal function (may produce diuresis with CrCl <20 ml/min)
Pharmacokinetics
PO: (Rapid acting) peak 2-4 hr, steady state within 4-5 days; (Slow acting) peak 8 hr; 50%-70% bound to erythrocytes, up to 33% bound to plasma proteins; 70%-95% excreted unchanged in urine by glomerular filtration and active tubular secretion; $t_{1/2}$ 8 hr

INDICATIONS AND USES: Slow acting: edema (CHF, nephrotic syndrome, hepatic cirrhosis, corticosteroid and estrogen therapy); potentiation of loop diuretics: concomitant with loop diuretic to induce diuresis in patients who did not respond to either diuretic alone; hypertension. Rapid acting: hypertension (not indicated for diuresis as dosage not established)
DOSAGE
NOTE: Equivalent hydrochlorothiazide dose: 5 mg-50 mg
Adult
• *Edema:* PO (Slow acting) 5-10 mg q AM; up to 20 mg qd may be required for edema associated with renal disease
• *Hypertension:* PO (Slow acting) 1.25-5 mg q AM; (Rapid acting) 0.5-1 mg q AM
Child
• PO (Slow acting) 0.2-0.4 mg/kg/day divided q12-24h
💲 AVAILABLE FORMS/COST OF THERAPY
• Tab, Uncoated—Oral: 0.5 mg, 100's: **$73.63-$124.04** (Mykrox)
• Tab, Uncoated—Oral: 2.5 mg, 100's: **$42.86-$94.30**; 5 mg, 100's: **$53.21-$107.16**; 10 mg, 100's: **$60.65-$591.40** (Zaroxolyn)
CONTRAINDICATIONS: Anuria, hepatic coma or pre-coma
PRECAUTIONS: Fluid and electrolyte imbalance (including sodium, potassium, chloride, magnesium, calcium), renal disease, hepatic disease, gout, COPD, lupus erythematosus, diabetes mellitus, hyperparathyroidism, vomiting, diarrhea, elevated cholesterol/triglycerides
PREGNANCY AND LACTATION: Pregnancy category B; therapy for preexisting hypertension can be continued throughout pregnancy with minimal risk; initiating for simple edema not recommended;

---

few unequivocal indications for diuretic therapy in pregnancy except for pulmonary edema or congestive heart failure; excreted into breast milk in small amounts; considered compatible with breast feeding

SIDE EFFECTS/ADVERSE REACTIONS

CNS: Anxiety, depression, *dizziness, drowsiness, fatigue, headache,* paresthesia, *weakness,* neuropathy

CV: Chest pain, irregular pulse, ***arrhythmias,*** orthostatic hypotension, palpitations, volume depletion

EENT: Blurred vision, dry mouth

GI: Abdominal bloating, *anorexia,* jaundice, cholecystitis, constipation, cramps, diarrhea, GI irritation, hepatitis, *nausea,* ***pancreatitis,*** *vomiting*

GU: Frequency, glucosuria, impotence, polyuria

HEME: **Agranulocytosis, aplastic anemia, leukopenia**

METAB: Hypercalcemia, hyperglycemia, hyperuricemia, hypochloremia, *hypokalemia,* hypomagnesemia, hyponatremia, increased creatinine, BUN

MS: Muscle cramps, joint pain

SKIN: Fever, photosensitivity, pruritis, purpura, *rash,* urticaria

INTERACTIONS

Drugs

❷ *Angiotensin-converting enzyme inhibitors:* Risk of postural hypotension when added to ongoing diuretic therapy; more common with loop diuretics; first dose hypotension possible in patients with sodium depletion or hypovolemia due to diuretics or sodium restriction; hypotensive response is usually transient; hold diuretic day of first dose

❸ *Calcium:* Milk-alkali syndrome

❸ *Carbenoxolone:* Enhanced hypokalemia

❸ *Cholestyramine, colestipol:* Reduced serum concentrations of metolazone

❸ *Corticosteroids:* Concomitant therapy may result in excessive potassium loss

❸ *Diazoxide:* Hyperglycemia

❸ *Digitalis glycosides:* Diuretic-induced hypokalemia may increase the risk of digitalis toxicity

❸ *Hypoglycemic agents:* Metolazone increases blood glucose

❸ *Lithium:* Increased serum lithium concentrations, toxicity may occur

❸ *Methotrexate:* Enhanced bone marrow suppression

❸ *Nonsteroidal antiinflammatory drugs:* Concurrent use may reduce diuretic and antihypertensive effects

SPECIAL CONSIDERATIONS

• More effective than other thiazide-type diuretics in patients with impaired renal function

• Metolazone formulations are not bioequivalent or therapeutically equivalent at the same doses. Mykrox is more rapidly and completely bioavailable; Don't interchange brands.

PATIENT/FAMILY EDUCATION

• Will increase urination; take early in the day to prevent sleep disturbance

• May cause sensitivity to sunlight; avoid prolonged exposure to the sun and other ultraviolet light

• May cause gout attacks; notify clinician if sudden joint pain occurs

MONITORING PARAMETERS

• Weight, urine output, serum electrolytes, BUN, creatinine, CBC, uric acid, glucose, lipids

M

---

italic = common side effects   ***bold italic*** = life-threatening reactions

metoprolol

(me-toe′pro-lole)

Rx: Lopressor, Toprol XL
Combinations
  Rx: with hydrochlorothiazide
    (Lopressor Hct)
Chemical Class: β_1-selective
(cardioselective) adrenoreceptor blocker
Therapeutic Class: Antihypertensive; antianginal;
postmyocardial infarction

CLINICAL PHARMACOLOGY

Mechanism of Action: PO competitive β-adrenergic antagonist; produces negative inotropic and chronotropic responses; slows AV nodal
conduction; decreases heart rate; decreases myocardial oxygen consumption; antiarrhythmic effects
(class II); reduction in platelet aggregation and blood viscosity; suppression of renin release; inhibition
of central sympathetic outflow; decreases presynaptic receptor neurotransmitter release; no intrinsic
sympathomimetic, weak membrane
stabilizing activity; moderate lipid
solubility

Pharmacokinetics

PO: Peak effect 1.5-4 hr, duration
10-20 hr (peak delayed with extended release)
IV: Peak effect 20 min, duration 5-8
hr
8%-12% bound to plasma proteins;
extensively metabolized in liver, excreted in urine (3%-10% unchanged); $t_{1/2}$ 3-4 hr

INDICATIONS AND USES: Glaucoma*, migraine headache*, hypertension, postmyocardial infarction,
supraventricular arrhythmias (atrial
fibrillation, atrial flutter, paroxysmal supraventricular tachycardia)*,
aggressive behavior*, angina pectoris, anxiety*, cataract extraction
prophylaxis*, congestive heart failure, neuroleptic-induced akathisia*,
retinal detachment*, tremor*, malignant vasovagal syncope or neuro-
cardiogenic syncope*

DOSAGE

Adult

• *Hypertension:* PO 100 mg/day in
single or divided doses, max 450
mg/day; Sus Action 50-100 mg qd,
max 400 mg/day

• *Angina pectoris:* PO 50 mg bid,
max 400 mg/day; Sus Action 100
mg qd, max 400 mg/day

• *MI:* (early treatment) IV 5 mg q2
min times 3 doses, then PO 25-50
mg q6h 15 min after last IV dose,
continue for 48 hr; maintenance 100
mg bid; (late treatment) 100 mg bid
as soon as clinical condition allows;
continue for at least 3 mo

• *Heart Failure:* Sus Action 25 mg
qd × 2 wk initially with NYHA class
II, 12.5 mg qd initially in more severe heart failure; double dose q2wk
to highest tolerated dose or 200 mg
max

**⑧ AVAILABLE FORMS/COST
OF THERAPY**

• Inj, Sol—IV: 5 mg/5 ml, 1's:
$3.14-$8.93

• Tab, Coated—Oral: 50 mg, 100's:
$41.75-$83.80; 100 mg, 100's:
$62.75-$125.83

• Tab, Coated, Sus Action—Oral: 25
mg, 100's: **$67.91**; 50 mg, 100's:
$67.91; 100 mg, 100's: **$102.04**;
200 mg, 100's: **$204.05**

CONTRAINDICATIONS: Bronchial
asthma, cardiogenic shock, overt
cardiac failure, 2nd and 3rd degree
AV block, severe sinus bradycardia,
heart rate <45 beats/min, systolic
BP <100 mm Hg

PRECAUTIONS: Anesthesia/sur-
gery (myocardial depression), avoid
abrupt withdrawal, bronchospastic
airways, congestive heart failure, di-

abetes mellitus, hyperthyroidism/thyrotoxicosis, concurrent clonidine (discontinue atenolol several days prior to withdrawal of clonidine), peripheral vascular disease, renal disease, impaired hepatic function

PREGNANCY AND LACTATION: Pregnancy category C; similar drug, atenolol, frequently used in the third trimester for treatment of hypertension (many studies of efficacy and safety of atenolol in pregnancy-induced hypertension); long-term use has been associated with intrauterine growth retardation; excreted into breast milk in insignificant concentrations; prudent to monitor infant for signs of β-blockade

SIDE EFFECTS/ADVERSE REACTIONS

CNS: Confusion, depression, *dizziness, fatigue,* headache, insomnia, memory loss, strange dreams

CV: Bradycardia, ***CHF,*** cold extremities, ***heart block,*** hypotension

EENT: Tinnitus, visual disturbances

GI: Constipation, *diarrhea,* dry mouth, heartburn, nausea

GU: Impotence, sexual dysfunction

*HEME: **Agranulocytosis** (rare)*

METAB: Hyperlipidemia (increased TG, total cholesterol, LDL; decreased HDL); masked hypoglycemic response to insulin (sweating excepted)

*RESP: **Bronchospasm (1%),** dyspnea*

SKIN: Alopecia, pruritis, rash

INTERACTIONS

Drugs

3 *α-adrenergic blockers:* Potential enhanced first dose response (marked initial drop in blood pressure) particularly on standing (especially prazosin)

3 *Amiodarone:* Bradycardia, cardiac arrest, or ventricular dysrhythmia

3 *Antidiabetics:* Altered response to hypoglycemia, prolonged recovery of normoglycemia, hypertension, blockade of tachycardia; may increase blood glucose and impair peripheral circulation

3 *Antipyrine:* Increased antipyrine concentrations

3 *Barbiturates:* Reduced β-blocker concentrations

2 *Beta agonists:* Antagonism of bronchodilating effect

3 *Bromazepam, diazepam, oxazepam:* Increased benzodiazepine effect (lorazepam and alprazolam unaffected)

3 *Cimetidine, etintidine, propafenone, propoxyphene, quinidine:* Increased plasma metoprolol concentration

3 *Clonidine:* Abrupt withdrawal of clonidine while on a β-blocker may exaggerate the rebound hypertension due to unopposed α stimulation

3 *Digoxin:* Additive prolongation of atrioventricular (AV) conduction time

3 *Dihydropyridines (nicardipine, nifedipine, felodipine, isradipine, nisoldipine):* Increased beta blocker effects

3 *Diltiazem:* Potentiates β-adrenergic effects; hypotension, left ventricular failure, and AV conduction disturbances problematic in elderly, patients with left ventricular dysfunction, aortic stenosis, or with large doses of either drug

3 *Dipyridamole, Tacrine:* Bradycardia

3 *Fluoxetine:* Enhanced effect of β-blocker

3 *Isoproterenol:* Potential reduction in effectiveness of isoproterenol in the treatment of asthma; less likely with cardioselective agents like metoprolol

M

🖪 *Local anesthetics:* Use of local anesthetics containing epinephrine may result in hypertensive reactions in patients taking β-blockers

🖪 *NSAIDs:* Reduced hypotensive effects of β-blockers

🖪 *Phenylephrine:* Enhanced pressor response to phenylephrine, particularly when it is administered IV

🖪 *Prazosin:* First-dose response to prazosin may be enhanced by β-blockade

🖪 *Quinolones:* Inhibition of β-blocker metabolism, increased β-blocker effects

🖪 *Rifampin:* Reduced plasma metoprolol concentration

🖪 *Theophylline:* Antagonistic pharmacodynamic effects

🖪 *Verapamil:* Potentiates β adrenergic effects; hypotension, left ventricular failure, and AV conduction disturbances problemmatic in elderly, patients with left ventricular dysfunction, aortic stenosis, or with large doses of either drug

SPECIAL CONSIDERATIONS
PATIENT/FAMILY EDUCATION
• Do not discontinue abruptly; may require taper; rapid withdrawal may produce rebound hypertension or angina
• Avoid driving or other activities requiring alertness until response to therapy is determined
• Take with or immediately following meals
• Extended release tablets are scored and can be divided; whole or half tablet should be swallowed whole and not chewed or crushed

MONITORING PARAMETERS
• Angina: Reduction in nitroglycerin usage; frequency, severity, onset, and duration of angina pain; heart rate
• Arrhythmias: heart rate

• Congestive heart failure: Functional status, cough, dyspnea on exertion, paroxysmal nocturnal dyspnea, exercise tolerance, and ventricular function
• Hypertension: Blood pressure
• Migraine headache: Reduction in the frequency, severity, and duration of attacks
• Postmyocardial infarction: Left ventricular function, lower resting heart rate
• Toxicity: Blood glucose, bronchospasm, hypotension, bradycardia, depression, confusion, hallucination, sexual dysfunction

---

metronidazole

(me-troe-ni′da-zole)

Rx: Flagyl, Flagyl ER, Metro IV, MetroCream, MetroGel, Metrolotion, Noritate, Protostat
Kit: Helidac (metronidazole, bismuth subsalicylate, tetracycline)
Chemical Class: Nitroimidazole derivative
Therapeutic Class: Antibiotic; antiprotozoal; anthelmintic

CLINICAL PHARMACOLOGY
Mechanism of Action: Reduced metronidazole, which is cytotoxic but short-lived, interacts with DNA to cause a loss of helical structure, strand breakage, and resultant inhibition of nucleic acid synthesis and cell death
Pharmacokinetics
PO: Peak 1-3 hr
IV: Onset immediate
VAG: 20%-25% systemic bioavailability

<20% bound to plasma proteins; metabolized in liver; eliminated via urine (60%-80%) and feces (6%-15%); $t_{\frac{1}{2}}$ 6-8 hr

INDICATIONS AND USES: Trichomoniasis, amebiasis, giardiasis,* anaerobic bacterial infections, perioperative prophylaxis during colorectal surgery, bacterial vaginosis (VAG and PO*), acne rosacea, *Helicobacter pylori* infection associated with peptic ulcer disease (as part of a multidrug regimen), pseudomembranous colitis,* hepatic encephalopathy,* Crohn's disease*

Antibacterial spectrum usually includes:
• Anaerobic Gram-negative bacilli: *Bacteroides* spp. including the *B. fragilis* group (*B. fragilis, B. distasonis, B. ovatus, B. thetaiotaomicron, B. vulgatus*), *Fusobacterium* spp.
• Anaerobic Gram-positive bacilli: *Clostridium* spp., susceptible strains of *Eubacterium*
• Anaerobic Gram-positive cocci: *Peptococcus* spp., *Peptostreptococcus* spp.
• Protozoa: *Entamoeba histolytica, Trichmonas vaginalis, Giardia lamblia, Balantidium coli*

DOSAGE
Adult
• *Amebiasis:* PO 500-750 mg q8h
• *Trichomoniasis:* PO 250 mg q8h for 7 days or 2 g as a single dose
• *Anaerobic infections:* PO/IV 7.5 mg/kg q6h; do not exceed 4 g/day
• *Pseudomembranous colitis:* PO 250-500 mg tid-qid for 10-14 days; IV 500 mg q8h for 10-14 days
• *Rosacea:* TOP apply to affected areas bid
• *Bacterial vaginosis:* Vag 5 g (1 applicatorful) bid for 5 days; PO 500 mg bid for 7-10 days

• *H. pylori:* PO 250 mg qid or 500 mg bid in combination with omeprazole and clarithromycin, omeprazole and amoxicillin or bismuth subsalicylate and clarithromycin

Child
• *Amebiasis:* PO 35-50 mg/kg/day divided q8h; do not exceed 4 g/day
• *Other parasitic infections:* PO 15-30 mg/kg/day divided q8h
• *Anaerobic infections:* PO/IV 30 mg/kg/day divided q6h; do not exceed 4 g/day
• *Pseudomembranous colitis:* PO 20 mg/kg/day divided q6h

$ **AVAILABLE FORMS/COST OF THERAPY**
• Cap, Gel—Oral: 375 mg, 50's: **$143.56**
• Cream—Top: 0.75%, 45 g: **$44.69-$54.88**
• Gel—Top: 0.75%, 28, 45 g: **$44.69-$54.88**/45 g
• Gel—Vag: 0.75%, 70 g: **$29.04-$48.87**
• Inj, Sol—IV: 500 mg/100 ml, 100 ml: **$2.29-$29.66**
• Kit, Blister card—Oral: : **$81.64**
• Lot—Top: 0.75%, 60 ml: **$57.06**
• Tab, Plain Coated—Oral: 250 mg, 100's: **$5.93-$190.13**; 500 mg, 100's: **$12.53-$346.37**
• Tab, Sus Action—Oral: 750 mg, 30's: **$209.41**

PRECAUTIONS: History of blood dyscrasias, severe hepatic impairment, CNS disease, severe renal failure

PREGNANCY AND LACTATION: Pregnancy category B; use in pregnancy controversial; use in 1st trimester and single-dose therapy often avoided; use with caution during breast feeding; if single-dose therapy is used, discontinue breast feeding for 12-24 hr to allow excretion of the drug

italic = common side effects   ***bold italic*** = life-threatening reactions

SIDE EFFECTS/ADVERSE REACTIONS

CNS: Ataxia, confusion, depression, dizziness, headache, incoordination, insomnia, irritability, peripheral neuropathy, *seizures,* vertigo, weakness

CV: T-wave flattening

EENT: Furry tongue, glossitis, stomatitis

GI: Abdominal discomfort, *anorexia,* constipation, diarrhea, *dry mouth,* epigastric distress, *metallic taste, nausea,* **pancreatitis** (rare), pseudomembranous colitis, vomiting

GU: Cystitis, decreased libido, discoloration of urine (IV), dyspareunia, dysuria, incontinence, polyuria, sense of pelvic pressure, urethral burning, vaginal dryness

HEME: Transient thrombocytopenia, leukopenia

MS: Fleeting joint pains

SKIN: Erythematous rash, flushing, pruritus, urticaria

INTERACTIONS

Drugs

🄳 *Carbamazepine:* Increased carbamazepine levels

🄳 *Cholestyramine, colestipol:* Reduced metronidazole absorption

🄳 *Disulfiram:* CNS toxicity

🄳 *Ethanol:* Disulfiram-like reaction

➋ *Fluorouracil:* Enhanced toxicity of fluorouracil

🄳 *IV phenytoin, phenobarbital, diazepam, nitroglycerine, trimethoprim-sulfamethoxazole:* Disulfiram-like reaction due to ethanol in IV preparations

➋ *Oral anticoagulants:* Increased hypoprothrombinemic response to warfarin

🄳 *Phenytoin:* Increased phenytoin levels

Labs

• *Interference:* Glucose

• *False decrease:* AST, zidovudine level

• *False positive increase:* Clindamycin, erythromycin, polymyxin, tetracycline, and trimethoprim assays

SPECIAL CONSIDERATIONS

• Treat sexual partner(s) for trichomoniasis

PATIENT/FAMILY EDUCATION

• Drug may cause GI upset; take with food

• Avoid alcoholic beverages during therapy and for at least 24 hr following last dose (disulfiram-like reaction possible)

• Drug may cause darkening of urine

• May cause an unpleasant metallic taste

• H_2 blocker must be prescribed with Helidac kit

MONITORING PARAMETERS

• CBC

---

metyrosine

(me-tye′roe-seen)

Rx: Demser

Chemical Class: α-methyl-L-tyrosine

Therapeutic Class: Agent for pheochromocytoma

CLINICAL PHARMACOLOGY

Mechanism of Action: Inhibitor of tyrosine hydroxylase, the rate-limiting step in catecholamine biosynthesis; decreases endogenous catecholamine concentrations by 35%-80%

Pharmacokinetics

PO: Peak 1-3 hr, onset within 1st 2 days of therapy; excreted unchanged in urine; $t_{1/2}$ 3.4-7.2 hr

INDICATIONS AND USES: Pheochromocytoma (preoperative preparation for surgery; patients in whom surgery is contraindicated;

chronic treatment in malignant neo-plasm), adjunct to neuroleptics in chronic schizophrenia*

DOSAGE

Adult and Child >12 yr

• PO 250 mg qid, may increase by 250-500 mg qd up to max of 4 g/day in divided doses

$ AVAILABLE FORMS/COST OF THERAPY

• Cap, Gel—Oral: 250 mg, 100's: **$170.00**

PRECAUTIONS: Impaired hepatic or renal function, children <12 yr

PREGNANCY AND LACTATION: Pregnancy category C

SIDE EFFECTS/ADVERSE REACTIONS

CNS: Anxiety, confusion, depression, disorientation, drooling, hallucinations, headache, insomnia and psychic stimulation upon drug withdrawal, parkinsonism, *sedation, speech difficulty,* tremor, trismus

CV: Peripheral edema

EENT: Nasal stuffiness

GI: Abdominal pain, *diarrhea (10%),* dry mouth, increased AST, nausea, vomiting

GU: Crystalluria, urolithiasis, failure to ejaculate, hematuria, impotence, transient dysuria

HEME: Anemia, eosinophilia, **thrombocytopenia,** thrombocytosis

METAB: Breast swelling, galactorrhea

MISC: Hypersensitivity reactions (urticaria, pharyngeal edema)

INTERACTIONS

Drugs

3 *Phenothiazines, haloperidol:* Potentiation of EPS

Labs

• *False increase:* Urinary catecholamines (due to presence of metyrosine metabolites)

SPECIAL CONSIDERATIONS

PATIENT/FAMILY EDUCATION

• Maintain a daily liberal fluid intake

• Avoid alcohol or CNS depressants

MONITORING PARAMETERS

• Blood pressure, ECG

---

mexiletine

(mex-il'e-teen)

Rx: Mexitil

Chemical Class: Lidocaine derivative

Therapeutic Class: Antidysrhythmic (Class IB)

CLINICAL PHARMACOLOGY

Mechanism of Action: Blocks the fast sodium channel in cardiac tissues; reducing rate of rise and amplitude of the action potential, and decreasing the effective refractory period in Purkinje fibers; does not significantly alter sinus node automaticity, left ventricular function, systolic arterial blood pressure, AV conduction velocity, QRS or QT intervals

Pharmacokinetics

PO: Onset 0.5-2 hr, peak 2-3 hr; 60%-75% bound to plasma proteins; metabolized in liver, eliminated via bile and urine; $t_{1/2}$ 10-12 hr (prolonged in hepatic or renal failure, reduced cardiac output, acute MI)

INDICATIONS AND USES: Documented, life-threatening ventricular dysrhythmia; diabetic neuropathy*

DOSAGE

Adult

• PO 200 mg q8h initially, adjust in 50-100 mg increments q2-3 days, do not exceed 1200 mg/day

Child

• PO 1.4-5 mg/kg/dose q8h

• *Dosing adjustment in renal impairment:* Administer 50%-75% of normal dose if CrCl <10 ml/min

---

italic = common side effects   ***bold italic*** = life-threatening reactions

• *Dosing adjustment in hepatic disease:* Administer 25%-30% of normal dose

$ AVAILABLE FORMS/COST OF THERAPY

• Cap, Gel—Oral: 150 mg, 100's: **$35.95-$115.45**; 200 mg, 100's: **$82.22-$137.41**; 250 mg, 100's: **$95.25-$158.30**

CONTRAINDICATIONS: Cardiogenic shock, pre-existing 2nd or 3rd degree AV block (if pacemaker not present)

PRECAUTIONS: Structural heart disease, hepatic disease, renal function impairment, children, 1st degree AV block, pre-existing sinus node dysfunction, intraventricular conduction abnormalities, hypotension, severe CHF, seizure disorder

PREGNANCY AND LACTATION: Pregnancy category C; limited data do not suggest significant risk to the fetus; compatible with breast feeding

SIDE EFFECTS/ADVERSE REACTIONS

CNS: Changes in sleep habits, confusion, *coordination difficulties,* depression, *dizziness,* fatigue, fever, hallucinations, headache, *lightheadedness,* nervousness, paresthesias, psychosis, **seizures,** short-term memory loss, speech difficulties, *tremor,* weakness

CV: Angina, atrial dysrhythmias, AV block, bradycardia, **cardiogenic shock,** chest pain, **CHF,** conduction disturbances, edema, hot flashes, hypertension, hypotension, **increased ventricular dysrhythmias,** palpitations, PVCs, syncope

EENT: Blurred vision, tinnitus

GI: Abdominal pain, altered taste, changes in appetite, constipation, diarrhea, dry mouth, dysphagia, esophageal ulceration, hepatitis, oral mucous membrane changes, peptic ulcer, pharyngitis, salivary changes, **upper GI bleeding,** upper GI distress (nausea, vomiting, heartburn, 40%)

GU: Decreased libido, impotence, urinary hesitancy

HEME: **Agranulocytosis, leukopenia,** positive ANA, **thrombocytopenia** (rare)

MS: Arthralgia

RESP: Dyspnea, hiccups

SKIN: Diaphoresis, dry skin, **exfoliative dermatitis,** hair loss, rash

INTERACTIONS

Drugs

3 *Acetazolamide, sodium bicarbonate:* Alkalinization of urine retards mexiletine elimination

3 *Phenytoin, rifampin:* Reduced mexiletine concentrations

3 *Quinidine:* Elevated mexiletine concentrations

2 *Theophylline:* Elevated theophylline serum concentrations and toxicity

SPECIAL CONSIDERATIONS

• Because of proarrhythmic effects, not recommended for non-life threatening arrhythmias

• Antiarrhythmic drugs have not been shown to increase survival of patients with ventricular arrhythmias

• Initiate therapy in facilities capable of providing continuous ECG monitoring and managing life-threatening dysrhythmias

PATIENT/FAMILY EDUCATION

• Take with food or antacid

MONITORING PARAMETERS

• Therapeutic mexiletine concentrations 0.5-2 µg/ml

mezlocillin

(mez'-loe-sill-in)
Rx: Mezlin
Chemical Class: Semisynthetic acylaminopenicillin
Therapeutic Class: Antibiotic

CLINICAL PHARMACOLOGY
Mechanism of Action: Inhibits bacterial cell wall synthesis; bactericidal

Pharmacokinetics
IM: Peak 45-90 min; 16%-42% bound to plasma proteins; 15% metabolized to inactive metabolites; excreted principally in urine by tubular secretion and glomerular filtration, partly excreted via bile; $t_{1/2}$ 0.7-1.3 hr (prolonged in severe renal impairment)

INDICATIONS AND USES: Treatment of infections caused by susceptible gram-negative aerobic bacilli and mixed aerobic-anaerobic bacterial infections including serious intra-abdominal infections, UTIs, gynecologic infections, respiratory tract infections, skin and skin stucture infections, bone and joint infections, and septicemia; uncomplicated gonorrhea; perioperative prophylaxis

Antibacterial spectrum usually includes:
• Gram-positive organisms: *Staphylococcus aureus* (non-penicillinase-producing strains), β-hemolytic streptococci (Groups A and B), *Streptococcus pneumoniae, S. faecalis* (enterococcus)
• Gram-negative organisms: *Escherichia coli, Klebsiella* spp. (including *K. pneumoniae*), *Proteus mirabilis, P. vulgaris, Enterobacter* spp., *Shigella* spp., *Morganella morganii, Pseudomonas aeruginosa, Providencia rettgeri, H. influenzae, H. parainfluenzae, Providen-cia stuartii, Citrobacter* spp., *Neisseria* spp., many strains of *Serratia, Salmonella,* and *Acinetobacter* are also susceptible
• Anaerobes: *Peptococcus* spp., *Peptostreptococcus* spp., *Clostridium* spp., *Bacteroides* sp. (including *B. fragilis* group), *Fusobacterium* spp., *Veillonella* spp., *Eubacterium* spp.

DOSAGE
Adult
• IM/IV 3 g q4h or 4 g q6h, do not exceed 24 g/day; IM doses should not exceed 2 g/injection
• *Uncomplicated UTI:* IM/IV 1.5-2 g q6h
• *Complicated UTI:* IM/IV 3 g q6h
• *Uncomplicated gonococcal urethritis:* IM/IV 1-2 g in conjunction with 1 g of probenecid
• *Perioperative prophylaxis:* IV 4 g 0.5-1.5 hr prior to surgery
Child 1 mo-12 yr
• IM/IV 50 mg/kg q4h

§ AVAILABLE FORMS/COST OF THERAPY
• Inj, Dry-Sol—IM, IV: 1 g/vial: **$4.94**; 2 g/vial: **$8.92**; 3 g/vial: **$13.84-$14.43**
• Inj, Dry-Sol—IV: 4 g/vial: **$17.95-$18.84**

PRECAUTIONS: Hypersensitivity to cephalosporins, renal insufficiency, prolonged or repeated therapy, sodium restricted patients

PREGNANCY AND LACTATION: Pregnancy category B; excreted into breast milk in low concentrations; no adverse effects have been observed

SIDE EFFECTS/ADVERSE REACTIONS
CNS: Fever, headache, neuromuscular hyperirritability, *seizures*
GI: Abdominal pain, colitis, *diarrhea,* glossitis; increased AST, ALT; *nausea,* **pseudomembranous colitis,** vomiting

---

italic = common side effects   **bold italic** = life-threatening reactions

GU: **Acute interstitial nephritis,** transient increases in serum creatinine and BUN

HEME: **Bleeding abnormalities, bone marrow depression,** eosinophilia

METAB: Hypernatremia, hypokalemia

RESP: **Respiratory distress**

SKIN: Erythema multiforme, pain at inj site, rash, urticaria

INTERACTIONS
Drugs
■ *Aminoglycosides:* Potential for inactivation of aminoglycosides in patients with severe renal impairment

■ *Chloramphenicol:* Possible inhibition of penicillin antibacterial activity

■ *Methotrexate:* Increased methotrexate concentrations, possible toxicity

Labs
• *False increase:* Urine glucose (with Clinitest; Diastix and TesTape do not interfere), urine protein

SPECIAL CONSIDERATIONS
MONITORING PARAMETERS
• Renal, hepatic, and hematologic systems during prolonged therapy
• Serum electrolytes

miconazole
(mi-kon´a-zole)
Rx: *IV:* Monistat
Top: Micatin, Monistat-Derm, Fungoid Tincture Nail Kit
Vag: Monistat 3, Monistat 5, Monistat 7, Monistat Dual-Pak, Femizol-7
Chemical Class: Imidazole derivative
Therapeutic Class: Antifungal

CLINICAL PHARMACOLOGY
Mechanism of Action: Alters permeability of fungal cell membrane
Pharmacokinetics
TOP: Small amounts absorbed systemically
IV: Onset immediate; distributed into inflamed joints, vitreous humor, peritoneal cavity; limited crossing of blood-brain barrier, terminal $t_{1/2}$ 24 hr; metabolized in liver, excreted in feces, urine (inactive metabolites); >90% protein binding

INDICATIONS AND USES: *IV:* Second line drug in treatment of severe systemic fungal infections such as coccidioidomycosis, candidiasis, cryptococcoses, paracoccidioidomycosis, fungal meningitis, fungal UTI; *TOP:* Tinea pedis, tinea cruris, tinea corporis, tinea versicolor; *Vag:* vulvovaginal candidiasis

DOSAGE
Adult
• IV INF initial test dose of 200 mg, then 200-3600 mg/day; may be divided in 3 INF 200-1200 mg/INF for 1-20 wk

• *Fungal meningitis:* Supplement IV INF with intrathecal miconazole 20 mg q3-7 days

• *Bladder mycoses:* Supplement IV INF with bladder irrigation of miconazole 200 mg bid-qid or as continuous INF

• *Vulvovaginal candidiasis:* Vag (cr) 1 applicatorful qhs for 7 days; (supp) 200 mg (1 supp) qhs for 3 days

• *Tinea:* Top apply to affected area bid for 2-4 wk

Child >1 yr

• IV 20-40 mg/kg/day, not to exceed 15 mg/kg/dose

• *Tinea:* Top same as adult

💲 AVAILABLE FORMS/COST OF THERAPY

• Aer, Spray—Top: 2%, 90, 105, 120 ml: **$4.74**/90 ml
• Cre—Top: 2%, 15, 30, 60, 85 g: **$2.35-$18.89**/15 g
• Cre—Vag: 2%, 45 g: **$4.79-$20.56**
• Inj, Sol—Intrathecal, IV: 10 mg/ml, 20 ml: **$192.35**
• Kit—Top Cre, Vag Supp: 100 mg: **$28.74**; 200 mg: **$11.75**
• Oint—Top: 2%, 150 g: **$9.31**
• Powder—Top: 2%, 90 g: **$4.00-$5.15**
• Supp—Vag: 100 mg, 7's: **$7.98-$16.22**; 200 mg, 3's: **$17.92-$35.06**
• Tampon—Vag: 100 mg, 5's: **$15.96**
• Tincture—Top: 2%, 30 ml: **$9.00-$12.25**

PRECAUTIONS: Renal disease, hepatic disease

PREGNANCY AND LACTATION: Pregnancy category C (Top category B); unknown if excreted into breast milk

SIDE EFFECTS/ADVERSE REACTIONS

CNS: Drowsiness, headache

CV: **Dysrhythmias** (rapid IV), tachycardia

GI: Anorexia, cramps, diarrhea, nausea, vomiting (IV)

GU: Hyponatremia, itching, pelvic cramps (topical forms), vulvovaginal burning

HEME: **Thrombocytopenia**

METAB: Hyperlipidemia (due to vehicle in IV prep)

SKIN: Fever, flushing, hives, *phlebitis* (IV), pruritus, rash

INTERACTIONS

• The base in suppository products may interfere with latex; do not use these with contraceptive diaphragms, condoms

Drugs

🔳 *Aminoglycosides:* Decreased antibiotic peak levels

❷ *Cisapride:* Increased cisapride concentrations, toxicity and arrhythmias

🔳 *Cyclosporine:* Possible increased cyclosporine levels

🔳 *Felodipine:* Enhanced vasodilation, hypotension

❷ *HMG-CoA reductase inhibitors (e.g. lovastatin):* Increased toxicity, rhabdomyolysis

🔳 *Loratadine:* Increased loratadine concentrations

🔳 *Midazolam:* Reduced midazolam metabolism

🔳 *Quinidine:* Increased quinidine concentrations

🔳 *Tacrolimus:* Possible increased tacrolimus levels

🔳 *Tolbutamide:* Inhibition of tolbutamide metabolism

🔳 *Triazolam:* Reduced triazolam metabolism

🔳 *Warfarin:* Enhanced anticoagulant effect

M

---

midazolam

(mid-az'zoe-lam)

Rx: Versed
Chemical Class: Benzodiaz-
epine
Therapeutic Class: Sedative
DEA Class: Schedule IV

CLINICAL PHARMACOLOGY

Mechanism of Action: CNS depression via facilitation of inhibitory
GABA at benzodiazepine receptor
sites (BZ_1—associated with sleep;
BZ_2—associated with memory, motor, sensory, and cognitive function); effects include muscle relaxation (spinal cord), anticonvulsant
activity (brain stem), ataxia (cerebellum), emotional behavior (limbic and cortical areas), and anxiolytic effects (separate from general
CNS depression)

Pharmacokinetics

IM: Onset 15 min, peak serum concentration ½-1 hr

IV: Onset 3-5 min, onset of anesthesia 1½-5 min

Protein binding 97%; $t_{1/2}$ 1.2-12.3 hr;
metabolized in liver, metabolites excreted in urine; crosses placenta,
blood-brain barrier

INDICATIONS AND USES: Preoperative sedation (IM); general anesthesia induction, sedation for diagnostic endoscopic procedures, intubation (IV)

DOSAGE

Adult

• *Preoperative sedation:* IM 70-80
µg/kg 30-60 min before general anesthesia

• *Conscious sedation:* IV using 1
mg/ml dilution, titrate slowly to desired effect (e.g., slurred speech);
give no more than 2.5 mg over at
least 2 min; wait at least 2 min to
fully evaluate effect; administer
small doses to appropriate level of
sedation prn

• *Induction of general anesthesia:*
IV 150-350 µg/kg over 30 sec, wait 2
min, follow with 25% of initial dose
if needed; use lower doses for patients who are >55 yr age, premedi-
cated, debilitated, or severe systemic disease

Child

• *Preoperative sedation:* IM 80-200
µg/kg

• *General anesthesia:* IV 50-200
µg/kg

$ AVAILABLE FORMS/COST OF THERAPY

• Inj, Sol—IM, IV: 1 mg/ml, 2, 5, 10
ml: **$1.43-$5.55**/2 ml; 5 mg/ml, 1, 2,
5, 10 ml: **$3.50-$55.68**/2 ml

• Syrup—Oral: 2 mg/ml, 118 ml:
$147.16

CONTRAINDICATIONS: Shock,
coma, alcohol intoxication, acute
narrow-angle glaucoma

PRECAUTIONS: COPD, CHF,
chronic renal failure, hepatic disease, elderly, debilitated, myasthenia gravis, other muscular dystro-
phies and myotonias

NOTE: Associated with respiratory
depression and respiratory arrest,
especially when used IV for conscious sedation; death and hypoxic
encephalopathy have resulted; reserve use for settings that provide
for continuous monitoring of respiratory and cardiac function and immediate availability of resuscitative
drugs, equipment, and personnel

PREGNANCY AND LACTATION:
Pregnancy category D; excreted in
breast milk, use with caution in nursing mothers

SIDE EFFECTS/ADVERSE REACTIONS

CNS: Anxiety, confusion, euphoria, headache, insomnia, paresthesia, retrograde amnesia, slurred speech, tremors, weakness

CV: Bigeminy, hypotension, nodal rhythm, PVCs, tachycardia

EENT: Blocked ears, blurred vision, diplopia, loss of balance, nystagmus

GI: Hiccups, increased salivation, nausea, vomiting

RESP: Apnea, ***bronchospasm,*** coughing, dyspnea, ***laryngospasm, respiratory depression***

SKIN: Pain, pruritus, rash, swelling at inj site, urticaria

INTERACTIONS

Drugs

3 *Calcium channel blockers, erythromycin, ketoconazole, itraconazole:* Increased midazolam levels; increased sedation; respiratory depression

3 Additive effects with other CNS depressants

---

midodrine

(mid'o-dreen)

Rx: ProAmatine

Chemical Class: Synthetic catecholamine

Therapeutic Class: α-adrenergic sympathomimetic; vasopressor

CLINICAL PHARMACOLOGY

Mechanism of Action: Long-acting, selective α-adrenergic agonist; activity in both venous and arterial systems

Pharmacokinetics

PO: Peak 30 min, onset 45-90 min, duration 4-6 hr

Rapid oral absorption; essentially a "pro-drug," i.e., hydrolyzed enzymatically to active metabolite (desg-lymidodrine: peak 1 hr); renal excretion; $t_{1/2}$'s, 0.5 hr and 3 hr (parent and metabolite, respectively)

INDICATIONS AND USES: Orthostatic hypotension, secondary hypotension,* ejaculation disorders,* female stress incontinence,* urinary incontinence

DOSAGE

Adult

• *Orthostatic hypotension:* 2.5 mg PO bid-tid, increasing gradually to a maximum recommended dose of 40 mg daily

• Give upon arising then q3-4 hr during daytime

• *Psychotropic drug-induced hypotension:* 7.5-15 mg/day

• *Ejaculatory incompetence:* 5 mg tid

🅂 AVAILABLE FORMS/COST OF THERAPY

• Tab—Oral: 2.5 mg, 100's: **$116.68**; 5 mg, 100's: **$234.91**

CONTRAINDICATIONS: Hypertension, severe organic heart disease or congestive heart failure, acute renal disease, acute nephritis, or urinary retention, pheochromocytoma, thyrotoxicosis

PREGNANCY AND LACTATION: Pregnancy category C; unknown if excreted in breast milk

SIDE EFFECTS/ADVERSE REACTIONS

CNS: Dizziness, drowsiness, excitability, headache, irritability, *paresthesia (18%)*, restlessness

CV: Supine hypertension (25%)

GI: Nausea, vomiting

GU: Dysuria, urinary frequency, urinary retention

METAB: Changes in blood glucose, increase in body weight

SKIN: Chills, diaphoresis, *paresthesia (18%)*, *piloerection (13%)*

---

italic = common side effects **bold italic** = life-threatening reactions

M

INTERACTIONS
Drugs
❷ *Alpha adrenergic agonists:* Enhanced pressor response

❸ *Alpha adrenergic antagonists:* Antagonism of midodrine's effects

❸ *Cardiac glycosides, Beta blockers:* Increased risk of bradycardia, AV block, arrhythmia

SPECIAL CONSIDERATIONS
• Advantages include rapid and nearly complete absorption, a long elimination $t_{1/2}$, lack of central nervous system (CNS) penetration, and minimal to no cardiac effects

• Supine hypertension has been a therapy-limiting complication

PATIENT/FAMILY EDUCATION
• To minimize supine hypertension, avoid taking drug after the evening meal

---

mifepristone
(miff-eh-pris´tone)
Rx: Mifeprex, RU-486
Chemical Class: Anti-progestational agent
Therapeutic Class: Abortifacient

CLINICAL PHARMACOLOGY
Mechanism of Action: Interacts competitively with progesterone at progesterone receptors. Weak antiglucocorticoid and antiandrogenic activity

Pharmacokinetics
PO: Rapidly absorbed, peak 90 min, hepatic metabolism by CYP450 3A4, $t_{1/2}$ 18 hours, excreted in feces (83%) and urine (9%)

INDICATIONS AND USES: In conjunction with misoprostol for medical termination of intrauterine pregnancy through day 49 of pregnancy (measured from last menstrual period and presuming 28 day cycle)

DOSAGE
Adult
• PO 600 mg as single dose, followed in 48 hr by 400 mg misoprostol unless confirmed abortion has occurred

💲 AVAILABLE FORMS/COST OF THERAPY
• Tab—Oral: 200 mg, 3's: **$250.00**

CONTRAINDICATIONS:
Confirmed or suspected ectopic pregnancy, undiagnosed adnexal mass, IUD in place, chronic adrenal failure, concurrent long-term corticosteroid therapy, anticoagulation, hemorrhagic disorders, inherited porphyrias, lack of access to medical facility equipped to provide emergency treatment of incomplete abortion

PRECAUTIONS:
Cardiovascular, hypertensive, hepatic, pulmonary or renal disease, Type 1 diabetes mellitus, severe anemia, heavy smoking, smokers aged ≥ 35 (no data on safety in these populations)

PREGNANCY AND LACTATION:
Pregnancy category X; excretion in human milk unknown but likely

SIDE EFFECTS/ADVERSE REACTIONS
CNS: Headache (31%), fatigue (10%), dizziness (12%)

GI: Nausea (61%), vomiting (26%) diarrhea (20%)

*GU: **Cramping and vaginal bleeding (96%), uterine hemorrhage (5%)***

INTERACTIONS
Drugs
❸ *Ketoconazole, itraconazole, erythromycin, grapefruit juice:* May inhibit mifepristone metabolism, raising serum levels

❸ *Rifampin, dexamethasone, St. John's Wort, phenytoin, phenobarbital, carbamazepine:* May induce mifepristone metabolism, lowering serum levels

---

* = non-FDA-approved use

SPECIAL CONSIDERATIONS

• Provided only to licensed physicians who sign and return a Prescriber's Agreement. Not available through pharmacies

• Patients should be given the Medication Guide and sign the Patient Agreement (Danco Laboratories, 1-877-432-7596)

• Provide medication for cramping and GI symptoms, instructions on what to do if significant bleeding or other adverse reactions occur

• Advise patient bleeding/spotting occur for average of 9-16 days; 8% have some bleeding for >30 days

• Expulsion occurs within the first 48hs in 6%, in 63-72% within 24 hr of misoprostol administration (most of these within 4 hr), surgical intervention in 4.5-8%

• Quantitative hCG levels not decisive until ≥10 days following mifepristone administration. Confirm continuing pregnancy by ultrasound scan. Uterine debris does not necessarily require surgical removal

• Report adverse events (blood transfusion, hospitalization, ongoing pregnancy) in writing to Medical Director, Danco Laboratories LLC, PO Box 4816, New York, NY 10185

• For 24 hr/day consultation contact Danco Laboratories at 1-877-432-7596

PATIENT/FAMILY EDUCATION

• Completing treatment schedule is important, including the 48 hr visit for misoprostol and the post treatment follow-up visit at 14 days

• Vaginal bleeding and uterine cramping will occur, but are not proof of complete expulsion

• There is a risk of fetal malformation if treatment fails

• Treatment failure is managed by surgical termination

• Contraception should be initiated as soon as pregnancy termination has been confirmed

---

miglitol

(mig-lee′tall)

Rx: Glyset

Chemical Class: Desoxynojirimycin derivative

Therapeutic Class: Antidiabetic; hypoglycemic, oral α-glucosidase inhibitor

CLINICAL PHARMACOLOGY

Mechanism of Action: Reversible inhibition of intestinal α-glucosidase, preventing breakdown of oligosaccharides and disaccharides to glucose and other monosaccharides, resulting in delayed absorption and lowering of postprandial hyperglycemia; does not enhance endogenous insulin secretion; minor inhibitory activity against lactase

Pharmacokinetics

PO: T_{max} 2-5 hr Absorption saturable (PO), with complete absorption of 25 mg dose, only 50-75% absorption of 100 mg dose; minimal protein binding (<4%); not metabolized; renal excretion (95% recovered in urine after 24 hr); $t_{1/2}$ 2 hr

INDICATIONS AND USES: Adjunct to diet and exercise in diabetes mellitus, type 2, alone or in combination with other hypoglycemics

DOSAGE

Adult

• Initial dose, 25 mg qd (with first bite of main meal); increase gradually to 25 mg tid to minimize gastrointestinal adverse effects; maintenance dose, 50-100 mg tid

---

italic = common side effects   ***bold italic*** = life-threatening reactions

💲 AVAILABLE FORMS/COST OF THERAPY

• Tab, Film-Coated—Oral: 25 mg, 100's: **$58.75**; 50 mg, 100's: **$64.61**; 100 mg, 100's: **$76.20**

CONTRAINDICATIONS: Diabetic ketoacidosis; inflammatory bowel disease, colonic ulceration, partial intestinal obstruction (or conditions that predispose to obstruction); chronic intestinal diseases associated with marked disorders of digestion or absorption; conditions that may deteriorate as a result of increased gas formation; hypersensitivity

PRECAUTIONS: Hypoglycemia (oral glucose [dextrose], whose absorption is not delayed by miglitol, should be used to treat mild to moderate hypoglycemia instead of sucrose [cane sugar])

PREGNANCY AND LACTATION: Pregnancy category B; small amounts excreted in human milk (0.4% of maternal dose)

SIDE EFFECTS/ADVERSE REACTIONS

GI: Abdominal pain (12%), diarrhea (29%), flatulence (42%) (incidence decreases with time)

SKIN: Rash (4%)

INTERACTIONS

Drugs

3 *β-blockers:* Antagonistic glycemic effects, prolong hypoglycemia, mask hypoglycemia symptoms

3 *Diazoxide:* Antagonistic effects (diazoxide causes hyperglycemia)

3 *Epinephrine:* Antagonistic effects; combination may decrease hypoglycemic efficacy

3 *MAOI:* MAOIs stimulate insulin secretion; additive effects; increased risk of hypoglycemia

3 *Hypoglycemics (sulfonylureas, bioguanides, insulin):* Combination increases risk of hypoglycemia

3 *Isoniazid:* Antagonistic effects; combination may decrease hypoglycemic efficacy

3 *Niacin:* Antagonistic effects; combination may decrease hypoglycemic efficacy

Labs

• *Iron:* Decreased; not associated with reduction in hemoglobin or other hematologic indices.

SPECIAL CONSIDERATIONS

• *Pharmacodynamics*

Expected drops in HbA1c: -0.25% to -1.0%; expected drops in fasting plasma glucose: 20-30 mg/dL

PATIENT/FAMILY EDUCATION

• Review prevalence and management of gastrointestinal adverse effects.

MONITORING PARAMETERS

• Self-monitored blood glucose, HbA1c, signs and symptoms of hyper- and hypoglycemia

---

milrinone

(mill're-none)

Rx: Primacor

Chemical Class: Bipyridine derivative

Therapeutic Class: Cardiac inotropic agent

CLINICAL PHARMACOLOGY

Mechanism of Action: Positive inotropic agent with vasodilator properties; selective inhibitor of peak III cAMP phosphodiesterase isozyme in cardiac and vascular muscle; reduces preload and afterload by direct relaxation of vascular smooth muscle

Pharmacokinetics

IV: Onset 2-5 min, peak 10 min, duration variable, $t_{1/2}$ 2-4 hr; metabolized in liver, excreted in urine as drug (83%) and metabolites

INDICATIONS AND USES: Short-term management of CHF not responsive to other medication (can be used with digitalis)

DOSAGE

Adult

• IV bolus 50 µg/kg given over 10 min; start INF of 0.375-0.75 µg/kg/min

• Reduced dose in renal impairment:

CREATININE CLEARANCE (ML/MIN/1.73 M 2)	INFUSION RATE (MG/KG/MIN)
5	0.20
10	0.23
20	0.28
30	0.33
40	0.38
50	0.43

$ AVAILABLE FORMS/COST OF THERAPY

• Inj, Sol—IV: 1 mg/ml, 5, 10 ml: **$35.10-$38.55**/5 ml

CONTRAINDICATIONS: Severe aortic stenosis, severe pulmonic stenosis, acute MI

PRECAUTIONS: Children, renal disease, hepatic disease; atrial flutter, fibrillation; outflow tract obstruction in hypertrophic subaortic stenosis, elderly

PREGNANCY AND LACTATION: Pregnancy category C; caution with breast feeding until more known about excretion in breast milk

SIDE EFFECTS/ADVERSE REACTIONS

CNS: Headache, tremor

CV: Chest pain, **dysrhythmias** (12%), hypotension

GI: Abdominal pain, anorexia, hepatotoxicity, jaundice, nausea, vomiting

HEME: **Thrombocytopenia**

METAB: Hypokalemia

SPECIAL CONSIDERATIONS

MONITORING PARAMETERS

• Fluid and electrolyte changes, renal function

• Improvement in cardiac output may increase diuresis, and K^+ loss

---

minocycline
(mi-noe-sye′kleen)
Rx: Dynacin, Minocin
Chemical Class: Semisynthetic tetracycline
Therapeutic Class: Antibiotic

CLINICAL PHARMACOLOGY

Mechanism of Action: Inhibits protein synthesis, phosphorylation in microorganisms by binding to 30S and possibly the 50S ribosomal subunits; bacteriostatic

Pharmacokinetics

PO: Peak 2-3 hr; $t_{1/2}$ 11-17 hr; biliary and urinary excretion; crosses placenta; excreted in breast milk; 76% protein bound

INDICATIONS AND USES: Syphilis; non-gonococcal urethritis; endocervical and rectal infections caused by *C. trachomatis, U. urealyticum,* gonorrhea; lymphogranuloma venereum; rickettsial infections (Rocky Mountain spotted fever, typhus fever, Q fever, rickettsialpox, tick fevers); inflammatory acne; skin granulomas caused by *Mycobacterium marinum,* respiratory tract infections caused by susceptible organisms; skin and skin structure infections; UTI; treatment of asymptomatic meningococcal carriers when rifampin contraindicated; tularemia; cholera; plague; chancroid; psittacosis; brucellosis (with streptomycin); yaws; anthrax; actinomycosis; trachoma, relapsing

---

italic = common side effects   ***bold italic*** = life-threatening reactions

fever, granuloma inguinale, listeriosis; sclerosing agent in malignant pleural effusions

Antibacterial spectrum usually includes:

• Gram-positive organisms: *Streptococcus pneumoniae, Str. pyogenes,* alpha hemolytic streptococci; many strains strep resistant, demonstrate susceptibility

• Gram-negative organisms: *Bartonella bacilliformis, Brucella, Campylobacter fetus, Francisella tularensis, Haemophilus influenzae, H. ducreyi, Listeria monocytogenes, Neisseria gonorrhea, Vibrio cholera, Yersinia pestis,* some strains of *E. coli, Klebsiella, Shigella, Bacteroides, Enterobacter aerogenes, Acinetobacter*

• Other organisms: *Bacillus anthracis, Balantidium coli, Borrelia recurrentis, Chlamydia psittoci, C. trachomatis, Clostridium, Fusobacterium fusiforme, Mycoplasma pneumoniae, Propionibacterium acnes, Rickettsiae, Treponema pallidum, Ureaplasma urealyticum*

DOSAGE

Adult

• PO/IV 200 mg, then 100 mg q12h or 50 mg q6h, not to exceed 400 mg/24h IV

• *Gonorrhea* (not drug of choice): PO 200 mg, then 100 mg q12h for 4 days

• *Chlamydia trachomatis, Ureaplasma urealyticum:* PO 100 mg bid for 7 days

• *Syphilis* (PCN allergic patients): PO 200 mg, then 100 mg q12h for 10-15 days

• *Acne:* PO 50 mg 1-3 times/day

• *Skin granulomas from M. marinum:* PO 100 mg bid for 6-8 wk

• *Sclerosing agent:* 300 mg diluted with 50 ml 0.9% NaCl inj instilled via thoracostomy tube

Child >8 yr

• PO/IV 4 mg/kg then 2 mg/kg q12h

§ AVAILABLE FORMS/COST OF THERAPY

• Cap, Gel—Oral: 50 mg, 100's: **$58.75-$223.44**; 75 mg, 100's: **$197.96-$291.81**; 100 mg, 100's: **$39.81-$186.11**

• Inj, Lyphl-Sol—IV: 100 mg/vial: **$44.43**

• Susp—Oral: 50 mg/5 ml, 60 ml: **$39.01**

CONTRAINDICATIONS: Children <8 yr

PRECAUTIONS: Hepatic disease

PREGNANCY AND LACTATION: Pregnancy category D; not recommended in last half of pregnancy secondary to adverse effects on fetal teeth; not recommended in breast feeding

SIDE EFFECTS/ADVERSE REACTIONS

CNS: Dizziness, fever, lightheadedness, pseudotumor cerebri, vertigo,

CV: Pericarditis

EENT: Decreased calcification of deciduous teeth, dysphagia, oral candidiasis

GI: Abdominal cramps, abdominal pain, anorexia, *diarrhea,* enterocolitis, epigastric burning, flatulence, glossitis, hepatotoxicity, *nausea,* stomatitis, *vomiting*

GU: Increased BUN

HEME: Eosinophilia, **hemolytic anemia, neutropenia, thrombocytopenia**

SKIN: Angioedema, blue-gray color of skin and mucous membranes, **exfoliative dermatitis,** *increased pigmentation, photosensitivity,* pruritus, *rash, urticaria*

INTERACTIONS

Drugs

3 *Antacids:* Decreased effect of minocycline

3 *Barbiturates:* Decreased effect of minocycline

---

* = non-FDA-approved use

❷ *Bismuth:* Inhibited antibiotic absorption

❸ *Carbamazepine:* Decreased effect of minocycline

❸ *Colestipol, cholestyramine:* Inhibited antibiotic absorption

❸ *Digoxin:* Increased digoxin levels in 10% of patients

❸ *Iron:* Decreased minocycline absorption

❷ *Methoxyflurane:* Renal toxicity

❸ *Oral contraceptives:* Decreased contraceptive efficacy

❸ *Penicillins:* Antagonizes antibacterial effect of penicillins

❸ *Warfarin:* Possible increase in hypoprothrombinemic response

SPECIAL CONSIDERATIONS
PATIENT/FAMILY EDUCATION
• May take with food
• Avoid sun exposure

---

minoxidil
(min-nox'i-dill)
Rx: *Oral:* Loniten
OTC: Rogaine
Chemical Class: Piperidinopyrimidine derivative
Therapeutic Class: Direct vasodilator: antihypertensive (oral use); hair growth stimulant (topical use)

CLINICAL PHARMACOLOGY
Mechanism of Action: Relaxes arteriolar smooth muscle, causes vasodilation with reflex increase in heart rate, cardiac output; increases cutaneous blood flow, stimulate hair follicles

Pharmacokinetics
PO: Onset 30 min, peak 2-3 hr, duration 24-48 hr, $t_{1/2}$ 4.2 hr; metabolized in liver, 97% renal excretion (metabolites); excreted in breast milk

TOP: Small amounts absorbed (0.3%-4.5%), absorption increased through inflamed skin; onset of action min 4 mo; growth peaks at 1 yr

INDICATIONS AND USES: Severe hypertension not responsive to other therapy, in conjunction with diuretic; topically to treat alopecia androgenetica (less effective in frontal hair loss), alopecia areata

DOSAGE
Adult and Adolescents
• PO 2.5-5 mg/day as single dose or divided bid not to exceed 100 mg/day, usual range 10-40 mg/day; double dose q3 days to appropriate response; for rapid control adjust q6h, monitor closely
• TOP 1 ml (2% sol) bid regardless of size of area, max 2 ml qd
Child <12 yr
• Initial dose PO 0.2 mg/kg/day (max 5 mg), effective range 0.25-1 mg/kg/day in 1 or 2 doses, max 50 mg/day

💲 **AVAILABLE FORMS/COST OF THERAPY**
• Sol—Top: 2%, 60 ml: **$7.75-$60.05**; 5%, 60 ml: **$14.16-$48.00**
• Tab, Uncoated—Oral: 2.5 mg, 100's: **$22.01-$79.84**; 10 mg, 100's: **$25.43-$175.41**

CONTRAINDICATIONS: Acute MI, dissecting aortic aneurysm, pheochromocytoma (PO)

PRECAUTIONS: Children, renal disease, CAD, CHF (PO)

PREGNANCY AND LACTATION: Pregnancy category C; compatible with breast feeding

SIDE EFFECTS/ADVERSE REACTIONS
CV: Angina, *CHF,* edema, **pericardial effusion, pericarditis, pulmonary edema,** severe rebound hypertension, sodium and water retention, tachycardia, *T wave changes* (direction and magnitude, 60%)
GI: Nausea, vomiting

---

italic = common side effects   ***bold italic*** = life-threatening reactions

M

GU: Breast tenderness, gynecomastia

HEME: Decreased Hct (hemodilution), *leukopenia, thrombocytopenia*

SKIN: Hypertrichosis (80% of patients, resolves 1-6 months after discontinuation of drug), pruritus, rash, *Stevens-Johnson syndrome*

SKIN: Contact dermatitis, hypertrichosis; irritant

INTERACTIONS

Drugs

❷ *Guanethidine:* Orthostatic hypotension, may be severe

• No known interactions with top sol

SPECIAL CONSIDERATIONS

• Must be used in conjunction with diuretic (except dialysis patients) and β-blocker or other sympathetic nervous system depressant (to prevent reflex tachycardia)

PATIENT/FAMILY EDUCATION

• At least 4 mo of bid application necessary before evidence of hair growth with topical solution

• Continued treatment necessary to maintain or increase hair growth with topical solution

---

mirtazapine

(mir-taz'a-peen)

Rx: Remeron

Chemical Class: Tetracyclic piperazino-azepine derivative

Therapeutic Class: Antidepressant

CLINICAL PHARMACOLOGY

Mechanism of Action: Enhances central noradrenergic and serotonergic activity by blocking central presynaptic α_2 inhibitory receptors and postsynaptic serotonin receptors; has anxiolytic properties; moderate anticholinergic and orthostatic hypotensive effects; high sedative activity

Pharmacokinetics

PO: Peak 2 hr, completely absorbed; elimination $t_{1/2}$ 20-40 hr (longer in females than males); 85% protein bound; extensive hepatic metabolism; excretion 75% by kidney, 15% in feces

INDICATIONS AND USES: Depression, preoperative insomnia/anxiety*

DOSAGE

Adult

• *Depression:* PO 15 mg qhs to start, increase q1-2 wk; effective dosage range 15-45 mg qd

• *Preoperative insomnia:* PO 15 mg

$ AVAILABLE FORMS/COST OF THERAPY

• Tab—Oral: 15 mg, 30's: **$86.61**; 30 mg, 30's: **$89.21**; 45 mg, 30's: **$90.94**

• Tab, Disintegrating—Oral: 15 mg, 30's: **$72.11**; 30 mg, 30's: **$74.28**; 45 mg, 30's: **$90.94**

CONTRAINDICATIONS: Concurrent MAO inhibitor therapy

PRECAUTIONS: Elderly, hepatic insufficiency, renal insufficiency, mania or hypomania, seizure disorder

PREGNANCY AND LACTATION: Unknown if excreted in breast milk

SIDE EFFECTS/ADVERSE REACTIONS

CNS: Abnormal dreams, anxiety, cerebral ischemia, confusion, *dizziness* (7%), *drowsiness* (54%), EPS, hallucinations, migraine, *seizures* (<0.01%), tremor, vertigo

CV: Angina, bradycardia, CHF, hypertension, hypotension, MI, syncope, ventricular extrasystoles

EENT: Dry mouth

GI: Constipation (13%), increased appetite, weight gain

HEME: **Agranulocytosis and neutropenia** (0.1%), anemia, lymphadenopathy, lymphocytosis, **pancytopenia,** thrombocytopenia
METAB: Elevated cholesterol

INTERACTIONS
Drugs
⚠ *MAOIs:* Possible serotonin syndrome (hyperthermia, autonomic instability, seizures, death)

SPECIAL CONSIDERATIONS
• Chemical structure unrelated to TCAs, SSRIs, MAOIs
• Shown to be an effective antidepressant in several trials but place in therapy not yet determined
• Manufacturer recommends stopping MAOI 14 days before initiating therapy secondary to interactions between MAOIs and other antidepressants

---

misoprostol
(me-soe-prost′ole)
Rx: Cytotec
Combinations
  Rx: with diclofenac (Arthrotec)
Chemical Class: Prostaglandin E_1 analog
Therapeutic Class: Gastrointestinal protectant; abortifacient

---

CLINICAL PHARMACOLOGY
Mechanism of Action: Inhibits gastric acid secretion; may protect gastric mucosa; can increase bicarbonate and mucus production; stimulates uterine contractions
Pharmacokinetics
PO: Rapidly metabolized to active metabolite; peak 12 min; plasma steady state achieved within 2 days; excreted in urine; $t_{1/2}$ 20-40 min; unknown if metabolite excreted in breast milk

INDICATIONS AND USES: Prevention of nonsteroidal anti-inflammatory drug (NSAID)-induced gastric ulcers; treatment of duodenal ulcer*; abortifacient in early pregnancies (with methotrexate or mifepristone)*; morning after contraception*

DOSAGE
Adult
• *Gastric ulcer prophylaxis:* PO 200 μg qid with food for duration of NSAID therapy; if drug not tolerated, decrease to 100 μg qid or 200 μg bid

💲 AVAILABLE FORMS/COST OF THERAPY
• Tab, Uncoated—Oral: 100 μg, 60's: **$41.93-$58.00**; 200 μg, 60's: **$53.51-$70.28**

CONTRAINDICATIONS: Pregnancy (unless used as abortifacient)
PRECAUTIONS: Women of childbearing age, children
PREGNANCY AND LACTATION: Pregnancy category X; do not use in breast feeding (possible diarrhea in infant)

SIDE EFFECTS/ADVERSE REACTIONS
CNS: Headache
GI: Abdominal pain, constipation, *diarrhea,* dyspepsia, flatulence, nausea, vomiting
GU: Cramps, spotting, vaginal bleeding

INTERACTIONS
Drugs
3 *Phenylbutazone:* Increase in adverse effects (headache, flushes, dizziness, nausea)

SPECIAL CONSIDERATIONS
• Reserve use for those patients at high risk for NSAID-induced ulcer (e.g., elderly, history of previous ulcer)
• Does not prevent NSAID-associated GI pain or discomfort

---

italic = common side effects   ***bold italic*** = life-threatening reactions

modanfinil
(moe-daf'ih-nil)
Rx: Provigil
Chemical Class: Benzhydryl-sulfinylacetamide compound; (bears a distant similarity to dextroamphetamine)
Therapeutic Class: Central nervous system stimulant

CLINICAL PHARMACOLOGY
Mechanism of Action: Mechanism of CNS stimulation unknown; does not bind to potentially relevant receptors (norepinephrine, serotonin, dopamine, GABA, adenosine, histamine₃, melatonin, or benzodiazepines); not a direct or indirect dopamine receptor or α_1 adrenergic agonist; no peripheral sympathomimetic effects as observed with amphetamines; however, does require an intact sympathomimetic nervous system for activity
Pharmacokinetics
PO: Peak conc 2-4 hr; absorption is rapid, not affected by food; metabolized by liver (metabolites inactive), protein binding 60%; Vd 0.9L/kg; metabolites renally excreted (10% unchanged in urine); $t_{1/2}$ 7.5-12 hr
INDICATIONS AND USES: Narcolepsy, idiopathic hypersomnia,* obstructive sleep apnea (hypopnea syndrome),* organic brain syndrome,* sleep deprevation
DOSAGE
Adult and child >16 yr
• *Narcolepsy:* 200 mg qam (400 mg daily doses fail to provide further benefits); *Idiopathic hypersomnia:* 200-300 mg qam (up to 500 mg)/day divided bid—qam and noon); reduce 50% for severe hepatic insufficiency

* = non-FDA-approved use

💲 AVAILABLE FORMS/COST OF THERAPY
• Tab—Oral: 100 mg, 100's: **$398.75**; 200 mg, 100's: **$551.25**
PRECAUTIONS: Cardiovascular disease (left ventricular hypertrophy, ischemic ECG changes, chest pain, arrhythmia, mitral valve prolapse, recent myocardial infarction, unstable angina); elderly patients (possible dose reductions); history of emotional instability, drug abuse or psychosis, hypertension (periodic monitoring is advised); severe hepatic disease (50% dose reduction); severe renal impairment; risk of pregnancy with concurrent oral contraceptives use
PREGNANCY AND LACTATION: Pregnancy category C; no mutagenic or clastogenic potential in several *in vitro* assays; *in vivo* mouse bone marrow micronucleus assays were also negative for mutagenicity; not fully evaluated; breast milk excretion unknown
SIDE EFFECTS/ADVERSE REACTIONS
CNS: Headache (50%) nervousness (8%), dizziness (5%), depression (4%), anxiety (4%), and insomnia (3%), delayed sleep; euphoria, motor excitation reported with 500 mg daily doses
CV: Minimal effects on blood pressure and pulse
GI: Hypersalivation, nausea (13%), diarrhea (8%), dry mouth (5%)
SPECIAL CONSIDERATIONS
• Comparisons of modanfinil with agents that have proven effective in narcolepsy, including methylphenidate, pemoline, and dextroamphetamine, are needed to clarify its relative safety and efficacy, and place in therapy

MONITORING PARAMETERS
• *Efficacy:* Daytime sleepiness, daytime sleep episodes, and overall daily performance
• *Toxicity:* Blood pressure

---

moexipril
(moe-ex'a-prile)
Rx: Univasc
Combinations
  Rx: with hydrochlorothiazide (Uniretic)
Chemical Class: Nonsulfhydryl angiotensin-converting enzyme (ACE) inhibitor
Therapeutic Class: Antihypertensive

CLINICAL PHARMACOLOGY
Mechanism of Action: Antihypertensive, hypoproliferative, and cardioprotective effects attributable to competitive inhibition of angiotensin-converting enzyme (ACE) yielding decreased plasma concentrations of angiotensin II, plasma aldosterone concentrations, systemic vascular resistance, blood pressure, preload, and afterload, not accompanied by changes in heart rate, pressor sensitivity to exogenous norepinephrine, or baroreceptor sensitivity
Pharmacokinetics
PO: Prodrug, requiring hepatic conversion to active metabolite (moexiprilat); bioavailability 13%; onset 1 hr, duration 24 hr; fecal excretion 50% (13% renal excretion); $t_{1/2}$ 2-10 hr

INDICATIONS AND USES: Hypertension, CHF (left ventricular dysfunction),* MI (left ventricular salvage),* erythrocytosis,* nephropathy,* retinopathy*

DOSAGE
Adult
• PO 7.5 mg (3.75 mg with concomitant diuretic) qd; maintenance 7.5-30 mg qd or divided bid
• *Dosage in renal failure:* PO 3.75 mg qd; max maintenance 15 mg/day
§ **AVAILABLE FORMS/COST OF THERAPY**
• Tab, Uncoated—Oral: 7.5, 15 mg, 100's: **$82.25**
PRECAUTIONS: History of anaphylaxis, renal insufficiency (<30 ml/min), hypotension (CHF, elderly, volume depletion—diuretics, dialysis, cirrhosis), aortic stenosis, hyperkalemia (potassium supplements, potassium-sparing diuretics, renal disease, diabetes), neutropenia (autoimmune diseases, collagen vascular, febrile illness, immunosuppressant drug therapy), proteinuria, renal artery stenosis, surgery/anesthesia (excessive hypotension, correctable with fluids)
PREGNANCY AND LACTATION: Pregnancy category D; ACE inhibitors can cause fetal and neonatal morbidity and death when administered to pregnant women; when pregnancy is detected, discontinue ACE inhibitors as soon as possible
SIDE EFFECTS/ADVERSE REACTIONS
CNS: Dizziness, fatigue, headache, insomnia, peripheral neuropathy
CV: *CHF, dysrhythmia, hypotension,* Raynaud's syndrome
GI: Abdominal pain, apthous ulcers, diarrhea, dysgeusia, gastric irritation, nausea, vomiting, weight loss
GU: Nephrotic syndrome, polyuria, proteinuria, renal insufficiency
HEME: *Agranulocytosis,* decreased hemoglobin, *neutropenia, pancytopenia, thrombocytopenia*
METAB: Electrolyte disturbance (hyperkalemia, hyponatremia)
RESP: *Cough*

SKIN: Alopecia, pemphigus, pruritus, rash, scalded-mouth sensation
INTERACTIONS
Drugs
❷ *Allopurinol:* Combination may predispose to hypersensitivity reactions

❸ α*-adrenergic blockers:* Exaggerated first dose hypotensive reactions when added to moexipril

❸ *Aspirin:* May reduce hemodynamic effects of moexipril; less likely at doses under 236 mg; less likely with nonacetylated salicylates

❸ *Azathioprine:* Increased myelosuppression

❸ *Cyclosporine:* Combination may cause renal insufficiency

❸ *Insulin:* Moexipril may enhance insulin sensitivity

❸ *Iron:* Moexipril may increase chance of systemic reaction to IV iron

❸ *Lithium:* Reduced lithium clearance

❸ *Loop diuretics:* Initiation of moexipril may cause hypotension and renal insufficiency in patients taking loop diuretics

❸ *NSAIDs:* May reduce hemodynamic effects of moexipril

❸ *Potassium-sparing diuretics:* Increased risk of hyperkalemia

❸ *Trimethoprim:* Additive risk of hyperkalemia, especially in patient predisposed to renal insufficiency
Labs
• ACE inhibition can account for approximately 0.5 mEq/L rise in serum potassium
SPECIAL CONSIDERATIONS
PATIENT/FAMILY EDUCATION
• Caution with salt substitutes containing potassium chloride
• Rise slowly to sitting/standing position to minimize orthostatic hypotension

• Dizziness, fainting, lightheadedness may occur during 1st few days of therapy
• May cause altered taste perception or cough; persistent dry cough usually does not subside unless medication is stopped; notify clinician if these symptoms persist
MONITORING PARAMETERS
• BUN, creatinine, potassium within 2 wk after initiation of therapy (increased levels may indicate acute renal failure)

---

molindone
(moe-lin′done)
Rx: Moban
Chemical Class: Dihydroindolone derivative
Therapeutic Class: Antipsychotic

CLINICAL PHARMACOLOGY
Mechanism of Action: Dopamine receptor antagonist, with higher affinity for D_2 over D_1 receptors, and variable selectivity among the cotical dopamine tracts; also activity on nondopaminergic sites, i.e., cholinergic, α_1-adrenergic and histamine receptors (explaining side effects); moderate risk extrapyramidal reactions and sedation; minimal orthostatic hypotension and anticholinergic effects
Pharmacokinetics
PO: Onset erratic, peak 1½ hr, duration 24-36 hr
Metabolized by liver (36 recognized metabolites); excreted in urine and feces; $t_{1/2}$ 1½ hr
INDICATIONS AND USES: Psychotic disorders
DOSAGE
NOTE: 10 mg equivalent to chlorpromazine 100 mg

Adult

• PO initial dose 50-75 mg/day increasing to 225 mg/day if needed; maintenance dose, mild, 5-15 mg tid-qid; moderate, 10-25 mg tid-qid; severe 225 mg/day may be required

$ **AVAILABLE FORMS/COST OF THERAPY**

• Conc—Oral: 20 mg/ml, 120 ml: **$190.00-$206.13**
• Tab, Uncoated—Oral: 5 mg, 100's: **$89.00-$120.00**; 10 mg, 100's: **$95.72-$172.50**; 25 mg, 100's: **$142.78-$257.31**; 50 mg, 100's: **$190.66-$343.69**; 100 mg, 100's: **$235.86-$254.71**

CONTRAINDICATIONS: Coma, children

PRECAUTIONS: Hypertension, hepatic disease, cardiac disease, Parkinson's disease, brain tumor, glaucoma, urinary retention, diabetes mellitus, respiratory disease, prostatic hypertrophy, geriatric patients

PREGNANCY AND LACTATION: Pregnancy category C

SIDE EFFECTS/ADVERSE REACTIONS

CNS: Akathisia, drowsiness, dystonia, extrapyramidal symptoms including pseudoparkinsonism, headache, *seizures,* tardive dyskinesia

CV: ***Cardiac arrest,*** ECG changes, hypertension, *orthostatic hypotension,* tachycardia

EENT: Blurred vision, glaucoma

GI: Anorexia, constipation, diarrhea, *dry mouth,* jaundice, *nausea, vomiting,* weight gain

GU: Amenorrhea, enuresis, gynecomastia, impotence, urinary frequency, urinary retention

HEME: ***Agranulocytosis, anemia, leukocytosis, leukopenia***

RESP: Dyspnea, ***laryngospasm, respiratory depression***

SKIN: Dermatitis, photosensitivity, rash

MISC: Decreased sweating

INTERACTIONS

Drugs

3 *Barbiturates:* Reduce serum levels of molindone

3 *Benztropine:* May inhibit therapeutic response to molindone

3 *Bromocriptine:* May inhibit therapeutic response to molindone; molindone may inhibit therapeutic effect of bromocriptine on hyperprolactinemia

3 *Carbamazepine:* Reduces serum levels of molindone

3 *Fluoxetine:* Increases serum levels of molindone

3 *Guanethidine:* Reduced antihypertensive effect of guanethidine

3 *Indomethacin:* May increase risk of CNS side effects of molindone

2 *Levodopa:* Molindone reduces antiparkinsonian effects of levodopa

3 *Lithium:* May reduce serum levels of lithium

3 *Orphenadrine:* Reduces serum levels of molindone

3 *Paroxetine:* Increases serum levels of molindone

3 *Quinidine:* Increases serum levels of molindone

3 *Trihexyphenidyl:* May inhibit therapeutic response to molindone

SPECIAL CONSIDERATIONS

• Neuroleptic structurally different from the phenothiazines, thioxanthenes, and butyrophenones

• High potency with high incidence of EPS, but a low incidence of sedation, anticholinergic effects, and cardiovascular effects

M

mometasone

(mo-met′a-sone)
Rx: Elocon, Nasonex
Chemical Class: Synthetic glucocorticoid
Therapeutic Class: Topical corticosteroid, intermediate potency; nasal corticosteroid

CLINICAL PHARMACOLOGY
Mechanism of Action: Depresses formation, release, and activity of endogenous mediators of inflammation such as prostaglandins, kinins, histamine, liposomal enzymes, and the complement system resulting in decreased edema, erythema, and pruritus
Pharmacokinetics
TOP: Absorbed systemically across stratum corneum, extent dependent on dosage form and condition of the skin; hepatic metabolism (resistant to skin metabolism)
INDICATIONS AND USES: Topical: symptomatic relief of inflammation and/or pruritus associated with acute and chronic corticosteroid-responsive skin disorders Nasal spray: prophylaxis and treatment of the nasal symptoms of allergic rhinitis
DOSAGE
Adult
• TOP apply qd-bid, rub completely into skin
• Nasal spray: 1 spray in each nostril qd-bid
⑤ AVAILABLE FORMS/COST OF THERAPY
• Cre—Top: 0.1%, 15, 45 g: **$20.19-$24.04**/15 g
• Lotion—Top: 0.1%, 30, 60 ml: **$25.34**/30 ml
• Oint—Top: 0.1%, 15, 45 g: **$23.36**/15 g
• Spray—Nasal: 0.05 mg/inh, 17 g: **$51.17-$62.60**

PRECAUTIONS: Skin lesions covering large surface areas or involving thin-skinned areas; children, adolescents, geriatrics
PREGNANCY AND LACTATION: Pregnancy category C; systemic corticosteroids are excreted into breast milk in quantities not likely to have deleterious effects in breastfeeding infants; no information on topical steroids
SIDE EFFECTS/ADVERSE REACTIONS
CV: Hypertension
EENT: Glaucoma, subcapsular cataracts
METAB: Cushing's syndrome, glucose intolerance, hypokalemic syndrome
SKIN: Acneiform eruptions, allergic contact dermatitis; folliculitis, furunculosis, *hair loss,* hyperesthesia, *hypopigmentation,* pustules, pyoderma, secondary skin infection, skin atrophy, *striae,* vesiculation
INTERACTIONS
Labs
• *Interference:* With adrenal function as assessed by corticotropin stimulation, 24-hr urine-free cortisol measurements; plasma cortisol

monobenzone

(mono-ben′zone)
Rx: Benoquin
Chemical Class: Hydroquinone derivative
Therapeutic Class: Depigmenting agent

CLINICAL PHARMACOLOGY
Mechanism of Action: Decreases the number of functional melanocytes and inhibits the process of pigmentation (inhibition of tyrosinase,

which catalyzes the oxidation of tyrosine to dihydroxyphenylalanine, a precursor of melanin)

Pharmacokinetics

TOP: Depigmentation is usually observed after 1-4 mo of therapy (discontinue if satisfactory results are not observed in 4 mo); complete depigmentation may require 9-12 mo

INDICATIONS AND USES: Final depigmentation in extensive vitiligo

DOSAGE

Adult

• TOP apply and rub into pigmented areas 2-3 times daily

Child

• Safety in children <12 not established

💲 **AVAILABLE FORMS/COST OF THERAPY**

• Cre—Top: 20%, 37.5 g: **$43.06**

CONTRAINDICATIONS: Freckling; hyperpigmentation due to photosensitization; melasma (cholasma) of pregnancy; cafe-au-lait spots; pigmented nevi; malignant melanoma; pigment resulting from pigments other than melanin (i.e., bile, silver)

PREGNANCY AND LACTATION: Pregnancy category C; excretion into breast milk unknown

SIDE EFFECTS/ADVERSE REACTIONS

SKIN: Burning, *dermatitis,* irritation

SPECIAL CONSIDERATIONS

PATIENT/FAMILY EDUCATION

• Drug is not a mild cosmetic bleach; treated areas should not be exposed to sunlight (protect with a topical sunscreen)

montelukast
(mon-te'loo-kast)

Rx: Singulair

Chemical Class: Cyclopropaneacetic acid derivative

Therapeutic Class: Antiasthmatic; leukotriene receptor antagonist

CLINICAL PHARMACOLOGY

Mechanism of Action: Inhibits the physiologic actions of leukotriene D_4; leukotriene D_4 increases airway reactivity and vascular permeability and causes bronchoconstriction

Pharmacokinetics

PO: Peak 3-4 hr (2-2.5 hr for chew tab); 64% bioavailability (63-73% for chew tab, lower end of range when taken with food); 99% bound to plasma proteins; extensively metabolized by the liver; 86% excreted in feces (via the bile), <0.2% in urine; $t_{1/2}$ 2.7-5.5 hr

INDICATIONS AND USES: Prophylaxis and chronic treatment of asthma in adults and pediatric patients 2 years of age and older

DOSAGE

Adult and Child >15 yr

• PO 10 mg qd in the evening

Child 6-14 yr

• PO 5 mg chew tab qd in the evening

Child 2-5 yr

• PO 4 mg chew tab qd in the evening

💲 **AVAILABLE FORMS/COST OF THERAPY**

• Tab, Coated—Oral: 10 mg, 100's: **$247.69**

• Tab, Chewable—Oral: 4 mg, 90's: **$226.69**; 5 mg, 100's: **$247.69**

PRECAUTIONS: Not for reversal of bronchospasm in acute asthma attacks; avoid abrupt substitution for inhaled or oral corticosteroids; not

M

---

italic = common side effects   ***bold italic*** = life-threatening reactions

for monotherapy in exercise-induced asthma; eosinophilic conditions; phenylketonuric patients (chew tabs contain phenylalanine); children <2 yr

PREGNANCY AND LACTATION: Pregnancy category B; excretion into breast milk unknown, use caution in nursing mothers

SIDE EFFECTS/ADVERSE REACTIONS

CNS: Dizziness, headache

EENT: Nasal congestion, rhinorrhea, ear pain, sneezing

GI: Abdominal pain; dyspepsia; increased ALT, AST

HEME: Eosinophilia

MS: Leg pain

RESP: Cough

SKIN: Rash, urticaria

MISC: Asthenia/fatigue, fever, thirst

SPECIAL CONSIDERATIONS

PATIENT/FAMILY EDUCATION

• Take regularly, even during symptom-free periods

MONITORING PARAMETERS

• Pulmonary function tests

---

moricizine

(mor-iss´i-zeen)

Rx: Ethmozine

Chemical Class: Phenothiazine derivative

Therapeutic Class: Antidysrhythmic (Class I)

CLINICAL PHARMACOLOGY

Mechanism of Action: Decreases rate of rise of action potential, prolongs refractory period, and shortens the action potential duration; depression of inward influx of sodium mediates these effects; slows atrial and AV nodal conduction; increase in resting blood pressure and heart rate; inhibits platelet aggregation; anticholinergic effects

Pharmacokinetics

PO: Peak 0.5-2.2 hr

Well absorbed; metabolized by the liver, metabolites are excreted in feces and urine; protein binding >90%; $t_{1/2}$ 1.5-3.5 hr

INDICATIONS AND USES: Symptomatic, life-threatening ventricular dysrhythmias

DOSAGE

Adult

• PO 600-900 mg/day in 2-3 divided doses; increase dosage in 150 mg increments at 3-day intervals up to 900 mg/day; decrease dose in patients with significant liver and renal dysfunction

$ AVAILABLE FORMS/COST OF THERAPY

• Tab, Coated—Oral: 200 mg, 100's: **$125.64**; 250 mg, 100's: **$137.14**; 300 mg, 100's: **$170.78**

CONTRAINDICATIONS: 2nd-3rd degree AV block; right bundle branch block when associated with left hemiblock (bifascicular block) unless a pacemaker is present; cardiogenic shock

PRECAUTIONS: CHF, hypokalemia, hyperkalemia, sick sinus syndrome, children, impaired hepatic and renal function, cardiac dysfunction

PREGNANCY AND LACTATION: Pregnancy category B; secreted into breast milk (1 patient); potential for serious adverse effects exists

SIDE EFFECTS/ADVERSE REACTIONS

CNS: Depression, *dizziness,* euphoria, fatigue, headache, nervousness, perioral numbness, sleep disorders, tinnitus

CV: Bradycardia, chest pain, *CHF, dysrhythmias,* hypertension, *MI, palpitations,* syncope, thrombophlebitis

GI: Abdominal pain, diarrhea, *nausea,* vomiting

GU: Difficult urination, dysuria, incontinence, sexual dysfunction
RESP: **Apnea,** asthma, cough, *dyspnea,* hyperventilation, pharyngitis
MISC: Musculoskeletal pain, sweating

INTERACTIONS
Drugs
3 *Cimetidine:* Increases serum moricizine concentrations
3 *Theophylline:* Reduces serum theophylline levels by increasing clearance

SPECIAL CONSIDERATIONS
• Antidysrhythmic therapy has not been proven to be beneficial in terms of improving survival among patients with asymptomatic or mildly symptomatic ventricular dysrhythmias
• Studied in the CAST (Cardiac Arrhythmia Suppression Trial, I and II) with findings of excessive cardiac mortality and no benefit on long-term survival compared to placebo
• Initiate therapy in facilities capable of providing continuous ECG monitoring and managing life threatening dysrhythmias

---

morphine
(mor'feen)
Rx: Astramorph, Duramorph, Infumorph, Kadian, MS Contin, MSIR, Oramorph SR, RMS, Roxanol
Chemical Class: Natural opium alkaloid; phenanthrene derivative
Therapeutic Class: Narcotic analgesic
DEA Class: Schedule II

CLINICAL PHARMACOLOGY
Mechanism of Action: Narcotic agonist with activity at µ-receptors (supraspinal analgesia, euphoria, respiratory and physical depression, miosis, and reduced GI motility), κ-receptors (pentazocine-like spinal analgesia, sedation, and miosis), and Δ-receptors (dysphoria, psychotomimetic effects [e.g., hallucinations]), and respiratory and vasomotor stimulation caused by drugs with antagonist activity); Standard pharmacologic comparator for analgesic, antitussive, constipation, respiratory depression, sedation, emesis, and physical dependence effects.

Pharmacokinetics
PO: 60 mg = 10 IM morphine; duration of action: 8-12 hr (Sus Action preps); 4-5 hr (other oral dosage forms)
SC: Onset 10-30 min, peak analgesia 50-90 min, duration 4-5 hr
IM: Onset 10-30 min, peak analgesia 30-60 min, duration 4.5 hr
IV: Peak analgesia 20 min
Metabolized by liver; 85% excreted by kidneys, 7%-10% biliary; $t_{1/2}$ 2½-3 hr

INDICATIONS AND USES: Severe pain; anesthesia (adjunct); diarrhea*; cough*; acute pulmonary edema*

DOSAGE
Adult
• *Chronic pain:* SC/IM 4-15 mg q4h prn; PO 5-30 mg q4h prn; Sus Action 15-60 mg q8-12h (base dose on 24-hr requirement of immediate-release morphine); PR 10-20 mg q4h prn
• IV 4-15 mg diluted in 4-5 ml H_2O for inj, over 5 min
Child
• *Analgesia:* SC 0.1-0.2 mg/kg, not to exceed 15 mg

S **AVAILABLE FORMS/COST OF THERAPY**
• Cap, Gel—Oral: 15 mg, 100's: **$37.19**; 30 mg, 100's: **$69.40**

---

italic = common side effects   **bold italic** = life-threatening reactions

• Cap, Sus Action—Oral: 20 mg, 100's: **$109.04**; 30 mg, 60's: **$119.00**; 50 mg, 100's: **$265.94**; 60 mg, 60's: **$227.39**; 100 mg, 100's: **$472.50**

• Inj, Sol—Epidural, Intrathecal, IV: 0.5 mg/ml, 2, 10 ml: **$2.31-$11.63**/10 ml; 1 mg/ml, 2, 10, 30, 60, 250, 720 ml: **$2.30-$92.20**/10 ml

• Inj, Sol—IM; IV; SC: 2 mg/ml, 1, 10, 60 ml: **$0.64-$1.18**/1 ml; 4 mg/ml, 1 ml: **$0.71-$1.24**; 5 mg/ml, 30 ml: **$2.53-$17.00**; 8 mg/ml, 1 ml: **$0.60-$1.24**; 10 mg/ml, 1, 3, 10, 20, 30 ml: **$0.60-$1.28**/1 ml; 15 mg/ml, 1, 10, 20 ml: **$0.67-$2.71**/1 ml

• Inj, Sol—IV: 25 mg/ml, 4 ml: **$11.33-$85.50**; 50 mg/ml, 10 ml: **$40.96-$286.75**

• Sol—Oral: 10 mg/5 ml, 500 ml: **$20.00-$31.20**; 20 mg/5 ml, 500 ml: **$56.70-$81.90**; 20 mg/ml, 120 ml: **$40.00-$52.61**

• Supp—Rect: 5 mg, 12's: **$12.49-$14.66**; 10 mg, 12's: **$14.39-$17.47**; 20 mg, 12's: **$17.02-$21.06**; 30 mg, 12's: **$29.44**

• Tab, Coated, Sus Action—Oral: 15 mg, 100's: **$89.17-$99.63**; 30 mg, 100's: **$169.46-$189.34**; 60 mg, 100's: **$330.61-$369.44**; 100 mg, 100's: **$489.56-$546.99**; 200 mg, 100's: **$896.53-$1,001.71**

• Tab, Soluable—IM, SC: 10 mg, 100's: **$25.79-$27.15**; 15 mg, 100's: **$36.51**

• Tab, Uncoated—Oral: 15 mg, 100's: **$12.15-$34.45**; 30 mg, 100's: **$23.08-$57.80**

CONTRAINDICATIONS: Respiratory depression, hemorrhage, acute asthma attack, paralytic ileus, convulsive states (injection)

PRECAUTIONS: Addictive personality, elderly, hepatic disease, renal disease, child <18 yr, head injury, acute abdominal conditions, hypothyroidism, prostatic hypertrophy, Addison's disease

PREGNANCY AND LACTATION: Pregnancy category B; trace amounts enter breast milk; compatible with breast feeding

SIDE EFFECTS/ADVERSE REACTIONS

CNS: Addiction, confusion, *dizziness, drowsiness,* euphoria, headache, *sedation*

CV: Bradycardia, *hypotension,* palpitations

EENT: Blurred vision, diplopia, *miosis,* tinnitus

GI: Anorexia, biliary tract pressure, *constipation,* cramps, *nausea,* vomiting

GU: Urinary retention

RESP: **Respiratory depression**

SKIN: Bruising, diaphoresis, flushing, pruritus, rash, urticaria

MISC: Histamine release (decreased blood pressure, fast heartbeat, increased sweating, redness or flushing of face, wheezing or troubled breathing)

INTERACTIONS

Drugs

3 *Amitryptylline:* Additive respiratory and CNS-depressant effects

3 *Antihistamines, chloroal hydrate, gluethimide, methocarbamol:* Enhanced depressant effects

3 *Barbiturates:* Additive respiratory and CNS-depressant effects

3 *Cimetidine:* Increased respiratory and CNS depression

3 *Cloimpramine:* Additive respiratory and CNS-depressant effects

3 *Ethanol:* Additive CNS effects

3 *MAOI's:* Markedly potentiate the actions of morphine

3 *Nortriptylline:* Additive respiratory and CNS-depressant effects

Labs

• *Increase:* Urine glucose, urine 17-ketosteroids

• False elevations of amylase and lipase

SPECIAL CONSIDERATIONS

• Treatment of overdose: Naloxone (Narcan) 0.2-0.8 mg IV

• Remains the strong analgesic of choice for acute, severe pain, acute MI pain, and the agent of choice for chronic cancer pain

• 200 mg Sus Action tablet for use only in opioid-tolerant patients

• Do not administer agonist/antagonist analgesics (i.e., pentazocine, nalbuphine, butorphanol, dezocine, buprenorphine) to patient who has received a prolonged course of morphine (a pure agonist). In opioid-dependent patients, mixed agonist/anagonist analgesics may precipitate withdrawal symptoms

PATIENT/FAMILY EDUCATION

• Change position slowly to avoid orthostasis

• Avoid alcohol and other CNS depressants

• Physical dependency may result

• Do not chew or crush Sus Action preparations

---

moxifloxacin
(moks-i-floks′a-sin)
Rx: Avelox
Chemical Class: Fluoroquinolone derivative
Therapeutic Class: Antibiotic

CLINICAL PHARMACOLOGY
Mechanism of Action: Inhibits DNA gyrase and topoisomerase 4, which are needed for the synthesis of bacterial DNA

Pharmacokinetics
PO: Peak 1-3 hr; bioavailability 90%; protein binding 50% (concentrated in lung and sinus tissue); 50% metabolized by liver (sulfoxide, major metabolite), also excreted in urine (20% unchanged) and feces (25% unchanged); elimination $t_{1/2}$ 12 hr

INDICATIONS AND USES: Infections of the upper (sinusitis) and lower (bronchitis, community acquired pneumonia) respiratory tract and skin caused by susceptible organisms; antibacterial spectrum usually includes:

• Gram-positive organisms: *Staphylococcus aureus* (methicillin-susceptible strains only), *Staphylococcus epidermidis* (methicillin-susceptible strains only), *Streptococcus agalactiae, Streptococcus pneumoniae* (penicillin-susceptible and penicillin-resistant strains), *Streptococcus pyogenes, Streptococcus viridans* group

• Gram-negative organisms: *Citrobacter freundii, Enterobacter cloacae, Escherichia coli, Haemophilus influenzae, Haemophilus parainfluenzae, Klebsiella oxytoca, Klebsiella pneumoniae, Legionella pneumophila, Moraxella catarrhalis, Proteus mirabilis*

• Anaerobes: *Fusobacterium* species, *Peptostreptococcus* species, *Prevotella* species

Other organisms: *Chlamydia pneumoniae, Mycoplasma pneumoniae*

DOSAGE
Adult and Child ≥18 yr

• *Bronchitis, acute bacterial exacerbation of chronic bronchitis:* PO 400 mg qd for 5 days

• *Pneumonia, community acquired:* PO 400 mg qd for 10 days

• *Sinusitis, acute bacterial:* PO 400 mg qd for 10 days

• *Skin and skin structure infections:* 400 mg qd for 7 days

🅂 AVAILABLE FORMS/COST OF THERAPY

• Tab, Coated—Oral: 400 mg, 10's: **$87.13**

---

italic = common side effects

bold italic = life-threatening reactions

PRECAUTIONS: May prolong the QT interval, avoid in patients with known prolongation of the QT interval, hypokalemia, or patients receiving class Ia (e.g., quinidine, procainamide) or class III (e.g., amiodarone, sotalol) antiarrhythmic agents, or cisapride, erythromycin, antipsychotics, and tricyclic antidepressants; bradycardia; acute myocardial infarction; known or suspected CNS disorders (e.g., severe cerebral arteriosclerosis, epilepsy) or in the presence of other risk factors that may predispose to seizures or lower the seizure threshold

PREGNANCY AND LACTATION: Pregnancy category C; excreted into breast milk, safety not established, allow 48 hr to elapse after last dose before resuming breast feeding

SIDE EFFECTS/ADVERSE REACTIONS

CNS: Anxiety, asthenia, confusion, dizziness (3%), depersonalization, headache (2%), incoordination, insomnia, somnolence, tremor, vertigo

CV: Edema, hypertension, hypotension, palpitation, tachycardia, vasodilatation

EENT: Taste perversion, tinnitus

GI: Abdominal pain (2%), *diarrhea* (6%), dyspepsia (1%), *nausea* (8%), vomiting (2%), abnormal liver function test (1%), increased amylase, *pseudomembranous colitis*

GU: Moniliasis, vaginitis, increase in BUN, creatinine

HEME: **Leukopenia,** prothrombin time decrease, prothrombin time increase, thrombocythemia, ***thrombocytopenia***

METAB: Hyperglycemia

MS: Arthralgia, myalgia, tendon inflammation, tendon rupture

RESP: Asthma, cough, increased dyspnea

SKIN: Urticaria, rash, pruritus, sweating

INTERACTIONS

Drugs

■ *Aluminum:* Reduced absorption of moxifloxacin; do not take within 4 hr of dose

■ *Antacids:* Reduced absorption of moxifloxacin; do not take within 4 hr of dose

■ *Antipyrine:* Inhibits metabolism of antipyrine; increased plasma antipyrine level

■ *Calcium:* Reduced absorption of moxifloxacin; do not take within 4 hr of dose

■ *Diazepam:* Inhibits metabolism of diazepam; increased plasma diazepam level

■ *Didanosine:* Markedly reduced absorption of moxifloxacin; take moxifloxacin 2 hr before didanosine

■ *Foscarnet:* Coadministration increases seizure risk

■ *Iron:* Reduced absorption of moxifloxacin; do not take within 4 hr of dose

■ *Magnesium:* Reduced absorption of moxifloxacin; do not take within 4 hr of dose

■ *Metoprolol:* Inhibits metabolism of metoprolol; increased plasma metoprolol level

■ *Morphine:* Reduced absorption of moxifloxacin; do not take within 2 hr of dose

■ *Pentoxifylline:* Inhibits metabolism of pentoxifylline; increased plasma pentoxifylline level

■ *Phenytoin:* Inhibits metabolism of phenytoin; increased plasma phenytoin level

■ *Propranolol:* Inhibits metabolism of propranolol; increased plasma propranolol level

■ *Ropinirole:* Inhibits metabolism of ropinirole; increased plasma ropinirole level

---

* = non-FDA-approved use

3 *Sodium bicarbonate:* Reduced absorption of moxifloxacin; do not take within 4 hr of dose

3 *Sucralfate:* Reduced absorption of moxifloxacin; do not take within 4 hr of dose

3 *Warfarin:* Inhibits metabolism of warfarin; increases hypoprothrombinemic response to warfarin

3 *Zinc:* Reduced absorption of moxifloxacin; do not take within 4 hr of dose

SPECIAL CONSIDERATIONS
PATIENT/FAMILY EDUCATION
• May be taken with or without meals
• Should be taken at least 4 hr before or 8 hr after multivitamins (containing iron or zinc), antacids (containing magnesium, calcium, or aluminum), sucralfate, or didanosine chewable/buffered tablets
• Discontinue treatment, rest and refrain from exercise, and inform prescriber if pain, inflammation, or rupture of a tendon occur
• Test reaction to this drug before operating an automobile or machinery or engaging in activities requiring mental alertness or coordination

---

mupirocin
(mew-per´o-sen)
Rx: Bactroban
Chemical Class: Pseudomonic acid derivative
Therapeutic Class: Topical antibiotic

CLINICAL PHARMACOLOGY
Mechanism of Action: Inhibits bacterial protein synthesis; shows no cross-resistance with chloramphenicol, erythromycin, fusidic acid, gentamicin, lincomycin, methicillin, neomycin, novobiocin, penicillin, streptomycin, and tetracycline

Pharmacokinetics
No measurable systemic absorption
INDICATIONS AND USES: Impetigo caused by *Staphylococcus aureus* (including methicillin-resistant and β-lactamase producing strains), *S. epidermidis, S. saprophyticus,* β-hemolytic *Streptococcus, Str. pyogenes,* eradication of nasal colonization with methicillin-resistant *S. aureus,* secondarily infected traumatic skin lesions

DOSAGE
Impetigo: TOP—Apply small amount to affected area tid
Nasal: Divide ½ the ointment from single-use tube between the nostrils and apply bid for 5 days

$ **AVAILABLE FORMS/COST OF THERAPY**
• Cre—Top: 2%, 15, 30 g: **$29.69/**15 g
• Oint—Nasal: 2%, 1 g, 10's: **$56.38**
• Oint—Top: 2%, 15, 30 g: **$16.55-$24.95**/15 g

PREGNANCY AND LACTATION: Pregnancy category B; excretion into breast milk unknown

SIDE EFFECTS/ADVERSE REACTIONS
SKIN: Burning, contact dermatitis, dry skin, erythema, increased exudate, *itching,* rash, *stinging,* swelling, tenderness

SPECIAL CONSIDERATIONS
• Comparable efficacy to systemic semisynthetic penicillins and erythromycin in impetigo and infected wounds

---

italic = common side effects   ***bold italic*** = life-threatening reactions

mycophenolate
(my-co-fen'o-late)
Rx: CellCept
Chemical Class: Mycophenolic acid derivative
Therapeutic Class: Immunosuppressant

CLINICAL PHARMACOLOGY
Mechanism of Action: Mycophenolic acid (MPA), the active metabolite, inhibits T- and B-lymphocytes by interfering with purine synthesis; prolongs the survival of allogeneic transplants and reverses ongoing acute rejection

Pharmacokinetics
PO: Peak 6 hr; rapid absorption (94% bioavailable); presystemic metabolism to MPA (active metabolite); MPAG (inactive metabolite) converted to MPA via enterohepatic recirculation; immediately posttransplant (<40 days), mean AUC, C_{max} approximately 50% lower than healthy volunteers or stable renal transplant patients; MPA 97% bound to plasma albumin; excreted as inactive metabolite in urine; not removed by hemodialysis; $t_{1/2}$ 17 hr

INDICATIONS AND USES: Primary maintenance immunosuppression and/or rescue or rejection therapy following renal, heart, and liver transplantation; rheumatoid arthritis*; psoriasis*

DOSAGE
Adult
• *Renal transplant:* PO/IV 1.0 g bid starting as soon as possible following transplantation; give PO on empty stomach, IV over not less than 2 hr; usually given with corticosteroids and cyclosporine
• *Cardiac transplant:* PO/IV 1.5 g bid
• *Hepatic transplant:* PO 1.5 g bid; IV 1.0 g bid
• *Renal impairment:* With severe chronic renal impairment (GFR <25 ml/min/1.73 m^2) outside of the immediate posttransplant period, doses >1 g should be avoided

Child
• *Renal transplant:* PO (oral suspension) 600 mg/m^2 bid; BSA 1.25-1.5 m^2 PO (capsules) 750 mg bid; BSA >1.5 m^2 (capsules or tablets) 1 g bid; max dose is 2 g/day; give PO on empty stomach as soon as possible following transplantation

💲 AVAILABLE FORMS/COST OF THERAPY
• Cap, Gel—Oral: 250 mg, 100's: **$276.93**
• Inj, Lyphl, Sol—IV: 500 mg vial, 4's: **$131.58**
• Susp—Oral: 200 mg/ml 175 ml: **$387.66**
• Tab—Oral: 500 mg, 100's: **$553.79**

CONTRAINDICATIONS: IV form is contraindicated in patients allergic to polysorbate 80

PRECAUTIONS: Pregnancy, peptic ulcer disease, history of GI bleeding, decreased renal function, phenylketonuria (susp contains aspartame), Lesch-Nyhan and Kelley-Seegmiller syndrome

PREGNANCY AND LACTATION: Pregnancy category C; mycophenolic acid excreted in milk; not recommended during breast feeding

SIDE EFFECTS/ADVERSE REACTIONS
CNS: Headache, pain
CV: Hypertension
GI: Constipation, *diarrhea,* dyspepsia, nausea, oral moniliasis, *vomiting*
GU: Hematuria, UTI
HEME: **Anemia,** leukocytosis, ***leukopenia, thrombocytopenia***

METAB: Fever, hypercholesteremia, hyperkalemia, hypokalemia, hypophosphatemia, peripheral edema
MS: Back pain
MISC: **Malignancy, infection (opportunistic), sepsis**

INTERACTIONS
Drugs

3 *Acyclovir:* Increased serum acyclovir and mycophenolate concentrations possible

3 *Antacids with magnesium and aluminum hydroxides:* Decreased mycophenolate bioavailability; separate administration times

3 *Azathioprine:* Due to potential bone marrow suppression, concomitant administration not recommended

3 *Cholestyramine:* Decreased mycophenolate bioavailability due to interruption of enterohepatic recirculation

3 *Ganciclovir:* Increased serum ganciclovir and mycophenolate concentrations possible

3 *Live vaccines:* Use of live attenuated vaccines should be avoided; vaccines may be less effective

3 *Probenecid:* Increased serum mycophenolate concentrations

SPECIAL CONSIDERATIONS

• Drug can be given concurrently with cyclosporine, which may enable reduced cyclosporine doses and lower toxicity, or potential cyclosporine substitute in patients developing cyclosporine toxicity

• Drug is less likely than azathioprine to induce severe bone marrow depression, and may replace azathioprine in conventional maintenance immunosuppression regimens

• IV can be administered for up to 14 days; switch to PO as soon as possible

PATIENT/FAMILY EDUCATION

• Women of childbearing potential should use effective contraception before and during therapy and 6 weeks after therapy has stopped

MONITORING PARAMETERS

• CBC qwk × 1 mo, then q2wk × 2 mo, then monthly

---

nabumetone
(na-byu′-me-tone)
Rx: Relafen
Chemical Class: Acetic acid derivative
Therapeutic Class: NSAID with analgesic and antipyretic activity

---

CLINICAL PHARMACOLOGY

Mechanism of Action: Reversible cyclooxygenase (i.e., prostaglandin synthetase) inhibitor; nonselectively decreases the formation of both prostaglandins and thromboxane A2; variable effects on lipoxygenase synthesis and subsequent leukotriene production; antiinflammatory, antipyretic, and analgesic activity; inhibits platelet aggregation

Pharmacokinetics

PO: Peak 2½-4 hr; plasma protein binding >99%; $t_{1/2}$ 22-30 hr; parent drug is a prodrug, which is metabolized in liver to active metabolite 6-methoxy-2-naphthylacetic acid (6 MNA); excreted in urine (metabolites)

INDICATIONS AND USES: Osteoarthritis; pain—mild to moderate; rheumatoid arthritis; soft tissue injuries*; prevention of cognitive decline*

DOSAGE
Adult

• PO 1 g as a single dose; may increase to 1.5-2 g/day if needed; may give qd or bid

---

$ AVAILABLE FORMS/COST OF THERAPY

• Tab, Uncoated—Oral: 500 mg, 100's: **$129.70-$149.88**; 750 mg, 100's: **$117.25-$177.00**

CONTRAINDICATIONS: Bronchospasm, nasal polyps, angioedema precipitated by aspirin or other NSAIDs

PRECAUTIONS: History of GI ulceration, bleeding, or perforation; renal dysfunction, hypertension or cardiac conditions aggravated by fluid retention and edema, history of liver dysfunction, history of coagulation

PREGNANCY AND LACTATION: Pregnancy category C; excretion into breast milk unknown, not recommended for use in nursing mothers

SIDE EFFECTS/ADVERSE REACTIONS

CNS: Anxiety, confusion, depression, dizziness, drowsiness, fatigue, headache, insomnia, nervousness, tremors

CV: **CHF, dysrhythmias,** edema, palpitations, peripheral, tachycardia

EENT: Blurred vision, hearing loss, tinnitus

GI: Anorexia, cholestatic hepatitis, constipation, cramps, diarrhea, dry mouth, flatulence, gastritis, jaundice, nausea, peptic ulcer, **perforation, ulceration,** vomiting

GU: Azotemia, cystitis, dysuria, hematuria, **nephrotoxicity,** oliguria

HEME: **Blood dyscrasias**

RESP: **Bronchospasm,** dyspnea, pharyngitis

SKIN: Photosensitivity, pruritus, purpura, rash, sweating

INTERACTIONS

Drugs

3 *Aminoglycosides:* Reduced clearance with elevated aminoglycoside levels and potential for toxicity (especially indomethacin in premature infants; other NSAIDs probably)

3 *Antihypertensives:* (alpha blockers, angiotensin converting enzyme inhibitors, angiotensin II receptor blockers, beta blockers, diuretics) inhibition of antihypertensive and other favorable hemodynamic effects

3 *Corticosteroids:* Increased risk of GI ulceration

3 *Cyclosporine:* Increased nephrotoxicity risk

3 *Lithium:* Decreased clearance of lithium (mediated via prostaglandins) resulting in elevated serum lithium levels and risk of toxicity

3 *Methotrexate:* Decreased renal secretion of methotrexate resulting in elevated methotrexate levels and risk of toxicity

3 *Phenylpropanolamine:* Possible acute hypertensive reaction

3 *Potassium-Sparing Diuretics:* Additive hyperkalemia potential

3 *Triamterene:* Acute renal failure reported with addition of indomethacin; caution with other NSAIDs

3 *Warfarin:* Transient increase in prothrombin time due to displaced protein binding; increased risk of GI bleeding although likely less risky than other NSAIDs due to preferential action on COX-2

SPECIAL CONSIDERATIONS

• No significant advantage over other NSAIDs; cost should govern use

MONITORING PARAMETERS

• Initial hemogram and fecal occult blood test within 3 months of starting regular chronic therapy; repeat every 6-12 months (more frequently in high risk patients (>65 years, peptic ulcer disease, concurrent steroids or anticoagulants); electrolytes, creatinine, and BUN within 3 months of starting regular chronic therapy; repeat every 6-12 months

---

nadolol

(nay-doe'lole)

Rx: Corgard
Combinations
  Rx: With Bendroflumenthiazide (Corzide)
Chemical Class: Nonselective, β-adrenergic blocker
Therapeutic Class: Antihypertensive; antianginal; antiglaucoma agent

---

CLINICAL PHARMACOLOGY
Mechanism of Action: PO: Competitive beta-adrenergic antagonist; produces negative inotropic and chronotropic responses; slows AV nodal conduction; decreases heart rate; decreases myocardial oxygen consumption; antiarrhythmic effects (class II); reduction in platelet aggregation and blood viscosity; suppression of renin release; inhibition of central sympathetic outflow; decreases presynaptic receptor neurotransmitter release; no intrinsic sympathomimetic or membrane stabilizing activity; low to moderate lipid solubility
Pharmacokinetics
PO: Onset variable, peak 3-4 hr, duration 17-24 hr, $t_{1/2}$ 16-20 hr; not metabolized, excreted in urine (unchanged)
INDICATIONS AND USES: Glaucoma,* migraine headache, hypertension, post-myocardial infarction, supraventricular arrhythmias (atrial fibrillation, atrial flutter, paroxysmal supraventricular tachycardia),* aggressive behavior,* angina pectoris, anxiety,* cataract extraction prophylaxis,* congestive heart fail-

ure,* hyperthyroidism,* neuroleptic-induced akathisia,* retinal detachment,* tremor,* gastrointestinal tract bleeding*

DOSAGE
Adult and child >16 yr
• *Angina Pectoris:* PO 40 mg qd; increase by 40-80 mg q3-7 days; maintenance 40-240 mg/day
• *Arrhythmias:* PO 60-160 mg qd for supraventricular arrhythmias
• *Hypertension:* PO 40 mg qd; increase by 40-80 mg q3-7 days; maintenance 40-320 mg qd
• *Hyperthyroidisms:* PO 80-160 mg qd
• *Migraine headache prophylaxis:* PO 80-240 mg qd
• *Tremor:* PO 80-240 mg qd
§ AVAILABLE FORMS/COST OF THERAPY
• Tab, Uncoated—Oral: 20 mg, 100's: **$72.40-$163.50**; 40 mg, 100's: **$40.04-$191.30**; 80 mg, 100's: **$111.90-$262.81**; 120 mg, 100's: **$151.68-$342.54**; 160 mg, 100's: **$168.70-$380.96**

CONTRAINDICATIONS: Bronchial asthma, cardiogenic shock, overt cardiac failure, second and third degree AV block, severe sinus bradycardia

PRECAUTIONS: Anesthesia-surgery (myocardial depression), avoid abrupt withdrawal, Bronchospastic airways, congestive heart failure, diabetes mellitus, hyperthyroidism/thyrotoxicosis, concurrent clonidine (discontinue nadolol several days prior to withdrawal of clonidine, peripheral vascular disease, renal disease

PREGNANCY AND LACTATION: Pregnancy category C; similar drug, atenolol, frequently used in the third trimester for treatment of hypertension (many studies of efficacy and safety of atenolol in pregnancy-induced hypertension); long-term use

N

---

italic = common side effects   ***bold italic*** = life-threatening reactions

has been associated with intrauterine growth retardation; mean milk: plasma ratio, 0.80 in one study; quantity of drug ingested by breast feeding infant unlikely to be therapeutically significant

SIDE EFFECTS/ADVERSE REACTIONS

CNS: Depression, dizziness, fatigue, hallucinations, headache, lethargy, paresthesias

CV: AV block, *bradycardia,* chest pain, **CHF,** conduction disturbances, edema, flushing, *hypotension,* palpitations, peripheral ischemia, vasodilation

EENT: Sore throat

GI: Colitis, constipation, cramps, diarrhea, dry mouth, flatulence, hepatomegaly, increased transaminases, serum alkaline phosphatase; nausea, pancreatitis, taste distortion, vomiting

HEME: **Agranulocytosis, thrombocytopenia**

METAB: Hyperkalemia, hyperuricemia

RESP: **Bronchospasm,** cough, dyspnea, **laryngospasm,** nasal stuffiness, pharyngitis, respiratory dysfunction, wheezing

SKIN: Fever, pruritus, rash

INTERACTIONS

Drugs

3 *Adenosine:* Bradycardia aggravated

3 *α-1 adrenergic blockers:* Potential enhanced first dose response (marked initial drop in blood pressure, particularly on standing (especially prazocin).

3 *Amiodarone:* Symptomatic bradycardia and sinus arrest; caution in patients with bradycardia, sick sinus syndrome, or partial AV block when either amiodarone or β-blocking drug is used

3 *Ampicillin:* Reduced nadolol bioavailability

3 *Antacids:* Reduced nadolol absorption

3 *Calcium channel blockers:* See dihydropyridine and verapamil

3 *Clonidine:* Exacerbation of rebound hypertension upon discontinuation of clonidine

3 *Digoxin:* Additive prolongation of atrioventricular (AV) conduction time

3 *Dihydropyridine calcium channel blockers:* Severe hypotension or impaired cardiac performance; most prevalent with impaired left ventricular function, cardiac arrhythmias, or aortic stenosis

3 *Diltiazem:* Potentiates beta-adrenergic effects; hypotension, left ventricular failure, and AV conduction disturbances problemmatic in elderly, patients with left ventricular dysfunction, aortic stenosis, or with large doses of either drug

3 *Dipyridamole:* Bradycardia aggravated

3 *Hypoglycemic agents:* Masked hypoglycemia, hyperglycemia

3 *Lidocaine:* Increased serum lidocaine concentrations possible

3 *Neostigmine:* Bradycardia aggravated

3 *NSAIDs:* Reduced antihypertensive effect of nadolol

3 *Physostigmine:* Bradycardia aggravated

3 *Prazosin:* First-dose response to prazosin may be enhanced by β-blockade

3 *Tacrine:* Bradycardia aggravated

❷ *Theophylline:* Antagonistic pharmacodynamic effects

3 *Verapamil:* Potentiates beta-adrenergic effects; hypotension, left ventricular failure, and AV conduction disturbances problemmatic in elderly, patients with left ventricular dysfunction, aortic stenosis, or with large doses of either drug

SPECIAL CONSIDERATIONS

• No unique advantage over less expensive β-blockers

PATIENT/FAMILY EDUCATION

• Do **not** discontinue abruptly; may require taper; rapid withdrawal may produce rebound hypertension or angina

MONITORING PARAMETERS

• Angina: reduction in nitroglycerin usage; frequency, severity, onset, and duration of angina pain; heart rate

• Arrhythmias: heart rate

• Congestive heart failure: functional status, cough, dyspnea on exertion, paroxysmal nocturnal dyspnea, exercise tolerance, and ventricular function

• Hypertension: Blood pressure

• Migraine headache: reduction in the frequency, severity, and duration of attacks

• Post myocardial infarction: left ventricular function, lower resting heart rate

• Toxicity: blood glucose, bronchospasm, hypotension, bradycardia, depression, confusion, hallucination, sexual dysfunction

---

nafarelin

(na-far´eh-lin)

Rx: Synarel

Chemical Class: Synthetic gonadotropin-releasing hormone analog

Therapeutic Class: Gonadotropin

CLINICAL PHARMACOLOGY

Mechanism of Action: Stimulates release of LH and FSH resulting in a temporary increase of ovarian steroidogenesis; repeated dosing abolishes stimulatory effects on the pituitary gland with decreased secretion of gonadal steroids and consequent pseudomenopause

Pharmacokinetics

NASAL: Peak 10-40 min, $t_{1/2}$ 3 hr; rapidly absorbed intranasally, 2.8% bioavailability; 80% bound to plasma proteins; metabolized and excreted in urine and feces

INDICATIONS AND USES: Endometriosis; central precocious puberty in both sexes

DOSAGE

Adult

• *Endometriosis:* 400 µg/day; 200 µg (1 spray) in 1 nostril q AM, 200 µg in other nostril q PM; start treatment between days 2 and 4 of menstrual cycle; may increase to 800 µg/day; recommended duration of treatment is 6 mo

Child

• *Central precocious puberty:* 1600 µg/day (2 sprays in each nostril bid); may increase to 1800 µg/day if adequate suppression is not achieved

$ **AVAILABLE FORMS/COST OF THERAPY**

• Sol—Nasal: 200 µg/inh, 10 ml: **$453.36** (30 day supply for endometriosis)

CONTRAINDICATIONS: Undiagnosed abnormal vaginal bleeding

PRECAUTIONS: Ovarian cysts, persistent menstruation (menstruation should cease during therapy for endometriosis), osteoporosis risk factors (chronic alcohol and/or tobacco use, strong family history of osteoporosis, or chronic use of drugs that can reduce bone mass such as anticonvulsants or corticosteroids)

PREGNANCY AND LACTATION: Pregnancy category X; not recommended in nursing mothers

SIDE EFFECTS/ADVERSE REACTIONS

CNS: Depression, emotional lability, flushing, headache, insomnia

N

---

italic = common side effects | **bold italic** = life-threatening reactions

EENT: Rhinitis

GU: Breast tenderness, decreased libido; increased pubic hair, transient breast enlargement, vaginal dryness, bleeding

METAB: Bone density changes (8.7% decrease in trabecular bone density after 6 mo), *hot flashes*

SKIN: Acne, increased body hair

MISC: Body odor, seborrhea

INTERACTIONS

Drugs

3 *Decongestants, nasal/topical:* Potential interference with absorption; allow 30 min after use of nafarelin before applying a topical decongestant

Labs

• *Interference:* Gonadal and gonadotropic function tests conducted during treatment and for 4-8 wk after treatment may be misleading

SPECIAL CONSIDERATIONS

• Alternative to danazol and oophorectomy in the treatment of endometriosis; more tolerable adverse effect profile compared to danazol for some patients

• Agent of choice in patients concerned about future fertility

• Benefits are temporary

---

nafcillin

(naf´sill´in)

Rx: Nallpen

Chemical Class: Semisynthetic penicillinase-resistant penicillin
Therapeutic Class: Antibiotic

CLINICAL PHARMACOLOGY

Mechanism of Action: Inhibits bacterial wall synthesis; bactericidal

Pharmacokinetics

IV: Peak 5 min

IM/PO: Peak 30-60 min, duration 4-6 hr

Poor/erratic oral absorption; 90% bound to plasma proteins; metabolized by the liver, elimination 30% as unchanged drug in urine, primarily eliminated by nonrenal routes (namely hepatic inactivation and excretion in bile); $t_{1/2}$ 1 hr

INDICATIONS AND USES: Infections caused by penicillinase-producing staphylococci, which have demonstrated sensitivity to the drug Antibacterial spectrum usually includes:

• Gram-positive organisms: *Staphylococcus aureus, Streptococcus pyogenes, S. viridans, S. bovis, S. pneumoniae,* including penicillinase producing strains

DOSAGE

Adult

• PO/IM/IV 2-6 g/day in divided doses q4-6h (IV doses should be administered over 60 min to minimize vein irritation)

Child

• IM 25 mg/kg q12h; PO 25-50 mg/kg/day in divided doses q6h

Neonates

• IM 10 mg/kg bid

⑤ AVAILABLE FORMS/COST OF THERAPY

• Cap, Gel—Oral: 250 mg, 100's: **$125.00**

• Inj, Dry-Sol—IM, IV: 500 mg: **$0.22**; 1 g: **$2.27-$11.50**; 2 g: **$0.67-$19.24**

PRECAUTIONS: Hypersensitivity to cephalosporins (5%-16% cross-allergenicity), neonates, hepatic and renal insufficiency

PREGNANCY AND LACTATION: Pregnancy category B; excreted into breast milk

SIDE EFFECTS/ADVERSE REACTIONS

CNS: Anxiety, coma, depression, hallucinations, lethargy, *seizures,* twitching

CV: Phlebitis or thrombophlebitis

GI: Abdominal pain, colitis, *diarrhea,* glossitis (black or hairy tongue), increased LFTs, *vomiting*
GU: Glomerulonephritis, hematuria, interstitial nephritis, *moniliasis,* oliguria, proteinuria, *vaginitis*
HEME: **Bone marrow depression,** increased bleeding time

INTERACTIONS
Drugs

🔳 *Chloramphenicol:* Inhibited antibacterial activity of nafcillin; administer nafcillin 3 hr before chloramphenicol

🔳 *Cyclosporine:* Reduced serum cyclosporine concentrations

🔳 *Macrolide antibiotics:* Inhibited antibacterial activity of nafcillin; administer nafcillin 3 hr before macrolides

🔳 *Methotrexate:* Increased serum methotrexate concentrations

🔳 *Oral contraceptives:* Occasional impairment of oral contraceptive efficacy; consider use of supplemental contraception during cycles in which nafcillin is used

🔳 *Tacrolimus:* Reduced serum tacrolimus concentrations

🔳 *Tetracyclines:* Inhibited antibacterial activity of nafcillin; administer nafcillin 3 hr before tetracyclines

🔳 *Warfarin:* May inhibit hypoprothrombinemic response to warfarin

Labs
• *Increase:* Serum protein

SPECIAL CONSIDERATIONS
MONITORING PARAMETERS
• Oral nafcillin absorption is erratic (consider alternate oral penicillinase-resistant penicillins)
• CBC, creatinine and UA for eosinophils during therapy to monitor for adverse effects

naftifine
(naf´te-feen)
Rx: Naftin
Chemical Class: Synthetic allylamine derivative
Therapeutic Class: Antifungal

CLINICAL PHARMACOLOGY
Mechanism of Action: Fungicidal, fungistatic; interferes with sterol biosynthesis by inhibiting the enzyme squalene 2,3-epoxidase
Pharmacokinetics
TOP: Systemic absorption 6% (cream), 4.2% (gel); excreted via urine and feces; $t_{1/2}$ 2-3 days
INDICATIONS AND USES: Topical fungal infections (i.e., tinea cruris, tinea corporis, tinea pedis) caused by the following susceptible organisms: *Trichophyton rubrum, T. mentagrophytes, T. tonsurans, Epidermophyton floccosum, Microsporum canis, M. audouini, M. gypseum,* fungistatic against *Candida* spp.

DOSAGE
Adult
• TOP apply qd (cream) or bid (gel) to affected area; reevaluate if no improvement after 4 wk of therapy

💲 AVAILABLE FORMS/COST OF THERAPY
• Cre—Top: 1%, 15, 30, 60 g: **$29.36**/30 g
• Gel—Top: 1%, 20, 40, 60 g: **$49.34**/40 g

PREGNANCY AND LACTATION: Pregnancy category B; excretion into breast milk unknown

SIDE EFFECTS/ADVERSE REACTIONS
SKIN: Burning, dryness, *itching,* local irritation, redness, *stinging*

SPECIAL CONSIDERATIONS
• First of a new class of antifungals (allylamine derivatives) unrelated to imidazoles

N

• Because of fungicidal activity at low concentrations may provide quicker onset of healing, enhance patient compliance with qd therapy

---

nalbuphine

(nal'byoo-feen)

Rx: Nubain

Chemical Class: Synthetic opiate derivative-Phenanthrene derivative

Therapeutic Class: Narcotic agonist-antagonist analgesic

CLINICAL PHARMACOLOGY

Mechanism of Action: Analgesia via µ-subclass opiate receptor binding in CNS; µ-receptors mediate morphine-like supraspinal analgesia, euphoria, and respiratory and physical depression; narcotic antagonist activity is approx. 10 × pentazocine

Pharmacokinetics

IV: Onset 2-3 min, duration 3-6 hr

SC/IM: Onset <15 min, duration, 3-6 hr

Metabolized by liver, excreted by kidneys; t₁/₂, 5 hr

INDICATIONS AND USES: Moderate to severe pain; can be used for supplement to balanced anesthesia, for preoperative and postoperative analgesia, and for obstetrical analgesia during labor and delivery

DOSAGE

NOTE: 3-6 mg IM is equivalent to 10 mg IM morphine

Adult

• *Pain:* SC/IM/IV 10-20 mg q3-6h prn, not to exceed 160 mg/day

• *Supplement to balanced anesthesia:* Induction 0.3-3 mg/kg IV administered over 10-15 min period; maintenance 0.25-0.50 mg/kg as required

💲 AVAILABLE FORMS/COST OF THERAPY

• Inj, Sol—IM, IV, SC: 10 mg/ml, 1 ml: **$1.14-$1.77**; 20 mg/ml, 1 ml: **$1.34-$2.28**

CONTRAINDICATIONS: Narcotic addiction

PRECAUTIONS: Addictive personality, increased intracranial pressure, MI (acute), severe heart disease, respiratory depression, hepatic disease, renal disease, sulfite sensitivity

PREGNANCY AND LACTATION: Pregnancy category B

SIDE EFFECTS/ADVERSE REACTIONS

CNS: Confusion, crying, *dizziness,* dreams, dysphoria (high doses), euphoria, *headache, sedation; vertigo*

CV: Bradycardia, change in blood pressure, palpitations

EENT: Blurred vision, diplopia, miosis, tinnitus

GI: Anorexia, constipation, cramps, dry mouth, nausea, vomiting

GU: Dysuria, increased urinary output, urinary retention, urinary urgency

RESP: Respiratory depression

SKIN: Bruising, diaphoresis, flushing, pruritus, *rash,* urticaria

MISC: Flushing, speech difficulty, warmth

INTERACTIONS

Drugs

🔢 *Barbiturates:* Additive respiratory and CNS depression

🔢 *Cimetidine:* Inhibition of narcotic hepatic metabolism; additive CNS effects

🔢 *Rifampin:* May reduce narcotic concentrations and precipitate withdrawal

Labs

• *Increase:* Amylase

---

* = non-FDA-approved use

SPECIAL CONSIDERATIONS

• Proposed, but not significant, advantages include low abuse potential, low respiratory depressant effects, low incidence of psychomimetic toxicity, and a lower incidence of hemodynamic toxicity

---

nalidixic acid

(nal-i-dix'ik)

Rx: NegGram
Chemical Class: Synthetic naphthyridine derivative
Therapeutic Class: Antibiotic

CLINICAL PHARMACOLOGY
Mechanism of Action: Inhibits DNA polymerization, primarily single-stranded DNA precursors in late stages of chromosomal replication; bactericidal
Pharmacokinetics
PO: Peak (serum) 1-2 hr, peak (urine) 3-4 hr; rapid absorption; 90% protein bound; metabolized in liver, excreted in urine (unchanged, hydroxynalidixic acid, similar antibacterial activity, and conjugates); serum $t_{1/2}$ 90 min, urine $t_{1/2}$ 6 hr; crosses placenta, enters breast milk
INDICATIONS AND USES: UTI caused by *E. coli, Klebsiella, Enterobacter, Proteus mirabilis, P. vulgaris, P. morganii*
DOSAGE
Adult
• PO 1 g qid × 1-2 wk, 2 g/day for long-term treatment
Child >3 mo
• PO 55 mg/kg/day in 4 divided doses for 1-2 wk; 33 mg/kg/day in 4 divided doses for long-term treatment
$ **AVAILABLE FORMS/COST OF THERAPY**
• Susp-Oral: 250 mg/5 ml, 480 ml: **$128.78**

• Tab, Uncoated—Oral: 250 mg, 56's: **$58.48**; 500 mg, 100's: **$43.45-$75.50**; 1 g, 100's: **$117.88-$260.30**
CONTRAINDICATIONS: Seizure disorder, infants <3 mo
PRECAUTIONS: Elderly, renal disease, hepatic disease, severe cerebral arteriosclerosis
PREGNANCY AND LACTATION: Pregnancy category B (safe last 2 trimesters); excreted into breast milk in low concentrations
SIDE EFFECTS/ADVERSE REACTIONS
CNS: Dizziness, drowsiness, *headache,* increased intracranial pressure, insomnia, ***seizures;*** toxic psychosis
EENT: Blurred vision, change in color perception, sensitivity to light
GI: Abdominal pain, diarrhea, increased transaminase levels, *nausea, vomiting*
SKIN: Photosensitivity, pruritus, rash, urticaria
INTERACTIONS
Drugs
3 *Warfarin:* Enhanced hypoprothrombinemic effects
Labs
• *False positive:* Urinary glucose
• *Increase:* Serum glucose, urine 17-ketogenic steroids, urine 17-ketosteroids, urine porphyrins, urine VMA
SPECIAL CONSIDERATIONS
• Resistance occurs in 2%-14% of patients during treatment

N

---

italic = common side effects   ***bold italic*** = life-threatening reactions

nalmefene

(nal'me-feen)
Rx: Revex
Chemical Class: Naltrexone
derivative
Therapeutic Class: Opiate anti-
dote

CLINICAL PHARMACOLOGY
Mechanism of Action: Prevents or
reverses the effects of opioids, including respiratory depression; no
opioid agonist activity
Pharmacokinetics
IV: Peak 5 min, duration is as long as
most opioids; distribution to CNS
rapid; 45% bound to plasma proteins; metabolized by the liver, excreted in urine; $t_{1/2}$ 9.4 hr
INDICATIONS AND USES: Complete or partial reversal of opioid
drug effects, including respiratory
depression; management of known
or suspected opioid overdose
DOSAGE
Adult
• *Postoperative opioid depression:*
Use 100 µg/ml dosage strength (blue
label): IV initial dose 0.25 µg/kg,
then 0.25 µg/kg incremental doses at
2-5 min intervals, stopping as soon
as the desired degree of opioid reversal is obtained; cumulative total
doses above 1 µg/kg do not provide
additional therapeutic effects
• *Management of known or suspected opioid overdose:* Use 1
mg/ml dosage strength (green label): IV initial dose 0.5 mg/70 kg,
then, if needed, a second dose of 1
mg/70 kg 2-5 min later (if a total
dose of 1.5 mg/70 kg has been administered without clinical response, additional drug is unlikely
to have an effect)

• *Reasonable suspicion of opioid
dependency:* Challenge dose of 0.1
mg/70 kg initially; if no evidence of
withdrawal in 2 min, follow recommended dosing
**§ AVAILABLE FORMS/COST
    OF THERAPY**
• Inj—Sol: 100 µg/ml, 1 ml (blue label): **$3.70**; 1 mg/ml, 2 ml (green la-
bel): **$47.78**
PRECAUTIONS: Pre-existing cardiac disease; known risk of precipitated withdrawal (like other opioid
antagonists, is known to produce
acute withdrawal symptoms and,
therefore, should be used with extreme caution in patients with
known physical dependence on
opioids or following surgery involving high doses of opioids)
PREGNANCY AND LACTATION:
Pregnancy category B; excretion
into breast milk unknown, use caution in nursing mothers
**SIDE EFFECTS/ADVERSE REAC-
    TIONS**
CNS: Dizziness, headache, postoperative pain, withdrawal syndrome
CV: Hypertension, tachycardia
GI: Nausea, vomiting
METAB: Chills, fever
SPECIAL CONSIDERATIONS
• Longer duration of action than
naloxone at fully reversing doses;
agent of choice in instances where
prolonged opioid effects are predicted, including overdose with
longer-acting opioids (e.g., methadone, propoxyphene), patients
given large doses of opioids, and
those with liver disease or renal failure (eliminating the need for continuous infusions of naloxone and
prolonged observation periods after
outpatient procedures)

naloxone

(nal-oks'one)

Rx: Narcan
Combinations
Rx: with pentazocine (Talwin NX)
Chemical Class: Thebaine derivative
Therapeutic Class: Opiate antidote

CLINICAL PHARMACOLOGY

Mechanism of Action: Prevents or reverses the effects of opioids, including respiratory depression; no opioid agonist activity

Pharmacokinetics

IV: Onset 2 min

SC/IM: Onset slightly less rapid than IV

Metabolized in liver, excreted in urine; t₁/₂ 64 min

INDICATIONS AND USES: Complete or partial reversal of narcotic depression, including respiratory depression; diagnosis of suspected acute opioid overdosage; reversal of alcoholic coma,* refractory shock,* Alzheimer's type dementia,* schizophrenia,* anaphylaxis*

DOSAGE

Adult

• *Narcotic overdose (known or suspected):* SC/IM/IV 0.4-2 mg initially, repeat at 2-3 min intervals up to 10 mg, if no response after 10 mg reevaluate diagnosis

• *Postoperative narcotic depression (partial reversal):* IV 0.1-0.2 mg at 2-3 min intervals to desired level of reversal (adequate ventilation and alertness without significant pain or discomfort); repeat doses may be required within 1-2 hr intervals

Child

• *Narcotic overdose (known or suspected):* SC/IM/IV 0.01 mg/kg initially, give subsequent doses of 0.01 mg/kg prn at 2-3 min intervals

• *Postoperative narcotic depression (partial reversal):* IV 0.005-0.01 mg q2-3 min to desired degree of reversal

💲 AVAILABLE FORMS/COST OF THERAPY

• Inj, Sol—IM, IV, SC: 0.02 mg/ml, 2 ml: **$1.14-$2.92**; 0.4 mg/ml, 1 ml: **$0.50-$5.25**; 1 mg/ml, 2 ml: **$4.75**

PRECAUTIONS: Physical narcotic dependency, pre-existing cardiovascular disorders

PREGNANCY AND LACTATION: Pregnancy category B; excretion into breast milk unknown, use caution in nursing mothers

SIDE EFFECTS/ADVERSE REACTIONS

CNS: **Seizures,** tremulousness

CV: Hypertension, hypotension, tachycardia, **ventricular dysrhythmia**

GI: Nausea, vomiting

RESP: **Pulmonary edema**

SKIN: Sweating

MISC: Reversal of analgesia

SPECIAL CONSIDERATIONS

• Duration of action of some narcotics may exceed that of naloxone; repeat doses prn

MONITORING PARAMETERS

• ECG, blood pressure, respiratory rate, mental status, pupil dilation

N

italic = common side effects   ***bold italic*** = life-threatening reactions

naltrexone

(nal-trex'one)
Rx: ReVia
Chemical Class: Thebaine derivative
Therapeutic Class: Opiate antidote; alcohol deterrent

CLINICAL PHARMACOLOGY

Mechanism of Action: Prevents or reverses the effects of opioids including respiratory depression; no opioid agonist activity; mechanism of action in alcoholism not understood, may block the effects of endogenous opioids; does not cause disulfiram-like reaction

Pharmacokinetics

PO: Peak 1 hr; duration: 50 mg blocks 25 mg IV heroin × 24 hr, 100-150 mg blocks narcotic doses × 48-72 hr; significant 1st-pass metabolism; 21% bound to plasma proteins; metabolized to active metabolite (6-β-naltrexol), excreted primarily by kidney; $t_{1/2}$ 10 hr (13 hr for 6-β-naltrexol)

INDICATIONS AND USES: Alcohol dependence, narcotic addiction, eating disorders,* postconcussional syndrome*

DOSAGE

Adult

• *Alcoholism:* PO 50 mg qd

• *Narcotic dependence:* PO 25 mg initially, observe for 1 hr, administer remaining 25 mg if no withdrawal signs occur (**do not attempt treatment until patient has remained opioid-free for 7-10 days; verify by analyzing urine for opioids and performing naloxone challenge test**); maintenance 50 mg qd or 100-150 mg q2-3 days

☒ **AVAILABLE FORMS/COST OF THERAPY**

• Tab, Uncoated—Oral: 50 mg, 100's: **$336.66-$508.16**

CONTRAINDICATIONS: Current use of opioid analgesics, opioid dependency, acute opioid withdrawal, positive urine screen for opioids, failed naloxone test, acute hepatitis, liver failure

PRECAUTIONS: Active liver disease, children

PREGNANCY AND LACTATION: Pregnancy category C

SIDE EFFECTS/ADVERSE REACTIONS

CNS: Anxiety, attempted suicide, chills, confusion, *depression, difficulty sleeping,* disorientation, dizziness, fatigue, feeling down, hallucinations, *headache,* irritability, *nervousness,* nightmares, paranoia, restlessness

CV: Edema, increased blood pressure, non-specific ECG changes, palpitations, phlebitis, tachycardia

EENT: Blurred vision, clogged ears, excess mucus or phlegm, itching, nasal congestion, nose bleeds, photophobia, rhinorrhea, sinus trouble, sneezing, sore throat, tinnitus

GI: Abdominal pain, constipation, *cramps,* diarrhea, excessive gas, hemorrhoids, *hepatotoxicity,* increased thirst, loss of appetite, *nausea,* ulcer, *vomiting*

GU: Delayed ejaculation; decreased potency, discomfort during urination; increased, decreased sexual interest; increased urinary frequency

MS: Joint, muscle pain, painful shoulders, legs, or knees

RESP: Cough, heavy breathing, hoarseness, shortness of breath

SKIN: Acne, alopecia, athlete's foot, cold sores, oily skin, pruritus, skin rash

* = non-FDA-approved use

SPECIAL CONSIDERATIONS
PATIENT/FAMILY EDUCATION
• Wear ID tag indicating naltrexone use
• Do not try to overcome reversal of opiate effects by self-administration of large doses of narcotic
• Do not exceed recommended dose
MONITORING PARAMETERS
• Liver function tests

---

nandrolone
(nan'droe-lone)
Rx: *Decanoate:*
Deca-Durabolin, Hybolin
Decanoate, Kabolin,
Nandrolone Decanoate
Chemical Class: Halogenated
testosterone derivative
Therapeutic Class: Androgen;
antineoplastic
DEA Class: Schedule III

CLINICAL PHARMACOLOGY
Mechanism of Action: Promotes body tissue-building processes and reverses catabolic processes when administered with adequate calories and protein; inhibits endogenous testosterone release
Pharmacokinetics
IM: Metabolized in liver, excreted in urine
INDICATIONS AND USES: Anemia of renal insufficiency
DOSAGE
Adult
• *Anemia of renal disease:* IM 50-100 mg qwk (women); 100-200 mg qwk (men)
Child 2-13 yr
• *Anemia of renal disease:* IM 25-50 mg q3-4 wk

💲 AVAILABLE FORMS/COST OF THERAPY
• Inj, Sol (decanoate)—IM: 50 mg/ml, 2 ml: **$4.90-$14.42**; 100 mg/ml, 2 ml: **$3.50-$30.61**; 200 mg/ml, 1 ml: **$21.24-$27.81**
CONTRAINDICATIONS: Male patients with prostate or breast cancer, hypercalcemia in females with breast cancer, nephrosis, nephrotic phase of nephritis, enhancement of physical appearance or athletic performance
PRECAUTIONS: Elderly, children, cardiac disease or risk factors for atherosclerosis, renal disease, hepatic disease, seizure disorder, migraine headache, diabetes
PREGNANCY AND LACTATION: Pregnancy category X, use extreme caution in nursing mothers
SIDE EFFECTS/ADVERSE REACTIONS
CNS: Choreiform movement, depression, excitation, habituation, insomnia
CV: Edema
EENT: Deepening of voice, hoarseness
GI: Cholestatic jaundice, diarrhea, ***hepatic necrosis, hepatocellular neoplasms,*** nausea, ***peliosis hepatis,*** vomiting
GU: Amenorrhea, clitoral hypertrophy, decreased breast size, decreased libido, testicular atrophy, vaginitis, virilization
METAB: Decreased glucose tolerance, decreased HDL cholesterol, increased LDL cholesterol, increased serum cholesterol, retention of sodium, chloride, water, potassium, phosphates, calcium
MS: Premature closure of epiphyses in children
SKIN: Acne, alopecia, flushing, hirsutism, rash, sweating

N

---

italic = common side effects   ***bold italic*** = life-threatening reactions

INTERACTIONS
Drugs
❸ *Antidiabetic agents:* Enhanced hypoglycemic effects

❷ *Cyclosporine:* Increased cyclosporine concentrations, potential for toxicity

❸ *HMG-CoA reductase inhibitors (lovastatin, pravastatin):* Myositis risk increased

❷ *Oral anticoagulants:* Enhanced hypoprothrombinemic response

❸ *Tacrolimus:* Increased tacrolimus concentrations, potential for toxicity

SPECIAL CONSIDERATIONS
• Anabolic steroids have potential for abuse, especially in the athlete

MONITORING PARAMETERS
• Women should be observed for signs of virilization
• Liver function tests, lipids, Hct
• Growth rate in children (X-rays for bone age q 6 mo)

---

naproxen
(na-prox'en)

Rx: *Sodium salt:* Anaprox, Anaprox DS, Naprelan
Rx: *EC-Naprosyn*
OTC: Aleve
Chemical Class: Propionic acid derivative
Therapeutic Class: NSAID with analgesic and antipyretic activity

---

CLINICAL PHARMACOLOGY
Mechanism of Action: Reversible cyclooxygenase (i.e., prostaglandin synthetase) inhibitor; non-selectively decreases the formation of both prostaglandins and thromboxane A2; variable effects on lipoxygenase synthesis and subsequent leukotriene production; antiinflammatory, antipyretic, and analgesic activity; inhibits platelet aggregation

Pharmacokinetics
PO: Onset 1 hr, peak 2-4 hr, duration up to 7 hr; >99% bound to plasma proteins; metabolized in liver, excreted by kidney; $t_{1/2}$ 12-15 hr

INDICATIONS AND USES: Bursitis, dysmenorrhea, ergotamine withdrawal,* erythema nodosum,* fever, gouty arthritis, headache, menorrhagia,* musculoskeletal disorders,* osteoarthritis, rheumatoid arthritis, soft tissue injuries,* ankylosing spondylitis, prevention of cognitive decline,* prevention of colon cancer,* pain—mild to moderate

DOSAGE
Adult
• *Arthritis:* PO 250-500 mg (275-550 mg naproxen sodium) bid, may increase to 1.5 g/day (1.65 g/day naproxen sodium) for limited periods; Sus Action PO 750-1000 mg qd; max 1000 mg/d

• *Acute gout:* PO 750 mg (825 mg naproxen sodium), followed by 250 mg (275 mg naproxen sodium) q8h until attack subsides; Sus Action PO 1000 mg qd, may increase to 1500 mg qd for brief period if needed

• *Mild to moderate pain, primary dysmenorrhea:* PO 500 mg (550 mg naproxen sodium) at earliest symptoms of menses, followed by 250 mg (275 mg naproxen sodium) q6-8h; do not exceed 1.25 g/day (1.375 g/day naproxen sodium)

• Minor aches and pains (OTC): PO 220 mg q12h prn

Child
• *Juvenile arthritis:* PO 10 mg/kg divided bid

---

* = non-FDA-approved use

AVAILABLE FORMS/COST OF THERAPY

Naproxen
• Susp—Oral: 125 mg/5 ml, 500 ml: **$38.23**
• Tab, Uncoated—Oral: 250 mg, 100's: **$9.30-$110.54**; 375 mg, 100's: **$16.99-$124.86**; 500 mg, 100's: **$104.30-$173.53**
• Tab, Enteric Coated—Oral: 375 mg, 100's: **$101.21-$134.24**; 500 mg, 100's: **$120.74-$163.94**

Naproxen Sodium (Naproxen)
• Tab, Uncoated—Oral: 220 mg (200 mg), 100's: **$8.25-$9.24**; 275 mg (250 mg), 100's: **$11.13-$105.10**; 550 mg (500 mg), 100's: **$90.00-$163.63**
• Tab, Enteric Coated—Oral: 412.5 mg (375 mg), 100's: **$127.94**; 550 mg (500 mg), 75's: **$117.02**

CONTRAINDICATIONS: Bronchospasm, nasal polyps, angioedema precipitated by aspirin or other NSAIDs

PRECAUTIONS: History of GI ulceration, bleeding, or perforation; renal dysfunction, hypertension or cardiac conditions aggravated by fluid retention and edema, history of liver dysfunction, history of coagulation disorders

PREGNANCY AND LACTATION: Pregnancy category B (category D if used in 3rd trimester); could cause constriction of the ductus arteriosus *in utero,* persistent pulmonary hypertension of the newborn, or prolonged labor; passes into breast milk in small quantities; compatible with breast feeding

SIDE EFFECTS/ADVERSE REACTIONS

CNS: Dizziness, drowsiness, headache, lightheadedness
CV: Chest pain, ***CHF, dysrhythmias, edema,*** hypertension, palpitation, tachycardia
EENT: Hearing disturbances, *tinnitus,* visual disturbances
GI: Abdominal cramps, *constipation, diarrhea, dyspepsia,* flatulence, **gastric or duodenal ulcer with bleeding or perforation,** *heartburn,* hepatitis, *nausea,* occult blood in stool, **pancreatitis,** *stomatitis,* vomiting
GU: **Acute renal failure**
HEME: **Agranulocytosis,** eosinophilia, **leukopenia, neutropenia, pancytopenia, thrombocytopenia**
METAB: Hyperglycemia, hyperkalemia, hypoglycemia, hyponatremia
RESP: **Bronchospasm,** dyspnea, pulmonary infiltrates
SKIN: Ecchymoses, photosensitivity, *pruritus, rash,* urticaria

INTERACTIONS

Drugs

3 *Aminoglycosides:* Reduced clearance with elevated aminoglycoside levels and potential for toxicity (especially indomethacin in premature infants; other NSAIDs probably)

3 *Anticoagulants:* Excessive hypoprothrombinemia, decreased platelet aggregation with increased risk of GI bleeding

3 *Antihypertensives (α-blockers, angiotensin-converting enzyme inhibitors, angiotensin II receptor blockers, β-blockers, diuretics):* Inhibition of antihypertensive and other favorable hemodynamic effects

3 *Corticosteroids:* Increased risk of GI ulceration

3 *Cyclosporine:* Increased nephrotoxicity risk

3 *Lithium:* Decreased clearance of lithium (mediated via prostaglandins) resulting in elevated serum lithium levels and risk of toxicity

N

■ *Methotrexate:* Decreased renal secretion of methotrexate resulting in elevated methotrexate levels and risk of toxicity

■ *Phenylpropanolamine:* Possible acute hypertensive reaction

■ *Potassium-sparing   diuretics:* Additive hyperkalemia potential

■ *Triamterene:* Acute renal failure reported with addition of indomethacin; caution with other NSAIDs

Labs

• *False increase:* Serum bicarbonate, urine 5-HIAA

SPECIAL CONSIDERATIONS

• No significant advantage over other NSAIDs; cost should govern use

PATIENT/FAMILY EDUCATION

• Avoid concurrent use of aspirin and alcoholic beverages

• Take with food, milk, or antacids to decrease GI upset

• Notify clinician if edema, black stools, or persistent headache occur

MONITORING PARAMETERS

• Initial hemogram and fecal occult blood test within 3 mo of starting regular chronic therapy; repeat every 6-12 mo (more frequently in high-risk patients (>65 years, peptic ulcer disease, concurrent steroids or anticoagulants); electrolytes, creatinine, and BUN within 3 mo of starting regular chronic therapy; repeat every 6-12 mo

---

naratriptan

(nare-a-trip'tan)

Rx: Amerge

Chemical Class: Serotonin derivative

Therapeutic Class: Antimigraine agent

CLINICAL PHARMACOLOGY

Mechanism of Action: Selectively activates vascular 5-HT_1-receptors in cranial arteries causing vasoconstriction and inhibition of proinflammatory neuropeptide release, actions correlating with the relief of migraine in humans

Pharmacokinetics

PO: 70% bioavailability, peak 2-3 hr, onset 3 hr; 28%-31% bound to plasma proteins; metabolized by various cytochrome P-450 isozymes to inactive metabolites; 50% excreted unchanged in urine; $t_{1/2}$ 6 hr (11 hr in moderate renal impairment; 16 hr in severe hepatic impairment)

INDICATIONS AND USES: Acute migraine headache with or without aura.

DOSAGE

Adult

• PO 1-2.5 mg at first sign of headache; may repeat after 4 hr if partial response or headache returns (max 5 mg/24 hr)

• Mild to moderate renal or hepatic impairment: Do not exceed 2.5 mg/24 hr

$ AVAILABLE FORMS/COST OF THERAPY

• Tab, Film Coated—Oral: 1 mg, 2.5 mg, 9's: **$173.06**

CONTRAINDICATIONS: Severe renal impairment (creatinine clearance <15 ml/min) or severe hepatic impairment; ischemic heart disease, hemiplegic or basilar migraine;

Prinzmetal's angina; uncontrolled hypertension; within 24 hr of ergotamine-containing products; concurrent use of MAO inhibitor therapy (or within 2 wk of discontinuing an MAO inhibitor)

PRECAUTIONS: Atypical headache; mild to moderate renal or hepatic impairment; elderly; children

PREGNANCY AND LACTATION: Pregnancy category C; use caution in nursing mothers

SIDE EFFECTS/ADVERSE REACTIONS

CNS: Paresthesia, dizziness, fatigue, drowsiness, vertigo, tremors, cognitive function disorders, sleep disorders, equilibrium disorders

CV: Palpitations, increased blood pressure, tachyarrhythmias, abnormal ECG, syncope

EENT: Photophobia, blurred vision, tinnitus

GI: Nausea, hyposalivation, vomiting, dyspeptic symptoms, diarrhea, constipation

GU: Bladder inflammation, polyuria, diuresis

HEME: Increased white cells

METAB: Thirst, polydipsia, dehydration, fluid retention

MS: Muscle pain, arthralgia, articular rheumatism, muscle cramps/spasms, joint/muscle stiffness, tightness, rigidity

RESP: Bronchitis, cough, pneumonia

SKIN: Sweating, rash, pruritus, urticaria

MISC: Pain/pressure sensations in neck/throat/jaw; chills, fever

INTERACTIONS

Drugs

⚠ *Ergotamine containing drugs:* Increased vasoconstriction

⚠ *MAO inhibitors:* Potential for decreased metabolism of naratriptan

❷ *Sibutramine:* Increased risk of serotonin syndrome

SPECIAL CONSIDERATIONS

• Longer acting than sumatriptan and zolmitriptan so recurrent headaches requiring a second dose less likely; slower onset than sumatriptan and zolmitriptan; should probably be reserved for patients who get recurrent headaches

• Safety of treating, on average, more than 4 headaches in a 30-day period has not been established

PATIENT/FAMILY EDUCATION

• Use only to treat migraine headache, not for prevention

---

natamycin

(na-ta-mye´sin)

Rx: Natacyn

Chemical Class: Tetraene polyene derivative

Therapeutic Class: Ophthalmic antifungal

CLINICAL PHARMACOLOGY

Mechanism of Action: Binds to fungal cell membrane, altering membrane permeability; depletes essential cellular constituents; fungicidal

Pharmacokinetics

OPHTHAL: Produces effective concentrations within corneal stroma; systemic absorption should not occur after topical administration

INDICATIONS AND USES: Fungal blepharitis, conjunctivitis, keratitis caused by susceptible organisms Antifungal spectrum usually includes: *Candida, Aspergillus, Cephalosporium, Fusarium, and Penicillium,* initial drug of choice in *Fusarium solani* keratitis

---

DOSAGE
Adult
• *Fungal keratitis:* 1 gtt into conjunctival sac q1-2h, decrease to 1 gtt 6-8 times/day after 3-4 days; continue therapy for 14-21 days
• *Fungal blepharitis, conjunctivitis:* 1 gtt 4-6 times/day

$ AVAILABLE FORMS/COST OF THERAPY
• Susp—Ophth: 5%, 15 ml: **$136.55**

PRECAUTIONS: Fungal endophthalmitis (effectiveness as single agent not established)

PREGNANCY AND LACTATION: Pregnancy category C

SIDE EFFECTS/ADVERSE REACTIONS
EENT: Conjunctival chemosis, conjunctival hyperemia

SPECIAL CONSIDERATIONS
PATIENT/FAMILY EDUCATION
• Shake well before using

MONITORING PARAMETERS
• Failure of keratitis to improve following 7-10 days of administration suggests infection not susceptible to natamycin

---

nateglinide
(na-teg'lin-ide)
Rx: Starlix
Chemical Class: Amino acid derivative
Therapeutic Class: Oral hypoglycemic/oral antidiabetic agent

CLINICAL PHARMACOLOGY
Mechanism of Action: Insulin secretagogue, dependent upon functioning beta-cells in the pancreatic islets; interacts with the ATP-sensitive potassium (K+ATP) channel on pancreatic beta-cells; subsequent depolarization opens calcium channel, producing calcium influx and insulin secretion; extent of release is glucose dependent and diminishes at low glucose levels; highly selective with low affinity for heart and skeletal muscle

Pharmacokinetics
PO: T_{max}, 1 hr post dose, rapidly absorbed; absolute bioavailability 73%, AUC unaffected by meals; T_{max} delayed and C_{max} decreased; Vd 10 L, 98% plasma protein bound; metabolized by mixed-function oxidase system (CYP2C9, CYP3A4) in liver (metabolites less potent), excreted in urine 80%, feces 10% (75% within 6 hr); $t_{1/2}$ 1.5 hr

INDICATIONS AND USES: Diabetes mellitus, type 2: Monotherapy or in combination with metformin

DOSAGE
Adult and Child >16 yr
• Monotherapy or in combination with metformin: 120 mg tid ac; 60 mg tid ac for patients with A1c near goal at initiation
• No dosage reductions for elderly, mild-severe renal insufficiency, mild hepatic insufficiency

$ AVAILABLE FORMS/COST OF THERAPY
• Tab—Oral: 60 mg, 100's: **$110.10**; 120 mg, 100's: **$104.00**

CONTRAINDICATIONS: Hypersensitivity; diabetes mellitus, type 1; diabetic ketoacidosis

PRECAUTIONS: Hypoglycemia, hepatic impairment (mod-sev disease), situations associated with loss of glucose control (infection, stress, trauma, surgery)

PREGNANCY AND LACTATION: Pregnancy category C (no adequate and well-controlled studies in pregnant women); excretion into human breast milk unknown

SIDE EFFECTS/ADVERSE REACTIONS
CNS: Dizziness

---

* = non-FDA-approved use

EENT: Flu symptoms, upper respiratory infection
METAB: **Hypoglycemia** (0.3%)
MS: Arthropathy, back pain
RESP: Bronchitis, coughing
MISC: Accidental trauma

INTERACTIONS
Drugs
3 *β-blockers:* Antagonistic glycemic effects, prolong hypoglycemia, mask hypoglycemia symptoms

3 *Diazoxide:* Antagonistic effects (diazoxide causes hyperglycemia)

3 *Epinephrine:* Antagonistic effects; combination may decrease hypoglycemic efficacy

3 *MAOI:* MAOIs stimulate insulin secretion; additive effects; increased risk of hypoglycemia

3 *Hypoglycemics (bioguanides, insulin):* Combination increases risk of hypoglycemia

3 *Isoniazid:* Antagonistic effects; combination may decrease hypoglycemic efficacy

3 *Niacin:* Antagonistic effects; combination may decrease hypoglycemic efficacy

Labs
• *Uric acid:* Increased

SPECIAL CONSIDERATIONS
• *Pharmacodynamics* (60-120 mg tid ac for 24 weeks): HbA1c change - 0.5%; fasting plasma glucose change - 15 mg/dL; weight change - 0.3-0.9 kg

PATIENT/FAMILY EDUCATION
• Review signs and symptoms and management of hypoglycemia
• Drug administration timing (i.e., before meals)

MONITORING PARAMETERS
• Home/self blood glucose monitoring, HbA1c, signs and symptoms of hyper/hypoglycemia, complete blood count, routine blood chemistry

---

nedocromil
(ned-oh-crow´mil)
Rx: *Oral:*Tilade *Ophth:*Alocril
Chemical Class: Pyranoquinoline dicarboxylic acid derivative
Therapeutic Class: Antiasthmatic, inhaled

CLINICAL PHARMACOLOGY
Mechanism of Action: Inhibits activation and release of inflammatory mediators from cells involved in asthmatic inflammation, including eosinophils, neutrophils, macrophages, mast cells, monocytes, and platelets; inhibits both early and late asthmatic responses to inhaled antigen and irritants
Pharmacokinetics
INH: Low systemic bioavailability; duration 4-6 hr; 89% bound to plasma proteins; excreted unchanged in urine; $t_{1/2}$ 1.5-3.3 hr

INDICATIONS AND USES: Maintenance therapy in mild to moderate bronchial asthma, pruritus associated with allergic conjunctivitis (Ophth), prevention of exercise-induced asthma,* prevention of acute bronchospasm induced by environmental pollutants*

DOSAGE
Adult and Child ≥6 yr
• INH 2 inhalations qid at regular intervals; may reduce to bid-tid in patients under good control
• OPHTH 1-2 gtts each eye bid

$ **AVAILABLE FORMS/COST OF THERAPY**
• Aer—INH: 1.75 mg/spray, 112 sprays: **$42.72**

PRECAUTIONS: Acute bronchospasm **(not a bronchodilator)**

PREGNANCY AND LACTATION: Pregnancy category B; excretion into breast milk unknown

---

SIDE EFFECTS/ADVERSE REACTIONS

CNS: Dizziness, *headache*

CV: Chest pain

EENT: Burning eyes, nasal congestion, *pharyngitis,* rhinitis, throat irritation, upper respiratory infection, photophobia

GI: Abdominal pain, diarrhea, dry mouth, dyspepsia, nausea, *unpleasant taste,* vomiting

RESP: **Bronchospasm,** *coughing*

SPECIAL CONSIDERATIONS

PATIENT/FAMILY EDUCATION

• Must be used regularly to achieve benefit, even during symptom-free periods

• Therapeutic effect may take up to 4 wk

• Not to be used to treat acute asthmatic symptoms

---

nefazodone

(neh-faz'oh-doan)

Rx: Serzone

Chemical Class: Phenylpiperazine derivative

Therapeutic Class: Antidepressant

CLINICAL PHARMACOLOGY

Mechanism of Action: Inhibits neuronal uptake of serotonin (significant) and norepinephrine (slight); antagonizes α_1-adrenergic receptors, minimal anticholinergic, moderate sedative, and slight orthostatic hypotensive effects

Pharmacokinetics

PO: Absolute bioavailability low (about 20%); peak 1 hr; >99% bound to plasma proteins; extensively metabolized (active metabolite hydroxynefazodone), $t_{1/2}$ 2-4 hr

INDICATIONS AND USES: Depression

DOSAGE

Adult

• PO 200 mg/day in 2 divided doses, increase in increments of 100-200 mg/day in intervals of no less than 1 wk; max dose, 600 mg/day

• *Elderly:* PO 100 mg/day bid with gradual titration

💲 AVAILABLE FORMS/COST OF THERAPY

• Tab, Uncoated—Oral: 50 mg, 60's: **$89.19**; 100 mg, 60's: **$87.79**; 150 mg, 60's: **$74.12**; 200 mg, 60's: **$94.79**; 250 mg, 60's: **$96.55**

PRECAUTIONS: Active liver disease, elevated serum transaminases, elderly, children, CV disease, cerebrovascular disease, dehydration, hypovolemia, history of mania, suicidal ideation, seizure disorder, visual disturbances

PREGNANCY AND LACTATION: Pregnancy category C; excretion into breast milk unknown, use caution in nursing mothers

SIDE EFFECTS/ADVERSE REACTIONS

CNS: Abnormal dreams, agitation, *asthenia,* ataxia, *confusion, dizziness, headache,* insomnia, *lightheadedness,* memory impairment, paresthesia, *somnolence,* tremor

CV: Peripheral edema, postural hypotension, sinus bradycardia

EENT: Abnormal vision, blurred vision, pharyngitis, taste perversion, tinnitus, visual field defect

GI: Constipation, diarrhea, dry mouth, dyspepsia, increased appetite, nausea

GU: Impotence, urinary frequency, urinary retention, vaginitis

RESP: Cough

SKIN: Pruritus, rash

---

* = non-FDA-approved use

INTERACTIONS
Drugs
❷ *Alprazolam:* Significant increase in serum alprazolam concentrations; if coadministered reduce alprazolam dose by 50%

❸ *Atorvastatin, lovastatin, simvastatin:* Potential for development of myositis with rhabdomyolysis

❸ *Buspirone:* Significant increase in serum buspirone concentrations

❷ *Carbamazepine:* 95% decrease in serum nefazodone concentrations; concomitant use contraindicated

▲ *Cisapride, pimozide:* Theoretical potential for QT prolongation and dysrhythmia; concomitant use contraindicated

❸ *Cyclosporine, tacrolimus:* Toxic blood levels of immunosuppressives have been reported; monitor levels and adjust immunosuppressive dosage as needed

❸ *Digoxin:* Increased serum digoxin concentrations

❷ *Triazolam:* Significant increase in serum triazolam concentrations; if coadministered reduce triazolam dose by 75%

❷ *MAOIs:* Serious adverse reactions possible including hyperthermia, rigidity, myoclonus, autonomic instability, mental status changes, seizures; observe a 14-day washout period between discontinuing one drug and starting the other

SPECIAL CONSIDERATIONS
• Priapism has been reported; educate and monitor appropriately

PATIENT/FAMILY EDUCATION
• Therapeutic effect may not be apparent for several weeks
• Drug may cause drowsiness, use caution driving or performing other tasks where alertness is required

nelfinavir
(nel-fin´eh-veer)
Rx: Viracept
Chemical Class: HIV protease inhibitor
Therapeutic Class: HIV infection

CLINICAL PHARMACOLOGY
Mechanism of Action: By inhibiting the HIV protease, nelfinavir causes immature and noninfectious virus to be produced
Pharmacokinetics
PO: Onset 1 hr, peak 2-4 hr, bioavailability better with food; 98% protein bound; metabolized in liver by cytochrome P450 system including CYP3A, some metabolites active; $t_{1/2}$ 3.5-5 hr, 98% excreted in feces as unchanged drug and metabolites
INDICATIONS AND USES: Combination therapy for HIV-1
DOSAGE
Adult and Child >14 yr
• PO: 750 mg tid with food
Child 2-13 yr
• PO: 20-30 mg per dose, taken tid with food
• Adjust dose when used with indinavir, rifabutin, ritonavir
• For latest treatment guidelines see www.hivatis.org
🆂 AVAILABLE FORMS/COST OF THERAPY
• Powder—Oral: 50 mg nelfinavir base per g, 144 g: **$66.48**
• Tab, Uncoated—Oral: 250 mg, 270's: **$609.12**
CONTRAINDICATIONS: Concurrent use of rifampin
PRECAUTIONS: Phenylketonuria, hepatic insufficiency, hemophilia; do not administer concurrently with cisapride; avoid coadministration with rifampin, midazolam, or triazolam

PREGNANCY AND LACTATION:
Pregnancy category B; excreted in
breast milk; breast feeding not recommended   for   HIV-infected
women

SIDE EFFECTS/ADVERSE REAC-
TIONS

CNS: Dizziness, headache

EENT: Iritis, rhinitis

GI: Diarrhea (20%), dyspepsia,
nausea

GU: Nephrolithiasis, sexual dysfunction

HEME: Anemia, leukopenia, thrombocytopenia

METAB: Hyperlipidemia, hyperuricemia, increased alkaline phosphatase, transaminases, CPK, LDH

MS: Arthralgia, myalgia, myopathy

RESP: Dyspnea

SKIN: Folliculitis, pruritus, rash

MISC: Weakness

INTERACTIONS

Drugs

3 *Barbiturates:* Increased clearance of nelfinavir; reduced clearance of barbiturates

2 *Carbamazepine:*   Increased
clearance of nelfinavir; reduced
clearance of carbamazepine

⚠ *Cisapride:* Increased plasma
levels of cisapride

⚠ *Ergot   alkaloids:* Increased
plasma levels of ergot alkaloids

3 *Erythromycin:* Reduced clearance of nelfinavir; nelfinavir reduces clearance of erythromycin

⚠ *Lovastatin:* Nelfinavir reduces
clearance of lovastatin

⚠ *Midazolam:* Increased plasma
levels of midazolam and prolonged
effect

3 *Nevirapine:* Reduces plasma
nelfinavir levels; increase nelfinavir
dose to 1000 mg tid

3 *Oral contraceptives:* Nelfinavir
may reduce efficacy

3 *Phenytoin:* Increased clearance
of nelfinavir; reduced clearance of
phenytoin

2 *Rifabutin:* Increased clearance
of nelfinavir; reduced clearance of
rifabutin—reduce rifabutin dose to
150 mg qd and increase nelfinavir
dose to 1000 mg tid

⚠ *Rifampin:* Increased clearance of
nelfinavir

3 *Ritonavir:* Decreased clearance
of nelfinavir; decrease nelfinavir
dose to 750 mg bid

3 *Saquinavir:* Decreased clearance of saquinavir; reduce dose of
Fortovase (saquinavir soft gel capsule) to 800 mg tid

⚠ *Simvastatin:* Nelfinavir reduces
clearance of simvastatin

⚠ *Triazolam:* Increased plasma
levels of triazolam and prolonged
effect

SPECIAL CONSIDERATIONS

• Positive results of treatment are
based on surrogate markers only

• Take with meal or snack

PATIENT/FAMILY EDUCATION

• Contains phenylalanine, take with
food

MONITORING PARAMETERS

• CBC, electrolytes, renal function,
liver enzymes, CPK

---

* = non-FDA-approved use

neomycin

(nee-oh-mye´sin)

Rx: (Oral): Mycifradin,
Neo-Fradin

OTC: (Topical): Myciguent
Combinations

Rx: with polymyxin B
(Neosporin G.U. irrigant)

OTC: with polymyxin B,
bacitracin (Neosporin, My-
citracin)

Chemical Class: Aminoglycoside

Therapeutic Class: Antibiotic

CLINICAL PHARMACOLOGY

Mechanism of Action: Interferes
with protein synthesis in bacterial
cell by binding to 30S ribosomal
subunit, which causes misreading of
genetic code, inaccurate peptide sequence forms in protein chain, causing bacterial death

Pharmacokinetics

PO: Poorly absorbed, small absorbed fraction rapidly excreted via
kidney, unabsorbed fraction eliminated unchanged in feces; intestinal
bacteria suppressed for 48-72 hr after oral administration

INDICATIONS AND USES: (Oral)
preoperative bowel preparation, adjunctive therapy of hepatic coma,
hypercholesterolemia*; (topical)
minor skin infections

Antibacterial spectrum usually includes:

• *E. coli* and the *Klebsiella-Entero-
bacter* group; no anaerobic coverage; minimal coverage of gram-
positive organisms

DOSAGE

Adult

• *Preoperative bowel preparation:*
PO 1 g q1h for 4 doses then 1 g q4h
for 5 doses; or 1 g at 1, 2, and 11 PM
on day preceding surgery as an adjunct to cathartics, enema, and oral
erythromycin; or 6 g/day divided
q4h for 2-3 days

• *Hepatic coma:* PO 4-12 g/day divided q4-6h

• TOP apply to affected area qd-tid

Child

• *Preoperative bowel preparation:*
PO 90 mg/kg/day divided q4h for 2
days; or 25 mg/kg at 1, 2, and 11 PM
on the day preceding surgery as an
adjunct to cathartics, enema, and
oral erythromycin

• *Hepatic coma:* 2.5-7 g/m²/day divided q4-6h for 5-6 days, not to exceed 12 g/day

• TOP apply to affected area qd-tid

$ **AVAILABLE FORMS/COST
OF THERAPY**

• Cre—Top: 0.5%, 15, 30 g:
$2.98/15 g

• Oint—Top: 0.5%, 15, 30 g:
$2.98/15 g

• Sol—Oral: 125 mg/5 ml, 480 ml:
$25.05-$31.34

• Tab, Uncoated—Oral: 500 mg,
100's: **$11.51-$124.57**

CONTRAINDICATIONS: Intestinal
obstruction, inflammatory or ulcerative gastrointestinal disease

PRECAUTIONS: Hepatic disease,
renal disease, prolonged treatment,
application to extensive burns or
large surface area, children <18 yr,
myasthenia gravis, parkinsonism

PREGNANCY AND LACTATION:
Pregnancy category D; ototoxicity
has not been reported as an effect of
in utero exposure; 8th cranial nerve
toxicity in the fetus is well known
following exposure to other aminoglycosides and could potentially
occur with neomycin

**SIDE EFFECTS/ADVERSE REAC-
TIONS**

EENT: Ototoxicity (prolonged and
high-dose therapy)

---

italic = common side effects   ***bold italic*** = life-threatening reactions

GI: Diarrhea, malabsorption syndrome has occurred during prolonged therapy; *nausea,* ***pseudomembranous colitis,*** *vomiting*

GU: ***Nephrotoxicity*** (prolonged and high-dose therapy)

SKIN: Sensitization (low-grade reddening with swelling, dry scaling, and itching or a failure to heal)

INTERACTIONS
Drugs
3 *Digitalis glycosides:* Reduced serum digoxin concentration

2 *Ethacrynic acid:* Increased risk of ototoxicity, especially in patients with renal impairment

3 *Oral anticoagulants:* Enhanced hypoprothrombinemic response; more common with large doses of neomycin, dietary vitamin K deficiency, impaired hepatic function

A *Methotrexate:* Oral absorption of methotrexate reduced 30%-50%

3 *Penicillin V:* Reduced concentrations of penicillin V, possible reduced efficacy

3 *Warfarin:* Enhanced hypoprothrombinemic response

SPECIAL CONSIDERATIONS
• Inform patient and family about possible toxic effects on the 8th cranial nerve; monitor for loss of hearing, ringing or roaring in ears, or a feeling of fullness in head

PATIENT/FAMILY EDUCATION
• Drink plenty of fluids

MONITORING PARAMETERS
• Renal function, audiometric testing during extended therapy or with application to extensive burns or large surface area

---

neostigmine
(neo-stig'meen)
Rx: Prostigmin
Chemical Class: Synthetic quaternary ammonium derivative
Therapeutic Class: Cholinergic

CLINICAL PHARMACOLOGY
Mechanism of Action: An acetylcholinesterase inhibitor, inhibits destruction of acetylcholine, facilitating transmission of impulses across myoneuronal junction

Pharmacokinetics
IM: Onset 20-30 min
IV: Onset 4-8 min
PO: Onset 45-75 min Duration 2-4 hr

INDICATIONS AND USES: Symptomatic control of myasthenia gravis; prevention and treatment of postoperative distention and urinary retention (after excluding mechanical obstruction); postoperative antidote for nondepolarizing neuromuscular blocking agents

DOSAGE
Adult
• *Myasthenia gravis*
• PO 15-375 mg/day; usual dose 150 mg given over 24 hr
• SC/IM 1 ml of 1:2000 sol (0.5 mg); individualize subsequent doses; reserve for myasthenic crisis when difficulty breathing and swallowing is present
• *Antidote for nondepolarizing neuromuscular blocking agents*
• IV 0.5-2 mg slow injection; doses greater than 5 mg rarely needed; give atropine sulfate 0.6-1.2 mg IV several min before neostigmine
• *Prevention of postoperative distention and urinary retention*
• SC/IM 1 ml of 1:4000 sol (0.25 mg) as soon as possible postoperatively; repeat q4-6h for 2-3 days

---

• *Treatment of postoperative distention*
• SC/IM 1 ml of 1:2000 sol (0.5 mg) prn
• *Treatment of urinary retention*
• SC/IM 1 ml of 1:2000 sol (0.5 mg); if patient unable to void within 1 hr, catheterize; after bladder has been emptied continue 0.5 mg injections q3h for at least 5 injections

Child
• *Myasthenia gravis*
• PO 2 mg/kg/day divided q3-4h; individualize interval between doses
• SC/IM/IV 0.01-0.04 mg/kg/dose q2-3h prn
• *Antidote for nondepolarizing neuromuscular blocking agents*
• IV 0.025-0.08 mg/kg/dose with atropine 0.01-0.03 mg/kg or glycopyrrolate 0.004-0.015 mg/kg

Infant
• *Antidote for nondepolarizing neuromuscular blocking agents*
• IV 0.025-0.01 mg/kg/dose with atropine 0.01-0.04 mg/kg or glycopyrrolate 0.004-0.02 mg/kg

$ **AVAILABLE FORMS/COST OF THERAPY**
• Inj, Sol—IM, IV, SC: 1:1000 (1 mg/ml), 10 ml: **$0.85-$16.08**; 1:2000 (0.5 mg/ml), 1, 10 ml: **$2.50-$12.19**/10 ml; 1:4000 (0.25 mg/ml), 1 ml: **$1.41**
• Tab—Oral: 15 mg, 100's: **$58.19**
CONTRAINDICATIONS: Urinary or intestinal obstruction
PRECAUTIONS: Seizure disorder, asthma, coronary occlusion, hyperthyroidism, dysrhythmias, peptic ulcer, bradycardia, hypotension, presence of other cholinergics (atropine should be available for cholinergic crisis)
PREGNANCY AND LACTATION: Pregnancy category C; transient muscle weakness occurred in 20% of infants born to mothers using neo-

stigmine and similar drugs; ionized at physiologic pH, would not be expected to be excreted in breast milk
SIDE EFFECTS/ADVERSE REACTIONS
CNS: Dizziness, drowsiness, headache, incoordination, ***loss of consciousness, paralysis, seizures***
CV: ***AV block,*** bradycardia, ***cardiac arrest, dysrhythmias, hypotension,*** non-specific ECG changes, tachycardia
EENT: Blurred vision, conjunctival hyperemia, diplopia, lacrimation, miosis, spasm of accommodation, visual changes
GI: *Cramps, diarrhea, dysphagia, increased gastric secretions, increased salivation, nausea, vomiting,* flatulence, increased peristalsis
GU: Urinary frequency, incontinence, urgency
MS: Arthralgia, fasciculation, muscle cramps and spasms, weakness
RESP: Bronchospasm, dyspnea, increased secretions, ***laryngospasm, respiratory arrest, respiratory depression***
SKIN: Rash, sweating, urticaria
INTERACTIONS
Drugs
3 *Tacrine:* Increased cholinergic effects
SPECIAL CONSIDERATIONS
MONITORING PARAMETERS
• *Myasthenia gravis*
• Therapeutic response: Increased muscle strength, improved gait, absence of labored breathing
• Toxicity: Narrow margin between first appearance of side effects and serious toxicity

N

---

nesiritide

(neh-sir'i-tide)

Rx: Natrecor

Chemical Class: Recombinant human peptide, cardiac hormone

Therapeutic Class: Natriuretic peptide

CLINICAL PHARMACOLOGY

Mechanism of Action: Increases intracellular concentrations of guanosine 3´5´-cyclic monophosphate (cGMP) resulting in smooth muscle relaxation; clinically, produces dose-dependent reductions in pulmonary capillary wedge pressure (PCWP) and systemic arterial pressure in patients with heart failure

Pharmacokinetics

IV: Plasma brain natiuretic peptide levels increase from baseline end ogenous levels by approx 3-6 fold post infusion doses of 0.01-0.13 µg/kg/min; 60% of effect on PCWP achieved within 15 minutes; hemodynamic effects may last up to 2-3 hr Volume of distribution (steady state) 0.19 L/kg, mean clearance 9.2 ml/min/kg, elimination via cellular internalization and lysosomal proteolysis, endopeptidases on vascular lumenal surface, and renal filtration; $t_{1/2}$ 18 min

INDICATIONS AND USES: Acutely decompensated congestive heart failure

DOSAGE

Adult

• IV 2 µg/kg bolus; follow with 0.01 µg/kg/min infusion

• *Renal insufficiency:* Dosage adjustment not required

💲 AVAILABLE FORMS/COST OF THERAPY

• Inj, Lyoph-powder—IV: 1.5 mg, single use vials: **$456.00**

CONTRAINDICATIONS: Hypersensitivity, cardiogenic shock, SBP <90 mm Hg

PRECAUTIONS: Low cardiac filling pressures, valvular stenosis, restrictive or obstructive cardiomyopathy, constrictive pericarditis, pericardial tamponade (i.e., conditions dependent on venous return), renal insufficiency

PREGNANCY AND LACTATION: Pregnancy category C (neither animal or human studies have been done); breast milk data unavailable

SIDE EFFECTS/ADVERSE REACTIONS

CNS: Anxiety, dizziness, headache (23%), insomnia

CV: Bradycardia, hypotension (25-50%), ventricular tachycardia, ventricular extrasystoles, angina pectoris

GI: Abdominal pain, nausea (24%), vomiting

GU: Renal insufficiency

MS: Back pain

INTERACTIONS

Drugs

❸ *Angiotensin-converting enzyme inhibitors:* Added hypotensive effects

❷ *Bumetanide:* Physically and/or chemically incompatible; should not be coadministered as infusions

❷ *Enalaprilat:* Physically and/or chemically incompatible; should not be coadministered as infusions

❷ *Ethacrynic acid:* Physically and/or chemically incompatible; should not be coadministered as infusions

❷ *Furosemide:* Physically and/or chemically incompatible; should not be coadministered as infusions

❷ *Heparin:* Physically and/or chemically incompatible; should not be coadministered as infusions

❷ *Hydralazine:* Physically and/or chemically incompatible; should not be coadministered as infusions

❷ *Insulin:* Physically and/or chemically incompatible; should not be coadministered as infusions

❷ *Sodium Metabisulfite (preservative):* Incompatible; flush line between administration

SPECIAL CONSIDERATIONS

• Limited experience in administration for longer than 48 hr

• If hypotension occurs, discontinue and subsequently restart at dose reduced dose by 30% (no bolus) once patient has stabilized

MONITORING PARAMETERS

• Plasma brain natriuretic peptide concentrations, plasma aldosterone, heart failure hemodynamic measurements, clinical symptoms of heart failure, routine blood chemistries, blood pressure

---

netilmicin

(ne-til-mye´sin)

Rx: Netromycin

Chemical Class: Aminoglycoside

Therapeutic Class: Antibiotic

CLINICAL PHARMACOLOGY

Mechanism of Action: Interferes with protein synthesis in bacterial cell by binding to 30S ribosomal subunit, which causes misreading of genetic code; inaccurate peptide sequence forms in protein chain, causing bacterial death

Pharmacokinetics

IM: Onset rapid, peak 30-60 min

IV: Onset immediate, peak 30 min after a 30 min inf

<30% bound to plasma proteins; duration 6-8 hr; not metabolized, eliminated unchanged in urine via glomerular filtration; plasma $t_{1/2}$ 2-3 hr; (antibacterial effect may persist after drug levels decline)

INDICATIONS AND USES: Serious or life-threatening bacterial infections of the urinary tract, skin and skin structures, lower respiratory tract, septicemia, intraabdominal infections

Antibacterial spectrum usually includes:

• Gram-positive organisms: *Staphylococcus* spp. (including penicillinase and non-penicillinase-producing strains), *Streptococcus faecalis* (in combination with cell wall synthesis inhibitor)

• Gram-negative organisms: *Acinetobacter* spp., *Escherichia coli, Proteus* spp. (indole-positive and indole-negative), *Pseudomonas aeruginosa, Klebsiella* spp., *Enterobacter* spp., *Serratia* spp., *Citrobacter* spp., *Providencia* spp., *Salmonella* spp., *Shigella* spp., *Yersinia pestis*

DOSAGE

Use ideal body weight for dosage calculations

Adult

• *Serious systemic infections:* IM/IV 1.3-2.2 mg/kg diluted in 50-100 ml NS or D_5W and infused over 30-60 min q8h or 2-3.25 mg/kg q12h; adjust dosage based on results of netilmicin serum peak and trough levels

• *Complicated UTI:* IM/IV 1.5-2 mg/kg q12h

Child 6 wk-12 yr

• IM/IV 1.8-2.7 mg/kg q8h or 2.7-4 mg/kg q12h

S AVAILABLE FORMS/COST OF THERAPY

• Inj, Sol—IM, IV: 100 mg/ml, 1.5 ml: **$15.70**

PRECAUTIONS: Neonates, renal disease, myasthenia gravis, hearing deficits, Parkinson's disease, elderly, dehydration, hypokalemia

---

italic = common side effects   **bold italic** = life-threatening reactions

PREGNANCY AND LACTATION: Pregnancy category D; ototoxicity has not been reported as an effect of *in utero* exposure; 8th cranial nerve toxicity in the fetus is well known following exposure to other aminoglycosides and could potentially occur with netilmicin; potentiation of magnesium sulfate-induced neuromuscular weakness in neonates has been reported, use caution during the last 32 hr of pregnancy; excreted in breast milk in small amounts

SIDE EFFECTS/ADVERSE REACTIONS

CNS: Confusion, depression, dizziness, muscle twitching, myasthenia gravis-like syndrome, neurotoxicity, numbness, *seizures,* tremors, vertigo

CV: Hypertension, palpitations

EENT: Deafness, ototoxicity, tinnitus, visual disturbances

GI: Anorexia, hepatomegaly, increased ALT, AST, bilirubin; *nausea,* splenomegaly, *vomiting*

GU: Azotemia, hematuria, *nephrotoxicity, oliguria, renal damage, renal failure*

HEME: Agranulocytosis, anemia, eosinophilia, *leukopenia, thrombocytopenia*

METAB: Decreased serum calcium, sodium, potassium, magnesium

RESP: Respiratory depression

SKIN: Alopecia, burning, dermatitis, *rash,* urticaria

INTERACTIONS

Drugs

3 *Amphotericin B:* Synergistic nephrotoxicity

2 *Atracurium:* Netilmicin potentiates respiratory depression by atracurium

3 *Carbenicillin:* Potential for inactivation of netilmicin in patients with renal failure

3 *Carboplatin:* Additive nephrotoxicity or ototoxicity

3 *Cephalosporins:* Increased potential for nephrotoxicity in patients with preexisting renal disease

3 *Cisplatin:* Additive nephrotoxicity or ototoxicity

3 *Cyclosporine:* Additive nephrotoxicity

2 *Ethacrynic acid:* Additive ototoxicity

3 *Indomethacin:* Reduced renal clearance of netilmicin in premature infants

3 *Methoxyflurane:* Additive nephrotoxicity

2 *Neuromuscular blocking agents:* Netilmicin potentiates respiratory depression by neuromuscular blocking agents

3 *NSAIDs:* May reduce renal clearance of netilmicin

3 *Penicillins (extended spectrum):* Potential for inactivation of netilmicin in patients with renal failure

3 *Piperacillin:* Potential for inactivation of netilmicin in patients with renal failure

2 *Succinylcholine:* Netilmicin potentiates respiratory depression by succinylcholine

3 *Ticarcillin:* Potential for inactivation of netilmicin in patients with renal failure

3 *Vancomycin:* Additive nephrotoxicity or ototoxicity

2 *Vecuronium:* Netilmicin potentiates respiratory depression by vecuronium

SPECIAL CONSIDERATIONS
PATIENT/FAMILY EDUCATION
• Inform patient and family about possible toxic effects on the 8th cranial nerve; monitor for dizziness, loss of hearing, ringing or roaring in ears, or feeling of fullness in head

MONITORING PARAMETERS
• Urinalysis for proteinuria, cells, casts; urine output

* = non-FDA-approved use

• Serum peak drawn at 30-60 min after IV inf or 60 min after IM inj, trough level drawn just before next dose; adjust dosage per levels usual therapeutic plasma levels; peak 4-12 µg/ml, trough ≤2 µg/ml

• Serum creatinine for CrCl calculation

• Serum calcium, magnesium, sodium

• Audiometric testing; assess hearing before, during, after treatment

---

nevirapine

(neh-veer´a-peen)
Rx: Viramune
Chemical Class: Dipyridodiazepinone derivative
Therapeutic Class: Antiviral

CLINICAL PHARMACOLOGY
Mechanism of Action: Directly reactive non-competitive inhibitor of HIV-1 reverse transcriptase; does not require intracellular phosphorylation; not active against HIV-2 reverse transcriptase
Pharmacokinetics
PO: Onset 15 min, peak 2 hr with 2nd peak at 3-14 hr due to enterohepatic circulation; elimination $t_{1/2}$ 20-40 hr; protein binding 50%-60%; distributed into CNS; metabolized in liver primarily by hydroxylation with enterohepatic recycling; self-induces cytochrome P450 isoenzymes over period of 2 wk; minimal excretion in urine

INDICATIONS AND USES: HIV-1 infection as part of a multidrug treatment regimen

DOSAGE
Adult
• PO 200 mg qd for 14 days, then 200 mg bid in combination with nucleoside analogue antiretroviral agents

• For latest treatment guidelines, see www.hivatis.org

§ AVAILABLE FORMS/COST OF THERAPY
• Cap—Oral: 200 mg, 100's: **$472.59**
• Susp—Oral: 50 mg/ml, 240 ml: **$69.05**

PRECAUTIONS: Stevens-Johnson syndrome, liver disease, CNS disorders

PREGNANCY AND LACTATION: Pregnancy category C; excreted in breast milk, breast feeding not recommended

SIDE EFFECTS/ADVERSE REACTIONS
CNS: Fatigue (63%), headache (33%), sedation
GI: Diarrhea (37%), increased GGTP levels (10%), nausea (20%)
*SKIN: Rash (17%), **Stevens-Johnson syndrome***
MISC: Fever (40%)

INTERACTIONS
Drugs
3 *Clarithromycin:* 26% increase in plasma nevirapine level by clarithromycin; 30% decrease in plasma clarithromycin level by nevirapine; dose adjustment not recommended
3 *Erythromycin:* Mild increase in plasma nevirapine level by erythromycin; dose adjustment not recommended
3 *Indinavir:* 28% decrease in indinavir AUC by nevirapine; dose adjustment not recommended
2 *Ketoconazole:* 63% reduction in plasma ketoconazole level by nevirapine; 15%-30% increase in plasma nevirapine level by ketoconazole; coadministration not recommended
3 *Methadone:* Marked decrease in methadone level by nevirapine; dose adjustment recommended

N

---

italic = common side effects   **bold italic** = life-threatening reactions

3 *Nelfinavir:* 10% increase in nelfinavir AUC by nevirapine; dose adjustment not recommended

3 *Rifabutin:* 16% reduction in plasma nevirapine level by rifabutin

2 *Rifampin:* 37% reduction in plasma nevirapine level by rifampin; coadministration not recommended

3 *Ritonavir:* 11% decrease in ritonavir AUC by nevirapine; dose adjustment not recommended

3 *Saquinavir:* 25% decrease in saquinavir AUC by nevirapine; dose adjustment not recommended

3 *Troleandomycin:* Mild increase in plasma nevirapine level by troleandomycin; dose adjustment not recommended

SPECIAL CONSIDERATIONS
• 2-week lead in period with qd dosing decreases the potential for development of rash; stop therapy in any patient developing a severe rash or rash with constitutional symptoms

MONITORING PARAMETERS
• CBC, ALT, AST, renal function

---

niacin (vitamin B₃; nicotinic acid)

(nye′a-sin)

Rx: Niacor, Niaspan, Nicolor; Combinations

  Rx: with lovastatin (Advicor)

OTC: Nia-Bid, Nia-C, Niacels, Nico-400, Nicotinex, Slo-Niacin

Chemical Class: B complex vitamin

Therapeutic Class: Vitamin; antilipemic

CLINICAL PHARMACOLOGY

Mechanism of Action: Necessary for lipid metabolism, tissue respiration, and glycogenolysis; lowers total serum cholesterol, low-density lipoprotein (LDL) cholesterol and triglyceride concentrations by inhibiting the synthesis of very-low-density lipoproteins (VLDL), which are precursors to the formation of cholesterol; raises high-density lipoprotein (HDL) cholesterol

Pharmacokinetics

PO: Readily absorbed from GI tract; peak 45 min; metabolized in liver, eliminated in urine (almost entirely as metabolites); $t_{1/2}$ 45 min

INDICATIONS AND USES: Vitamin deficiency (pellagra); types IIa, IIb, IV and V, hyperlipidemia as an adjunct to a low-cholesterol diet; to reduce risk of recurrent MI in patients with history of MI and hypercholesterolemia; reduction of atherosclerotic disease in patients with a history of CAD

DOSAGE

Adult

• *Recommended daily allowance PO:* Males 19-50 yr 19 mg/day; males >51 yr 15 mg/day; females 11-50 yr 15 mg/day; females >51 yr 13 mg/day

• *Pellagra:* PO 50-100 mg tid-qid; max 500 mg/day

• *Niacin deficiency:* PO 10-20 mg/day; max 100 mg/day

• *Hyperlipidemia:* PO 1.5-6 g/day divided bid-tid with or after meals (start at 100-250 mg/day and titrate gradually)

Child

• *Recommended daily allowance PO:* 0-0.5 yr 5 mg/day; 0.5-1 yr 6 mg/day; 1-3 yr 9 mg/day; 4-6 yr 12 mg/day; 7-10 yr 13 mg/day; males 11-14 yr 17 mg/day; males 15-18 yr 20 mg/day

• *Pellagra:* PO 50-100 mg tid

🆂 AVAILABLE FORMS/COST OF THERAPY

• Cap, Gel, Sus Action—Oral: 125 mg, 100's: **$4.05-$6.15**; 250 mg, 100's: **$2.90-$8.42**; 400 mg, 100's: **$4.31-$8.75**; 500 mg, 100's: **$3.99-$98.79**

• Elixir—Oral: 50 mg/5 ml, 480 ml: **$8.25**

• Tab, Uncoated—Oral: 50 mg, 100's: **$0.64-$4.02**; 100 mg, 100's: **$0.74-$4.21**; 250 mg, 100's: **$3.24-$3.39**; 500 mg, 100's: **$1.99-$70.66**

• Tab, Sus Action—Oral: 500 mg, 100's: **$3.45-$79.20**; 750 mg, 100's: **$7.42-$112.96**; 1000 mg, 100's: **$8.25-$141.48**

CONTRAINDICATIONS: Hepatic dysfunction, active peptic ulcer, severe hypotension, hemorrhage

PRECAUTIONS: Unstable CAD, gallbladder disease, history of jaundice or liver disease, history of peptic ulcer, history of arterial bleeding, gout, diabetes mellitus, tartrazine sensitivity

PREGNANCY AND LACTATION: Pregnancy category A (category C if used in doses greater than recommended daily allowance); actively excreted in human breast milk; recommended daily allowance during lactation is 18-20 mg

SIDE EFFECTS/ADVERSE REACTIONS

CNS: Transient headache

CV: Atrial fibrillation, hypotension, orthostasis

EENT: Cystoidmacular edema, toxic amblyopia

GI: Abdominal pain, activation of peptic ulcer, diarrhea, *GI distress,* **hepatotoxicity** (more common with sustained-release formulations), *nausea,* vomiting

METAB: Decreased glucose tolerance, hyperuricemia

MS: Myopathy, myositis, ***rhabdomyolysis***

SKIN: Dry skin, keratosis nigricans, *pruritus, sensation of warmth, severe generalized flushing,* skin rash, tingling

INTERACTIONS

Drugs

🅱 *Lovastatin:* Isolated cases of myopathy and rhabdomyolysis have occurred, causality not established

Labs

• *Interference:* Plasma and urine catecholamines, urine glucose with Benedict's reagent

SPECIAL CONSIDERATIONS

• In 1 g doses: 10%-20% reduction of total plus LDL-cholesterol, 30%-70% reduction in triglycerides, and a 20%-35% increase in HDL-cholesterol

• Increased risk of hepatotoxicity with sustained release products

PATIENT/FAMILY EDUCATION

• Gradual dosage titration lessens flushing, adverse effects

• Avoid alcohol and hot beverages (increases flushing)

• Administer with meals and 2 glasses of water

• 125-350 mg of aspirin 20-30 min prior to dose may lessen flushing

• Do not miss any doses (flushing may return)

MONITORING PARAMETERS

• Liver function tests, blood glucose, uric acid regularly

• Fasting lipid profile q3-6 mo

N

---

nicardipine
(nye-card´i-peen)
Rx: Cardene, Cardene SR
Chemical Class: Dihydropyridine
Therapeutic Class: Calcium channel blocker: antihypertensive; antianginal

CLINICAL PHARMACOLOGY
Mechanism of Action: Inhibits calcium ion influx across cell membrane in vascular smooth muscle and cardiac muscle; produces relaxation of coronary and peripheral vascular smooth muscle; slight increase in AV conduction; hemodynamics: no effect on myocardial contractility; increases cardiac output; significantly decreases peripheral vascular resistance

Pharmacokinetics
PO: Onset 20 min, peak serum concentration 0.5-2 hr; >95% bound to plasma proteins, significant 1st-pass effect (35% systemic bioavailability); kinetics nonlinear; excreted in urine (60%) and feces (35%); $t_{1/2}$ 8.6 hr (steady state)

INDICATIONS AND USES: Chronic stable angina,* hypertension, Raynaud's disease*

DOSAGE
Adult
• *Angina:* PO 20 mg tid, may increase after 3 days to 40 mg tid
• *Hypertension:* PO 20 mg tid, may increase to 40 mg tid; SR 30 mg bid, may increase to 60 mg bid; IV INF 5 mg/hr initially, may be increased by 2.5 mg/hr q5-15 min up to maximum of 15 mg/hr; following achievement of goal blood pressure, decrease inf rate to 3 mg/hr, then adjust rate as needed to maintain desired response

* = non-FDA-approved use

💲 **AVAILABLE FORMS/COST OF THERAPY**
• Cap—Oral: 20 mg, 100's: **$39.25-$58.11**; 30 mg, 100's: **$62.42-$69.35**
• Cap, Gel, Sus Action—Oral: 30 mg, 60's: **$54.49**; 45 mg, 60's: **$86.51**; 60 mg, 60's: **$103.55**
• Inj, Sol—IV: 25 mg/10 ml ampul: **$26.84**

CONTRAINDICATIONS: Advanced aortic stenosis
PRECAUTIONS: CHF, hypotension, hepatic insufficiency, renal function impairment, aortic stenosis, elderly, children
PREGNANCY AND LACTATION: Pregnancy category C; significant excretion into rat maternal milk

SIDE EFFECTS/ADVERSE REACTIONS
CNS: Anxiety, *asthenia,* depression, *dizziness,* fatigue, *headache,* insomnia, malaise, nervousness, paresthesia, somnolence, tremor
CV: Angina, bradycardia, **dysrhythmia,** hypotension, palpitations, *peripheral edema,* syncope, tachycardia
GI: Abdominal cramps, constipation, diarrhea, dry mouth, flatulence, gastric upset, nausea, vomiting
GU: Nocturia, polyuria
SKIN: Hair loss, pruritus, rash, urticaria
MISC: Cough, epistaxis, flushing, muscle cramps, nasal congestion, sexual dysfunction, shortness of breath, sweating, tinnitus, weight gain

INTERACTIONS
Drugs
3 *Cyclosporine, tacrolimus:* Increased blood concentrations of these drugs, increased risk of toxicity
3 *Histamine H_2-antagonists:* Increased blood levels of nicardipine with cimetidine and ranitidine

3 *Fentanyl:* Severe hypotension or increased fluid volume requirements

3 *Neuromuscular blocking agents:* Prolongation of neuromuscular blockade

---

nicotine

(nik´o-teen)

Rx: *Nasal Spray:* Nicotrol NS; Inhaler: Nicotrol Inhaler
OTC: *Chewing Gum:* Nicorette; *Transdermal:* Nicoderm CQ, Nicotrol, Habitrol
Chemical Class: Pyridine alkaloid
Therapeutic Class: Smoking deterrent

CLINICAL PHARMACOLOGY
Mechanism of Action: Agonist at the nicotinic receptors at the autonomic ganglia in the adrenal medulla, at neuromuscular junctions, and in the brain, producing reinforcing properties: stimulating effect (locus ceruleus)—increased alertness and cognitive performance; reward effect (limbic system); stimulant effects predominate at low doses; at high doses, reward effects predominate
Pharmacokinetics
BUCCAL: Peak 15-30 min, $t_{1/2}$ 30-60 min
TOP: Peak 4-9 hr, $t_{1/2}$ 3-4 hr
NASAL SPRAY: Peak 4-15 min, $t_{1/2}$ 2 hr
INH: 50% bioavailable (absorbed activity); peak 15 min, $t_{1/2}$ 2 hr
<5% bound to plasma proteins, metabolized by liver to cotinine and nicotine-*N*-oxide, eliminated in urine (10%-30% as unchanged drug)

INDICATIONS AND USES: Smoking cessation (temporary adjunct in conjunction with behavior modification), hemidystonia,* ulcerative colitis*

DOSAGE
Adult
• *Gum:* Chew 9-12 pieces of gum (2 mg for regular smokers, 4 mg for heavy smokers) at 1-2 hr intervals daily; do not exceed 80 mg/day; gradually reduce number of pieces/day; use longer than 3 mo is discouraged
• *Transdermal systems:* Apply qd, discard system in use and apply new system at different site; wear for 16 hr (Nicotrol) or 24 hr (Habitrol, Nicoderm CQ); initiate therapy at highest available dosage of nicotine for all patients except those weighing <45 kg, those who smoke <10 cigarettes/day, and/or those who have cardiovascular disease (should receive lower initial doses); maintain initial dose for 4-12 wk; reduce doses for 1 or more periods of therapy in patients who have abstained from smoking over next 2-8 wk
• *Nasal spray:* One dose = 1 mg (1 spray in each nostril); individualize dose; 1-2 doses/hr to a max of 5 doses/hr or 40 doses/day; duration of treatment should not exceed 3 months
• *Inhaler:* 10 inhalations provide approx the same amount of nicotine as one puff on average cigarette; continuous puffing × 20 min—6-16 cartridges/day × 12 wk; then gradual tapering over 12 wk; individualize dose to control "urge to smoke"; recommended max cartridges/day:16

N

$ AVAILABLE FORMS/COST OF THERAPY

• Aerosol—INH: 4 mg delivered (10 mg/cartridge), 42's: **$40.80** (Nicotrol Inhaler)
• Film, Cont Rel—Percutaneous: 7, 14, 21 mg/24 hr, 7's, all: **$24.21** (Nicoderm CQ-OTC); 7 mg/24 hr, 30's: **$109.61** (Habitrol); 14 mg/24 hr, 30's: **$115.70** (Habitrol); 15 mg/16 hr, 7's: **$24.71-$25.76** (Nicotrol-OTC); 21 mg/24 hr, 30's: **$121.75** (Habitrol)
• Sol—Nasal Spray: 0.5 mg/Inh, 10 mg/ml, 10 ml: **$40.80** (Nicotrol NS)
• Tab, Chewing Gum—Buccal: 2 mg, 48's: **$23.36-$27.36** (Nicorette-OTC); 4 mg, 48's: **$26.17-$74.59** (Nicorette-OTC)

CONTRAINDICATIONS: Temporomandibular joint disease (chewing gum)

PRECAUTIONS: Cardiovascular disease (history of MI, angina pectoris), serious cardiac dysrhythmias or vasospastic diseases, hypertension, hyperthyroidism, pheochromocytoma, insulin-dependent diabetes; hepatic, renal function impairment; elderly, children, oral or pharyngeal elimination (chewing gum), esophagitis, peptic ulcer disease, skin disease (transdermal), dental problems (chewing gum)

PREGNANCY AND LACTATION: Pregnancy category D; use of nicotine gum during last trimester has been associated with decreased fetal breathing movements; passes freely into breast milk; however, lower concentrations in milk can be expected with transdermal systems than cigarette smoking when used as directed

SIDE EFFECTS/ADVERSE REACTIONS

CNS: Abnormal dreams, confusion, depression, *dizziness,* euphoria, *headache,* impaired concentration, insomnia, lightheadedness, *nervousness,* numbness, paresthesia, *seizures,* syncope, weakness

CV: Edema, flushing, hypertension, palpitations, tachycardia, *tachydysrhythmias*

EENT: Pharyngitis, *sinusitis,* tinnitus

GI: Abdominal pain, altered liver function tests, anorexia, aphthous ulcers (chewing gum); *constipation, diarrhea,* dry mouth, *dyspepsia,* eructation secondary to air swallowing, gingivitis, glossitis, jaw ache, *nausea,* stomatitis, *taste perversion,* traumatic injury to oral mucosa or teeth, vomiting

GU: Dysmenorrhea

MS: Arthralgia, *asthenia, back pain, myalgia*

RESP: Breathing difficulty, *cough, hiccups,* hoarseness, sneezing, wheezing

SKIN: Burning at application site, erythema, itching, *pruritus,* rash, sweating, urticaria

INTERACTIONS

Drogs

3 *Adenosine:* Increased hemodynamic and AV blocking effects of adenosine

3 *Cimetidine:* Increased blood nicotine concentration, may reduce the amount of gum or patches needed

3 *Coffee, cola:* Reduced absorption of nicotine from chewing gum

SPECIAL CONSIDERATIONS

• Drugs that may require dosage reduction with smoking cessation: acetaminophen, caffeine, imipramine, oxazepam, pentazocine, propranolol, theophylline, insulin, prazocin, labetalol

• Drugs that may require an increase in dose with smoking cessation: isoproterenol, phenylephrine

PATIENT/FAMILY EDUCATION

• Chew gum slowly until burning or tingling sensation is felt, then park gum between cheek and gum until tingling sensation goes away

• Chew <30 min/piece

• Avoid coffee and cola drinks while chewing gum or using inhaler

• **Do not smoke while utilizing nicotine replacement therapy**

• Apply new transdermal system daily

• Rotate sites; apply to non-hairy area on upper torso

---

nifedipine

(nye-fed'i-peen)

Rx: Adalat, Adalat CC, Procardia; Procardia XL

Chemical Class: Dihydropyridine

Therapeutic Class: Calcium channel blocker: antihypertensive; antianginal

CLINICAL PHARMACOLOGY

Mechanism of Action: Inhibits calcium ion influx across cell membrane in vascular smooth muscle and cardiac muscle; produces relaxation of coronary and peripheral vascular smooth muscle; hemodynamics: decreases myocardial contractility; increases cardiac output; significantly decreases peripheral vascular resistance

Pharmacokinetics

PO: Peak serum concentration 30 min, onset within 20 min (1-5 min if capsule bitten and swallowed)

SUS ACTION: Peak 6 hr

50%-60% bioavailable, 92%-98% bound to plasma proteins; metabolized by liver to inactive V_d 14-2.2 L/kg metabolites, excreted by kidneys; $t_{1/2}$ 2-5 hr

INDICATIONS AND USES: Vasospastic (Prinzmetal's or variant) angina, chronic stable angina, hypertension, prevention of migraine headache,* preterm labor,* primary pulmonary hypertension,* esophageal disorders,* high altitude pulmonary edema*; Raynaud's disease,* CHF,* cardiomyopathy (diastolic dysfunction)

DOSAGE

Adult

• PO 10 mg tid initially, usual range 10-20 mg tid; doses >120 mg/day are rarely necessary; PO XL 30-60 mg qd, titration to doses >120 mg/day is not recommended; PO CC 30 mg qd, titration to doses >90 mg/day not recommended

Child

• *Hypertensive urgencies:* PO 0.25-0.5 mg/kg/dose

⑤ AVAILABLE FORMS/COST OF THERAPY

• Cap, Gel—Oral: 10 mg, 100's: **$7.88-$74.59**; 20 mg, 100's: **$69.00-$134.20**

• Tab, Coated, Sus Action—Oral: 30 mg, 100's: **$93.95-$182.54**; 60 mg, 100's: **$152.81-$321.57**; 90 mg, 100's: **$254.54-$302.75**

CONTRAINDICATIONS: Use of immediate-release preparations in patients with severe obstructive CAD or recent MI, hypertensive emergencies

PRECAUTIONS: CHF, hypotension, hepatic insufficiency, renal function impairment, aortic stenosis, elderly, children, recent β-blocker withdrawal

PREGNANCY AND LACTATION: Pregnancy category C; has been used for tocolysis and as an antihypertensive agent in pregnant women; compatible with breast feeding

---

italic = common side effects   **bold italic** = life-threatening reactions

SIDE EFFECTS/ADVERSE REACTIONS

(NOTE: Usually less frequent with extended-release preparations)

CNS: Anxiety, asthenia, depression, *dizziness,* fatigue, *headache,* insomnia, malaise, nervousness, paresthesia, somnolence, tremor

CV: Bradycardia, **dysrhythmia,** *hypotension,* palpitations, *peripheral edema,* syncope, tachycardia

GI: Abdominal cramps, constipation, diarrhea, dry mouth, flatulence, gastric upset, *nausea,* vomiting

GU: Nocturia, polyuria

SKIN: Hair loss, pruritus, rash, urticaria

MISC: Cough, epistaxis, *flushing,* muscle cramps, nasal congestion, sexual dysfunction, shortness of breath, sweating, tinnitus, weight gain

INTERACTIONS

Drugs

3 *Barbiturates, rifampin, rifabutin:* Reduced plasma concentrations of nifedipine

3 *Beta-blockers:* Enhanced effects of β-blockers, hypotension; increased metoprolol and propanolol concentrations; additive negative effects on myocardial contractility

3 *Cimetidine, ranitidine, famotidine:* Increased nifedipine concentrations possible

3 *Digitalis glycosides:* Increased digitalis levels; increased risk of toxicity

3 *Diltiazem:* Increased serum concentrations of nifedipine

3 *Doxazosin:* Enhanced hypotensive effects

3 *Fentanyl:* Severe hypotension or increased fluid volume requirements

3 *Food:* Increased absorption of Adalat CC

3 *Grapefruit juice:* Increased serum nifedipine concentrations

3 *Histamine H₂-antagonists:* Increased blood levels of nifedipine with cimetidine

3 *Lansoprazole:* Increased nifedipine absorption

3 *Magnesium:* Potential for transient hypotensive effect

3 *Phenytoin:* Increased phenytoin concentration

3 *Quinidine:* Reduced blood concentrations of quinidine

3 *Vincristine:* Marked increase in vincristine half-life, clinical significance unknown

SPECIAL CONSIDERATIONS

• Given the seriousness of the reported adverse events and the lack of any clinical documentation attesting to a benefit, the use of nifedipine capsules for hypertensive urgencies or emergencies should be abandoned (*JAMA* 1996; 276:1328-1331)

PATIENT/FAMILY EDUCATION

• Administer Adalat CC on an empty stomach

• Do not crush or chew sustained release dosage forms

• Empty Procardia XL tablets may appear in stool, this is no cause for concern

---

nimodipine

(nye-mode´i-peen)
Rx: Nimotop
Chemical Class: Dihydropyridine
Therapeutic Class: Calcium channel blocker: cerebral vasodilator

---

CLINICAL PHARMACOLOGY

Mechanism of Action: Inhibits calcium ion influx across membranes of vascular smooth muscle; greater effect on cerebral arteries

Pharmacokinetics

PO: Peak 1 hr; >95% bound to plasma proteins; extensively metabolized in liver to inactive metabolites, excreted in urine (50%) and feces (32%); t½ 1.7-9 hr

INDICATIONS AND USES: Subarachnoid hemorrhage, acute ischemic stroke,* prevention of migraine headache*

DOSAGE

Adult

• *Subarachnoid hemorrhage:* PO 60 mg q4h for 21 consecutive days beginning within 96 hr of occurrence of hemorrhage, reduce to 30 mg q4h in patients with hepatic failure; for patients unable to swallow oral capsules, the capsule may be punctured at both ends with an 18-gauge needle and the contents emptied directly into nasogastric tube, which is then flushed with 30 ml of normal saline

• *Prevention of migraine headache*
PO 120 mg/day in divided doses; response may not be apparent for 1-2 mo

$ **AVAILABLE FORMS/COST OF THERAPY**

• Cap, Elastic—Oral: 30 mg, 100's: **$729.14**

PRECAUTIONS: Impaired hepatic, renal function; children <18 yr

PREGNANCY AND LACTATION: Pregnancy category C

SIDE EFFECTS/ADVERSE REACTIONS

CNS: Dizziness, headache, lightheadedness, mental depression
CV: ECG abnormalities, edema, flushing, hypotension, palpitations
GI: Constipation, hepatitis, jaundice, lower abdominal discomfort
HEME: Anemia, ***thrombocytopenia***
MS: Muscle pain
RESP: Dyspnea
SKIN: Rash

INTERACTIONS

Drugs

3 *Cimetidine:* Increased serum nimodipine concentrations
3 *Omeprazole:* Increased serum nimodipine concentrations
3 *Valproic acid:* Increased oral bioavailability of nimodipine

SPECIAL CONSIDERATIONS

MONITORING PARAMETERS

• Blood pressure

---

nisoldipine

(nye-sold'i-peen)
Rx: Sular
Chemical Class: Dihydropyridine
Therapeutic Class: Calcium channel blocker: antihypertensive

CLINICAL PHARMACOLOGY

Mechanism of Action: Inhibits calcium ion influx across cell membrane in vascular smooth muscle and cardiac muscle; produces relaxation of coronary and peripheral vascular smooth muscle; hemodynamics: no effect on myocardial contractility and cardiac output; significantly decreases peripheral vascular resistance

Pharmacokinetics

PO: Systemic bioavailability 5% significant 1st pass metabolism; peak serum concentration, 1.5 hr; high-fat meal increases peak concentration by ~300%; highly metabolized in liver, excreted in urine; t½ 2-14 hr

INDICATIONS AND USES: Hypertension

DOSAGE

Adult

• PO 20 mg qd; may increase by 10 mg/wk or longer intervals to maximum of 60 mg/day

---

italic = common side effects   ***bold italic*** = life-threatening reactions

$ AVAILABLE FORMS/COST OF THERAPY
• Tab, Coated—Oral: 10, 20, 30, 40 mg, 100's: **$109.53**

PRECAUTIONS: CHF, hypotension, following myocardial infarction, hepatic insufficiency, aortic stenosis, elderly, children

PREGNANCY AND LACTATION: Pregnancy category C

SIDE EFFECTS/ADVERSE REACTIONS

CNS: Anxiety, asthenia, depression, dizziness, fatigue, *headache,* insomnia, malaise, nervousness, paresthesia, somnolence, tremor

CV: Bradycardia, **dysrhythmia,** flushing, hypotension, palpitations, *peripheral edema,* syncope, tachycardia

EENT: Epistaxis, nasal congestion, sore throat, tinnitus

GI: Abdominal cramps, constipation, diarrhea, dry mouth, flatulence, gastric upset, nausea, vomiting

GU: Nocturia, polyuria, sexual dysfunction

MS: Muscle cramps

RESP: Cough, shortness of breath

SKIN: Hair loss, pruritus, sweating, urticaria

MISC: Weight gain

INTERACTIONS

Drugs

🔳 *Beta-adrenergic blockers:* Increased propranolol concentration

🔳 *Cimetidine, famotidine, nizatidine, omeprazole, ranitidine:* Increased nisoldipine concentrations possible

🔳 *Fentanyl:* Severe hypotension or increased fluid volume requirements

🔳 *Food:* Increased absorption with high-fat meal or grapefruit juice

SPECIAL CONSIDERATIONS
• No significant advantages over other dihydropyridine calcium channel blockers

PATIENT/FAMILY EDUCATION
• Do not take with high-fat meal or grapefruit juice

---

nitrofurantoin
(nye-troe-fyoor´an-toyn)
Rx: Furadantin, Macrodantin
Combinations
  Rx: nitrofurantoin macrocrystals with nitrofurantoin monohydrate (Macrobid)
Chemical Class: Synthetic nitrofuran derivative
Therapeutic Class: Antibiotic

CLINICAL PHARMACOLOGY

Mechanism of Action: May inhibit acetylcoenzyme A, interfering with bacterial carbohydrate metabolism; may also disrupt bacterial cell wall formation; bactericidal in urine at therapeutic doses

Pharmacokinetics

PO: Therapeutic concentrations achieved only in urine, macrocrystalline formulation slows absorption causing less GI irritation, food increases absorption, 60% bound to plasma proteins, partially inactivated in most body tissues, eliminated in urine (30%-50% unchanged), $t_{1/2}$ 20-60 min

INDICATIONS AND USES: UTIs

Antibacterial spectrum usually includes:

• Gram-positive organisms: *Staphylococcus aureus, S. saprophyticus, Enterococcus faecalis, Streptococcus agalactiae,* group D streptococci, viridans streptococci, *Corynebacterium*

• Gram-negative organisms: *Citrobacter amalonaticus, C. diversus, C. freundii, Klebsiella oxytoca, K. ozaenae, Enterobacter, Escherichia coli, Neisseria, Salmonella, Shigella*

---

* = non-FDA-approved use

• NOTE: Not active against *Proteus* spp., *Serratia* spp., or *Pseudomonas* spp.

DOSAGE

Adult

• PO 50-100 mg qid; (Macrobid) 100 mg bid with food; for long-term suppressive therapy, 50-100 mg qhs

Child >1 mo

• PO 5-7 mg/kg/day divided qid × 1 week; for long-term suppressive therapy 1 mg/kg/day divided qd-bid

$ AVAILABLE FORMS/COST OF THERAPY

• Cap, Gel—Oral: 25 mg, 100's: **$41.70-$83.18**; 50 mg, 100's: **$58.20-$109.53**; 100 mg, 100's: **$98.50-$186.01**

• Cap—Oral: 100 mg, 100's: **$188.39** (Macrobid)

CONTRAINDICATIONS: CrCl <60 ml/min (inadequate antibacterial concentrations achieved in urine), children <1 mo, during labor and delivery (glutathione instability)

PRECAUTIONS: G-6-PD deficiency, renal impairment, anemia, diabetes, electrolyte imbalance, vitamin B deficiency, debilitating disease

PREGNANCY AND LACTATION: Pregnancy category B; compatible with breast feeding in infants >1 mo

SIDE EFFECTS/ADVERSE REACTIONS

CNS: Asthenia, chills, confusion, depression, dizziness, drowsiness, euphoria, headache, nystagmus, peripheral neuropathy (including optic neuritis), psychotic reactions (rare), vertigo

CV: ECG changes

GI: Abdominal pain, anorexia, cholestatic jaundice, chronic active hepatitis, diarrhea, **hepatic necrosis,** hepatitis, *nausea,* **pancreatitis,** parotitis, *vomiting*

GU: Superinfection of GU tract

HEME: **Agranulocytosis, aplastic anemia,** eosinophilia, **granulocytopenia, hemolytic anemia, leukopenia, megaloblastic anemia, thrombocytopenia**

MS: Arthralgia, myalgia

RESP: **Acute and chronic pulmonary hypersensitivity reactions** (dyspnea, chest pain, cough, pulmonary infiltration)

SKIN: Angioedema, **erythema multiforme, exfoliative dermatitis,** pruritus, rash, transient alopecia, urticaria

INTERACTIONS

Labs

• *Interference:* Urine alkaline phosphatase, urine lactate dehydrogenase

• *False positive:* Urine glucose (not with glucose enzymatic tests)

• *False increase:* Serum bilirubin, serum creatinine

• *False decrease:* Serum unconjugated bilirubin

SPECIAL CONSIDERATIONS

PATIENT/FAMILY EDUCATION

• Food or milk may decrease GI upset

• May cause brown discoloration of urine

MONITORING PARAMETERS

• Periodic liver function tests during prolonged therapy

• CBC with differential and platelets during prolonged therapy

• Pulmonary review of systems

N

---

italic = common side effects   **bold italic** = life-threatening reactions

nitrofurazone

(nye-troe-fyoor'a-zone)

Rx: Furacin

Chemical Class: Synthetic nitrofuran derivative

Therapeutic Class: Topical antibiotic

CLINICAL PHARMACOLOGY

Mechanism of Action: Exact mechanism of action unknown; appears to inhibit bacterial enzymes involved in carbohydrate metabolism; antibacterial action inhibited by organic matter (e.g., blood, pus, serum) and *p*-aminobenzoic acid

INDICATIONS AND USES: Topical adjunct in 2nd and 3rd degree burns when bacterial resistance is a potential problem; prevention of infection of skin grafts and/or donor sites prior to or following surgery

Antibacterial spectrum usually includes:

• *S. aureus, Streptococcus, E. coli, Clostridium perfringens, Aerobacter aerogens, Proteus* spp.

DOSAGE

Adult and Child

• TOP apply to affected area qd or every few days, depending on dressing technique; apply directly or place on gauze; flushing with sterile saline facilitates removal

$ AVAILABLE FORMS/COST OF THERAPY

• Cre—Top: 0.2%, 28, 454 g: **$8.26**/454 g

• Oint—Top: 0.2%, 30, 454 g: **$6.38–$98.11**/454 g

• Sol—Top: 0.2%, 480 ml: **$6.48**

PRECAUTIONS: Renal function impairment (ointment contains polyethylene glycol); children; superinfection with non-susceptible organisms possible; no evidence of efficacy in minor burns, surface bacterial infection involving wounds, cutaneous ulcers, or the various pyodermas

PREGNANCY AND LACTATION: Pregnancy category C; excretion into breast milk unknown

SIDE EFFECTS/ADVERSE REACTIONS

SKIN: Contact dermatitis (rash, pruritus, local edema)

INTERACTIONS

Labs

• *False increase:* Urine creatinine, urine glucose via Benedict's reagent

nitroglycerin

(nye-troe-gli'ser-in)

Rx: (Translingual): *Buccal/ Sublingual/Translingual:* Nitrolingual, Nitroquick, Nitrostat

Oral: Nitro-Bid, Nitrocap TD, Nitrocine, Nitrogard, Nitroglyn, Nitrong, Nitro TD, Nitro-Time

Topical: Nitr-Bid, Nitrol

Transdermal: Deponit, Minitran, Nitrodisc, Nitro-Dur, Transderm-Nitro

IV: Nitro-Bid, Nitrostat IV, Tridil

Chemical Class: Organic nitrate

Therapeutic Class: Vasodilator: antianginal

CLINICAL PHARMACOLOGY

Mechanism of Action: Stimulation of c-GMP production yields vascular smooth muscle relaxation; venous dilation predominates but dose-dependent dilation of arterial beds occurs; dilation of postcapillary vessels promotes venous pooling, decreases venous return to the heart, reducing left ventricular end-diastolic pressure (preload); arteriolar relaxation reduces systemic vascular resistance and arterial pressure (afterload); myocardial oxygen consumption/demand is decreased; blood pressure decreases with reflex tachycardia; dilates coronary arteries and improves collateral flow to ischemic regions

Pharmacokinetics

SL: Onset 1-3 min, peak 4-8 min, duration 30-60 min

LINGUAL SPRAY: Onset 2 min, peak 4-10 min, duration 30-60 min

BUCCAL: Onset 2-5 min, peak 4-10 min, duration 2 hr

PO: Onset 20-45 min, peak 45-120 min, duration 4-8 hr

TOP: Onset 15-60 min, peak 30-120 min, duration 2-12 hr

TRANSDERMAL: Onset 40-60 min, peak 60-180 min, duration 8-24 hr

IV: Onset immediate, peak immediate, duration 3-5 min

60% bound to plasma proteins, metabolized by liver to inorganic nitrate (extensive 1st-pass effect), eliminated in urine; $t_{1/2}$ 1-4 min

INDICATIONS AND USES: Acute angina (SL, translingual spray, buccal), angina prophylaxis (top, transdermal, translingual spray, buccal, oral), perioperative hypertension (IV), congestive heart failure associated with MI (IV), unresponsive angina pectoris (IV), acute MI (SL, top),* Raynaud's disease (top),* hypertensive crisis (IV)*

DOSAGE

Adult

• BUCCAL 1 mg q3-5h while awake initially, titrate dosage upward if angina occurs with tab in place

• PO 2.5-9 mg bid-qid, up to 26 mg qid

• IV 5 µg/min via continuous inf, increase by 5 µg/min q3-5 min to 20 µg/min; if no response, increase by 10 µg/min q3-5 min up to 200 µg/min

• TOP 1-2 inches q8h, up to 4-5 inches q4h

• TRANSDERMAL 0.2-0.4 mg/hr initially, titrate to 0.4-0.8 mg/hr; apply new patch daily; tolerance is minimized by removing patch for 10-12 hr/day

• SL 0.2-0.6 mg q5 min for max of 3 doses in 15 min; may also use prophylactically 5-10 min prior to activities that provoke angina attack

• TRANSLINGUAL 1-2 sprays under tongue q3-5 min for max of 3 doses in 15 min; may also use prophylactically 5-10 min prior to activities that provoke angina attack

Child

• IV 0.25-0.5 µg/kg/min, titrate by 0.5-1 µg/kg/min q3-5 min prn; usual dose 1-3 µg/kg/min; max 20 µg/kg/min

💲 AVAILABLE FORMS/COST OF THERAPY

• Aer Spray—Oral: 0.4 mg/spray, 14.49 g: **$31.22**

• Cap, Gel, Sus Action—Oral: 2.5 mg, 100's: **$3.95-$14.20**; 6.5 mg, 100's: **$3.95-$18.25**; 9 mg, 100's: **$8.25-$24.90**

• Inj, Sol—IV: 5 mg/ml, 10 ml: **$1.13-$15.00**

• Oint—Percutaneous: 2%; 1, 3, 30, 60 g: **$6.48-$16.33/60 g**

• Tab, Uncoated, Sus Action—Buccal: 1 mg, 100's: **$37.87**; 2 mg, 100's: **$40.09**; 3 mg, 100's: **$43.33**

• Tab—SL: 0.3 mg, 100's: **$6.76-$10.78**; 0.4 mg, 100's: **$7.09-$11.08**; 0.6 mg, 100's: **$7.09-$11.36**

• Transdermal: 0.1 mg/hr, 30's: **$42.74-$57.93**; 0.2 mg/hr, 30's: **$32.18-$78.30**; 0.3 mg/hr, 30's: **$48.61-$65.86**; 0.4 mg/hr, 30's:

$38.49-$87.36; 0.6 mg/hr, 30's: **$46.00-$71.46**; 0.8 mg/hr, 30's: **$68.29-$71.46**

CONTRAINDICATIONS: Severe anemia, closed-angle glaucoma, postural hypotension, early MI (SL), head trauma, cerebral hemorrhage, hypotension or uncorrected hypovolemia, inadequate cerebral circulation, increased intracranial pressure, constrictive pericarditis, pericardial tamponade (IV)

PRECAUTIONS: Early days of MI, hypertrophic cardiomyopathy; severe hepatic, renal disease; children, glaucoma, abrupt withdrawal, continuous delivery (tolerance develops rapidly, IV excepted)

PREGNANCY AND LACTATION: Pregnancy category C; use of SL for angina during pregnancy without fetal harm has been reported

SIDE EFFECTS/ADVERSE REACTIONS

CNS: Agitation, anxiety, apprehension, confusion, *dizziness,* dyscoordination, *headache,* hypoesthesia, hypokinesia, insomnia, nervousness, nightmares, restlessness, vertigo, weakness

CV: Atrial fibrillation, *collapse,* crescendo angina, *dysrhythmias,* palpitations, *postural hypotension,* premature ventricular contractions, rebound hypertension, retrosternal discomfort, syncope, tachycardia

EENT: Blurred vision

GI: Abdominal pain, diarrhea, dyspepsia, fecal incontinence, nausea, tenesmus, tooth disorder, vomiting

GU: Dysuria, impotence, urinary frequency

HEME: **Hemolytic anemia, methemoglobinemia**

MS: Arthralgia

SKIN: Allergic reactions (ointment), contact dermatitis (transdermal), crusty skin lesions, *cutaneous vasodilation with flushing,* **exfoliative dermatitis,** pallor, pruritus, rash, sweating

INTERACTIONS

Drugs

❷ *Ergot alkaloids:* Opposition to coronary vasodilatory effects of nitrates

❸ *Ethanol:* Additive vasodilation could cause hypotension

❸ *Metronidazole:* Ethanol contained in IV nitroglycerine preparations could cause disulfiram-like reaction in some patients

❸ *Sildenafil:* Excessive hypotensive effects

Labs

• *False increase:* Serum triglycerides

SPECIAL CONSIDERATIONS

• 10-12 hr drug-free intervals prevent development of tolerance

PATIENT/FAMILY EDUCATION

• Avoid alcohol

• Notify clinician if persistent headache occurs

• Take oral nitrates on empty stomach with full glass of water

• Keep tablets and capsules in original container, keep container closed tightly

• Dissolve SL tablets under tongue, lack of burning does not indicate loss of potency, use when seated, take at 1st sign of anginal attack, activate emergency response system if no relief after 3 tablets spaced 5 min apart

• Spray translingual spray onto or under tongue, do not inhale spray

• Place buccal tablets under upper lip or between cheek and gum, permit to dissolve slowly over 3-5 min, do not chew or swallow

• Spread thin layer of ointment on skin using applicator or dose-measuring papers, do not use fingers, do not rub or massage

---

* = non-FDA-approved use

• Apply transdermal systems to non-hairy area on upper torso, remove for 10-12 hr/day (usually hs)

MONITORING PARAMETERS
• Blood pressure, heart rate at peak effect times

---

nitroprusside
(nye-troe-pruss'ide)
Rx: Nitropress
Chemical Class: Cyanonitrosylferrate derivative
Therapeutic Class: Antihypertensive

CLINICAL PHARMACOLOGY
Mechanism of Action: Relaxes vascular smooth muscle and dilates peripheral arteries and veins; more active on veins than arteries; reduces left ventricular end-diastolic pressure and pulmonary capillary wedge pressure (preload); reduces systemic vascular resistance, systolic arterial pressure, and mean arterial pressure (afterload); dilates coronary arteries

Pharmacokinetics
IV: Onset immediate; rapidly metabolized by interaction with sulfhydryl groups in erythrocytes and tissues (cyanogen is produced and converted to thiocyanate in liver), eliminated via urine (metabolites); circulating $t_{1/2}$ 2 min

INDICATIONS AND USES: Hypertensive crisis, controlled hypotension during surgery, severe refractory congestive heart failure (in combination with dopamine),* acute MI*

DOSAGE
Adult and Child
• IV INF 0.25-0.3 µg/kg/min initially, gradually increase every few minutes to desired blood pressure control or max rate of 10 µg/kg/min;

average dose is 3 µg/kg/min; if adequate blood pressure control is not achieved after 10 min of 10 µg/kg/min discontinue infusion; cyanide toxicity more likely when >500 µg/kg is administered faster than 2 µg/kg/min

§ AVAILABLE FORMS/COST OF THERAPY
• Inj, Lyphl-Sol—IV: 50 mg/vial: **$3.90-$12.48**

CONTRAINDICATIONS: Decreased cerebral perfusion, arteriovenous shunt or coarctation of the aorta (i.e., compensatory hypertension), congenital (Leber's) optic atrophy, tobacco amblyopia

PRECAUTIONS: Hepatic disease, decreased renal function, prolonged infusion, elevated intracranial pressure, anemia, hypovolemia, poor surgical risks, hypothyroidism, hyponatremia

PREGNANCY AND LACTATION: Pregnancy category C; exretion into breast milk is unknown, use caution in nursing mothers

SIDE EFFECTS/ADVERSE REACTIONS
CNS: Apprehension, *dizziness, headache,* increased intracranial pressure
CV: Bradycardia, ECG changes, hypotension, palpitations, retrosternal discomfort, tachycardia
GI: Abdominal pain, ileus, nausea, retching
HEME: Decreased platelet aggregation, ***methemoglobinemia***
METAB: Hypothyroidism
MS: Muscle twitching
SKIN: Diaphoresis, flushing, irritation at INF site, rash
MISC: ***Thiocyanate or cyanide toxicity***

INTERACTIONS
Drugs
§ *Clonidine:* Severe hypotensive reactions have been reported

---

italic = common side effects   ***bold italic*** = life-threatening reactions

3 *Diltiazem:* Reduction in the dose of nitroprusside required to produce hypotension

3 *Guanabenz, guanfacine:* Potential for severe hypotensive reactions

SPECIAL CONSIDERATIONS
MONITORING PARAMETERS

• Blood pressure, arterial blood gases, oxygen saturation, cyanide and thiocyanate concentrations, anion gap, lactate levels

---

nizatidine

(ni-za'ti-deen)

Rx: Axid

OTC: Axid AR

Chemical Class: Ethenediamine derivative

Therapeutic Class: Gastrointestinal antiulcer agent

CLINICAL PHARMACOLOGY

Mechanism of Action: Competitive, reversible inhibitor of histamine at gastric H_2-receptors; reduces gastric acid secretion

Pharmacokinetics

PO: Onset 30-60 min, peak 0.5 to 3 hr, duration 4-8 hr, oral bioavailability 70%; protein binding 35%; metabolized in liver, 60% of drug excreted unchanged in urine, 6% eliminated in feces; $t_{1/2}$ 1-2 hr

INDICATIONS AND USES: Short-term treatment of duodenal and benign gastric ulcers; maintenance therapy for duodenal ulcer; gastroesophageal reflux disease (GERD); heartburn, acid indigestion, sour stomach due to overindulgence (OTC); gastritis*

DOSAGE

Adult

• *Heartburn, acid indigestion, sour stomach due to overindulgence:* PO 75 mg bid (OTC)

• *Active duodenal or benign gastric ulcer:* PO 300 mg hs or 150 mg bid × 4-8 wk

• *Maintenance of healed duodenal ulcer:* PO 150 mg hs

• *Gastroesophageal reflux disease:* PO 150 mg bid

• Dosage adjustment for renal insufficiency (active ulcer disease), CrCl 20-50 ml/min, 150 mg qd; CrCl <20 ml/min, 150 mg qod

§ AVAILABLE FORMS/COST OF THERAPY

• Cap, Gel—Oral: 75 mg, 30's (OTC): **$9.36**; 150 mg, 60's: **$120.15**; 300 mg, 30's: **$125.37**

PRECAUTIONS: Renal insufficiency

PREGNANCY AND LACTATION: Pregnancy category B; excreted in breast milk (0.1% of dose)

SIDE EFFECTS/ADVERSE REACTIONS

CNS: Dizziness, drowsiness, headache

CV: Bradycardia, palpitation, tachycardia

EENT: Rhinitis

GI: Constipation, diarrhea, flatulence, hepatitis, nausea

HEME: Anemia, *thrombocytopenia*

METAB: Gynecomastia, hyperuricemia

MS: Myalgia

SKIN: Acne, pruritus, sweating, urticaria

INTERACTIONS

Drugs

3 *Cefpodoxime, cefuroxime; enoxacin; ketoconazole:* Reduction in gastric acidity reduces absorption, decreases plasma levels, potential for therapeutic failure

3 *Glipizide, glyburide tolbutamide:* Increased absorption of these drugs, potential for hypoglycemia

3 *Nifedipine; Nitrendipine; nisoldipine:* Increased concentrations of these drugs

---

* = non-FDA-approved use

SPECIAL CONSIDERATIONS
• No advantage over other agents of this class, base selection on cost

PATIENT/FAMILY EDUCATION
• Stagger doses of nizatidine and antacids

---

norepinephrine
(nor-ep-i-nef'rin)
Rx: Levophed
Chemical Class: Synthetic catecholamine
Therapeutic Class: α- & β-Adrenergic sympathomimetic; vasopressor

---

CLINICAL PHARMACOLOGY
Mechanism of Action: Stimulates β_1- and α-adrenergic receptors causing increased myocardial contractility and heart rate as well as vasoconstriction; increases blood pressure and coronary artery blood flow; marked pressor effect primarily due to increased peripheral resistance

Pharmacokinetics
IV: Onset rapid, duration 1-2 min after INF discontinued; metabolized in liver and other tissues by monoamine oxidase (MAO) and catechol-*O*-methyltransferase (COMT) to inactive metabolites; pharmacologic action terminated mainly by uptake and metabolism in sympathetic nerve endings; excreted in urine (metabolites)

INDICATIONS AND USES: Acute hypotensive states, adjunct in treatment of cardiac arrest and profound hypotension

DOSAGE
Adult
• IV INF 8-12 µg/min; initiate at 4 µg/min and titrate to desired response

Child
• IV INF 0.05-0.1 µg/kg/min initally, titrate to desired effect

$ **AVAILABLE FORMS/COST OF THERAPY**
• Inj, Sol—IV: 0.1%, 4 ml: **$11.01-$16.63**

CONTRAINDICATIONS: Hypotension from blood volume deficits (except as an emergency measure until volume replacement can be completed), mesenteric or peripheral vascular thrombosis, cyclopropane and halothane anesthesia

PRECAUTIONS: Atherosclerosis, arteriosclerosis, diabetic endarteritis, Buerger's disease, elderly, extravasation (may cause necrosis and sloughing of surrounding tissue), sulfite sensitivity

PREGNANCY AND LACTATION: Pregnancy category D

SIDE EFFECTS/ADVERSE REACTIONS
CNS: Anxiety, *headache*
CV: Bradycardia, ***cardiac dysrhythmias***, *chest pain*, hypertension, palpitations, tachycardia
EENT: Photophobia
GI: Nausea, vomiting
RESP: Respiratory distress
SKIN: Diaphoresis, gangrene, necrosis and sloughing following extravasation, pallor
MISC: Organ ischemia (due to vasocontriction of renal and mesenteric arteries)

INTERACTIONS
Drugs
❷ *Amitriptyline, desipramine, imipramine, protriptyline:* Marked enhancement of pressor response to norepinephrine
❸ *Guanadrel, guanethidine:* Exaggerated pressor response to norepinephrine
❸ *MAOIs:* Slight increase in the pressor response to norepinephrine

---

italic = common side effects   ***bold italic*** = life-threatening reactions

3 *Methyldopa:* Prolongation in the pressor response to norepinephrine

SPECIAL CONSIDERATIONS

• Antidote for extravasation ischemia: infiltrate with 10-15 ml of saline containing 5-10 mg of phentolamine

MONITORING PARAMETERS

• Blood pressure, heart rate, ECG, urine output, peripheral perfusion

---

norethindrone

(nor-eth′in-drone)

Rx: Micronor, Nor-Q.D.;

Acetate: Aygestin

Combinations

  Rx: with ethinyl estradiol (see oral contraceptives)

Chemical Class: 19-nortestosterone derivative

Therapeutic Class: Progestin; contraceptive

CLINICAL PHARMACOLOGY

Mechanism of Action: Exerts a progestational effect on the endometrium, alters cervical mucus, suppresses ovulation in some patients, renders the endometrium hostile to implantation

Pharmacokinetics

PO: 80% bound to plasma proteins; metabolized in liver; $t_{1/2}$ 10 hr

INDICATIONS AND USES: Prevention of conception, secondary amenorrhea, abnormal uterine bleeding, endometriosis, prevention of endometrial hyperplasia during postmenopausal estrogen therapy

DOSAGE

Adult and Adolescents

• *Amenorrhea and abnormal uterine bleeding:* PO 2.5-10 mg acetate on days 5-25 of menstrual cycle **or** to induce optimum secretory transformation of estrogen-primed endometrium 2.5-10 mg of acetate for 5-10 days during the latter half of menstrual cycle

• *Endometriosis:* PO 5 mg acetate qd for 14 consecutive days; increase by 2.5 mg/day at 14 day intervals until max 15 mg/day is reached; daily therapy may then be continued consecutively (no drug-free intervals) for 6-9 mo

• *Contraception:* PO 0.35 mg qd beginning on first day of menses

• *Prevention of endometrial hyperplasia in conjunction with estrogen:* 5 mg × 10-13 days/mo

5 AVAILABLE FORMS/COST OF THERAPY

• Tab, Uncoated—Oral: 0.35 mg, 28's: **$36.53-$39.65**

• Tab, Uncoated (acetate)—Oral: 5 mg, 50's: **$69.18-$80.73**

CONTRAINDICATIONS: Active thrombophlebitis or thromboembolic disorders, cerebral hemorrhage, impaired liver function or disease, breast cancer, undiagnosed vaginal bleeding, missed abortion, use as a diagnostic test for pregnancy

PRECAUTIONS: Asthma, cardiac or renal dysfunction, depression, diabetes, epilepsy, migraine

PREGNANCY AND LACTATION: Pregnancy category X; compatible with breast feeding

SIDE EFFECTS/ADVERSE REACTIONS

CNS: Depression, dizziness, fatigue, headache

CV: Edema

GI: Anorexia, ***cholestatic jaundice,*** cramps, increased weight, *nausea,* vomiting

GU: Amenorrhea, breakthrough bleeding, spotting, breast changes, dysmenorrhea, endometriosis

METAB: Hyperglycemia

SKIN: Acne, alopecia, hirsutism, melasma, rash

SPECIAL CONSIDERATIONS
PATIENT/FAMILY EDUCATION
• Missed dose: one tablet—Take as soon as remembered, or take 2 tablets at next regular time
• Missed 2 consecutive tablets—take 2 tablets at next 2 regular times
• Three missed tablets—Discontinue, restart after menses appear or pregnancy is ruled out
NOTE: Use an additional method of contraception if 2 or more tablets are missed until menses appear or pregnancy ruled out
• Progestin only pills have slightly higher failure rate than combination oral contraceptives
• When used as contraceptive, menstrual cycle may be disrupted and irregular and unpredictable bleeding or spotting may result

---

norfloxacin
(nor-flox′a-sin)
Rx: Noroxin; (Ophthalmic): Chibroxin
Chemical Class: Fluoroquinolone derivative
Therapeutic Class: Antibiotic

CLINICAL PHARMACOLOGY
Mechanism of Action: Interferes with the enzyme DNA gyrase needed for the synthesis of bacterial DNA; bactericidal
Pharmacokinetics
PO: Peak 1-2 hr; 10%-15% bound to plasma proteins; partially metabolized, excreted in urine (60%) and feces (30%); t₁/₂ 3-4 hr
INDICATIONS AND USES: Complicated and uncomplicated UTIs, uncomplicated gonorrhea (urethral, cervical), conjunctivitis (ophth), gastroenteritis,* travelers' diarrhea* Antibacterial spectrum usually includes:

• Gram-positive organisms: *Enterococcus faecalis, Staphylococcus aureus, S. epidermidis, S. saprophyticus, Streptococcus agalactiae*
• Gram-negative organisms: *Citrobacter freundii, Enterobacter aerogenes, E. cloacae, Escherichia coli, Klebsiella pneumoniae, Neisseria gonorrhoeae, Proteus mirabilis, P. vulgaris, Pseudomonas aeruginosa, Serratia marcescens* Conjunctivitis due to *Acinetobacter calcoaceticus,*Aeromonas hydrophila,* Haemophilus influenzae, Proteus mirabilis,* Serratia marcescens,* Staphylococcus aureus, Staphylococcus epidermidis, Staphylococcus warnerii,* Streptococcus pneumoniae*

DOSAGE
Adult
• *Urinary tract infection:* PO 400 mg bid on an empty stomach for 3-10 days (uncomplicated) or 10-21 days (complicated)
• *Gonorrhea:* PO 800 mg as a single dose followed by doxycycline 100 mg bid for 7 days
• *Gastroenteritis:* PO 400 mg bid for 5 days
• *Travelers' diarrhea:* PO 400 mg bid for up to 3 days until symptoms resolve
• Dosage in renal impairment, administer 400 mg qd in patients with CrCl <30 ml/min/1.73 m²
• *Conjunctivitis:* Ophth 1 drop qid

$ **AVAILABLE FORMS/COST OF THERAPY**
• Sol—Ophth: 0.3%, 5 ml: **$22.54**
• Tab, Plain Coated—Oral: 400 mg, 100's: **$380.70**
PRECAUTIONS: Children (potential for arthropathy and osteochondrosis), elderly, renal disease, seizure disorders, dehydration (potential for crystalluria)

---

italic = common side effects   ***bold italic*** = life-threatening reactions

PREGNANCY AND LACTATION: Pregnancy category C; excretion into breast milk unknown; due to the potential for arthropathy and osteochondrosis use extreme caution in nursing mothers

SIDE EFFECTS/ADVERSE REACTIONS

CNS: Anxiety, depression, dizziness, fatigue, headache, insomnia, *seizures,* somnolence

EENT: Visual disturbances

GI: Abdominal pain, anorexia, diarrhea, dry mouth, flatulence, heartburn, increased AST, ALT; *nausea, pseudomembranous colitis,* vomiting

GU: Crystalluria

HEME: Eosinophilia, *leukopenia*

SKIN: Photosensitivity, pruritus, rash

INTERACTIONS

Drugs

⬛ *Aluminum:* Reduced absorption of norfloxacin; do not take within 4 hr of dose

⬛ *Antacids:* Reduced absorption of norfloxacin; do not take within 4 hr of dose

⬛ *Antipyrine:* Inhibits metabolism of antipyrine; increased plasma antipyrine level

⬛ *Caffeine:* Inhibits metabolism of caffeine; increased plasma caffeine level

⬛ *Calcium:* Reduced absorption of norfloxacin; do not take within 4 hr of dose

⬛ *Diazepam:* Inhibits metabolism of diazepam; increased plasma diazepam level

⬛ *Didanosine:* Markedly reduced absorption of norfloxacin; take norfloxacin 2 hr before didanosine

⬛ *Foscarnet:* Coadministration increase seizure risk

⬛ *Iron:* Reduced absorption of norfloxacin; do not take within 4 hr of dose

⬛ *Magnesium:* Reduced absorption of norfloxacin; do not take within 4 hr of dose

⬛ *Metoprolol:* Inhibits metabolism of metoprolol; increased plasma metoprolol level

⬛ *Pentoxifylline:* Inhibits metabolism of pentoxifylline; increased plasma pentoxifylline level

⬛ *Phenytoin:* Inhibits metabolism of phenytoin; increased plasma phenytoin level

⬛ *Propranolol:* Inhibits metabolism of propranolol; increased plasma propranolol level

⬛ *Ropinirole:* Inhibits metabolism of ropinirole; increased plasma ropinirole level

⬛ *Sodium bicarbonate:* Reduced absorption of norfloxacin; do not take within 4 hr of dose

⬛ *Sucralfate:* Reduced absorption of norfloxacin; do not take within 4 hr of dose

⬛ *Theobromine:* Inhibits metabolism of theobromine; increased plasma theobromine level

⬛ *Theophylline:* Inhibits metabolism of theophylline; cut maintenance theophylline dose in half during therapy with norfloxacin

⬛ *Warfarin:* Inhibits metabolism of warfarin; increases hypoprothrombinemic response to warfarin

⬛ *Zinc:* Reduced absorption of norfloxacin; do not take within 4 hr of dose

Labs

• *False increase:* Uroporphyrin

SPECIAL CONSIDERATIONS

PATIENT/FAMILY EDUCATION

• Administer on an empty stomach (1 hr before or 2 hr after meals)

• Drink fluids liberally

• Do not take antacids containing magnesium or aluminum or products containing iron or zinc within 4 hr before or 2 hr after dosing

• Avoid excessive exposure to sunlight

norgestrel

(nor-jess'trel)

Rx: Ovrette
Combinations
  Rx: with ethinyl estradiol (see oral contraceptives)
Chemical Class: 19-nortestosterone derivative
Therapeutic Class: Progestin; contraceptive

CLINICAL PHARMACOLOGY

Mechanism of Action: Exerts a progestational effect on the endometrium, alters cervical mucus, suppresses ovulation in some patients, renders the endometrium hostile to implantation

Pharmacokinetics

PO: 93%-95% bound to plasma proteins; metabolized in liver, excreted in urine and feces; $t_{1/2}$ 11-45 hr

INDICATIONS AND USES: Prevention of conception; emergency contraception* (morning-after pill)

DOSAGE

Adult

• *Contraception:* PO 0.075 mg qd beginning on 1st day of menses
• *Emergency contraception:* 2 doses, 1st dose within 72 hr of unprotected intercourse, 2nd dose 12 hr later:

FORMULATION	TABLETS/DOSE
Norgestrel 0.5 mg + ethinyl estradiol 50 µg (Ovral)	2
Levonorgestrel 0.15 mg or norgestrel 0.3 mg + ethinyl estradiol 30 µ (Nordette, Lo/Ovral, Levlen, Levora)	4
Norgestrel 0.075 mg (Ovrette)	20

AVAILABLE FORMS/COST OF THERAPY

• Tab, Uncoated—Oral: 0.075 mg, 28's: **$21.90**

CONTRAINDICATIONS: Active thrombophlebitis or thromboembolic disorders, cerebral hemorrhage, impaired liver function or disease, breast cancer, undiagnosed vaginal bleeding, missed abortion, use as a diagnostic test for pregnancy

PRECAUTIONS: Epilepsy, migraine, asthma, cardiac or renal dysfunction, depression, diabetes

PREGNANCY AND LACTATION: Pregnancy category X; compatible with breast feeding

SIDE EFFECTS/ADVERSE REACTIONS

CNS: Depression, dizziness, fatigue, headache, migraines

CV: Edema

GI: Anorexia, ***cholestatic jaundice,*** cramps, increased weight, *nausea,* vomiting

GU: Amenorrhea, breakthrough bleeding, breast changes, dysmenorrhea, spotting

METAB: Hyperglycemia

SKIN: Acne, alopecia, hirsutism, melasma, rash

SPECIAL CONSIDERATIONS
PATIENT/FAMILY EDUCATION

• Missed dose: One tablet—Take as soon as remembered, take next tablet at regular time; Two consecutive tablets—Take 1 of the missed tablets, discard the other
• Three missed tablets—Discontinue
• Use an additional method of contraception if 2 or more tablets are missed until menses appear or pregnancy ruled out.
• Progestin only pills have slightly higher failure rate than combination oral contraceptives
• Take with food if GI upset occurs

N

• Menstrual cycle may be disrupted and irregular and unpredictable bleeding or spotting can result
• Based on WHO study, norgestrel (levonorgestrel) only pills preferred emergency contraception; equal efficacy and 50% less nausea, vomiting compared to combined regimen

---

nortriptyline

(nor-trip′ti-leen)

Rx: Aventyl, Pamelor
Chemical Class: Dibenzocycloheptene derivative: secondary amine
Therapeutic Class: Tricyclic antidepressant

CLINICAL PHARMACOLOGY
Mechanism of Action: Inhibits reuptake of norepinephrine and serotonin (blocking activity moderate and high, respectively) at the presynaptic neuron prolonging neuronal activity; inhibits histamine and acetylcholine activity; mild peripheral vasodilator effects and possible "quinidine-like" actions on cardiac conduction, moderate anticholinergic and sedative, slight orthostatic hypotensive side effects
Pharmacokinetics
PO: Peak 7-8.5 hr; 93%-95% bound to plasma proteins; metabolized in liver, excreted in urine, small amounts excreted in bile; $t_{1/2}$ 28-31 hr
INDICATIONS AND USES: Depression, panic disorder,* premenstrual depression,* dermatologic disorders (chronic urticaria and angioedema, nocturnal pruritis in atopic eczema),* nocturnal enuresis*

DOSAGE
Adult
• PO 25 mg qhs initially, increase at 3-5 day increments to 75-150 mg/day divided qd-qid
Elderly and Adolescents
• PO 30-50 mg/day in divided doses
Child
• *Nocturnal enuresis:* PO, 6-7 yr 10 mg/day; 8-11 yr 10-20 mg/day; >11 yr 25-35 mg/day

💲 **AVAILABLE FORMS/COST OF THERAPY**
• Cap, Gel—Oral: 10 mg, 100's: **$35.05-$70.16**; 25 mg, 100's: **$6.95-$140.00**; 50 mg, 100's: **$14.71-$263.81**; 75 mg, 100's: **$200.97-$402.13**
• Sol—Oral: 10 mg/5 ml, 480 ml: **$42.95-$80.49**

CONTRAINDICATIONS: Acute recovery phase of MI, concurrent use of MAOIs
PRECAUTIONS: Suicidal patients, convulsive disorders, prostatic hypertrophy, psychiatric disease, severe depression, increased intraocular pressure, narrow-angle glaucoma, urinary retention, cardiac disease, hepatic disease, renal disease, hyperthyroidism, electroshock therapy, elective surgery, elderly, abrupt discontinuation
PREGNANCY AND LACTATION: Pregnancy category D; effect on nursing infant unknown but may be of concern, especially after prolonged exposure
SIDE EFFECTS/ADVERSE REACTIONS
CNS: Anxiety, confusion (especially in elderly), *dizziness,* extrapyramidal symptoms (elderly), fatigue, headache, increased psychiatric symptoms, insomnia, memory impairment, nervousness, nightmares, panic, *seizures,* stimulation, tremors, weakness

---

* = non-FDA-approved use

*CV: **Dysrhythmias,*** ECG changes, hypertension, *orthostatic hypotension,* palpitations, syncope, tachycardia

EENT: Blurred vision, mydriasis, nasal congestion, ophthalmoplegia, tinnitus

GI: Constipation, cramps, diarrhea, *dry mouth,* epigastric distress, hepatitis, increased appetite, jaundice, nausea, paralytic ileus, stomatitis, vomiting

GU: Urinary retention

*HEME: **Agranulocytosis,*** eosinophilia, ***leukopenia, thrombocytopenia***

SKIN: Photosensitivity, pruritus, rash, sweating, urticaria

INTERACTIONS

Drugs

🔢 *Anticholinergics:* Excessive anticholinergic effects

🔢 *Barbiturates:* Reduced serum concentrations of cyclic antidepressants

🔢 *Carbamazepine, rifampin:* Reduced cyclic antidepressant serum concentrations

🔢 *Chlorpropamide:* Enhanced by hypoglycemic effects of chlorpropamide

🔢 *Cimetidine:* Increased serum nortriptyline concentrations

🔢 *Clonidine:* Reduced antihypertensive response to clonidine; enhanced hypertensive response with abrupt clonidine withdrawal

❷ *Epinephrine:* Markedly enhanced pressor response to IV epinephrine

🔢 *Ethanol:* Additive impairment of motor skills; abstinent alcoholics may eliminate cyclic antidepressants more rapidly than non-alcoholics

🔢 *Fluoxetine:* Marked increases in cyclic antidepressant plasma concentrations

❷ *Guanethidine:* Inhibited antihypertensive response to guanethidine

❷ *Moclobemide:* Potential association with fatal or non-fatal serotonin syndrome

⚠ *MAOIs:* Excessive sympathetic response, mania or hyperpyrexia possible

🔢 *Neuroleptics:* Increased therapeutic and toxic effects of both drugs

❷ *Norepinephrine:* Markedly enhanced pressor response to norepinephrine

🔢 *Phenylephrine:* Enhanced pressor response to IV phenylephrine

🔢 *Propoxyphene:* Enhanced effect of cyclic antidepressants

🔢 *Quinidine:* Increased cyclic antidepressant serum concentrations

Labs

• *False increase:* Serum carbamazepine

SPECIAL CONSIDERATIONS

PATIENT/FAMILY EDUCATION

• Therapeutic effects may take 2-3 wk

• Avoid rising quickly from sitting to standing, especially elderly

• Avoid alcohol and other CNS depressants

• Do not discontinue abruptly after long-term use

• Wear sunscreen or large hat to prevent sunburn

MONITORING PARAMETERS

• CBC, weight, ECG, mental status (mood, sensorium, affect, suicidal tendencies)

• Determination of nortriptyline plasma concentrations is not routinely recommended but may be useful in identifying toxicity, drug interactions, or noncompliance (adjustments in dosage should be made according to clinical response not plasma concentrations), therapeutic range 50-150 ng/ml

---

italic = common side effects   ***bold italic*** = life-threatening reactions

nystatin
(nye-stat´in)
Rx: (Troche): Mycostatin; (Oral): Mycostatin, Nilstat, Nystex
(Topical): Mycostatin, Nystex, Nystop, Pedi-Dry
Combinations
  Rx: (Topical) with triamcinolone (Mycolog-II, Mycomer, Mycasone, Myco Biotic II, Tri-Statin II, Mytrex, Myco-Triacet II, Mycogen II)
Chemical Class: Amphoteric polyene macrolide
Therapeutic Class: Antifungal

CLINICAL PHARMACOLOGY
Mechanism of Action: Binds to sterols in the fungal cell membrane, which results in loss of potassium and other cellular constituents; fungicidal/static

Pharmacokinetics
PO: Poorly absorbed; excreted almost entirely in feces as unchanged drug
TOP: Not absorbed from intact skin or mucous membranes

INDICATIONS AND USES: Cutaneous, mucocutaneous, and oral cavity candidal infections; candidal vulvovaginitis; intestinal candidiasis

DOSAGE
Adult
• *Oral candidiasis:* PO 400,000-600,000 U susp, swish and swallow qid; Troche 200,000-400,000 U 4-5 times/day
• *Cutaneous candidal infections:* Top apply ointment, cream, or powder to affected area tid-qid
• *Intestinal candidal infections:* PO 500,000-1,000,000 U q8h
• *Vaginal candidal infections:* Insert 1-2 vaginal tablets qhs for 2 wk

Child
• *Oral candidiasis:* PO 200,000 U qid or 100,000 U to each side of mouth qid
• *Cutaneous candidal infections:* Top apply ointment, cream, or powder to affected area tid-qid
Neonate
• *Oral candidiasis:* PO 100,000 U qid or 50,000 U to each side of mouth qid

💲 AVAILABLE FORMS/COST OF THERAPY
• Cap, Gel—Oral: 500,000 U 100's: **$31.40**; 1,000,000 U 100's: **$78.00**
• Cre—Top: 100,000 U/g 15, 30 g: **$2.80-$29.71**/30 g
• Lozenge—Oral: 200,000 U, 30's: **$31.40**
• Oint—Top: 100,000 U/g, 15, 30 g: **$3.00-$6.77**/30 g
• Powder—Top: 100,000 U/g, 15, 60 g: **$26.58-$30.51**/15 g
• Susp—Oral: 100,000 U/ml, 60, 480 ml: **$4.50-$32.29**/60 ml
• Tab, Plain Coated—Oral: 500,000 U, 100's: **$17.36-$71.55**
• Tab, Uncoated—Vag: 100,000 U, 15's: **$5.50-$43.31**

PREGNANCY AND LACTATION: Pregnancy category A/C; due to poor bioavailability, serum and breast milk levels do not occur

SIDE EFFECTS/ADVERSE REACTIONS
GI: Diarrhea, GI distress, nausea, vomiting
SKIN: Burning, rash, stinging, urticaria

SPECIAL CONSIDERATIONS
PATIENT/FAMILY EDUCATION
• Do not use troches in child <5 yr

octreotide

(ok-tree′oh-tide)

Rx: Sandostatin, Sandostatin Lar Depot

Chemical Class: Somatostatin analog

Therapeutic Class: Antidiarrheal; acromegaly agent

CLINICAL PHARMACOLOGY

Mechanism of Action: Actions similar to somatostatin; inhibits growth hormone, glucagon, and insulin more than somatostatin; suppresses LH response to gonadotropin releasing hormone; decreases splanchnic blood flow; inhibits release of serotonin, gastrin, vasoactive intestinal peptide (VIP), secretin, motilin, and pancreatic polypeptide

Pharmacokinetics

SC: Onset 0.4 hr, duration 12 hr; IV and SC doses bioequivalent; 65% protein bound; elimination $t_{1/2}$ 1.7 hr; metabolized by liver, 32% of dose excreted unchanged in urine; in dialysis patients, clearance is half of normals

IM: Intragluteal (depot): onset 1 hr; steady-state serum concentrations achieved after 3rd injection; plateau concentrations maintained 2-3 weeks; relative biavailability of long-acting vs. immediate release is 60-63%

INDICATIONS AND USES: Acromegaly, carcinoid syndrome (associated with metastatic carcinoid tumors), vasoactive intestinal peptide tumors (VIPomas), insulinoma,* HIV-associated secretory diarrhea,* cryptosporidiosis in HIV-infected persons,* control of bleeding esophageal varices,* irritable bowel syndrome,* dumping syndrome*

DOSAGE

Adult

• *Acromegaly:* SC or IV 0.05-0.1 mg tid

• *Carcinoid syndrome:* SC or IV 0.1-0.6 mg/day in 2-4 divided doses (mean daily dosage is 0.3 mg; max daily dose 1.5 mg)

• *VIPomas:* SC or IV 0.2-0.3 mg/day in 2-4 divided doses (range 0.15-0.75 mg)

• *HIV-associated diarrhea:* SC or IV 0.15-1.8 mg/day in 2-4 divided doses

• *Bleeding esophageal varices:* IV 0.05-0.1 mg bolus then 0.025-0.05 mg/hr continuous INF; 0.1 mg q8h as adjunct to sclerotherapy

• *Depot: Acromegaly:* Intragluteal 20 mg q4wk, assess dose at 3 mo; growth hormone (GH) <2.5 ng/ml, somatomedin C (IGF-1) normal, asymptomatic, continue 20 mg q4wk; GH >2.5 ng/ml, IGF-1 elevated and/or symptomatic, 30 mg q4wk; GH <1 ng/ml, IGF-1 normal, asymptomatic, 10 mg q4wk; max dose 40 mg q4wk; *Carcinoid syndrome and VIPomas:* Intragluteal 20 mg q4wk, at 2 mo may increase to 30 mg q4wk if symptomatic or decrease to 10 mg q4wk for trial period if asymptomatic

Child

• SC 0.001-0.01 mg/kg/day in 2-4 divided doses

• For IV use, may be diluted in 50-200 ml of D_5NS and given IV over 15-30 min or given by IV push over 3 min

💲 AVAILABLE FORMS/COST OF THERAPY

• Inj, Sol—IM: 10 mg, 20 mg: **$1,535.23**; 20 mg, 30 mg: **$1,763.18**

• Inj, Sol—SC, IV: 0.05 mg/ml, 1 ml: **$8.89**; 0.1 mg/ml, 1 ml: **$17.25**; 0.5 mg/ml, 1 ml: **$83.20**

---

italic = common side effects   ***bold italic*** = life-threatening reactions

PRECAUTIONS: Gallbladder disease (stones or sludge in 48% of patients treated for 12 mo; in 2% of patients treated for 1 mo); may affect glycemic control in diabetics; may cause hypothyroidism; worsening of CHF; altered absorption of dietary fats; depressed vitamin B_{12} levels

PREGNANCY AND LACTATION: Pregnancy category B; breast milk excretion unknown

SIDE EFFECTS/ADVERSE REACTIONS

CNS: Dizziness, fatigue, headache, weakness

CV: Bradycardia (21% in acromegalies), conduction abnormalities, dysrhythmias

GI: Abdominal discomfort, *constipation,* diarrhea, distension, flatulence, nausea, ***pancreatitis,*** vomiting

HEME: Vitamin B_{12} deficiency

METAB: Goiter, hyperglycemia, hypoglycemia, *hypothyroidism*

MS: Bell's palsy, leg cramps

SKIN: Alopecia

MISC: Local pain on inj

INTERACTIONS

Drugs

❷ *Cyclosporine:* Decreased serum cyclosporine concentrations

❸ *Oral hypoglycemic agents, insulin:* Octreotide can alter glycemic control, dose adjustment of antidiabetic agents may be necessary

SPECIAL CONSIDERATIONS

• Octreotide is incompatible in TPN solutions

• Patient tolerance to ocreotide should be determined with 2 weeks SC/IV therapy before switching to depot therapy

• Only give depot intragluteally, avoid deltoid injections due to pain at injection site

• Withdraw octreotide yearly for 4 wk in acromegaly patients who have received irradiation to assess disease activity

MONITORING PARAMETERS

• Thyroid function, serum glucose (especially in drug-treated diabetics), vitamin B_{12} levels

• Heart rate (especially in persons taking β-blockers and calcium channel blockers)

• Periodic zinc levels in patients receiving TPN

---

ofloxacin

(o-flox′a-sin)
Rx: (Oral): Floxin;
(Ophthalmic): Ocuflox
Chemical Class: Fluoroquinolone derivative
Therapeutic Class: Antibiotic

CLINICAL PHARMACOLOGY

Mechanism of Action: Interferes with the enzyme DNA gyrase needed for the synthesis of bacterial DNA; bactericidal

Pharmacokinetics

PO: Peak 1-2 hr; 98% oral bioavailability; 32% bound to plasma proteins; excreted primarily unchanged in urine; $t_{1/2}$ 5-10 hr

INDICATIONS AND USES: Lower respiratory tract infections, uncomplicated urethral and cervical gonorrhea; non-gonococcal urethritis, cervicitis; skin and skin structure infections, UTIs, prostatitis; superficial ocular infections involving the conjunctiva or cornea (ophthalmic preparation)

Antibacterial spectrum usually includes:

• Gram-positive organisms: *Staphylococcus aureus, S. epidermidis, S. saprophyticus, Enterococcus faecalis*

---

* = non-FDA-approved use

• Gram-negative organisms: *Acinetobacter* spp., *Aeromonas* spp., *Campylobacter* spp., *Citrobacter* spp., *Enterobacter* spp., *Escherichia coli, Haemophilus influenzae, H. parainfluenzae, Klebsiella pneumoniae, Klebsiella* spp., *Legionella* spp., *Listeria monocytogenes, Moraxella catarrhalis, Morganella morganii, Neisseria gonorrhoeae, N. meningitidis, Plesiomonas shigelloides, Proteus mirabilis, P. vulgaris, Providencia rettgeri, P. stuartii, Pseudomonas aeruginosa, P. fluorescens, Salmonella* spp., *Serratia* spp., *Shigella* spp., *Vibro* spp., *Xanthomonas maltophilia, Yersinia enterocolitica*

DOSAGE

Adult

• *Lower respiratory tract infections:* PO/IV 400 mg q12h for 10 days
• *Uncomplicated gonorrhea:* PO 400 mg as a single dose plus doxycycline 100 mg bid for 7 days
• *Nongonococcal urethritis, cervicitis:* PO/IV 300 mg q12h for 7 days
• *Skin and skin structure infections:* PO/IV 400 mg q12h for 10 days
• *UTI:* PO/IV 200 mg q12h for 3-10 days
• *Prostatitis:* PO/IV 300 mg q12h for 6 wk (do not continue IV therapy for >10 days, switch to PO)
• *Renal function impairment:* CrCl 10-50 ml/min use 24 hr dosage interval; CrCl <10 ml/min, 50% of recommended dose given q24h
• *Superficial ocular infections:* Ophth 1 gtt q2-4h for 1st 2 days, then qid for additional 5 days

Child >1 yr

• *Superficial ocular infections:* Ophth 1 gtt q2-4h for 1st 2 days, then qid for additional 5 days

💲 AVAILABLE FORMS/COST OF THERAPY

• Inj, Sol—IV: 40 mg/ml, 10 ml: **$26.40**

• Sol—Ophth: 0.3%, 5, 10 ml: **$24.55**/5 ml
• Tab, Plain Coated—Oral: 200 mg, 100's: **$225.94**; 300 mg, 100's: **$268.88**; 400 mg, 100's: **$567.13**

PRECAUTIONS: Children (potential for arthropathy and osteochondrosis), elderly, renal disease, seizure disorders

PREGNANCY AND LACTATION: Pregnancy category C; excreted into breast milk in quantities approximating maternal plasma concentrations; due to the potential for arthropathy and osteochondrosis, use extreme caution in nursing mothers

SIDE EFFECTS/ADVERSE REACTIONS

CNS: Anxiety, depression, dizziness, fatigue, headache, insomnia, ***seizures,*** somnolence
EENT: Dizziness, visual disturbances
GI: Abdominal pain, anorexia, diarrhea, dry mouth; flatulence, heartburn, increased AST, ALT; *nausea,* ***pseudomembranous colitis,*** vomiting
SKIN: Photosensitivity, pruritus, rash

INTERACTIONS

Drugs

🔳 *Aluminum:* Reduced absorption of ofloxacin; do not take within 4 hr of dose
🔳 *Antacids:* Reduced absorption of ofloxacin; do not take within 4 hr of dose
🔳 *Calcium:* Reduced absorption of ofloxacin; do not take within 4 hr of dose
🔳 *Iron:* Reduced absorption of ofloxacin; do not take within 4 hr of dose
🔳 *Magnesium:* Reduced absorption of ofloxacin; do not take within 4 hr of dose

■ *Procainamide:* Ofloxacin competitively inhibits renal tubular excretion of procainamide

■ *Sodium bicarbonate:* Reduced absorption of ofloxacin; do not take within 4 hr of dose

■ *Sucralfate:* Reduced absorption of ofloxacin; do not take within 4 hr of dose

■ *Warfarin:* Inhibits metabolism of warfarin; increases hypoprothrombinemic response to warfarin

■ *Zinc:* Reduced absorption of ofloxacin; do not take within 4 hr of dose

Labs

• *False increase:* Uroporphyrin

SPECIAL CONSIDERATIONS

PATIENT/FAMILY EDUCATION

• Administer on an empty stomach (1 hr before or 2 hr after meals)
• Drink fluids liberally
• Do not take antacids containing magnesium or aluminum or products containing iron or zinc within 4 hr before or 2 hr after dosing
• Avoid excessive exposure to sunlight

---

olanzapine

(oh-lan′za-peen)

Rx: Zyprexa
Chemical Class: Thienbenzodiazepine derivative
Therapeutic Class: Antipsychotic

CLINICAL PHARMACOLOGY

Mechanism of Action: Serotonin 5-HT$_2$ > dopamine-(D$_2$-) receptor antagonist; activity against several neurotransmitter systems: selective antagonist at limbic dopamine receptors (D$_1$, D$_2$, D$_4$, D$_5$) and serotonin receptors (5-HT$_2$, 5-HT$_6$, 5-HT$_7$); antagonism at α-$_1$-adrenergic receptors; and activity at musca-

rinic, histamine H$_1$, or nicotinic receptors; high sedation and anticholinergic effects; moderate orthostatic hypotension and weight gain risk; minimal risk of extrapyramidal symptoms

Pharmacokinetics

PO: Peak 6 hr, extensive first pass metabolism (40%), absorption unaffected by food; 93% bound to plasma proteins; highly metabolized by the liver; excreted in urine (57%) and feces (30%); t$_{1/2}$ 30 hr (21-54 hr)

INDICATIONS AND USES: Management of psychotic disorders

DOSAGE

Adult

• PO 5-10 mg qd; dosage may be increased in 5 mg/day increments if needed in intervals not <1 wk; maximum 20 mg/day; initiate with 5 mg qd in debilitated patients

■ **AVAILABLE FORMS/COST OF THERAPY**

• Tab, Film-Coated—Oral: 2.5 mg, 60's: **$324.18**; 5 mg, 60's: **$382.89**; 7.5 mg, 60's: **$422.21**; 10 mg, 60's: **$582.00**; 15 mg, 100's: **$1,455.00**; 20 mg, 60's: **$1,164.00**
• Tab, Disintegrating—Oral: 5 mg, 30's: **$228.58**; 10 mg, 30's: **$328.23**; 15 mg, 100's: **$471.38**; 20 mg, 30's: **$617.63**

PRECAUTIONS: Hepatic function impairment; children <18 yr; history of myocardial infarction, heart failure, cardiac conduction abnormalities; cerebrovascular disease; seizure disorders; patients at risk for aspiration pneumonia; prostatic hypertrophy, narrow-angle glaucoma, history of paralytic ileus

PREGNANCY AND LACTATION: Pregnancy category C; excretion into human breast milk unknown; excreted in the milk of treated rats

---

SIDE EFFECTS/ADVERSE REACTIONS

CNS: Agitation, *akathisia,* amnesia, *anxiety,* articulation impairment, *dizziness,* euphoria, *headache, hostility,* hypertonia, *insomnia, nervousness, somnolence,* stuttering, tardive dyskinesia, tremor

CV: Chest pain, edema, hypotension, *postural hypotension,* tachycardia

EENT: Amblyopia, blepharitis, pharyngitis, *rhinitis*

GI: Abdominal pain, *constipation, dry mouth,* increased appetite, transaminase elevations

GU: Premenstrual syndrome

METAB: Weight gain

MS: Back pain, joint pain, twitching

SKIN: Rash

MISC: Fever, ***neuroleptic malignant syndrome***

INTERACTIONS

Drugs

3 *Carbamazepine:* Decreased olanzapine concentrations

3 *Levodopa:* Antagonism of the effects of levodopa due to dopamine receptor blockade

SPECIAL CONSIDERATIONS

PATIENT/FAMILY EDUCATION

• Avoid exposure to extreme heat

MONITORING PARAMETERS

• Periodic assessment of liver transaminases in patients with significant hepatic disease

olsalazine

(ohl-sal'ah-zeen)
Rx: Dipentum
Chemical Class: Salicylate derivative
Therapeutic Class: GI anti-inflammatory agent

CLINICAL PHARMACOLOGY

Mechanism of Action: Bioconverted by colonic bacteria to 5-aminosalicylic acid (mesalamine), which may act by blocking cyclooxygenase and inhibiting prostaglandin production in the colon; local, mucosal anti-inflammatory effect in patients with chronic inflammatory bowel disease

Pharmacokinetics

PO: Limited systemic bioavailability (2.4% of 1 g dose absorbed); peak 1 hr; >99% bound to plasma proteins; <1% recovered in urine; serum $t_{1/2}$ 0.9 hr

INDICATIONS AND USES: Maintenance of remission of ulcerative colitis in patients intolerant of sulfasalazine

DOSAGE

Adult

• PO 1 g/day in 2 evenly divided doses

$ AVAILABLE FORMS/COST OF THERAPY

• Cap, Gel—Oral: 250 mg, 100's: **$107.74**

PRECAUTIONS: Children, preexisting renal disease

PREGNANCY AND LACTATION: Pregnancy category C; mesalamine has produced adverse effects in a nursing infant and should be used with caution during breast feeding, observe nursing infant closely for changes in stool consistency

---

italic = common side effects   ***bold italic*** = life-threatening reactions

SIDE EFFECTS/ADVERSE REACTIONS

CNS: Depression, drowsiness, headache

GI: Anorexia, bloating, *cramping, diarrhea,* dyspepsia, nausea, stomatitis, vomiting

MS: Arthralgia

SKIN: Itching, rash

SPECIAL CONSIDERATIONS
PATIENT/FAMILY EDUCATION
• Take with food. Notify clinician if diarrhea occurs

MONITORING PARAMETERS
• BUN, urinalysis, serum creatinine in patients with pre-existing renal disease

---

omeprazole

(om-eh-pray′zole)

Rx: Prilosec

Chemical Class: Benzimidazole derivative

Therapeutic Class: Gastrointestinal antisecretory agent

CLINICAL PHARMACOLOGY

Mechanism of Action: Irreversibly inactivates proton pump in gastric parietal cells, which blocks the final step in secretion of hydrochloric acid; acid secretion is inhibited until additional enzyme is synthesized; inhibits basal and stimulated gastric acid secretion

Pharmacokinetics

PO: Peak 0.5-3½ hr; 95% bound to plasma proteins; metabolized in liver to inactivate metabolites, excreted in urine (77%) and feces (23%); t½ ½-1 hr (does not reflect duration of acid suppression)

INDICATIONS AND USES: Active duodenal ulcer; short-term treatment of active benign gastric ulcers, in combination with clarithromycin for the treatment of *H. pylori;* gastroesophageal reflux disease (GERD) (including maintenance therapy); erosive esophagitis (including maintenance therapy); pathological hypersecretory conditions (e.g., Zollinger-Ellison syndrome, multiple endocrine adenomas, systemic mastocytosis); NSAID-induced ulcer*; posterior laryngitis*; treatment of steatorrhea in cystic fibrosis patients (enhances efficacy of pancreatic enzymes)*

DOSAGE
Adult

• *Active duodenal ulcer:* PO 20 mg qd for 4-8 wk

• *H. Pylori:* PO 20 mg bid in combination with clarithromycin 500 mg bid and amoxicillin 1 g bid for 7 days (other regimens have also been used)

• *Gastric ulcer:* PO 40 mg qd for 4-8 wk

• *GERD:* PO 20 mg qd for 4-8 wk

• *Maintenance of healing in erosive esophagitis:* 10-20 mg qd

• *Pathological hypersecretory conditions:* PO 60 mg qd initially, doses up to 120 mg tid have been administered (administer doses >80 mg/day in divided doses)

Ⓢ AVAILABLE FORMS/COST OF THERAPY

• Cap, Gel, Sus Action—Oral: 10 mg, 100's: **$337.56**; 20 mg, 100's: **$413.93**; 40 mg, 100's: **$594.00**

PRECAUTIONS: Not for maintenance therapy of duodenal ulcer or GERD; elderly; children; symptomatic response does not preclude gastric malignancy

PREGNANCY AND LACTATION: Pregnancy category C; suppression of gastric acid secretion is potential effect in nursing infant, clinical significance unknown

SIDE EFFECTS/ADVERSE REACTIONS

CNS: Asthenia, dizziness, headache

---

* = non-FDA-approved use

GI: Abdominal pain, constipation, diarrhea, flatulence, nausea
MS: Back pain
RESP: Cough
SKIN: Rash

INTERACTIONS

Drugs

3 *Carbamazepine, diazepam, digoxin, glipizide, glyburide, nifedipine, nimodipine, nisoldipine, nitrendipine:* Increased concentrations of these drugs

3 *Cefpodoxime, cefuroxime, enoxacin, ketoconazole:* Decreased concentrations of these drugs

3 *Glipizide, glyburide, tolbutamide:* Increased absorption of these drugs, potential of hypoglycemia

3 *Methotrexate:* Case report of elevated methotrexate concentration

3 *Phenytoin:* Increased phenytoin concentration

SPECIAL CONSIDERATIONS

• Some patients on maintenance therapy may respond to 10 mg qd or 20 mg qod

PATIENT/FAMILY EDUCATION

• Take before eating
• Swallow capsule whole; do not open, chew, or crush

---

ondansetron

(on-dan-seh'tron)
Rx: Zofran, Zofran ODT
Chemical Class: Carbazole derivative
Therapeutic Class: Antiemetic

CLINICAL PHARMACOLOGY

Mechanism of Action: Selectively blocks the action of serotonin at 5-HT$_3$ receptors; cytotoxic chemotherapy appears to be associated with release of serotonin from enterochromaffin cells of the small intestine which may stimulate vagal afferents through 5-HT$_3$ receptors, initiating the vomiting reflex

Pharmacokinetics

IV: Peak immediate
PO: Peak 1.7-2 hr; bioavailability 56%

70%-76% bound to plasma proteins; extensively metabolized, excreted in urine and feces (metabolites); t$_{1/2}$ 4 hr (2-3 hr in children <15 yr; 5.5 hr in adults >75 yr)

INDICATIONS AND USES: Prevention of nausea and vomiting associated with emetogenic cancer chemotherapy, total body irradiation, and postoperative nausea and vomiting

DOSAGE

Adult

• *Emetogenic chemotherapy:* PO 8 mg 30 min before chemotherapy, repeat 8 hr after initial dose; then bid for 1-2 days after completion of chemotherapy; IV 0.15 mg/kg/dose infused 30 min before start of chemotherapy, repeat 4 and 8 hr after initial dose, or single 32 mg dose beginning 30 min before chemotherapy

• *Total body irradiation:* PO 8 mg 1-2 hr before each fraction of radiotherapy administered qd

• *Postoperative nausea or vomiting:* IV 4 mg over ≥30 sec immediately prior to induction of anesthesia or postoperatively; PO 16 mg as a single dose 1 hr prior to induction of anesthesia

Child

• PO 4 mg 30 min before chemotherapy, repeat 4 and 8 hr after initial dose then tid for 1-2 days after completion of chemotherapy; IV 0.15 mg/kg/dose infused 30 min before start of chemotherapy, repeat 4 and 8 hr after initial dose

---

italic = common side effects **bold italic** = life-threatening reactions

AVAILABLE FORMS/COST OF THERAPY

• Inj, Sol—IV: 2 mg/ml, 20 ml: **$267.09**; 32 mg/50 ml, 50 ml: **$1,238.46**
• Sol—Oral: 4 mg/5 ml, 50 ml: **$184.26**
• Tab Coated—Oral: 4 mg, 30's: **$479.20**; 8 mg, 30's: **$903.50**
• Tab ODT (dissolving)—Oral: 4 mg, 30's: **$542.43**; 8 mg, 30's: **$914.00**

PRECAUTIONS: Abdominal surgery (may mask ileus or gastric distension), children ≤3 yr

PREGNANCY AND LACTATION: Pregnancy category B; has been used in the treatment of hyperemesis gravidarum

SIDE EFFECTS/ADVERSE REACTIONS

CNS: Headache, lightheadedness, *seizures*

CV: Angina, bradycardia, syncope, tachycardia

EENT: Blurred vision

GI: Constipation, diarrhea, transient elevation in liver enzymes

METAB: Hypokalemia

RESP: Bronchospasm

SKIN: Rash

opium

(oh´pee-um)
Rx: Opium Tincture
Combinations
   Rx: with belladonna alkaloids (B&O Suppositories)
Chemical Class: Natural alkaloid
Therapeutic Class: Narcotic analgesic; antidiarrheal
DEA Class: Schedule II

CLINICAL PHARMACOLOGY

Mechanism of Action: Narcotic agent with some activity at μ-receptors (supraspinal analgesia, euphoria, respiratory and physical depression, miosis, and reduced GI motility), κ-receptors (pentazocine-like spinal analgesia, sedation, and miosis), and Δ-receptors (dysphoria, psychotomimetic effects [e.g., hallucinations], and respiratory and vasomotor stimulation caused by drugs with antagonist activity); standard pharmacologic comparator for analgesic, antitussive, constipation, respiratory depression, sedation, emesis, and phyiscal dependence effects

GI: Decreases gastric motility; decreases biliary, pancreatic, and intestinal secretions and delays digestion of food in the small intestine; resting tone increases and periodic spasms occur; decreases propulsive peristaltic waves in the large intestine; constricts sphincter of Oddi

Pharmacokinetics

PO: Variably absorbed from GI tract; metabolized in liver, excreted in urine

INDICATIONS AND USES: Symptomatic treatment of diarrhea; relief of severe pain in place of morphine; narcotic abstinence syndrome suppressant in neonates*

---

* = non-FDA-approved use

DOSAGE
Adult
• PO (tincture) 0.6 ml qid
Child
• PO (tincture) for diarrhea 0.005-0.01 ml/kg/dose q3-4h; for analgesia 0.01-0.02 ml/kg/dose q3-4h

💲 AVAILABLE FORMS/COST OF THERAPY
• Tincture—Oral: 10%, 118 ml: **$49.29**

CONTRAINDICATIONS: Acute bronchial asthma, upper airway obstruction, glaucoma, respiratory depression, acute alcoholism, delerium tremens, premature labor

PRECAUTIONS: Head injury, increased intracranial pressure, acute abdominal conditions, elderly, severe impairment of hepatic or renal function, hypothyroidism, Addison's disease, prostatic hypertrophy, urethral stricture, history of drug abuse; seizure disorder

PREGNANCY AND LACTATION: Pregnancy category B (category D if used for prolonged periods or in high doses at term); compatible with breast feeding

SIDE EFFECTS/ADVERSE REACTIONS
CNS: Agitation, dependency, dizziness, *drowsiness,* lethargy, restlessness, *sedation*

CV: Bradycardia, orthostatic hypotension, palpitations, tachycardia

GI: Anorexia, constipation, dry mouth, *nausea, vomiting*

GU: Urinary retention

*RESP: **Respiratory depression, respiratory paralysis***

SKIN: Flushing, rash, urticaria

INTERACTIONS
Drugs
🔢 *Barbiturates:* Additive CNS depression

🔢 *Cimetidine:* Increased effect of narcotic analgesics

🔢 *Ethanol:* Additive CNS effects

🔢 *Neuroleptics:* Hypotension and excessive CNS depression

Labs
• *False increase:* Amylase and lipase

SPECIAL CONSIDERATIONS
• Opium has been replaced by safer, more effective analgesics and sedative/hypnotics for diagnostic or operative medication; useful as an antidiarrheal

• Do not administer agonist/antagonist analgesics (i.e., pentazocine, nalbuphine, butorphanol, dezocine, buprenorphine) to patient who has received a prolonged course of opium (a pure agonist). In opioid-dependent patients, mixed agonist/antagonist analgesics may precipitate withdrawal symptoms

PATIENT/FAMILY EDUCATION
• Drug may be addictive if used for prolonged periods

---

orlistat
(ohr'lih-stat)
Rx: Xenical
Chemical Class: Lipase inhibitor
Therapeutic Class: Weight loss

CLINICAL PHARMACOLOGY
Mechanism of Action: Nonsystemic reversible inhibition of lipases in the lumen of the stomach and small intestine; inhibited enzyme no longer able to hydrolyze dietary fat into absorbable free fatty acids, resulting in caloric deficit and potential for subsequent weight loss

Pharmacokinetics
PO: Peak 8 hr, barely detectable (at the limits of detection) Minimal systemic absorption (PO) - <2% bioavailable; metabolized in the gut

---

wall (2 metabolites-inconsequential), excreted in feces (97%; 83% unchanged after 3-5 days); $t_{1/2}$, 1-2 hr

INDICATIONS AND USES: Management of obesity (i.e., initial body mass index (BMI) 30 kg/m^2, or 27 kg/m^2 in the presence of other risk factors e.g., hypertension, diabetes, dyslipidemia) including weight loss, weight maintenance, with a reduced-calorie diet; hyperlipidemia*

DOSAGE

Adult and Child >16 yr

• PO 120 mg tid with each meal containing fat (during or within 1 hour after the meal)

§ AVAILABLE FORMS/COST OF THERAPY

• Cap—Oral: 120 mg, 90's: **$118.80**

CONTRAINDICATIONS: Chronic malabsorption syndrome or cholestasis

PRECAUTIONS: Fat soluble vitamin, vitamin D, beta-carotene deficiency; history of hyperoxaluria or calcium oxalate nephrolithiasis; anorexia nervosa or bulimia

PREGNANCY AND LACTATION: Pregnancy category B

SIDE EFFECTS/ADVERSE REACTIONS

CNS: Anxiety, depression

CV: Edema, hypertension

GI: Manifestation of mechanism of action: oily spotting, flatus with discharge, fecal urgency, fatty/oily stool, oily evacuation, increased defecation, fecal incontinence , abdominal pain/discomfort, gingival disorder, infectious diarrhea, nausea, vomiting

GU: Menstrual irregularity

SKIN: Rash, dry skin

INTERACTIONS

Drugs

❷ *Fat-soluble vitamins:* pharmacokinetic interaction resulting in 30-60% reduction in beta-carotene, vitamin E

❷ *Warfarin:* because fat soluble vitamins may be depleted; an exaggerated hypoprothrombinemic effect is possible

SPECIAL CONSIDERATIONS

• Standard weight loss maintained over 2 years is approximately 10% of initial weight

PATIENT/FAMILY EDUCATION

• If a meal contains no fat, the dose of orlistat can be omitted

• Supplement with fat soluble vitamin, vitamin D, and beta-carotene

• Psyllium laxative may decrease GI adverse effects

MONITORING PARAMETERS

• Lipids, weight, plasma levels of vitamins A, D, E

---

orphenadrine

(or-fen′a-dreen)

Rx: Antiflex, Banflex, Mio-rel, Myotrol, Norflex, Orfro, Orphenate

Combinations

Rx: with aspirin, caffeine (Norgesic, Norgesic Forte, Orphengesic, Orphengesic Forte)

Chemical Class: Tertiary amine

Therapeutic Class: Skeletal muscle relaxant

CLINICAL PHARMACOLOGY

Mechanism of Action: Probable central action at brain stem; does not directly relax tense skeletal muscle; possesses anticholinergic actions

Pharmacokinetics

PO: Peak 2 hr, duration 4-6 hr; metabolized to 8 known metabolites, excreted in urine and feces; $t_{1/2}$ 14 hr

INDICATIONS AND USES: Adjunctive therapy to rest and physical therapy for painful acute musculoskeletal conditions, quinine-resistant leg cramps*

---

* = non-FDA-approved use

DOSAGE

Adult

• PO 100 mg bid; IM/IV 60 mg, may repeat q12h prn

💲 **AVAILABLE FORMS/COST OF THERAPY**

• Inj, Sol—IM, IV: 30 mg/ml, 10 ml: **$6.25-$29.90**

• Tab, Plain Coated, Sus Action—Oral: 100 mg, 100's: **$9.50-$257.25**

CONTRAINDICATIONS: Glaucoma, pyloric or duodenal obstruction, stenosing peptic ulcer, prostatic hypertrophy, obstruction of bladder neck, cardiospasm, myasthenia gravis

PRECAUTIONS: Children, cardiac decompensation, coronary insufficiency, cardiac dysrhythmia, tachycardia, sulfite sensitivity

PREGNANCY AND LACTATION: Pregnancy category C; excretion into breast milk unknown, use caution in nursing mothers

SIDE EFFECTS/ADVERSE REACTIONS

CNS: Agitation, confusion, *dizziness, drowsiness,* hallucinations, headache, *lightheadedness,* tremor, weakness

CV: Palpitation, tachycardia, transient syncope

EENT: Blurred vision, increased ocular tension, pupil dilation

GI: Constipation, dry mouth, gastric irritation, nausea, vomiting

GU: Urinary hesitancy, urinary retention

*HEME: **Aplastic anemia** (rare)

SKIN: Urticaria and other dermatoses

INTERACTIONS

Drugs

🔳 *Neuroleptics:* Lower serum neuroleptic concentrations, excessive anticholinergic effects

oseltamivir

(ah-suhl-tahm'ah-veer)

Rx: Tamiflu

Chemical Class: Carboxylic acid ethyl ester

Therapeutic Class: Antiviral

CLINICAL PHARMACOLOGY

Mechanism of Action: Inhibits influenza virus neuraminidase; may alter virus particle aggregation and release

Pharmacokinetics

PO: Peak 1 hr; oral bioavailability 75%; converted by hepatic esterase hydrolysis to the active form, oseltamivir carboxylate with $t_{1/2}$ 1-3 hr; oseltamivir 42% protein bound, oseltamivir carboxylate 3% protein bound; oseltamivir carboxylate excreted in urine with $t_{1/2}$ 6-10 hr; crosses placenta, excreted in breast milk

INDICATIONS AND USES: Treatment of uncomplicated influenza infection in adults who have been symptomatic for no more than 2 days; reduces median time to improvement of symptoms by 1.3 days

DOSAGE

Adult and child >16 yr

• PO 75 mg bid for 5 days; dose adjustment for renal insufficiency: if CrCl < 30 ml/min, give 75 mg q day for 5 days

💲 **AVAILABLE FORMS/COST OF THERAPY**

• Cap—Oral: 75 mg, 10's: **$59.54**

• Powder, Reconst—Oral: 12 mg/ml, 25, 75 ml: **$32.88**/25 ml

PRECAUTIONS: Children under age 18 yr, renal insufficiency

PREGNANCY AND LACTATION: Pregnancy category C; excreted in breast milk of animals

SIDE EFFECTS/ADVERSE REACTIONS

CNS: Insomnia, vertigo
GI: Nausea (10%)

SPECIAL CONSIDERATIONS
PATIENT/FAMILY EDUCATION

• May administer without regard for food
• When started within 40 hr of onset of symptoms, there was a 1.3 day reduction in the median time to improvement in influenza-infected subjects receiving osteltamivir compared to subjects receiving placebo

---

oxacillin

(ox-a-sill'in)
Rx: Bactrocill
Chemical Class: Semisynthetic penicillin, (penicillinase-resistant)
Therapeutic Class: Antibiotic

CLINICAL PHARMACOLOGY

Mechanism of Action: Inhibits bacterial wall synthesis; bactericidal
Pharmacokinetics
PO: Peak 0.5-2 hr, duration 4-6 hr
IM: Peak 30 min, duration 4-6 hr
89%-94% bound to plasma proteins; partially metabolized to active and inactive metabolites, rapidly excreted in urine; $t_{1/2}$ 0.3-0.8 hr

INDICATIONS AND USES: Infections of the upper and lower respiratory tract, skin and skin structures, bones and joints; meningitis, septicemia, and endocarditis caused by penicillinase-producing staphylococci; perioperative prophylaxis*
Antibacterial spectrum usually includes:

• Gram-positive organisms: penicillinase-producing and non-penicillinase-producing strains of *Staphylococus aureus, S. epidermidis, S.*

saprophyticus; groups A, B, C, and G streptococci; *Streptococcus pneumoniae,* some viridans streptococci, *Bacillus anthracis*

DOSAGE
Adult
• PO 500-1000 mg q4-6h; IM/IV 250-1000 mg q4-6h; max 12 g/day
Child
• PO/IM/IV 50-100 mg/kg/day divided q4-6h; max 300 mg/kg/day

🔢 AVAILABLE FORMS/COST OF THERAPY

• Cap, Gel—Oral: 250 mg, 100's: **$20.95-$37.43**; 500 mg, 100's: **$33.15-$57.00**
• Inj, Dry-Sol—IM, IV: 500 mg/vial: **$1.37-$3.17**; 1 g/vial: **$2.79-$15.00**; 2 g/vial: **$0.79-$25.28**; 4 g/vial: **$11.38**
• Powder, Reconst—Oral: 250 mg/5 ml, 100 ml: **$3.75-$14.58**

PRECAUTIONS: Hypersensitivity to cephalosporins, renal insufficiency, prolonged or repeated therapy, neonates

PREGNANCY AND LACTATION: Pregnancy category B; potential exists for modification of bowel flora in nursing infant, allergy or sensitization, and interference with interpretation of culture results if fever workup required

SIDE EFFECTS/ADVERSE REACTIONS

CNS: Chills, fever, headache
CV: Phlebitis, thrombophlebitis
GI: Increased AST, ALT
GU: Hemorrhagic cystitis, interstitial nephritis, nephropathy
HEME: Eosinophilia, *bone marrow suppression,* positive Coombs test, *thrombocytopenia*
MS: Myalgia
SKIN: Pain at inj site, pruritus, rash, sterile abscess at inj site
MISC: Serum sickness-like reactions

---

* = non-FDA-approved use

INTERACTIONS
Drugs
▣ *Chloramphenicol:* Inhibited antibacterial activity of oxacillin, ensure adequate amounts of both agents are given and administer oxacillin a few hours before chloramphenicol

▣ *Methotrexate:* Increased serum methotrexate concentrations

▣ *Tetracyclines:* Inhibited antibacterial activity of oxacillin, ensure adequate amounts of both agents are given and administer oxacillin a few hours before tetracycline

SPECIAL CONSIDERATIONS
• Sodium content of 1 g = 2.8-3.1 mEq

PATIENT/FAMILY EDUCATION
• Administer on an empty stomach (1 hr before or 2 hr after meals)

MONITORING PARAMETERS
• Urinalysis, BUN, serum creatinine, CBC with differential, periodic liver function tests

---

oxamniquine
(ox-am′ni-kwin)
Rx: Vansil
Chemical Class: Tetrahydroquinoline derivative
Therapeutic Class: Anthelmintic

CLINICAL PHARMACOLOGY
Mechanism of Action: Dislodges schistosomes from usual site of residence in mesenteric veins to liver where they are retained and subsequently killed by host tissue reactions; causes contraction and paralysis of musculature and subsequent immobilization of the worm's suckers; laying of eggs by females ceases within 24-48 hr substantially reducing egg load and eliminating principal cause of pathology associated with schistosomal infection

Pharmacokinetics
PO: Peak 1-1½ hr; extensively metabolized to inactive metabolites, excreted in urine; $t_{\frac{1}{2}}$ 1-2½ hr

INDICATIONS AND USES: All stages of *Schistosoma mansoni* infection; single-dose treatment of neurocysticercosis (in combination with praziquantel)*

DOSAGE
Adult
• PO 12-15 mg/kg as a single dose (Western Hemisphere strains of *Schistosoma mansoni*); 30-60 mg/kg given in 2-4 equally divided doses of 15 mg/kg bid for 1-2 days (African and Middle Eastern strains of *Schistosoma mansoni*)

Child <30 kg
• PO 20 mg/kg given in 2 divided doses of 10 mg/kg with 2-8 hr between doses

▣ **AVAILABLE FORMS/COST OF THERAPY**
• Cap, Gel—Oral: 250 mg, 24's: **$130.61**

PRECAUTIONS: Seizure disorder

PREGNANCY AND LACTATION: Pregnancy category C

SIDE EFFECTS/ADVERSE REACTIONS
CNS: Dizziness, drowsiness, headache, ***seizures (rare)***

GI: Abdominal pain, anorexia, mild to moderate liver enzyme elevations, nausea, vomiting

GU: Orange-red discoloration of urine

SKIN: Urticaria

SPECIAL CONSIDERATIONS
• Alternate to praziquantel for *Schistosoma mansoni,* little effect against other *Schistosoma*

PATIENT/FAMILY EDUCATION
• Take with food

• May cause orange-red discoloration of urine

---

oxandrolone

(ox-an'droe-lone)

Rx: Oxandrin

Chemical Class: Halogenated testosterone derivative

Therapeutic Class: Androgen

DEA Class: Schedule III

CLINICAL PHARMACOLOGY

Mechanism of Action: Promotes body tissue-building processes and reverses catabolic processes when administered with adequate calories and protein; inhibits endogenous testosterone release

Pharmacokinetics

PO: Metabolized in liver, excreted in urine

INDICATIONS AND USES: Promotion of weight gain following extensive surgery, chronic infection, or severe trauma; protein catabolism associated with prolonged administration of corticosteroids; bone pain associated with osteoporosis; alcololic hepatitis;* short stature associated with Turner's syndrome;* HIV wasting syndrome and HIV-associated muscle weakness;* constitutional delay of growth and puberty,* severe refractory hypertriglyceridemia*

DOSAGE

Adult

• PO 2.5 mg bid-qid for 2-4 wk; repeat intermittently prn; range of effective doses 2.5-20 mg/day

Child

• PO total daily dose is ≤0.1 mg/kg or ≤0.045 mg/lb; repeat intermittently prn

$ **AVAILABLE FORMS/COST OF THERAPY**

• Tab, Uncoated—Oral: 2.5 mg, 100's: **$427.50**

CONTRAINDICATIONS: Male patients with prostate or breast cancer, hypercalcemia in females with breast cancer, nephrosis, nephrotic phase of nephritis, hypercalcemia, enhancement of physical appearance or athletic performance

PRECAUTIONS: Elderly, children, cardiac disease, renal disease, hepatic disease, seizure disorder, migraine headache, diabetes

PREGNANCY AND LACTATION: Pregnancy category X; use extreme caution in nursing mothers

SIDE EFFECTS/ADVERSE REACTIONS

CNS: Choreiform movement, depression, excitation, habituation, insomnia

CV: Edema, **CHF**

EENT: Deepening of voice, hoarseness

GI: Cholestatic jaundice, diarrhea, **hepatic necrosis, hepatocellular neoplasms,** nausea, **peliosis hepatis,** vomiting

GU: Amenorrhea, clitoral hypertrophy, decreased breast size, decreased libido, menstrual irregularities, testicular atrophy, vaginitis, virilization

METAB: Decreased glucose tolerance, decreased HDL, increased LDL, increased serum cholesterol, retention of sodium, chloride, water, potassium, phosphates, calcium

MS: Premature closure of epiphyses in children

SKIN: Acne, alopecia, flushing, hirsutism, male pattern baldness, rash, sweating

INTERACTIONS

Drugs

3 *Antidiabetic agents:* Enhanced hypoglycemic effects

---

* = non-FDA-approved use

❷ *Cyclosporine:* Increased cyclosporine concentrations, toxicity

❸ *HMG-CoA reductase inhibitors (lovastatin, pravastatin):* Myositis risk increased

❸ *Tacrolimus:* Increased tacrolimus concentrations, toxicity

❷ *Oral anticoagulants:* Enhanced hypoprothrombinemic response

SPECIAL CONSIDERATIONS
• Anabolic steroids have potential for abuse, especially in the athlete

PATIENT/FAMILY EDUCATION
• Adequate dietary intake of calories and protein essential for successful treatment

MONITORING PARAMETERS
• LFTs, lipids
• Growth rate in children (X-rays for bone age q 6 mo)
• Serum calcium in breast cancer patients

oxaprozin

(ox-a-pro′zin)
Rx: Daypro
Chemical Class: Propionic acid derivative
Therapeutic Class: NSAID with analgesic and antipyretic activity

CLINICAL PHARMACOLOGY
Mechanism of Action: Reversible cyclooxygenase (i.e., prostaglandin synthetase) inhibitor; nonselectively decreases the formation of both prostaglandins and thromboxane A2; variable effects on lipoxygenase synthesis and subsequent leukotriene production; antiinflammatory, antipyretic, and analgesic activity; inhibits platelet aggregation

Pharmacokinetics
PO: Peak 3-5 hr; 99.9% bound to plasma proteins; metabolized in liver to inactive metabolites, excreted in urine (65%) and feces (35%); $t_{1/2}$ 42-50 hr

INDICATIONS AND USES: Osteoarthritis, rheumatoid arthritis, prevention of cognitive decline,* acute gout,* pain—mild to moderate, tendonitis/bursitis*

DOSAGE
Adult
• PO 600-1200 mg qd, individualize dosage to lowest effective dose; max 1800 mg/day or 26 mg/kg/day, whichever is lower

AVAILABLE FORMS/COST OF THERAPY
• Tab, Uncoated—Oral: 600 mg, 100's: **$148.11-$181.79**

CONTRAINDICATIONS: Bronchospasm, nasal polyps, angioedema precipitated by aspirin or other NSAIDs

PRECAUTIONS: History of GI ulceration, bleeding, or perforation; renal dysfunction, hypertension or cardiac conditions aggravated by fluid retention and edema, history of liver dysfunction, history of coagulation disorders

PREGNANCY AND LACTATION: Pregnancy category C (category D if used in 3rd trimester); could cause constriction of the ductus arteriosus *in utero,* persistent pulmonary hypertension of the newborn, or prolonged labor

SIDE EFFECTS/ADVERSE REACTIONS
CNS: Dizziness, headache, lightheadedness
CV: Chest pain, ***CHF, dysrhythmias,*** edema, hypertension, hypotension, palpitation, tachycardia
EENT: Dry eyes, hearing disturbances, photophobia, tinnitus, visual disturbances

italic = common side effects   ***bold italic*** = life-threatening reactions

GI: Abdominal cramps, constipation, diarrhea, *dyspepsia,* flatulence, **gastric or duodenal ulcer with bleeding or perforation,** hepatitis, *nausea,* occult blood in stool, ***pancreatitis,*** vomiting

GU: ***Acute renal failure***

HEME: **Agranulocytosis,** eosinophilia, **leukopenia, neutropenia, pancytopenia, thrombocytopenia**

METAB: Hyperglycemia, hyperkalemia, hypoglycemia, hyponatremia

RESP: **Bronchospasm,** dyspnea, pulmonary infiltrates

SKIN: Photosensitivity, rash, urticaria

INTERACTIONS

Drugs

❸ *Aminoglycosides:* Reduced clearance with elevated aminoglycoside levels and potential for toxicity (especially indomethacin in premature infants; other NSAIDs probably)

❸ *Anticoagulants:* Excessive hypoprothrombinemia, decreased platelet aggregation with increased risk of GI bleeding

❸ *Antihypertensives (α-blockers, angiotensin-converting enzyme inhibitors, angiotensin II receptor blockers, β-blockers, diuretics):* Inhibition of antihypertensive and other favorable hemodynamic effects

❸ *Corticosteroids:* Increased risk of GI ulceration

❸ *Cyclosporine:* Increased nephrotoxicity risk

❸ *Lithium:* Decreased clearance of lithium (mediated via prostaglandins) resulting in elevated serum lithium levels and risk of toxicity

❸ *Methotrexate:* Decreased renal secretion of methotrexate resulting in elevated methotrexate levels and risk of toxicity

❸ *Phenylpropanolamine:* Possible acute hypertensive reaction

❸ *Potassium-sparing diuretics:* Additive hyperkalemia potential

❸ *Triamterene:* Acute renal failure reported with addition of indomethacin; caution with other NSAIDs

SPECIAL CONSIDERATIONS

• No significant advantage over other NSAIDs; cost should govern use

PATIENT/FAMILY EDUCATION

• Avoid aspirin and alcoholic beverages

• Take with food, milk, or antacids to decrease GI upset

MONITORING PARAMETERS

• Initial hemogram and fecal occult blood test within 3 mo of starting regular chronic therapy; repeat every 6-12 mo (more frequently in high-risk patients (>65 years, peptic ulcer disease, concurrent steroids or anticoagulants); electrolytes, creatinine, and BUN within 3 mo of starting regular chronic therapy; repeat every 6-12 mo

---

oxazepam

(ox-a′ze-pam)

Rx: Serax

Chemical Class: Benzodiazepine

Therapeutic Class: Anxiolytic

DEA Class: Schedule IV

CLINICAL PHARMACOLOGY

Mechanism of Action: CNS depressant via facilitation of inhibitory GABA at benzodiazepine receptor sites (BZ_1—associated with sleep; BZ_2—associated with memory, motor, sensory, and cognitive function); effects include muscle relaxation (spinal cord), anticonvulsant activity (brain stem), ataxia (cerebellum), emotional behavior (limbic and cortical areas), and anxiolytic effects (separate from general CNS depression)

Pharmacokinetics

PO: Peak 2-4 hr, onset of action intermediate compared to other benzodiazepines; 86%-96% bound to plasma proteins; metabolized via conjugation to inactive metabolites, excreted in urine as unchanged drug (50%) and metabolites; $t_{1/2}$ 5-15 hr

INDICATIONS AND USES: Anxiety disorders; anxiety associated with depression; management of anxiety, tension, agitation, irritability in older patients; alcohol withdrawal; irritable bowel*

DOSAGE

Adult

• PO 10-30 mg tid-qid

ⓢ AVAILABLE FORMS/COST OF THERAPY

• Cap, Gel—Oral: 10 mg, 100's: **$16.50-$96.86**; 15 mg, 100's: **$23.80-$122.30**; 30 mg, 100's: **$33.80-$176.89**

• Tab, Uncoated—Oral: 15 mg, 100's: **$26.45-$117.64**

CONTRAINDICATIONS: Narrowangle glaucoma, psychosis

PRECAUTIONS: Elderly, debilitated, hepatic disease, renal disease, history of drug abuse, abrupt withdrawal, respiratory depression

PREGNANCY AND LACTATION: Pregnancy category D; may cause fetal damage when administered during pregnancy; excreted into breast milk, may accumulate in breast-fed infants and is therefore not recommended

SIDE EFFECTS/ADVERSE REACTIONS

CNS: Abnormal thinking, agitation, amnesia, anxiety, apathy, *asthenia,* ataxia, decreased libido, decreased reflexes, emotional lability, hang-

over, hostility, *hypokinesia,* neuritis, seizure, sleep disorder, *somnolence,* stupor, twitch

CV: **Dysrhythmia,** syncope

EENT: Ear pain; epistaxis, eye irritation, pain, pharyngitis, photophobia, rhinitis, sinusitis, swelling

GI: Abdominal pain, decreased, increased appetite; dyspepsia; enterocolitis, flatulence, gastritis, melena, mouth ulceration

GU: Frequent urination, hematuria, itching; menstrual cramps; nocturia, oliguria, penile discharge, urinary hesitancy, urgency; urinary incontinence, vaginal discharge

HEME: **Agranulocytosis**

MS: Back pain, lower extremity pain

RESP: Asthma, cold symptoms, cough, dyspnea, hyperventilation

SKIN: Acne, dry skin, photosensitivity, urticaria

INTERACTIONS

Drugs

🔒 *Ethanol:* Enhanced adverse psychomotor effects of benzodiazepines

Labs

• *False increase:* Serum glucose

SPECIAL CONSIDERATIONS

• Niche compared to other benzodiazepines: treatment of anxiety in patients with hepatic disease; consider for alcohol withdrawal

• Tablet form contains tartrazine; risk of allergic-type reactions especially in patients with aspirin hypersensitivity

PATIENT/FAMILY EDUCATION

• Avoid alcohol and other CNS depressants

• Do not discontinue abruptly after prolonged therapy

• Inform clinician if planning to become pregnant, pregnant, or become pregnant while taking this medicine

• May be habit forming

MONITORING PARAMETERS
• Periodic CBC, UA, blood chemistry analyses during prolonged therapy

---

oxcarbazepine

(oks-kar-bays'uh-peen)
Rx: Trileptal
Chemical Class: Dibenzazepine
Therapeutic Class: Antiepileptic

CLINICAL PHARMACOLOGY
Mechanism of Action: Blockade of voltage-sensitive sodium channels, resulting in stabilization of hyperexcited neural membranes, inhibition of repetitive neuronal firing, and diminution of propagation of synaptic impulses, actions important in the prevention of seizure spread
Pharmacokinetics
PO: Peak: T_{max} 4.5 hr (parent and major metabolite) Completely absorbed (PO), tablets and suspension, equal bioavailability, no food effect on absorption; Vd of major metabolite, 10-monohydroxy oxcarbazepine (MHD) 49 L, 40% bound to plasma proteins; oxcarbazepine is essentially a prodrug, rapidly converted to 10-monohydroxy metabolite [MHD], 95% of drug excreted in urine as metabolites (1% as unchanged drug); $t_{1/2}$ of oxcarbazepine 2 hr; $t_{1/2}$ of MHD 9 hr
INDICATIONS AND USES: Epilepsy, monotherapy and adjunctive use for partial seizures; bipolar disorder*; panic disorder*; spasticity*; trigeminal neuralgia*

DOSAGE
Adult and Child >16 yr
• *Monotherapy:* initial: 300 mg bid; increase at 2 week intervals by up to 600 mg/day; maintenance 2400 mg/day
• Conversion from another antiepileptic drug (AED) initiate with 300 mg bid; simultaneously, reduction of the concomitant AED should begin; increase oxcarbazepine dose at weekly intervals (600 mg/day increments) to a maximum of 2400 mg/day in 2-4 weeks; terminate concomitant AED over 3-6 weeks; monitor closely
• *Trigeminal neuralgia:* 300 mg bid-qid; dosage increases weekly until pain control achieved; max 2400 mg/day
• *Dosage in renal failure:* CrCl <30 ml/min: 150 mg bid (½ dose); increase slowly based on response
• *Dosage in geriatric patients:* Plasma conc and AUC 30-60% higher (presumable due to age-related reductions in creatinine clearance); initiate at low dosage and titrate slowly to response
Child 4-16 yr
• *Note:* PK parameters in children over 8 years of age are similar to those in adults, but clearance in younger children is approximately 30-40% greater than in older children and adults
• *Adjunctive therapy:* 4-5 mg/kg bid, not to exceed 600 mg/day; maintenance dose should be attained within 2 weeks: 20-29 kg - 900 mg/day; 29.1-39 kg - 1200 mg/day; >39 kg - 1800 mg
• *Monotherapy:* Titrate up to 30 mg/kg/day divided bid over 1-3 weeks

💲 AVAILABLE FORMS/COST OF THERAPY
• Liq—Oral: 300 mg/5 ml, 250 ml: **$92.65**

---

* = non-FDA-approved use

• Tab, Coated—Oral: 150 mg (yellow-ovaloid) 100's: **$100.23**; 300 mg (yellow-ovaloid) 100's: **$183.03**; 600 mg (yellow-ovaloid) 100's: **$336.39**

CONTRAINDICATIONS: Hypersensitivity

PRECAUTIONS: Alcohol, CNS adverse effects, hormonal contraceptives, hypothyroidism, rapid withdrawal may precipitate seizures

PREGNANCY AND LACTATION: Pregnancy category C, increased incidence of fetal structural abnormalities and other manifestation of developmental toxicity have been observed in the offspring of animals; no adequate and well-controlled data in humans; oxcarbazepine and MHD both excreted in human breast milk; milk:plasma ratio: 0.5 (both)

SIDE EFFECTS/ADVERSE REACTIONS

CNS: Concentration difficulties, coordination abnormalities (ataxia, gait disturbances), cognitive symptoms, fatigue (15%), headache, insomnia, nystagmus, psychomotor slowing, speech or language problems, somnolence, tremor

EENT: Diplopia, abnormal vision

GI: Abdominal pain, dyspepsia, nausea, vomiting

GU: UTI, micturition frequency, vaginitis

METAB: Hyponatremia

SKIN: Rash

INTERACTIONS

Drugs

• *Note:* Oxcarbazepine is an inhibitor of CYP2C19 and an inducer of CYP3A4 and CYP3A5

3 *Alcohol:* Additive CND depression and psychomotor impairment

3 *Barbiturates:* Decreases oxcarbazepine levels

3 *Benzodiazepines:* Additive CNS effects

3 *Calcium channel blockers (dihydropyridines):* Induction of antihypertensive metabolism; decreased antihypertensive efficacy

3 *Estradiol, oral contraceptives:* Induction of hepatic metabolism; decreased hormonal efficacy

3 *Medroxyprogesterone:* Induction of hepatic metabolism; decreased hormonal efficacy

3 *Lamotrigine:* Induction of hepatic metabolism; decreased lamotrigine levels by 30%

3 *Phenytoin:* Alterations in hepatic metabolism resulting in increases in phenytoin levels/risk of toxicity and decreases in oxcarbazepine

3 *Verapamil:* Decreased plasma oxcarbazepine concetrations

Labs

• *Thyroid levels:* Decreased

• *Serum sodium:* Decreased; increased risk of hyponatremia

SPECIAL CONSIDERATIONS

• Considered an alternative to carbamazepine in intolerant patients

PATIENT/FAMILY EDUCATION

• Review and reinforce prevalence of CNS adverse effects early in treatment (reason for gradual titration regimens) with tolerance developing with continued adherence

• Risk of recurrent seizures with missed doses

MONITORING PARAMETERS

• Seizure frequency and electroencephalogram changes in patients with seizure disorder; a reduction or elimination of pain in patients with trigeminal neuralgia; therapeutic serum levels not adequately established - estimates of therapeutic serum concentrations of the active metabolite (MHD) in the 50-110 µmol range; serum electrolytes (especially sodium), LFTs, blood counts, serum lipids

oxiconazole

(ox-i-con´a-zole)
Rx: Oxistat
Chemical Class: Synthetic imidazole derivative
Therapeutic Class: Antifungal

CLINICAL PHARMACOLOGY
Mechanism of Action: Alteration of the fungal cell membrane, which allows leakage of essential intracellular components
Pharmacokinetics
TOP: Low systemic absorption
INDICATIONS AND USES: Tinea pedis (athlete's foot), tinea cruris (jock itch), and tinea corporis (ringworm) due to *Trichophyton rubrum, T. mentagrophytes,* and *Epidermophyton floccosum,* tinea (pityriasis) versicolor
DOSAGE
Adult and Child
• TOP apply to affected area(s) qd for 2 wk (jock itch, ringworm) or 4 wk (athlete's foot)
$ AVAILABLE FORMS/COST OF THERAPY
• Cre—Top: 1%, 15, 30, 60 g: **$35.24**/30 g
• Lotion—Top: 1% 30 ml: **$28.73**
PREGNANCY AND LACTATION: Pregnancy category B; excreted in breast milk
SIDE EFFECTS/ADVERSE REACTIONS
SKIN: Burning, contact dermatitis, dyshidrotic eczema, erythema, fissuring, folliculitis, irritation, maceration, nodules, pain, papules, pruritus, rash, scaling, stinging, tingling
SPECIAL CONSIDERATIONS
• Niche: once daily imadazole; base choice on cost and convenience
PATIENT/FAMILY EDUCATION
• For external use only, avoid contact with eyes or vagina

oxtriphylline

(ox-trye´fi-lin)
Rx: Choledyl SA
Chemical Class: Xanthine derivative (64% theophylline)
Therapeutic Class: Antiasthmatic, bronchodilator; COPD agent

CLINICAL PHARMACOLOGY
Mechanism of Action: Directly relaxes bronchial and pulmonary blood vessel smooth muscle; stimulates CNS; induces diuresis; increases gastric acid secretion, lowers lower esophageal sphincter pressure; is a central respiratory stimulant; exact mechanism unproven but may involve antagonism of pulmonary adenosine receptors
Pharmacokinetics
PO: Peak 4 hr; metabolized by liver, excreted in urine; $t_{1/2}$ 3-12 hr; $t_{1/2}$ increased in geriatric patients, hepatic disease, cor pulmonale, and CHF, decreased in children and smokers
INDICATIONS AND USES: Asthma, reversible bronchospasm associated with chronic bronchitis and emphysema
DOSAGE
Adult
• PO 800-1200 mg/d divided q12h; smokers may require more frequent dosing; adjust dose based on measurement of serum theophylline concentrations
$ AVAILABLE FORMS/COST OF THERAPY
• Tab, Enteric Coated—Oral: 200 mg, 100's: **$28.88**
• Tab, Coated, Sus Action—Oral: 400 mg, 100's: **$39.19**; 600 mg, 100's: **$47.02**

---

* = non-FDA-approved use

CONTRAINDICATIONS: Active peptic ulcer, underlying seizure disorder (not on anticonvulsant therapy)

PRECAUTIONS: Elderly, CHF, cor pulmonale, hepatic disease, pre-existing dysrhythmias, hypertension, hypoxemia, sustained high fever, history of peptic ulcer, alcoholism

PREGNANCY AND LACTATION: Pregnancy category C; pharmacokinetics of theophylline may be altered during pregnancy, monitor serum concentrations carefully; excreted into breast milk, may cause irritability in the nursing infant, otherwise compatible with breast feeding

SIDE EFFECTS/ADVERSE REACTIONS

CNS: Anxiety, *dizziness,* headache, insomnia, lightheadedness, muscle twitching, reflex hyperexcitability, restlessness, *seizures*

CV: **Circulatory failure,** extrasystoles, flushing, hypotension, *palpitations, sinus tachycardia,* **ventricular dysrhythmias**

GI: Anorexia, bitter taste, diarrhea, dyspepsia, epigastric pain, esophageal reflux, hematemesis, *nausea, vomiting*

GU: Proteinuria, urinary frequency

METAB: Hyperglycemia

RESP: Tachypnea

SKIN: Alopecia, urticaria

INTERACTIONS

Drugs

3 *Adenosine:* Inhibited hemodynamic effects of adenosine

3 *Allopurinol, amiodarone, cimetadine, ciprofloxacin, disulfiram, erythromycin, interferon alfa, isoniazid, methimazole, metoprolol, norfloxacin, pefloxacin, pentoxifylline, propafenone, propylthiouracil, radioactive iodine, tacrine, thiabendazole, ticlopidine, verapamil:* Increased theophylline concentrations

3 *Aminoglutethimide, barbiturates, carbamazepine, moricizine, phenytoin, rifampin, ritonavir, thyroid hormone:* Reduced theophylline concentrations; decreased serum phenytoin concentrations

2 *Enoxacin, fluvoxamine, mexiletine, propanolol, troleandomycin:* Increased theophylline concentrations

3 *Imipenem:* Some patients on oxtriphylline have developed seizures following the addition of imipenem

3 *Lithium:* Reduced lithium concentrations

3 *Smoking:* Increased oxtriphylline dosing requirements

Labs

• *False increase:* Serum barbiturate concentrations, urinary uric acid

• *False decrease:* Serum bilirubin

• *Interference:* Plasma somatostatin

SPECIAL CONSIDERATIONS

• Touted to produce less GI side effects; if dosed equipotently based on theophylline equivalents (oxtriphylline = 64% theophylline) no difference; compare costs as well as other characteristics

PATIENT/FAMILY EDUCATION

• Avoid large amounts of caffeine-containing products (tea, coffee, chocolate, colas)

MONITORING PARAMETERS

• Serum theophylline concentrations (therapeutic level is 8-20 µg/ml); toxicity may occur with small increase above 20 µg/ml, especially in the elderly

oxybutynin
(ox-i-byoo´ti-nin)
Rx: Ditropan, Ditropan XL
Chemical Class: Synthetic tertiary amine
Therapeutic Class: Genitourinary muscle relaxant; GI antispasmodic

CLINICAL PHARMACOLOGY
Mechanism of Action: Exerts direct antispasmodic effect on smooth muscle and inhibits action of acetylcholine at postganglionic cholinergic sites; increases bladder capacity and delays initial desire to void by reducing number of motor impulses reaching the detrusor muscle
Pharmacokinetics
PO: Peak 3-6 hr, onset ½-1 hr, duration 6-10 hr; metabolized in liver, eliminated via kidneys

INDICATIONS AND USES: Antispasmodic in uninhibited neurogenic or reflex neurogenic bladder, primary nocturnal enuresis,* antispasmodic in various GI disorders,* diabetic diarrhea,* postgustatory sweating*

DOSAGE
Adult
• PO 5 mg bid-tid; do not exceed 5 mg qid; Sus Action PO 5 mg qd, titrate by 5 mg weekly to effective dose; max 30 mg/day
Child
• PO 1-5 yr 0.2 mg/kg/dose divided bid-qid; >5 yr 5 mg bid, up to 5 mg tid

⑤ AVAILABLE FORMS/COST OF THERAPY
• Syr—Oral: 5 mg/5 ml, 473 ml: **$33.80-$94.75**
• Tab, Uncoated—Oral: 5 mg, 100's: **$15.28-$64.32**
• Tab, Uncoated—Oral: 5 mg, 100's: **$256.25**; 10 mg, 100's: **$278.75**; 15 mg, 100's: **$308.75**

CONTRAINDICATIONS: Angle-closure glaucoma, myasthenia gravis, partial or complete obstruction of the GI tract, adynamic ileus, megacolon, severe colitis, intestinal atony, obstructive uropathy, unstable cardiovascular status

PRECAUTIONS: Elderly, autonomic neuropathy, hepatic or renal disease, hyperthyroidism, CHD, prostatic hypertrophy, reflux esophagitis, ulcerative colitis

PREGNANCY AND LACTATION: Pregnancy category B; may suppress lactation

SIDE EFFECTS/ADVERSE REACTIONS
CNS: Asthenia, dizziness, *drowsiness,* hallucinations, insomnia, restlessness
CV: Palpitations, tachycardia, vasodilation
EENT: Amblyopia, blurred vision, cycloplegia, decreased lacrimation, mydriasis
GI: Constipation, decreased GI motility, *dry mouth,* nausea, vomiting
GU: Impotence, urinary hesitancy and retention
METAB: Suppression of lactation
SKIN: Decreased sweating, rash

SPECIAL CONSIDERATIONS
• Reported anticholinergic side effects not clinically or significantly different from other agents (i.e., propantheline); compare costs

PATIENT/FAMILY EDUCATION
• Avoid prolonged exposure to hot environments, heat prostration may result
• Use caution in driving or other activities requiring alertness
• Swallow extended release tablets whole, do not chew or crush
• Extended release tablet shell not absorbable

* = non-FDA-approved use

oxycodone
(ox-ee-koe´done)

Rx: Oxycontin, Oxy IR, Percolone Oxyfast, Roxicodone

Combinations

Rx: with aspirin (Percodan, Endodan, Roxiprin); with acetaminophen (Percocet, Endocet, Tylox, Roxicet, Roxilox)

Chemical Class: Semisynthetic opium alkaloid; phenanthrene derivative

Therapeutic Class: Narcotic analgesic

DEA Class: Schedule II

CLINICAL PHARMACOLOGY

Mechanism of Action: Narcotic agonist with activity at μ-receptors (supraspinal analgesia, euphoria, respiratory and physical depression, miosis, and reduced GI motility), κ-receptors (pentazocine-like spinal analgesia, sedation, and miosis), and Δ-receptors (dysphoria, psychotomimetic effects [e.g., hallucinations], and respiratory and vasomotor stimulation caused by drugs with antagonist activity); compared to morphine, equal analgesic, antitussive, constipation, respiratory depression, sedation, emesis, and physical dependence effects

Pharmacokinetics

PO: Onset 10-15 min, peak 30-60 min, duration 3-6 hr; metabolized in liver and kidneys, excreted primarily in urine

INDICATIONS AND USES: Moderate to moderately severe pain

DOSAGE

Adult

• PO 5 mg q6h prn

• Sus Action: PO (opioid-naive patients) 10 mg q12h, titrate to adequate pain relief; (patients on fixed ratio opioid/APAP or ASA combinations) 10-20 mg q12h (if taking 1-5 tabs/caps daily of fixed ratio drug), 20-30 mg q12h (6-9 tabs/caps each day), 30-40 mg q12h (10-12 tabs/caps each day), titrate to adequate pain relief; (patients currently on opioid therapy) calculate the total mg amount of current opioid and convert to oxycodone equivalent using conversion chart supplied by manufacturer; (patients on transdermal fentanyl therapy) 18 hours after stopping transdermal fentanyl, initiate 10 mg q12h for every 25 μg/hr fentanyl patch, titrate to adequate pain relief

Child

• PO 6-12 yr 1.25 mg q6h prn; >12 yr 2.5 mg q6h prn

$ **AVAILABLE FORMS/COST OF THERAPY**

• Cap—Oral: 5 mg, 100's: **$29.30-$36.97**

• Sol—Oral: 5 mg/5 ml, 500 ml: **$41.65**; 20 mg/ml, 30 ml: **$33.75-$40.78**

• Tab, Uncoated—Oral: 5 mg, 100's: **$27.00-$68.75**; 15 mg, 100's: **$110.00**; 30 mg, 100's: **$212.00**

• Tab, Sus Action—Oral: 10 mg, 100's: **$129.21**; 20 mg, 100's: **$247.28**; 40 mg, 100's: **$438.75**; 80 mg, 100's: **$825.08**; 160 mg, 100's: **$1,555.71**

CONTRAINDICATIONS: Acute bronchial asthma, upper airway obstruction

PRECAUTIONS: Head injury, increased intracranial pressure, acute abdominal conditions, elderly, severe impairment of hepatic or renal function, hypothyroidism, Addison's disease, prostatic hypertrophy, urethral stricture, history of drug abuse

PREGNANCY AND LACTATION: Pregnancy category B (category D if used for prolonged periods or in high doses at term); excreted into breast milk

SIDE EFFECTS/ADVERSE REACTIONS

CNS: Agitation, dependency, dizziness, *drowsiness,* lethargy, restlessness, *sedation*

CV: Bradycardia, orthostatic hypotension, palpitations, tachycardia

GI: Anorexia, constipation, nausea, vomiting

GU: Urinary retention

*RESP: **Respiratory depression, respiratory paralysis***

SKIN: Flushing, rash, urticaria

INTERACTIONS

Drugs

⬛ *Amitriptylline:* Additive respiratory and CNS-depressant effects

⬛ *Antihistamines, chloral hydrate, glutethimide, methocarbamol:* Enhanced depressant effects

⬛ *Barbiturates:* Additive respiratory and CNS depressant effects

⬛ *Cimetidine:* Increased respiratory and CNS depression

⬛ *Clomipramine:* Additive respiratory and CNS depressant effects

⬛ *Ethanol:* Additive CNS effects

⬛ *MAOI's:* Markedly potentiate the actions of morphine

⬛ *Nortriptylline:* Additive respiratory and CNS depressant effects

⬛ *Protease inhibitors:* Increased CNS and respiratory depression

Labs

• *False increase:* Amylase and lipase

SPECIAL CONSIDERATIONS

PATIENT/FAMILY EDUCATION

• Physical dependency may result when used for extended periods

• Change position slowly, orthostatic hypotension may occur

• Do not administer agonist/antagonist analgesics (i.e., pentazocine, nalbuphine, butorphanol, dezocine, buprenorphine) to patient who has received a prolonged course of oxycodone (a pure agonist). In opioid-dependent patients, mixed agonist/antagonist analgesics may precipitate withdrawal symptoms

---

oxymetazoline
(ox-ee-met-az´oh-leen)

OTC: (Nasal): 4-way long lasting, Afrin 12-Hour, Benzedrex 12 hr, Cheracol, Dristan 12-hour, Duramist Plus, Duration, Genasal, Neo-Synephrine 12-Hour, Oxymata 12, Vicks Sinex 12-Hour Ultra Fine Mist; (Ophthalmic): Ocu Clear, Visine L.R.

Chemical Class: Imidazoline derivative

Therapeutic Class: Decongestant

CLINICAL PHARMACOLOGY

Mechanism of Action: Local α-adrenergic-mediated vasoconstriction on dilated conjunctival and nasal mucosal blood vessels

Pharmacokinetics

TOP: Onset 5-10 min, duration 5-6 hr; some systemic absorption

INDICATIONS AND USES: Nasal congestion; eye redness due to minor eye irritations

DOSAGE

Adult and Child ≥6 yr

• NASAL 2-3 gtt or sprays of 0.05% sol instilled into each nostril bid; do not exceed 3-5 days duration

• CONJUNCTIVAL 1 gtt q6h; do not exceed 3-4 days duration

Child 2-5 yr

• NASAL 2-3 gtt of 0.025% sol instilled into each nostril bid; do not exceed 3-5 days duration

💲 **AVAILABLE FORMS/COST OF THERAPY**

• Sol—Nasal: 0.025%, 20 ml: **$3.52-$4.82**; 0.05%, 15, 30 ml: **$1.84**/30 ml

• Spray—Nasal: 0.05%, 15, 30 ml: **$0.76-$7.24**/30 ml

• Sol—Ophth: 0.025%, 15, 30 ml: **$3.89-$5.42**/30 ml

CONTRAINDICATIONS: Angle-closure glaucoma

PRECAUTIONS: Children <2 yr, hyperthyroidism, heart disease, hypertension, diabetes mellitus

PREGNANCY AND LACTATION: Pregnancy category C

SIDE EFFECTS/ADVERSE REACTIONS

CNS: Dizziness, headache, nervousness, weakness

CV: Cardiac irregularities, hypertension

EENT: Anosmia; blurred vision, dryness, increased or decreased intraocular pressure; irritation, mild transient stinging, mydriasis, rebound congestion/hyperemia ("rhinitis medicamentosa"), sneezing, stinging, transient burning, ulceration of nasal mucosa

GI: Nausea

SKIN: Sweating

SPECIAL CONSIDERATIONS

• Manage rebound congestion by stopping oxymetazoline: one nostril at a time, substitute systemic decongestant, substitute inhaled steroid

PATIENT/FAMILY EDUCATION

• Do not use for > 3-5 days or rebound congestion may occur

oxymetholone

(ox-ee-meth′oh-lone)

Rx: Anadrol-50

Chemical Class: Halogenated testosterone derivative

Therapeutic Class: Androgen; hematopoietic agent

DEA Class: Schedule III

CLINICAL PHARMACOLOGY

Mechanism of Action: Promotes body tissue-building processes and reverses catabolic processes when administered with adequate calories and protein; inhibits endogenous testosterone release

Pharmacokinetics

PO: Metabolized in liver, excreted in urine

INDICATIONS AND USES: Anemias caused by deficient red cell production, acquired or congenital aplastic anemia, myelofibrosis and hypoplastic anemias due to administration of myelotoxic drugs

DOSAGE

Adult

• PO 1-5 mg/kg/day

💲 **AVAILABLE FORMS/COST OF THERAPY**

• Tab, Uncoated—Oral: 50 mg, 100's: **$1,488.66**

CONTRAINDICATIONS: Hypersensitivity, male patients with prostate or breast cancer, hypercalcemia in females with breast cancer, nephrosis, nephrotic phase of nephritis, enhancement of physical appearance or athletic performance

PRECAUTIONS: Elderly, children, cardiac disease, renal disease, hepatic disease, seizure disorder, migraine headache, diabetes

PREGNANCY AND LACTATION: Pregnancy category X; use extreme caution in nursing mothers

---

italic = common side effects   ***bold italic*** = life-threatening reactions

SIDE EFFECTS/ADVERSE REACTIONS

CNS: Choreiform movement, depression, excitation, habituation, insomnia

CV: Edema, **CHF**

EENT: Deepening of voice, hoarseness

GI: Cholestatic jaundice, diarrhea, **hepatic necrosis, hepatocellular neoplasms,** nausea, **peliosis hepatis,** vomiting

GU: Amenorrhea, clitoral hypertrophy, decreased breast size, decreased libido, testicular atrophy, vaginitis, virilization

HEME: **Leukemia** (observed in several patients with aplastic anemia, role of oxymetholone unclear)

METAB: Decreased glucose tolerance, decreased HDL cholesterol, increased LDL cholesterol, increased serum cholesterol; retention of sodium, chloride, water, potassium, phosphates, calcium

MS: Premature closure of epiphyses in children

SKIN: Acne, alopecia, flushing, hirsutism, rash, sweating

INTERACTIONS

Drugs

3 *Antidiabetic agents:* Enhanced hypoglycemic effects

2 *Cyclosporine:* Increased cyclosporine concentrations, toxicity

3 *HMG-CoA reductase inhibitors (lovastatin, prevastatin):* Myositis risk increased

3 *Tacrolimus:* Increased tacrolimus concentrations, potential for toxicity

2 *Oral anticoagulants:* Enhanced hypoprothrombinemic response

SPECIAL CONSIDERATIONS

• Anabolic steroids have potential for abuse, especially in the athlete

• Comparative advantages include less potential for virilization in women, convenience of oral administration; disadvantage includes increased risk of hepatotoxicity

PATIENT/FAMILY EDUCATION

• Hematologic response is often not immediate, needs minimum trial of 3-6 mo

MONITORING PARAMETERS

• LFTs, lipids, Hct

• Serum calcium in breast cancer patients

• Growth rate in children (X-rays for bone age q 6 mo)

---

oxymorphone

(ox-ee-mor′fone)

Rx: Numorphan

Chemical Class: Synthetic opium alkaloid; phenanthrene derivative

Therapeutic Class: Narcotic analgesic

DEA Class: Schedule II

CLINICAL PHARMACOLOGY

Mechanism of Action: Narcotic agonist with activity at μ-receptors (supraspinal analgesia, euphoria, respiratory and physical depression, miosis, and reduced GI motility), κ-receptors (pentazocine-like spinal analgesia, sedation, and miosis), and Δ-receptors (dysphoria, psychotomimetic effects [e.g., hallucinations], and respiratory and vasomotor stimulation caused by drugs with antagonist activity); compared to morphine, equal analgesia, and constipation; less antitussive; more emesis, respiratory depression, and physical dependence

Pharmacokinetics

PR: Onset 15-30 min, duration 3-6 hr

IV: Onset 5-10 min, duration 3-6 hr

SC/IM: Onset 10-15 min, duration 3-6 hr

Metabolized primarily in liver, excreted mainly in urine

INDICATIONS AND USES: Moderate to severe pain, preoperative sedation, analgesia during labor, pulmonary edema (not arising from chemical respiratory irritant)

DOSAGE

Adult

• SC/IM 1-1.5 mg q4-6h prn; IV 0.5 mg; PR 5 mg q4-6h prn

• *Analgesia during labor:* IM 0.5-1 mg

$ AVAILABLE FORMS/COST OF THERAPY

• Inj, Sol—IM, IV, SC: 1 mg/ml, 1 ml: **$3.88**; 1.5 mg/ml, 10 ml: **$49.00**

• Supp—Rect: 5 mg, 6's: **$27.50**

CONTRAINDICATIONS: Acute bronchial asthma, upper airway obstruction

PRECAUTIONS: Head injury, increased intracranial pressure, acute abdominal conditions, elderly, severe impairment of hepatic or renal function, hypothyroidism, Addison's disease, prostatic hypertrophy, urethral stricture, history of drug abuse, children

PREGNANCY AND LACTATION: Pregnancy category B (category D if used for prolonged periods or in high doses at term); use during labor produces neonatal respiratory depression

SIDE EFFECTS/ADVERSE REACTIONS

CNS: Agitation, dependency, dizziness, *drowsiness,* lethargy, restlessness, *sedation*

CV: Bradycardia, orthostatic hypotension, palpitations, tachycardia

GI: Anorexia, constipation, nausea, vomiting

GU: Urinary retention

*RESP: **Respiratory depression, respiratory paralysis***

SKIN: Flushing, rash, urticaria

INTERACTIONS

Drugs

❸ *Barbiturates:* Additive CNS depression

❸ *Cimetidine:* Increased effect of narcotic analgesics

❷ *Ethanol:* Additive CNS effects

❸ *Neuroleptics:* Hypotension and excessive CNS depression

Labs

• *False increase:* Amylase and lipase

SPECIAL CONSIDERATIONS

• Do not administer agonist/antagonist analgesics (i.e., pentazocine, nalbuphine, butorphanol, dezocine, buprenorphine) to patient who has received a prolonged course of oxymorphone (a pure agonist). In opioid-dependent patients, mixed agonist/antagonist analgesics may precipitate withdrawal symptoms.

PATIENT/FAMILY EDUCATION

• Physical dependency may result when used for extended periods

• Change position slowly, orthostatic hypotension may occur

---

oxytetracycline
(ox′ee-tet-tra-sye′kleen)
Rx: Terramycin
Combinations
  Rx: with polymyxin (Terek); with phenazopyridine, sulfamethizole (Urobiotic-250, Tija)
Chemical Class: Tetracycline derivative
Therapeutic Class: Antibiotic

CLINICAL PHARMACOLOGY
Mechanism of Action: Inhibits protein synthesis in microorganisms by binding at the bacterial 30S ribosomal subunit; bacteriostatic

---

italic = common side effects   ***bold italic*** = life-threatening reactions

Pharmacokinetics

PO: Peak 2-4 hr; absorption 50%, decreased by food; 20%-40% protein bound; $t_{1/2}$ 6-10 hr; excreted in urine, bile, feces in active form

INDICATIONS AND USES: Treatment of infections caused by the following susceptible organisms:

• Gram-positive organisms: *Streptococcus* spp. (44%-74% resistant), *Diplococcus pneumoniae*

• Gram-negative organisms: *E. coli, Enterobacter aerogenes, Shigella* spp., *Actinobacter calcoaceticus, Haemophilus influenzae, H. ducreyi, Klebsiella* spp., *Yersinia pestis, Francisella tularensis, Bartonella bacilliformis, Bacteroides* spp., *Campylobacter fetus, Brucella* spp. (in conjunction with streptomycin)

• Miscellaneous organisms: *Treponema pallidum, T. pertenue* (syph- ilis and yaws), *Chlamydia trachomatis,* agents of lymphogranuloma venereum and granuloma inguinale, rickettsial infections, agents of psittacosis and ornithosis, *Mycoplasma pneumoniae, Borrelia recurrentis, Neisseria gonorrhoeae, N. meningitidis* (IV only), *Listeria monocytogenes, Clostridium* spp., *Bacillus anthracis, Fusobacterium fusiforme, Actinomyces* spp.

DOSAGE

Adult

• *Moderate to severe infections:* PO 250-500 mg q6h; IM 100 mg q8h or 150 mg q12h

• *Gonorrhea:* PO 1.5 g, then 500 mg qid for a total of 9 g

• *Chlamydia trachomatis:* PO 500 mg qid × 7 days

• *Syphilis:* PO 2-3 g in divided doses × 10-15 days up to 30-40 g total (not agent of first choice)

• *Acne:* PO 250 mg qid × 2 wk; then 250-500 mg qd

• Dosage adjustment necessary in renal impairment

Child >8 yr

• *Moderate to severe infections:* PO 25-50 mg/kg/day in divided doses q6h; IM 15-25 mg/kg/day in divided doses q8-12h

$ **AVAILABLE FORMS/COST OF THERAPY**

• Cap—Oral: 250 mg, 100's: **$87.72**

• Inj, Sol—IM: 50 mg/ml, 10 ml, 5's: **$51.70**

PRECAUTIONS: Renal disease, hepatic disease, last trimester of pregnancy, neonatal period and early childhood (may cause permanent tooth discoloration in children <8 yr), direct sunlight exposure, outdated products (have been associated with Fanconi's syndrome), sulfite sensitivity, hiatal hernia

PREGNANCY AND LACTATION: Pregnancy category D; excreted into breast milk; milk:plasma ratio: 0.6-0.8; theoretically, may cause dental staining, but usually undetectable in infant serum (<0.05 µg/ml)

SIDE EFFECTS/ADVERSE REACTIONS

CNS: Fever, pseudotumor cerebri

CV: Pericarditis

EENT: Decreased calcification of deciduous teeth, dysphagia, glossitis, oral candidiasis

GI: Abdominal cramps, abdominal pain, anorexia, black, hairy tongue; *diarrhea,* dysphagia, enterocolitis, epigastric burning, fatty liver, flatulence, ***hepatotoxicity,*** nausea, proctitis, pruritus ani, sore throat; stomatitis, vomiting

GU: Increased BUN

HEME: Eosinophilia, ***hemolytic anemia, leukocytosis, neutropenia, thrombocytopenia***

---

* = non-FDA-approved use

SKIN: Angioedema, ***exfoliative dermatitis,*** increased pigmentation, onycholysis and discoloration of nails, pain at inj site, *photosensitivity,* pruritus, *rash, urticaria*

MISC: Tooth discoloration in children <8 yr

INTERACTIONS
Drugs
❷ *Antacids:* Reduced absorption of oxytetracycline

❸ *Bismuth salts:* Reduced absorption of oxytetracycline

❸ *Calcium:* See antacids

❸ *Food:* Reduced absorption of oxytetracycline

❸ *Iron:* Reduced absorption of oxytetracycline

❸ *Magnesium:* See antacids

❷ *Methoxyflurane:* Increased risk of nephrotoxicity

❸ *Oral contraceptives:* Interruption of enterohepatic circulation of estrogens, reduced oral contraceptive effectiveness

❸ *Zinc:* Reduced absorption of oxytetracycline

Labs
• *False negative:* Urine glucose with Clinistix or TesTape

• *Interference:* Uroporphyrin

• *False increase:* Urinary and plasma catecholamines, serum bilirubin, CFS protein, urine glucose, serum uric acid, urine vanillylmandelic acid

SPECIAL CONSIDERATIONS
• Offers no significant advantage over tetracycline; shares similar spectrum of activity (may be slightly less active than tetracycline and has longer dosage interval)

PATIENT/FAMILY EDUCATION
• Avoid milk products, take with a full glass of water

oxytocin
(ox-ee-toe′sin)
Rx: Pitocin, Syntocinon
Chemical Class: Synthetic polypeptide
Therapeutic Class: Oxytocic, galactokinetic

CLINICAL PHARMACOLOGY
Mechanism of Action: Produced by the posterior pituitary, augments the number of contracting myofibrils in the uterus, producing contraction; induces alveolar milk ejection (not production); has weak antidiuretic effects

Pharmacokinetics
IM: Onset 3-5 min, duration 3-5 hr

IV: Onset immediate, duration 30-60 min

Not absorbed orally; $t_{1/2}$<10 min; elimination via liver, kidneys, and oxytocinase

INDICATIONS AND USES: Induction and augmentation of labor; missed or incomplete abortion (adjunctive); postpartum bleeding; postpartum breast engorgement,* antepartum fetal heart rate testing (oxytocin challenge test)*

DOSAGE
Adult
• *Labor induction:* IV dilute 10 U/L of 0.9% NS or D_5NS, run at 1-2 mU/min at 15-30 min intervals to begin normal labor

• *Augmentation of labor:* IV INF in D_5W or 0.9% NaCl at 1-2 mU/min; may increase q15-30 min; not to exceed 20 mU/min

• *Incomplete abortion:* IV INF 10 U/500 ml D_5W or 0.9% NaCl given at 20-40 mU/min

• *Control of postpartum bleeding:* IV dilute 10-40 U/L, run at 10-20 mU/min, adjust rate as needed; IM 10 U following delivery of placenta

$ AVAILABLE FORMS/COST OF THERAPY

• Inj, Sol—IM, IV: 10 U/ml, 1 ml: **$1.12-$3.50**

CONTRAINDICATIONS: Cephalopelvic disproportion; fetal distress where delivery is not imminent; hypertonic uterus, contraindication to vaginal delivery (i.e., active herpes genitalis, placenta previa, cord presentation, or prolapse)

PRECAUTIONS: Cervical or uterine surgery, uterine sepsis, fetal distress, partial placenta previa, prematurity, cyclopropane anesthesia (maternal bradycardia), water intoxication

PREGNANCY AND LACTATION: Nasal oxytocin contraindicated during pregnancy; only minimal amounts pass into breast milk

SIDE EFFECTS/ADVERSE REACTIONS

CNS: Hypertension, *seizures,* tetanic contractions

CV: Bradycardia, *dysrhythmias,* hypotension, increased pulse, premature ventricular contractions, tachycardia

FETUS: Dysrhythmias, hypoxia, intracranial hemorrhage, jaundice

GI: Anorexia, constipation, nausea, vomiting

GU: Abruptio placentae, decreased uterine blood flow

METAB: Anuria, confusion, drowsiness, headache, water intoxication

RESP: Asphyxia

SKIN: Rash

SPECIAL CONSIDERATIONS

• Routinely used for the induction of labor at term and postpartum for the control of uterine bleeding; not the drug of choice for induction of labor for abortion

MONITORING PARAMETERS

• Continuous monitoring necessary for IV use (length, intensity, duration of contractions); fetal heart rate—acceleration, deceleration, fetal distress

---

pamidronate

(pam-id'drow-nate)

Rx: Aredia

Chemical Class: Synthetic analog of pyrophosphate

Therapeutic Class: Bisphosphonate

CLINICAL PHARMACOLOGY

Mechanism of Action: Binds to hydroxyapatite at sites of bone resorption, inhibiting normal and abnormal bone resorption ("crystal poison"); minimal secondary reduction in bone formation (resorption coupled to formation)

Pharmacokinetics

IV: Taken up by bones (49% of dose); 51% excreted unchanged in urine within 72 hr; $t_{1/2}$ 27.2 hr

INDICATIONS AND USES: Paget's disease; hypercalcemia of malignancy; osteolytic bone lesions of multiple myeloma;* heterotropic ossification caused by spinal cord injury or complicating total hip replacement,* hyperparathyroidism,* bone pain in prostatic carcinoma and metastatic breast cancer,* prevention of glucocorticoid-induced osteoporosis*

DOSAGE

Adult

• *Severe hypercalcemia of malignancy* (corrected serum calcium >13.5 mg/dl): IV INF 90 mg over 24 hr

---

* = non-FDA-approved use

• *Moderate hypercalcemia of malignancy* (corrected serum calcium 12-13.5 mg/dl): IV INF 60 mg over at least 4 hr or 90 mg over 24 hr
• *Paget's disease:* IV INF 30 mg over 4 hr on 3 consecutive days (total 90 mg)
• *Osteolytic bone lesions of multiple myeloma:* IV 90 mg over 4 hr once monthly

§ AVAILABLE FORMS/COST OF THERAPY
• Inj, Sol—IV: 30 mg, 1's: **$291.53**; 60 mg, 1's: **$428.97**; 90 mg, 1's: **$787.11**

PRECAUTIONS: Renal dysfunction
PREGNANCY AND LACTATION: Pregnancy category C; caution with administration to a nursing mother
SIDE EFFECTS/ADVERSE REACTIONS
CNS: Headache, *seizures*
CV: Hypertension
EENT: Iritis, uveitis
GI: Abdominal pain, anorexia, constipation, nausea, vomiting
GU: Fluid overload, UTI
HEME: Anemia
METAB: Hyperpyrexia, hypokalemia, hypomagnesemia, hypophosphatemia
MS: Bone pain
SKIN: Induration, pain on palpitation at site of catheter insertion, redness, swelling

SPECIAL CONSIDERATIONS
• "Second-generation" bisphosphonate that offers potential advantages over etidronate (as does alendronate) in that it inhibits bone resorption at doses that do not impair bone mineralization, and is less likely than etidronate to produce osteomalacia
• Allow at least 7 days between initial treatment for patients requiring retreatment for hypercalcemia

pancrelipase
(pan-kre-li′pase)
Rx: Cotazym, Cotazym-S, Creon, Ilozyme, Ku-Zyme HP, Lipram, Pancrease, Pancrease MT, Protilase, Ultrase MT, Viokase, Zymase
Chemical Class: Pancreatic enzymes
Therapeutic Class: Digestant

CLINICAL PHARMACOLOGY
Mechanism of Action: Pancreatic enzymes: hydrolyze fats to glycerol and fatty acids; change protein to proteoses; convert starch into dextrins and sugars
INDICATIONS AND USES: Exocrine pancreatic secretion insufficiency due to cystic fibrosis (digestive aid), chronic pancreatitis, postpancreatectomy, ductal obstructions caused by cancer; steatorrhea due to malabsorption syndrome and postgastrectomy, or post-GI surgery
DOSAGE
Adjust dosage according to severity of symptoms (steatorrhea)
Adult
• 4000-48,000 U lipase with each meal/snack; may increase to 64,000-80,000 U with meals or increase to hourly intervals in severe deficiencies provided adverse GI effects do not occur; powder 0.7 g with meals and snacks
Child
• 6 mo-1 yr, 2000 U lipase per meal
• 1-6 yr, 4000-8000 U lipase with each meal; 4000 U with snacks
• 7-12 yr, 4000-12,000 U lipase with each meal and snacks

§ AVAILABLE FORMS/COST OF THERAPY
• Cap, Enteric Coated—Oral: 4000 U lipase/12,000 U protease/12,000 U amylase, 100's: **$27.35**; 4000/

25,000/20,000, 100's: **$25.30-$35.73**; 5000/20,000/20,000, 100's: **$30.25**; 8000/30,000/30,000, 100's: **$22.36-$57.21**; 10,000/30,000/30,000, 100's: **$72.95**; 12,000/24,000/24,000, 100's: **$66.39**; 12,000/39,000/39,000, 100's: **$74.55-$93.19**; 16,000/48,000/48,000, 100's: **$93.33-$151.99**; 20,000/65,000/65,000, 100's: **$129.17-$161.45**; 20,000/75,000/66,400, 100's: **$146.97-$179.56**

• Powder—Oral: 16,800 U lipase/70,000 U protease/70,000 U amylase, 8 oz: **$118.15-$159.35**

• Tab, Uncoated—Oral: 8000 U lipase/30,000 U protease/30,000 U amylase, 100's: **$12.81-$38.78**; 11,000/30,000/30,000, 250's: **$139.23**

CONTRAINDICATIONS: Hypersensitivity to pork, acute pancreatitis and exacerbations of chronic pancreatic disease

PREGNANCY AND LACTATION: Pregnancy category C

SIDE EFFECTS/ADVERSE REACTIONS

EENT: Buccal soreness

GI: Anal soreness, anorexia, diarrhea, glossitis, nausea, vomiting

METAB: Hyperuricemia, hyperuricuria

SKIN: Rash

SPECIAL CONSIDERATIONS

• Substitution at dispensing should be avoided

• Enteric-coated pancreatic enzymes are more effective than regular formulations; individual variations may require trials with several enzymatic preparations

• For patients who do not respond appropriately, adding antacid or H₂-antagonist may provide better results

• Preparations high in lipase concentration seem to be more effective for reducing steatorrhea

PATIENT/FAMILY EDUCATION

• Advise patient to take before or with meals

• Protect enteric coating; advise patient not to crush or chew microspheres in caps or tabs

MONITORING PARAMETERS

• Growth curves in children

---

pantoprazole

(pan-toe-pra´zole)

Rx: Protonix

Chemical Class: Substituted benzimidazole

Therapeutic Class: Gastrointestinal antiulcer agent

CLINICAL PHARMACOLOGY

Mechanism of Action: Suppresses gastric acid secretion by inhibiting the parietal cell H^+/K^+ ATP pump

Pharmacokinetics

PO: Bioavailability 77%; 98% bound to plasma proteins; extensively metabolized by liver cytochrome P450 enzymes (CYP2C19, CYP3A4); metabolites primarily eliminated in the urine; $t_{1/2}$ 2 hr (does not reflect duration of acid suppression)

INDICATIONS AND USES: Short-term treatment of duodenal ulcers; short-term treatment of gastric ulcers; moderate to severe GERD; eradication of *H. pylori* infection (in combination with clarithromycin and metronidazole)

DOSAGE

Adult

• PO 40 mg qd taken before or with breakfast

• IV 40 mg qd

AVAILABLE FORMS/COST OF THERAPY

• Tab, Sust Action—Oral: 20 mg, 40 mg, 90's: **$293.63**

---

* = non-FDA-approved use

• Inj, powder—IV: 40 mg/vial, 25's: *Cost not available*

PRECAUTIONS: Symptomatic response does not rule out gastric malignancy; hepatic insufficiency

PREGNANCY AND LACTATION: Pregnancy category B; excretion into breast milk unknown, use caution in nursing mothers

SIDE EFFECTS/ADVERSE REACTIONS

CNS: Headache, dizziness, depression

CV: Edema

EENT: Visual disturbances

GI: Diarrhea, nausea, abdominal pain, flatulence

SKIN: Rash, pruritis

MISC: Fever

INTERACTIONS

Drugs

3 *Ketoconazole:* Decreased bioavailability of ketoconazole

SPECIAL CONSIDERATIONS
PATIENT/FAMILY EDUCATION

• Caution patients not to split, crush or chew delayed-release tablets; swallow whole

MONITORING PARAMETERS

• Symptom relief, mucosal healing

---

papaverine

(pa-pav´er-een)

Rx: Papacon, Pavabid Plateau, Pava-Time S.R., Pavacot, Pavagen T.D.
Chemical Class: Benzylisoquinoline alkaloid
Therapeutic Class: Peripheral vasodilator

CLINICAL PHARMACOLOGY

Mechanism of Action: Relaxes all smooth muscle; inhibits cyclic nucleotide phosphodiesterase, which increases intracellular cAMP, causing vasodilation; increases cerebral blood flow and decreases cerebral vascular resistance in normal subjects

Pharmacokinetics

SUS ACTION: Poor and erratic absorption; oral bioavailability 54%; 90% bound to plasma proteins; metabolized in liver, excreted in urine (inactive metabolites) $t_{1/2}$ varies widely; peak plasma levels 1-2 hr

INDICATIONS AND USES: Arterial spasm resulting in cerebral and peripheral ischemia*; myocardial ischemia associated with vascular spasm or dysrhythmias*

DOSAGE

Adult

• PO Sus Action 150-300 mg q8-12h

$ AVAILABLE FORMS/COST OF THERAPY

• Cap, Gel, Sus Action—Oral: 150 mg, 100's: **$6.75-$11.35**

• Inj, Sol: 30 mg/ml, 2 ml: **$3.75-$10.00**

CONTRAINDICATIONS: Complete AV heart block

PRECAUTIONS: Cardiac dysrhythmias, glaucoma

PREGNANCY AND LACTATION: Pregnancy category C

SIDE EFFECTS/ADVERSE REACTIONS

CNS: Dizziness, drowsiness, headache, malaise, sedation, vertigo

CV: Increased blood pressure, tachycardia

GI: Abdominal pain, altered liver enzymes, anorexia, constipation, diarrhea, hepatotoxicity, jaundice, nausea

RESP: Increased depth of respirations

SKIN: Flushing, rash, *sweating*

INTERACTIONS

Drugs

3 *Levodopa:* Loss of control of Parkinson's disease

---

italic = common side effects   ***bold italic*** = life-threatening reactions

SPECIAL CONSIDERATIONS
• No objective evidence of *any* therapeutic value

---

paregoric
(par-e-gor´ik)
Rx: Paregoric
Chemical Class: Opiate (most preparations also contain camphor and ethanol)
Therapeutic Class: Antidiarrheal
DEA Class: Schedule III

CLINICAL PHARMACOLOGY
Mechanism of Action: Direct effect on circular smooth muscle of the bowel that prolongs GI transit time; reduces GI secretions

Pharmacokinetics
PO: Onset 20-30 min, peak 60 min, duration 4 hr; metabolized in liver by glucuronidation; metabolites excreted in urine (90% within 24 hr), 10% excreted in bile

INDICATIONS AND USES: Diarrhea; neonatal opioid withdrawal syndrome*

DOSAGE
Adult
• PO 5-10 ml up to qid
Child
• *Antidiarrheal:* Age >2 yr, PO 0.25-0.5 ml/kg up to qid
• *Opioid withdrawal syndrome:* Neonate, PO 0.2 ml q3h, increase dose by 0.05 ml q3h until symptoms controlled (max dose of 0.7 ml)
NOTE: 4 ml of paregoric equal to 2.5 mg diphenoxylate, 1.6 mg morphine sulfate

🛈 AVAILABLE FORMS/COST OF THERAPY
• Liq—Oral: 0.4 mg/ml, 480 ml: **$8.95-$10.13**

CONTRAINDICATIONS: Diarrhea due to poisoning, infectious diarrhea

PRECAUTIONS: Respiratory disease, elderly patients

PREGNANCY AND LACTATION: Pregnancy category B; excreted in breast milk

SIDE EFFECTS/ADVERSE REACTIONS
CNS: Depression, *dizziness, drowsiness,* fatigue, restlessness, withdrawal syndrome (with prolonged use at high dose)
CV: Hypotension, orthostatic hypotension
EENT: Miosis
GI: Abdominal cramping, *constipation*
GU: Urinary retention
RESP: Respiratory depression
SKIN: Pruritus

INTERACTIONS
Drugs
🛈 *Barbiturates, rifampin:* Increased metabolism of paregoric
🛈 *Cimetidine:* Decreased metabolism of paregoric

SPECIAL CONSIDERATIONS
• Contains ethanol

---

paricalcitol
(pare-i-cal´sih-tal)
Rx: Zemplar
Chemical Class: Synthetic vitamin D analog
Therapeutic Class: Fat-soluble vitamin

CLINICAL PHARMACOLOGY
Mechanism of Action: Suppresses parathyroid hormone (PTH) levels in patients with chronic renal failure (CRF)

---

* = non-FDA-approved use

Pharmacokinetics

IV: Peak 5 min; approximately 50% metabolized; eliminated primarily by hepatobiliary excretion, 74% of dose recovered in feces, 16% recovered in urine; $t_{1/2}$ 15 hr

INDICATIONS AND USES: Prevention and treatment of secondary hyperparathyroidism associated with CRF

DOSAGE

Adult

• IV bolus 0.04 to 0.2 µg/kg no more frequently than qod at any time during dialysis; max 0.24 µg/kg if satisfactory response not observed, dose may be increased by 2-4 µg at 2-4 wk intervals

$ **AVAILABLE FORMS/COST OF THERAPY**

• Inj—IV: 2 µg/ml, 1 ml: **$11.13**; 5 µg/ml, 1 ml: **$6.95**

CONTRAINDICATIONS: Evidence of vitamin D toxicity, hypercalcemia

PRECAUTIONS: Children

PREGNANCY AND LACTATION: Pregnancy category C; use caution in nursing mothers

SIDE EFFECTS/ADVERSE REACTIONS

CNS: Lightheadedness
CV: Palpitation, edema
GI: **GI bleeding,** *nausea,* vomiting, dry mouth
RESP: Pneumonia
MISC: Chills, feeling unwell, fever, flu, sepsis

INTERACTIONS

Drugs

3 *Digoxin:* Hypercalcemia produced by paricalcitol may potentiate digoxin toxicity

SPECIAL CONSIDERATIONS

• Phosphate-binding compounds may be needed to control serum phosphorus levels

PATIENT/FAMILY EDUCATION

• Adhere to a dietary regimen of calcium supplementation and phosphorus restriction; avoid excessive use of aluminum-containing compounds

MONITORING PARAMETERS

• Serum calcium and phosphorus twice weekly during initial phase of therapy, then at least monthly once dosage has been established; if an elevated calcium level or a Ca × P product > 75 is noted, immediately reduce or interrupt dosage until parameters are normalized, then reinitiate at lower dose; intact PTH assay every 3 mo (target range in CRF patients ≤ 1.5-3 × the nonuremic upper limit of normal)

---

paromomycin

(par-oh-moe-mye´sin)
Rx: Humatin
Chemical Class: Aminoglycoside
Therapeutic Class: Amebicide; antibiotic

P

CLINICAL PHARMACOLOGY
Mechanism of Action: Direct action in intestinal lumen
Pharmacokinetics
PO: Poor absorption; 100% excreted in feces

INDICATIONS AND USES: Intestinal amebiasis; adjunct in hepatic coma; other parasitic infections* *(Dientamoeba fragilis, Diphyllobothrium latum, Taenia saginata, T. solium, Dipylidium caninum, Hymenolepis nana)*

DOSAGE

Adult

• *Intestinal amebiasis:* PO 25-35 mg/kg/day in 3 divided doses pc for 5-10 days

---

italic = common side effects   ***bold italic*** = life-threatening reactions

• *Hepatic coma:* 4 g qd in divided doses for 5-6 days

Child

• *Intestinal amebiasis:* PO 25-35 mg/kg/day in 3 divided doses pc for 5-10 days

💲 AVAILABLE FORMS/COST OF THERAPY

• Cap, Gel—Oral: 250 mg, 100's: **$190.08-$262.44**

CONTRAINDICATIONS: GI obstruction

PRECAUTIONS: GI ulcerations, superinfection

PREGNANCY AND LACTATION: Pregnancy category C; poor oral bioavailability and lipid solubility limit passage into breast milk

SIDE EFFECTS/ADVERSE REACTIONS

EENT: Ototoxicity

GI: Anorexia, diarrhea, epigastric distress, nausea, pruritus ani, steatorrhea, *vomiting*

GU: Hematuria, **nephrotoxicity**

---

paroxetine

(par-ox'e-teen)

Rx: Paxil, Paxil CR
Chemical Class: Phenylpiperidine
Therapeutic Class: Selective serotonin reuptake inhibitor (SSRI) antidepressant

---

CLINICAL PHARMACOLOGY

Mechanism of Action: Inhibits CNS neuronal uptake of serotonin (5HT); no significant activity for histaminergic, α- or β-adrenergic, muscarinic, or dopaminergic receptors

Pharmacokinetics

PO: Peak 5.2 hr; protein binding 93%-95%; metabolized in liver (CYP2D6), unchanged drugs and metabolites excreted in feces (36%) and urine (64%); $t_{1/2}$ 21 hr

INDICATIONS AND USES: Major depressive disorder; obsessive-compulsive disorder; panic disorder; social anxiety disorder; generalized anxiety disorder; posttraumatic stress disorder

DOSAGE

Adult

• *Depression:* PO 20 mg qd in AM; after 4 wk if no clinical improvement is noted, dose may be increased by 10 mg/day qwk to desired response, not to exceed 50 mg/day; Sus Action PO 25 mg qd in AM, dose may be increased by 12.5 mg/day qwk, max 62.5 mg/day

• *Generalized anxiety disorder:* PO 20 mg qd, increase by 10 mg/day q wk prn; usual dose 20-50 mg/day

• *Obsessive-compulsive disorder:* PO 20 mg qd, increase in 1 wk increments by 10 mg/day; usual dose requirement 40 mg/day, maximum 60 mg/day

• *Panic disorder:* PO 10 mg qd, increase by 10 mg/day qwk prn; max 60 mg/day; Sus Action PO 12.5 mg qd in AM, dose may be increased by 12.5 mg/day qwk, max 75 mg/day

• *Posttraumatic stress disorder:* PO 20 mg qd, increase by 10 mg/day q wk prn; usual dose 20-50 mg/day

• *Social anxiety disorder:* PO 20 mg qd; max 60 mg/day

• *Elderly, severe renal or hepatic impairment:* PO 10 mg qd initially, increase by 10 mg/day q wk as indicated; Doses should not exceed 40 mg/day; Sus Action PO 12.5 mg qd initially, increase by 12.5 mg/day qwk if indicated, doses should not exceed 50 mg/day

---

💲 AVAILABLE FORMS/COST OF THERAPY

• Susp—Oral: 10 mg/5 ml, 250 ml: **$135.09**
• Tab, Coated—Oral: 10 mg, 30's: **$69.95**; 20 mg, 100's: **$220.05**; 30 mg, 30's: **$72.37**; 40 mg, 30's: **$79.40**
• Tab, Sus Action—Oral: 12.5 mg, 25 mg, 37.5 mg, all 30's: *Cost not available*

CONTRAINDICATIONS: Patients taking MAOIs (or within 14 days of discontinuing an MAOI), concomitant use with thioridazine (see drug interactions)

PRECAUTIONS: History of mania, seizure disorder, suicide ideation, narrow angle glaucoma, renal and hepatic disease, abrupt discontinuation

PREGNANCY AND LACTATION: Pregnancy category B; limited information; milk concentrations similar to plasma following a single oral dose; thus <1% of the daily dose would be transferred to a breast-feeding infant

SIDE EFFECTS/ADVERSE REACTIONS

CNS: Agitation, *anxiety,* asthenia, delusions, dizziness, euphoria, fatigue, hallucinations, headache, insomnia, myoclonus, nervousness, psychosis, sedation, tremor
CV: Palpitations, postural hypotension, vasodilation
EENT: Pharyngitis, visual changes
GI: Anorexia, constipation, cramps, *decreased appetite,* diarrhea, dry mouth, dyspepsia, flatulence, *nausea,* taste changes, vomiting
GU: Abnormal ejaculation, urinary frequency
MS: Arthritis, myalgia, myasthenia, myopathy, pain
RESP: Cough, dyspnea, infection, nasal congestion, pharyngitis, sinus headache, sinusitis
SKIN: Rash, sweating
MISC: Fever

INTERACTIONS
Drugs
🔳 *Beta-blockers (metroprolol, propranolol, sotalol):* Inhibition of metabolism (CYP2D6) leads to increased plasma concentrations of selective beta blockers and potential cardiac toxicity; atenolol may be safer choice
🔳 *Cimetidine:* Increased plasma paroxetine concentrations
🔳 *Cyproheptadine:* Serotonin antagonist may partially reverse antidepressant and other effects
❷ *Dexfenfluramine:* Duplicate effects on inhibition of serotonin reuptake; inhibition of dexfenfluramine metabolism (CYP2D6) exaggerates effect; both mechanisms increase risk of serotonin syndrome
🔳 *Dextromethorphan:* Inhibition of dextromethorphan's metabolism (CYP2D6) by paroxetine and additive serotonergic effects
🔳 *Diuretics, loop (bumetanide, furosemide, torsemide):* Possible additive hyponatremia; two fatal case reports with furosemide and paroxetine
❷ *Fenfluramine:* Duplicate effects on inhibition of serotonin reuptake; inhibition of dexfenfluramine metabolism (CYP2D6) exaggerates effect; both mechanisms increase risk of serotonin syndrome
🔳 *Haloperidol:* Inhibition of haloperidol's metabolism (CYP2D6) may increase risks of extrapyramidal symptoms
🔳 *Lithium:* Neurotoxicity (tremor, confusion, ataxia, dizziness, dysarthria, and absence seizures) reported in patients receiving this combination; mechanism unknown

P

▲ *MAOI's (isocarboxazid, phenelzine, tranylcypromine):* Increased CNS serotonergic effects have been associated with severe or fatal reactions with this combination

3 *Phenobarbital:* Decreased plasma paroxetine concentrations

3 *Phenytoin:* Decreased plasma paroxetine concentrations

3 *Selegiline:* Sporadic cases of mania and hypertension

3 *Sumatriptan:* Increased incidence of adverse effects

3 *Theophylline:* Elevated theophylline levels have been reported

▲ *Thioridazine:* Increased plasma thioridazine concentrations; increased risk of ventricular arrhythmias

3 *Tricyclic antidepressants (clomipramine, desipramine, doxepin, imipramine, nortriptyline, trazodone):* Marked increases in tricyclic antidepressant levels due to inhibition of metabolism (CYP2D6)

2 *Tryptophan:* Additive serotonergic effects

3 *Warfarin:* Increased risk of bleeding

SPECIAL CONSIDERATIONS

• Somewhat sedating compared to fluoxetine and sertraline

PATIENT/FAMILY EDUCATION

• Avoid alcohol

• May take 1-4 wk to see improvement of symptoms

pemoline
(pem´oh-leen)
Rx: Cylert
Chemical Class: Oxazolidine derivative
Therapeutic Class: CNS stimulant; anorexiant
DEA Class: Schedule IV

CLINICAL PHARMACOLOGY
Mechanism of Action: Cerebral stimulation via dopaminergic mechanisms; minimal sympathomimetic effects
Pharmacokinetics
PO: Peak 2-4 hr, duration 8 hr, gradual onset of action (3-4 wk to effect); 50% protein bound; metabolized (50%) by liver, excreted (40%) by kidneys; $t_{1/2}$ 12 hr
INDICATIONS AND USES: Attention deficit disorder with hyperactivity; narcolepsy*
DOSAGE
Child >6 yr
• *Attention deficit disorder:* 37.5 mg in AM, increasing by 18.75 mg/wk, not to exceed 112.5 mg/day
⑤ AVAILABLE FORMS/COST OF THERAPY
• Tab, Chewable—Oral: 37.5 mg, 100's: **$136.81-$198.08**
• Tab, Uncoated—Oral: 18.75 mg, 100's: **$87.07-$115.60**; 37.5 mg, 100's: **$136.88-$181.70**; 75 mg, 100's: **$236.28-$313.76**
CONTRAINDICATIONS: Hepatic insufficiency
PRECAUTIONS: Renal disease, drug abuse, child <6 yr
PREGNANCY AND LACTATION: Pregnancy category B
SIDE EFFECTS/ADVERSE REACTIONS
CNS: Aggressiveness, depression, dizziness, drowsiness, dyskinetic movements, Gilles de la Tourette's

disorder, hallucinations, headache, *hyperactivity, insomnia,* irritability, *restlessness, seizures,* stimulation

GI: Abdominal pain, anorexia, diarrhea, hepatitis, increased liver enzymes, jaundice, nausea

MISC: Growth suppression in children, rashes

SPECIAL CONSIDERATIONS
MONITORING PARAMETERS
• LFTs periodically

---

penbutolol
(pen-bute′o-loll)
Rx: Levatol
Chemical Class: Nonselective β-adrenergic blocker
Therapeutic Class: Antihypertensive; antianginal

CLINICAL PHARMACOLOGY
Mechanism of Action: Competitive, nonselective, β-receptor antagonist; some intrinsic sympathomimetic activity; no membrane stabilizing activity; high lipid solubility

Pharmacokinetics
PO: Peak 1½-3 hr, duration >20 hr; absorption 100% bioavailability; metabolized by hepatic conjugation and oxidation; 80%-98% protein bound; metabolites excreted mainly in urine; $t_{\frac{1}{2}}$ 5 hr

INDICATIONS AND USES: Hypertension; angina pectoris*; MI*; migraine (prophylaxis)*; alcohol withdrawal syndrome*; aggressive behavior*; antipsychotic-induced akathisia*

DOSAGE
Adult
• *Hypertension:* 20 mg qd (flat dose-response curve)

§ AVAILABLE FORMS/COST OF THERAPY
• Tab, Uncoated—Oral: 20 mg, 100′s: **$124.10**

CONTRAINDICATIONS: Cardiogenic shock, sinus bradycardia, 2nd and 3rd degree atrioventricular conduction block, asthma

PRECAUTIONS: Anesthesia and major surgery; diabetes mellitus; abrupt withdrawal with concurrent CAD or thyrotoxicosis

PREGNANCY AND LACTATION: Pregnancy category C

SIDE EFFECTS/ADVERSE REACTIONS
CNS: Dizziness, fatigue, headache, insomnia
CV: Bradycardia, CHF
GI: Diarrhea, dyspepsia, nausea
GU: Impotence
RESP: Cough, dyspnea
SKIN: Excessive sweating

INTERACTIONS
Drugs
§ *Adenosine:* Bradycardia aggravated
§ *Amiodarone:* Bradycardia, cardiac arrest, ventricular arrhythmia risk after initiation of penbutolol
§ *Antacids:* Reduced penbutolol absorption
§ *Calcium channel blockers:* See dihydropyridine calcium channel blockers and verapamil
§ *Clonidine, guanabenz, guanfacine:* Exacerbation of rebound hypertension upon discontinuation of clonidine
§ *Cocaine:* Cocaine-induced vasoconstriction potentiated; reduced coronary blood flow
§ *Contrast media:* Increased risk of anaphylaxis
§ *Digitalis:* Enhances bradycardia
§ *Dihydropyridine, calcium channel blockers:* Additive pharmacodynamic effects

P

---

italic = common side effects   ***bold italic*** = life-threatening reactions

3 *Dipyridamole:* Bradycardia aggravated

3 *Epinephrine, isoproterenol, phenylephrine:* Potentiates pressor response; resultant hypertension and bradycardia

3 *Flecainide:* Additive negative inotropic effects

3 *Fluoxetine:* Increased β-blockade activity

3 *Fluoroquinolones:* Reduced clearance of penbutolol

3 *Insulin:* Altered response to hypoglycemia; increased blood glucose concentrations; impaired peripheral circulation

3 *Lidocaine:* Increased serum lidocaine concentrations possible

3 *Neostigmine:* Bradycardia aggravated

3 *Neuroleptics:* Both drugs inhibit each other's metabolism; additive hypotension

3 *NSAIDs:* Reduced antihypertensive effect of penbutolol

3 *Physostigmine:* Bradycardia aggravated

3 *Prazosin:* First-dose response to prazosin may be enhanced by β-blockade

3 *Tacrine:* Bradycardia aggravated

2 *Terbutaline:* Antagonized bronchodilating effects of terbutaline

2 *Theophylline:* Antagonistic pharmacodynamic effects

3 *Verapamil:* Enhanced effects of both drugs; particularly AV nodal conduction slowing; reduced penbutolol clearance

SPECIAL CONSIDERATIONS
• Exacerbation of ischemic heart disease following abrupt withdrawal due to hypersensitivity to catecholamines possible

• Comparative trials indicate that penbutolol is as effective as propranolol and atenolol in the treatment of hypertension; may have fewer adverse CNS effects than propranolol

---

penciclovir
(pen-sye´kloe-veer)
Rx: Denavir
Chemical Class: Synthetic acyclic guanine derivative
Therapeutic Class: Antiviral

CLINICAL PHARMACOLOGY
Mechanism of Action: Inhibitory activity against herpes simplex virus types 1 (HSV-1) and 2 (HSV-2); phosphorylated to penciclovir triphosphate in HSV-infected cells, inhibiting viral DNA synthesis to penciclovir triphosphate
Pharmacokinetics
TOP: Measurable concentrations not found in plasma or urine
INDICATIONS AND USES: Recurrent herpes labialis (cold sores)
DOSAGE
Adult
• TOP apply to affected area q2h during waking hours for 4 days; start treatment as early as possible (i.e., during prodrome or when lesions first appear)
S **AVAILABLE FORMS/COST OF THERAPY**
• Cre—Top: 10 mg/g (1%), 2 g: **$22.90**
PRECAUTIONS: Immunocompromised patients
PREGNANCY AND LACTATION: Pregnancy category B; no data in nursing mothers, but milk concentrations should be low due to apparent lack of systemic absorption

---

SIDE EFFECTS/ADVERSE REACTIONS

SKIN: Application site reaction, pruritus, rash

SPECIAL CONSIDERATIONS

• In clinical trials, shortened the duration of lesions by approximately ½ day compared to placebo (4½ vs. 5 days); duration of pain was also shortened by approximately ½ day

---

penicillamine

(pen-i-sill´a-meen)

Rx: Cuprimine, Depen

Chemical Class: Thiol derivative

Therapeutic Class: Heavy metal antidote; disease-modifying antiarthritic drug (DMARD)

CLINICAL PHARMACOLOGY

Mechanism of Action: Binds with ions of lead, mercury, copper, iron, zinc to form a water-soluble complex excreted by kidneys; improves lymphocyte function, markedly reduces IgM rheumatoid factor and immune complexes, depresses T-cell but not B-cell activity; combines with cystine to form disulfide, which is more soluble, reduces excess cystine excretion in cystinuria

Pharmacokinetics

PO: Peak 1 hr, onset of action (Wilson's disease, 1-3 mo, rheumatoid arthritis, 2-3 mo); metabolized in liver; renal and fecal elimination

INDICATIONS AND USES: Wilson's disease; rheumatoid arthritis; cystinuria; lead poisoning,* primary biliary cirrhosis,* scleroderma*

DOSAGE

Adult

• *Wilson's disease:* PO 250 mg tid-qid, maximum 2 g/day

• *Rheumatoid arthritis:* PO 125-250 mg/day, increase 250 mg q2-3 mo prn, max 1 g/day; doses >500 mg/d should be administered in divided doses

• *Cystinuria:* PO 250 mg qid ac, not to exceed 5 g/day

Child

• *Chelating agent and cystinuria:* PO 20-30 mg/kg/day in divided doses qid ac

💲 **AVAILABLE FORMS/COST OF THERAPY**

• Cap, Gel—Oral: 125 mg, 100's: **$81.19**; 250 mg, 100's: **$115.93**

• Tab, Coated—Oral: 250 mg, 100's: **$264.89**

CONTRAINDICATIONS: Penicillamine-related aplastic anemia or agranulocytosis; severe renal disease; pregnancy (except Wilson's disease or certain cases of cystinuria)

PRECAUTIONS: Renal insufficiency

PREGNANCY AND LACTATION: Pregnancy category D (continued therapy in Wilson's disease and cystinuria probably OK, not rheumatoid arthritis)

SIDE EFFECTS/ADVERSE REACTIONS

CV: Hypotension, tachycardia

EENT: Optic neuritis, tinnitus

GI: Abdominal cramping, anorexia, *diarrhea,* hepatotoxicity, *nausea,* pain, peptic ulcer, *vomiting*

*GU: **Glomerulonephritis, nephrotic syndrome,** proteinuria*

*HEME: **Aplastic anemia,** eosinophilia, **granulocytopenia, hemolytic anemia,** increased sedimentation rate, **leukopenia,** lupus syndrome, **thrombocytopenia***

MS: Arthralgia

RESP: Asthma, pneumonitis, ***pulmonary fibrosis***

SKIN: Alopecia, ecchymosis, *erythema,* fever, *pruritus, urticaria*

---

italic = common side effects   **bold italic** = life-threatening reactions

INTERACTIONS
Drugs
3 *Antacids:* Magnesium-aluminum hydroxides reduce bioavailability

3 *Digoxin:* Reduced digoxin concentrations

3 *Iron:* Oral iron substantially reduces plasma penicillamine concentration, with reduced therapeutic response

Labs
• *Cholesterol:* Decreased serum levels

• *Fructoseamine:* Decreased serum levels

• *Iron:* Decreased serum levels

• *Ketones:* Increased false-positive reactions with legal reaction

SPECIAL CONSIDERATIONS
• Because penicillamine can cause severe adverse reactions, restrict its use in rheumatoid arthritis to patients who have severe, active disease and who have failed to respond to an adequate trial of conventional therapy

PATIENT/FAMILY EDUCATION
• Should be administered on empty stomach, ½-1 hr before meals or at least 2 hr after meals

• Urine may become discolored (red)

• Patients with cystinuria should drink large amounts of water

• Therapeutic effect may take 1-3 mo

MONITORING PARAMETERS
• Hepatic, renal studies: CBC, urinalysis, skin for rash

• Urinary copper excretion

---

penicillin
(pen-i-sill'in)
Rx: *Penicillin G (Aqueous Pen G):* Pfizerpen
Rx: *Penicillin G:* Pentids
Rx: *Penicillin V:*
(Phenoxy-methyl Penicillin),
Beepen VK, Pen-V, Pen-Vee K,
Truxcillin VK, Veetids
Rx: *Penicillin G Benzathine:*
Bicillin L-A, Permapen
Rx: *Penicillin G Procaine:*
Crysticillin, Wycillin
Rx: *Penicillin G Benzathine and Procaine combined:*
Bicillin C-R
Chemical Class: Natural penicillin
Therapeutic Class: Antibiotic

CLINICAL PHARMACOLOGY
Mechanism of Action: Inhibits bacterial wall synthesis; bactericidal
Pharmacokinetics
Excreted in urine and breast milk, crosses placenta
Penicillin G: IV immediate peak; IM peak 15-30 min; PO duration 6 hr, peak 1 hr
Penicillin V: PO peak 30-60 min, duration 6-8 hr, $t_{1/2}$ 30 min
Benzathine Penicillin: IM very slow absorption, duration 21-28 days, $t_{1/2}$ 30-60 min
Procaine Penicillin: IM peak 1-4 hr, duration 15 hr

INDICATIONS AND USES: For infections caused by susceptible organisms: *Penicillin G:* meningococcal meningitis, syphilis, anthrax, streptococcal infections, botulism, diphtheria, listeria, pasteurella infections, Lyme disease*; *Penicillin V:* scarlet fever; erysipelas; skin and soft-tissue infections; Vincent's gingivitis and pharyngitis; strep pharyngitis; rheumatic fever pro-

---

* = non-FDA-approved use

phylaxis; endocarditis prophylaxis; *Benzathine penicillin:* Group A strep respiratory tract infection; syphilis, yaws; prophylaxis of rheumatic fever and/or chorea; *Procaine penicillin:* otitis media; skin and soft-tissue infections; scarlet fever; erysipelas; Vincent's gingivitis and pharyngitis; syphilis; gonorrhea; endocarditis prophylaxis; yaws; anthrax; erysipeloid; *Benzathine and procaine penicillin combined:* moderately severe streptococcal and pneumococcal infections. Do not use for severe infections, syphilis, gonorrhea, or yaws.

Antibacterial spectrum includes non–penicillinase-producing strains of:

• Gram-positive organisms: *Staphylococcus aureus, Streptococcus pyogenes, Str. viridans, Str. faecalis, Str. bovis, Str. pneumoniae, Bacillus anthracis, Listeria monocytogenes, Corynebacterium diphtheriae*

• Gram-negative organisms: *Neisseria gonorrhoeae, N. meningitidis, E. coli, Proteus mirabilis, Salmonella, Shigella, Enterobacter, S. moniliformis*

• Anaerobes: *Clostridium* sp., *Peptococcus* sp., *Peptostreptococcus* sp., *Bacteroides* sp. (except *B. fragilis*), *Fusobacterium* sp., *Eubacterium* sp.,

• Other organisms: *Treponema pallidum, Actinomyces bovis*

DOSAGE
PENICILLIN G (AQUEOUS)
Adult
• *Moderate to severe infections:* IM/IV 12-30 million U/day in divided doses q4h
• *Endocarditis prophylaxis:* IM/IV 2 million U 30-60 min before dental procedure; 1 million U 6 hr after procedure

Child
• *Moderate to severe infections:* IM/IV 25,000-300,000 U/day in divided doses q4-12h
PENICILLIN G
Adult
• *Pneumococcal/streptococcal infections:* PO 400,000-500,000 U q6-8h for 10 days
• *Rheumatic fever prophylaxis:* PO 200,000-250,000 U bid continuously
• *Meningococcal meningitis:* IM 1-2 million U q2h; IV 20-30 million U/day continuous drip for 14 day or until afebrile for 7 day
• *Pneumococcal empyema:* IV 5-24 million U/day in divided doses q4-6h
• *Pneumococcal meningitis:* IV 20-24 million U/day in divided doses q4-6h for 14 day
• *Pasturella infections:* IV 4-6 million U/day in divided doses for 2 wk
• *Listeria infections:* IV 15-20 million U/day in divided doses for 2 wk (meningitis) or 4 wk (endocarditis)
• *Neurosyphilis:* IV 2-4 million U q4h for 10-14 days (many recommend following with Pen G Benzathine 2.4 million U IM qwk for 3 doses)

Child
• *Pneumococcal/streptococcal infections:* PO 25,000-90,000 U/kg/day in 3-6 divided doses
• *Rheumatic fever prophylaxis:* PO 25,000-90,000 U/kg/day in 3-6 divided doses; IV 100,000-250,000 U/kg/day in divided doses q4h
Infant (use larger doses for meningitis)
• >7 days and >2000 g, IV 100,000-200,000 U/kg/day in divided doses q6h
• >7 days and <2000 g, IV 75,000-150,000 U/kg/day in divided doses q8h

• <7 days and >2000 g, IV 50,000-150,000 U/kg/day in divided doses q8h

• <7 days and <2000 g, IV 50,000-100,000 U/kg/day in divided doses q12h

PENICILLIN V

Adult

• *Pneumococcal infections:* PO 250-500 mg q6h

• *Streptococcal infections:* PO 125-250 mg q6-8h for 10 days

• *Strep pharyngitis:* PO 500 mg bid for 10 days

• *Rheumatic fever prophylaxis:* PO 125-250 mg bid continuously

Child

• PO 15-50 mg/kg/day in divided doses q6h

BENZATHINE PENICILLIN

Adult

• *Early syphilis:* IM 2.4 million U in single dose

• *Syphilis >1 yr duration:* IM 2.4 million U in single dose

• *Neurosyphilis:* To follow up treatment with Pen G procaine or Pen G potassium as below

• *Group A strep URI:* IM 1.2 million U in single dose

• *Rheumatic fever:* IM 1.2 million U in single dose q mo or 600,000 U q2 wk

Child

• *Congenital syphilis (<2 yr):* IM 50,000 U/kg in single dose

• *Rheumatic fever/glomerulonephritis prophylaxis (<60 lb):* IM 600,000 U in single dose

• *Group A strep URI (>27 kg):* IM 900,000 U in single dose; (<27 kg) 50,000 U/kg in single dose

PROCAINE PENICILLIN

Adult

• *Moderate to severe infections:* IM 600,000-1.2 million U/day in divided doses

• *Gonorrhea:* IM 4.8 million U in two inj given 30 min after probenecid 1 g

• *Syphilis (primary, secondary, latent with neg CSF):* IM 600,000 U/day for 8 days

• *Neurosyphilis:* IM 2-4 million U/day with probenecid 500 mg qid for 10-14 days (many recommend following with Pen G benzathine 2.4 million U q wk for 3 doses)

Child

• *Moderate to severe infections:* Same as adult; avoid in newborn (risk procaine toxicity, sterile abscess)

• *Congenital syphilis:* IM 50,000 U/kg qd for 10-14 days

BENZOTHAINE AND PROCAINE PENICILLIN COMBINED

Adult

• *Moderate infections:* 2.4 million U IM once or q2-3 days until temperature normalizes

Child

• *Moderate infections:* (30-60 pounds) 900,000-1.2 million U; (<30 pounds) 600,000 units U once or q2-3 days until temperature normalizes

$ **AVAILABLE FORMS/COST OF THERAPY**

Penicillin G (aqueous)

• Inj, Sol—IV: 1,000,000 U/vial, 50 ml, 1500 ml: **$13.20**; 2,000,000 U, 50 ml, 1500 ml: **$13.74**; 3,000,000 U, 50 ml, 1500 ml: **$14.26**; 5,000,000 U/vial: **$1.91-$10.03**; 10,000,000 U/vial: **$6.66-$40.55**; 20,000,000 U/vial: **$5.30-$23.98**

Penicillin G

• Inj, Dry-Sol—IM, IV: 5,000,000 U/vial: **$41.27-$66.00**

Penicillin V

• Powder, Reconst—Oral: 125 mg/5 ml, 100, 200 ml: **$1.74-$6.25**/100 ml; 250 mg/5 ml, 100, 150, 200 ml: **$2.18-$5.31**/100 ml

• Tab, Uncoated—Oral: 250 mg, 100's: **$5.34-$23.96**; 500 mg, 100's: **$9.05-$48.41**
Benzathine Penicillin G
• Inj, Susp—IM: 300,000 U/ml, 1 ml: **$3.87**; 600,000 U/ml, 1 ml: **$9.01-$14.75**
Procaine Penicillin G
• Inj, Sol—IM: 150,000 U/ml, 10 ml: **$16.46-$21.85**; 300,000 U/ml, 1 ml: **$6.13-$9.26**; 600,000 U/ml, 1 ml: **$3.30-$9.53**
Benzathine and Procaine Penicillin G Combined
• Inj, Susp—IM: 150,000 U/150,000 U/ml, 10 ml: **$16.46-$21.85**; 300,000 U/300,000 U/ml, 2 ml: **$10.37-$20.36**; 900,000 U/300,000 U/2 ml, 2 ml: **$12.52-$21.19**
PRECAUTIONS: Hypersensitivity to cephalosporins
PREGNANCY AND LACTATION: Pregnancy category B; may cause diarrhea, candidiasis, or allergic response in nursing infant
SIDE EFFECTS/ADVERSE REACTIONS
CNS: Anxiety, coma, depression, hallucinations, lethargy, *seizures,* twitching
GI: Abdominal pain, colitis, *diarrhea,* glossitis, *nausea, vomiting*
GU: Glomerulonephritis, hematuria, oliguria, proteinuria, vaginitis
HEME: **Bone marrow depression,** increased bleeding time
METAB: Alkalosis, hyperkalemia, hypernatremia, hypokalemia
SKIN: Rash
MISC: Jarisch-Herxheimer reaction (Benzathine penicillin)
INTERACTIONS
Drugs
🖪 *Chloramphenicol:* Inhibited antibacterial activity of penicillin; administer penicillin 3 hr before chloramphenicol

🖪 *Macrolide antibiotics:* Inhibited antibacterial activity of penicillin; administer penicillin 3 hr before macrolides
🖪 *Methotrexate:* Penicillin in large doses may increase serum methotrexate concentrations
🖪 *Oral contraceptives:* Occasional impairment of oral contraceptive efficacy; consider use of supplemental contraception during cycles in which penicillin is used
🖪 *Tetracyclines:* Inhibited antibacterial activity of penicillin; administer penicillin 3 hr before tetracyclines
Labs
• *Albumin:* Decreased serum levels at very high penicillin levels
• *Aminoglycosides:* Decreased serum levels if specimen stored for a prolonged period of time
• *Folate:* Decreased serum levels
• *17-ketogenic steroids:* Increased urine concentrations
• *17-ketosteroids:* Increased urine concentrations
• *Protein:* Increased CSF concentrations
• *Protein electrophoresis:* False positives; causes bisalbuminemia
• *Sugar:* False positive with copper reduction procedures
• *Piperacillin:* False positive in the presence of penicillin V
• *Amdinocillin:* False positive in the presence of penicillin G
• *Methicillin:* False positive in the presence of penicillin G
SPECIAL CONSIDERATIONS
• Cross reactivity with cephalosporins is approx 10%

pentamidine

(pen-tam'i-deen)
Rx: NebuPent, Pentam
Chemical Class: Aromatic diamidine derivative
Therapeutic Class: Antiprotozoal

CLINICAL PHARMACOLOGY

Mechanism of Action: Interferes with protozoal nuclear metabolism; inhibits RNA/DNA, phospholipid, and protein synthesis

Pharmacokinetics

INH: Peak plasma levels minimally detected; bronchoalveolar lavage levels > than those obtained by injection (5-43 ng/ml vs. 1.5-4.0 ng/ml)

IV/IM: peak within 60 min
69% bound to plasma proteins; 33%-66% excreted in urine unchanged; $t_{1/2}$ 6.4-9.4 hr

INDICATIONS AND USES: Treatment of *Pneumocystis carinii* pneumonia (PCP) (IM/IV); prevention of PCP in high-risk, HIV-infected patients with a history of ≥1 episode of PCP and/or peripheral CD4+ lymphocyte count ≤200/mm³ (INH); trypanosomiasis*; visceral leishmaniasis*; amebic meningoencephalitis*; babesiosis*

DOSAGE

Adult

• *Treatment:* IM/IV 4 mg/kg qd for 14 days (reduce dosage, use a longer infusion time, or extend dosing interval in renal failure)

• *Prevention:* INH 300 mg q4 wk via Respirgard II nebulizer by Marquest

Child

• *Treatment:* IM/IV 4 mg/kg qd for 10-14 days

• *Prevention:* IM/IV 4 mg/kg q2-4 wk; INH (≥5 yr) 300 mg q3 wk via Respirgard II nebulizer

* = non-FDA-approved use

§ AVAILABLE FORMS/COST OF THERAPY

• Aer—INH: 300 mg, 1's: **$98.75**
• Inj, Sol—IV: 300 mg, 1's: **$91.84-$98.75**

PRECAUTIONS: Children (INH), hypertension, hypotension, hypoglycemia, hyperglycemia, hypocalcemia, leukopenia, thrombocytopenia, anemia, hepatic or renal dysfunction, ventricular tachycardia, pancreatitis, Stevens-Johnson syndrome

PREGNANCY AND LACTATION: Pregnancy category C; since aerosolized pentamidine results in very low systemic concentrations, fetal exposure to the drug is probably negligible; breast milk levels following aerosolized administration are likely nil

SIDE EFFECTS/ADVERSE REACTIONS

CNS: (Inj) Confusion/hallucination, dizziness, fever, neuralgia; (INH) anxiety, *chills,* confusion, depression, *dizziness,* drowsiness, emotional lability, *fatigue,* hallucination, headache, insomnia, memory loss, neuralgia, neuropathy, paranoia, paresthesia, *seizures,* tremors, unsteady gait, vertigo

CV: (Inj) hypotension, *ventricular tachycardia;* (INH) *chest pain/congestion,* **CVA,** edema, hypertension, palpitations, syncope, tachycardia, vasculitis, vasodilation

EENT: (INH) Blepharitis, blurred vision, conjunctivitis, eye discomfort, loss of taste or smell, *pharyngitis*

GI: (Inj) Anorexia, bad taste in mouth, diarrhea, elevated liver function tests nausea; (INH) abdominal pain, colitis, diarrhea, dry mouth, dyspepsia, esophagitis, gastric ulcer, gastritis, gingivitis, hematochezia, hepatic dysfunction, hepatitis, hepatomegaly, hypersalivation, melena, *nausea,* oral ulcer, **pancreatitis,** splenomegaly

GU: (Inj) Flank pain, *increased serum creatinine,* nephritis, **renal failure**

HEME: (Inj and INH) **Anemia, leukopenia, thrombocytopenia**

METAB: (Inj) Hyperkalemia, hypocalcemia, hypoglycemia

MS: (INH) arthralgia, myalgia

RESP: (INH) **Bronchospasm,** cough, cyanosis, hemoptysis, hyperventilation, pleuritis, pneumonitis, pneumothorax, rales, *shortness of breath,* tachypnea

SKIN: (Inj) Rash, sterile abscess and pain at IM inj site; **Stevens-Johnson syndrome;** (INH) desquamation, dry skin, erythema, pruritis, rash, urticaria

SPECIAL CONSIDERATIONS

• Considered 2nd line for *P. carinii* pneumonia, following cotrimoxazole (unresponsive to or intolerant of cotrimoxazole)

MONITORING PARAMETERS

• BUN, serum creatinine, blood glucose daily

• CBC and platelets; liver function tests, including bilirubin, alkaline phosphatase, AST, and ALT; and serum calcium before, during, and after therapy

• ECG at regular intervals

pentazocine

(pen-taz′oh-seen)

Rx: Talwin, Talwin NX (with Naloxone)

Combinations

Rx: with ASA (Talwin Compound)

with APAP (Talacen)

Chemical Class: Synthetic opiate of benzomorphan series

Therapeutic Class: Narcotic agonist-antagonist analgesic

DEA Class: Schedule IV

CLINICAL PHARMACOLOGY

Mechanism of Action: Has analgesic and very weak opiate antagonistic effects; binds to opiate receptors in the CNS causing inhibition of ascending pain pathways, altering the perception of and response to pain; believed to be a competitive antagonist at μ opiate receptors and an agonist at κ and σ opiate receptors

Pharmacokinetics

PO: Onset 15-30 min, duration 4-5 hr

IM/SC: Onset 15-30 min, duration 2-3 hr

IV: Onset 2-3 min, duration 2-3 hr 61% bound to plasma proteins, large 1st-pass effect, metabolized in liver, eliminated mainly in urine, small amounts eliminated in feces, $t_{1/2}$ 2-3 hr (prolonged in hepatic failure)

INDICATIONS AND USES: Moderate to severe pain

DOSAGE

Adult

• PO 50 mg q3-4h prn, may increase to 100 mg/dose prn, do not exceed 600 mg/day; IM/SC 30-60 mg q3-4h prn, do not exceed 360 mg/day; IV 30 mg q3-4h prn, do not exceed 360 mg/day

P

Child
• PO (>12 yr) same as adult; IM/SC (5-8 yr) 15 mg; (8-14 yr) 30 mg

$ **AVAILABLE FORMS/COST OF THERAPY**
• Inj, Sol—IV, IM, SC: 30 mg/ml, 10 ml: **$33.41-$41.75**
• Tab, Uncoated—Oral: 50 mg pentazocine/0.5 mg naloxone, 100's: **$93.99-$126.55**

PRECAUTIONS: Head injury, increased intracranial pressure, acute abdominal conditions, elderly, severe impairment of hepatic or renal function, hypothyroidism, Addison's disease, prostatic hypertrophy, urethral stricture, history of drug abuse, impaired respiration, bronchial asthma, cyanosis, obstructive respiratory conditions, acute MI (see Special Considerations), chronic opiate use (may precipitate withdrawal symptoms), children

PREGNANCY AND LACTATION: Pregnancy category B (category D if used for prolonged periods or in high doses at term); use during labor may produce neonatal respiratory depression

SIDE EFFECTS/ADVERSE REACTIONS

CNS: Agitation, dependency, *dizziness, drowsiness, euphoria,* lethargy, restlessness, *sedation*
CV: Circulatory depression, increased blood pressure, **shock,** tachycardia
EENT: Blurred vision, diplopia, miosis, nystagmus
GI: Anorexia, constipation, nausea, vomiting
GU: Urinary retention
HEME: Eosinophilia, **granulocytopenia, leukopenia**
RESP: **Respiratory depression, respiratory paralysis**
SKIN: Flushing, rash, urticaria

INTERACTIONS
Drugs
3 *Aspirin:* Increased risk of papillary necrosis
3 *Barbiturates:* Additive CNS depression
3 *Phenothiazines:* Additive CNS depression
Labs
• *Increase:* Amylase

SPECIAL CONSIDERATIONS
• Naloxone 0.5 mg added to oral tablets to discourage misuse via parenteral inj
• Less effective compared to morphine, but less respiratory depression and opposite cardiovascular pharmacodynamics; increases pulmonary, arterial, and central venous pressure

PATIENT/FAMILY EDUCATION
• Report any symptoms of CNS changes, allergic reactions
• Physical dependency may result when used for extended periods
• Change position slowly, orthostatic hypotension may occur
• Avoid hazardous activities if drowsiness or dizziness occurs
• Avoid alcohol, other CNS depressants unless directed by clinician

---

pentobarbital
(pen-toe-bar′bi-tal)
Rx: Nembutal
Chemical Class: Barbituric acid derivative
Therapeutic Class: Sedative/hypnotic; anticonvulsant
DEA Class: Schedule II (oral, parenteral), schedule III (rectal)

CLINICAL PHARMACOLOGY
Mechanism of Action: CNS depressant: depresses the sensory cortex, decreases motor activity, alters cerebellar function, produces drowsi-

ness, sedation, and hypnosis; little analgesic action at subanesthetic doses (may increase reaction to painful stimuli); anticonvulsant activity in anesthetic doses; dose-dependent respiratory depression (hypnotic doses produce respiratory depression similar to physiologic sleep)

Pharmacokinetics
PO: Onset 15-60 min, peak 30-60 min, duration 3-4 hr
PR: Onset 20-60 min, peak, duration 3-4 hr
IM: Onset 10-25 min
IV: Onset 1 min, duration 15 min
35%-45% bound to plasma proteins; metabolized in liver, excreted in urine (metabolites); $t_{1/2}$ 22-50 hr

INDICATIONS AND USES: Insomnia (short term), status epilepticus, facilitation of intubation and anesthesia, increased intracranial pressure,* cerebral ischemia,* drownings,* emesis,* psychiatric interviews*

DOSAGE
Adult
• *Hypnotic:* PO 100-200 mg hs or 20 mg tid-qid for daytime sedation; IM 150-200 mg; IV 100 mg initially, may repeat q1-3 min up to 200-500 mg total; PR 120-200 mg hs
• *Preoperative sedation:* IM 150-200 mg
• *Pentobarbital coma for increased intracranial pressure:* IV 10-15 mg/kg over 1-2 hr loading dose, then 1 mg/kg/hr INF, increase to 2-3 mg/kg/hr if necessary; maintain burst suppression on EEG
Child
• *Sedative:* PO 2-6 mg/kg/day divided tid; max 100 mg/day
• *Hypnotic:* IM 2-6 mg/kg; max 100 mg/dose; PR <4 yr 3-6 mg/kg/dose, >4 yr 1.5-3 mg/kg/dose

• *Preoperative sedation:* PO/IM/PR 2-6 mg/kg; max 100 mg/dose; IV 1-3 mg/kg to a max of 100 mg until asleep
• *Pentobarbital coma for increased intracranial pressure:* Same as adult

💲 AVAILABLE FORMS/COST OF THERAPY
• Cap, Gel—Oral: 50 mg, 100's: **$42.82**; 100 mg, 100's: **$67.08**
• Inj, Sol—IM, IV: 50 mg/ml, 2 ml: **$2.73-$3.68**
• Supp—Rect: 30 mg, 12's: **$44.58**; 60 mg, 12's: **$62.53**; 120 mg, 12's: **$58.33**; 200 mg, 12's: **$85.75**

CONTRAINDICATIONS: Respiratory depression, severe liver impairment, porphyria

PRECAUTIONS: Myasthenia gravis, myxedema, anemia, hepatic disease, renal disease, hypertension, elderly, acute or chronic pain, mental depression, history of drug abuse, abrupt discontinuation, children, hyperthyroidism, fever, diabetes

PREGNANCY AND LACTATION: Pregnancy category D; excreted in breast milk; effect on nursing infant unknown

P

SIDE EFFECTS/ADVERSE REACTIONS
CNS: CNS depression, dizziness, *drowsiness, hangover,* headache, *lethargy,* lightheadedness, mental depression, physical dependence, slurred speech, stimulation in the elderly and children, vertigo
CV: Bradycardia, hypotension
GI: Constipation, diarrhea, nausea, vomiting
HEME: **Agranulocytosis, megaloblastic anemia** (long-term treatment), **thrombocytopenia**
RESP: **Apnea, bronchospasm, depression, laryngospasm**

---

italic = common side effects   **bold italic** = life-threatening reactions

SKIN: Abscesses at inj site, *angioedema,* erythema multiforme, pain, *rash,* **Stevens-Johnson syndrome,** thrombophlebitis, urticaria

MISC: Osteomalacia (prolonged use), rickets

INTERACTIONS
Drugs

3 *Acetaminophen:* Enhanced hepatotoxic potential of acetaminophen overdoses

3 *Antidepressants, cyclic:* Reduced serum concentrations of cyclic antidepressants

3 *β-adrenergic blockers:* Reduced serum concentrations of β-blockers which are extensively metabolized

3 *Calcium channel blockers:* Reduced serum concentrations of verapamil and dihydropyridines

3 *Chloramphenicol:* Increased barbiturate concentrations; reduced serum chloramphenicol concentrations

3 *Corticosteroids:* Reduced serum concentrations of corticosteroids; may impair therapeutic effect

3 *Cyclosporine:* Reduced serum concentration of cyclosporine

3 *Digitoxin:* Reduced serum concentration of digitoxin

3 *Disopyramide:* Reduced serum concentration of disopyramide

3 *Doxycycline:* Reduced serum doxycycline concentrations

3 *Estrogen:* Reduced serum concentration of estrogen

3 *Ethanol:* Excessive CNS depression

3 *Griseofulvin:* Reduced griseofulvin absorption

3 *Methoxyflurane:* Enhanced nephrotoxic effect

3 *MAOIs:* Prolonged effect of barbiturates

3 *Narcotic analgesics:* Increased toxicity of meperidine; reduced effect of methadone; additive CNS depression

3 *Neuroleptics:* Reduced effect of either drug

2 *Oral anticoagulants:* Decreased hypoprothrombinemic response to oral anticoagulants

3 *Oral contraceptives:* Reduced efficacy of oral contraceptives

3 *Phenytoin:* Unpredictable effect on serum phenytoin levels

3 *Propafenone:* Reduced serum concentration of propafenone

3 *Quinidine:* Reduced quinidine plasma concentration

3 *Tacrolimus:* Reduced serum concentration of tacrolimus

3 *Theophylline:* Reduced serum theophylline concentrations

3 *Valproic acid:* Increased serum concentrations of amobarbital

3 *Warfarin:* See oral anticoagulants

SPECIAL CONSIDERATIONS
PATIENT/FAMILY EDUCATION

• Avoid driving or other activities requiring alertness

• Avoid alcohol ingestion or CNS depressants

• Do not discontinue medication abruptly after long-term use

MONITORING PARAMETERS

• Excessive usage; hypnotic hangover

---

pentosan polysulfate
(pen´toe-san)

Rx: Elmiron

Chemical Class: Sulfated glycosaminoglycan (heparin derivative)

Therapeutic Class: Anticoagulant, fibrinolytic

CLINICAL PHARMACOLOGY
Mechanism of Action: Anticoagulant, fibrinolytic and anti-inflammatory effects; biochemical properties of sulfated glycosaminoglycans

---

may replace or augment natural surface glycosaminoglycans in interstitial cystitis patients

Pharmacokinetics
PO: Poorly/erratically absorbed (bioavailability 3%); metabolized in liver and excreted in urine; $t_{1/2}$ 1 hr after IV dose

INDICATIONS AND USES: Interstitial cystitis, urolithiasis,* nonbacterial prostatitis,* prophylaxis of DVT*

DOSAGE
Adult
• *Interstitial cystitis:* PO 100 mg tid with water on an empty stomach

§ AVAILABLE FORMS/COST OF THERAPY
• Cap—Oral: 100 mg, 100's: **$162.24**

PRECAUTIONS: Bleeding complications, thrombocytopenia, hepatic insufficiency, transient elevations in liver transaminases

PREGNANCY AND LACTATION: Pregnancy category B; no data in nursing mothers

SIDE EFFECTS/ADVERSE REACTIONS
CNS: Dizziness, headache (3%)
EENT: Amblyopia, conjunctivitis, optic neuritis, tinnitus
GI: Abdominal pain, diarrhea (4%), dyspepsia, LFT abnormalities, nausea (4%)
HEME: Anemia, ecchymosis, ***leukopenia,*** prolonged PT and PTT, ***thrombocytopenia***
RESP: Dyspnea, epistaxis, pharyngitis, rhinitis
SKIN: Alopecia (4%), pruritus, rash, urticaria
MISC: Peripheral edema

---

pentoxifylline
(pen-tox-if'ih-lin)
Rx: Trental
Chemical Class: Dimethylxanthine derivative
Therapeutic Class: Hemorheologic agent

CLINICAL PHARMACOLOGY
Mechanism of Action: Thought to improve blood flow by decreasing blood viscosity and improving erythrocyte flexibility; increases blood flow to affected microcirculation, enhancing tissue oxygenation

Pharmacokinetics
PO: Peak 1 hr; undergoes 1st-pass metabolism in liver to active metabolites; excreted mainly in urine (95%) and feces (5%); $t_{1/2}$ 24-48 min (metabolites 60-96 min)

INDICATIONS AND USES: Intermittent claudication, cerebrovascular insufficiency,* diabetic angiopathies and neuropathies,* transient ischemic attack,* leg ulcers,* sickle cell thalassemias,* stroke,* high-altitude sickness,* asthenozoospermia,* acute and chronic hearing disorders,* eye circulation disorders,* Raynaud's phenomenon,* apththous ulcers*

DOSAGE
Adult
• PO 400 mg tid with meals; decrease to 400 mg bid if GI and CNS side effects occur

§ AVAILABLE FORMS/COST OF THERAPY
• Tab, Coated, Sus Action—Oral: 400 mg, 100's: **$45.00-$86.63**

PRECAUTIONS: Impaired renal function, children, chronic occlusive arterial disease of limbs

PREGNANCY AND LACTATION: Pregnancy category C; excreted in breast milk

P

---

italic = common side effects   ***bold italic*** = life-threatening reactions

SIDE EFFECTS/ADVERSE REAC-TIONS

CNS: Anxiety, confusion, dizziness, headache, tremor

CV: Angina or chest pain, dyspnea, edema, hypotension

EENT: Blurred vision, conjunctivitis, earache, epistaxis, laryngitis, nasal congestion, scotomata, sore throat, swollen neck glands

GI: Anorexia, bad taste, belching, bloating, cholecystitis, constipation, dry mouth, dyspepsia, excessive salivation, flatus, nausea, thirst, vomiting

HEME: **Leukopenia**

SKIN: Brittle fingernails, pruritus, rash, urticaria

MISC: Malaise, weight change

INTERACTIONS
Drugs

3 *Fluoroquinolones (ciprofloxin, enoxacin, norfloxacin, pefloxacin, pipemidic acid):* Increased pentoxyphylline concentrations with subsequent side effects

3 *Theophylline:* Increased plasma theophylline concentrations

SPECIAL CONSIDERATIONS
• Statistically, but not always, clinically significant effects in intermittent claudication, however, other drugs less impressive; will not replace surgical options

PATIENT/FAMILY EDUCATION
• Therapeutic effect may require 2-4 wk
• Stop smoking

---

pergolide
(per´go-lide)
Rx: Permax
Chemical Class: Ergoline derivative
Therapeutic Class: Antiparkinson's agent, dopaminergic

CLINICAL PHARMACOLOGY
Mechanism of Action: Potent dopamine receptor agonist at both D_1- and D_2-receptor sites; directly stimulates postsynaptic dopamine receptors in nigrostriatal system; inhibits prolactin

Pharmacokinetics

PO: 90% bound to plasma proteins; metabolized to at least 10 metabolites (some with dopamine agonist activity), excreted by kidney

INDICATIONS AND USES: Parkinson's disease (adjunct to levodopa/carbidopa)

DOSAGE
Adult

• PO 0.05 mg qd for 1st 2 days; increase gradually by 0.1 or 0.15 mg/day every 3rd day over next 12 days; subsequent increases by 0.25 mg/day every 3rd day until optimal therapeutic response obtained; divide total daily dose tid; doses >5 mg/day have not been systematically evaluated

$ **AVAILABLE FORMS/COST OF THERAPY**
• Tab, Uncoated—Oral: 0.05 mg, 30's: **$35.60**; 0.25 mg, 100's: **$188.18**; 1 mg, 100's: **$381.34**

PRECAUTIONS: Hypotension, children, cardiac dysrhythmia, preexisting dyskinesia; coadministration with drugs affecting protein binding

PREGNANCY AND LACTATION: Pregnancy category B; may interfere with lactation

---

SIDE EFFECTS/ADVERSE REACTIONS

CNS: Akathisia, anxiety, confusion, *dizziness, dyskinesia,* dystonia, *hallucination, insomnia,* personality disorder, psychosis, somnolence, uncoordination

CV: Hypertension, hypotension, palpitation, peripheral edema, postural hypotension, syncope, vasodilation

EENT: Epistaxis, *rhinitis*

GI: Anorexia, *constipation,* diarrhea, dry mouth, *dyspepsia, nausea*

GU: Hematuria

RESP: Abnormal vision, dyspnea, hiccups

SKIN: Rash

MISC: Pain

INTERACTIONS

Drugs

3 *Lisinopril:* Additive hypotension

3 *Neuroleptics:* Potentially antagonistic pharmacodynamic effects

SPECIAL CONSIDERATIONS

• Adjunct to levodopa/carbidopa in Parkinson's disease; longer acting than bromocriptine

PATIENT/FAMILY EDUCATION

• Hypotensive cautions

---

perindopril

(per-in´doh-pril)

Rx: Aceon

Chemical Class: Nonsulfhydryl angiotensin-converting enzyme (ACE) inhibitor

Therapeutic Class: Antihypertensive

CLINICAL PHARMACOLOGY

Mechanism of Action: Prodrug for perindoprilat, which inhibits angiotensin converting enzyme, thus preventing conversion of angiotensin I to angiotensin II; angiotensin II is a potent vasoconstrictor and stimulates retention of sodium and water

Pharmacokinetics

PO: Peak 1 hr; well absorbed (PO), absolute bioavailability 75%; concomitant food reduces bioavailability 35%; extensively metabolized by liver (30-50% to perindoprilat - major metabolite with 25% bioavailability, peak 3-7 hr); excreted exclusively in urine (metabolites and parent; $t_{1/2}$ 0.8-1 hr (perindoprilat $t_{1/2}$ 3-10 hr); no accumulation with every day administration with normal renal function; crosses placenta

INDICATIONS AND USES: Hypertension, alone or in combination with other antihypertensives; CHF, microalbuminuria

DOSAGE

Adult and Child >16 yr

• PO 2 mg bid or 4 mg qd; titrate to max 16 mg qd (Note: previous diuretic use, suspend diuretic for 2-3 days or proceed cautiously, with close follow-up of renal function (BUN, serum creatinine)

Renal Impairment

• PO CrCl <30 ml/min, not recommended; CrCl >30 ml, 2 mg qd; titrate to max PO 8 mg qd

Elderly

• 8 mg qd

$ **AVAILABLE FORMS/COST OF THERAPY**

• Tab, Scored—Oral: 2 mg, 4 mg, 30's: **$108.62**; 8 mg, 30's: **$155.97**

CONTRAINDICATIONS: History of ACE-inhibitor associated angioedema; pregnancy (2nd and 3rd trimesters)

PRECAUTIONS: Renal or hepatic impairment, salt/volume depletion; hypertension with renal artery stenosis (increases in BUN and serum creatinine); monitor for neutropenia in concomitant renal or collagen vascular disease; watch for

P.

---

hyperkalemia in diabetes; dialysis, surgery; additional warnings: increased susceptibility to anaphylactoid reactions, angioedema, hypotension, neutropenia, agranulocytosis

PREGNANCY AND LACTATION: Pregnancy category C (1st trimester); category D (2nd and 3rd trimesters); associated with fetal and neonatal injury including hypotension, neonatal skull hypoplasia, anuria, reversible or irreversible renal effects and death; oligohydramnios; possibly hypoplastic lung development, IUGR, PDA

SIDE EFFECTS/ADVERSE REACTIONS

CNS: Headache, dizziness, hypertonia, somnolence

CV: Palpitations, orthostatic hypotension

EENT: Sinusitis, viral infection

GI: Dyspepsia

GU: Proteinuria

HEME: Neutropenia (0.1%)

METAB: Electrolyte disturbances

MS: Upper extremity pain

RESP: Cough

MISC: Anaphylactic reaction, facial edema, angioedema (0.1%), fever, malaise

INTERACTIONS

Drugs

3 *Azathioprine:* Increased myelosuppression

3 *Cyclosporine, tacrolimus:* Additive effects; increased risk of hyperkalemia, nephrotoxicity

3 *Diuretics:* Excessive hypotension, hypoperfusion

3 *Heparin:* Hyperkalemia

3 *Insulin, sulfonylureas:* Additive hypoglycemia

3 *Lithium:* Increase lithium levels

3 *Nonsteroidal antiinflammatory drugs:* Decreased antihypertensive efficacy, increased risk of nephrotoxicity

2 *Potassium supplements, potassium sparing diuretics, potassium salt substitutes:* Hyperkalemia

3 *Trimethoprim:* Additive risk of hyperkalemia, especially in patient predisposed to renal insufficiency

3 *Interferon alfa 2a:* Increased myelosuppression

Labs

• ACE inhibition can account for an approximately 0.5 mEq/L rise in serum potassium

SPECIAL CONSIDERATIONS

PATIENT/FAMILY EDUCATION

• Caution with salt substitutes containing potassium chloride

• Rise slowly to sitting/standing position to minimize orthostatic hypotension

• Dizziness, fainting, lightheadedness may occur during 1st few days of therapy

• May cause altered taste perception or cough; persistent dry cough usually does not subside unless medication is stopped; notify clinician if these symptoms persist

• Warnings regarding angioedema (swelling of face, extremities, eyes, lips, tongue, hoarseness, or difficulty swallowing or breathing) especially following first dose

MONITORING PARAMETERS

• Baseline electrolytes, renal function tests, and urinalysis baseline and at least BUN, creatinine, potassium within 2 weeks after initiation of therapy (increased levels may indicate acute renal failure)

• Serial orthostatic blood pressures and pulse rates

permethrin
(per-meth´ren)
Rx: Acticin, Elimite
OTC: Nix
Chemical Class: Synthetic pyrethroid derivative
Therapeutic Class: Pediculicide; scabicide

CLINICAL PHARMACOLOGY
Mechanism of Action: Acts on parasite nerve cell membranes; disrupts sodium channel current; delays repolarization and paralyzes pest; pediculicidal and ovicidal activity
Pharmacokinetics
TOP: Less than 2% of amount applied systemically absorbed; rapidly metabolized to inactive metabolites, excreted in urine; residual detectable on hair for at least 10 days following single application

INDICATIONS AND USES: Single application treatment of infestation with *Pediculus humanus capitis* (head louse) and its nits, or *Sarcoptes scabiei* (scabies)

DOSAGE
Adult and Child
• *Head lice (1%):* Top apply after hair has been shampooed, rinsed, and towel dried; apply sufficient volume of liquid to saturate hair and scalp; leave on hair for 10 min before rinsing with water; remove remaining nits; may repeat in 1 wk if necessary (1 application generally sufficient)
• *Scabies (5%):* Top apply cream from head to toe; leave on for 8-14 hr before washing off with water; may repeat in 1 wk if live mites reappear

AVAILABLE FORMS/COST OF THERAPY
• Cre—Top: 5%, 60 g: **$25.72-$32.75**
• Liq—Top: 1%, 60 ml: **$8.19**
PRECAUTIONS: Children <2 mo
PREGNANCY AND LACTATION: Pregnancy category B; excretion into breast milk unknown

SIDE EFFECTS/ADVERSE REACTIONS
SKIN: Edema, numbness, *pruritus* (difficult to distinguish from infestation itself), rash, tingling, transient burning and stinging, transient erythema

SPECIAL CONSIDERATIONS
PATIENT/FAMILY EDUCATION
• For external use only; shake well
• Avoid contact with eyes, mucous membranes
• Itching may be temporarily aggravated following application
• Do not repeat administration sooner than 1 wk
• Itching from allergic reaction caused by mite may persist for several weeks even though infestation is cured

perphenazine
(per-fen´a-zeen)
Rx: Trilafon
Chemical Class: Piperazine phenothiazine derivative
Therapeutic Class: Antipsychotic; antiemetic

CLINICAL PHARMACOLOGY
Mechanism of Action: Dopamine receptor antagonist, with higher affinity for D_2- over D_1-receptors, and variable selectivity among the cortical dopamine tracts; also activity on nondopaminergic sites, i.e., cholinergic, α_1-adrenergic and histamine receptors (explaining side effects); moderate incidence of sedation and extrapyramidal reactions; minimal orthostatic hypotension and anticholinergic effects

P

Pharmacokinetics

PO: Onset ½-1 hr, peak 4-8 hr

IM: Onset 10 min, peak 1-2 hr, duration 6 hr

90% bound to plasma proteins; metabolized in liver, excreted in urine and bile; $t_{1/2}$ 9 hr

INDICATIONS AND USES: Psychotic disorders, severe nausea and vomiting,* intractable hiccups,* hemiballismus,* aggressive behavior,* tricyclic-induced tremor,* organic mental syndromes*

DOSAGE

NOTE: 10 mg equivalent to chlorpromazine 100 mg

Adult

• *Psychosis:* PO 4-16 mg bid-qid; do not exceed 64 mg/day; IM 5 mg q6h up to 15 mg/day in ambulatory patients, 30 mg/day in hospitalized patients

• *Nausea/vomiting:* PO 8-16 mg/day in divided doses up to 24 mg/day; IM 5-10 mg q6h up to 15 mg/day in ambulatory patients, 30 mg/day in hospitalized patients; IV 1 mg at 1-2 min intervals up to 5 mg total

Child

• Not established <12 yr; use lowest adult dose >12 yr

• *Nausea/vomiting:* IM 5 mg q6h

$ **AVAILABLE FORMS/COST OF THERAPY**

• Inj, Sol—IM, IV: 5 mg/ml, 1 ml: **$7.83**

• Liq—Oral: 16 mg/5 ml, 120 ml: **$44.64**

• Tab, Coated—Oral: 2 mg, 100's: **$7.81-$86.03**; 4 mg, 100's: **$10.69-$117.71**; 8 mg, 100's: **$12.23-$142.81**; 16 mg, 100's: **$21.55-$192.13**

CONTRAINDICATIONS: Severe toxic CNS depression, coma, subcortical brain damage, bone marrow depression

PRECAUTIONS: Children <12 yr, elderly, prolonged use, severe cardiovascular disorders, epilepsy, hepatic or renal disease, glaucoma, prostatic hypertrophy, severe asthma, emphysema, hypocalcemia (increased susceptibility to dystonic reactions), COPD

PREGNANCY AND LACTATION: Pregnancy category C; has been used as an antiemetic during normal labor without producing any observable effect on newborn; excreted into human breast milk; effects on nursing infant unknown, but may be of concern

SIDE EFFECTS/ADVERSE REACTIONS

CNS: Agitation, anxiety, catatonic-like behavioral states, confusion, depression, *drowsiness, EPS (pseudoparkinsonism, akathisia, dystonia,* tardive dyskinesia), euphoria, exacerbation of psychotic symptoms including hallucinations, *headache,* heat or cold intolerance, insomnia, lethargy, *neuroleptic malignant syndrome,* restlessness, *seizures,* vertigo

CV: ECG changes, hypotension, *tachycardia*

EENT: Blurred vision, cataracts, dry eyes, glaucoma, pigmentation of retina or cornea, retinopathy

GI: Anorexia, constipation, diarrhea, *dry mouth,* dyspepsia, hypersalivation, increased LFTs, *nausea,* vomiting

GU: Priapism, urinary retention

HEME: **Agranulocytosis,** anemia, **aplastic anemia, hemolytic anemia,** leukocytosis, minimal decreases in red blood cell counts, transient leukopenia

METAB: Breast engorgement, gynecomastia, hyperglycemia, hypoglycemia, hyponatremia, impotence, increased libido, lactation, mastalgia, menstrual irregularities

RESP: Bronchospasm, increased depth of respiration, laryngospasm
SKIN: Diaphoresis, loss of hair, maculopapular and acneiform skin reactions, photosensitivity

INTERACTIONS

Drugs

3 *Amodiaquine, chloroquine, sulfadoxine-pyrimethamine:* Increased neuroleptic concentrations

3 *Anticholinergics:* May inhibit neuroleptic response; excess anticholinergic effects

3 *Antidepressants:* Potential for increased therapeutic and toxic effects from increased levels of both drugs

3 *Barbiturates:* Decreased neuroleptic levels

3 *Clonidine, guanadrel, granethidine:* Severe hypotensive episodes possible

3 *Epinephrine:* Blunted pressor response to epinephrine

3 *Ethanol:* Additive CNS depression

2 *Levodopa:* Inhibited antiparkinsonian effect of levodopa

3 *Lithium:* Lowered levels of both drugs, rarely neurotoxicity in acute mania

3 *Narcotic analgesics:* Hypotension and increased CNS depression

3 *Orphenadrine:* Lowered neuroleptic concentrations, excessive anticholinergic effects

3 *Propranolol:* Increased plasma

Labs

• *Creatinine:* Decreased serum levels

SPECIAL CONSIDERATIONS

PATIENT/FAMILY EDUCATION

• Arise slowly from reclining position
• Do not discontinue abruptly
• Use a sunscreen during sun exposure to prevent burns, take special precautions to stay cool in hot weather

• Concentrate may be diluted just prior to administration with distilled water, acidified tap water, orange or grape juice

MONITORING PARAMETERS

• Observe closely for signs of tardive dyskinesia (abnormal involuntary movement scale)
• Periodic CBC with platelets during prolonged therapy

---

phenazopyridine

(fen-az′o-peer′i-deen)
Rx: Azo-Standard, Baridium, Eridium, Geridium, Phenazodine, Pyridiate, Pyridium, Urodine, Urogesic, Viridium
Combinations
  Rx: with sulfamethoxazole (Azo-Gantanol); with sulfisoxazole (Azo-Gantrisin)
Chemical Class: Azo dye
Therapeutic Class: Urinary tract analgesic

CLINICAL PHARMACOLOGY

Mechanism of Action: Exerts topical analgesic effect on urinary tract mucosa

Pharmacokinetics

PO: Rapidly excreted by kidneys, 65% excreted unchanged in urine

INDICATIONS AND USES: Symptomatic relief of urinary burning, itching, frequency, and urgency associated with UTI, or following urologic procedures

DOSAGE

Adult

• PO 100-200 mg tid after meals; do not exceed 2 days when used concomitantly with antibacterial agents for UTI

---

italic = common side effects   ***bold italic*** = life-threatening reactions

Child
• PO 12 mg/kg/day divided tid after meals

💲 AVAILABLE FORMS/COST OF THERAPY
• Tab, Coated—Oral: 100 mg, 100's: **$1.49-$69.48**; 200 mg, 100's: **$2.09-$133.90**

CONTRAINDICATIONS: Renal insufficiency

PRECAUTIONS: Chronic use in undiagnosed urinary tract pain, children <12 yr

PREGNANCY AND LACTATION: Pregnancy category B

SIDE EFFECTS/ADVERSE REACTIONS
CNS: Headache
EENT: Staining of contact lenses, yellowish tinge of sclera
GI: GI disturbances, **hepatitis,** jaundice
GU: Orange-red discoloration of urine, renal stones, **transient acute renal failure**
HEME: **Hemolytic anemia, methemoglobinemia**
SKIN: Pruritus, rash, yellowish tinge of skin
MISC: **Anaphylactoid-like reaction**

INTERACTIONS
Labs
• *Albumin:* Increased serum concentrations
• *Bacteria:* False negatives on Microstix
• *Bile:* False positive with Ictotest, BiliLabstix
• *Bilirubin, conjugated:* False elevations in serum
• *Bilirubin, unconjugated:* False serum concentration elevations
• *BSP Retention:* False negatives
• *Cholinesterase:* Adds 34% negative bias to Ectachem method
• *Urine:* Yellow-orange color
• *Feces:* Orange-red color
• *Glucose:* Decreased serum levels

• *17-ketogenic steroids:* False positives in urine
• *Ketones:* Nitroprusside reactions masked by color; false negatives
• *17-ketosteroids:* Increase in urine
• *Porphyrins:* False positive
• *Pregnanediol:* Increased urine levels
• *Protein:* Increased serum levels
• *PSP excretion:* False positive in alkaline pH
• *Urobilinogen:* False positive urine test
• *Vanillylmandelic acid:* Increased urine concentrations
• *Xylose excretion:* Increased urine concentrations

SPECIAL CONSIDERATIONS
PATIENT/FAMILY EDUCATION
• May cause GI upset
• Take after meals
• May cause reddish-orange discoloration of urine; may stain fabric; may also stain contact lenses

---

phendimetrazine
(fen-dye-me′tra-zeen)
Rx: Adipost, Bontril, Dital Rexigen, Dyrexan-OD, Melfiat-105, Plegine, Prelu-2
Chemical Class: Morpholine
Therapeutic Class: Anorexiant
DEA Class: Schedule III

CLINICAL PHARMACOLOGY
Mechanism of Action: Acts on adrenergic and dopaminergic pathways, directly stimulating the satiety center in the hypothalamic and limbic regions
Pharmacokinetics
PO: Onset 30 min, peak 1-3 hr, duration 4-20 hr; metabolized by liver, excreted by kidneys; $t_{1/2}$ 2-10 hr
INDICATIONS AND USES: Exogenous obesity (as a short-term adjunct to caloric restriction)

DOSAGE
Adult
• PO 35 mg bid-tid, 1 hr ac, not to exceed 70 mg tid; PO Sus Action 105 mg q AM before breakfast

💲 AVAILABLE FORMS/COST OF THERAPY
• Cap, Gel, Sus Action—Oral: 105 mg, 100's: **$20.75-$120.32**
• Tab, Uncoated—Oral: 35 mg, 100's: **$5.00-$80.96**

CONTRAINDICATIONS: Moderate to severe hypertension, children, glaucoma, history of drug abuse, cardiovascular disease, advanced arteriosclerosis, agitated states, hyperthyroidism, within 14 days of MAOI administration

PRECAUTIONS: Diabetes mellitus, convulsive disorders, mild hypertension

PREGNANCY AND LACTATION: Pregnancy category C

SIDE EFFECTS/ADVERSE REACTIONS
CNS: Dizziness, drowsiness, dysphoria, exacerbation of schizophrenia, headache, *insomnia,* mental depression, *nervousness, overstimulation, restlessness,* shivering, tremor, weakness

CV: Chest pain, palpitation, ***tachycardia***

GI: Constipation, diarrhea, dry mouth, nausea, unpleasant taste

GU: Impotence, testicular pain, urinary hesitancy

SKIN: Clamminess, excessive sweating, pallor, rash

SPECIAL CONSIDERATIONS
PATIENT/FAMILY EDUCATION
• May cause insomnia; avoid taking late in the day
• Weight reduction requires strict adherence to caloric restriction
• Do not discontinue abruptly

phenelzine
(fen'el-zeen)
Rx: Nardil
Chemical Class: Hydrazine derivative
Therapeutic Class: Monoamine oxidase (MAO) inhibitor antidepressant

CLINICAL PHARMACOLOGY
Mechanism of Action: MAOI resulting in increased endogenous concentrations of serotonin, norepinephrine, epinephrine, and dopamine in the CNS; chronic administration results in down regulation (desensitization) of α_2- or β-adrenergic and serotonin receptors, which may correlate with antidepressant activity

Pharmacokinetics
PO: Onset of action 4-8 wk, duration of MAO inhibition at least 10 days, peak serum concentration 2-4 hr, metabolized in liver, excreted in urine as metabolites and unchanged drug

INDICATIONS AND USES: Treatment-resistant depression, including patients characterized as atypical, nonendogenous, or neurotic

DOSAGE
Adult
• PO 15 mg tid initially, increase as tolerated to 60-90 mg/day; following achievement of maximal benefit, reduce dosage slowly over several weeks to lowest effective dose that maintains response

💲 AVAILABLE FORMS/COST OF THERAPY
• Tab, Sugar Coated—Oral: 15 mg, 100's: **$54.15**

CONTRAINDICATIONS: Pheochromocytoma, congestive heart failure, liver disease, severe renal function impairment, cerebrovascu-

P

---

italic = common side effects   ***bold italic*** = life-threatening reactions

lar defect, cardiovascular disease, hypertension, history of headache, age >60 yr

PRECAUTIONS: Children <16 yr, hypotension, bipolar affective disorder, agitation, schizophrenia, hyperactivity, diabetes mellitus, seizure disorder, angina, hyperthyroidism, suicidal ideation

PREGNANCY AND LACTATION: Pregnancy category C

SIDE EFFECTS/ADVERSE REACTIONS

CNS: Agitation, akathisia, ataxia, chills, coma, confusion, *dizziness, drowsiness,* euphoria, fatigue, headache, hyperreflexia, hypomania, jitteriness, mania, memory impairment, muscle twitching, myoclonic movements, neuritis, overactivity, overstimulation, restlessness, *seizures,* sleep disturbance, tremors, vertigo, weakness

CV: **Dysrhythmias,** edema, **hypertension,** orthostatic hypotension, palpitations, tachycardia

EENT: Blurred vision, glaucoma, nystagmus

GI: Abdominal pain, anorexia, black tongue, constipation, diarrhea, dry mouth, elevated transaminases, hepatitis, nausea

GU: Dysuria, incontinence, sexual disturbance, urinary retention

HEME: **Agranulocytosis,** anemia, spider telangiectases, **thrombocytopenia**

METAB: Hypermetabolic syndrome, hypernatremia, SIADH-like syndrome

SKIN: Hyperhydrosis, photosensitivity, rash

MISC: Weight gain

INTERACTIONS

Drugs

⚠ *Amphetamines, alcoholic beverages containing tyramine, metaraminol, phenylephrine, phenyl-* *propanolamine, pseudoephedrine, tyramine:* Severe hypertensive reaction

❷ *Antidepressants, cyclic:* Excessive sympathetic response, mania, hyperpyrexia

❸ *Barbiturates:* Prolonged effect of some barbiturates

⚠ *Clomipramine:* Death

⚠ *Dexfenfluramine, dextromethorphan, fenfluramine, meperidine:* Agitation, blood pressure changes, hyperpyrexia, convulsions

⚠ *Fluoxetine, Sertraline:* Hypomania, confusion, hypertension, tremor

⚠ *Food:* Foods containing large amounts of tyramine can result in hypertensive reactions

❸ *Guanadrel, guanethidine:* May inhibit antihypertensive effects

❸ *Levodopa:* Severe hypertensive reaction

❷ *Lithium:* Malignant hyperpyrexia

❸ *Neuromuscular blocking agents:* Prolonged muscle relaxation caused by succinylcholine

❸ *Reserpine:* Hypertensive reaction

❸ *Sumatriptan:* Increased sumatriptan plasma concentrations

Labs

• *Aspartate aminotransferase:* Increased serum levels

• *Bilirubin:* False–positive increases in serum

• *Uric acid:* False–positive increases in serum

SPECIAL CONSIDERATIONS

PATIENT/FAMILY EDUCATION

• Avoid tyramine-containing foods, beverages, and OTC products containing decongestants or dextromethorphan and products such as diet aids

• May cause drowsiness, dizziness, blurred vision

• Use caution driving or performing other tasks requiring alertness

• Arise slowly from reclining position

• Therapeutic effect may require 4-8 wk

---

phenobarbital

(fee-noe-bar´bi-tal)
Rx: Bellatal, Luminal, Solfoton
Combinations
  Rx: with atropine, hyoscyamine, scopolamine (Donnatal); with belladonna, ergotamine (Bellergal Spacetabs)
Chemical Class: Barbituric acid derivative
Therapeutic Class: Sedative/hypnotic; anticonvulsant
DEA Class: Schedule IV

CLINICAL PHARMACOLOGY
Mechanism of Action: CNS depressant: depresses the sensory cortex, decreases motor activity, alters cerebellar function, produces drowsiness, sedation, and hypnosis; little analgesic action at subanesthetic doses (may increase reaction to painful stimuli); anticonvulsant activity in subhypnotic doses; dose-dependent respiratory depression (hypnotic doses produce respiratory depression similar to physiologic sleep)
Pharmacokinetics
PO: Onset 20-60 min, peak 1-6 hr, duration 10-16 hr
IV: Onset within 5 min, peak effect within 30 min, duration 4-10 hr 20%-50% bound to plasma proteins; metabolized in liver, excreted in urine (20%-50% unchanged); t₁/₂ 53-140 hr (prolonged in overdose)

INDICATIONS AND USES: Routine and preoperative sedation, tonic-clonic (grand mal) seizures, partial seizures, prevention of febrile seizures (controversial), status epilepticus (not 1st line), neonatal hyperbilirubinemia,* congenital nonhemolytic unconjugated hyperbilirubinemia,* chronic intrahepatic cholestasis*

DOSAGE
Adult
• *Anticonvulsant:* PO/IV 1-3 mg/kg/day in divided doses or 50-100 mg bid-tid
• *Status epilepticus:* IV 300-800 mg initially followed by 120-240 mg at 20 min intervals until seizures are controlled or a total dose of 1-2 g
• *Sedation:* PO/IM 30-120 mg/day in 2-3 divided doses
• *Hypnotic:* PO/IM/IV/SC 100-320 mg/kg hs
• *Preoperative sedation:* IM 100-200 mg 1-1½ hr before procedure
Child
• *Anticonvulsant:* PO/IV neonates 2-4 mg/kg/day in 1-2 divided doses; infants 5-8 mg/kg/day in 1-2 divided doses; 1-5 yr 6-8 mg/kg/day in 1-2 divided doses; 5-12 yr 4-6 mg/kg/day in 1-2 divided doses
• *Status epilepticus:* IV neonates 15-20 mg/kg in a single or divided dose; infants and children 10-20 mg/kg in a single or divided dose, may give additional 5 mg/kg/dose q15-30 min until seizure is controlled or a total dose of 40 mg/kg is reached
• *Sedation:* PO 2 mg/kg tid
• *Hypnotic:* IM/IV/SC 3-5 mg/kg hs
• *Preoperative sedation:* PO/IM/IV 1-3 mg/kg 1-1½ hr before procedure

⑤ AVAILABLE FORMS/COST OF THERAPY
• Elixir—Oral: 20 mg/5 ml, 480 ml: **$3.65-$12.42**

---

italic = common side effects   ***bold italic*** = life-threatening reactions

• Inj, Sol—IM, IV: 30 mg/ml, 1 ml: **$2.24-$2.99**; 60 mg/ml, 1 ml: **$2.55-$3.35**; 65 mg/ml, 1 ml: **$1.70**; 130 mg/ml, 1 ml: **$3.67-$4.11**

• Tab, Uncoated—Oral: 15 mg, 100's: **$0.54-$7.37**; 30 mg, 100's: **$0.64-$5.31**; 60 mg, 100's: **$2.66-$5.34**; 100 mg, 100's: **$3.31-$3.34**

• Tab—Oral: 16.2 mg, 100's: **$2.90-$3.34**; 32.4 mg, 100's: **$2.68**; 64.8 mg, 100's: **$4.40**; 97.2 mg, 100's: **$5.63**

CONTRAINDICATIONS: Respiratory depression, severe liver impairment, porphyria

PRECAUTIONS: Myasthenia gravis, myxedema, anemia, hepatic disease, renal disease, hypertension, elderly, acute or chronic pain, mental depression, history of drug abuse, abrupt discontinuation, children, hyperthyroidism, fever, diabetes

PREGNANCY AND LACTATION: Pregnancy category D; risks to fetus include minor congenital defects, hemorrhage at birth, addiction; risk to mother may be greater if seizure control is lost due to stopping drug; use at lowest possible level to control seizures; excreted into breast milk, has caused major adverse effects in some nursing infants, use caution in nursing women

SIDE EFFECTS/ADVERSE REACTIONS

CNS: CNS depression, dizziness, *drowsiness, hangover,* headache, *lethargy,* lightheadedness, mental depression, physical dependence, slurred speech, stimulation in the elderly and children, vertigo

CV: Bradycardia, hypotension

GI: Constipation, diarrhea, nausea, vomiting

HEME: **Agranulocytosis, megaloblastic anemia** (long-term treatment), **thrombocytopenia**

RESP: **Apnea, bronchospasm, depression, laryngospasm**

SKIN: Abscesses at injection site, **angioedema,** erythema multiforme, pain, *rash,* **Stevens-Johnson syndrome,** thrombophlebitis, urticaria

MISC: Osteomalacia (prolonged use), rickets

INTERACTIONS

Drugs

🔢 *Acetaminophen:* Enhanced hepatotoxic potential of acetaminophen overdoses

🔢 *Antidepressants:* Reduced serum concentrations of cyclic antidepressants

🔢 *Beta-blockers:* Reduced serum concentrations of β-blockers, which are extensively metabolized (metoprolol, propranolol, sotalol)

🔢 *Calcium channel blockers:* Reduced concentrations of verapamil and nifedipine

🔢 *Chloramphenicol:* Increased barbiturate concentrations; reduced serum chloramphenicol concentrations

🔢 *Corticosteroids:* Reduced serum concentrations of corticosteroids, may impair therapeutic effect

🔢 *Cyclosporine:* Reduced serum concentration of cyclosporine

🔢 *Digitoxin:* Reduced serum concentration of digitoxin

🔢 *Disopyramide:* Reduced serum concentration of disopyramide

🔢 *Doxycycline:* Reduced serum doxycycline concentrations

🔢 *Estrogen:* Reduced serum concentration of estrogen

🔢 *Ethanol:* Excessive CNS depression

🔢 *Felbamate:* Increased phenobarbital concentrations; increased risk of toxicity

🔢 *Furosemide:* Decreased diuretic effect

🔢 *Griseofulvin:* Reduced griseofulvin absorption

3 *Lamotrigine:* Lower lamotrigine plasma levels and decreased elimination t½

3 *Methoxyflurane:* Enhanced nephrotoxic effect

3 *Narcotic analgesics:* Increased toxicity of meperidine; reduced effect of methadone; additive CNS depression

3 *Neuroleptics:* Reduced effect of either drug

2 *Oral anticoagulants:* Decreased hypoprothrombinemic response to oral anticoagulants

3 *Oral contraceptives:* Reduced efficacy of oral contraceptives

3 *Phenytoin:* Unpredictable effect on serum phenytoin levels

3 *Primidone:* Excessive phenobarbital concentrations

3 *Propafenone:* Reduced serum concentration of propafenone

3 *Quinidine:* Reduced quinidine plasma concentration

3 *Tacrolimus:* Reduced serum concentration of tacrolimus

3 *Theophylline:* Reduced serum theophylline concentrations

3 *Valproic acid:* Increased serum phenobarbital concentrations

Labs
• *Amino acids:* Increase in urine collection measurements
• *Calcium:* False increases with Technicon SRA-2000
• *Glucose:* False negatives with Clinistix, Diastix
• *5-Hydroxyindoleacetic acid:* False high colorimetric values
• *Lactate dehydrogenase:* Increased serum levels
• *Protein:* False elevations at high concentrations

SPECIAL CONSIDERATIONS
PATIENT/FAMILY EDUCATION
• Avoid driving or other activities requiring alertness
• Avoid alcohol ingestion or CNS depressants
• Do not discontinue medication abruptly after long-term use

MONITORING PARAMETERS
• Periodic CBC, liver and renal function tests, serum folate, vitamin D during prolonged therapy
• Serum phenobarbital concentration (therapeutic range for seizure disorders 20-40 µg/ml)

---

phenoxybenzamine
(fen-ox-ee-ben′za-meen)
Rx: Dibenzyline
Chemical Class: Haloalkylamine derivative
Therapeutic Class: Sympatholytic: Agent for pheochromocytoma

CLINICAL PHARMACOLOGY
Mechanism of Action: Irreversible α-adrenergic receptor (both pre- and postsynaptic) blocker; produces "chemical sympathectomy"; increases blood flow to skin, mucosa, abdominal viscera; lowers supine and standing blood pressure

Pharmacokinetics
PO: Incomplete oral absorption (20%-30%) onset gradual over several hours, duration 3-4 days; metabolized via dealkylation, excreted in urine and bile; t½ 24 hr

INDICATIONS AND USES: Pheochromocytoma (control of episodes of hypertension and sweating), micturition disorders (neurogenic bladder, functional outlet obstruction, partial prostatic obstruction),* peripheral vasospastic disorders*

DOSAGE
Adult
• PO 10 mg bid initially, increase dosage qod until optimal response obtained as judged by blood pressure; usual dosage range 20-40 mg bid-tid

P

Child
• PO 1-2 mg/kg/day divided q6-8h

$ **AVAILABLE FORMS/COST OF THERAPY**
• Cap, Gel—Oral: 10 mg, 100's: **$631.04**

CONTRAINDICATIONS: Conditions where a fall in blood pressure may be undesirable

PRECAUTIONS: Marked cerebral or coronary arteriosclerosis, renal damage, respiratory infection

PREGNANCY AND LACTATION: Pregnancy category C; indicated in hypertension secondary to pheochromocytoma during pregnancy, especially after 24 wk gestation when surgical intervention is associated with high rates of maternal and fetal mortality; no adverse fetal effects due to this treatment have been observed

SIDE EFFECTS/ADVERSE REACTIONS

CNS: Confusion, *dizziness,* drowsiness, sedation

CV: Palpitations, *postural hypotension, tachycardia*

EENT: Miosis, nasal congestion

GI: GI irritation, nausea, vomiting

GU: Inhibition of ejaculation

MISC: Fatigue

SPECIAL CONSIDERATIONS
PATIENT/FAMILY EDUCATION
• Avoid alcohol; avoid sudden changes in posture, dizziness may result
• Avoid cough, cold, or allergy medications containing sympathomimetics

---

phentermine
(fen´ter-meen)
Rx: Adipex-P, Fastin, Ionamin, Obe-Nix, Supramine, Tara-30, T-Diet, Teramin, Termene, Tora, Umi-Pex 30, Zantryl
Chemical Class: Phenethylamine analog (amphetamine-like
Therapeutic Class: Anorexiant
DEA Class: Schedule IV

CLINICAL PHARMACOLOGY
Mechanism of Action: Acts on adrenergic and dopaminergic pathways, directly stimulating the satiety center in the hypothalamic and limbic regions

Pharmacokinetics
PO-SUS REL: Duration 10-14 hr; metabolized by liver, excreted by kidney

INDICATIONS AND USES: Exogenous obesity

DOSAGE
Adult (>16 years)
• PO 8 mg tid ½ hr ac, or 15-37.5 mg as single daily dose before breakfast or 10-14 hr before retiring

$ **AVAILABLE FORMS/COST OF THERAPY**
• Cap, Sus Action—Oral: 15 mg, 100's: **$125.37-$226.64**; 18.75 mg, 100's: **$28.95-$47.80**; 30 mg, 100's: **$5.78-$112.80**; 37.5 mg, 100's: **$13.46-$169.67**
• Tab, Uncoated—Oral: 8 mg, 100's: **$54.07**
• Tab, Sus Action—Oral: 37.5 mg, 100's: **$12.08-$166.68**

CONTRAINDICATIONS: Glaucoma, history of drug abuse, cardiovascular disease, moderate to severe hypertension, advanced arteriosclеrosis, agitated states, hyperthyroidism, within 14 days of MAOI administration

PRECAUTIONS: Diabetes mellitus, convulsive disorders, hypertension, children

PREGNANCY AND LACTATION: Pregnancy category C

SIDE EFFECTS/ADVERSE REACTIONS

CNS: Dizziness, drowsiness, *dysphoria,* exacerbation of schizophrenia, headache, *insomnia,* mental depression, *nervousness, overstimulation, restlessness,* shivering, tremor, weakness

CV: Chest pain, palpitation, ***tachycardia***

GI: Constipation, diarrhea, dry mouth, nausea, unpleasant taste

GU: Impotence, testicular pain, urinary hesitancy

SKIN: Clamminess, excessive sweating, pallor, rash

INTERACTIONS

Drugs

3 *Furazolidone:* Increased pressor response

3 *Guanethidine:* Decreased hypotensive effect

A *MAO Inhibitors:* Increased pressor response

3 *Tricyclic antidepressants:* Decreased anorexiant effect

Labs

• *Drugs of abuse:* Urine screen; false positive for amphetamines

• *Phenmetrazine:* False positive urine

• *Quinine:* False positive urine

SPECIAL CONSIDERATIONS

PATIENT/FAMILY EDUCATION

• May cause insomnia, avoid taking late in the day

• Weight reduction is facilitated by adherence to caloric restriction and exercise

phentolamine

(fen-tole´a-meen)

Rx: Regitine
Chemical Class: Imidazoline
Therapeutic Class: Sympatholytic: Agent for pheochromocytoma

CLINICAL PHARMACOLOGY

Mechanism of Action: α-adrenergic receptor (both pre- and postsynaptic) blocker; produces immediate onset and short duration "chemical sympathectomy"; acts at both the arterial and venous level; lowers supine and standing blood pressure; causes cardiac stimulation

Pharmacokinetics

IV: Onset of action immediate, duration 10-15 min

IM: Onset 15-20 min, duration 3-4 hr
Metabolized in liver, excreted in urine (10% as unchanged drug)

INDICATIONS AND USES: Diagnosis of and treatment of hypertension associated with pheochromocytoma, treatment of dermal necrosis following extravasation of α-adrenergic drugs (norepinephrine, epinephrine, dobutamine, dopamine), hypertensive crises secondary to MAOI or sympathomimetic amine interactions and rebound hypertension on withdrawal of antihypertensives,* with papaverine as intracavernous injection for impotence*

DOSAGE

Adult

• *Diagnosis of pheochromocytoma:* IM/IV 5 mg

• *Hypertension, surgery for pheochromocytoma:* IM/IV 5 mg 1-2 hr before procedure, repeat q2-4h as needed

---

italic = common side effects   ***bold italic*** = life-threatening reactions

• *Drug extravasation:* Dilute 5-10 mg in 10 ml NS, infiltrate area with sol within 12 hr (blanching resolves within 1 hr if successful)

Child

• *Diagnosis of pheochromocytoma:* IM/IV 0.05-0.1 mg/kg/dose, max single dose 5 mg

• *Hypertension, surgery for pheochromocytoma:* IM/IV 0.05-0.1 mg/kg/dose 1-2 hr before procedure, repeat q2-4h as needed

• *Drug extravasation:* 0.1-0.2 mg/kg diluted in 10 ml NS infiltrated into area of extravasation within 12 hr

$ AVAILABLE FORMS/COST OF THERAPY

• Inj, Sol—IM, IV: 5 mg/ml; 1 ml vial: **$35.00**

CONTRAINDICATIONS: Angina, MI

PRECAUTIONS: Peptic ulcer disease (may exacerbate)

PREGNANCY AND LACTATION: Pregnancy category C; unknown if excreted in breast milk

SIDE EFFECTS/ADVERSE REACTIONS

CNS: **Cerebrovascular occlusion,** dizziness, flushing, severe headache, weakness

CV: Angina, **dysrhythmias,** *hypotension,* **MI,** *reflex tachycardia*

EENT: Nasal congestion

GI: Abdominal pain, diarrhea, dry mouth, nausea, vomiting

INTERACTIONS

Drugs

3 *Epinepherine, ephedrine:* Vasoconstricting and hypertensive effects of these drugs are antagonized

Labs

• *5-hydroxyindoleacetic acid:* Urine, falsely high colorimetric values

SPECIAL CONSIDERATIONS

• Urinary catecholamines preferred over phentolamine for screening for pheochromocytoma

---

phenylephrine (systemic)

(fen-ill-ef′rin)

Rx: Neo-Synephrine, AH-Chew D

Combinations

Rx: with chlorpheniramine (Ed A-Hist, Prehist, Histatab); with brompheniramine (Dimetane); with chlorpheniramine, phenylpropanolamine (Hista-Vadrin); with chlorpheniramine, phenyltoloxamine (Comhist); with brompheniramine, phenylpropanolamine (Bromophen T.D., Tamine S.R.); with chlorpheniramine, phenyltoloxamine, phenylpropanolamine (Decongestabs, Naldecon, Nalgest, Triphen, Uni-decon); with chlorpheniramine, pyrilamine, phenylpropanolamine (Vanex, Histalet); with chlorpheniramine, pyrilamine (R-tannate, Rhinatate, R-tannamine, Rynatan, Tanoral, Triotann, Tritan, Tri-tannate)

Chemical Class: Substituted phenylethylamine

Therapeutic Class: Vasopressor

CLINICAL PHARMACOLOGY

Mechanism of Action: Selective postsynaptic α_1-receptor agonist; causes vasoconstriction with increase in blood pressure and reflex bradycardia

---

* = non-FDA-approved use

Pharmacokinetics

IV: Duration 20-30 min

IM/SC: Duration 45-60 min

PO: Biodegraded in gut wall (c-o-methyltransferase); essentially, not bioavailable

Excreted in urine; $t_{1/2}$ 2½ hr

INDICATIONS AND USES: Hypotension, shock, paroxysmal supraventricular tachycardia (PSVT), prolongation of spinal anesthesia, vasoconstriction in regional analgesia

DOSAGE

Adult

• *Decongestant:* PO 10 mg q4-6hr, PRN

• *Hypotension:* SC/IM 2-5 mg, may repeat q10-15 min if needed; IV 0.1-0.5 mg, may repeat q10-15 min if needed; IV INF 10 mg/500 ml D_5W given 100-180 gtt/min (based on 20 gtt/ml), then 40-60 gtt/min titrated to BP

• *PSVT:* IV bolus 0.5 mg given rapidly; subsequent doses should not exceed previous dose by >0.1-0.2 mg; max single dose 1 mg

• *Prolongation of spinal anesthesia:* Add 2-5 mg to anesthetic solution; increases duration of block by 50%

• *Prevention of hypotension in spinal anesthesia:* SC/IM 2-3 mg 3-4 min before anesthetic inj

• *Vasoconstriction in regional anesthesia:* Add 1 mg to 20 ml anesthetic sol

Child

• *Hypotension:* SC/IM 0.1 mg/kg/dose q1-2h (max 5 mg); IV bolus 5-20 µg/kg/dose q10-15 min; IV INF 0.1-0.5 µg/kg/min

• *PSVT:* IV 5-10 µg/kg/dose over 20-30 sec

• *Prevention of hypotension in spinal anesthesia:* SC/IM 0.05-0.1 mg/kg/dose

💲 AVAILABLE FORMS/COST OF THERAPY

• Inj, Sol—IM, IV, SC: 10 mg/ml, 1 ml: **$0.75-$4.39**

• Liq—Oral: 5 mg/5 ml, 120 ml: **$10.98**

• Supp—Rect: 0.25% 12's: **$5.50**

• Tab, chewable—Oral: 10 mg, 100's: **$69.60**

CONTRAINDICATIONS: Ventricular fibrillation/tachycardia, pheochromocytoma, narrow-angle glaucoma, severe hypertension

PRECAUTIONS: Arterial embolism, peripheral vascular disease, elderly, hyperthyroidism, bradycardia, myocardial disease, severe arteriosclerosis

PREGNANCY AND LACTATION: Pregnancy category C; unknown if excreted in breast milk

SIDE EFFECTS/ADVERSE REACTIONS

CNS: Anxiety, dizziness, headache, insomnia, tremor

CV: Angina, ectopic beats, hypertension, palpitations, reflex bradycardia, tachycardia

GI: Nausea, vomiting

SKIN: **Gangrene,** necrosis, tissue sloughing with extravasation

INTERACTIONS

Drugs

❸ *Beta-Blockers (non-selective):* Predisposed to hypertensive episodes

❸ *Guanethidine:* Enhanced pupillary response to phenylephrine

❸ *Imipramine:* Enhanced pressor response

⚠ *MAOIs:* Hypertensive episodes

Labs

• *Amino acids:* Increased in urine

• *Metanephrines, total:* Increased in urine

SPECIAL CONSIDERATIONS

• Antidote to extravasation: 5-10 ml phentolamine in 10-15 ml saline infiltrated throughout ischemic area

---

italic = common side effects   ***bold italic*** = life-threatening reactions

• Not indicated for hypotension secondary to hypovolemia

• As not bioavailable orally (see pharmacokinetics), combination products essentially lack decongestant. Only available by prescription, as lack effectiveness data required by FDA OTC panels

---

phenylephrine (topical)

(fen-ill-ef′rin)

Rx: *Ophthalmic:* Ak-Dilate, Ak-Nefrin, Mydfrin, Neo-Synephrine, Prefrin Liquifilm, Relief
OTC: *Nasal:* Alconefrin, Alconefrin, Neo-Synephrine, Nostril, Rhinall, Sinex, *Anorectal:* Medicone, Hem-Prep,
Combinations
  Rx: (Nasal): with zinc (Zincfrin); with pheniramine (Dristan Nasal);
  Rx: (Ophthalmic); with tropicamide (Diophenyl-t); with pyrilamine (Prefrin-A)
Chemical Class: Substituted phenylethylamine
Therapeutic Class: Decongestant; mydriatic

CLINICAL PHARMACOLOGY
Mechanism of Action: Postsynaptic α-receptor agonist; produces vasoconstriction (rapid, long-acting) of arterioles, decreasing fluid exudate, mucosal engorgement; stimulation of α-adrenergic receptors of the dilator muscle of the pupil, produce contraction, thus pupillary dilation
Pharmacokinetics
NASAL: May be systemically absorbed; duration of action 30 min-4 hr

OPHTH: Peak effect of mydriasis 15-60 min (2.5% sol), 10-90 min (10% sol); duration of action 3 hr (2.5% sol), 3-7 hr (10% sol)
INDICATIONS AND USES: Nasal congestion; mydriasis, uveitis with synechiae, and ocular decongestion; regional anesthesia; decongestant
DOSAGE
Adult
• *Nasal:* Instill 2-3 gtt or sprays to nasal mucosa bid (0.25% sol, use 0.5%-1% sol in resistant only)
• *Ophth:* Mydriasis: 1 gtt to conjunctival sac (2.5% or 10% sol) after giving top anesthetic; ocular decongestant: 1 gtt to conjunctiva q3-4 hr as needed (0.12% sol)
• *Anorectal:* Apply PR after bowel movement, or bid
Child
• *Nasal:* 6-12 yr instill 1-2 gtt or sprays (0.25%) q3-4h prn; <6 yr instill 2-3 gtt or sprays (0.125%) q3-4h prn
• *Ophth:* 1 gtt of 2.5% sol to conjunctiva; ocular decongestant: 1 gtt to conjunctiva q3-4 hr as needed (0.08%-0.12% sol)
💲 AVAILABLE FORMS/COST OF THERAPY
• Sol—Nasal: 0.125% drops, 15 ml: **$3.38**; 0.25% drops, 15 ml: **$4.99**; 0.5% spray, 15 ml: **$4.54**; 1% drops, 15 ml: **$3.76**
• Sol—Ophth: 0.125%, 15 ml: **$3.56-$10.00**; 2.5%, 5 ml: **$2.63-$19.50**; 10%, 5 ml: **$3.00-$26.16**
CONTRAINDICATIONS: Ten percent ophth sol not recommended in infants (hypertension)
PRECAUTIONS: Child <6 yr, elderly, diabetes, cardiovascular disease, hypertension, hyperthyroidism, increased intracranial pressure, prostatic hypertrophy, glaucoma
PREGNANCY AND LACTATION: Pregnancy category C; no breast feeding data, use caution

---

* = non-FDA-approved use

SIDE EFFECTS/ADVERSE REACTIONS

CNS: Anxiety, dizziness, fever, headache, insomnia, restlessness, tremors, weakness

EENT: Burning, dryness, irritation, rebound congestion, sneezing, stinging, visual blurring (ophth)

GI: Anorexia, nausea, vomiting

SKIN: Contact dermatitis

INTERACTIONS

• See interactions under systemic phenylephrine; interactions less likely than with systemic administration if given in proper dosage

SPECIAL CONSIDERATIONS

• Do not administer for more than 3-5 days (nasal product) or 2-3 days (ocular product used as decongestant) due to rebound congestion

---

phenytoin
(fen´i-toy-in)
Rx: Dilantin
fosphenytoin
(foss-fen´i-toy-in)
Rx: Cerebyx
Chemical Class: Hydantoin derivative
Therapeutic Class: Anticonvulsant

CLINICAL PHARMACOLOGY

Mechanism of Action: Inhibits spread of seizure activity in motor cortex by promoting sodium efflux, which stabilizes the threshold against hyperexcitability; fosphenytoin is pro-drug form of phenytoin; see Special Considerations

Pharmacokinetics

PO: Slow and variable absorption among products; peak 1½-3 hr (prompt cap), 4-12 hr (extended cap)

IV: (As phenytoin): Immediate onset

IM: (As phenytoin): Slow but complete (92%) absorption

IM/IV: (As fosphenytoin): Completely bioavailable after IM Inj; 95-99% protein bound (decreases as plasma concentrations increase); conversion to phenytoin is complete; conversion $t_{1/2}$, 15 min

$t_{1/2}$ changes with dose and serum concentration secondary to saturation of hepatic metabolic enzyme systems; (mean, 12-28 hr) biotransformation increased in younger children, pregnant women, trauma; metabolites excreted in urine

INDICATIONS AND USES: Generalized tonic-clonic seizures; simple or complex partial seizures (psychomotor or temporal lobe); status epilepticus; nonepileptic seizures associated with Reye's syndrome or after head trauma; fosphenytoin—substitute for oral phenytoin when PO administration not feasible; migraines; trigeminal neuralgia*; Bell's palsy; ventricular dysrhythmias, especially related to digitalis toxicity*; epidermolysis bullosa*; diabetic neuropathy pain*

DOSAGE

NOTE: Fosphenytoin 75 mg equivalent to 50 mg phenytoin, after administration; the dose of IV fosphenytoin is expressed as phenytoin equivalents (PE) to avoid the need to perform molecular weight-based adjustments when converting between fosphenytoin and phenytoin doses

Adult

Phenytoin:

• *Seizures:* IV loading dose 15-20 mg/kg based on recent dosing history and serum levels, followed by 100 mg PO or IV q6-8h; PO loading dose 1 g divided 400 mg, 300 mg, 300 mg given q2h; if load not necessary, may give 100 mg tid, follow levels; maintenance dose: 300

---

italic = common side effects   ***bold italic*** = life-threatening reactions

mg/day or 5-6 mg/kg/day in divided doses; once dosage established may use extended caps and dose qd
• *Neuritic pain:* PO 200-400 mg/day
Fosphenytoin
• *Status epilepticus:* IV 15-20 mg PE/kg loading dose administered at 100-150 mg PE/min
• *Nonemergent and maintenance dosing:* IM/IV 10-20 mg PE/kg loading dose administered at a rate ≤150 mg PE/min: maintenance 4-6 mg PE/kg/day
Child
Phenytoin:
• *Seizures:* IV loading dose 15-20 mg/kg in divided doses of 5-10 mg/kg; PO 5 mg/kg/day in 2 or 3 divided doses to max 300 mg/day; daily maintenance dose 4-8 mg/kg

💲 AVAILABLE FORMS/COST OF THERAPY
Phenytoin
• Cap, Gel—Oral: 100 mg, 100's: **$7.13-$24.50**
• Cap, Sus Action: 30 mg, 100's: **$25.76**; 100 mg, 100's: **$26.97-$44.90**
• Inj, Sol—IM, IV: 50 mg/ml, 2 ml: **$1.29-$4.93**
• Susp—Oral: 125 mg/5 ml, 240 ml: **$31.15**
• Tab, Chewable—Oral: 50 mg, 100's: **$26.71**
Fosphenytoin
• Sol—IV, IM: 150 mg (100 mg phenytoin sodium)/2 ml: **$20.71**
CONTRAINDICATIONS: Bradycardia, 2nd and 3rd degree AV block, Stokes-Adams syndrome, sinoatrial block
PRECAUTIONS: Hepatic disease, renal disease, diabetes mellitus
PREGNANCY AND LACTATION: Pregnancy category D (risk of congenital defects increased 2-3 times; fetal hydantoin syndrome includes craniofacial abnormalities, hypoplasia, ossification of distal phalanges; may also be transplacental carcinogen); compatible with breast feeding

SIDE EFFECTS/ADVERSE REACTIONS
CNS: Ataxia, confusion, *dizziness, drowsiness,* fatigue, headache, insomnia, nystagmus, paresthesias, *psychiatric changes, slurred speech*
CV: ***CV collapse*** (when drug administered too rapidly IV), hypotension, ***ventricular fibrillation***
EENT: Blurred vision, diplopia, *gingival hyperplasia,* nystagmus
GI: Anorexia, *constipation,* **hepatitis,** jaundice, *nausea, vomiting,* weight loss
GU: **Nephritis**
HEME: **Agranulocytosis, aplastic anemia, leukopenia,** lymphadenopathy, **megaloblastic anemia, thrombocytopenia**
METAB: Hyperglycemia
SKIN: Alopecia, hirsutism, **lupus erythematosus,** rash, **Stevens-Johnson syndrome**

INTERACTIONS
Drugs
🔢 *Acetaminophen:* Enhances the hepatotoxic potential of acetaminophen overdoses; may reduce the therapeutic response to acetaminophen
🔢 *Acetazolamide:* Osteomalacia
🔢 *Amiodarone:* Increased phenytoin levels; decreased amiodarone levels
🔢 *Azole-antifungals (fluconazole):* Phenytoin induces metabolism (CYP3A4) reducing antifungal effects
🔢 *Benzodiazepines (alprazolam, diazepam, midazolam, triazolam):* Enhanced metabolism (CYP3A4) phenytoin reduces benzodiazepine effects
🔢 *Carbamazepine:* Combined use usually decreases levels of both drugs

❸ *Chloramphenicol, disulfiram, fluoxetine, isoniazid, omeprazole, sulfonamides:* Increased phenytoin levels

❸ *Cimetidine, cisplatin, diazoxide, folate, rifampin:* Decreased phenytoin levels

❸ *Clozapine:* Reduced levels via phenytoin induced enhanced metabolism

❸ *Corticosteroids:* Decreased therapeutic effect of steroids

❸ *Cyclic antidepressants:* Increased antidepressant levels

❸ *Cyclosporine:* Reduced cyclosporine levels

❸ *Dicumarol:* Increased anticoagulant effect, increased phenytoin levels

❸ *Digitalis glycosides:* Lower digitalis levels

❸ *Disopyramide:* Reduced efficacy, increased toxicity of disopyramide

❸ *Dopamine:* More susceptible to hypotension after IV phenytoin

❸ *Doxycycline:* Reduced doxycycline concentrations

❸ *Felbamate:* Felbamate consistently increases phenytoin levels

❸ *Furosemide:* Decreased diuretic effect

❷ *Itraconazole:* Phenytoin induces metabolism (CYP3A4) reducing antifungal effects

❸ *Lamotrigine:* Phenytoin stimulates metabolism-lower plasma levels; decreased $t_{1/2}$

❸ *Levodopa:* Decreased antiparkinsonian effect

❸ *Lithium:* Increased risk of lithium intoxication; causal explanation not known

❷ *Mebendazole in high doses:* Decreased mebendazole levels

❷ *Methadone:* Withdrawal

❸ *Metyrapone:* Invalidates test

❸ *Mexiletine:* Decreased mexiletine levels

❸ *Oral contraceptives:* Decreased contraceptive effect

❸ *Primidone:* Enhanced conversion to phenobarbital

❸ *Pyridoxine:* Large doses may decrease phenytoin levels

❸ *Quinidine:* Decreased quinidine levels

❸ *Quinolone antibiotics (ciprofloxacin, enoxacin, norfloxacin, pefloxacin):* Elevates phenytoin concentrations

❸ *Sucralfate:* Phenytoin reduces GI absorption

❸ *Tacrolimus:* Reduced tacrolimus levels

❸ *Theophylline:* Reduced theophylline levels

❸ *Thyroid hormone:* Increased thyroid replacement dose requirements

❸ *Tolbutamide:* Phenytoin inhibits insulin release, may result in hyperglycemia; tolbutamide displaces phenytoin from protein-binding sites; monitor for alterations in glucose control

❸ *Trimethoprim:* Increased phenytoin concentrations

❸ *Valproic acid:* Variable effects on phenytoin levels; decreased valproic acid levels

❸ *Warfarin:* Transient increased hypoprothrombinemic response followed by inhibition of hypoprothrombinemic response

Labs
• *False positive:* Barbiturates, urine
• *Increased:* Cholesterol, serum; thyroxine, serum

SPECIAL CONSIDERATIONS
• Pro-drug, fosphenytoin rapidly converted to phenytoin *in vivo:* minimal activity before conversion; water soluble, thus more suitable for parenteral applications: doesn't require cardiac monitoring; can be administered at faster rate; no IV filter

required; compatible with both saline and dextrose mixtures; requires refrigeration

MONITORING PARAMETERS

• Therapeutic range 10-20 μg/ml; nystagmus appears at 20 μg/ml, ataxia at 30 μg/ml, dysarthria and lethargy at levels above 40 μg/ml; lethal dose 2-5 g

phosphorated carbohydrate solution

OTC: Emetrol, Nausea Relief, Nausetrol

Chemical Class: Hyperosmolar carbohydrate with phosphoric acid

Therapeutic Class: Antiemetic

CLINICAL PHARMACOLOGY

Mechanism of Action: Reduces smooth muscle contraction by direct local action on the wall of the GI tract

INDICATIONS AND USES: Relief of nausea caused by upset stomach from intestinal flu, stomach flu and food or drink indiscretions; regurgitation in infants;* morning sickness;* motion sickness;* nausea and vomiting caused by drug therapy or inhalation anesthesia*

DOSAGE

Adult and Child >12 yr

• Nausea: PO 15-30 ml repeated every 15 min until distress subsides; max 5 doses; do not use for >1 hr

• Morning sickness: PO 15-30 ml on arising; repeat q3h or when nausea threatens

Child 2-12 yr

• Nausea: PO 5-10 ml repeated every 15 min until distress subsides; max 5 doses; do no use for >1 hr

Infants

• Regurgitation in infants: PO 5-10 ml, 10-15 min before each feeding; may use 10-15 ml, 30 min before feeding in refractory cases

$ **AVAILABLE FORMS/COST OF THERAPY**

• Sol—Oral: 1.87 g dextrose/1.87 g fructose/21.5 mg phosphoric acid; 118, 120, 236, 240, 473, 480 ml: **$1.02-$5.30**/120 ml

PRECAUTIONS: Diabetes (contains significant amount of sugar); hereditary fructose intolerance

PREGNANCY AND LACTATION: Pregnancy category B; used to treat morning sickness

SIDE EFFECTS/ADVERSE REACTIONS

GI: Abdominal pain, diarrhea

SPECIAL CONSIDERATIONS

PATIENT/FAMILY EDUCATION

• Seek medical attention if symptoms are not relieved or recur frequently

physostigmine

(fi-zoe-stig′meen)

Rx: Antilirium

Chemical Class: Alkaloid; cholinesterase inhibitor

Therapeutic Class: Antiglaucoma agent; miotic; cholinergic

CLINICAL PHARMACOLOGY

Mechanism of Action: Inactivates acetylcholinesterase, potentiates acetylcholine at sites of cholinergic transmission; results in miosis, which increases outflow of aqueous humor, fall in intraocular pressure, and potentiation of accommodation; antagonizes anticholinergics

Pharmacokinetics

OPHTH: Onset 20-30 min, duration 12-36 hr (miosis); peak 2-6 hr, duration 12-36 hr (intraocular pressure)

* = non-FDA-approved use

IV/IM: Crosses blood- brain barrier; peak effect 20-30 min (IM), 5 min (IV); duration of action 30-60 min; destroyed in body by hydrolysis, very small amounts excreted in urine

INDICATIONS AND USES: Open-angle glaucoma (ophth), treatment of anticholinergic toxicity (systemic, including tricyclic antidepressants)

DOSAGE

Adult

• *Glaucoma:* Instill ¼ inch strip of 0.25% oint in conjunctival sac qd-tid; instill 1 gtt of a 0.25%-0.5% sol in conjunctival sac qd-qid

• *Anticholinergic toxicity:* IM/IV 0.5 mg-2 mg given at rate not greater than 1 mg/min; repeat q 20-30 min; max single dose 4 mg, as needed

Child

• *Glaucoma:* See adult

• *Anticholinergic toxicity:* IV 0.02 mg (20 µg)/kg over at least 1 min; may repeat q5-10min; max dose 2 mg

$ **AVAILABLE FORMS/COST OF THERAPY**

• Inj, Sol—IM, IV: 1 mg/ml, 2 ml: **$7.32-$11.11**

• Oint—Ophth: 0.25%, 3.5 g: **$1.62-$6.25**

CONTRAINDICATIONS: Inflammatory disease of iris or ciliary body, newborn (parenteral solution contains benzyl alcohol, toxic to neonate), organophosphate poisoning, intestinal or urogenital tract obstruction, asthma, diabetes mellitus, patients receiving choline esters or depolarizing neuromuscular blocking agents (decamethonium, succinylcholine)

PRECAUTIONS: Epilepsy, parkinsonism, bradycardia, bronchitis, CV disease

PREGNANCY AND LACTATION: Pregnancy category C; no data on breast feeding available

SIDE EFFECTS/ADVERSE REACTIONS

CNS: Anxiety, delirium, disorientation, hallucinations, headache, hyperactivity, ***seizures***

CV: Bradycardia, hypertension, hypotension, irregular pulse

EENT: Blurred vision, conjunctivitis, decreased secretion in salivary and sweat glands; decreased secretions in pharynx, nasal passages, lacrimation, rhinorrhea, salivation, twitching of eyelids

GI: Abdominal cramps, diarrhea, nausea, vomiting

RESP: ***Bronchospasm,*** decreased bronchial secretions, dyspnea, ***pulmonary edema***

MISC: Hyperpyrexia

INTERACTIONS

Drugs

3 *β-blockers:* Additive bradycardia

SPECIAL CONSIDERATIONS

• Atropine is antidote

P

---

phytonadione (vitamin K$_1$)

(fye-toe-na-dye′one)

Rx: AquaMEPHYTON, Mephyton

Chemical Class: Naphthoquinone fat-soluble vitamin

Therapeutic Class: Vitamin, antihemorrhagic

CLINICAL PHARMACOLOGY

Mechanism of Action: Normally synthesized by intestinal flora; promotes hepatic formation of clotting factors II, VII, IX, and X and anticoagulants protein C and protein S

---

italic = common side effects   **bold italic** = life-threatening reactions

Pharmacokinetics

PO, INJ: Readily absorbed from normal duodenum, bile salts required; rapid hepatic metabolism; onset of action 6-12 hr oral, 1-2 hr IV; prothrombin time normalizes in 12-14 hr following administration of adequate doses; excreted in urine, bile

INDICATIONS AND USES: Vitamin K malabsorption; hypoprothrombinemia; hemorrhagic disease of the newborn (prophylaxis); does not reverse hypoprothrombinemia due to hepatocellular damage

DOSAGE

Adult

• *Hypoprothrombinemia:* PO 2.5-10 mg (up to 25 mg) may repeat in 12 hr; IV/SC 1-10 mg (up to 25 mg), may repeat in 6-8 hr;

NOTE: overzealous use during anticoagulant therapy may restore conditions which originally permitted thromboembolic phenomena, use doses >2.5 mg only if prothrombin time severely elevated, or if active bleeding present

• *Hypoprothrombinemia prevention during total parenteral nutrition:* IM 5-10 mg qwk

Child

• *Hypoprothrombinemia:* PO/IV/SC 1-10 mg;

NOTE: overzealous use during anticoagulant therapy may restore conditions which originally permitted thromboembolic phenomena

• *Hypoprothrombinemia prevention during total parenteral nutrition:* IV 2-5 mg q wk

Infants

• *Hypoprothrombinemia:* PO/IV/SC 1-2 mg

• *Prevention of hemorrhagic disease of the newborn (HDN):* IM/SC 0.5-1 mg after birth, repeat in 6-8 hr if required (e.g., mother received anticonvulsants, rifampin, isoniazid during pregnancy)

§ AVAILABLE FORMS/COST OF THERAPY

• Inj, Emulsion—IM, IV, SC: 1 mg/0.5 ml: **$2.79-$5.00**; 10 mg/ml, 1 ml: **$4.80-$5.02**

• Tab, Uncoated—Oral: 5 mg, 100's: **$65.33**

CONTRAINDICATIONS: Severe hepatic disease

PRECAUTIONS: G-6-PD deficiency; premature infants; correction of anticoagulant-induced hypoprothrombinemia in patients with continued needs for anticoagulation should be approached cautiously; consider mini-dosing (1-2.5 mg)

PREGNANCY AND LACTATION: Pregnancy category C; oral supplementation of women on anticonvulsants during last 2 weeks of pregnancy has been done to prevent HDN, but effectiveness unproven; compatible with breast feeding

SIDE EFFECTS/ADVERSE REACTIONS

CNS: Headache, *kernicterus* (premature infants, high doses)

HEME: **Hemoglobinuria, hemolytic anemia, hyperbilirubinemia** (newborn)

SKIN: Flushing sensation, rash, urticaria

MISC: **Anaphylaxis**

INTERACTIONS

Drugs

3 *Oral anticoagulants:* Decreased anticoagulant effect

SPECIAL CONSIDERATIONS

• IV doses should be diluted and infused slowly over 20-30 min

---

* = non-FDA-approved use

pilocarpine

(pye-loe-kar´peen)

Rx: *Ophthalmic:* Akarpine, Isopto Carpine, Ocu-Carpine, Ocusert, Pilocar, Pilopine-HS, Piloptic
Oral: Salagen
Combinations
  Rx: with epinephrine (E-Pilo-6)
Chemical Class: Choline ester
Therapeutic Class: Miotic; ophthalmic cholinergic; antiglaucoma agent; salivation stimulant

CLINICAL PHARMACOLOGY

Mechanism of Action: Produces pupillary constriction by duplicating muscarinic effects of acetylcholine; increases aqueous humor outflow, intraocular pressure (IOP) decreases; orally increases exocrine gland secretion

Pharmacokinetics

OPHTH: Onset 10-30 min, duration 4-8 hr (sol, gel); Ocusert system onset 1½-2 hr, duration 7 days

PO: Onset 20 min, peak 1 hr, duration 3-5 hr; excreted in urine

INDICATIONS AND USES: Ophth:open-angle glaucoma, chronic angle-closure glaucoma, acute angle-closure glaucoma (in combination with other agents to decrease IOP before surgery), reversal of mydriasis, pre- and postoperative increased IOP; oral: xerostomia from salivary gland hypofunction secondary to radiotherapy for head and neck cancer

DOSAGE
Adult
• *Glaucoma:* Instill 1-2 gtt of 1% or 2% sol in eye q6-8h; instill 20-40 µg/hr (Ocusert) in cul-de-sac of eye, replace q7d; instill ½ inch ribbon of gel in conjunctival sac qhs
• *Xerostomia:* PO 5-10 mg tid

$ AVAILABLE FORMS/COST OF THERAPY
• Gel—Ophth: 4%, 3.5 g: **$35.75**
• Insert—Ophth: 20 µg/hr, 8's: **$43.32**; 40 µg/hr, 8's: **$43.32**
• Sol, Ophth: 0.25%, 15 ml: **$14.75**; 0.5%, 15 ml: **$1.68-$14.75**; 1.0%, 15 ml: **$1.95-$21.62**; 2.0%, 15 ml: **$2.02-$22.00**; 3.0%, 15 ml: **$2.17-$16.13**; 4.0%, 15 ml: **$2.35-$23.25**; 5.0%, 15 ml: **$2.60-$11.88**; 6.0%, 15 ml: **$2.95-$25.56**; 8.0%, 15 ml: **$28.06**; 10%, 15 ml: **$22.88**
• Tab, Coated—Oral: 5 mg, 100's: **$128.59**

CONTRAINDICATIONS: Acute iritis, or other condition where acute miosis undesirable

PRECAUTIONS: Bronchial asthma, hypertension, bradycardia, hyperthyroidism, CV disease, biliary disease, renal colic (nephrolithiasis), epilepsy, parkinsonism, asthma

PREGNANCY AND LACTATION: Pregnancy category C

SIDE EFFECTS/ADVERSE REACTIONS

CNS: Headache
CV: AV block, bradycardia, ***dysrhythmia,*** hypertension, hypotension, ***shock,*** tachycardia
EENT: Blurred vision, conjunctival irritation (Ocusert), eye pain with change in focus, retinal detachment, stinging, tearing, twitching of eyelids
GI: Abdominal cramps, diarrhea, nausea, vomiting
GU: Bladder tightness, frequency, urgency
RESP: ***Bronchospasm***

---

italic = common side effects   **bold italic** = life-threatening reactions

SPECIAL CONSIDERATIONS
• Antidote is atropine
PATIENT/FAMILY EDUCATION
• Miotics cause poor dark adaptation, use caution with night driving

---

pimozide
(pi′moe-zide)
Rx: Orap
Chemical Class: Diphenylbutylpiperidine derivative
Therapeutic Class: Antipsychotic

CLINICAL PHARMACOLOGY
Mechanism of Action: Dopamine receptor antagonist, with higher affinity for D_2- over D_1-receptors, and variable selectivity among the cortical dopamine tracts; also activity on nondopaminergic sites, i.e., cholinergic, α_1-adrenergic and histaminic receptors (explaining side effects); high risk extrapyramidal reactions; minimal orthostatic hypotension; moderate sedation and anticholinergic effects
Pharmacokinetics
PO: $t_{1/2}$ 19-39 hr, peak 4-12 hr
50% absorbed; hepatic metabolism, excreted in urine and stool
INDICATIONS AND USES: Gilles de la Tourette's syndrome (patients nonresponsive to haloperidol), chronic schizophrenia without excitement, agitation, or hyperactivity*
DOSAGE
NOTE: 0.3-0.5 mg equivalent to chlorpromazine 100 mg
Adult
• *Tourette's:* PO 1-2 mg qd in divided doses, increase qod as needed (usual dose 200 µg/kg/day or 10 mg qd, whichever is less); max 300 µg/kg/day or 20 mg qd

• *Psychotic disorders:* PO 2-4 mg qd, increase qwk by 2-4 mg qd
§ AVAILABLE FORMS/COST OF THERAPY
• Tab, Uncoated—Oral: 1 mg, 100's: **$65.29**; 2 mg, 100's: **$87.06**
CONTRAINDICATIONS: Simple tics other than Tourette's, history of cardiac dysrhythmias
PRECAUTIONS: Breast cancer (increased prolactin levels), liver disease, renal disease, hypokalemia (dysrhythmias), sensitivity to other neuroleptics
PREGNANCY AND LACTATION: Pregnancy category C
SIDE EFFECTS/ADVERSE REACTIONS
CNS: Akathisia, dizziness, *drowsiness, extra-pyramidal effects,* headache, mood or behavior changes, ***neuroleptic malignant syndrome, parkinsonism, tardive dyskinesia***
CV: Hypotension, ***prolonged QT interval,*** tachycardia, ***ventricular dysrhythmias***
EENT: Blurred vision, dryness of mouth
GI: Anorexia, *constipation,* diarrhea, nausea, obstructive jaundice, vomiting
GU: Loss of bladder control
HEME: ***Blood dyscrasias***
SKIN: Itching, rash
MISC: Galactorrhea, mastalgia
INTERACTIONS
Drugs
3 *Anticholinergics (benztropine, trihexyphenidyl):* Antagonistic pharmacodynamic effects; excessive anticholinergic effects
3 *Bromocriptine:* Antagonistic pharmacodynamic effects
3 *Carbamazepine:* Decreased antipsychotic drug concentrations; decreased therapeutic response
3 *Clonidine:* Exaggerated hypotension

---

* = non-FDA-approved use

🔳 *Fluoxetine:* Increased risk of extrapyramidal symptoms

🔳 *Indomethacin:* Exaggerated side effects: drowsiness, tiredness, confusion

❷ *Levodopa:* Antagonistic effects on the antiparkinsonian effects

🔳 *Lithium:* Reduced serum concentrations of both drugs; neurotoxic reactions reported in manic patients (delirium, seizures, encephalopathy, extrapyramidal symptoms)

🔳 *Meperidine:* Excessive hypotension and CNS depression

🔳 *Paroxetine:* Increased risk of extrapyramidal symptoms

🔳 *Phenobarbital:* Reduced pimozide concentrations; increased risk of hyperthermia associated with phenobarbital withdrawal

🔳 *Quinidine:* Increased pimozide concentrations and risk or subsequent toxicity

🔳 *Trazodone:* Additive hypotension

---

pindolol

(pin´doe-loll)
Rx: Visken
Chemical Class: Nonselective β-adrenergic blocker
Therapeutic Class: Antihypertensive; antianginal

CLINICAL PHARMACOLOGY

Mechanism of Action: Competitive, nonselective, β-adrenergic antagonist at β-receptors; produces negative inotropic and chronotropic responses; slows AV nodal conduction; decreases heart rate; decreases myocardial oxygen consumption; antiarrhythmic effects (class II); reduction in platelet aggregation and blood viscosity; suppression of renin release; inhibition of central sympathetic outflow; decreases presynaptic receptor neurotransmitter release; high intrinsic sympathomimetic activity; low membrane stabilizing activity; moderate lipid solubility

Pharmacokinetics

PO: Incomplete GI absorption (40%-60% bioavailable); peak serum concentrations, 2-4 hr; not metabolized by liver; excreted unchanged in urine and feces; $t_{1/2}$ 6-7 hr; crosses placenta in measurable, but not significant concentrations

INDICATIONS AND USES: Hypertension, angina pectoris,* migraine headache,* postmyocardial infarction,* alcohol withdrawal syndrome,* hyperthyroidism,* syncope, neuroleptic-induced akathesia*

DOSAGE

Adult and Child >16 yr

• *Hypertension:* PO 5-30 mg bid
• *Angina pectoris:* PO 2.5-5 mg/day initially; titrate gradually to 10-40 mg divided bid
• *Hyperthyroidism:* 15-30 mg/day

Child

• PO initial 1-1.2 mg/kg/dose qd; maximum 2 mg/kg/day qd

💲 **AVAILABLE FORMS/COST OF THERAPY**

• Tab, Uncoated—Oral: 5 mg, 100's: **$58.00-$116.12**; 10 mg, 100's: **$17.46-$153.78**

CONTRAINDICATIONS: Cardiogenic shock; 2nd, 3rd degree heart block; severe bradycardia; overt cardiac failure; bronchial asthma

PRECAUTIONS: Anesthesia/surgery (myocardial depression), avoid abrupt withdrawal, bronchospastic airways, congestive heart failure, diabetes mellitus, concurrent clonidine (discontinue pindolol several days prior to withdrawal of clonidine), peripheral vascular disease, renal disease

P

---

italic = common side effects   **bold italic** = life-threatening reactions

PREGNANCY AND LACTATION:
Pregnancy category B; similar drug, atenolol, frequently used in the third trimester for treatment of hypertension (many studies of efficacy and safety of atenolol in pregnancy-induced hypertension; long-term use has been associated with intrauterine growth retardation; enters breast milk in measurable amounts; observe for signs of β-blockade

SIDE EFFECTS/ADVERSE REACTIONS

CNS: Anxiety, *dizziness,* fatigue, hallucinations, *insomnia*

CV: **AV block,** bradycardia, chest pain, **CHF,** claudication, edema, hypotension, palpitation, tachycardia

EENT: Double vision, dry burning eyes, sore throat, *visual changes*

GI: Abdominal pain, diarrhea, **ischemic colitis, mesenteric arterial thrombosis,** nausea, vomiting

GU: Frequency, impotence

HEME: **Agranulocytosis, purpura, thrombocytopenia**

RESP: **Bronchospasm,** cough, *dyspnea,* rales

SKIN: Alopecia, pruritus, rash

MISC: Fever, joint pain, muscle pain

INTERACTIONS

Drugs

3 *Adenosine:* Bradycardia aggravated

• *Amiodarone:* Additive prolongation of atrioventricular (AV) conduction time; symptomatic bradycardia and sinus arrest

3 *Antacids:* Reduced pindolol absorption

3 *Calcium channel blockers:* See dihydropyridine calcium channel blockers and verapamil

3 *Cimetidine:* Renal clearance reduced; AUC increased with cimetidine coadministration

3 *Clonidine, guanabenz, guanfacine:* Exacerbation of rebound hypertension upon discontinuation of clonidine

3 *Cocaine:* Cocaine-induced vasoconstriction potentiated; reduced coronary blood flow

3 *Contrast media:* Increased risk of anaphylaxis

3 *Digitalis:* Enhances bradycardia:

3 *Digoxin:* Additive prolongation of atrioventricular (AV) conduction time

3 *Dihydropyridine calcium channel blockers:* Additive pharmacodynamic effects:

3 *Disopyramide:* Additive decreases in cardiac output

3 *Dipyridamole:* Bradycardia aggravated

3 *Diltiazem:* Potentiates pharmacologic effects of β-adrenergic blocker, hypotension, left ventricular failure, and AV conduction disturbances reported; more likely in the elderly and in patients with left ventricular dysfunction, aortic stenosis, or large doses

3 *Epinephrine, isoproterenol, phenylephrine:* Potentiates pressor response; resultant hypertension and bradycardia

3 *Flecainide:* Additive negative inotropic effects

3 *Fluoxetine:* Increased β-blockade activity

3 *Fluoroquinolones:* Reduced clearance of pindolol

3 *Insulin:* Altered response to hypoglycemia; increased blood glucose concentrations; impair peripheral circulation

3 *Lidocaine:* Increased serum lidocaine concentrations possible

3 *Neostigmine:* Bradycardia aggravated

3 *Neuroleptics:* Both drugs inhibit each other's metabolism; additive hypotension

---

* = non-FDA-approved use

NSAIDs: Reduced antihypertensive effect of pindolol

Physostigmine: Bradycardia aggravated

Prazosin: First-dose response to prazosin may be enhanced by β-blockade

Prazosin, terazosin, doxazosin: Potential enhanced first dose response (marked initial drop in blood pressure) particularly on standing (especially prazosin)

Tacrine: Bradycardia aggravated

Terbutaline: Antagonized bronchodilating effects of terbutaline

Theophylline: Antagonistic pharmacodynamic effects

Verapamil: Enhanced effects of both drugs; particularly AV nodal conduction slowing; reduced pindolol clearance

Labs
• *Alkaline phosphatase:* Increased serum levels
• *Aspartate aminotransferase:* Decreased serum levels
• *Bilirubin:* Decreased serum level
• *Creatine kinase:* Decreased serum level

SPECIAL CONSIDERATIONS
• Abrupt discontinuation may precipitate angina; taper over 1-2 wk
• Effective antihypertensive and probably antianginal agent (though not approved for this indication), especially for patients who develop symptomatic bradycardia with β-blockade

MONITORING PARAMETERS
• Angina: Reduction in nitroglycerin usage; frequency, severity, onset, and duration of angina pain; heart rate
• Hypertension: Blood pressure
• Toxicity: Blood glucose, bronchospasm, hypotension, bradycardia, depression, confusion, hallucination, sexual dysfunction

pioglitazone
(pye-oh-gli'ta-zone)
Rx: Actos
Chemical Class: Thiazolidinedione
Therapeutic Class: Oral hypoglycemic; insulin resistance reducer

CLINICAL PHARMACOLOGY
Mechanism of Action: Potent and selective agonist for peroxisome proliferator-activated receptor-gamma (PPARγ) which regulates the control of glucose production, transport, and utilization as well as fatty acid metabolism; improves glycemic control and reduces circulating insulin levels via improving sensitivity to insulin in muscle and adipose tissue and inhibiting hepatic glyconeogenesis

Pharmacokinetics
PO: Bioavailability unknown (PO), animal data reflects 50%; 99% protein bound to albumin; extensively metabolized (CYP2C8 and CYP3A4) in the liver (both active and inactive metabolites); renal (15-30% - primarily metabolites), bile and feces are major routes of excretion; $t_{1/2}$ 3-7 hr

INDICATIONS AND USES: Diabetes mellitus, type 2, alone or in combination with sulfonylureas, metformin, or insulin; Werner syndrome;* polycystic ovary syndrome*

DOSAGE
Adult and Child >18 yr
• PO 15-30 mg qd (maximum dose 45 mg/day)

Hepatic Impairment
• Avoid use with concurrent liver dysfunction

P

💲 AVAILABLE FORMS/COST OF THERAPY

• Tab, Coated—Oral: 15 mg, 90's: **$276.89**; 30 mg, 90's: **$443.35**; 45 mg, 90's: **$480.92**

CONTRAINDICATIONS: Diabetes mellitus, type 1; diabetic ketoacidosis; hepatic function impairment or clinical evidence of active liver disease (transaminase elevation >2.5 times upper limit of normal), hypersensitivity, uncompensated CHF

PRECAUTIONS: Congestive heart failure (NYHA III, IV), anemia, premenopausal anovulatory patients with insulin resistance (ovulation may resume and pregnancy may occur if not protected)

PREGNANCY AND LACTATION: Pregnancy category C; abnormally high glucose levels during pregnancy associated with higher incidence of congenital anomalies, morbidity, and mortality; insulin monotherapy or sulfonylurea preferred agents; breast milk excretion unknown

SIDE EFFECTS/ADVERSE REACTIONS

CNS: Headache, paresthesia
CV: Edema
EENT: Aggravation of retinopathy, sinusitis, pharyngitis
GI: Abdominal discomfort, hepatotoxicity (incidence, 0.25%)
HEME: Anemia (2-4% drop in hematocrit over 12 weeks)
METAB: Hypoglycemia (with sulfonylurea or insulin)
MS: Myalgia, elevated CK

INTERACTIONS

Drugs
🔳 *Combination oral contraceptives:* May reduce estrogen and progestin levels (another thiazolidinedione reduced both hormones 30%)

🔳 *Fenugreek, ginseng, glucomannan, guar gum:* Pharmacodynamic interaction as both pioglitazone and listed natural products both possess hypoglycemic effects

Labs
• Possible elevations of AST, ALT, bilirubin, LDH; increases in LDL-cholesterol (15%) and HDL-cholesterol (15%); decreased in hematocrit, hemoglobin; decreased alkaline phosphatase

SPECIAL CONSIDERATIONS

• Expected hypoglycemic effects: Decreases in serum glucose: 50-75 mg/dL; decreases in hemoglobin A1c: 1.2-1.5%

PATIENT/FAMILY EDUCATION

• Caloric restriction, weight loss, and exercise are essential adjuvant therapy
• Blood draws for LFT monitoring along with routine diabetes mellitus labs. Review symptoms of hepatitis (unexplained nausea, vomiting, abdominal pain, fatigue, anorexia or dark urine)
• Notify clinician for rapid increases in weight or edema or symptoms of heart failure (shortness of breath, nocturia)
• Review hypoglycemia risks and symptoms when added to other hypoglycemic agents

MONITORING PARAMETERS

• Diabetes mellitus symptoms, periodic serum glucose and HbA1c measurements; LFT (AST, ALT) prior to initiation of therapy and periodically thereafter; hemoglobin/hematocrit

---

* = non-FDA-approved use

piperacillin; piperacillin/ tazobactam

(pi-per'a-sill-in; taz'o-bac-tam)

Rx: Pipracil (piperacillin); Zosyn, (piperacillin/ tazobactam)

Chemical Class: Aminobenzyl penicillin, penicillin derivative/ β-lactamase inhibitor (tazobactam)

Therapeutic Class: Antibiotic

CLINICAL PHARMACOLOGY

Mechanism of Action: Inhibits bacterial wall synthesis; bactericidal; tazobactam protects piperacillin from degradation by β-lactamase enzymes, extending the spectrum of activity

Pharmacokinetics

IM: Peak 30-50 min

IV: Peak 20-30 min

$t_{1/2}$ 0.7-1.33 hr; 33% protein bound; excreted in urine, bile; crosses placenta

INDICATIONS AND USES: Infections of the respiratory and genitourinary tract, bone; skin and intraabdominal infections; gonococcal infections; septicemia caused by susceptible organisms; combination with tazobactam effective against β-lactamase producing strains, moderate to severe nosocomial pneumonia

Antibacterial spectrum usually includes:

• Gram-positive organisms: *S. aureus, S. pyogenes, S. viridans, S. faecalis, S. bovis, S. pneumoniae, Clostridium perfringens, C. tetani*

• Gram-negative organisms: *N. gonorrhoeae, N. meningitidis, Bacteroides, Fusobacterium nucleatum, E. coli, Klebsiella, P. vulgaris, Proteus mirabilis, Morganella morganii,* *Enterobacter, Citrobacter, Pseudomonas aeruginosa, Serratia, Acinetobacter, Peptococcus, Peptostreptococcus, Eubacterium*

• Anaerobes: *Bacteroides* sp., *Clostridium difficile*

DOSAGE

Adult

• *Systemic infections:* Piperacillin IM/IV 100-300 mg/kg/day in divided doses q4-6h; piperacillin/ tazobactam IV INF 12-15 g/day given as 3.375 g q6hr over 30 min × 7-10 days

• *Prophylaxis of surgical infections:* IV 2 g ½-1 hr before procedure; may be repeated during surgery or after surgery

• *Uncomplicated gonorrhea:* IM 2 g as a single dose with 1 g probenecid 30 min before

• *Renal insufficiency:* Reduce dosage to degree of impairment; hemodialysis removes 40% of dose over 4 hr

Child >12 yr

• *Systemic infections:* IM/IV 100-300 mg/kg/day in divided doses q4-6h

• *Child* (doses are suggested but not established)

• IV 200-300 mg/kg/d (max daily dose 24 g) divided q4-6h

Neonate (term)

• IV 75 mg/kg q8h 1st week of life, q6h in 2nd week

Neonate (<36 wks)

• IV 75 mg/kg q12h 1st week of life, q8h in 2nd week

$ **AVAILABLE FORMS/COST OF THERAPY**

Piperacillin

• Inj, Lyphl-Sol—IM, IV: 2 g/vial: **$11.76**; 3 g/vial: **$19.88**; 4 g/vial: **$26.50**

Piperacillin/Tazobactam

• Inj, Sol—IV: 2 g/0.25 mg: **$10.80**; 3 g/0.375 mg: **$16.21**; 4 g/0.5 mg: **$20.53**

italic = common side effects   ***bold italic*** = life-threatening reactions

PRECAUTIONS: Hypersensitivity to cephalosporins; CHF; children <12 yr

PREGNANCY AND LACTATION: Pregnancy category B; excreted in breast milk in small concentrations

SIDE EFFECTS/ADVERSE REACTIONS

CNS: Anxiety, coma, depression, hallucinations, lethargy, seizures, twitching

GI: Abdominal pain, colitis, *diarrhea,* glossitis, increased AST, ALT; *nausea, vomiting*

GU: **Glomerulonephritis,** hematuria, *moniliasis,* oliguria, proteinuria, *vaginitis*

HEME: Anemia, **bone marrow depression,** increased bleeding time

METAB: Hypernatremia, hypokalemia

INTERACTIONS

Drugs

🔳 *Aminoglycosides:* Carbenicillin and other piperacillins can inactivate aminoglycosides in vitro and in certain patients with renal dysfunction

🔳 *Chloramphenicol:* Inhibited antibacterial activity of piperacillin; administer piperacillin 3 hr before chloramphenicol

🔳 *Macrolide antibiotics:* Inhibited antibacterial activity of piperacillin; administer piperacillin 3 hr before macrolides

🔳 *Methotrexate:* Piperacillin in large doses may increase serum methotrexate concentrations

🔳 *Oral contraceptives:* Occasional impairment of oral contraceptive efficacy; consider use of supplemental contraception during cycles in which piperacillin is used

🔳 *Tetracyclines:* Inhibited antibacterial activity of piperacillin; administer piperacillin 3 hr before tetracyclines

Labs

• *Cephalothin:* False positive serum
• *Penicillin G:* False positive serum
• *Protein:* False positive urine

SPECIAL CONSIDERATIONS

• Preferred over mezlocillin, more effective against *Pseudomonas,* reserve for carbenicillin- or ticarcillin-resistant *P. aeruginosa* infections in combination with an aminoglycoside

---

pirbuterol
(purr-byoo´ter-ole)
Rx: Maxair
Chemical Class: Sympathomimetic amine; β-adrenergic agonist
Therapeutic Class: Antiasthmatic, bronchodilator

CLINICAL PHARMACOLOGY
Mechanism of Action: Causes bronchodilation by β_2-stimulation, resulting in relaxation of bronchial smooth muscle; inhibits mast cell degranulation; stimulates cilia to remove secretions

Pharmacokinetics
INH: Onset 3 min, peak ½-1 hr, duration 5 hr, $t_{1/2}$ 2 hr

INDICATIONS AND USES: Prevention and reversal of bronchospasm including patients with asthma

DOSAGE
Adult and Child >12 yr
• MDI 1-2 puffs q4-6h, not to exceed 12 puffs/day

🔳 **AVAILABLE FORMS/COST OF THERAPY**
• MDI—INH: 0.2 mg/puff, 2.8 g: **$10.08**; 0.2 mg/puff, 14 g: **$40.75**; 0.2 mg/puff, 25.6 g: **$26.64**

PRECAUTIONS: Ischemic heart disease, cardiac dysrhythmias, hyperthyroidism, diabetes mellitus, prostatic hypertrophy, hypertension

---

* = non-FDA-approved use

PREGNANCY AND LACTATION:
Pregnancy category C
SIDE EFFECTS/ADVERSE REACTIONS
CNS: Anxiety, dizziness, drowsiness, hallucinations, headache, irritability, insomnia, restlessness, stimulation, tremors
CV: Angina, *dysrhythmias,* hypertension, hypotension, palpitations, tachycardia
EENT: Dry nose and mouth; irritation of nose, throat
GI: Anorexia, gastritis, nausea, vomiting
MS: Muscle cramps
RESP: **Bronchospasm,** coughing, dyspnea
INTERACTIONS
Drugs
❷ *Beta-blockers:* Decreased action of pirbuterol, cardioselective agents preferable if concurrent use necessary
❸ *Furosemide:* Potential for additive hypokalemia
SPECIAL CONSIDERATIONS
• No significant advantage over other selective β₂-agonists
PATIENT/FAMILY EDUCATION
• Initial and periodic reviews of metered dose inhaler technique

---

piroxicam
(peer-ox′i-kam)
Rx: Feldene
Chemical Class: Oxicam derivative
Therapeutic Class: NSAID with analgesic and antipyretic activity

---

CLINICAL PHARMACOLOGY
Mechanism of Action: Reversible cyclooxygenase (i.e., prostaglandin synthetase) inhibitor; nonselectively decreases the formation of both prostaglandins and thromboxane A2; variable effects on lipoxygenase synthesis and subsequent leukotriene production; antiinflammatory, antipyretic, and analgesic activity; inhibits platelet aggregation
Pharmacokinetics
PO: Peak concentration 3-5 hr, analgesic onset 1 hr, duration 48-72 hr, antirheumatic onset 7-12 days, peak 2-3 wk, $t_{1/2}$ 30-86 hr; metabolized in liver, excreted in urine (metabolites); excreted in breast milk; 99% protein binding
INDICATIONS AND USES: Osteoarthritis, rheumatoid arthritis, ankylosing spondylitis,* prevention of cognitive decline,* prevention of colon cancer,* dysmenorrhea,* erythromelalgia,* acute gout,* pain* (dental, cancer, episiotomy, postoperative, sickle cell disease), soft tissue injury*
DOSAGE
Adult
• 20 mg qd or 10 mg bid
🖻 **AVAILABLE FORMS/COST OF THERAPY**
• Cap, Gel—Oral: 10 mg, 100's: **$86.39-$179.66**; 20 mg, 100's: **$10.90-$316.69**
CONTRAINDICATIONS: Bronchospasm, nasal polyps and angioedema precipitated by aspirin or other NSAIDs
PRECAUTIONS: History of GI ulceration, bleeding, or perforation; renal dysfunction, hypertension or cardiac conditions aggravated by fluid retention and edema, history of liver dysfunction, history of coagulation
PREGNANCY AND LACTATION: Pregnancy category B (avoid administration near term); excreted into breast milk; approximately 1% of mother's serum levels; should not present a risk to nursing infant

SIDE EFFECTS/ADVERSE REACTIONS

CNS: Anxiety, confusion, depression, dizziness, *drowsiness,* fatigue, *headache,* insomnia, tremors

CV: **Dysrhythmias,** palpitations, peripheral edema, tachycardia

EENT: Blurred vision, hearing loss, tinnitus

GI: Anorexia, **bleeding,** cholestatic hepatitis, constipation, cramps, *diarrhea,* dry mouth, flatulence, jaundice, *nausea,* **perforation, ulceration,** *vomiting*

GU: **Nephrotoxicity**

HEME: **Blood dyscrasias**

SKIN: Photosensitivity, pruritus, purpura, rash, sweating

INTERACTIONS

Drugs

3 *Aminoglycosides:* Reduced clearance with elevated aminoglycoside levels and potential for toxicity (especially indomethacin in premature infants; other NSAIDs probably)

3 *Anticoagulants:* Excessive hypoprothrombinemia, decreased platelet aggregation with increased risk of GI bleeding

3 *Antihypertensives (α-blockers, angiotensin-converting enzyme inhibitors, angiotensin II receptor blockers, β-blockers, diuretics):* Inhibition of antihypertensive and other favorable hemodynamic effects

3 *Corticosteroids:* Increased risk of GI ulceration

3 *Cyclosporine:* Increased nephrotoxicity risk

3 *Lithium:* Decreased clearance of lithium (mediated via prostaglandins) resulting in elevated serum lithium levels and risk of toxicity

3 *Methotrexate:* Decreased renal secretion of methotrexate resulting in elevated methotrexate levels and risk of toxicity

3 *Phenylpropanolamine:* Possible acute hypertensive reaction

3 *Potassium-sparing diuretics:* Additive hyperkalemia potential

3 *Triamterene:* Acute renal failure reported with addition of indomethacin; caution with other NSAIDs

SPECIAL CONSIDERATIONS

• Similar in efficacy to the other NSAIDs but has the advantage and disadvantage of an extended $t_{1/2}$; high GI toxicity potential

MONITORING PARAMETERS

• Initial hemogram and fecal occult blood test within 3 mo of starting regular chronic therapy; repeat every 6-12 mo (more frequently in high-risk patients (>65 years, peptic ulcer disease, concurrent steroids or anticoagulants); electrolytes, creatinine, and BUN within 3 mo of starting regular chronic therapy; repeat every 6-12 mo

---

plicamycin (mithramycin)

(plik-a-mi′sin)

Rx: Mithracin

Chemical Class: Crystalline aglycone

Therapeutic Class: Antineoplastic; antihypercalcemic

CLINICAL PHARMACOLOGY

Mechanism of Action: Inhibits DNA, RNA, protein synthesis; derived from *Streptomyces plicatus;* replication is decreased by binding to DNA; demonstrates calcium-lowering effect not related to its tumoricidal activity; also acts on osteoclasts and blocks action of parathyroid hormone

Pharmacokinetics

IV: Rapidly cleared from blood in 2 hr; 90% excretion in 24 hr; crosses blood-brain barrier

---

* = non-FDA-approved use

INDICATIONS AND USES: Testicular cancer; hypercalcemia and hypercalciuria of malignancy

DOSAGE

Adult

• *Testicular tumors:* IV 25-30 μg/kg/day × 8-10 days, not to exceed 30 μg/kg/day

• *Hypercalcemia/hypercalciuria:* IV 25 μg/kg/day × 3-4 days, repeat at intervals of 1 wk

$ AVAILABLE FORMS/COST OF THERAPY

• Inj, Lyphl-Sol—IV: 2.5 mg: **$105.94**

CONTRAINDICATIONS: Thrombocytopenia, bone marrow depression, bleeding disorders

PRECAUTIONS: Renal disease, hepatic disease, electrolyte imbalances

PREGNANCY AND LACTATION: Pregnancy category X

SIDE EFFECTS/ADVERSE REACTIONS

CNS: Depression, drowsiness, fever, flushing, headache, lethargy, weakness

GI: Anorexia, diarrhea, increased liver enzymes, *nausea, stomatitis, vomiting*

GU: Increased BUN, creatinine; proteinuria

HEME: **Hemorrhage, neutropenia, thrombocytopenia**

METAB: Decreased serum calcium, phosphate, potassium

SKIN: Cellulitis, extravasation, facial flushing, *rash*

INTERACTIONS

Drugs

3 *Bisphosphonates, calcitonin, foscarnet, glucagon:* Additive hypocalcemic effect

SPECIAL CONSIDERATIONS

• Effective but also toxic; use is therefore limited; additive with other calcium lowering therapies

MONITORING PARAMETERS

• CBC, differential, platelet count q wk; withhold drug if WBC is <4000/mm^3 or platelet count is <50,000/mm^3

• Renal function studies: BUN, serum uric acid, urine CrCl, electrolytes, input and output ratio

• Liver function tests: bilirubin, AST, ALT, alk phosphatase before and during therapy

---

podofilox
(po-doe-fil'ox)
Rx: Condylox
Chemical Class: Podophyllum and Juniperus derivative
Therapeutic Class: Keratolytic

CLINICAL PHARMACOLOGY

Mechanism of Action: Exact mechanism unknown; results in necrosis of visible wart tissue

Pharmacokinetics

TOP: Application of 0.1-1.5 ml yields peak serum levels of 1-17 ng/ml in 1-2 hr; t$_{1/2}$ 1-4½ hr; no accumulation with multiple applications

INDICATIONS AND USES: Condyloma acuminatum (perianal, external genital)

DOSAGE

Adult

• TOP apply (cotton-tipped applicator) q12h for 3 consecutive days, then hold for 4 days; repeat 1 wk cycle until wart gone; if incomplete response after 4 cycles, consider alternate treatment; limit treatment to <10 cm^2 of wart tissue and no more than 0.5 ml of sol/day

$ AVAILABLE FORMS/COST OF THERAPY

• Gel—Top: 0.5%, 3.5 g: **$127.11**

• Sol—Top: 0.5%, 3.5 ml: **$110.53**

CONTRAINDICATIONS: Mucous membrane warts

P

PRECAUTIONS: External use only
PREGNANCY AND LACTATION: Pregnancy category C
SIDE EFFECTS/ADVERSE REACTIONS

CNS: Dizziness, insomnia, tingling
GI: Vomiting
GU: Hematuria
HEME: Bleeding
SKIN: Burning, chafing, crusting, edema, *erosion, inflammation, itching, pain,* scarring, tenderness, ulceration, vesicle formation
MISC: Malodor, pain with intercourse

SPECIAL CONSIDERATIONS
• Safety preferred over podophyllum resin

---

podophyllum
(poe-dah'fil-um)
Available in combination with benzoin
Rx: Podocon-25 (75% benzoin), Pododerm (10% benzoin)
Chemical Class: Podophyllum derivative
Therapeutic Class: Keratolytic

CLINICAL PHARMACOLOGY
Mechanism of Action: Arrests mitosis in metaphase by binding to tubulin, protein subunit of spindle microtubules
INDICATIONS AND USES: Condyloma acuminatum, multiple superficial epitheliomatoses and keratoses
DOSAGE
Adults
• *Warts:* TOP apply sparingly to wart using applicator, cover with wax paper, bandage for 1-4 hr, wash, may repeat qwk if needed
• *Keratosis, epitheliomatoses:* TOP apply qd with applicator, let dry, remove tissue, may reapply if needed

§ AVAILABLE FORMS/COST OF THERAPY
• Liq—Top: 25%, 5, 15, 30 ml: **$26.00-$47.69**/15 ml
CONTRAINDICATIONS: Bleeding warts or moles, birthmarks, moles with hair growing from them, poor blood circulation, diabetes
PRECAUTIONS: Avoid application on inflamed or irritated tissue
PREGNANCY AND LACTATION: Pregnancy category X; excretion into breast milk unknown, use caution in nursing mothers
SIDE EFFECTS/ADVERSE REACTIONS

CNS: Coma, confusion, dizziness, paresthesia, peripheral neuropathy, *seizures,* stupor
HEME: Leukopenia, thrombocytopenia
SKIN: Irritation of unaffected areas
MISC: Abdominal pain, diarrhea, nausea, vomiting

SPECIAL CONSIDERATIONS
• Not to be dispensed to the patient, professional application only
• Because of the potential for toxicity, cryotherapy should be attempted 1st or podofilox substituted

---

* = non-FDA-approved use

polymyxin B
(pol-ee-mix'in)

Rx: Aerosporin

Combinations

Rx: *Ophthal:* with bacitracin (Polysporin); with dexamethasone, neomycin (Dexacidin, Maxitrol); with hydrocortisone, neomycin (Cortisporin); with neomycin, bacitracin (Neosporin, Ocutricin); with neomycin, gramicidin (Neosporin); with oxytetracycline (Terak); with prednisolone, neomycin (Poly-Pred); with trimethoprim (Polytrim); *Topical:* with bacitracin, hydrocortisone, neomycin (Cortisporin); with dexamethasone, neomycin (Dioptrol, Maxitrol); with hydrocortisone, neomycin (Cortisporin)

OTC: *Topical:* with bacitracin (Bacimyxin, Polysporin); with bacitracin, neomycin (Neosporin, Triple Antibiotic); with bacitracin, neomycin, lidocaine (Lanabiotic, Spectrocin); with gramicidin (Polysporin); with gramicidin, lidocaine (Lidosporin, Polysporin Burn Formula); with gramicidin, neomycin (Neosporin)

Chemical Class: Polymyxin derivative

Therapeutic Class: Antibiotic; ophthalmic antibiotic

CLINICAL PHARMACOLOGY

Mechanism of Action: Interferes with membrane phospholipids and increases membrane permeability; bactericidal

Pharmacokinetics

PO: Not absorbed from the GI tract
IM/IV/IT: (intrathecal): Repeated injections accumulate; tissue diffusion poor; does not cross blood-brain barrier; $t_{1/2}$ 4½-6 hr; excreted slowly in urine unchanged (60%)

INDICATIONS AND USES: Serious infections (bacteremia) caused by susceptible strains of *Pseudomonas aeruginosa, E. aerogenes, Klebsiella pneumoniae, E. coli, Haemophilus influenzae* when other antibiotics cannot be used; in meningeal infections, polymyxin B must be given intrathecally; ophth: superficial external ocular infections

DOSAGE

Adult

• IV INF 15,000-25,000 U/kg/day in divided doses q12h, or 25,000 U/kg/day in divided doses q4-8h; reduce dosage with renal dysfunction

• IM pain at inj site; reconstitute with procaine 1%; 25,000-30,000 U/kg/day divided q4-6h; reduce dosage with renal dysfunction

• IT 50,000 U qd for 3-4 days, then 50,000 qod for 2 wk after cultures negative and CSF glucose normalized

Child

• IV INF 15,000-25,000 U/kg/day in divided doses q12h, or 25,000 U/kg/day in divided doses q4-8h; infants <2 yr, up to 40,000 U/day

• IM not recommended, severe pain at inj site; reconstitute with procaine 1%; 25,000-30,000 U/kg/day q4-6h; reduce dosage with renal dysfunction; infants <2 yr up to 40,000 U/day

• IT 50,000 U qd for 3-4 days, then 50,000 qod for 2 wk after cultures negative and CSF glucose normalized; infants <2 yr up to 20,000U/day × 3-4 days, then 25,000 U qod for 2 wk after cultures negative

💲 AVAILABLE FORMS/COST OF THERAPY

• Inj, Dry-Sol—IM, IV, IT: 500,000 U/vial: **$5.25-$9.00**

CONTRAINDICATIONS: Severe renal disease

PRECAUTIONS: Renal dysfunction, neurologic or neuromuscular deficits

PREGNANCY AND LACTATION: Pregnancy category B

SIDE EFFECTS/ADVERSE REACTIONS

CNS: Coma, confusion, dizziness, drowsiness, headache, paresthesia, **seizures,** slurred speech, stiff neck, weakness

EENT: Overgrowth of nonsusceptible organisms, poor corneal wound healing, temporary visual haze

GU: Azotemia, hematuria, leukocyturia, proteinuria

RESP: **Apnea** (concurrent use of other neurotoxic drugs or inadvertant overdosage)

SKIN: Urticaria

INTERACTIONS

Drugs

❷ *Anesthetics, neuromuscular blockers (e.g., gallamine, pancuronium, succinylcholine, tubocurarine):* Increased skeletal muscle relaxation

SPECIAL CONSIDERATIONS

• Generally replaced by the aminoglycosides or extended-spectrum penicillins for serious infections; still used for bladder irrigation and gut decontamination; used in combination with other antibiotics and/or corticosteroids topically to treat infections of the eye and skin

MONITORING PARAMETERS

• Intake and output, BUN, creatinine, urinalysis

---

polythiazide

(poly-thi'a-zide)

Rx: Renese

Combinations

   Rx: with prazosin (Minizide); with reserpine (Renese-R)

Chemical Class: Sulfonamide derivative

Therapeutic Class: Thiazide diuretic antihypertensive

CLINICAL PHARMACOLOGY

Mechanism of Action: Inhibits reabsorption of sodium and chloride in cortical thick ascending limb of the loop of Henle and the early distal tubules—increasing the urinary excretion of sodium and chloride; sulfonamide moiety provides some carbonic anhydrase inhibition activity; other actions—increased potassium and bicarbonate excretion; decreased calcium excretion; uric acid retention; antihypertensive action dependent on sodium depletion, drop in peripheral vascular resistance, and reduction in extracellular volume

Pharmacokinetics

PO: Onset 2 hr, peak 6 hr, duration 24-48 hr, $t_{1/2}$ 25.7 hr

INDICATIONS AND USES: Edema (CHF, hepatic cirrhosis, corticosteroid and estrogen therapy, nephrotic syndrome, acute glomerulonephritis), hypertension, calcium nephrolithiasis,* prevention of osteoporosis,* diabetes insipidus*

DOSAGE

NOTE: Equivalent hydrochlorothiazide dose 2 mg = 50 mg

Adult

• PO 1-4 mg qd

$ AVAILABLE FORMS/COST OF THERAPY

• Tab, Uncoated—Oral: 1 mg, 100's: **$49.29**; 2 mg, 100's: **$64.50**; 4 mg, 100's: **$101.34**

CONTRAINDICATIONS: Anuria, renal decompensation

PRECAUTIONS: Fluid and electrolyte imbalance (including sodium, potassium, magnesium calcium), renal disease, hepatic disease, gout, COPD, lupus erythematosus, diabetes mellitus, hyperparathyroidism, vomiting, diarrhea, elevated cholesterol/triglycerides, tartrazine sensitivity

PREGNANCY AND LACTATION: Pregnancy category D. Therapy for preexisting hypertension can be continued throughout pregnancy with minimal risk; initiating for simple edema not recommended; few unequivocal indications for diuretic therapy in pregnancy except for pulmonary edema or congestive heart failure; excreted in breast milk in low concentrations; compatible with breast feeding

SIDE EFFECTS/ADVERSE REACTIONS

CNS: Dizziness, headache, paresthesias, vertigo, xanthopsia

CV: Arrhythmias, orthostatic hypotension

GI: Anorexia, constipation, cramping, diarrhea, gastric irritation, jaundice (intrahepatic cholestatic jaundice), nausea, *pancreatitis,* vomiting

HEME: **Agranulocytosis, aplastic anemia, leukopenia, thrombocytopenia**

METAB: Glycosuria, hyperglycemia, hyperuricemia, lipid abnormalities (increased total and LDL cholesterol, triglycerides)

MS: Muscle spasm, weakness

SKIN: Cutaneous vasculitis, necrotizing angitis, photosensitivity, purpura, rash, urticaria, vasculitis

INTERACTIONS

Drugs

❷ *Angiotensin-converting enzyme inhibitors:* Risk of postural hypotension when added to ongoing diuretic therapy; more common with loop diuretics; first dose hypotension possible in patients with sodium depletion or hypovolemia due to diuretics or sodium restriction; hypotensive response is usually transient; hold diuretic day of first dose

🔳 *Calcium:* With large doses can result in milk-alkali syndrome

🔳 *Carbenoxolone:* Additive potassium wasting; severe hypokalemia

🔳 *Cholestyramine, colestipol:* Reduced absorption

🔳 *Corticosteroids:* Concomitant therapy may result in excessive potassium loss

🔳 *Diazoxide:* Hyperglycemia

🔳 *Digitalis glycosides:* Diuretic-induced hypokalemia increases risk of digitalis toxicity

🔳 *Hypoglycemic agents:* Increased dosage requirements due to increased glucose levels

🔳 *Lithium:* Increased lithium levels, potential toxicity

🔳 *Methotrexate:* Additive bone marrow suppression

🔳 *Nonsteroidal antiinflammatory drugs:* Concurrent use may reduce diuretic and antihypertensive effects

Labs

• *False decrease:* Urine estriol

SPECIAL CONSIDERATIONS

• Doses above 1 mg provide no further blood pressure reduction, but are more likely to induce metabolic disturbance (i.e., hypokalemia, hyperuricemia, etc.)

• May protect against osteoporotic hip fractures

P

---

italic = common side effects   ***bold italic*** = life-threatening reactions

- Loop diuretics or metolazone more effective if CrCl <40-50 ml/min

PATIENT/FAMILY EDUCATION

- Will increase urination temporarily (approx. 3 wk); take early in the day to prevent sleep disturbance
- May cause sensitivity to sunlight; avoid prolonged exposure to the sun and other ultraviolet light
- May cause gout attacks; notify clinician if sudden joint pain occurs

MONITORING PARAMETERS

- Weight, urine output, serum electrolytes, BUN, creatinine, CBC, uric acid, glucose, lipids

---

poractant alfa
(poor-ak'tant)
Rx: Curosurf
Chemical Class: Phospholipid
Therapeutic Class: Porcine lung surfactant

CLINICAL PHARMACOLOGY
Mechanism of Action: Maintains lung inflation by lowering surface tension
Pharmacokinetics
Administered intratracheally; distributed to all lobes, distal airways, and alveolar spaces; biological $t_{1/2}$ 36 hr

INDICATIONS AND USES: Treatment (rescue) of respiratory distress syndrome (RDS) in premature infants

DOSAGE
Infant

- Intratracheal 100 mg/kg, followed by 2 additional 100 mg/kg doses at 12 and 24 hr in neonates still requiring mechanical ventilation with supplemental oxygen; a dose of 200 mg/kg within 10 min of delivery, followed prn by a 2nd mg/kg dose 6-24 hr later has been used for prophylaxis against neonatal RDS

§ AVAILABLE FORMS/COST OF THERAPY

- Susp—Intratracheal: 120 mg/1.5 ml, vial: **$312.00**; 240 mg/3 ml, vial: **$610.80**

PRECAUTIONS: Infants born after >3 wk following ruptured membranes; intraventricular hemorrhage; major congenital malformations

SIDE EFFECTS/ADVERSE REACTIONS
CV: Patent ductus arteriosus, hypotension (transient)
RESP: Apnea
SKIN: Flushing
MISC: Antibody formation

SPECIAL CONSIDERATIONS
MONITORING PARAMETERS

- Continuous ECG and transcutaneous O_2 saturation; pCO_2; lung compliance; respiratory rate

---

potassium iodide
Rx: Pima, SSKI, Strong Iodine Solution (Lugol's Solution)
Chemical Class: Iodine product
Therapeutic Class: Expectorant; antithyroid agent

CLINICAL PHARMACOLOGY
Mechanism of Action: Reduces viscosity of mucus by increasing respiratory tract secretions; inhibits the release and synthesis of thyroid hormone
Pharmacokinetics
PO: Accumulates in thyroid gland; onset (antithyroid effects) 24-48 hr, peak effect (antithyroid effects) 10-15 days after continuous therapy; excreted mainly by the kidneys

INDICATIONS AND USES: Expectorant; preoperative reduction of thyroid gland vascularity prior to thyroidectomy, thyrotoxic crisis (in conjunction with other antithyroid agents), persistent or recurrent hyperthyroidism; radiation emergencies (to prevent uptake of radioactive isotopes of iodine); cutaneous sporotrichosis*

DOSAGE

Adult

• *Expectorant:* PO 300-650 mg tid-qid

• *Preoperative thyroidectomy:* PO 50-250 mg (1-5 gtt SSKI; 3-5 gtt Lugol's solution) tid for 10-14 days prior to surgery

• *Thyrotoxic crisis:* PO 300-500 mg (6-10 gtt SSKI; 1 ml Lugol's solution) tid

• *Cutaneous sporotrichosis:* PO 65-325 mg tid

• *Radiation emergency:* PO 130 mg qd for 10 days

Child

• *Expectorant:* PO 60-250 mg qid; max 500 mg/day

• *Preoperative thyroidectomy:* PO 50-250 mg (1-5 gtt SSKI; 3-5 gtt Lugol's solution) tid for 10-14 days prior to surgery

• *Thyrotoxic crisis:* PO <1 yr 65 mg qd for 10 days; older children 130 mg qd for 10 days

• *Radiation emergency:* PO <1 yr, 65 mg qd for 10 days; older children, 130 mg qd for 10 days

$ AVAILABLE FORMS/COST OF THERAPY

• Sol—Oral: 15 g/15 ml, 30 ml: **$5.87-$12.10**

• Syr—Oral: 325 mg/5 ml, 480 ml: **$22.90**

CONTRAINDICATIONS: Tuberculosis, acute bronchitis, hyperkalemia

PRECAUTIONS: Hypocomplementemic vasculitis, goiter, autoimmune thyroid disease, sulfite sensitivity (increased risk for iodine-induced adverse effects)

PREGNANCY AND LACTATION: Pregnancy category D; use of iodides as expectorants during pregnancy is contraindicated; concentrated in breast milk, may affect infant's thyroid activity but considered compatible with breast feeding

SIDE EFFECTS/ADVERSE REACTIONS

CNS: Fever, headache

*CV: **Angioedema***

EENT: Rhinitis

GI: GI upset, metallic taste, soreness of teeth and gums

HEME: Cutaneous and mucosal hemorrhage, eosinophilia

METAB: Goiter, hypothyroidism

MS: Arthralgia

SKIN: Acne, urticaria

MISC: Lymph node enlargement

INTERACTIONS

Drugs

3 *Lithium:* Increased likelihood of hypothyroidism

SPECIAL CONSIDERATIONS

PATIENT/FAMILY EDUCATION

• Dilute sol with water or fruit juice to improve taste, drink sol through straw

• Administer with food or milk

MONITORING PARAMETERS

• Thyroid function tests if used for thyroid-related conditions

P

---

potassium salts

(po-taah'see-um)

Rx: *Potassium chloride:*
Cena-K, Gen K, K+ Care,
K+10, Kaochlor, Kaon-Cl,
Kato, Kay Ciel, K-Dur, K-Lease,
K-lor, Klor-Con, Klorvess,
Klotrix, K·lyte/Cl, K-Norm,
K-tab, Micro-K, Potasalan,
Rum-K, Slow-K, Ten-K

Rx: *Potassium gluconate:*
Kaon, Kaylixir, K-G Elixer

Rx: *Combinations of
potassium salts:* Effer-K,
K·Lyte, Klor-Con EF (as
bicarbonate, citrate), K+ Care
ET (as bicarbonate), Klorvess
Effervescent Granules (as
bicarbonate, chloride,
citrate); K-Lyte/Cl (as
bicarbonate, chloride),
Kolyum (as chloride,
gluconate); Tri-K, (as acetate,
bicarbonate, citrate); Twin-K
(as gluconate, citrate)
Chemical Class: Potassium salt
Therapeutic Class: Electrolyte
supplement

CLINICAL PHARMACOLOGY
Mechanism of Action: Principal intracellular cation of most body tissues; necessary for maintenance of intracellular tonicity and proper relationships with sodium across cell membranes; needed for adequate nerve transmission, cardiac, skeletal, and smooth muscle contraction, renal function, and acid-base balance

Pharmacokinetics
PO/IV: Primarily renal excretion (90%); fecal (10%)

INDICATIONS AND USES: Prevention and treatment of hypokalemia; with alkalosis (i.e., due to diuretics), use potassium chloride salt; when acidosis present, use potassium acetate, bicarbonate, citrate, or gluconate salts; hypertension*

DOSAGE
Individualize dosage up to 400 mEq/day (usually not more than 3 mEq/kg/day): 10-30 mEq/day for prevention; 40-100 mEq/day for treatment

mEq/g of potassium salts

K^+ Salt	mEq/g
gluconate	4.3
citrate	9.8
bicarbonate	10
acetate	10.2
chloride	13.4

Adult

• *Potassium acetate:* Serum potassium >2.5 mEq/L: IV INF up to 200 mEq/day in concentration <40 mEq/L at rate of 10 mEq/hr; serum potassium <2.0 mEq/L: IV INF up to 400 mEq/day in concentration <80 mEq/L and rate up to 40 mEq/hr

• *Potassium bicarbonate:* PO dissolve 25-50 mEq in water qd-bid up to 100 mEq/d

• *Potassium chloride:* PO 10-100 mEq/d divided qd-tid; IV serum potassium >2.5 mEq/L: IV up to 200 mEq/day in concentration <40 mEq/L at a rate not exceeding 10 mEq/hr; serum potassium <2.0 mEq/L: IV up to 400 mEq/day in concentration <80 mEq/L and rate of 40 mEq/hr

• *Potassium gluconate:* PO 20 mEq in divided doses bid-qid

Child

• *Potassium acetate:* IV up to 3 mEq/kg or 40 mEq/m^2 per day

• *Potassium chloride:* PO sol 15-40 mEq/m^2 or 1-3 mEq/kg/day in divided doses diluted in water or juice; IV up to 3 mEq/kg or 40 mEq/m^2 per day

---

* = non-FDA-approved use

• *Potassium gluconate:* PO 20-40 mEq/m^2 or 2-3 mEq/kg per day in divided doses

🛐 AVAILABLE FORMS/COST OF THERAPY

Potassium Acetate
• Inj, Sol—IV: 2 mEq/ml, 20 ml: **$1.60-$2.39**; 4 mEq/ml, 50 ml: **$5.00-$6.46**

Potassium Bicarbonate
• Tab, Effervescent—Oral: 25 mEq, 30's: **$6.06-$19.00**

Potassium Chloride
• Cap, Gel, Sus Action—Oral: 8 mEq, 100's: **$10.75-$28.94**; 10 mEq, 100's: **$14.20-$32.04**
• Inj, Conc—Sol: 1.5 mEq/ml, 20 ml: **$4.92-$8.78**; 2 mEq/ml, 10 ml: **$0.54-$3.40**
• Liq—Oral: 20 mEq/15 ml, 480 ml: **$1.49-$48.00**; 30 mEq/15 ml, 480 ml: **$23.60**; 40 mEq/15 ml, 480 ml: **$2.59-$26.94**
• Powder, Reconst—Oral: 20 mEq/pkg, 30's: **$3.95-$53.26**; 25 mEq/pkg, 30's: **$7.41**
• Tab, Coated, Sus Action—Oral: 8 mEq, 100's: **$9.79-$36.00**; 10 mEq, 100's: **$9.92-$49.93**; 20 mEq, 100's: **$41.12-$60.90**
• Tab, Effervescent—Oral: 25 mEq, 30's: **$17.48-$39.93**; 50 mEq, 30's: **$77.51**

Potassium Gluconate
• Elixir—Oral: 20 mEq/15 ml, 480 ml: **$5.49-$29.90**

CONTRAINDICATIONS: Renal disease (severe), severe hemolytic disease, Addison's disease, hyperkalemia, acute dehydration, extensive tissue breakdown

PRECAUTIONS: Cardiac disease, potassium-sparing diuretic therapy, systemic acidosis

SIDE EFFECTS/ADVERSE REACTIONS

CNS: Confusion

*CV: **Arrest,** bradycardia, cardiac depression, **dysrhythmias,** lowered R and depressed RST, peaking T waves, prolonged P-R interval, widened QRS complex

GI: Cramps, diarrhea, nausea, pain, ulceration of small bowel, *vomiting*

GU: Oliguria

SKIN: Cold extremities, rash

INTERACTIONS

Drugs

🖪 *ACE inhibitors:* Hyperkalemia

🖪 *Disopyramide:* Increased potassium concentrations can enhance disopyramide effects

🖪 *Hypoglycemics:* Correction of hypokalemia may result in hypoglycemia

❷ *Potassium-sparing diuretics:* Hyperkalemia

SPECIAL CONSIDERATIONS

• Avoid use of compressed tablets or enteric-coated tablets (i.e., non-sustained release or effervescent tablets for sol) due to significant ulcerogenic tendency and propensity to cause significant local tissue destruction

• Sol, powder, and oral susp: dilute or dissove in 120 ml cold water or juice

• Extended release caps and tabs: do not crush; take with food; swallow with full glass of liquid

• Injectable potassium products must be diluted prior to administration; direct inj of potassium concentrate may be fatal

• Central line preferable for IV infusions concentrated >40 mEq/L

MONITORING PARAMETERS

• ECG monitoring advisable for IV infusion rate >10 mEq/hr

• Normal serum potassium level 3.5-5.0 mEq/L (higher, to 7.7 mEq/L in neonates)

italic = common side effects   ***bold italic*** = life-threatening reactions

pralidoxime

(pra-li-dox′eem)
Rx: Protopam
Chemical Class: Quaternary
ammonium derivative
Therapeutic Class: Anticho-
linesterase antidote

CLINICAL PHARMACOLOGY

Mechanism of Action: Reactivates
cholinesterase inactivated by exposure to organophosphate pesticides
or related compounds by displacing
the enzyme from its receptor sites;
most effective if administered
within 24 hr of exposure

Pharmacokinetics

IM/IV: Peak 5-15 min, not bound to
plasma proteins; metabolized in
liver, excreted rapidly in urine (metabolite and unchanged drug); $t_{1/2}$ 1.7
hr (repeated doses may be needed)

INDICATIONS AND USES: Antidote
in poisonings due to organophosphate pesticides and related compounds; control of overdosage by
anticholinesterase drugs used to
treat myasthenia gravis

DOSAGE

Use in conjunction with atropine

Adult

• *Organophosphate poisoning:*
IM/IV 1-2 g, repeat in 1-2 hr if muscle weakness has not resolved, then
at 10-12 hr intervals if cholinergic
signs reappear

• *Anticholinesterase overdosage:*
IV 1-2 g, followed by 250 mg q5 min
until desired response

Child

• *Organophosphate poisoning:*
IM/IV 20-50 mg/kg/dose, repeat in
1-2 hr if muscle weakness has not resolved, then at 10-12 hr intervals if
cholinergic signs reappear

$ **AVAILABLE FORMS/COST
OF THERAPY**

• Inj, Lyphl-Sol—IM, IV, SC: 50
mg/ml, 20 ml: **$108.37**

PRECAUTIONS: Rapid IV inj, impaired renal function, myasthenia
gravis, carbamate poisoning (less
effective than with organophosphate
poisoning)

PREGNANCY AND LACTATION:
Pregnancy category C

**SIDE EFFECTS/ADVERSE REAC-
TIONS**

CNS: Dizziness, drowsiness, headache

CV: Tachycardia

EENT: Blurred vision, diplopia, impaired accommodation

GI: Transaminase elevations (return
to normal within 2 wk), nausea

MS: Muscular weakness

RESP: Hyperventilation

SKIN: Pain at inj site (IM)

**SPECIAL CONSIDERATIONS
MONITORING PARAMETERS**

• CBC; plasma cholinesterase activity may help confirm diagnosis and
follow course of illness

pramipexole

(pram-eh-pex′ol)
Rx: Mirapex
Chemical Class: Non-ergoline;
a propylaminobenzothiazole
Therapeutic Class: Anti-Par-
kinson's agent, dopaminergic

CLINICAL PHARMACOLOGY

Mechanism of Action: Dopamine
D_2-receptor agonist, with activity at
both presynaptic and postsynaptic
receptor sites; D_3-receptor subtype
affinity greater than D_2-, D_4-recep-
tor subtypes (different from other
dopamine-receptor agonists); moderate affinity for alpha-2 adrenoceptors; low affinity for alpha-1, beta-

adrenoceptors, serotonin, acetylcholine, and D_1 receptors; in Parkinson's disease, stimulates caudate neurons via D_3-receptor agonist mechanism

Pharmacokinetics

PO: Peak 1-3 hr; well absorbed (PO); minimally metabolized by liver, protein binding less than 20%, excreted renally, unchanged after 24 hr; $t_{1/2}$ 8-14 hr; crosses placenta

INDICATIONS AND USES: Treatment of signs and symptoms of idiopathic Parkinson's disease

DOSAGE

Adult

• *Parkinson's disease:* PO 0.125 mg tid initially increase gradually at 5-7 day intervals (max 1.5 mg tid); discontinue over a 1 wk period

• *Renal failure and geriatric patients:* Reduce dose according to CrCl; starting dose and (maximal dose) shown below

• CrCl >60 ml/min: 0.125 mg tid (1.5 mg tid)

• CrCl 35 to 59 ml/min: 0.125 mg bid (1.5 mg bid)

• CrCl 15 to 34 ml/min: 0.125 mg qd (1.5 mg qd)

• Ccr <15 ml/min and hemodialysis: avoid use of pramipexole

$ AVAILABLE FORMS/COST OF THERAPY

• Tab—Oral: 0.125 mg, 63's: **$53.97**; 0.25 mg, 90's: **$102.34**; 0.5 mg, 1 mg, 1.5 mg, 90's: **$193.09**

PRECAUTIONS: Hypersensitivity history or other untoward effects related to use of other dopamine agonists, psychotic disorders, dementia (potential for exacerbation), cardiovascular disease (postural hypotensive effects, increases in heart rate, and possibly hypertension), renal impairment (dose reductions are indicated), worsening of dyskinesia with advanced Parkinson's disease; abrupt withdrawal of treatment (taper down over 1 wk)

PREGNANCY AND LACTATION: Pregnancy category C; inhibits prolactin secretion; excretion into breast milk unknown

SIDE EFFECTS/ADVERSE REACTIONS

CNS: Akathesia, amnesia, asthenia, confusion, *dizziness, drowsiness,* dyskinesia, dystonia, hallucinations, hypesthesia, *insomnia,* restlessness, *somnolence (13%)*

CV: **Dysrhythmias,** chest pain, hypertension, *orthostatic hypotension* (domperidone may prevent), palpitations, syncope, tachycardia

EENT: Blurred vision

GI: Anorexia, *constipation (7%), dry mouth (10%),* dyspepsia, dysphagia, flatulence, *nausea (20%)*

GU: Impotence, urinary frequency

METAB: Decreases prolactin, thyrotropin levels; increases growth hormone, cortisol; peripheral edema, weight loss

MS: Increased CPK, leg cramps

SKIN: Diaphoresis, generalized rash, pruritus

INTERACTIONS

Drugs

▣ *Cimetidine:* 50% increase in pramipexole AUC and 40% increase in $t_{1/2}$

▣ *Dopamine antagonists (phenothiazines, butyrophenones, thioxanthenes, metoclopropamide):* May diminish effectiveness of pramipexole

▣ *Levodopa:* 40% increase in levodopa concentrations

SPECIAL CONSIDERATIONS

• At least as effective as bromocriptine in the treatment of advanced parkinsonian patients with levodopa-related motor fluctuations; adverse effects similar in incidence and severity; appears to lack

P

---

italic = common side effects   ***bold italic*** = life-threatening reactions

some of the toxicity seen with bromocriptine, pergolide, and cabergoline (e.g., pleuropulmonary disease); may be a useful alternative in patients with intolerable adverse effects due to ergot derivatives

MONITORING PARAMETERS
• United Parkinson's Disease Rating Scale (UPDRS) useful for monitoring efficacy endpoints

pramoxine
(pra-mox'een)
OTC: Itch-X, PrameGel, Prax, ProctoFoam-NS, Tronolane, Tronothane
Chemical Class: Dyclonine derivative
Therapeutic Class: Topical anesthetic

CLINICAL PHARMACOLOGY
Mechanism of Action: Decreases the neuronal membrane's permeability to sodium ions thus inhibiting depolarization; blocks initiation and conduction of nerve impulses
Pharmacokinetics
TOP: Onset 2-5 min. duration may be several days

INDICATIONS AND USES: Temporary relief of pain and itching associated with dermatoses, minor burns, anogenital pruritus or irritation, anal fissures, hermorrhoids

DOSAGE
Adult
• TOP apply tid-qid: PR apply up to 5 times daily; apply 1 applicatorful of aerosol foam bid-tid after bowel movements

§ AVAILABLE FORMS/COST OF THERAPY
• Aer Foam Susp—Rect, Top: 1%, 15 g: **$26.37**
• Cre—Rect, Top: 1%, 30, 60 g: **$10.00**/30 g
• Cre—Top: 1%, 30 g: **$10.58**
• Gel—Top: 1%, 35.4, 120 g: **$6.59/** 120 g
• Lotion—Top: 1%, 15, 120, 240 ml: **$3.66**/15 ml
• Spray—Top: 1%, 59 ml: **$4.32**
• Supp—Rect: 1%, 10's: **$3.41**

PRECAUTIONS: Prolonged use, rectal bleeding, children, denuded skin

PREGNANCY AND LACTATION: Pregnancy category C; excretion into breast milk unknown

SIDE EFFECTS/ADVERSE REACTIONS
SKIN: Burning, irritation, rash, stinging

SPECIAL CONSIDERATIONS
• Cross-sensitization with other local anesthetics unlikely

PATIENT/FAMILY EDUCATION
• Do not use near eyes or nose
• Contact clinician if condition fails to improve after 3-4 days or worsens
• Do not apply to large areas
• Do not apply to unaffected areas

pravastatin
(prav-i-sta'tin)
Rx: Pravachol
Chemical Class: Substituted hexahydronaphthalene
Therapeutic Class: Antilipemic (HMG-CoA reductase inhibitor); "statin"

CLINICAL PHARMACOLOGY
Mechanism of Action: Competitively inhibits 3-hydroxy-3-methyl-glutaryl-coenzyme A (HMG-CoA) reductase, an early rate-limiting step in cholesterol biosynthesis; increases HDL cholesterol mildly (7-12%), significant decreases in total and LDL cholesterol

(16-25%, 22-34%, respectively), moderate lowering effect on triglycerides (11-24%)

Pharmacokinetics

PO: Peak 1-1½ hr; absolute bioavailability 17%; 50% bound to plasma proteins; metabolized in liver, excreted in urine (20%) and feces (70%); t½ 77 hr

INDICATIONS AND USES: Elevated triglyceride levels (Fredrickson Type IV), primary dysbetalipoproteinemia (Fredrickson Type III), primary prevention of coronary events, and secondary prevention of cardiovascular events

DOSAGE

Adult

• PO 10-20 mg qhs, may increase to 40 mg qhs if needed

• *Significant renal or hepatic dysfunction:* PO 10 mg qhs initially

🅢 AVAILABLE FORMS/COST OF THERAPY

• Tab, Uncoated—Oral: 10 mg, 100's: **$168.79**; 20 mg, 100's: **$181.75**; 40 mg, 80 mg, 90's: **$391.19**

CONTRAINDICATIONS: Active liver disease, unexplained persistent elevated liver function tests

PRECAUTIONS: History of liver disease, renal function impairment, elderly, children <18 yr, alcoholism; risk factors predisposing to the development of renal failure secondary to rhabdomyolysis (severe acute infection, trauma, hypotension, uncontrolled seizure disorder, severe metabolic disorders, electrolyte imbalance)

PREGNANCY AND LACTATION: Pregnancy category X; small amounts excreted in breast milk; should probably not be used by women who are nursing

SIDE EFFECTS/ADVERSE REACTIONS

CNS: Dizziness, headache

CV: Chest pain

GI: Abdominal pain, anorexia, cholestatic jaundice, cirrhosis, constipation, fatty change in liver, flatulence, heartburn, hepatitis, increased serum transaminase levels, nausea, ***pancreatitis,*** vomiting

GU: Erectile dysfunction, loss of libido

MS: Arthralgia, localized pain, myalgia, myopathy, ***rhabdomyolysis***

SKIN: Alopecia, photosensitivity, pruritus, rash

MISC: Fatigue, gynecomastia

INTERACTIONS

Drugs

❷ *Azole antifungals (fluconazole, itraconazole, ketoconazole, miconazole):* Increased plasma pravastatin levels via inhibition of metabolism with increased risk of rhabdomyolysis

❸ *Cholestyramine:* Reduced bioavailability of pravastatin

❸ *Clarithromycin:* Increased plasma pravastain levels via inhibition of metabolism with increased risk of rhabdomyolysis

❷ *Clofibrate:* Small increased risk of myopathy with combination

❸ *Colestipol:* Reduced bioavailability of pravastatin

❸ *Cyclosporine:* Concomitant administration increases risk of severe myopathy or rhabdomyolysis

❸ *Danazol:* Increased plasma pravastatin levels via inhibition of metabolism with increased risk of rhabdomyolysis

❸ *Erythromycin:* Increased pravastatin levels via inhibition of metabolism with increased risk of rhabdomyolysis

P

❸ *Fluoxetine:* Increased pravastatin levels via inhibition of metabolism with increased risk of rhabdomyolysis

❷ *Gemfibrozil:* Small increased risk of myopathy with combination, especially at high doses of statin

❸ *Isradipine:* May decrease pravastatin plasma concentrations

❸ *Niacin:* Concomitant administration increases risk of severe myopathy or rhabdomyolysis

❸ *Nefazodone:* May inhibit hepatic metabolism of pravastatin with risk of rhabdomyolysis

❸ *Troleandomycin:* Increased pravastatin levels via inhibition of metabolism with increased risk of rhabdomyolysis

SPECIAL CONSIDERATIONS

• Statin selection based on lipid-lowering prowess, cost, and availability

PATIENT/FAMILY EDUCATION

• Avoid prolonged exposure to sunlight and other UV light
• Promptly report any unexplained muscle pain, tenderness, or weakness, especially if accompanied by fever or malaise
• Strictly adhere to low cholesterol diet
• Take daily doses in the evening for increased effect

MONITORING PARAMETERS

• ALT and AST at baseline, and at 12 weeks of therapy. If no change at 12 weeks, no further monitoring necessary (discontinue if elevations persist at >3 times upper limit of normal)
• CPK in any patient complaining of diffuse myalgia, muscle tenderness, or weakness
• Fasting lipid profile

---

praziquantel
(pray-zi-kwon'tel)
Rx: Biltricide
Chemical Class: Pyrazinoisoquinoline derivative
Therapeutic Class: Anthelmintic

CLINICAL PHARMACOLOGY
Mechanism of Action: Increases cell membrane permeability in worm causing a loss of intracellular calcium, massive contractions and paralysis of worm musculature leading to detachment of suckers from blood vessel walls and dislodgment; also results in vacuolization and disintegration of the schistosome in tegument, followed by attachment of phagocytes and death
Pharmacokinetics
PO: Rapidly absorbed, peak 1-3 hr; significant 1st-pass biotransformation; metabolites excreted primarily in urine; $t_{1/2}$ 0.8-1½ hr

INDICATIONS AND USES: Schistosomiasis caused by *Schistosoma* spp. pathogenic to humans, clonorchiasis and opisthorchiasis (liver flukes), cysticercosis,* tissue fluke infections,* intestinal fluke infections,* intestinal cestode (tapeworm) infections*

DOSAGE
Adult and Child
• *Schistosomiasis:* PO 20 mg/kg/dose 2-3 times/day for 1 day at 4-6 hr intervals
• *Clonorchiasis and opisthorchiasis:* PO 75 mg/kg/day divided q8h for 1-2 days
• *Cysticercosis:* PO 50 mg/kg/day divided q8h for 14 days (administer steroids prior to starting praziquantel for neurocysticercosis)

---

* = non-FDA-approved use

• *Cestodes:* PO 10-20 mg/kg as a single dose (25 mg/kg for *Hymenolepsis nana*)

$ AVAILABLE FORMS/COST OF THERAPY

• Tab, Plain Coated—Oral: 600 mg, 6's: **$74.39**

CONTRAINDICATIONS: Ocular cysticercosis

PRECAUTIONS: Children <4 yr, cerebral cysticercosis (hospitalize patient for duration of therapy)

PREGNANCY AND LACTATION: Pregnancy category B; do not nurse on day of treatment and during the subsequent 72 hr

SIDE EFFECTS/ADVERSE REACTIONS

CNS: Dizziness, drowsiness, fever, headache

GI: Abdominal discomfort, minimal increases in liver enzymes

SKIN: Urticaria

MISC: Malaise

INTERACTIONS

Drugs

3 *Chloroquine and hydroxychloroquine:* Reduces plasma level of praziquantel

3 *Cimetidine:* Increases plasma level of praziquantel

SPECIAL CONSIDERATIONS

PATIENT/FAMILY EDUCATION

• Swallow tablets unchewed with some liquid during meals

• May cause drowsiness

• Use caution driving or performing other tasks requiring alertness

prazosin
(pra'zoe-sin)

Rx: Minipress

Combinations

  Rx: with polythiazide (Minizide)

Chemical Class: Quinazoline derivative

Therapeutic Class: α_1-adrenergic blocker: antihypertensive; symptomatic benign prostatic hypertrophy

CLINICAL PHARMACOLOGY

Mechanism of Action: Selectively blocks postsynaptic α_1-adrenergic receptors; dilates both arterioles and veins, reducing peripheral vascular resistance and blood pressure; no reflex tachycardia or changes in renin release; blockade of α_1-adrenoceptors in bladder neck and prostate; relaxes smooth muscle, improving urine flow rates in benign prostatic hypertrophy

Pharmacokinetics

PO: Oral bioavailability 48%-68%, peak 1-3 hr, duration of antihypertensive effect 10 hr; 92%-97% bound to plasma proteins; extensively metabolized to active metabolites, excreted in bile (90%) and urine (10%); $t_{1/2}$ 2-3 hr

INDICATIONS AND USES: Hypertension, benign prostatic hyperrophy,* Raynaud's vasospasm,*

DOSAGE

Adult

• PO 1 mg bid-tid, give 1st dose at bedtime; increase as needed to 6-15 mg/day in divided doses; doses >20 mg/day usually do not increase efficacy

Child

• PO 0.5-7 mg tid

☒ AVAILABLE FORMS/COST OF THERAPY

• Cap, Gel—Oral: 1 mg, 100's: **$8.25-$48.04**; 2 mg, 100's: **$9.32-$72.41**; 5 mg, 100's: **$15.77-$72.16**

PRECAUTIONS: Children, hepatic disease

PREGNANCY AND LACTATION: Pregnancy category C

SIDE EFFECTS/ADVERSE REACTIONS

CNS: Anxiety, asthenia, ataxia, depression, *dizziness,* fever, *headache,* hypertonia, insomnia, nervousness, paresthesia, somnolence

CV: Chest pain, dysrhythmia, edema, *"1st-dose" syncope,* flushing, palpitations, postural hypotension, tachycardia

EENT: Abnormal vision, tinnitus, vertigo

GI: Abdominal discomfort, constipation, diarrhea, dry mouth, flatulence, nausea, vomiting

GU: Incontinence, polyuria

MS: Arthralgia, myalgia

RESP: Dyspnea

SKIN: Pruritus, rash

INTERACTIONS

Drugs

☒ *ACE inhibitors:* Exaggerated first-dose response to prazosin

☒ *β-adrenergic blockers:* Exaggerated first-dose response to prazosin

☒ *NSAIDs:* Inhibits antihypertensive response to prazosin

☒ *Verapamil:* Reduces first pass metabolism of prazosin

Labs

• False positive urinary metabolites of norepinephrine and VMA

• No effect on prostate specific antigen (PSA)

SPECIAL CONSIDERATIONS

• The doxazosin arm of the ALLHAT study was stopped early; the doxazosin group had a 25% greater risk of combined cardiovascular disease events which was primarily accounted for by a doubled risk of CHF vs the chlorthalidone group; doxazosin was also found to be less effective at controlling systolic BP an average of 3 mm Hg; may want to consider primary antihypertensives in addition to alpha blockers for BPH symptoms

• Use as single antihypertensive agent limited by tendency to cause sodium and water retention and increased plasma volume

PATIENT/FAMILY EDUCATION

• Alert patients to the possibility of syncopal and orthostatic symptoms, especially with the 1st dose ("1st-dose syncope")

• Initial dose should be administered at bedtime in the smallest possible dose

---

prednisolone

(pred-niss'oh-lone)

Rx: Prelone; (acetate) Key-Pred, Predacort, Key-Pred-SP (sodium phosphate), Pediapred; Ophthalmic: (acetate) Econopred, Econopred Plus, Pred Mild, Pred Forte; (sodium phosphate) AK-Pred, Inflamase Mild, Inflamase Forte, Prednisol

Chemical Class: Glucocorticoid

Therapeutic Class: Systemic corticosteroid; ophthalmic corticosteroid

CLINICAL PHARMACOLOGY

Mechanism of Action: Decreases inflammation by depressing migration of polymorphonuclear leukocytes and activity of endogenous mediators of inflammation; has many profound metabolic effects, possesses mineralocorticoid activity

Pharmacokinetics

PO: Peak 1-2 hr, duration 2 days

IM: Peak 3-45 hr

Metabolized in most tissues but primarily in liver, excreted in urine; $t_{1/2}$ 115-212 min (biologic 18-36 hr)

INDICATIONS AND USES: Anti-inflammatory or immunosuppressant agent in the treatment of a variety of diseases of hematologic, allergic, inflammatory, neoplastic, and autoimmune origin; (ophth) steroid-responsive inflammatory conditions of the palpebral and bulbar conjunctiva, lid, cornea, and anterior segment of the globe, corneal injury (chemical, radiation, or thermal burns or penetration of foreign bodies)

DOSAGE

Adult

• PO 5-60 mg/day; IM (acetate) 4-60 mg/day

• *Multiple sclerosis (acute exacerbations):* PO 200 mg qd for 1 wk, followed by 80 mg qod for 1 mo

• *OPHTH* apply 1gtt q1h during day, q2h during night until favorable response, then 1 gtt q4h

Child

• *Acute asthma:* PO 1-2 mg/kg/day divided 1-2 times/day for 3-5 days

• *Anti-inflammatory/immunosuppressive:* PO 0.1-2 mg/kg/day divided qd-qid

• *OPHTH* apply 1 gtt q1h during day, q2h during night until favorable response, then 1 gtt q4h

S **AVAILABLE FORMS/COST OF THERAPY**

• Inj, Susp—IM (acetate): 25 mg/ml, 10, 30 ml: **$6.45-$13.60**/30 ml; 50 mg/ml, 10, 30 ml: **$6.95-$19.20**/30 ml

• Liq—Oral (sodium phosphate): 5 mg/5 ml, 120 ml: **$15.49-$28.52**

• Sol—Ophth (sodium phosphate): 0.125%, 5, 10 ml: **$1.73-$18.56**/5 ml; 1%, 5, 10, 15 ml: **$1.72-$18.38**/5 ml

• Susp—Ophth (acetate): 0.12%, 5, 10 ml: **$17.25-$24.78**/5 ml; 0.125%, 5, 10 ml: **$4.75-$25.96**/5 ml; 1%, 5, 10, 15 ml: **$1.80-$29.81**/5 ml

• Syr—Oral: 15 mg/5 ml, 30, 60, 120, 160, 240, 480 ml: **$11.81-$21.35**/60 ml

• Tab, Uncoated—Oral: 5 mg, 100's: **$2.66-$13.75**

CONTRAINDICATIONS: Systemic fungal infections; (ophth): acute superficial herpes simplex keratitis and other viral diseases of the cornea and conjunctiva; fungal diseases of ocular structures; ocular TB; following uncomplicated removal of a superficial corneal foreign body

PRECAUTIONS: Psychosis, cerebral malaria, elderly, AIDS, latent tuberculosis or amebiasis (reactivation of disease), diabetes mellitus, glaucoma, osteoporosis, ulcerative colitis (intestinal perforation), CHF, myasthenia gravis, renal disease, esophagitis, peptic ulcer, hypertension; (ophth): infections of the eye, glaucoma

PREGNANCY AND LACTATION: Pregnancy category B; compatible with breast feeding

SIDE EFFECTS/ADVERSE REACTIONS

CNS: Depression, headache, *mood changes,* **seizures,** vertigo

CV: CHF, hypertension, tachycardia, **thromboembolism,** thrombophlebitis

EENT: Systemic: Cataracts, glaucoma, increased intraocular pressure, optic nerve damage, papilledema; Ophthalmic: Blurred vision, burning with administration, cataracts, corneal infection, decreased visual acuity and visual fields, glaucoma exacerbation, increased in-

P

traocular pressure, optic nerve damage, poor corneal wound healing, stinging with administration

GI: Abdominal distension, diarrhea, **GI hemorrhage,** increased appetite, *nausea,* **pancreatitis**

METAB: Cushingoid state, decreased glucose tolerance, growth suppression in children, *HPA axis suppression,* hypercalciuria, hypokalemia

MS: Aseptic necrosis of femoral and humeral heads, fractures, muscle mass loss, osteoporosis, weakness

SKIN: Acne, *ecchymosis,* petechiae, striae, *poor wound healing,* suppression of skin test reactions, *thin fragile skin*

INTERACTIONS
Drugs
🖪 *Aminoglutethamide:* Increased clearance of prednisolone; doubling of dose may be required

🖪 *Antidiabetics:* Increased blood glucose

🖪 *Barbiturates:* Increased clearance of prednisolone

🖪 *Cholestyramine, colestipol:* Reduced absorption of prednisolone

🖪 *Clarithromycin, erythromycin, troleandomycin, ketoconazole:* Possible enhanced steroid effect

🖪 *Estrogens, oral contraceptives:* Enhanced effects of corticosteroids

🖪 *Intrauterine devices:* Decreased contraceptive effect (possibly secondary inhibition of inflammatory reaction)

🖪 *Isoniazid:* Reduced plasma concentrations of isoniazid; (rapid isoniazid acetylators at increased risk)

🖪 *NSAIDs:* Increased risk GI ulceration

🖪 *Rifampin:* May reduce hepatic clearance of prednisolone

🖪 *Salicylates:* Increased salicylate clearance

Labs
• *False increase:* Cortisol, digoxin, theophylline

• *False decrease:* Urine glucose (Clinistix, Diastix only, Testape no effect)

• *False negative:* Skin allergy tests

SPECIAL CONSIDERATIONS
PATIENT/FAMILY EDUCATION
• May cause GI upset

• Take single daily doses in AM

• Increased dose of rapidly acting corticosteroids may be necessary in patients subjected to unusual stress

• Signs of adrenal insufficiency include fatigue, anorexia, nausea, vomiting, diarrhea, weight loss, weakness, dizziness, and low blood sugar

• Avoid abrupt withdrawal of therapy following high-dose or long-term therapy. Relative insufficiency may exist for up to 1 yr after discontinuation

• Patients on chronic steroid therapy should wear medical alert bracelet

• Do not give live virus vaccines to patients on prolonged therapy

MONITORING PARAMETERS
• Potassium and blood sugar during long-term therapy

• Edema, blood pressure, cardiac symptoms, mental status, weight

• Observe growth and development of infants and children on prolonged therapy

• Check intraocular pressure and lens frequently during prolonged use of ophthalmic preparations

---

* = non-FDA-approved use

Pharmacokinetics

PO: Peak 1-3 hr; widely distributed in the body; rapidly metabolized in liver, excreted in urine (metabolites); $t_{1/2}$ 3.7-9.6 hr

INDICATIONS AND USES: Radical cure of vivax malaria, prevention of relapse in vivax malaria, following termination of chloroquine phosphate suppressive therapy in areas where vivax malaria is endemic, *Pneumocystis carinii* pneumonia (PCP) associated with AIDS (with clindamycin)*

DOSAGE

Adult

• *Vivax malaria:* PO 26.3 mg (15 mg base) qd for 14 days; patients suffering an attack of vivax malaria or having parasitized red blood cells should also receive a course of chloroquine phosphate; as follow-up therapy in areas where vivax malaria is endemic, begin therapy during the last 2 wk of, or following a course of, suppression with chloroquine or a comparable drug

• *PCP associated with AIDS:* PO 26.3-52.6 mg (15-30 mg base) qd (with clindamycin IV 1.8-3.6 g/day divided tid-qid or PO 1.2-3.6 g/day divided tid-qid) for 21 days

Child

• PO 0.5 mg/kg/day (0.3 mg base/kg/day; max 15 mg base/dose) for 14 days

💲 AVAILABLE FORMS/COST OF THERAPY

• Tab, Uncoated—Oral: 26.3 mg, 100's: **$90.38**

CONTRAINDICATIONS: Concomitant administration with quinacrine, acutely ill patients with a tendency to granulocytopenia (rheumatoid arthritis, systemic lupus erythematosus), concurrent administration of other potentially hemolytic drugs or bone marrow suppressants

PRECAUTIONS: G-6-PD deficiency, NADH methemoglobin reductase deficiency, large doses

PREGNANCY AND LACTATION: Pregnancy category C; if possible, withhold until after delivery; however, if prophylaxis or treatment is required, primaquine should not be withheld

SIDE EFFECTS/ADVERSE REACTIONS

CNS: Headache

EENT: Interference with visual accommodation

GI: Abdominal cramps, epigastric distress, *nausea, vomiting*

HEME: **Hemolytic anemia in G-6-PD deficient patients, leukopenia, methemoglobinemia in NADH methemoglobin reductase-deficient patients**

SKIN: Pruritus

SPECIAL CONSIDERATIONS
PATIENT/FAMILY EDUCATION

• Take with food if GI upset occurs, notify clinician if GI distress continues

• Urine may turn brown

MONITORING PARAMETERS

• CBC periodically during therapy, discontinue if marked darkening of urine or sudden decrease in hemoglobin concentrations or leukocyte count occurs

P

---

italic = common side effects   ***bold italic*** = life-threatening reactions

probenecid

(proe-ben´e-sid)

Rx: Benemid, Probalan
Combinations
  Rx: with colchicine (Colben-
  emid Proben-C); with
  ampicillin (Polycillin-PRB,
  Probampacin)
Chemical Class: Sulfonamide
derivative
Therapeutic Class: Antigout
agent; uricosuric

CLINICAL PHARMACOLOGY
Mechanism of Action: Uricosuric
inhibits tubular reabsorption of
urate; increasing urinary excretion
of uric acid; inhibits tubular secretion and increases plasma concentrations of most penicillins and
cephalosporins
Pharmacokinetics
PO: Peak 2-4 hr; 85%-95% bound to
plasma proteins; hydroxylated in
liver to active metabolites, excreted
in urine (metabolites); $t_{1/2}$ 4-17 hr
INDICATIONS AND USES: Hyperuricemia associated with gout and
gouty arthritis, antibiotic adjuvant:
elevates and prolongs penicillin and
cephalosporin serum concentrations; calcinosis,* diagnostic aid
(differentiation between Parkinsonism and depressive syndromes)
DOSAGE
Adult
• *Hyperuricemia:* PO 250 mg bid for
1 wk; increase to 500 mg bid; increase q4 wk prn to max of 2-3
g/day; begin therapy 2-3 wk following acute gout attack
• *Penicillin or cephalosporin
therapy:* PO 500 mg qid

Child 2-14 yr
• *Penicillin or cephalosporin
therapy:* PO 25 mg/kg/dose initially; 40 mg/kg/day divided qid as
maintenance dose
**§ AVAILABLE FORMS/COST
OF THERAPY**
• Tab, Plain Coated—Oral: 500 mg,
100's: **$9.00-$210.40**
• Tab, Uncoated—Oral: 0.5 mg
colchicine/500 mg probenecid
100's: **$16.65-$84.34**
CONTRAINDICATIONS: Children
<2 yr, blood dyscrasias, uric acid
kidney stones, initiation of therapy
during acute gouty attack, moderate
to severe renal impairment (CrCl
<10 ml/min)
PRECAUTIONS: History of peptic
ulcer; renal insufficiency (CrCL
<30 ml/min)
PREGNANCY AND LACTATION:
Pregnancy category B; has been
used during pregnancy without
causing adverse effects in fetus or in-
fant
**SIDE EFFECTS/ADVERSE REAC-
TIONS**
CNS: Dizziness, headache
GI: Anorexia, nausea, sore gums,
vomiting
GU: Costovertebral pain, hematuria,
nephrotic syndrome, renal colic,
uric acid stones, urinary frequency
HEME: Anemia, **aplastic anemia,
hemolytic anemia (possibly related
to G-6-PD deficiency)**
METAB: Exacerbation of gout
SKIN: Flushing, rash
MISC: Hypersensitivity reactions
INTERACTIONS
Drugs
§ *Dapsone:* Increased serum dap-
sone concentrations
§ *Dyphylline:* Increased serum dy-
phylline concentrations
❷ *Methotrexate:* Marked increases
in serum methotrexate concentrations

3 *Salicylates:* Inhibition of uricosuric effect if used regularly

3 *Thiopental:* Prolonged anesthesia

3 *Zidovudine:* Increased plasma zidovudine concentrations

Labs

• *False positive:* Urine glucose (Ames Clinitest tablet, no effect on Ames Keto-Diastix, Diastix, Multistix, Clinistix)

• *False increase:* Free T_4 (Boehringer-Mannheim Enzymum procedure)

SPECIAL CONSIDERATIONS
PATIENT/FAMILY EDUCATION

• Avoid aspirin or other salicylates
• Take with food or antacids
• Drink 48-64 oz water daily to prevent development of kidney stones

MONITORING PARAMETERS

• Serum uric acid concentrations: continue the probenecid dose that maintains normal concentrations
• Renal function tests

---

procainamide

(proe-kane'a-mide)

Rx: Procan SR, Pronestyl, Pronestyl-SR

Chemical Class: P-aminobenzamide derivative

Therapeutic Class: Antidysrhythmic (Class IA)

CLINICAL PHARMACOLOGY

Mechanism of Action: Decreases myocardial excitability and conduction velocity; may depress myocardial contractility; increases threshold potential of ventricle, His-Purkinje system; prolongs effective refractory period and increases action potential duration in atrial and ventricular muscle; possesses anticholinergic properties, which may modify direct myocardial effects

Pharmacokinetics

IM: Onset 10-30 min, peak 15-60 min

PO: Peak 0.75-2.5 hr

15%-20% bound to plasma proteins; metabolized via acetylation in liver to N-acetyl procainamide (NAPA), which is a Class III antidysrhythmic; excreted in urine (25% as NAPA); $t_{1/2}$ 2.5-4.7 hr (NAPA 6-8 hr)

INDICATIONS AND USES: Life-threatening ventricular dysrhythmias, less severe but symptomatic ventricular dysrhythmias in select patients, maintenance of sinus rhythm following cardioversion in atrial fibrillation and/or flutter,* suppression of recurrent paroxysmal atrial fibrillation*

DOSAGE

Adult

• PO 250-500 mg q3-6h; PO SR 500-1000 mg q6h, usual dose 50 mg/kg/24 hr, max 4 g/24hr; IM 0.5-1 g q4-8h until PO therapy possible; IV 1 g INF over 25-30 min or 100-200 mg/day repeated q5 min as needed to total dose of 1 g as a loading dose, followed by continuous INF of 1-6 mg/min, titrate to patient response

Child

• PO 15-50 mg/kg/24 hr divided q3-6h, max 4 g/24 hr; IM 20-30 mg/kg/24 hr divided q4-6h, max 4 g/24 hr; IV 3-6 mg/kg INF over 5 min not to exceed 100 mg/day as a loading dose, then 20-80 µg/kg/min as a continuous INF, max 4 g/24 hr

$ AVAILABLE FORMS/COST OF THERAPY

• Cap, Gel—Oral: 250 mg, 100's: **$7.20-$88.21**; 375 mg, 30's: **$9.30-$88.00**; 500 mg, 100's: **$9.20-$121.55**

• Inj, Sol—IM, IV: 100 mg/ml, 10 ml: **$4.00-$53.40**; 500 mg/ml, 2 ml: **$1.81-$5.63**

P

---

italic = common side effects   ***bold italic*** = life-threatening reactions

• Tab, Sugar Coated—Oral: 250 mg, 100's: **$60.65**; 375 mg, 100's: **$77.78**; 500 mg, 100's: **$100.99**

• Tab, Coated, Sus Action—Oral: 250 mg, 100's: **$13.70-$35.69**; 500 mg, 100's: **$11.20-$86.78**; 750 mg, 100's: **$29.90-$94.60**; 1000 mg, 100's: **$47.50-$150.00**

CONTRAINDICATIONS: Complete heart block, lupus erythematosus, torsade de pointes

PRECAUTIONS: Following MI, 1st-degree AV block (unless ventricular rate controlled by pacemaker), asymptomatic premature ventricular contractions, digitalis intoxication, CHF, myasthenia gravis, renal insufficiency, children

PREGNANCY AND LACTATION: Pregnancy category C; compatible with breast feeding, however long-term effects in nursing infant unknown

SIDE EFFECTS/ADVERSE REACTIONS

CNS: Depression, *dizziness,* giddiness, hallucinations, headache, psychosis, weakness

CV: Hypotension, **2nd-degree heart block, ventricular arrhythmias** (more common with IV administration)

GI: Abdominal pain, anorexia, bitter taste, diarrhea, hepatomegaly, nausea, vomiting

HEME: **Agranulocytosis, hemolytic anemia (rare), neutropenia, thrombocytopenia**

SKIN: **Angioneurotic edema,** flushing, pruritus, rash, urticaria

MISC: *Lupus erythematosus-like syndrome* (arthralgia, pleural or abdominal pain, arthritis, pleural effusion, pericarditis, fever, chills, rash) in up to 30% on long-term therapy

INTERACTIONS

Drugs

3 *Amiodarone, cimetidine, trimethoprim:* Increased procainamide concentrations

3 *Cholinergic drugs:* Antagonism of cholinergic actions on skeletal muscle

3 *Procaine:* Interferes with procainamide concentration assay

Labs

• *False decrease:* Cholinesterase

• *False increase:* Potassium

SPECIAL CONSIDERATIONS

PATIENT/FAMILY EDUCATION

• Strict compliance to dosage schedule imperative

• Empty wax core from sustained release tablets may appear in stool; this is harmless

• Initiate therapy in facilities capable of providing continuous ECG monitoring and managing life-threatening dysrhythmias

MONITORING PARAMETERS

• CBC with differential and platelets qwk for 1st 3 mo, periodically thereafter

• ECG: R/O overdosage if QRS widens >25% or QT prolongation occurs; reduce dosage if QRS widens >50%

• ANA titer increases may precede clinical symptoms of lupoid syndrome

• Serum creatinine, urea nitrogen

• Plasma procainamide concentration (therapeutic range 3-10 µg/ml; 10-30 µg/ml NAPA)

procaine

(proe'kane)

Rx: Novocain, Mericaine
Chemical Class: Benzoic acid
derivative
Therapeutic Class: Local anesthetic

CLINICAL PHARMACOLOGY

Mechanism of Action: Blocks generation and conduction of nerve impulses; the order of loss of nerve function is: (1) pain, (2) temperature, (3) touch, (4) proprioception, and (5) skeletal muscle tone

Pharmacokinetics

INJ: Onset 2-5 min (15-25 min epidural), duration 0.25-1 hr (0.5-1.5 epidural); rapidly hydrolyzed by plasma pseudocholinesterase to *p*-aminobenzoic acid and diethylaminoethanol; excreted in urine; $t_{1/2}$ 7.7 min

INDICATIONS AND USES: Infiltration anesthesia, peripheral or sympathetic nerve block, spinal anesthesia, intractable pain (IV),* pruritus caused by jaundice (IV)*

DOSAGE

Dose varies with procedure, depth of anesthesia, vascularity of tissues, duration of anesthesia, and condition of patient

Adult

• *Infiltration anesthesia:* Inj 350-600 mg of 0.25%-0.5%

• *Peripheral nerve block:* Inj up to 200 ml of 0.5% or 100 ml of 1% or 50 ml of 2%

💲 AVAILABLE FORMS/COST OF THERAPY

• Inj, Sol—Infiltration: 1%, 30 ml: **$3.50-$18.60**; 2%, 30 ml: **$1.89-$21.45**

• Inj, Sol—IV: 10%, 2 ml: **$2.04-$7.29**

CONTRAINDICATIONS: Myasthenia gravis (IV), severe shock, impaired cardiac conduction, inj into inflamed or infected tissue

PRECAUTIONS: Cardiac disease, hyperthyroidism, endocrine disease, liver disease, elderly, low plasma pseudocholinesterase concentrations, sulfite sensitivity, use in head and neck area, retrobulbar blocks

PREGNANCY AND LACTATION: Pregnancy category C; use caution in nursing mothers

SIDE EFFECTS/ADVERSE REACTIONS

CNS: Anxiety, disorientation, drowsiness, loss of consciousness, restlessness, *seizures,* shivering, tremors

CV: Bradycardia, ***cardiac arrest, dysrhythmias,*** fetal bradycardia, hypertension, hypotension, ***myocardial depression***

EENT: Blurred vision, pupil constriction, tinnitus

GI: Nausea, vomiting

*RESP: **Anaphylaxis, respiratory arrest***

SKIN: Allergic reactions, burning, edema, rash, skin discoloration at inj site, tissue necrosis, urticaria

INTERACTIONS

Drugs

🖪 β-*blockers:* Acute discontinuation of β-blockers before local anesthesia increases the risk of hypertensive reactions

Labs

• *False increase:* CSF protein, urine porpholinogen, urobilinogen

SPECIAL CONSIDERATIONS

• Esther-type local anesthetic

MONITORING PARAMETERS

• Blood pressure, pulse, respiration during treatment, ECG

• Fetal heart tones if used during labor

prochlorperazine
(proe-klor-per'a-zeen)
Rx: Compazine
Chemical Class: Piperazine phenothiazine derivative
Therapeutic Class: Antiemetic; antipsychotic

CLINICAL PHARMACOLOGY
Mechanism of Action: Dopamine antagonist directly affects medullary chemoreceptor trigger zone (CTZ); antipsychotic effects similar to those of chlorpromazine; weak anticholinergic effects, moderate sedative effects, strong extrapyramidal effects

Pharmacokinetics
PO: Onset 30-40 min, duration 3-4 hr (extended release 10-12 hr)
IM: Onset 10-20 min, duration 12 hr
PR: Onset 60 min, duration 3-4 hr
Metabolized in liver, excreted in urine and through enterohepatic circulation

INDICATIONS AND USES: Severe nausea and vomiting, psychotic disorders

DOSAGE
Adult
• *Antiemetic:* PO 5-10 mg tid-qid, usual max 40 mg/day; PO extended release 10 mg bid or 15 mg qd; IM 5-10 mg q3-4h, usual max 40 mg/day; IV 2.5-10 mg q3-4h, max 10 mg/dose, 40 mg/day; PR 25 mg bid
• *Psychosis:* PO 5-10 mg tid-qid, increase dose prn, max 150 mg/day; IM 10-20 mg q4h prn, convert to PO as soon as possible

Child
• *Antiemetic:* PO/PR 9-14 kg: 2.5 mg q12-24h, max 7.5 mg/day; 14-18 kg: 2.5 mg q8-12h, max 10 mg/day; 18-39 kg: 2.5 mg q8h or 5 mg q12h,

max 15 mg/day; IM 0.1-0.15 mg/kg/dose, convert to PO as soon as possible; IV not recommended
• *Psychosis:* PO/PR 2-12 yr: 2.5 mg bid-tid, increase dose prn, max 20 mg/day; 2-5 yr: 25 mg/day; IM 6-12 yr: 0.13 mg/kg/dose, convert to PO as soon as possible

$ AVAILABLE FORMS/COST OF THERAPY
• Cap, Gel, Sus Action—Oral: 10 mg, 50's: **$67.45**; 15 mg, 50's: **$100.25**
• Inj, Sol—IM, IV: 5 mg/ml, 2 ml: **$1.83-$4.11**
• Supp—Rect: 2.5 mg, 12's: **$24.90**; 5 mg, 12's: **$27.70**; 25 mg, 12's: **$34.00-$35.46**
• Syr—Oral: 5 mg/5 ml, 120 ml: **$24.29**
• Tab, Plain Coated—Oral: 5 mg, 100's: **$12.50-$95.00**; 10 mg, 100's: **$17.50-$102.24**; 25 mg, 100's: **$19.50**

CONTRAINDICATIONS: Severe toxic CNS depression, coma, subcortical brain damage, bone marrow depression, severe liver or cardiac disease, narrow-angle glaucoma, pediatric surgery
PRECAUTIONS: Children <5 yr, elderly, prolonged use, cardiovascular disease, epilepsy, hepatic or renal disease, glaucoma, prostatic hypertrophy, severe asthma, emphysema, hypocalcemia (increased susceptibility to dystonic reactions), thyrotoxicosis, tartrazine sensitivity
PREGNANCY AND LACTATION: Pregnancy category C; majority of evidence indicates safety for both mother and fetus if used occasionally in low doses; excretion into breast milk should be expected; sedation is a possible effect in nursing infant

SIDE EFFECTS/ADVERSE REACTIONS

CNS: Agitation, anxiety, catatonic-like behavioral states, confusion, depression, *drowsiness, EPS (pseudoparkinsonism, akathisia, dystonia,* tardive dyskinesia), euphoria, exacerbation of psychotic symptoms including hallucinations, *headache,* heat or cold intolerance, insomnia, lethargy, **neuroleptic malignant syndrome,** restlessness, **seizures,** vertigo

CV: ECG changes, hypertension, hypotension, tachycardia

EENT: Blurred vision, cataracts, dry eyes, *dry mouth,* glaucoma, pigmentation of retina or cornea, retinopathy

GI: Anorexia, constipation, diarrhea, dyspepsia, hypersalivation, *nausea,* vomiting

GU: Priapism, urinary retention

HEME: **Agranulocytosis,** anemia, **aplastic anemia, hemolytic anemia** leukocytosis, transient leukopenia

METAB: Breast engorgement, gynecomastia, hyperglycemia, hyperprolactinemia, hypoglycemia, hyponatremia, impotence, increased libido, lactation, mastalgia, menstrual irregularities

RESP: Bronchospasm, increased depth of respiration, laryngospasm

SKIN: Diaphoresis, loss of hair, maculopapular and acneiform skin reactions, photosensitivity

INTERACTIONS

Drugs

3 *Anticholinergics:* Inhibited therapeutic response to antipsychotic; enhanced anticholinergic side effects

3 *Antidepressants:* Increased serum concentrations of some cyclic antidepressants

3 *Attapulgite:* Inhibition of phenothiazine absorption

3 *Barbiturates:* Reduced effect of antipsychotic

3 *Beta-blockers:* Enhanced effects of both drugs (interaction less likely with atenolol, nadolol)

3 *Bromocriptine, lithium:* Reduced effects of both drugs

3 *Chloroquine, amodiaquine, pyrimethamine:* Possible increased phenothiazine concentrations

3 *Cigarettes:* Possible enhanced metabolism of neuroleptic

3 *Clonidine:* Possible enhanced hypotensive effect

3 *Epinephrine:* Reversed pressor response to epinephrine

3 *Ethanol:* Enhanced ethanol effects

3 *Guanethidine:* Inhibited antihypertensive response to guanethidine

3 *Indomethacin:* Possible increased CNS effects, other NSAIDs less likely to have effect

❷ *Levodopa:* Inhibited effect of levodopa on Parkinson's disease

3 *Narcotic analgesics:* Excessive CNS depression, hypotension, respiratory depression

3 *Orphenadrine:* Reduced serum neuroleptic concentrations, excessive anticholinergic effects

3 *Procarbazine:* Increased sedation, EPS effects

3 *SSRIs:* Increased risk EPS effects

3 *Trazadone:* Possible increased risk hypotension

Labs

• *False positive:* Phenylketones

SPECIAL CONSIDERATIONS

PATIENT/FAMILY EDUCATION

• Arise slowly from reclining position

• Do not discontinue abruptly

• Use a sunscreen during sun exposure to prevent burns; take special precautions to stay cool in hot weather

• May cause drowsiness

P

MONITORING PARAMETERS
• Observe closely for signs of tardive dyskinesia
• Treat acute dystonic reactions with parenteral diphenhydramine (2 mg/kg to max 50 mg) or benztropine (2 mg)
• Periodic CBC with platelets during prolonged therapy

---

procyclidine
(proe-sye′kli-deen)
Rx: Kemadrin
Chemical Class: Synthetic tertiary amine
Therapeutic Class: Anticholinergic, antiparkinson's agent

CLINICAL PHARMACOLOGY
Mechanism of Action: Blocks striatal cholinergic receptors, which helps balance cholinergic and dopaminergic activity
Pharmacokinetics
PO: Peak 1.1-2 hr, $t_{1/2}$ 11.5-12.6 hr
INDICATIONS AND USES: Adjunctive treatment of all forms of Parkinson's disease; drug-induced extrapyramidal symptoms
DOSAGE
Adult
• *Parkinsonism:* PO 2.5 mg tid after meals initially, increase to 5 mg tid gradually; may occasionally administer additional dose hs if necessary
• *Drug-induced extrapyramidal symptoms:* PO 2.5 mg tid initially, increase by 2.5 mg/day increments until relief of symptoms obtained; usual dose 10-20 mg/day
$ AVAILABLE FORMS/COST OF THERAPY
• Tab, Uncoated—Oral: 5 mg, 100's: **$45.85**

CONTRAINDICATIONS: Narrow-angle glaucoma, myasthenia gravis, GI/GU obstruction, peptic ulcer, megacolon, prostatic hypertrophy
PRECAUTIONS: Elderly, tachycardia, liver, kidney disease, drug abuse history, dysrhythmias, hypotension, hypertension, psychiatric patients, children, tardive dyskinesia
PREGNANCY AND LACTATION: Pregnancy category C; nursing infants may be particularly sensitive to anticholinergic effects
SIDE EFFECTS/ADVERSE REACTIONS
CNS: Anxiety, *confusion,* delusions, *depression,* dizziness, *hallucinations,* headache, incoherence, irritability, memory loss, restlessness, sedation
CV: Flushing, hypotension, mild bradycardia, palpitations, postural hypotension, tachycardia
EENT: Angle-closure glaucoma, blurred vision, difficulty swallowing, dilated pupils, dry eyes, *dry mouth,* increased intraocular tension, mydriasis, photophobia
GI: Abdominal distress, *constipation,* epigastric distress, nausea, *paralytic ileus,* vomiting
GU: Dysuria, erectile dysfunction, hesitancy, retention
MS: Cramping, muscular weakness
SKIN: Rash, urticaria, other dermatoses
MISC: Decreased sweating, heat stroke, hyperthermia, increased temperature, numbness of fingers
INTERACTIONS
Drugs
3 *Amantadine:* Potentiates CNS side effects of amantadine
3 *Anticholinergic:* Increased anticholinergic side effects
3 *Antipsychotic agents:* Possible worsening of psychosis, increased anticholinergic side effects

---

* = non-FDA-approved use

3 *Digoxin (slow dissolution tab):* Increased digoxin concentration

3 *Tacrine:* Reduced therapeutic effects of both drugs

SPECIAL CONSIDERATIONS
PATIENT/FAMILY EDUCATION
• Do not discontinue this drug abruptly
• Hard candy, frequent drinks, sugarless gum to relieve dry mouth
• Take with or after meals to prevent GI upset
• Use caution in hot weather, may increase susceptibility to heat stroke

---

progesterone
(proe-jess´ter-one)
Rx: Crinone (gel), Progestasert, (IUD)
Chemical Class: Natural progestin
Therapeutic Class: Progestin; contraceptive

CLINICAL PHARMACOLOGY
Mechanism of Action: Exerts a progestational effect on the endometrium, alters cervical mucus, suppresses ovulation in some patients, renders the endometrium hostile to implantation

Pharmacokinetics
Hepatic metabolism, mostly renal excretion

IM: Rapidly absorbed, $t_{1/2}$ is a few minutes; Gel: Absorption $t_{1/2}$ 25-50 hr

INDICATIONS AND USES: Amenorrhea, dysfunctional uterine bleeding; as an intrauterine device (IUD) for contraception in women with at least 1 child in mutually monogamous relationships; Gel: Luteal phase deficiency in women undergoing assisted reproductive technology (ART) therapy for infertility

DOSAGE
Adult
• *Amenorrhea:* IM 5-10 mg qd for 6-8 days; if ovarian activity has produced a proliferative endometrium, expect withdrawal bleeding 48-72 hr after last inj

• *Dysfunctional uterine bleeding:* IM 5-10 mg qd for 6 doses; bleeding should cease within 6 days; when used with estrogen, begin progesterone after 2 wk of estrogen therapy; discontinue inj when menstrual flow begins

• *Contraception:* Insert 1 system into uterine cavity; replace after 1 yr
• *ART:* 1 applicator (90 g) in vagina QD (BID in ovarian failure) × 10-12 wk if pregnancy achieved

$ AVAILABLE FORMS/COST OF THERAPY
• Inj, Sol—IM: 50 mg/ml, 10 ml: **$8.50-$44.53**
• Insert, Sus Action—Intrauterine: 38 mg: **$127.82**
• Gel (Crinone)—Vag: 4% 6 applicators: **$30.00**; 8% 6 applicators: **$60.00**

CONTRAINDICATIONS: Active thrombophlebitis or thromboembolic disorders, cerebral hemorrhage, impaired liver function or disease, breast cancer, undiagnosed vaginal bleeding, missed abortion, use as a diagnostic test for pregnancy; *IUD:* patients at risk for pelvic infection, previous ectopic pregnancy, genital actinomycosis, increased susceptibility to infection (e.g., leukemia, diabetes, AIDS), IV drug use
PRECAUTIONS: Epilepsy, migraine, asthma, cardiac or renal dysfunction, depression, diabetes; (intrauterine system) history of menorrhagia or hypermenorrhea, valvular or congenital heart disease

P

PREGNANCY AND LACTATION:
Pregnancy category D. Possible increase in limb reduction defects, hypospadias in male fetuses and mild virilization of female fetuses

SIDE EFFECTS/ADVERSE REACTIONS

CNS: Depression, fatigue, insomnia
CV: Fluid retention
GI: Increased weight, *nausea*
GU: Amenorrhea, breast changes, galactorrhea, breakthrough bleeding, spotting
IUD: Amenorrhea or delayed menses, anemia, cramping, difficult removal, dyspareunia, *ectopic pregnancy,* endometritis, intermenstrual spotting, pain, pelvic infection, *perforation of uterus and cervix,* prolongation of menstrual flow, *septic abortion, septicemia, spontaneous abortion,* uterine embedment
METAB: Hyperglycemia
SKIN: Acne, irritation at inj site, melasma, rash, changes in hair growth

INTERACTIONS

Drugs

3 *Aminoglutethimide:* Possible decreased progestin effect

Labs

• *Increase:* Alk phosphatase, pregnanediol, liver function tests
• *Decrease:* Glucose tolerance test, HDL

SPECIAL CONSIDERATIONS

• Gel provides enhanced uterine delivery compared with IM administration

PATIENT/FAMILY EDUCATION

• Diabetic patients may note decreased glucose tolerance
• No evidence that use for habitual or threatened abortion is effective
• Notify clinician of abnormal or excessive bleeding, severe cramping, abnormal or odorous vaginal discharge, missed period (IUD)

• Cost and risk of infection (greatest in first months after insertion) less for non hormonal IUDs (e.g. ParaGard)

---

promethazine

(proe-meth´a-zeen)
Rx: Anergan, Autineus 50, Phenergan, Promet, Promacot, Promethegan, Prorex
Combinations
  Rx: with codeine (Phenergan with Codeine Syrup); with dextromethorphan (Phenergan with Dextromethorphan Syrup)
Chemical Class: Ethylamine phenothiazine derivative
Therapeutic Class: Antihistamine; antiemetic; sedative; antitussive; antivertigo agent

---

CLINICAL PHARMACOLOGY

Mechanism of Action: Acts as antihistamine by blocking H_1-receptors; antiemetic effects by inhibition of medullary chemoreceptor trigger zone (CTZ); anticholinergic activity produces sedation and antivertigo/motion sickness effects

Pharmacokinetics

PO/IM/PR: Onset 20 min, duration 6-12 hr (sedative effects 2-8 hr)
IV: Onset 3-5 min, duration 6-12 hr (sedative effects 2-8 hr)
Metabolized in liver, excreted in urine and feces (inactive metabolites)

INDICATIONS AND USES: Symptomatic treatment of various allergic conditions; active and prophylactic treatment of motion sickness; preoperative, postoperative, or obstetric sedation; nausea and vomiting associated with anesthesia and surgery; adjunct to analgesic for control of postoperative pain

DOSAGE

Adult

• *Antihistamine:* PO/PR 12.5 tid and 25 mg qhs; IM/IV 25 mg, repeated in 2 hr if necessary, convert to PO as soon as possible

• *Antiemetic:* PO/IM/IV/PR 12.5-25 mg q4h prn

• *Motion sickness:* PO/PR 25 mg 30-60 min prior to departure, then q12h prn

• *Sedation:* PO/IM/IV/PR 25-50 mg/day

Child

• *Antihistamine:* PO/PR 0.1 mg/kg/dose q6h during the day and 0.5 mg/kg qhs prn

• *Antiemetic:* PO/IM/IV/PR 0.25-1 mg/kg q4-6h prn

• *Motion sickness:* PO/PR 0.5 mg/kg/dose 30-60 min prior to departure, then q12h prn

• *Sedation:* PO/IM/IV/PR 0.5-1 mg/kg/dose q6h prn

⑤ AVAILABLE FORMS/COST OF THERAPY

• Inj, Sol—IM, IV: 25 mg/ml, 1, 10 ml: **$0.65-$3.09**/ml; 50 mg/ml, 1, 10 ml: **$1.00-$3.83**/ml

• Supp—Rect: 12.5 mg, 12's: **$30.50-$47.41**; 25 mg, 12's: **$33.25-$54.38**; 50 mg, 12's: **$44.81-$69.65**

• Syr—Oral: 6.25 mg/5 ml, 120, 480, 3840 ml: **$1.80-$33.94**/480 ml; 25 mg/5 ml, 480 ml: **$10.99-$73.07**

• Tab, Uncoated—Oral: 12.5 mg, 100's: **$6.50-$30.08**; 25 mg, 100's: **$0.88-$53.14**; 50 mg, 100's: **$4.65-$81.44**

CONTRAINDICATIONS: Narrow-angle glaucoma

PRECAUTIONS: Acute asthma, bladder neck obstruction, prostatic hypertrophy, predisposition to urinary retention, cardiovascular disease, glaucoma, hepatic function impairment, hypertension, history of peptic ulcer, seizure disorder, intestinal obstruction

PREGNANCY AND LACTATION: Pregnancy category C; passage of drug into breast milk should be expected

SIDE EFFECTS/ADVERSE REACTIONS

CNS: Anxiety, confusion, *dizziness, drowsiness,* EPS reactions, paradoxical hyperexcitability (children, relative overdose), euphoria, fatigue, poor coordination

CV: Hypotension, palpitations, tachycardia

EENT: Blurred vision, dilated pupils, dry nose, nasal stuffiness, tinnitus

GI: Anorexia, cholestatic jaundice, *constipation,* diarrhea, dry mouth, nausea, vomiting

GU: Amenorrhea, dysuria, galactorrhea, gynecomastia, impotence, *urinary retention*

HEME: **Agranulocytosis, hemolytic anemia, thrombocytopenia**

METAB: Hyperprolactinemia

RESP: Chest tightness, increased thick secretions, wheezing

SKIN: Photosensitivity, rash, urticaria

INTERACTIONS

Drugs

❸ *CNS depressants:* Additive sedative action

Labs

• *False increase:* Tricyclic antidepressant

SPECIAL CONSIDERATIONS
PATIENT/FAMILY EDUCATION

• Avoid prolonged exposure to sunlight

P

---

propafenone

(proe-pa-fen'one)

Rx: Rythmol

Chemical Class: 3-Phenylpro-
piophenone derivative

Therapeutic Class: Antidysrhythmic (Class IC)

CLINICAL PHARMACOLOGY

Mechanism of Action: Local anesthetic effects and direct stabilizing
action on myocardial membranes;
reduces upstroke velocity (Phase O)
of the monophasic action potential;
reduces fast inward current carried
by sodium ions in Purkinje fibers,
and to a lesser extent myocardial fibers; increases diastolic excitability
threshold, prolongs effective refractory period, reduces spontaneous
automaticity, and depresses trig-
gered activity; weak β-blocking activity

Pharmacokinetics

PO: Bioavailability 3.4%-10.6%;
metabolized in liver to 5-hydroxy-
propafenone and N-depropylpro-
pafenone (active), excreted in urine;
$t_{1/2}$ 2-10 hr in >90% of patients
(10-32 hr in slow metabolizers)

INDICATIONS AND USES: Documented life-threatening ventricular
dysrhythmias (e.g., sustained ventricular tachycardia), supraventricular tachycardias including atrial fibrillation and flutter,* dysrhythmias
associated with Wolff-Parkinson-
White syndrome*

DOSAGE

Adult

• PO 150 mg q8h initially; increase
at 3-4 day intervals to 225 mg q8h
and, if necessary, to 300 mg q8h; do
not exceed 900 mg/day

**$ AVAILABLE FORMS/COST
OF THERAPY**

• Tab, Coated—Oral: 150 mg,
100's: **$142.25-$189.23**; 225 mg,
100's: **$232.93-$269.71**; 300 mg,
100's: **$296.99-$343.31**

CONTRAINDICATIONS: Uncontrolled CHF, cardiogenic shock, disorders of impulse generation or conduction in the absence of an artificial
pacemaker, bradycardia, marked
hypotension, bronchospastic disorders, electrolyte imbalance

PRECAUTIONS: Non-life-threatening dysrhythmias, recent MI, hepatic and renal function impairment,
elderly, children

PREGNANCY AND LACTATION:
Pregnancy category C

**SIDE EFFECTS/ADVERSE REAC-
TIONS**

CNS: Anxiety, ataxia, *dizziness,*
drowsiness, fatigue, headache, insomnia, tremor

CV: Angina, atrial fibrillation, *AV
block,* bradycardia, bundle branch
block, chest pain, *congestive heart
failure* (due to negative ionotrope
effects), edema, hypotension, *intraventricular conduction delay,* palpitations, premature ventricular contractions, *prodysrhythmia,* syncope, *ventricular tachycardia,* widened QRS complex

EENT: Blurred vision, *unusual taste*

GI: Abdominal pain, anorexia, *constipation,* diarrhea, dry mouth, dyspepsia, flatulence, liver abnormalities, *nausea, vomiting*

HEME: **Agranulocytosis,** anemia,
granulocytopenia, increased bleeding time, **leukopenia,** positive
ANA, purpura, ***thrombocytopenia***

MS: Arthralgia, weakness

RESP: Dyspnea

SKIN: Diaphoresis, rash

INTERACTIONS
Drugs
3 *Beta-blockers:* Increased metoprolol or propranolol concentrations

3 *Cimetidine:* Increased propafenone concentrations

3 *Digitalis glycosides:* Increased serum digoxin concentrations

3 *Food:* Increased peak serum propafenone concentrations

3 *Oral anticoagulants:* Increased serum warfarin concentrations, prolonged protime

3 *Quinidine:* Increased propafenone concentrations but reduced concentrations of its active metabolite; net effect uncertain (toxicity vs reduced efficacy)

3 *Rifampin, phenobarbital, rifabutin:* Reduced serum propafenone concentrations

3 *Theophylline:* Increased plasma theophylline concentrations

SPECIAL CONSIDERATIONS
PATIENT/FAMILY EDUCATION
• Signs of overdosage include hypotension, excessive drowsiness, decreased heart rate, or abnormal heartbeat

MONITORING PARAMETERS
• ECG, consider dose reduction in patients with significant widening of the QRS complex or 2nd- or 3rd-degree AV block

• ANA, carefully evaluate abnormal ANA test, consider discontinuation if persistent or worsening ANA titers are detected

propantheline
(proe-pan´the-leen)
Rx: Propantheline
Chemical Class: Synthetic quaternary ammonium derivative
Therapeutic Class: GI antispasmodic; GI antiulcer agent (adjunctive)

CLINICAL PHARMACOLOGY
Mechanism of Action: Inhibits GI motility and diminishes gastric acid secretion
Pharmacokinetics
PO: Incompletely absorbed, extensive metabolism in upper small intestine prior to absorption; peak 2-6 hr; metabolized in GI tract/liver, excreted in urine; $t_{1/2}$ 1.6-9 hr

INDICATIONS AND USES: Peptic ulcer disease (in combination with other drugs); irritable bowel syndrome,* urinary incontinence due to uninhibited hypertonic neurogenic bladder*

DOSAGE
Adult
• PO 7.5-15 mg 30 min ac and 30 min hs
Child
• *Antisecretory:* PO 1.5 mg/kg/day divided tid-qid
• *Antispasmodic:* PO 2-3 mg/kg/day divided q4-6h and hs

$ **AVAILABLE FORMS/COST OF THERAPY**
• Tab, Sugar Coated—Oral: 7.5 mg, 100's: **$42.66**; 15 mg, 100's: **$3.67-$83.58**

CONTRAINDICATIONS: Narrow-angle glaucoma, obstructive uropathy (e.g., bladder neck obstruction due to prostatic hypertrophy), obstructive disease of the GI tract (e.g., pyloroduodenal stenosis), paralytic ileus, intestinal atony, unstable cardiovascular status in acute hemor-

P

rhage, severe ulcerative colitis, toxic megacolon complicating ulcerative colitis, myasthenia gravis

PRECAUTIONS: Hyperthyroidism, CAD, dysrhythmias, CHF, ulcerative colitis, hypertension, hiatal hernia, hepatic disease, renal disease, urinary retention, prostatic hypertrophy, elderly

PREGNANCY AND LACTATION: Pregnancy category C; excretion into breast milk unknown, although would be expected to be minimal due to quaternary structure

SIDE EFFECTS/ADVERSE REACTIONS

CNS: Anxiety, confusion, dizziness, drowsiness, hallucination, headache, insomnia, stimulation (especially in elderly), weakness

CV: Palpitations, tachycardia

EENT: Blurred vision, cycloplegia, increased ocular tension, mydriasis, photophobia

GI: Absence of taste, *constipation, dry mouth,* dysphagia, heartburn, nausea, *paralytic ileus,* vomiting

GU: Hesitancy, impotence, retention

SKIN: Allergic reactions, anhidrosis, fever, pruritus, rash, urticaria

INTERACTIONS

Drugs

3 *Tricyclic antidepressants:* Additive anticholinergic effects

Labs

• *False increase:* Bicarbonate, chloride

SPECIAL CONSIDERATIONS

PATIENT/FAMILY EDUCATION

• Avoid driving or other hazardous activities until stabilized on medication

• Avoid alcohol or other CNS depressants

• Avoid hot environments, heat stroke may occur

• Use sunglasses when outside to prevent photophobia, may cause blurred vision

---

propoxyphene

(proe-pox′i-feen)

Rx: Darvon, Dolene; Darvon-N

Combinations

  Rx: with acetaminophen (Darvocet, Propacet, Wygesic)

Chemical Class: Synthetic opium alkaloid; diphenylheptane derivative

Therapeutic Class: Narcotic analgesic

DEA Class: Schedule IV

CLINICAL PHARMACOLOGY

Mechanism of Action: Narcotic agonist with activity at Mu receptors (supraspinal analgesia, euphoria, respiratory and physical depression, miosis, and reduced GI motility), Kappa receptors (pentazocine-like spinal analgesia, sedation, and miosis), and Delta receptors (dysphoria, psychotomimetic effects [e.g., hallucinations] and respiratory and vasomotor stimulation caused by drugs with antagonist activity); compared to morphine, less analgesia, respiratory depression, sedation, emesis, and physical dependence

Pharmacokinetics

PO: Onset 15-60 min, peak 2-2½ hr (3 hr napsylate), duration 4-6 hr; metabolized in liver (25% to norpropoxyphene), excreted in urine; $t_{1/2}$ 6-12 hr

INDICATIONS AND USES: Mild to moderate pain

DOSAGE

Adult

• PO 65 mg (100 mg napsylate) q4h prn; max 390 mg/day (600 mg/day napsylate)

• Cap, Gel—Oral (hydrochloride): 65 mg, 100's: **$6.61-$49.84**
• Tab, Uncoated—Oral (napsylate): 100 mg, 100's: **$72.49**

PRECAUTIONS: History of drug abuse, suicidal ideation, hepatic or renal function impairment, children

PREGNANCY AND LACTATION: Pregnancy category C (category D if used for prolonged periods or in high doses at term); withdrawal could theoretically occur in infants exposed *in utero* to prolonged maternal ingestion; compatible with breast feeding

SIDE EFFECTS/ADVERSE REACTIONS

CNS: Dizziness, dysphoria, euphoria, headache, lightheadedness, *sedation*
EENT: Visual disturbances
GI: Abdominal pain, abnormal liver function, constipation, *nausea,* reversible jaundice (rare), *vomiting*
RESP: Respiratory depression
SKIN: Rashes
MISC: Weakness

INTERACTIONS

Drugs

🔳 *Anticoagulants:* Potentiation of warfarin's anticoagulant effect
🔳 *Antidepressants:* Increased cyclic antidepressant serum concentrations
🔳 *Antihistamines, chloral hydrate, glutethimide, methocarbamol:* Enhanced depressant effects
🔳 *Barbiturates:* Additive respiratory and CNS depressant effects
🔳 *Beta-blockers:* Increased concentrations of highly metabolized β-blockers (metoprolol, propranolol)
❷ *Carbamazepine:* Marked increases in plasma carbamazepine concentrations

🔳 *Ethanol:* Additive CNS effects
🔳 *Protease inhibitors:* Increased respiratory and CNS depression

Labs

• *False increase:* Amylase and lipase

SPECIAL CONSIDERATIONS
PATIENT/FAMILY EDUCATION

• May cause drowsiness, dizziness or blurred vision
• Use caution driving or engaging in other activities requiring alertness
• Avoid alcohol

---

propranolol

(proe-pran′oh-lole)

Rx: Betachron, Inderal, Inderal LA
Combinations
   Rx: with HCTZ (Inderide)
Chemical Class: Nonselective β-adrenergic blocker
Therapeutic Class: Antihypertensive; antianginal; antimigraine agent; antidysrhythmic (class II); postmyocardial infarction; antiglaucoma agent

P

CLINICAL PHARMACOLOGY
Mechanism of Action: PO competitive β-adrenergic antagonist; produces negative inotropic and chronotropic responses; slows AV nodal conduction; decreases heart rate; decreases myocardial oxygen consumption; antiarrhythmic effects (class II); reduction in platelet aggregation and blood viscosity; suppression of renin release; inhibition of central sympathetic outflow; decreases presynaptic receptor neurotransmitter release; no intrinsic sympathomimetic or membrane stabilizing activity; low to moderate

---

italic = common side effects   ***bold italic*** = life-threatening reactions

lipid solubility; OPHTH: reduces intraocular pressure via reduction in production of aqueous humor

Pharmacokinetics

PO: Peak 60-90 min (L-A 6 hr), extensive 1st-pass effect

IV: Onset immediate

High lipid solubility; >90% bound to plasma proteins; metabolized in liver to active and inactive metabolites, excreted in urine; $t_{1/2}$ 4-6 hr (L-A 8-11 hr)

INDICATIONS AND USES: Glaucoma, migraine headache, hypertension, postmyocardial infarction, supraventricular arrhythmias (atrial fibrillation, atrial flutter, paroxysmal supraventricular tachycardia), ventricular arrhythmias, aggressive behavior,* angina pectoris, anxiety,* cataract extraction prophylaxis,* congestive heart failure,* hyperthyroidism,* neuroleptic-induced akathisia,* retinal detachment,* tremor, hypertrophic obstructive cardiomyopathy, hypertrophic subaortic stenosis, pheochromocytoma, portal hypertension, Wolff-Parkinson-White syndrome, Alzheimer's disease,* ascites,* carcinoid syndrome,* resistant giardiasis,* menopausal symptoms,* mitral valve prolapse,* priapism secondary to chronic antipsychotic medications,* restless leg syndrome,* schizophrenia,* tardive dyskinesia,* tetanus,* Tourette's syndrome,* withdrawal syndromes*

DOSAGE

Adult and Child >16 yr

• *Hypertension:* PO 40 mg bid (L-A 80 mg qd) initially, usual range 120-240 mg/day divided bid-tid (L-A 120-160 mg qd), max 640 mg/day

• *Dysrhythmias:* PO 10-30 mg tid-qid; IV (reserve for life-threatening situations or dysrhythmias occurring during anesthesia) 0.5-3 mg, at

a rate not exceeding 1 mg/min, a 2nd dose may be administered after 2 min prn, additional doses at intervals no less than 4 hr until desired response obtained

• *Angina pectoris:* PO 10-20 mg tid-qid (L-A 80 mg qd) initially, usual range 160-240 mg/day divided tid-qid, maximum 320 mg/day

• *Hypertrophic subaortic stenosis:* PO 20-40 mg tid-qid (L-A 80-160 mg qd)

• *Pheochromocytoma:* PO 30 mg/day in divided doses (in conjunction with α-adrenergic blocking agent)

• *Migraine prophylaxis:* PO 80 mg/day in divided doses (L-A 80 mg qd) initially, increase to optimal prophylaxis, usual range 160-240 mg/day

• *MI:* PO 180-240 mg/day divided bid-qid beginning 5-21 days after MI

• *Essential tremor:* PO 40 mg bid initially, usual range 120-320 mg/day divided tid

• *Gastrointestinal bleeding:* PO 40 to 360 mg qd titrated to reduce the resting heart rate by 25%

• *Thyroid storm:* IV 1 mg/min to max 10 mg; repeat in 4-6 hr; PO 40 to 80 mg q6h, following IV

Child

• *Dysrhythmias:* IV 0.1 mg/kg/dose up to a max of 1 mg/dose (slow infusion over 5 min); PO 2 to 6 mg/kg/day divided q6-8h (max 60 mg/day)

• *Hypertension:* PO 0.5-1 mg/kg/day divided q6-12h, increase dose at 3-7 day intervals, usual range 1-5 mg/kg/day

• *Migraine prophylaxis:* PO 0.6-1.5 mg/kg/day in divided doses

• *Tetralogy of Fallot* (acute treatment of spells): IV 0.15-0.25 mg/kg/dose (slowly—1 mg/min.);

repeated once after 15 min; PO (maintenance) 1 to 2 mg/kg q6h; increase in increments; max 5 mg/kg

• *Thyrotoxicosis:* PO 2 mg/kg/day, given q6h

§ AVAILABLE FORMS/COST OF THERAPY

• Cap, Gel, Sus Action—Oral: 60 mg, 100's: **$62.55-$131.79**; 80 mg, 100's: **$73.55-$145.19**; 120 mg, 100's: **$90.90-$145.19**; 160 mg, 100's: **$118.90-$228.83**

• Inj, Sol—IV: 1 mg/ml, 1 ml: **$4.25-$18.56**

• Sol—Oral: 20 mg/5 ml, 500 ml: **$31.79**; 40 mg/5 ml, 500 ml: **$49.51**; 80 mg/ml, 30 ml: **$33.53**

• Tab, Uncoated—Oral: 10 mg, 100's: **$2.25-$43.30**; 20 mg, 100's: **$2.01-$60.79**; 40 mg, 100's: **$2.93-$78.89**; 60 mg, 100's: **$4.25-$109.13**; 80 mg, 100's: **$2.25-$121.10**

CONTRAINDICATIONS: Bronchial asthma, cardiogenic shock, overt cardiac failure, 2nd and 3rd degree AV block, severe sinus bradycardia

PRECAUTIONS: Anesthesia/surgery (myocardial depression), avoid abrupt withdrawal, bronchospastic airways, congestive heart failure, diabetes mellitus, hyperthyroidism/thyrotoxicosis (atenolol, unlike propranolol, does not decrease T_3 levels), concurrent clonidine (discontinue atenolol several days prior to withdrawal of clonidine), peripheral vascular disease, renal disease

PREGNANCY AND LACTATION: Pregnancy category C; similar drug, atenolol, frequently used in the third trimester for treatment of hypertension (many studies of efficacy and safety of atenolol in pregnancy-induced hypertension); long-term use has been associated with intrauterine growth retardation; milk levels approximately half of peak plasma levels; considered insignificant; compatible with breast feeding

SIDE EFFECTS/ADVERSE REACTIONS

CNS: Depression, *dizziness,* drowsiness, *fatigue,* hallucinations, insomnia, *lethargy,* memory loss, mental changes, strange dreams

CV: Bradycardia, **CHF,** cold extremities, postural hypotension, profound hypotension, *2nd or 3rd degree heart block*

EENT: Dry, burning eyes; sore throat; visual disturbances

GI: Diarrhea, dry mouth, elevated LFTs, *ischemic colitis, mesenteric arterial thrombosis,* nausea, vomiting

GU: Impotence, sexual dysfunction

HEME: **Agranulocytosis, thrombocytopenia**

METAB: Hyperglycemia, hyperlipidemia (increased TG, total cholesterol, LDL; decreased HDL), masked hypoglycemic response to insulin (sweating excepted)

RESP: **Bronchospasm,** dyspnea

SKIN: Alopecia, pruritis, rash

INTERACTIONS

Drugs

3 *α-1 adrenergic blockers:* Potential enhanced first dose response (marked initial drop in blood pressure), particularly on standing (especially prazosin)

3 *Amiodarone:* Bradycardia, cardiac arrest, ventricular dysrhythmia shortly after initiation of β-blocker

3 *Antidiabetics:* Masked symptoms of hypoglycemia, prolonged recovery of normoglycemia

3 *Antipyrine:* Increased antipyrine concentrations

3 *Barbiturates, rifampin:* Reduced concentrations of propranolol

3 *β-agonists:* Antagonistic effects

P

3 *Calcium channel blockers:* Increased concentrations of propranolol; increased bioavailability of nifedipine

3 *Chlorpromazine:* Additive hypotensive effects and grand mal seizures; chlorpromazine decreases the clearance of oral propranolol by 25% to 32%, resulting in increased propranolol bioavailability

3 *Cimetidine, etintidine, fluoxetine, propoxyphene, propafenone, quinidine, quinolones:* Increased propranolol concentrations

3 *Clonidine, guanabenz, guanfacine:* Exacerbation of hypertension upon withdrawal of clonidine

3 *Cocaine:* Potentiation of cocaine-induced coronary vasospasm

3 *Contrast media:* Increased risk anaphylaxis

3 *Digitalis glycosides:* Increased digoxin concentrations

3 *Dihydroergotamine, ergotamine:* May result in excessive vasconstriction

3 *Fluvoxamine:* Increased propranolol serum concentrations; increased risk of bradycardia and hypotension

3 *Epinephrine:* Enhanced pressor response to epinephrine

3 *Flecainide:* Increased propranolol and flecainide concentrations; additive negative inotropic effects

3 *Hydralazine:* Increases oral bioavailability of propranolol (high clearance and lipophilic β-blockers) increasing risk of adverse effects

3 *Hydrochlorothiazide:* Exaggerated hyperglycemic response

3 *Lidocaine:* Increased lidocaine concentrations

3 *Local anesthetics:* Enhanced sympathomimetic side effects of epinephrine-containing local anesthetics

3 *Neostigmine, physostigmine, tacrine:* Additive bradycardia

3 *Neuroleptics:* Increased plasma concentrations of both drugs

3 *NSAIDs:* Reduced hypotensive effect of propranolol

3 *Phenylephrine:* Predisposition to acute hypertensive episodes

2 *Theophylline:* Increased theophylline concentrations; antagonistic pharmacodynamic effects

Labs

• *False increase:* Bilirubin

SPECIAL CONSIDERATIONS
PATIENT/FAMILY EDUCATION

• Do not discontinue abruptly, may require taper; rapid withdrawal may produce rebound hypertension or angina

MONITORING PARAMETERS

• Angina: Reduction in nitroglycerin usage; frequency, severity, onset, and duration of angina pain; heart rate

• Arrhythmias: Heart rate

• Congestive heart failure: Functional status, cough, dyspnea on exertion, paroxysmal nocturnal dyspnea, exercise tolerance, and ventricular function

• Hypertension: Blood pressure

• Migraine headache: Reduction in the frequency, severity, and duration of attacks

• Postmyocardial infarction: Left ventricular function, lower resting heart rate

• Toxicity: Blood glucose, bronchospasm, hypotension, bradycardia, depression, confusion, hallucination, sexual dysfunction

---

* = non-FDA-approved use

propylthiouracil

(proe-pill-thye-oh-yoor'a-sill)
Chemical Class: Thioamide
derivative
Therapeutic Class: Antithyroid
agent

CLINICAL PHARMACOLOGY

Mechanism of Action: Inhibits synthesis of thyroid hormones by interfering with the incorporation of iodine into tyrosyl residues of thyroglobulin; does not inhibit action of already formed or exogenously administered thyroid hormones; partially inhibits peripheral conversion of T_4 to T_3

Pharmacokinetics

PO: Bioavailability 80%-95%; 75%-80% bound to plasma proteins; metabolized in liver, excreted in urine (35% unchanged); $t_{1/2}$ 1-2 hr

INDICATIONS AND USES: Hyperthyroidism, preparation for thyroidectomy or radioactive iodine therapy, thyrotoxic crisis, alcoholic liver disease*

DOSAGE

Adult

• PO 300-450 mg/day divided q8h initially (doses of 600-1200 mg/day may be required); maintenance dose 100-150 mg/day divided q8-12h

Child

• PO 5-7 mg/kg/day divided q8h initially; maintenance dose ⅓-⅔ of initial dose divided q8-12h

• Dose in renal impairment: PO CrCl 10-50 ml/min, decrease recommended dose by 25%; CrCl <10 ml/min, decrease recommended dose by 50%

§ AVAILABLE FORMS/COST OF THERAPY

• Tab, Uncoated—Oral: 50 mg, 100's: **$2.25-$15.75**

PRECAUTIONS: Infection, bone marrow depression, hepatic disease, children (hepatotoxicity has occurred), thyroid storm

PREGNANCY AND LACTATION: Pregnancy category D; considered drug of choice for medical treatment of hyperthyroidism during pregnancy; excreted into breast milk in low amounts; compatible with breast feeding

SIDE EFFECTS/ADVERSE REACTIONS

CNS: CNS stimulation, depression, drowsiness, headache, neuritis, neuropathies, paresthesias, vertigo

CV: Edema

GI: Epigastric distress, hepatitis, jaundice, loss of taste, nausea, sialadenopathy, vomiting

GU: Nephritis

*HEME: **Agranulocytosis, aplastic anemia, granulocytopenia, hypoprothrombinemia, leukopenia,** lymphadenopathy, splenomegaly, **thrombocytopenia***

METAB: Insulin autoimmune syndrome (may result in ***hypoglycemic coma***)

MS: Arthralgia, myalgia

RESP: Interstitial pneumonitis

SKIN: Abnormal hair loss, erythema nodosum, ***exfoliative dermatitis,*** lupus-like syndrome, pruritis, skin pigmentation, urticaria, rash

INTERACTIONS

Drugs

3 *Oral anticoagulants:* Reduced hypoprothrombinemic response to oral anticoagulants

3 *Theophylline:* Physiologic response to antithyroid drug will increase theophylline concentrations via decreased clearance

Labs

• *False increase:* Glucose

---

italic = common side effects   ***bold italic*** = life-threatening reactions

P

SPECIAL CONSIDERATIONS
PATIENT/FAMILY EDUCATION
• Notify clinician of fever, sore throat, unusual bleeding or bruising, rash, yellowing of skin, vomiting
MONITORING PARAMETERS
• CBC periodically during therapy (especially during initial 3 mo), TSH

---

protamine
(proe´ta-meen)
Rx: Protamine
Chemical Class: Basic protein
Therapeutic Class: Heparin antidote

CLINICAL PHARMACOLOGY
Mechanism of Action: Forms a stable salt with unfractionated heparin (strongly acidic) resulting in loss of anticoagulant activity of both drugs
Pharmacokinetics
IV: Rapid onset of action, unfractionated heparin neutralized within 5 min, duration 2 hr; metabolic fate of unfractionated heparin-protamine complex unknown
INDICATIONS AND USES: Unfractionated heparin overdose
DOSAGE
Adult and Child
• IV 1 mg neutralizes 90 USP units of lung tissue-derived unfractionated heparin and 115 USP units of intestinal mucosa-derived unfractionated heparin; administer slowly over 10 min (for SC unfractionated heparin overdose, a portion of the total protamine dose should be administered by continuous INF over 8-16 hr), do not exceed 50 mg in a 10 min period; dose requirement decreases rapidly with time elapsed since IV unfractionated heparin inj; guide dosage by blood coagulation studies

AVAILABLE FORMS/COST OF THERAPY
• Inj, Sol—IV: 10 mg/ml, 25 ml: **$12.49-$23.36**
PRECAUTIONS: Rapid administration (hypotension, anaphylactoid reactions), previous protamine exposure, fish allergy
PREGNANCY AND LACTATION: Pregnancy category C
SIDE EFFECTS/ADVERSE REACTIONS
CNS: Lassitude
CV: Bradycardia, *circulatory collapse,* flushing, hypotension
GI: Nausea, vomiting
RESP: Dyspnea, *pulmonary edema, pulmonary hypertension*
MISC: Hypersensitivity reactions
SPECIAL CONSIDERATIONS
• Will not reliably inactivate low-molecular-weight heparin
MONITORING PARAMETERS
• Activated partial thromboplastin time (aPTT) or protamine activated clotting time (ACT) 15 min after dose, then in several hr

---

protriptyline
(proe-trip´ti-leen)
Rx: Vivactil
Chemical Class: Dibenzolcycloheptene derivative: secondary amine
Therapeutic Class: Tricyclic antidepressant

CLINICAL PHARMACOLOGY
Mechanism of Action: Inhibits the reuptake of norepinephrine (very high) and serotonin (moderate) at the presynaptic neuron; inhibition of histamine and acetylcholine activity; mild peripheral vasodilator effects and possible quinidine-like actions on cardiac conduction high an-

ticholinergic activity; slight sedative and orthostatic hypotensive activity

Pharmacokinetics

PO: Peak 24-30 hr, therapeutic response 2-4 wk; metabolized by liver, excreted by kidneys; $t_{1/2}$ 67-89 hr

INDICATIONS AND USES: Depression, obstructive sleep apnea*

DOSAGE

Adult

• PO 15-40 mg/day divided tid-qid; may increase to 60 mg/day; make increases in AM dosage (mild stimulant effect)

Geriatric/Adolescent

• PO 5 mg tid, increase gradually if needed; use caution if dose >20 mg/day

💲 AVAILABLE FORMS/COST OF THERAPY

• Tab, Plain Coated—Oral: 5 mg, 100's: **$39.95-$82.19**; 10 mg, 100's: **$57.80-$80.36**

CONTRAINDICATIONS: Acute recovery phase of MI; concurrent use of MAOIs

PRECAUTIONS: Suicidal patients, seizure disorders, prostatic hypertrophy, increased intraocular pressure, narrow-angle glaucoma, urinary retention, cardiac disease, hepatic or renal disease, hyperthyroidism, electroshock therapy, elective surgery, elderly, abrupt discontinuation

PREGNANCY AND LACTATION: Pregnancy category C

SIDE EFFECTS/ADVERSE REACTIONS

CNS: Anxiety, confusion (especially in elderly), *dizziness,* extrapyramidal symptoms (elderly), fatigue, headache, increased psychiatric symptoms, insomnia, memory impairment, nervousness, nightmares, panic, sedation, stimulation, tremors, weakness

CV: ***Dysrhythmias, ECG changes,*** hypertension, *orthostatic hypotension,* palpitations, syncope, tachycardia

EENT: Blurred vision, dry mouth, mydriasis, nasal congestion, ophthalmoplegia, tinnitus

GI: Constipation, cramps, diarrhea, epigastric distress, hepatitis, increased appetite, jaundice, nausea, ***paralytic ileus,*** stomatitis, vomiting

GU: Urinary retention

HEME: ***Agranulocytosis,*** eosinophilia, ***leukopenia, thrombocytopenia***

SKIN: Photosensitivity, pruritus, rash, sweating, urticaria

INTERACTIONS

Drugs

3 *Altretamine:* Orthostatic hypotension

3 *Amphetamines:* Theoretical increase in effect of amphetamines, clinical evidence lacking

3 *Antidiabetics:* Monitor for enhanced hypoglycemia

3 *Barbiturates, rifampin, carbamazepine:* Reduced cyclic antidepressant concentrations

3 *Beta agonists (especially isoproterenol):* Cardiac arrhythmia risk increased

2 *Bethanidine, clonidine, guanethidine, guanabenz, guanfacine, guanadrel, debrisoquen:* Reduced antihypertensive effect

2 *Epinephrine, norepinephrine:* Markedly enhanced pressor response to IV administration

3 *Ethanol:* Additive impairment of motor skills; abstinent alcoholics may eliminate cyclic antidepressants more rapidly than non-alcoholics

3 *Fluoxetine, paroxetine:* Marked increases in cyclic antidepressant plasma concentrations

P

---

italic = common side effects   ***bold italic*** = life-threatening reactions

3 *H₂ blockers (especially cimetidine), calcium channel blockers:* Increased cyclic concentrations

3 *Lithium:* Increased risk neurotoxicity (especially in elderly)

3 *MAOIs:* Excessive sympathetic response, mania, or hyperpyrexia possible

3 *Neuroleptics:* Increased therapeutic and toxic effects of both drugs

3 *Phenylephrine:* Enhanced pressor response

3 *Propantheline:* Enhanced anticholinergic effects

3 *Propoxyphene:* Enhanced effect of cyclic antidepressants

3 *Quinidine:* Increased cyclic antidepressant serum concentrations

3 *Ritonavir, indinavir:* Possible increased cyclic concentrations, toxicity

Labs

• *Increase:* Serum bilirubin, blood glucose, alk phosphatase

• *Decrease:* VMA, 5-HIAA

• *False increase:* Urinary catecholamines

SPECIAL CONSIDERATIONS
PATIENT/FAMILY EDUCATION

• Therapeutic effects may take 2-3 wk

• Use caution in driving or other activities requiring alertness

• Avoid rising quickly from sitting to standing, especially elderly

• Avoid alcohol and other CNS depressants

• Do not discontinue abruptly after long-term use

• Wear sunscreen or large hat to prevent photosensitivity

MONITORING PARAMETERS

• CBC, weight, ECG, mental status (mood, sensorium, affect, suicidal tendencies)

pseudoephedrine
(soo-doe-e-fed′rin)

OTC: Cenafed, Decofed, Efidac Genaphed, PediaCare Infants' Decongestant, Seudotabs, Sudafed, Sudafed 12 Hour Caplets (Pseudoephedrine is available in many prescription and over-the-counter combinations; the following list is not all-inclusive)

Combinations

Rx: with azatadine (Trinalin Repetabs); brompheniramine (Bromfed); carbinoxamine (Rondec); chlorpheniramine (Deconamine SR, Novafed A); codeine (Nucofed); guaifenesin and codeine (Novagest Expectorant); loratadine (Claritin-D)

OTC: with acetaminophen (Dristan Cold); chlorpheniramine (Chlor-Trimeton 12 Hour Relief); dexbrompheniramine (Drixoral Cold and Allergy); dextromethorphan (Thera-Flu Non-Drowsy Formula); diphenhydramine (Actifed Allergy); ibuprofen (Advil Cold & Sinus, Dristan Sinus); triprolidine (Actifed)

Chemical Class: Sympathomimetic amine

Therapeutic Class: Decongestant

CLINICAL PHARMACOLOGY
Mechanism of Action: Directly-stimulates α-adrenergic receptors in respiratory tract mucosa causing

vasoconstriction; direct stimulation of β-adrenergic receptors causes increased heart rate and contractility

Pharmacokinetics

PO: Onset 15-30 min, duration 4-6 hr (extended release 12 hr); partially metabolized in liver to inactive metabolite, excreted in urine (55%-75% unchanged)

INDICATIONS AND USES: Nasal decongestion associated with common cold, allergies, and sinusitis; promotes nasal or sinus drainage

DOSAGE

Adult

• PO 60 mg q4-6h; PO Sus Action 120 mg q12h or 240 mg qd (Efidac); max 240 mg/day

Child

• PO 6-11 yr 30 mg q4-6h, max 120 mg/day; 2-5 yr 15 mg q4-6h, max 60 mg/day; <2 yr 4 mg/kg/day divided q6h

💲 AVAILABLE FORMS/COST OF THERAPY

• Drops—Oral: 7.5 mg/0.8 ml, 15 ml: **$3.47-$5.18**
• Syr—Oral: 15 mg/5 ml, 120 ml: **$2.50-$4.50**; 30 mg/5 ml, 480 ml: **$5.25-$7.42**
• Tab, Chewable—Oral: 15 mg, 24's: **$4.44**
• Tab, Uncoated—Oral: 30 mg, 100's: **$1.35-$21.95**; 60 mg, 100's: **$1.24-$20.38**
• Tab, Sus Action—Oral: 120 mg, 20's: **$6.76**; 240 mg, 12's: **$6.77**

CONTRAINDICATIONS: Hypersensitivity to sympathomimetics, severe hypertension, severe CAD

PRECAUTIONS: Heart disease, coronary insufficiency, dysrhythmias, angina, hyperthyroidism, diabetes mellitus, prostatic hypertrophy, increased intracranial pressure, hypovolemia, mild to moderate hypertension

PREGNANCY AND LACTATION: Pregnancy category C; compatible with breast feeding

SIDE EFFECTS/ADVERSE REACTIONS

CNS: Anxiety, confusion, dizziness, drowsiness, hallucinations, headache, insomnia, *tremors*
CV: Chest pain, ***dysrhythmias,*** palpitations, tachycardia
GI: Anorexia, nausea, vomiting
GU: Dysuria, urinary retention
METAB: Hyperglycemia

INTERACTIONS

Drugs

🛑 *Antacids:* Sodium bicarbonate doses sufficient to alkalinize urine can inhibit elimination of pseudoephedrine

⚠ *MAOIs:* Hypertensive crisis

Labs

• *False increase:* Theophylline

SPECIAL CONSIDERATIONS
PATIENT/FAMILY EDUCATION

• May cause wakefulness or nervousness
• Take last dose 4-6 hr prior to hs, notify clinician of insomnia, dizziness, weakness, tremor, or irregular heart beat

P

---

italic = common side effects   ***bold italic*** = life-threatening reactions

psyllium

(sill´ee-yum)

OTC: Fiberall, Hydrocil, Konsyl, Metamucil, Modane Bulk, Perdiem Fiber, Reguloid, Serutan, Syllact, V-Lax

Combinations

OTC: with senna (Perdiem)

Chemical Class: Psyllium colloid

Therapeutic Class: Bulk laxative

CLINICAL PHARMACOLOGY

Mechanism of Action: Adsorbs water in intestine; promotes peristalsis and reduces GI transit time

Pharmacokinetics

PO: Generally not absorbed, onset 12-24 hr (may be as long as 2-3 days)

INDICATIONS AND USES: Constipation, irritable bowel syndrome, diverticular disease, spastic colon, hemorrhoids, hypercholesterolemia*

DOSAGE

Adult

• PO 1-2 rounded teaspoonfuls or 1-2 packets in 8 oz glass of liquid 1-4 times/day; 1-2 wafers with 8 oz glass of liquid 1-4 times/day

Child 6-11 yr

• PO ½ to 1 rounded teaspoonful in 4 oz glass of liquid 1-3 times/day

$ **AVAILABLE FORMS/COST OF THERAPY**

• Granules—Oral: 2.5-4.03 g/rounded teaspoon, 100, 180, 250, 480, 540 g: **$12.63/250 g**

• Powder, Effervescent—Oral: 3.4 g/dose, 30's (packets) and 300 g (bulk): **$5.83-$7.60**

• Powder, Hydrophilic—Oral: 3.5 g/rounded teaspoon, 210, 300, 420, 630 g: **$5.83-$9.22**

• Powder—Oral: 50% psyllium and 50% dextrose/dose, 120, 396, 420, 480, 630 g: **$3.50-$8.86**

• Tab—Oral: 500 mg, 200's: **$5.99**

• Wafer, Chewable—Oral: 1.7-3.4 g, 24's: **$3.92-$4.17**

CONTRAINDICATIONS: Intestinal obstruction, fecal impaction

PRECAUTIONS: Phenylketonurics (sugar-free preparations may contain aspartame), abdominal pain, nausea or vomiting

PREGNANCY AND LACTATION: Pregnancy category C; not systemically absorbed; exposure of fetus or nursing infant unlikely

SIDE EFFECTS/ADVERSE REACTIONS

GI: Anorexia, bloating, constipation, cramping, diarrhea, *esophageal or bowel obstruction,* flatulence, nausea, vomiting

SPECIAL CONSIDERATIONS
PATIENT/FAMILY EDUCATION

• Maintain adequate fluid consumption

• Do not use in presence of abdominal pain, nausea, or vomiting

• Avoid inhaling dust from powder preparations; can cause runny nose, watery eyes, wheezing

pyrantel

(pye-ran´tel)

OTC: Antiminth, Pin-Rid, Pin-X, Reese's Pinworm

Chemical Class: Pyrimidine derivative

Therapeutic Class: Anthelmintic

CLINICAL PHARMACOLOGY

Mechanism of Action: Spasmic paralysis of worm results from depolarizing neuromuscular blockade; worms expelled via normal peristalsis

---

* = non-FDA-approved use

Pharmacokinetics

PO: Poorly absorbed, achieves low systemic levels of unchanged drug; 50% excreted unchanged in feces, ≤7% found in urine (unchanged drug and metabolites)

INDICATIONS AND USES: Ascariasis (roundworm infection), enterobiasis (pinworm infection), hookworm infection,* trichostrongyliasis*

DOSAGE

Adult and Child

• *Roundworm, pinworm, trichostrongyliasis:* PO 11 mg/kg as a single dose; max 1 g/dose; repeat in 2 wk for pinworm infection

• *Hookworm:* PO 11 mg/kg qd for 3 days

$ AVAILABLE FORMS/COST OF THERAPY

• Susp—Oral: 144 mg/ml, 30, 60, 240 ml: **$7.74-$9.49**/30 ml

• Tab—Oral: 180 mg, 24's: **$5.78**

CONTRAINDICATIONS: Hepatic disease

PRECAUTIONS: Child <2 yr

PREGNANCY AND LACTATION: Pregnancy category C

SIDE EFFECTS/ADVERSE REACTIONS

CNS: Dizziness, drowsiness, headache, insomnia

GI: Abdominal cramps, anorexia, diarrhea, elevated liver enzymes, *nausea, vomiting*

SKIN: Rash

INTERACTIONS

Drugs

❷ *Piperazine:* Mutual antagonism

SPECIAL CONSIDERATIONS

PATIENT/FAMILY EDUCATION

• Take with food or milk

• Using a laxative to facilitate expulsion of worms is not necessary

• All family members in close contact with patient should be treated

• Strict hygiene is essential to prevent reinfection

• Shake suspension well before pouring

---

pyrazinamide

(pye-ra-zin´a-mide)

Rx: Pyrazinamide

Chemical Class: Niacinamide derivative

Therapeutic Class: Antituberculosis agent

CLINICAL PHARMACOLOGY

Mechanism of Action: Converted to pyrazinoic acid (POA) by susceptible strains of *Mycobacterium tuberculosis:* POA has specific antimycobacterial activity against *M. tuberculosis* and may lower environmental pH below that necessary for growth of the organism

Pharmacokinetics

PO: Peak 2 hr (POA 4-8 hr); 17% bound to plasma proteins; widely distributed in body tissues and fluids; metabolized in liver to POA (active), excreted in urine (4%-14% unchanged); $t_{1/2}$ 9-10 hr

INDICATIONS AND USES: Active tuberculosis (as part of a 6 mo regimen consisting of isoniazid, rifampin, and pyrazinamide given for 2 mo, followed by isoniazid and rifampin for 4 mo); after treatment failure with other primary drugs in any form of active tuberculosis

DOSAGE

Adult

• PO 15-30 mg/kg qd for 1st 2 mo of 6 mo regimen with isoniazid and rifampin or as part of an individualized regimen for drug-resistant disease, max 2 g/day; alternatively 50-70 mg/kg can be given twice weekly to improve compliance (base dosage calculations on lean body weight)

P

Child
• PO 15-40 mg/kg/day divided q12-24 hr, max 2 g/day; alternatively 50-70 mg/kg based on lean body weight twice weekly, max 3 g/dose

§ AVAILABLE FORMS/COST OF THERAPY
• Tab, Uncoated—Oral: 500 mg, 100's: **$87.38-$112.38**

CONTRAINDICATIONS: Severe liver disease, acute gout

PRECAUTIONS: History of gout, renal and hepatic function impairment, alcoholism, elderly, HIV infection (may require longer courses of therapy), diabetes mellitus

PREGNANCY AND LACTATION: Pregnancy category C; excreted into human milk

SIDE EFFECTS/ADVERSE REACTIONS
CNS: Fever
GI: Anorexia, hepatotoxicity, nausea, vomiting
GU: Dysuria, interstitial nephritis (rare)
HEME: Blood clotting abnormalities, increased serum iron concentration, porphyria, *sideroblastic anemia, thrombocytopenia*
METAB: Gout, *hyperuricemia*
MS: Arthralgia, *myalgia*
SKIN: Acne, photosensitivity, pruritus, rash, urticaria

INTERACTIONS
Drugs
3 *Cyclosporine:* Decreased concentrations cyclosporine
3 *Tacrolimus:* Decreased concentrations of tacrolimus
Labs
• *False positive:* Urine ketone tests

SPECIAL CONSIDERATIONS
PATIENT/FAMILY EDUCATION
• Compliance with full course is essential

• Notify clinician of fever, loss of appetite, malaise, nausea and vomiting, darkened urine, yellowish discoloration of skin and eyes, pain or swelling of joints

MONITORING PARAMETERS
• Liver function tests, serum uric acid at baseline and periodically throughout therapy

---

pyridostigmine
(peer-id-oh-stig′meen)
Rx: Mestinon, Mestinon Timespan, Regonol
Chemical Class: Synthetic quaternary ammonium compound
Therapeutic Class: Cholinergic

CLINICAL PHARMACOLOGY
Mechanism of Action: An acetylcholinesterase inhibitor; inhibits destruction of acetylcholine, facilitating transmission of impulses across myoneural junction
Pharmacokinetics
PO: Poorly absorbed, onset 30-45 min, duration 3-6 hr
IV: Onset 2-5 min, duration 2-3 hr
IM: Onset 15 min
Hydrolyzed by cholinesterases and metabolized by microsomal enzymes in liver, excreted in urine

INDICATIONS AND USES: Myasthenia gravis, reversal of non-depolarizing neuromuscular blocking agents after surgery

DOSAGE
Adult
• *Myasthenia gravis:* PO 600 mg/day divided to provide max relief; usual range 60-1500 mg/day, individualize dosage; PO Sus Action 180-540 mg qd-bid, individualize dosage, use dosage intervals of at least 6 hr; IM/IV 1/30th PO dose, inj IV very slowly

---

• *Reversal of non-depolarizing neuromuscular blockade:* IV 10-20 mg; give atropine 0.6-1.2 mg IV immediately prior to pyridostigmine to minimize side effects

Child

• *Myasthenia gravis:* PO 7 mg/kg/day divided into 5-6 doses; IM/IV 0.05-0.15 mg/kg/dose; max 10 mg/dose, inj IV very slowly

• *Reversal of non-depolarizing neuromuscular blockade:* IV 0.1-0.25 mg/kg/dose preceded by atropine or glycopyrrolate

$ AVAILABLE FORMS/COST OF THERAPY

• Inj, Sol—IM; IV: 5 mg/ml, 2 ml: **$1.76-$5.04**

• Syr—Oral: 60 mg/5 ml, 480 ml: **$52.81**

• Tab, Uncoated—Oral: 60 mg, 100's: **$54.80**

• Tab, Coated, Sus Action—Oral: 180 mg, 100's: **$95.50**

CONTRAINDICATIONS: Mechanical obstruction of intestinal or urinary tracts, hypersensitivity to bromides (pyridostigmine bromide)

PRECAUTIONS: Seizure disorder, bronchial asthma, bradycardia, recent coronary occlusion, vagotonia, hyperthyroidism, cardiac dysrhythmias, peptic ulcer, large oral doses in megacolon and decreased GI motility (accumulation and toxicity may occur when motility is restored), anticholinesterase insensitivity (reduce or withhold dosages until patient again becomes sensitive)

PREGNANCY AND LACTATION: Pregnancy category C; would not be expected to cross the placenta because it is ionized at physiologic pH; although apparently safe for the fetus, may cause transient muscle weakness in the newborn; compatible with breast feeding

SIDE EFFECTS/ADVERSE REACTIONS

CNS: Dizziness, drowsiness, headache, incoordination, *loss of consciousness, paralysis, seizures*

CV: AV block, bradycardia, *cardiac arrest, dysrhythmias,* hypotension, nodal rhythm, non-specific ECG changes, syncope, tachycardia

EENT: Blurred vision, conjunctival hyperemia, diplopia, lacrimation, miosis, spasm of accommodation, visual changes

GI: Cramps, diarrhea, dysphagia, flatulence, *increased gastric secretions,* increased peristalsis, *increased salivation, nausea, vomiting*

GU: Frequency, incontinence, urgency

MS: Arthralgia, fasciculation, muscle cramps and spasms, weakness

RESP: Bronchospasm, dyspnea, increased secretions, *laryngospasm, respiratory arrest, respiratory depression*

SKIN: Rash, sweating, urticaria

INTERACTIONS

Drugs

3 *Beta blockers:* Additive bradycardia

3 *Tacrine:* Increased anticholinergic effects

Labs

• *False increase:* Serum bicarbonate, chloride

SPECIAL CONSIDERATIONS

PATIENT/FAMILY EDUCATION

• Do not crush or chew sustained release preparations

MONITORING PARAMETERS

• Therapeutic response: increased muscle strength, improved gait, absence of labored breathing (if severe)

• Appearance of side effects (narrow margin between 1st appearance of side effects and serious toxicity)

---

italic = common side effects   ***bold italic*** = life-threatening reactions

• Symptoms of increasing muscle weakness may be due to cholinergic crisis (overdosage) or myasthenic crisis (increased disease severity). If crisis is myasthenia, patient will improve after 1-2 mg edrophonium; if cholinergic withdraw pyridostigmine and administer atropine

---

pyridoxine (vitamin B₆)

(peer-i-dox'een)
Rx: Doxine, Rodex, Vitabee 6 (Injection)
OTC: Nestrex
Chemical Class: B complex vitamin
Therapeutic Class: Vitamin; hydralazine/isoniazid antidote

CLINICAL PHARMACOLOGY
Mechanism of Action: Coenzyme in metabolism of protein, carbohydrates, and fat
Pharmacokinetics
PO: Readily absorbed; metabolized in liver to 4-pyridoxic acid, excreted in urine; biologic $t_{1/2}$ 15-20 days
INDICATIONS AND USES: Pyridoxine deficiency including inadequate diet and drug-induced (e.g., isoniazid, hydralazine, penicillamine, cycloserine, oral contraceptives); inborn errors of metabolism such as B₆-dependent seizures or B₆-responsive anemia; hydralazine or isoniazid poisoning,* premenstrual syndrome (PMS),* hyperoxaluria type I (and oxalate kidney stones); nausea and vomiting in pregnancy*; in conjunction with folic acid to reduce levels of homocysteine*
DOSAGE
Adult
• *Dietary deficiency:* PO 10-20 mg qd for 3 wk, then 2-5 mg/day

• *Drug-induced deficiency:* PO 100-200 mg/day
• *Prophylaxis of drug-induced deficiency:* PO 25-100 mg/day
• *Recommended daily allowance (RDA):* PO 1.6-2 mg
• *Isoniazid poisoning:* IV 4 g followed by 1 g IM q30 min to equal amount of isoniazid consumed; doses of 70-357 mg/kg have been administered without incident
Child
• *Dietary deficiency:* PO 5-25 mg/day for 3 wk, then 1.5-2.5 mg/day
• *Drug-induced deficiency:* PO 10-50 mg/day
• *Prophylaxis of drug-induced deficiency:* PO 1-2 mg/kg/day
• *Recommended daily allowance (RDA):* PO 1-3 yr 0.9 mg; 4-6 yr 1.3 mg; 7-10 yr 1.6 mg
§ AVAILABLE FORMS/COST OF THERAPY
• Inj, Sol—IM, IV: 100 mg/ml, 10, 30 ml: **$2.95-$8.25**/10 ml
• Tab—Oral: 10, 25, 50, 100, 200, 250, 500 mg, 100's, all: **$1.10-$12.50**
PREGNANCY AND LACTATION: Pregnancy category A (category C if used in doses above RDA); deficiency during pregnancy is common in unsupplemented women; excreted in human breast milk; RDA for lactating women is 2.3-2.5 mg
SIDE EFFECTS/ADVERSE REACTIONS
CNS: Awkwardness of hands, decreased sensation to touch/temperature/vibration, headache, numb feet, paresthesia, perioral numbness, *seizures* (following very large IV doses), sensory neuropathic syndromes, somnolence, unstable gait
GI: Increased AST, nausea
HEME: Low serum folic acid levels
RESP: Respiratory distress
SKIN: Burning or stinging at inj site

---

* = non-FDA-approved use

MISC: Allergic reactions
INTERACTIONS
Drugs
3 *Levodopa:* Inhibited antiparkinsonian effect of levodopa; concurrent use of carbidopa negates the interaction
3 *Phenytoin:* Reduced phenytoin concentrations
SPECIAL CONSIDERATIONS
PATIENT/FAMILY EDUCATION
• Avoid doses exceeding RDA unless directed by clinician
MONITORING PARAMETERS
• Respiratory rate, heart rate, blood pressure during large IV doses

---

pyrimethamine
(pye-ri-meth′a-meen)
Rx: Daraprim
Combinations
  Rx: with sulfadoxine (Fansidar)
Chemical Class: Synthetic aminopyrimidine derivative
Therapeutic Class: Antimalarial

CLINICAL PHARMACOLOGY
Mechanism of Action: Inhibits dihydrofolate reductase, which catalyzes the reduction of dihydrofolate to tetrahydrofolate; highly selective against plasmodia and *Toxoplasma gondii*
Pharmacokinetics
PO: Peak 2-6 hr; 87% bound to plasma proteins; metabolized in liver, excreted in urine; $t_{1/2}$ 4 days (7 days for sulfadoxine) (suppressive concentrations are maintained for approximately 2 wk)
INDICATIONS AND USES: Chemoprophylaxis of malaria due to susceptible strains of plasmodia; toxoplasmosis (in combination with sulfonamide); combination therapy

with quinine and sulfadiazine for uncomplicated attack of chloroquine-resistant *P. falciparum* malaria; initiation of transmission control and suppressive cure in conjunction with fast-acting schizonticide
DOSAGE
Adult
• *Malaria prophylaxis:* PO 25 mg qwk; begin 2 wk before entering areas where chloroquine-resistant *P. falciparum* exists, continue for at least 6-10 wk after leaving endemic area; in combination with sulfadoxine PO 1 tab qwk 1-2 days before departure, continue × 4-6 wk after return
• *Chloroquine-resistant P. falciparum malaria (with quinine and sulfadiazine):* PO 25 mg bid for 3 days or (use in combination with sulfadoxine) PO 2-3 tabs in single dose
• *Toxoplasmosis (with sulfadiazine):* PO 50-75 mg/day with 1-4 g of sulfonamide for 1-3 wk, reduce dose by 50% and continue for 4-5 wk; alternatively 25-50 mg/day for 3-4 wk
Child
• *Malaria prophylaxis:* PO 0.5 mg/kg qwk, do not exceed 25 mg/dose; begin 2 wk before entering areas where chloroquine-resistant *P. falciparum* exists, continue for at least 6-10 wk after leaving endemic area; in combination with sulfadoxine begin 1-2 days before departure, continue × 4-6 wk after return; PO ¾ tab qwk (9-14 yr), PO ½ tab qwk (4-8 yr), PO ¼ tab qwk (<4 yr)
• *Chloroquine-resistant P. falciparum malaria (with quinine and sulfadiazine):* PO <10 kg, 6.25 mg qd for 3 days; 10-20 kg 12.5 mg qd for 3 days; 20-40 kg 25 mg qd for 3 days or (in combination with sulfadoxine) PO 2 tabs in single dose

italic = common side effects   ***bold italic*** = life-threatening reactions

(9-14 yr), PO 1 tab in single dose (4-8 yr), PO ½ tab in single dose (<4 yr)

• *Toxoplasmosis (with sulfadiaz-ine):* PO 2 mg/kg/day divided q12h for 3 days followed by 1 mg/kg/day divided qd-bid for 4 wk

$ AVAILABLE FORMS/COST OF THERAPY

• Tab, Uncoated—Oral: 25 mg, 100's: **$41.29**
• Tab, Uncoated—Oral: 25 mg/500 mg sulfadoxine, 25's: **$98.08**

CONTRAINDICATIONS: Megalo-blastic anemia secondary to folate deficiency; infants <2 mo

PRECAUTIONS: Malabsorption syndrome, alcoholism, pregnancy (increased risk folate deficiency); renal or hepatic function impair-ment; seizure disorder; G-6-PD de-ficiency

PREGNANCY AND LACTATION: Pregnancy category C; most studies have found pyrimethamine to be safe in pregnancy; folic acid supple-mentation should be given to pre-vent folate deficiency; compatible with breast feeding

SIDE EFFECTS/ADVERSE REAC-TIONS

CNS: Depression, fever, headache, insomnia, lightheadedness, *seizures*
CV: Cardiac rhythm disturbance (large doses)
EENT: Dry throat
GI: Anorexia, atrophic glossitis, di-arrhea, dry mouth, *nausea, vomiting* (large doses)
GU: Hematuria (large doses)
HEME: Decreased folic acid, *hemo-lytic anemia, leukopenia, megalo-blastic anemia, pancytopenia, thrombocytopenia*
RESP: Pulmonary eosinophilia
SKIN: Abnormal skin pigmentation, dermatitis, **Stevens-Johnson syn-drome, toxic epidermal necrolysis**

INTERACTIONS
Drugs
❷ *Folic acid:* Decreased efficacy of pyrimethamine

SPECIAL CONSIDERATIONS

• Discontinue if folate deficiency develops; administer leucovorin 5-15 mg IM qd for ≥3 days when re-covery slow

PATIENT/FAMILY EDUCATION

• Take with food
• Discontinue at 1st sign of rash

MONITORING PARAMETERS

• CBC with platelets semi-weekly during therapy for toxoplasmosis, less frequently for malaria-related indications

---

quazepam
(kway'ze-pam)
Rx: Doral
Chemical Class: Benzodiaz-epine
Therapeutic Class: Hypnotic
DEA Class: Schedule IV

CLINICAL PHARMACOLOGY
Mechanism of Action: CNS depres-sant via facilitation of inhibitory GABA at benzodiazepine receptor sites (BZ$_1$—associated with sleep; BZ$_2$—associated with memory, mo-tor, sensory, and cognitive func-tion); effects include muscle relax-ation (spinal cord), anticonvulsant activity (brain stem), ataxia (cer-ebellum), emotional behavior (lim-bic and cortical areas), and anxi-olytic effects (separate from general CNS depression); decreases sleep latency, the number of awakenings, and the time spent in stage 0 (awake) sleep; stage 2 (unequivocal sleep) is increased; in sum, sleep time in-creased

Pharmacokinetics

PO: Peak 2 hr; 95% bound to plasma proteins; metabolized in liver to 2-oxoquazepam and N-desalkyl-2-oxoquazepam (both active), excreted in urine (31%) and feces (23%); $t_{1/2}$ 25-41 hr (metabolites 40-114 hr)

INDICATIONS AND USES: Short-term management of insomnia

DOSAGE

Adult ≥18 yr

• PO 7.5-15 mg hs; reduce dose after 1-2 nights if possible

$ AVAILABLE FORMS/COST OF THERAPY

• Tab, Coated—Oral: 7.5 mg, 100's: **$282.47**; 15 mg, 100's: **$308.70**

CONTRAINDICATIONS: Narrow-angle glaucoma, psychosis, pregnancy

PRECAUTIONS: Elderly, debilitated, hepatic disease, renal disease, history of drug abuse, abrupt withdrawal, respiratory depression, prolonged use, sleep apnea

PREGNANCY AND LACTATION: Pregnancy category X; may cause fetal damage when administered during pregnancy; excreted into breast milk; may accumulate in breast-fed infants and is therefore not recommended

SIDE EFFECTS/ADVERSE REACTIONS

CNS: Abnormal thinking, agitation, amnesia, anxiety, apathy, *asthenia,* ataxia, decreased libido, decreased reflexes, emotional lability, falling (especially elderly), hangover, hostility, *hypokinesia,* **seizure,** sleep disorder, *somnolence,* stupor

CV: Palpitations, syncope

EENT: Ear pain; epistaxis, eye irritation, pain, pharyngitis, photophobia, rhinitis, sinusitis, swelling

GI: Abdominal pain, anorexia, constipation, diarrhea, heartburn, increased AST, jaundice, nausea, vomiting

HEME: **Granulocytopenia, leukopenia**

RESP: Dyspnea

SKIN: Dermatitis

INTERACTIONS

Drugs

3 *Cimetidine:* Increased plasma levels of quazepam

3 *Clozapine:* Isolated cases of cardiorespiratory collapse have been reported, causal relationship to benzodiazepines has not been established

3 *Disulfiram:* Increased serum quazepam concentrations

3 *Ethanol:* Enhanced adverse psychomotor side effects of benzodiazepines

3 *Levodopa:* Possible exacerbation of parkinsonism

3 *Neuroleptics:* Increased sedation, respiratory depression

3 *Omeprazole, macrolides, azole antifungals, isoniazid, digoxin, SSRI's, quinolones:* Possible increased benzodiazepine concentrations

3 *Rifampin:* Reduced serum quazepam concentrations

SPECIAL CONSIDERATIONS

PATIENT/FAMILY EDUCATION

• Avoid alcohol and other CNS depressants

• Do not discontinue abruptly after prolonged therapy

• May cause daytime sedation, use caution while driving or performing other tasks requiring alertness

• Inform clinician if planning to become pregnant, or are pregnant, or if you become pregnant while taking this medicine

• May be habit forming

---

italic = common side effects   **bold italic** = life-threatening reactions

quetiapine
(kwe-tye′a-peen)
Rx: Seroquel
Chemical Class: Dibenzothiaz-
epine derivative
Therapeutic Class: Antipsychotic

CLINICAL PHARMACOLOGY
Mechanism of Action: Serotonin
5-HT$_2$ >dopamine (D$_2$)-receptor
antagonist; activity at several neurotransmitter systems: selective antagonist at limbic dopamine recep-
tors (D$_1$, D$_2$, D$_4$, D$_5$) and serotonin
receptors (5-HT$_2$, 5-HT$_6$, 5-HT$_7$);
antagonism at α_1-adrenergic receptors; and activity at muscarinic, histamine H$_1$, or nicotinic receptors;
moderate sedation and orthostatic
hypotension; minimal risk of ex-
trapyrimadal symptoms or weight
gain; no anticholinergic effects
Pharmacokinetics
PO: Peak 1.5 hr, onset of therapeutic
effect 7-14 days, bioavailability
15%; metabolic pathways in humans have not been adequately studied; mainly eliminated unchanged in
the urine; t$_{1/2}$ 3-3.5 hr
INDICATIONS AND USES: Schizophrenia
DOSAGE
Adult
• PO 25 mg bid initially, increase
25-50 mg bid or tid on second and
third day as tolerated to target dose
of 300-400 mg daily in two or three
divided doses by fourth day; adjust
dose at intervals of no less than 2
days; doses >750 mg have not been
studied
• *Hepatic impairment:* 25 mg qd initially, increase daily by 25-50
mg/day to effective dose based on
response and tolerability

**§ AVAILABLE FORMS/COST
OF THERAPY**
• Tab, Uncoated—Oral: 25 mg,
100's: **$153.40**; 100 mg, 100's:
$279.18; 200 mg, 100's: **$526.68**
CONTRAINDICATIONS: Severe
CNS depression
PRECAUTIONS: Neuroleptic malignant syndrome, hepatic disease,
cardiovascular disease, cerebrovascular disease, conditions that predispose to hypotension (dehydration,
hypovolemia, antihypertensive
medications), history of seizure disorder, thyroid disorders, hyperprolactinemia, patients at risk for aspiration pneumonia (dysphagia), suicide ideation
PREGNANCY AND LACTATION:
Pregnancy category C; excretion
into breast milk unknown, breast
feeding is not recommended
**SIDE EFFECTS/ADVERSE REAC-
TIONS**
CNS: Agitation, dizziness, dystonia
and other extrapyramidal symptoms, *headache,* hostility, *insomnia,
somnolence*
CV: Increased heart rate, orthostatic
hypotension
GI: Abdominal pain, asymptomatic
elevations of serum transaminases,
constipation, *dry mouth,* dyspepsia
METAB: Weight gain
INTERACTIONS
Drugs
3 *Antihypertensives:* Increased
risk of hypotension
3 *CYP3A inhibitors (Azole antifungals, macrolide antibiotics):* Increased plasma quetiapine concentrations
3 *Lorazepam:* Increased plasma
lorazepam concentrations
3 *Phenytoin, carbamazepine, barbiturates, rifampin, glucocorticoids
(enzyme inducers):* Decreased
plasma quetiapine concentrations

---

* = non-FDA-approved use

3 *Thioridazine:* Decreased plasma quetiapine concentrations

SPECIAL CONSIDERATIONS

• Limited clinical experience, but similar to clozapine and risperidone; may be effective for negative symptoms of schizophrenia; so far no agranulocytosis reported with quetiapine

PATIENT/FAMILY EDUCATION

• Avoid alcohol

---

quinapril

(kwin′na-pril)

Rx: Accupril

Chemical Class: Nonsulfhydryl angiotensin-converting enzyme (ACE) inhibitor

Therapeutic Class: Antihypertensive

CLINICAL PHARMACOLOGY

Mechanism of Action: Antihypertensive, hypoproliferative, and cardioprotective effects attributable to competitive inhibition of angiotensin-converting enzyme (ACE) yielding decreased plasma concentrations of angiotensin II, plasma aldosterone concentrations, systemic vascular resistance, blood pressure, preload, and afterload, not accompanied by changes in heart rate, pressor sensitivity to exogenous norepinephrine, or baroreceptor sensitivity

Pharmacokinetics

PO: Onset 1 hr, duration 24 hr; has little pharmacologic activity until metabolized to active metabolite (quinaprilat), excreted in urine (60%) and feces (37%); t$_{1/2}$ (quinaprilat) 2 hr

INDICATIONS AND USES: Hypertension, CHF (left ventricular dysfunction), MI, erythrocytosis,* nephropathy,* retinopathy*

DOSAGE

Adult and Child >16 yr

• *Hypertension:* PO 10 mg qd (5 mg if on concomitant diuretics); titrate according to response at 2 wk intervals; usual dose, 20-80 mg in 1-2 divided doses

• *Congestive heart failure:* PO 5 mg initially, then, if tolerated (excessive hypotension or deterioration in renal function) 5 mg bid with further dose adjustments titrated at weekly intervals up to 20 mg bid

• *Renal insufficiency:* Usual dosing for CrCl >60 ml/min; 5 mg qd for CrCl 30-60 ml/min; 2.5 mg qd for CrCl 10-30 ml/min

$ **AVAILABLE FORMS/COST OF THERAPY**

• Tab, Uncoated—Oral: 5, 10, 20, 40 mg, 90's, all: **$101.30**

PRECAUTIONS: History of anaphylaxis, renal insufficiency (<30 ml/min), hypotension (CHF, elderly, volume depletion—diuretics, dialysis, cirrhosis), aortic stenosis, hyperkalemia (potassium supplements, potassium-sparing diuretics, renal disease, diabetes), neutropenia (autoimmune diseases, collagen vascular diseases, febrile illness, immunosuppressant drug therapy), proteinuria, renal artery stenosis, surgery/anesthesia (excessive hypotension, correctable with fluids)

PREGNANCY AND LACTATION: Pregnancy category D; ACE inhibitors can cause fetal and neonatal morbidity and death when administered to pregnant women; when pregnancy is detected, discontinue ACE inhibitors as soon as possible

SIDE EFFECTS/ADVERSE REACTIONS

CNS: Dizziness, fatigue, *headache*

CV: Angina, palpitations, postural hypotension, syncope (especially with 1st dose)

---

italic = common side effects　　　***bold italic*** = life-threatening reactions

GI: Abdominal pain, constipation, nausea, vomiting

GU: Decreased libido, impotence, increased BUN, creatinine

HEME: **Agranulocytosis, neutropenia, thrombocytopenia**

METAB: Hyperkalemia, hyponatremia, hypoglycemia

MS: Arthralgia, arthritis, myalgia

RESP: Asthma, bronchitis, cough

SKIN: Angioedema, pruritis, rash, sweating

INTERACTIONS

Drugs

❷ *Allopurinol:* Predisposition to hypersensitivity reactions

❸ *Alpha adrenergic blockers:* Exaggerated 1st dose hypotensive response

❸ *Aspirin:* Reduced hemodynamic effects; less likely with nonacetylated salicylates

❸ *Azathioprine:* Increased myelosuppression

❸ *Cyclosporine:* Renal insufficiency

❸ *Insulin:* Enhanced hypoglycemic response

❸ *Iron (parenteral):* Increased risk systemic reaction

❸ *Lithium:* Increased risk of serious lithium toxicity

❸ *Loop diuretics:* Initiation of ACE inhibitor therapy may cause hypotension and renal insufficiency

❸ *NSAIDs:* Inhibition of the antihypertensive response

❸ *Potassium, potassium-sparing diuretics:* Increased risk for hyperkalemia

❸ *Trimethoprim:* Additive risk of hyperkalemia, especially in patient predisposed to renal insufficiency

Labs

• ACE inhibition can account for approximately 0.5mEq/L rise in serum potassium

SPECIAL CONSIDERATIONS

PATIENT/FAMILY EDUCATION

• Caution with salt substitutes containing potassium chloride

• Rise slowly to sitting/standing position to minimize orthostatic hypotension

• Dizziness, fainting, lightheadedness may occur during 1st few days of therapy

• May cause altered taste perception or cough; persistent dry cough usually does not subside unless medication is stopped; notify clinician if these symptoms persist

MONITORING PARAMETERS

• BUN, creatinine, potassium within 2 wk after initiation of therapy (increased levels may indicate acute renal failure)

---

quinidine

(kwin'i-deen)

Rx: Quinaglute Dura-Tabs, Quinalan, (gluconate); Cardioquin (polygalacturonate); Quinidex Extentabs, Quinora (sulfate)

Chemical Class: Dextrorotatory isomer of quinine

Therapeutic Class: Antidysrhythmic (Class IA); antimalarial

CLINICAL PHARMACOLOGY

Mechanism of Action: Decreases the rate of rise of diastolic (Phase 4) depolarization, thereby depressing automaticity in ectopic foci; slows depolarization, repolarization, and amplitude of the action potential leading to an increase in the refractoriness of atrial and ventricular tissue; exerts indirect anticholinergic effects through blockade of vagal innervation, which may facilitate con-

---

* = non-FDA-approved use

duction in the atrioventricular junction; in patients with malaria acts primarily as an intra-erythrocytic schizonticide with little effect upon sporozites or upon pre-erythrocytic parasites, gametocidal to *Plasmodium vivax* and *P. malariae,* but not to *P. falciparum*

Pharmacokinetics

PO: Peak 3-4 hr (gluconate), 1-1½ hr (sulfate), 6 hr (polygalacturonate); duration 6-8 hr (Sus Action tab 12 hr)

IM: Peak ½-1½ hr

80%-90% bound to plasma proteins; metabolized in liver, excreted in urine (10%-50% unchanged); $t_{1/2}$ 6 hr

INDICATIONS AND USES: PO: Premature ventricular contractions, ventricular tachycardia (when not associated with complete heart block), junctional (nodal) dysrhythmias, AV junctional premature complexes, paroxysmal junctional tachycardia, premature atrial contractions, paroxysmal atrial tachycardia, atrial flutter, atrial fibrillation (chronic and paroxysmal); IM/IV when PO therapy not feasible or when rapid therapeutic effect is required, life-threatening *Plasmodium falciparum* malaria

DOSAGE

Adult

• Give 200 mg test dose PO/IM several hr before full dosage to determine possibility of idiosyncratic reaction

• PO (sulfate) 100-600 mg q4-6h, initiate at 200 mg/dose and adjust dose to maintain desired therapeutic effect, max 3-4 g/d; Sus Action 300-600 mg q8-12h

• PO (gluconate) 324-972 mg q8-12h

• PO (polygalacturonate) 275 mg q8-12h

• IM 400 mg q4-6h

• IV 200-400 mg diluted and infused at a rate ≤10 mg/min

Child

• Give 2 mg/kg test dose PO/IM several hr before full dosage to determine possibility of idiosyncratic reaction

• PO (sulfate) 15-60 mg/kg/day divided into 4-5 doses or 6 mg/kg q4-6h; usual 30 mg/kg/day or 900 mg/m²/day given in 5 doses/day

🔢 **AVAILABLE FORMS/COST OF THERAPY**

Quinidine Gluconate

• Inj, Sol—IM;IV: 80 mg/ml, 10 ml: **$21.39**

• Tab, Uncoated, Sus Action—Oral: 324 mg, 100's: **$29.34-$69.04**

Quinidine Polygalacturonate

• Tab, Uncoated—Oral: 275 mg, 100's: **$144.59**

Quinidine Sulfate

• Tab, Uncoated—Oral: 200 mg, 100's: **$4.25-$20.79**; 300 mg, 100's: **$18.62-$66.81**

• Tab, Coated, Sus Action—Oral: 300 mg, 100's: **$64.85-$109.80**

CONTRAINDICATIONS: Digitalis intoxication manifested by AV condition disorders, complete AV block with an AV nodal or idioventricular pacemaker, left bundle branch block, or other severe intraventricular condition defects with marked QRS widening, ectopic impulses, and abnormal rhythms due to escape mechanisms, history of drug-induced torsade de pointes, history of long QT syndrome, myasthenia gravis

PRECAUTIONS: Treatment of atrial flutter without prior medication to control ventricular rate (e.g., digoxin, verapamil, diltiazem, beta-blocker), marginally compensated cardiovascular disease, incomplete AV block, digitalis intoxication, hyperkalemia, renal, or hepatic insufficiency

---

italic = common side effects   ***bold italic*** = life-threatening reactions

PREGNANCY AND LACTATION: Pregnancy category C; use during pregnancy has been classified in reviews of cardiovascular drugs as relatively safe for the fetus; high doses can produce oxytocic properties and potential for abortion; excreted in breast milk; compatible with breast feeding

SIDE EFFECTS/ADVERSE REACTIONS

CNS: Apprehension, ataxia, confusion, delirium, dementia, depression, *dizziness,* excitement, fever, *headache,* vertigo

CV: Angioedema, arterial embolism, *bradycardia,* **complete AV block,** hypotension, prolonged QT interval, syncope, **torsade de pointes,** ventricular extrasystoles, ventricular flutter, **ventricular tachycardia and fibrillation,** widening of the QRS complex

EENT: Disturbed hearing (tinnitus, decreased auditory acuity), disturbed vision (mydriasis, blurred vision, disturbed color perception, photophobia, diplopia, night blindness, scotomata), optic neuritis, reduced visual field

GI: Abdominal pain, anorexia, *diarrhea,* esophagitis, hepatotoxicity, nausea, vomiting

HEME: **Acute hemolytic anemia, agranulocytosis,** leukocytosis, **neutropenia, thrombocytopenia,** thrombocytopenic purpura

MS: Arthralgia, increase in serum skeletal muscle creatine phosphokinase, myalgia

SKIN: Abnormalities of pigmentation, cutaneous flushing with intense pruritus, eczema, exfoliative eruptions, photosensitivity, psoriasis, purpura, rash, urticaria, vasculitis

MISC: Cinchonism (tinnitus, headache, nausea, visual changes), lupus nephritis, positive ANA, systemic lupus erythematosus

INTERACTIONS

Drafts
Drugs

3 *Acetazolamide, antacids, sodium bicarbonate, thiazide diuretics:* Alkalinization of urine increases plasma quinidine concentrations

3 *Amiloride:* Increased risk of arrhythmias in patients with ventricular tachycardia

3 *Amiodarone, cimetidine, verapamil:* Increased plasma quinidine concentrations

3 *Azole antifungals:* Inhibition of quinidine metabolism (CYP3A4), increased concentrations

3 *Barbiturates, nifedipine, kaolin-pectin, phenytoin, rifampin, rifabutin:* Decreased plasma quinidine concentrations

3 *Beta-blockers:* Increased concentrations of metoprolol, propranolol, and timolol

3 *Cholinergic agents:* Reduced therapeutic effects of cholinergic drugs

2 *Codeine:* Inhibition of codeine to its active metabolite, diminished analgesia

3 *Cyclic antidepressants:* Increased imipramine, nortriptyline and desipramine concentrations

3 *Dextromethorphan:* Increased dextromethorphan concentrations, toxicity may result

3 *Digitalis glycosides:* Increased digoxin and digitoxin concentrations, toxicity may result

3 *Encainide:* Increased encainide serum concentrations in rapid encainide metabolizers

3 *Haloperidol:* Increased haloperidol concentrations, toxicity

3 *Macrolides:* Increased quinidine concentrations with erythromycin, troleandomycin, clarithromycin due to CYP34A inhibition

3 *Mexiletine:* Increased mexiletine concentrations

3 *Neuromuscular blocking agents:* Enhanced effects of neuromuscular blocking agents

3 *Nifedipine:* Increased serum nifedipine concentrations, decreased serum quinidine concentrations

3 *Procainamide:* Marked increased procainamide concentrations

3 *Propafenone:* Increased propafenone concentrations and decreased concentrations of its active metabolite; net effect unknown

3 *Warfarin:* Enhanced anticoagulant response

Labs
• *False increase:* Urine 17-ketosteroids

SPECIAL CONSIDERATIONS
• 267 mg gluconate=275 mg polygalacturonate=200 mg sulfate

PATIENT/FAMILY EDUCATION
• Take with food to decrease GI upset
• Do not crush or chew sustained release tablets

MONITORING PARAMETERS
• Plasma quinidine concentration (therapeutic range 2-6 μg/ml)
• ECG
• Liver function tests during the 1st 4-8 weeks
• CBC periodically during prolonged therapy

quinine
(kwye´nine)
Rx: Quinine
Chemical Class: Cinchona alkaloid
Therapeutic Class: Antimalarial

CLINICAL PHARMACOLOGY
Mechanism of Action: Exact antimalarial mechanism of action unknown, appears to interfere with plasmodial DNA function; increases the refractory period of skeletal muscle by direct action on the muscle fiber, decreases the excitability of the motor endplate, and affects the distribution of calcium within the muscle fiber

Pharmacokinetics
PO: Peak 1-3 hr; 70% bound to plasma proteins; metabolized in liver, excreted in urine; $t_{1/2}$ 4-5 hr

INDICATIONS AND USES: Chloroquine-resistant *falciparum* malaria (alone or in combination with pyrimethamine and a sulfonamide or with a tetracycline),* alternative for chloroquine-sensitive strains of *P. falciparum, P. malariae, P. ovale* and *P. vivax,* * nocturnal leg cramps*

DOSAGE
Adult
• *Chloroquine-resistant malaria:* PO 650 mg q8h for 5-7 days
• *Chloroquine-sensitive malaria:* PO 600 mg q8h for 5-7 days
• *Nocturnal leg cramps:* PO 260-300 mg hs

Child
• *Chloroquine-resistant malaria:* PO 25 mg/kg/day divided q8h for 5-7 days
• *Chloroquine-sensitive malaria:* PO 10 mg/kg q8h for 5-7 days

💲 AVAILABLE FORMS/COST OF THERAPY

• Cap, Gel—Oral: 200 mg, 100's: **$8.93-$22.94**; 325 mg, 100's: **$5.05-$52.60**
• Tab, Uncoated—Oral: 260 mg, 100's: **$9.95-$63.00**

CONTRAINDICATIONS: G-6-PD deficiency, optic neuritis, tinnitus, history of blackwater fever, thrombocytopenic purpura (associated with previous quinine ingestion), pregnancy

PRECAUTIONS: Cardiac dysrhythmias, myasthenia gravis

PREGNANCY AND LACTATION: Pregnancy category X; excreted into breast milk; compatible with breast feeding; use caution in infants at risk for G-6-PD deficiency

SIDE EFFECTS/ADVERSE REACTIONS

CNS: Apprehension, confusion, fever, headache, restlessness, vertigo
CV: Anginal symptoms, syncope
EENT: Blurred vision, deafness, diminished visual field, *diplopia,* disturbed color vision, photophobia, tinnitus, visual disturbances
GI: Epigastric pain, **hepatitis,** *nausea, vomiting*
HEME: **Acute hemolysis, agranulocytosis, hypoprothrombinemia,** thrombocytopenic purpura
RESP: Asthmatic symptoms
SKIN: Cutaneous rashes, edema of the face, flushing, pruritus, sweating
MISC: Cinchonism (tinnitus, headache, nausea, disturbed vision)

INTERACTIONS

Drugs
❸ *Digitalis glycosides:* Increased digoxin concentrations (especially at high quinine doses)
❸ *Smoking:* Reduced serum quinine concentrations
Labs
• *False increase:* 17-ketosteroids

SPECIAL CONSIDERATIONS
PATIENT/FAMILY EDUCATION

• Take with food
• May cause blurred vision, use caution driving
• Discontinue drug if flushing, itching, rash, fever, stomach pain, difficult breathing, ringing in ears, visual disturbances occur

---

quinupristin/ dalfopristin

(kwin-yoo′pris-tin/dal′foh-pris-tin)
Rx: Synercid
Chemical Class: Streptogramin combination
Therapeutic Class: Antibiotic

CLINICAL PHARMACOLOGY

Mechanism of Action: Inhibits bacterial protein synthesis by binding to a site on the 50S subunit of bacterial ribosomal RNA; composed of 30% quinupristin and 70% dalfopristin; individually, these are bacteriostatic but in combination are synergistic and bactericidal

Pharmacokinetics
IV: Peak 1 hr; quinupristin 30% protein bound, dalfopristin 55% protein bound; 95% metabolized in blood and liver by conjugation and hydrolysis; 75% excreted in feces as metabolites, 20% in urine as metabolites, and 5% in urine as unchanged drugs; $t_{1/2}$ 1.4 hr

INDICATIONS AND USES: Vancomycin-resistant *Enterococcus faecium* infections including bacteremia, nosocomial or community acquired pneumonia, complicated skin and skin structure infections caused by susceptible organisms
Antibacterial spectrum usually includes:

• Gram-positive organisms: *Enterococcus faecalis* (including vancomycin-resistant strains), *Listeria monocytogenes, Staphylococcus aureus* (including methicillin-resistant strains), *Staphylococcus epidermidis* (including methicillin-resistant strains), *Streptococcus pneumoniae* (penicillin-susceptible and penicillin-resistant strains), *Streptococcus pyogenes,* Viridans group streptococci

• Gram-negative organisms: *Legionella pneumophila, Moraxella catarrhalis, Neisseria gonorrhoeae*

• Anaerobes: Clostridium (not difficile) species

• Other organisms: Chlamydia species, *Mycoplasma pneumoniae*

DOSAGE

Adult and child ≥16 yr

• *Vancomycin-resistant Enterococcus faecium infections including bacteremia:* IV 7.5 mg/kg q8h for 14-28 days

• *Complicated skin and skin structure infections:* IV 7.5 mg/kg q12h for 7 days

• *Peritonitis associated with chronic ambulatory peritoneal dialysis:* IV 5-10 mg/kg q12h for 14 days

💲 AVAILABLE FORMS/COST OF THERAPY

• Inj, Lyphl-Sol—IV: 500 mg (150 mg/350 mg): **$107.43**

PRECAUTIONS: Renal disease, hepatic disease, co-administration with medications metabolized by CYP 3A4 isoform

PREGNANCY AND LACTATION: Pregnancy category B; breast milk excretion unknown

SIDE EFFECTS/ADVERSE REACTIONS

CNS: Headache

GI: Diarrhea, *hyperbilirubinemia (unconjugated, 25%),* increased transaminase levels, nausea *, pseudomembranous colitis,* vomiting

METAB: Hyponatremia

MS: Arthralgia, myalgia

SKIN: Infusion site irritation (40%), phlebitis (5%)

INTERACTIONS

Drugs

❷ *Antihistamines (astemizole, terfenadine):* Reduced antihistamine metabolism by CYP3A4 inhibition, possible prolonged QT interval

❸ *Antineoplastic agents (docetaxel, paclitaxel, vinca alkaloids):* Reduced antineoplastic metabolism by CYP3A4 inhibition

❸ *Benzodiazepines (diazepam, midazolam):* Reduced benzodiazepine metabolism by CYP3A4 inhibition

❸ *Calcium channel blockers (amlodipine, diltiazem, felodipine, isradipine, nicardipine, nifedipine, nimodipine, nisoldipine, verapamil):* Reduced calcium channel blocker metabolism by CYP3A4 inhibition

❸ *Carbamazepine:* Reduced carbamazepine metabolism by CYP3A4 inhibition

❷ *Cisapride:* Reduced cisapride metabolism by CYP3A4 inhibition, possible prolonged QT interval

❸ *Digoxin:* Decreased digoxin metabolism by GI bacteria may increase digoxin levels

❷ *Disopyramide:* Reduced disopyramide metabolism by CYP3A4 inhibition, possible prolonged QT interval

❸ *HMG-CoA reductase inhibitors (atorvastatin, fluvastatin, lovastatin, pravastatin, simvastatin):* Reduced statin metablolism by CYP3A4 inhibition

❷ *Immunosuppressives (cyclosporine, tacrolimus):* Reduced immunosuppressive metabolism by CYP3A4 inhibition

3 *Non-nucleoside reverse transcriptase inhibitors (delavirdine, nevirapine):* Reduced NNRTI metabolism by CYP3A4 inhibition

3 *Protease inhibitors (indinavir, ritonavir):* Reduced PI metabolism by CYP3A4 inhibition

❷ *Quinidine:* Reduced quinidine metabolism by CYP3A4 inhibition, possible prolonged QT interval

SPECIAL CONSIDERATIONS

• Most appropriate use is when Vancomycin-resistant *Enterococcus faecium* infection is documented or strongly suspected, or for therapy of methicillin resistant *Staphylococcus aureus* infection

PATIENT/FAMILY EDUCATION

• Due to high chance of drug interactions by inhibiting CYP 3A4, check with prescriber before taking any new medications

MONITORING PARAMETERS

• CBC, ALT, AST, bilirubin, renal function

---

rabeprazole

(rab-eh-pra´zole)
Rx: Aciphex
Chemical Class: Substituted benzimidazole
Therapeutic Class: Gastrointestinal antiulcer agent

CLINICAL PHARMACOLOGY

Mechanism of Action: Suppresses gastric acid secretion by inhibiting the parietal cell H^+/K^+ ATP pump

Pharmacokinetics

PO: Peak 2-5 hr, bioavailability 52%; 96% bound to plasma proteins; extensively metabolized by CYP3A and 2C19; 90% eliminated as metabolites in the urine; $t_{1/2}$ 1-2 hr (increased with hepatic disease)

INDICATIONS AND USES: Short-term (4-8 wk) treatment of erosive or ulcerative gastroesophageal reflux disease (GERD); maintenance therapy in erosive or ulcerative GERD; short-term (up to 4 wk) treatment of duodenal ulcers; long-term treatment of pathological hypersecretory conditions, including Zollinger-Ellison syndrome

DOSAGE

Adult

• *GERD:* PO 20 mg qd for 4-8 wk; maintenance: 20 mg qd

• *Duodenal ulcer:* PO 20 mg qd after breakfast for 4 wk

• *Hypersecretory conditions:* PO 60 mg qd; dose may need to be adjusted prn; doses as high as 100 mg qd and 60 mg bid have been used

$ **AVAILABLE FORMS/COST OF THERAPY**

• Tab, Sus Action—Oral: 20 mg, 30's: **$113.99**

PRECAUTIONS: Severe hepatic impairment

PREGNANCY AND LACTATION: Pregnancy category B; excretion into breast milk unknown, use caution in nursing mothers

SIDE EFFECTS/ADVERSE REACTIONS

CNS: Headache, delirium, twitching, insomnia, anxiety, dizziness, depression, somnolence, hypertonia, neuralgia, vertigo, *seizure,* abnormal dreams, decreased libido, neuropathy, paresthesia, tremor, agitation, amnesia, confusion, extrapyramidal reaction, hyperkinesia

CV: Chest pain, hypertension, *myocardial infarction,* syncope, angina, bundle branch block, palpitation, bradycardia, tachycardia, SVT, *pulmonary embolus,* thrombophlebitis, vasodilation, QT prolongation, *ventricular tachycardia,* ecchymosis, lymphadenopathy, peripheral edema

---

* = non-FDA-approved use

EENT: Cataract, amblyopia, glaucoma, dry eyes, abnormal vision, tinnitus, otitis media, corneal opacity, blurred vision, eye pain, retinal degeneration, strabismus

GI: Diarrhea, nausea, abdominal pain, vomiting, dyspepsia, flatulence, constipation, dry mouth, eructation, gastroenteritis, rectal hemorrhage, melena, anorexia, cholelithiasis, stomatitis, dysphagia, gingivitis, cholecystitis, increased appetite, colitis, esophagitis, glossitis, ***pancreatitis,*** proctitis, cholangitis, duodenitis, hepatitis, hepatic encephalopathy, fatty liver, salivary gland enlargement, increased transaminases

GU: Urinary frequency, cystitis, dysmenorrhea, dysuria, renal calculus, menorrhagia, polyuria, breast enlargement, impotence, hematuria, leukorrhea, orchitis, urinary incontinence

HEME: **Agranulocytosis, hemolytic anemia, leukopenia, pancytopenia, thrombocytopenia,** anemia

METAB: Hyperammonemia, elevated TSH, hyperthyroidism, hypothyroidism, gout

MS: Myalgia, arthritis, leg cramps, bone pain, bursitis

RESP: Dyspnea, asthma, epistaxis, laryngitis, hiccup, hyperventilation, apnea, hypoventilation

SKIN: Dermatologic eruptions, photosensitivity, rash, pruritus, sweating, urticaria, alopecia, dry skin, herpes zoster, psoriasis

MISC: Coma, jaundice, rhabdomyolysis, weakness, fever, chills, malaise, thirst, weight gain, dehydration, weight loss

INTERACTIONS
Drugs

3 *Cyclosporine:* Potential for increased cyclosporine concentrations

3 *Digoxin:* Increased serum concentrations of digoxin possible

3 *Ketoconazole:* Decreased bioavailability of ketoconazole

SPECIAL CONSIDERATIONS
PATIENT/FAMILY EDUCATION
• Sus action tablets should be swallowed whole, do not chew, crush, or split the tablets

MONITORING PARAMETERS
• Symptom relief, mucosal healing
• Symptomatic response does not rule out gastric malignancy

---

raloxifene
(ra-lox′-i-feen)
Rx: Evista
Chemical Class: Benzothiophene, selective estrogen receptor modulator (SERM)
Therapeutic Class: Antiosteoporotic

CLINICAL PHARMACOLOGY
Mechanism of Action: Binds to estrogen receptors, reducing resorption of bone, decreasing bone turnover. Estrogen-like effect on bone and lipids, lacks estrogen effects in uterine and breast tissues

Pharmacokinetics

PO: 60% of dose rapidly absorbed, undergoes extensive presystemic glucuronide conjugation. Absolute bioavailability 2%. Extensive protein binding but does not bind to sex steroid binding globulin. Not metabolized by cytochrome P450 pathways. Excreted in feces. $t_{1/2}$ 32 hr

INDICATIONS AND USES: Prevention and treatment of osteoporosis. Not indicated in premenopausal women.

DOSAGE
Adult
• PO 60 mg qd

---

italic = common side effects   **bold italic** = life-threatening reactions

$ AVAILABLE FORMS/COST OF THERAPY
• Tab, Coated—Oral: 60 mg, 100's: **$242.16**

CONTRAINDICATIONS: Pregnancy, women at risk for pregnancy, history of thromboembolism

PRECAUTIONS: Hepatic insufficiency

PREGNANCY AND LACTATION: Pregnancy category X. Abortion and fetal anomalies noted in animal studies. Unknown if excreted in milk.

SIDE EFFECTS/ADVERSE REACTIONS
CNS: Depression, insomnia
EENT: Sinusitis
GI: Nausea (8% incidence same as placebo), dyspepsia, vomiting
GU: Vaginitis, leukorrhea
*HEME: **Thromboembolism***
METAB: Weight gain, peripheral edema, *decreased total cholesterol (6%), decreased LDL-C (11%),* no effect on HDL-C or triglycerides
MS: Leg cramps (6%)
SKIN: Hot flashes (25%, vs 18% with placebo)

INTERACTIONS
Drugs
❷ *Cholestyramine:* Decreased absorption and enterohepatic cycling of raloxifene
❸ *Clofibrate, indomethacin, naproxen, ibuprofen, diazepam, diazoxide:* Possible displacement of these highly protein-bound drugs
❸ *Warfarin:* Decreased PT

SPECIAL CONSIDERATIONS
• Shown to preserve bone mass and increase bone mineral density relative to calcium alone at 24 mo, relationship to skeletal fracture rates not yet established
• Ensure adequate dietary or supplemental calcium, vitamin D

• Not associated with endometrial proliferation; however, investigate uterine bleeding
• Has not been adequately studied with concomitant use of estrogen or in women with prior history of breast cancer
• Risk of thromboembolic events greatest in first 4 mo, discontinue at least 72 hr prior to surgery involving immobilization. Resume when patient fully ambulatory

PATIENT/FAMILY EDUCATION
• May be taken without regard to meals
• Engage in weight-bearing exercises, do not smoke or use alcohol excessively
• Report leg pain or swelling, sudden chest pain, shortness of breath, vision changes
• Avoid restrictions of movement during travel. Discontinue if at bed rest.

MONITORING PARAMETERS
• Bone density tests (e.g., DEXA scan)

---

ramipril
(ram´i-pril)
Rx: Altace
Chemical Class: Nonsulfhydryl angiotensin-converting enzyme (ACE) inhibitor
Therapeutic Class: Antihypertensive

CLINICAL PHARMACOLOGY
Mechanism of Action: Antihypertensive, hypoproliferative, and cardioprotective effects attributable to competitive inhibition of angiotensin-converting enzyme (ACE) yielding decreased plasma concentrations of angiotensin II, plasma aldosterone concentrations, systemic vascular resistance, blood pressure,

---

* = non-FDA-approved use

preload, and afterload, not accompanied by changes in heart rate, pressor sensitivity to exogenous norepinephrine, or baroreceptor sensitivity

Pharmacokinetics

PO: Onset 1-2 hr, duration 24 hr; 73% bound to plasma proteins; has little pharmacologic activity until metabolized to active metabolite (ramiprilat), excreted in urine (60%) and feces (40%); $t_{1/2}$ (ramiprilat) 13-17 hr

INDICATIONS AND USES: Hypertension, CHF (left ventricular dysfunction), MI (left ventricular function salvage), erythrocytosis,* nephropathy,* retinopathy*

DOSAGE

Adult and Child >16 yr

• *Hypertension:* PO 2.5 mg qd initially (1.25 mg if on concomitant diuretic); usual maintenance dose, 2.5-20 mg qd

• *Congestive heart failure (left ventricular dysfunction):* PO 1.25-2.5 mg bid; max daily dose, 10 mg, usually divided

• *Myocardial infarction:* PO 1.25 mg initially, followed by 2.5 mg 12 hr later and full titration to 10 mg qd begun within 24 hr

• *Dosage in renal failure:* PO 25%-50% dosage reduction for CrCl 10-50 ml/min; 50%-75% reduction for CrCl <10 ml/min

§ AVAILABLE FORMS/COST OF THERAPY

• Cap, Gel—Oral: 1.25 mg, 100's: **$76.48**; 2.5 mg, 100's: **$89.79**; 5 mg, 100's: **$96.11**; 10 mg, 100's: **$111.36**

PRECAUTIONS: Renal insufficiency (<30 ml/min), hypotension (CHF, elderly, volume depletion—diuretics, dialysis, cirrhosis), aortic stenosis, hyperkalemia (potassium supplements, potassium-sparing diuretics, renal disease, diabetes), neutropenia (autoimmune diseases, collagen vascular, febrile illness, immunosuppressant drug therapy), proteinuria, renal artery stenosis, surgery/anesthesia (excessive hypotension, correctable with fluids)

PREGNANCY AND LACTATION: Pregnancy category D; ACE inhibitors can cause fetal and neonatal morbidity and death when administered to pregnant women; when pregnancy is detected, discontinue ACE inhibitors as soon as possible

SIDE EFFECTS/ADVERSE REACTIONS

CNS: Anxiety, dizziness, fatigue, *headache,* insomnia, paresthesia

CV: Angina, hypotension, palpitations, postural hypotension, syncope (especially with 1st dose)

GI: Abdominal pain, constipation, impaired taste sensation, nausea, pancreatitis, vomiting

GU: Decreased libido, impotence, renal insufficiency

HEME: **Agranulocytosis, neutropenia, thrombocytopenia**

METAB: Hyperkalemia, hyponatremia, hypoglycemia

MS: Arthralgia, arthritis, myalgia

RESP: Asthma, bronchitis, *cough,* dyspnea, sinusitis

SKIN: Angioedema, flushing, rash, sweating

INTERACTIONS

Drugs

❷ *Allopurinol:* Predisposition to hypersensitivity reactions

❸ *Alpha adrenergic blockers:* Exaggerated 1st dose hypotensive response

❸ *Aspirin:* Reduced hemodynamic effects; less likely with nonacetylated salicylates

❸ *Azathioprine:* Increased myelosuppression

❸ *Cyclosporine:* Renal insufficiency

R

▣ *Insulin:* Enhanced hypoglycemic response

▣ *Iron (parenteral):* Increased risk of systemic reaction

▣ *Lithium:* Increased risk of serious lithium toxicity

▣ *Loop diuretics:* Initiation of ACE inhibitor therapy may cause hypotension and renal insufficiency

▣ *NSAIDs:* Inhibition of the antihypertensive response to ACE inhibitors

▣ *Potassium, potassium-sparing diuretics:* Increased risk for hyperkalemia

▣ *Trimethoprim:* Additive risk of hyperkalemia, especially in patient predisposed to renal insufficiency

Labs

• ACE inhibition can account for approx 0.5mEq/L rise in serum potassium

SPECIAL CONSIDERATIONS
PATIENT/FAMILY EDUCATION

• Caution with salt substitutes containing potassium chloride

• Rise slowly to sitting/standing position to minimize orthostatic hypotension

• Dizziness, fainting, lightheadedness may occur during 1st few days of therapy

• May cause altered taste perception or cough; persistent dry cough usually does not subside unless medication is stopped; notify clinician if these symptoms persist

MONITORING PARAMETERS

• BUN, creatinine, potassium within 2 wk after initiation of therapy (increased levels may indicate acute renal failure)

• Potassium levels, although hyperkalemia rarely occurs

---

ranitidine
(ra-ni′ti-deen)
Rx: Zantac, Zantac EFFERdose, Zantac GELdose;
OTC: Zantac 75
Chemical Class: Aminoalkyl furan derivative
Therapeutic Class: Gastrointestinal antiulcer agent

CLINICAL PHARMACOLOGY
Mechanism of Action: Competitive, reversible inhibitor of histamine at gastric H_2-receptors; reduces gastric acid secretion

Pharmacokinetics

PO: Peak 1-3 hr

IM: Peak 0.25 hr

15% bound to plasma proteins; metabolized in liver, excreted in urine (30% of PO dose, 70% of IV dose unchanged) and bile; $t_{1/2}$ 2-2½ hr (prolonged in renal impairment)

INDICATIONS AND USES: Short-term treatment and maintenance of duodenal and benign gastric ulcers; pathological hypersecretory conditions (e.g., Zollinger-Ellison syndrome, systemic mastocytosis); gastroesophageal reflux disease (GERD); erosive esophagitis; heartburn, acid indigestion and sour stomach (OTC); stress ulcer prophylaxis,* chronic idiopathic urticaria (in combination with H_1-receptor antagonists),* acute upper GI bleeding*

DOSAGE
Adult

• *Duodenal and gastric ulcer:* PO 150 mg bid or 300 mg qhs for 4-8 wk, maintenance 150 mg qhs

• *GERD:* PO 150 mg bid

• *Erosive esophagitis:* PO 150 mg qid, maintenance 150 mg bid

---

* = non-FDA-approved use

• *Pathological hypersecretory conditions:* PO 150 mg bid initially, titrate to desired response up to 6 g/day; IV INF start at 1 mg/kg/hr, increase by 0.5 mg/kg/hr intervals q4h prn up to 2.5 mg/kg/hr

• IM/IV 50 mg q6-8h, do not exceed 400 mg/day; IV INF 6.25 mg/hr

• *Renal impairment (CrCl <50 ml/min):* PO 150 mg qd; IV/IM 50 mg q18-24 hr

Child

• PO 1.25-2.5 mg/kg q12h, max 300 mg/day; IM/IV 0.75-1.5 mg/kg q6-8h, max 6 mg/kg/day or 300 mg/day; IV INF 0.1-0.25 mg/kg/hr

💲 AVAILABLE FORMS/COST OF THERAPY

• Cap, Gel—Oral: 150 mg, 60's: **$101.52**; 300 mg, 100's: **$320.00**

• Granule, Effervescent—Oral: 150 mg, 60's: **$115.51**

• Inj, Sol—IM, IV: 25 mg/ml, 2 ml: **$4.16**

• Syr—Oral: 15 mg/ml, 480 ml: **$200.16**

• Tab, Coated—Oral: 75 mg, 30's: **$6.99**; 150 mg, 100's (OTC): **$10.49-$174.70**; 300 mg, 100's: **$267.19-$273.00**

• Tab, Effervescent—Oral: 150 mg, 60's: **$115.51**

PRECAUTIONS: Renal and hepatic function impairment, elderly, gastric malignancy, rapid IV administration, immunocompromised patients

PREGNANCY AND LACTATION: Pregnancy category B; compatible with breast feeding

SIDE EFFECTS/ADVERSE REACTIONS

CNS: Dizziness, insomnia, malaise, somnolence, vertigo

CV: Atrioventricular block, bradycardia, premature ventricular beats, tachycardia

GI: Abdominal discomfort or pain, constipation, diarrhea, hepatitis, increased liver function tests, nausea, pancreatitis (rare), vomiting

HEME: **Granulocytopenia, leukopenia, thrombocytopenia**

MS: Arthralgias, myalgias

SKIN: Alopecia, **erythema multiforme** (rare), rash

INTERACTIONS

Drugs

🔳 *Cefuroxine; cefpodoxime; enoxacin; ketoconazole:* Reduction in gastric acidity reduces absorption, decreased plasma levels, potential for therapeutic failure

🔳 *Glipizide; glyburide; tolbutamide:* Increased absorption of these drugs, potential for hypoglycemia

🔳 *Nifedipine, nitrendipine, nisoldipine:* Increased concentrations of these drugs

Labs

• *False positive:* Urine drugs of abuse screen

SPECIAL CONSIDERATIONS

• No advantage over other agents in this class, base selection on cost

PATIENT/FAMILY EDUCATION

• Stagger doses of ranitidine and antacids

• Dissolve effervescent tablets and granules in 6-8 oz water before drinking

MONITORING PARAMETERS

• Intragastric pH when used for stress ulcer prophylaxis, titrate dose to maintain pH >4

R

---

italic = common side effects   ***bold italic*** = life-threatening reactions

repaglinide

(re-pag'lih-nide)

Rx: Prandin

Chemical Class: Meglitinide

Therapeutic Class: Oral hypoglycemic agent

CLINICAL PHARMACOLOGY

Mechanism of Action: Stimulates insulin secretion via inhibition (closing) of ATP-sensitive potassium channels in β-cells (resultant increases in β-cell calcium influx)—lowers postprandial blood sugars

Pharmacokinetics

PO: Peak onset, 30-90 min (when administered 15 min ac); 4 hr duration, rapidly absorbed (PO bioavailability, 56%); >98% plasma protein bound; complete hepatic metabolism—CYP3A4 (no active metabolites); excreted predominantly in feces (unchanged after 24 hr); elimination $t_{1/2}$ <1 hr

INDICATIONS AND USES: Oral hypoglycemic adjunct to diet and exercise; as monotherapy and combination therapy with metformin in patients with type 2 diabetes mellitus; affects primarily postprandial blood glucose; minimal effects on fasting blood glucose were observed

DOSAGE

Adult and Child >16 yr

• 0.5 mg—4 mg tid (30 min ac); (0.5 mg initial dose when glycosylated hemoglobin <8%); 1-2 mg initial dose for patients who received other glucose-lowering agents (start morning after previous agent stopped) or had glycosylated hemoglobin >8%; max total daily dose should not exceed 16 mg; dosage adjustments should be made at inter-vals of at least 1 wk (slower in patients with moderate to severe hepatic failure)

$ AVAILABLE FORMS/COST OF THERAPY

• Tab, Coated—Oral: 0.5 mg, 100's: **$96.20**; 1 mg, 2 mg, 100's: **$96.60**

CONTRAINDICATIONS: Type 1 diabetes mellitus, ketoacidosis

PRECAUTIONS: Hypoglycemia; insulin replacement may be necessary during stress (infection, fever, trauma, surgery)

PREGNANCY AND LACTATION: Pregnancy category C

SIDE EFFECTS/ADVERSE REACTIONS

GI: Nausea, diarrhea, constipation, vomiting, dyspepsia

METAB: Hypoglycemia

INTERACTIONS

Drugs

3 *Aspirin, β-blockers, sulfa drugs, chloramphenicol, warfarin, MAO inhibitors:* hypoglycemia

3 *Ketoconazole, miconazole, erythromycin, troglitazone, rifampicin, carbamazepine, phenobarbital, butalbital, secobarbital, or primidone:* potential increased repaglinide metabolism secondary to cytochrome P450 enzyme induction

3 *Thiazide diuretics, calcium channel blockers, beta blockers, cough, cold, or hay fever medicines, estrogen, birth control pills, corticosteroids, thyroid medicine, phenytoin, isoniazid, or nicotinic acid:* hyperglycemia

SPECIAL CONSIDERATIONS

PATIENT/FAMILY EDUCATION

• Skip the dose of this medication if you skip a meal; take an extra dose with extra meal

• Recognize and treat hypoglycemia; maintain ready supply of glucose (glucose tablets or gel)

MONITORING PARAMETERS

• Blood glucose—biggest effect noted on postprandial values (50-75 mg/dL reductions expected); minimal effect on fasting blood glucose

• Glycosylated hemoglobin (1% to 2% reductions expected); hyperglycemia/hypoglycemia signs and symptoms

---

reserpine

(re-ser'peen)

Rx: Eskaserp, Lemiserp, Reserpoid, Resine, Serpalan, Serpasil, Unitensin-R
Combinations

Rx: with thiazide diuretics: i.e., bendroflumethazide (flumethiazide), chlorothiazide, chlorthalidone (Regreton), hydrochlorothiazide (Hydropres, Hydroserpalan, Hydroserpine, Mallopress), hydroflumethiazide (Salutensin), polythiazide (Reneese), quinethazone (Hydromox R), trichloromethiazide (Metatensin, Naquival), hydrochlorothiazide and hydralazine (Hyserp, Lo-Ten, Marpres, Ser-A-Gen, Seralazide, Ser-Ap-Es, Unipres, Uni-Serp)

Chemical Class: Rauwolfia alkaloid
Therapeutic Class: Antihypertensive; postganglionic adrenergic neuron inhibitor antipsychotic

---

CLINICAL PHARMACOLOGY

Mechanism of Action: Depletes stores of catecholamines and 5-hydroxytryptamine in the CNS and other organs; tissue catecholamines restored slowly, thus accumulative effect; blood pressure reduction results from a decrease in peripheral resistance and reduced cardiac output; sedative and tranquilizing properties also related to depletion of catecholamines and 5-hydroxytryptamine from the brain in higher doses

Pharmacokinetics

PO: Peak serum concentration 3.5 hr;slow onset of action (days), sustained duration of effect (1-6 wk; persistent hypotensive effects post discontinuation); 96% bound to plasma proteins; extensive hepatic metabolism; 90% excreted as metabolites—30% to 60% in feces, 1% unchanged in urine; $t_{1/2}$ 50-100 hr

INDICATIONS AND USES: Hypertension, agitated psychotic states in patients unable to tolerate phenothiazines, hyperthyroidism,* migraine,* progressive systemic sclerosis,* Raynaud's disease,* tardive dyskinesia*

DOSAGE

Adult

• *Hypertension:* PO 0.05 mg qd for 1-2 wk, then 0.1-0.25 mg qd; higher doses increase incidence of mental depression and serious side effects

• *Psychotic states:* PO 0.5 mg qd, range 0.1-1 mg/day

Child

• PO 20 μg/kg/day, max 0.25 mg/day

💲 AVAILABLE FORMS/COST OF THERAPY

• Tab, Uncoated—Oral: 0.1 mg, 100's: **$2.95-$29.28**; 0.25 mg, 100's: **$3.50-$34.70**

CONTRAINDICATIONS: Current depression or history of depression, active peptic ulcer, ulcerative colitis, patients receiving electroconvulsive therapy

PRECAUTIONS: History of peptic ulcer (increases GI motility and secretion), history of gallstones, renal function impairment, children

PREGNANCY AND LACTATION: Pregnancy category C; excreted into breast milk, no clinical reports of adverse effects in nursing infants have been located

SIDE EFFECTS/ADVERSE REACTIONS

CNS: Depression, *dizziness, drowsiness,* dull sensorium, *fatigue,* headache, *lethargy,* nervousness, nightmares, paradoxical anxiety, parkinsonian syndrome and other extrapyramidal tract symptoms (rare)

CV: Angina-like symptoms, *bradycardia,* **dysrhythmias** (particularly when used concurrently with digitalis or quinidine), edema, syncope

EENT: Conjunctival injection, deafness, epistaxis, glaucoma, nasal congestion, optic atrophy, uveitis

GI: Anorexia, diarrhea, dryness of mouth, hypersecretion, nausea, vomiting

GU: Decreased libido, dysuria, impotence

METAB: Breast engorgement, elevated prolactin, gynecomastia, pseudolactation, weight gain

MS: Muscular aches

RESP: Dyspnea

SKIN: Pruritus, purpura, rash

INTERACTIONS

Drugs

3 *Non-selective MAOIs:* Hypertensive reactions

Labs

• *False increase:* Serum bilirubin, urine creatinine

• *False positive:* Guiacols spot test

SPECIAL CONSIDERATIONS

• Only remaining rauwolfia derivative available

PATIENT/FAMILY EDUCATION

• May cause drowsiness or dizziness, use caution driving or participating in other activities requiring alertness

• Therapeutic effect may take 2-3 wk

MONITORING PARAMETERS

• Blood pressure, edema, drowsiness, despondency or self-depreciation, early morning insomnia, CNS depression, hypothermia, extrapyramidal tract effects

---

reteplase
(reh´te-place)
Rx: Retavase
Chemical Class: Tissue plasminogen activator
Therapeutic Class: Antithrombotic

CLINICAL PHARMACOLOGY

Mechanism of Action: Promotes thrombolysis by converting endogenous plasminogen to plasmin

Pharmacokinetics

IV: Fibrinogen levels fall below 100 mg/dl 2 hr following double-bolus administration, mean fibrinogen level back to normal by 48 hr; coronary artery patency is usually achieved within 30-90 min; $t_{1/2}$ 13-16 min; cleared by liver and kidney

INDICATIONS AND USES: Acute myocardial infarction

DOSAGE

Adult

• IV: 10 + 10 U double-bolus injection, each bolus is administered over 2 min, 30 min apart

⑤ AVAILABLE FORMS/COST OF THERAPY

• Inj—Lyphl sol: kit (2×10 U plus syringes, needles, etc.): **$2,640.00**

CONTRAINDICATIONS: Active internal bleeding, history of cerebrovascular accident, recent intracranial or intraspinal surgery or trauma, intracranial neoplasm, arteriovenous malformation or aneurysm, known bleeding diathesis, severe uncontrolled hypertension

PRECAUTIONS: Recent major surgery, previous puncture of noncompressible vessels, cerebrovascular disease, recent gastrointestinal or genitourinary bleeding, recent trauma; hypertension: systolic BP ≥180 mm Hg and/or diastolic BP ≥110 mm Hg; high likelihood of left heart thrombus; acute pericarditis, subacute bacterial endocarditis, hemostatic defects including those secondary to severe hepatic or renal disease, severe hepatic or renal dysfunction, pregnancy, diabetic hemorrhagic retinopathy or other hemorrhagic ophthalmic conditions, septic thrombophlebitis, advanced age, patients currently receiving oral anticoagulants, any other condition in which bleeding constitutes a significant hazard

PREGNANCY AND LACTATION: Pregnancy category C

SIDE EFFECTS/ADVERSE REACTIONS

CV: Cardiac tamponade, electromechanical dissociation, reinfarction
HEME: Bleeding
SKIN: Allergic reactions
MISC: Fever

INTERACTIONS

Drugs

❷ *Heparin, oral anticoagulants, drugs that alter platelet function (i.e., aspirin, dipyridamole, abciximab, eptifibitide, tirofiban):* May increase the risk of bleeding

SPECIAL CONSIDERATIONS

• No other IV medications should be administered in the same line

---

ribavirin

(rye-ba-vye′rin)
Rx: *Inhalation:*Virazole
*Oral:*Rebetol
Combinations
   Rx: with interferon alfa-2b
   (Rebetron)
Chemical Class: Nucleoside analog
Therapeutic Class: Antiviral

CLINICAL PHARMACOLOGY

Mechanism of Action: Inhibits RNA and/or DNA synthesis by respiratory syncytial virus (RSV), influenza virus (types A and B), and many other RNA and DNA viruses

Pharmacokinetics

PO: Onset 30 min, peak 1-2 hr; well absorbed

INH: Aerosol has systemic absorption; respiratory tract secretion concentration much higher than plasma concentration; $t_{1/2}$ in respiratory tract secretion 1.4-2.5 hr

Metabolized in liver and erythrocytes; plasma $t_{1/2}$ 9.5 hr; accumulates in erythrocytes, concentration plateaus at 4 days; elimination $t_{1/2}$ from erythrocytes 40 days; excreted in urine and feces

INDICATIONS AND USES: Severe lower respiratory tract infection by RSV in children (if begun within 1st 3 days of infection), influenza A,* influenza B,* hepatitis C (combination with interferon alfa-26), Lassa fever,* hantavirus-associated hemorrhagic fever*

DOSAGE

Adult

• *Influenza A or B:* INH sol of 6 g in 300 ml additive free sterile water administered by small particle aerosol generator for 18 hr then 4 hr tid per day for 3 days

---

italic = common side effects   ***bold italic*** = life-threatening reactions

• *Lassa fever:* Treatment, IV 30 mg/kg load, then in 6 hr, 16 mg/kg q6h for 4 days; then 8 mg/kg q8h for 6 days; prevention in high-risk contacts, PO 500 mg q6h for 7-10 days

• *Hantavirus-associated hemorrhagic fever:* Treatment, IV 33 mg/kg (max 2000 mg) load, then in 6 hr, 16 mg/kg (max 1000 mg) q6h for 15 doses, then 8 mg/kg (max 500 mg) q8h for 9 doses

Child

• *RSV infection:* INH sol of 6 g in 300 ml additive free sterile water administered by small particle aerosol generator for 12-18 hr per day for 3-7 days

• *Lassa fever:* Prevention in high-risk contacts, age >9 yr, PO 500 mg q6h for 7-10 days; age 6-9 yr, PO 400 mg q6h for 7-10 days

$ AVAILABLE FORMS/COST OF THERAPY

• Aer, Sol—INH: 6 g, 4's: **$5,499.38**
• Cap—Oral: 200 mg, 84's: **$861.00**

CONTRAINDICATIONS: Pregnancy and females of childbearing age

PRECAUTIONS: Patients receiving mechanical ventilation

PREGNANCY AND LACTATION: Pregnancy category X, teratogenic in animals; contraindicated in lactating women

SIDE EFFECTS/ADVERSE REACTIONS

CNS: Headache, *seizures (systemic administration only)*

CV: Cardiac arrest, hypotension

EENT: Conjunctivitis

GI: Anorexia, increased transaminases (systemic administration only), nausea

HEME: Anemia, reticulocytosis

RESP: Apnea, bacterial pneumonia, *pneumothorax, worsening of respiratory status*

SKIN: Rash

SPECIAL CONSIDERATIONS
PATIENT/FAMILY EDUCATION

• Female health care workers who are pregnant or may become pregnant should avoid exposure to ribavirin

MONITORING PARAMETERS

• Hematocrit

---

rifabutin

(rif'a-byoo-ten)

Rx: Mycobutin
Chemical Class: Semisynthetic rifamycin S derivative
Therapeutic Class: Antibiotic

CLINICAL PHARMACOLOGY

Mechanism of Action: Inhibits DNA-dependent RNA polymerase in susceptible strains of *Escherichia coli* and *Bacillus subtilis* but not in mammalian cells; it is not known if DNA-dependent RNA polymerase is inhibited in *M. avium* complex (MAC) (*Mycobacterium avium* and *M. intracellulare*)

Pharmacokinetics

PO: Peak 2-4 hr; high lipophilicity; 85% bound to plasma proteins; metabolized to active and inactive metabolites, excreted in feces (30%) and urine (53%); $t_{1/2}$ 45 hr

INDICATIONS AND USES: Prevention of disseminated MAC disease in patients with advanced HIV infection; (not drug of choice; macrolides are first-line)

DOSAGE

Adult

• PO 300 mg qd; if GI upset occurs, can be administered 150 mg bid with food

Child

• PO 5 mg/kg/day has been administered to small numbers of HIV-positive children

💲 AVAILABLE FORMS/COST OF THERAPY
• Cap, Gel—Oral: 150 mg, 100's: **$387.80**

CONTRAINDICATIONS: Hypersensitivity to rifamycins

PRECAUTIONS: Active tuberculosis (may lead to resistant strains), children

PREGNANCY AND LACTATION: Pregnancy category B

SIDE EFFECTS/ADVERSE REACTIONS
GI: Abdominal pain, *anorexia,* dyspepsia, eructation, flatulence, hepatitis, *nausea,* taste perversion, *vomiting*

GU: Discolored urine (30%)

HEME: **Leukopenia, neutropenia, thrombocytopenia**

MS: Mylagia

SKIN: Rash

INTERACTIONS
Drugs

3 *Acetaminophen:* Enhanced hepatotoxicity (overdoses and possibly large therapeutic doses)

3 *Cyclosporine:* Reduced concentration of cyclosporine

3 *Delavirdine:* Reduced concentration of delavirdine

3 *Eprosartan:* Reduced concentration of eprosartan

3 *Nifedipine:* Reduced nifedipine concentrations

3 *Oral contraceptives:* Menstrual irregularities, contraceptive failure

3 *Oral hypoglycemics:* Reduced hypoglycemic activity

3 *Propafenone:* Lowered propafenone concentrations, loss of antiarrhythmic efficacy

2 *Protease inhibitors:* Increased clearance (CYP3A4 induction) and decreased protease inhibitor efficacy

3 *Quinidine:* Marked reduction quinidine levels

3 *Tacrolimus:* Reduced concentration of tacrolimus

SPECIAL CONSIDERATIONS
• Has liver enzyme-inducing properties similar to rifampin although less potent
• Unlike rifampin, does not appear to alter the acetylation of isoniazid

PATIENT/FAMILY EDUCATION
• May discolor bodily secretions brown-orange, soft contact lenses may be permanently stained

MONITORING PARAMETERS
• Periodic CBC with differential and platelets
• Liver function tests

---

rifampin
(rye′fam-pin)
Rx: Rifadin, Rimactane
Chemical Class: Semisynthetic rifamycin B derivative
Therapeutic Class: Antituberculosis agent; antibiotic

CLINICAL PHARMACOLOGY
Mechanism of Action: Suppresses initiation of chain formation for RNA synthesis in susceptible bacteria by inhibiting DNA-dependent RNA polymerase

Pharmacokinetics
PO: Peak 2-4 hr; widely distributed into most body tissues and fluids; 84%-91% bound to plasma proteins; metabolized in liver to active metabolite, excreted mainly in bile; $t_{1/2}$ 3 hr

INDICATIONS AND USES: All forms of tuberculosis (in combination with at least 1 other antituberculosis drug), asymptomatic *Neisseria meningitidis* carriers, prophylaxis of meningitis due to *Hemophilus influenzae,** infections caused by *Staphylococcus aureus* and *S. epider-*

---

midis,* Legionella when not responsive to erythromycin,* leprosy (in combination with dapsone)*

Antibacterial spectrum usually includes: *Mycobacterium tuberculosis, M. bovis, M. marinum, M. kansasii;* some strains of *M. fortuitum, M. avium,* and *M. intracellulare; Staphylococcus aureus, Hemophilus influenzae, Legionella pneumophilia*

DOSAGE

Adult

• *Tuberculosis:* PO/IV 600 mg in a single daily dose for 6-9 mo (in combination with at least 1 other antituberculosis agent)

• *Meningococcal carriers:* PO 600 mg bid for 2 days

• *H. influenzae prophylaxis:* PO 600 mg q24h for 4 days

Child

• *Tuberculosis:* PO/IV 10-20 mg/kg, not to exceed 600 mg/day

• *Meningococcal carriers:* PO (>1 mo) 10 mg/kg q12h for 2 days; (<1 mo) 5 mg/kg q12h for 2 days

• *H. influenzae prophylaxis:* PO (<1 mo) 10 mg/kg q24h for 4 days; (>1 month) 20 mg/kg q24h for 4 days; do not exceed 600 mg/dose

💲 AVAILABLE FORMS/COST OF THERAPY

• Cap, Gel—Oral: 150 mg, 30's: **$40.23**; 300 mg, 100's: **$134.10-$233.20**

• Inj, Sol—IV: 600 mg/vial, 1's: **$77.50**

CONTRAINDICATIONS: Hypersensitivity to rifamycins

PRECAUTIONS: Hepatic dysfunction, porphyria, avoid extravasation

PREGNANCY AND LACTATION: Pregnancy category C; compatible with breast feeding

SIDE EFFECTS/ADVERSE REACTIONS

CNS: Ataxia, behavioral changes, confusion, dizziness, drowsiness, fatigue, fever, headache

EENT: Visual disturbances

GI: Abnormal liver function tests, anorexia, cramps, diarrhea, epigastric distress, flatulence, heartburn, hepatitis, jaundice, nausea, **pseudomembranous colitis,** vomiting

GU: **Acute renal failure,** elevations in BUN, hematuria, hemoglobinuria, hemolysis, interstitial nephritis, menstrual disturbances, renal insufficiency

HEME: Eosinophilia, **hemolytic anemia, thrombocytopenia, transient leukopenia**

MS: Generalized numbness, muscular weakness, pains in extremities

SKIN: Pemphigoid reaction, pruritus, rash, urticaria

MISC: "Flu" syndrome (fever, chills, headache, dizziness, bone pain)

INTERACTIONS

Drugs

🛂 *Acetaminophen:* Enhanced hepatotoxicity (overdoses and possibly large therapeutic doses)

🛂 *Aminosalicylic acid:* Reduced serum concentrations of rifampin

🛂 *Antidiabetics:* Diminished hypoglycemic activity of sulfonylureas

🛂 *Azole antifungals, barbiturates, benzodiazepines, beta-blockers (except nadolol), calcium channel blockers, chloramphenicol, clofibrate, cyclic antidepressants, dapsone, digitalis glycosides, disopyramide, lorcainide, methadone, mexiletine, nortriptyline, phenytoin, pirmenol, propafenone, quinidine, tocainide, theophylline, zidovudine:* Reduced serum concentrations of these drugs

🛂 *Corticosteroids:* Reduced effect of corticosteroids

---

* = non-FDA-approved use

❷ *Cyclosporine, tacrolimus:* Reduced concentrations of these drugs, possible therapeutic failure

❸ *Isoniazid:* Increased hepatotoxic potential of isoniazid in slow acetylators or patients with pre-existing liver disease

❷ *Oral anticoagulants:* Reduced hypoprothrombinemic effect of oral anticoagulants

❸ *Oral contraceptives:* Menstrual irregularities, contraceptive failure

❷ *Protease inhibitors:* Increased clearance (CYP3A4 induction) and decreased protease inhibitor efficacy

❸ *Thyroid:* Increased elimination, increased thyroid requirements

Labs
• *Increase:* Liver function tests, uric acid
• *Interference:* Folate, vitamin B$_{12}$, BSP, gallbladder studies
• *False decrease:* Serum bilirubin, ALT, AST (by some methods), cholesterol, triglycerides
• *False increase:* Serum bilirubin (some methods, may also be true physiologic increase), glucose, iron, LDH, uric acid, metronidazole, phosphate, tetracycline, trimethoprim
• *False positive:* Clindamycin, erythromycin, polymyxin

SPECIAL CONSIDERATIONS
PATIENT/FAMILY EDUCATION
• Take on empty stomach, at least 1 hr before or 2 hr after meals
• May cause reddish-orange discoloration of bodily secretions, may permanently discolor soft contact lenses

MONITORING PARAMETERS
• Liver function tests at baseline and q2-4 wk during therapy
• CBC with differential and platelets at baseline and periodically throughout treatment

rifapentine
(rif-a-pen′-teen)
Rx: Priftin
Chemical Class: Semisynthetic rifamycin B derivative
Therapeutic Class: Antituberculous agent

CLINICAL PHARMACOLOGY
Mechanism of Action: Suppresses initiation of chain formation for RNA synthesis in susceptible bacteria by inhibiting DNA-dependent RNA polymerase; bactericidal for intracellular and extracellular *M. tuberculosis* organisms

Pharmacokinetics
PO: Peak 5 hr; 70% bioavailable, increased by food; 93%-98% protein bound; metabolized by liver to active metabolite, 25-desacetyl rifapentine; metabolites excreted in stool (70%) and urine (17%); t$_{1/2}$ 13 hr; crosses placenta

INDICATIONS AND USES: Pulmonary tuberculosis (combination therapy)

DOSAGE
Adult and Child >16 yr
• PO 600 mg twice weekly with at least 72 hr between doses. After 2 mo, selected patients (e.g., clinically stable, adherent, and not HIV coinfected) may go to weekly dosing

⑧ AVAILABLE FORMS/COST OF THERAPY
• Tab, Coated—Oral: 150 mg, 32's: **$87.96**

CONTRAINDICATIONS: Hypersensitivity to any rifamycin (rifampin, rifabutin)

PRECAUTIONS: Alcoholism, liver disease, pregnancy (bleeding disorders in mother and newborn when taken in late pregnancy)

PREGNANCY AND LACTATION: Pregnancy category C (teratogenic in rats); excreted in breast milk, but compatible with breast feeding

SIDE EFFECTS/ADVERSE REACTIONS

CNS: Anorexia, headache, dizziness

CV: Hypertension

GI: Diarrhea, dyspepsia, *increased transaminases (20%), nausea, vomiting*

GU: Hematuria (13%), proteinuria (17%), pyuria, urinary casts

HEME: **Anemia, lymphopenia (16%), neutropenia (18%), thrombocytopenia**

MS: Arthralgia (9%)

SKIN: Rash (13%)

INTERACTIONS

Drugs

3 *Acetaminophen:* Enhanced hepatotoxicity

3 *Aminosalicylic acid:* Reduced plasma concentrations of rifapentine

3 *Azole antifungals, barbiturates, benzodiazepines, beta-blockers, calcium channel blockers, chloramphenicol, clofibrate, cyclic antidepressants, dapsone, digitalis glycosides, disopyramide, lorcainide, methadone, mexiletine, phenytoin, pirmenol, propafenone, quinidine, tocainide, theophylline, zidovudine:* Reduced plasma concentrations of these drugs

3 *Corticosteroids:* Reduced effect of corticosteroids

2 *Cyclosporine:* Reduced plasma concentration of cyclosporine

3 *Isoniazid:* Increased hepatotoxic potential of isoniazid in slow acetylators or patients with preexisting liver disease

3 *Oral contraceptives:* Reduced plasma levels of these drugs with menstrual irregularity and contraceptive failure

2 *Protease inhibitors:* Increased clearance and decreased protease inhibitor efficacy

3 *Sulfonylureas:* Diminished hypoglycemic activity of sulfonylureas

2 *Tacrolimus:* Reduced plasma concentration of tacrolimus

3 *Thyroid:* Increased clearance of thyroid hormone with increased dose requirement

2 *Warfarin:* Reduced hypoprothrombinemic effect of warfarin

Labs

• *Interference:* Folate and vitamin B_{12} levels by microbiologic assay

SPECIAL CONSIDERATIONS

PATIENT/FAMILY EDUCATION

• Use an alternative method of contraception if taking oral contraceptives concurrently

• Avoid alcoholic beverages concurrently with this medication

• Rifapentine causes urine, stool, saliva, sputum, sweat, and tears to turn reddish-orange to reddish-brown and may also permanently discolor soft contact lenses; avoid wearing soft contact lenses

MONITORING PARAMETERS

• ALT, AST, alkaline phosphate, bilirubin, and CBC prior to treatment and monthly during treatment

---

riluzole

(rye´loo-zole)

Rx: Rilutek

Chemical Class: Benzothiazole derivative

Therapeutic Class: Amyotrophic lateral sclerosis (ALS) agent

CLINICAL PHARMACOLOGY

Mechanism of Action: Mode of action unknown, but may involve an inhibitory effect on glutamate release, inactivation of voltage-dependent sodium channels, and the ability to interfere with intracellular events that follow transmitter binding at excitatory amino acid receptors

Pharmacokinetics

PO: Bioavailability 60%, reduced by high-fat meal; 96% bound to plasma proteins; extensively metabolized (some metabolites active) by liver, excreted mainly in urine (90%) and feces (5%); $t_{1/2}$ 12 hr

INDICATIONS AND USES: Amyotrophic lateral sclerosis (ALS; Lou Gehrig's disease); extends survival and/or time to tracheostomy

DOSAGE

Adult

• PO 50 mg q12h on an empty stomach

$ AVAILABLE FORMS/COST OF THERAPY

• Tab—Oral: 50 mg, 60's: **$899.72**

PRECAUTIONS: Abnormal liver function, renal insufficiency, elderly

PREGNANCY AND LACTATION: Pregnancy category C; excretion into breast milk unknown, use caution in nursing mothers

SIDE EFFECTS/ADVERSE REACTIONS

CNS: Asthenia, circumoral paresthesia, *dizziness, headache,* malaise, somnolence

CV: Hypertension, peripheral edema, phlebitis, postural hypotension

EENT: Vertigo

GI: Abdominal pain, anorexia, diarrhea, dyspepsia, flatulence, *nausea,* oral moniliasis, stomatitis, tooth disorder, vomiting, AST/ALT elevation

HEME: Anemia, **neutropenia**

GU: Dysuria

MS: Arthralgia, back pain

RESP: Decreased lung function, increased cough, *rhinitis*

SKIN: Alopecia, eczema, **exfoliative dermatitis,** pruritus

INTERACTIONS

Drugs

3 *Caffeine, theophylline, amitriptyline, quinolones (CYP1A2 inhibitors):* Possible decreased riluzole elimination

3 *Cigarette smoking, rifampin, omeprazole (CYP1A2 inducers):* Possible increased riluzole elimination

SPECIAL CONSIDERATIONS

MONITORING PARAMETERS

• ALT, AST qmo for 3 mo, q3mo for 1 yr, then periodically thereafter; discontinue treatment if ALT or AST increases to >5 times upper limit of normal

---

rimantadine

(ri-man'ti-deen)

Rx: Flumadine

Chemical Class: Substituted amine

Therapeutic Class: Antiviral agent

CLINICAL PHARMACOLOGY

Mechanism of Action: Inhibits growth of influenza A virus, possibly by inhibiting the uncoating of the virus

Pharmacokinetics

PO: Onset 3 hr; peak 5-7 hr; 40% protein bound; metabolized by liver ($t_{1/2}$ doubled in severe hepatic dysfunction), 25% of dose excreted in urine as unchanged drug; $t_{1/2}$ 19-31 hr (20-48 hr if age >70 yr)

INDICATIONS AND USES: Prevention and treatment (within 48 hr of onset of illness) of influenza A

R

DOSAGE

Adult

• *Prevention:* PO 100 mg bid; if age >65 yr or with severe hepatic or renal dysfunction (CrCl ≤10 ml/min), reduce dose to 100 mg qd

• *Treatment:* PO 100 mg bid; if age >65 yr or with severe hepatic or renal dysfunction (CrCl ≤10 ml/min), reduce dose to 100 mg qd

Child

• *Prevention:* Age >10 yr, PO 100 mg bid; age <10 yr, 5 mg/kg qd as single dose (max dose 150 mg)

$ AVAILABLE FORMS/COST OF THERAPY

• Syr—Oral: 50 mg/5 ml, 240 ml: **$41.58**

• Tab, Plain Coated—Oral: 100 mg, 100's: **$183.16-$212.23**

CONTRAINDICATIONS: Hypersensitivity to amantadine

PRECAUTIONS: Lactation

PREGNANCY AND LACTATION: Pregnancy category C; concentrated in breast milk

SIDE EFFECTS/ADVERSE REACTIONS

CNS: Asthenia, ataxia, depression, dizziness, insomnia, tremor

CV: Hypertension

GI: Abdominal pain, anorexia, constipation, diarrhea, nausea, vomiting

RESP: Bronchospasm, cough

SKIN: Rash

INTERACTIONS

Drugs

3 *Triamterene:* Increased concentrations, toxicity rimantadine

3 *Trihexyphenidyl:* Increased CNS effects

SPECIAL CONSIDERATIONS

PRECAUTIONS

• Resistant strains may develop during treatment (10%-30%)

---

risedronate

(rye-se-droe'nate)

Rx: Actonel

Chemical Class: Synthetic analog of pyrophosphate

Therapeutic Class: Bisphosphonate; bone resorption inhibitor

CLINICAL PHARMACOLOGY

Mechanism of Action: Binds to hydroxyapatite at sites of bone resorption, inhibiting normal and abnormal bone resorption ("crystal poison"); minimal secondary reduction in bone formation (resorption coupled to formation)

Pharmacokinetics

PO: Peak 1 hr; (A significant decrease in, or normalization of, serum calcium has been reported after one week of oral risedronate administration in patients with primary hyperparathyroidism); poor PO absorption (1%); food reduces absorption further 50%; 60% bound to bone in 12-24 hr; not metabolized; remainder excreted in urine; $t_{1/2}$, 220 hr (representing dissociation of risedronate from bone surface)

INDICATIONS AND USES: Paget's disease, hyperparathyroidism,* hypercalcemia of malignancy,* osteoporosis,* osteoporosis—glucocorticoid induced*

DOSAGE

Adult and Child >16 yr

• Paget's Disease: PO 30 mg qd × 2 months

• Osteoporosis (prophylaxis): PO 2.5-5 mg qd

• Postmenopausal osteoporosis (treatment): PO 35 mg q wk

• Primary hyperparathyroidism: PO 20 mg qd

---

* = non-FDA-approved use

• Tab, Coated—Oral: 5 mg, 30's: **$67.32**; 30 mg, 30's: **$474.65**

CONTRAINDICATIONS: Hypocalcemia

PRECAUTIONS: Renal impairment, congestive heart failure, hyperphosphatemia (potential for increased tubular reabsorption of phosphate), liver disease, fever

PREGNANCY AND LACTATION: Pregnancy category C; breast milk excretion unknown

SIDE EFFECTS/ADVERSE REACTIONS

CV: Chest pain
EENT: Iritis, dry eyes
GI: Diarrhea (20%); epigastric pain (rarely)
MS: Arthralgias, myesthenia

INTERACTIONS

Drugs

3 *Antacids, calcium:* decreased absorption of risedronate

3 *Food:* decreases bioavailability of risedronate by 50%

SPECIAL CONSIDERATIONS
PATIENT/FAMILY EDUCATION
• Administer 30 minutes before the first food/beverage/medication of the day, with 6-8 oz plain water

MONITORING PARAMETERS
• Albumin-adjusted serum calcium; N-telopeptide, alkaline phosphatase, phosphorus, osteocalcin, DEXA scan, bone and joint pain, fractures on x-ray (osteoporosis, Paget's disease)

risperidone
(ris-per'i-done)
Rx: Risperdal
Chemical Class: Benzisoxazole derivative
Therapeutic Class: Antipsychotic

CLINICAL PHARMACOLOGY
Mechanism of Action: Serotonin 5-HT$_2$ >dopamine-(D$_2$-) receptor antagonist; activity against several neurotransmitter systems: selective antagonist at limbic dopamine receptors (D$_1$, D$_2$, D$_4$, D$_5$) and serotonin receptors (5-HT$_2$, 5-HT$_6$, 5-HT$_7$); antagonism at α_1-adrenergic receptors; and activity at muscarinic, histamine H$_1$, or nicotinic receptors; minimal sedation, orthostatic hypotension, and weight gain; no anticholinergic effects; mild to moderate extrapyramidal symptoms (at higher doses, i.e., >10 mg) extrapyramidal reaction risk becomes similar to typical antipsychotics

Pharmacokinetics
PO: Peak level 1 hr; metabolized by liver to active metabolite, 9-hydroxyrisperidone (8% of Caucasians are poor metabolizers); mean elimination t$_{1/2}$ of total risperidone and 9-hydroxyrisperidone 20 hr; excreted in urine and feces; protein binding 85%

INDICATIONS AND USES: Psychotic disorders

DOSAGE
Adult
• PO: 1 mg bid, increase to 2 mg bid on 2nd day and 3 mg bid on 3rd day, then increase weekly as needed (usual effective dose 4-8 mg daily; max daily dose 16 mg; can be dosed either qd or bid); initial dose 0.5 mg

bid increasing to 1.5 mg bid by 3rd day in elderly or those with severe renal or hepatic impairment

$ AVAILABLE FORMS/COST OF THERAPY

• Sol—Oral: 1 mg/ml, 100 ml: **$273.16**

• Tab, Coated—Oral: 0.25 mg, 60's: **$152.00**; 0.5 mg, 60's: **$174.24**; 1 mg, 60's: **$174.24**; 2 mg, 60's: **$256.53**; 3 mg, 60's: **$342.48**; 4 mg, 60's: **$438.15**

PRECAUTIONS: Neuroleptic malignant syndrome, tardive dyskinesia, prolonged QT interval, seizures

PREGNANCY AND LACTATION: Pregnancy category C; excreted in breast milk

SIDE EFFECTS/ADVERSE REACTIONS

CNS: Aggressive reaction, *anxiety, decreased libido,* dizziness, *EPS (frequency is dose related), increased dream activity,* insomnia, *somnolence*

CV: Orthostatic hypotension, tachycardia

EENT: Abnormal vision (accommodation), *dry mouth*

GI: Abdominal pain, *constipation, dyspepsia,* nausea, vomiting

GU: Menorrhagia, polyuria, sexual (erectile and orgasmic) dysfunction, urinary retention, *vaginal dryness*

HEME: Anemia

METAB: Amenorrhea, galactorrhea, gynecomastia, hyponatremia

MS: Arthralgia, back pain, chest pain

RESP: Cough, dyspnea, pharyngitis, *rhinitis,* sinusitis

SKIN: Dry skin, *increased pigmentation, photosensitivity,* rash, seborrhea

MISC: Fatigue, fever

INTERACTIONS

Drugs

3 *Levodopa, dopamine agonists:* Risperidone may antagonize effect

SPECIAL CONSIDERATIONS

PATIENT/FAMILY EDUCATION

• Risk of orthostatic hypotension, especially during the period of initial dose titration

• Do not operate machinery during dose titration period

---

ritonavir

(ri-tone′a-veer)

Rx: Norvir

Chemical Class: HIV Protease inhibitor

Therapeutic Class: HIV infection

CLINICAL PHARMACOLOGY

Mechanism of Action: Protease inhibitor of HIV; antiretroviral effects via interference with protease enzyme processing of Gag-Pol polyproteins, resulting in budding of immature noninfectious particles; inhibits both acutely and chronically infected cells

Pharmacokinetics

PO: Peak levels at 2-4 hr (>2 μg/ml at doses of 800 mg/day— *in vivo* effective vs. HIV-1); well absorbed; metabolized by CYP3A (primary) and CYP2D6 (minor); $t_{1/2}$ 3.5 hr; 98-99% protein bound

INDICATIONS AND USES: In combination with other antiretroviral agents for the treatment of HIV infection

DOSAGE

Adult

• *HIV infection:* PO 600 mg bid in combination with nucleoside analogues (to reduce nausea at initiation of therapy, prescribe 300 mg bid for 1 day, 400 mg bid for 2 days, 500 mg bid for 1 day, and finally 600 mg bid thereafter)

• Adjust dose when used with indinavir, nelfinavir, saquinavir

---

* = non-FDA-approved use

Child

• *HIV infection:* PO 400 mg/m^2 not to exceed 600 mg bid; start at 250 mg/m^2 and increase every 2-3 days by 50 mg/m^2 twice daily. If 400 mg/m^2 is not tolerated, the highest tolerated dose should be used for maintenance in combination with nucleoside analogues

• For latest treatment guidelines, see www.hivatis.org

💲 AVAILABLE FORMS/COST OF THERAPY

• Cap—Oral: 100 mg, 120's: **$257.17**
• Sol—Oral: 80 mg/ml, 240 ml: **$335.14**

PRECAUTIONS: Liver disease, hypertriglyceridemia, diabetes mellitus, hemophilia type A and B

PREGNANCY AND LACTATION: Pregnancy category B; breast milk excretion unknown; breast feeding by HIV+ mothers not recommended

SIDE EFFECTS/ADVERSE REACTIONS

CNS: Abnormal dreams, *abnormal thinking,* agitation, amnesia, anxiety, aphasia, *asthenia (9%-14%),* ataxia, *circumoral paresthesia (15%),* confusion, convulsion, depression, diplopia, *dizziness,* euphoria, hallucinations, *headache,* hyperesthesia, incoordination, *insomnia, malaise,* nervousness, neuralgia, neuropathy, paralysis, personality disorder, peripheral neuropathy, *peripheral paresthesia (6%), somnolence,* tremor, vertigo

CV: Hemorrhage, hypotension, migraine, orthostatic hypotension, palpitations, peripheral vascular disorder, syncope, tachycardia, *vasodilation (2%)*

EENT: Abnormal electro-oculogram, abnormal electroretinogram, abnormal vision, blurred vision, blepharitis, eye pain, iritis, photophobia, uveitis, visual field defect

GI: Abdominal pain (7%), anorexia (6%), cheilitis, colitis, constipation, *diarrhea (12%-18%),* dry mouth, dyspepsia, dysphagia, elevations in liver transaminases (2%-15%), eructation, esophagitis, flatulence, gastritis, gastroenteritis, GI bleeding, gingivitis, hepatitis, hepatomegaly, ileitis, local throat irritation, *nausea (23%-26%),* oral candidiasis, pancreatitis, periodontal disease, *taste perversion (5%-10%), vomiting (12%-15%)*

GU: Decreased libido, dysuria, hematuria, impotence, kidney calculus, kidney failure, kidney pain, nocturia, polyuria, pyelonephritis, urethritis, urinary frequency, urinary retention

HEME: Anemia, ecchymosis, leukopenia, lymphadenophaty, lymphocytosis, thrombocytopenia

METAB: Avitaminosis, chills, dehydration, diabetes mellitus, edema, fever, gout, glycosuria, hypercholesterolemia, hyperlipidemia, hypothermia, increased phosphokinase, increased serum cholesterol, peripheral edema, sweating, thirst, triglycerides, weight loss

MS: Arthralgia, arthrosis, joint disorder, muscle cramps, muscle weakness, *myalgia,* myositis, twitching

RESP: Asthma, cough, dyspnea, epistaxis, hiccup, hypoventilation, interstitial pneumonia, *pharyngitis,* rhinitis

SKIN: Acne, contact dermatitis, dry skin, eczema, folliculitis, maculopapular rash, molluscum contagiosum, pruritus, psoriasis, *rash,* seborrhea, urticaria, vesiculobullous rash

R

---

italic = common side effects   **bold italic** = life-threatening reactions

INTERACTIONS
Drugs

▲ *Amiodarone:* Increased plasma levels of amiodarone

❷ *Atorvastatin:* Increased risk of myopathy possible

▲ *Astemizole:* Increased plasma levels of astemizole

❸ *Barbiturates:* Increased clearance of ritonavir; reduced clearance of barbiturates

▲ *Bepredil:* Increased plasma levels of bepredil

▲ *Bupropion:* Increased plasma levels of bupropion

❷ *Carbamazepine:* Increased clearance of ritonavir; reduced clearance of carbamazepine

❷ *Cerivastatin:* Increased risk of myopathy possible

▲ *Cisapride:* Increased plasma levels of cisapride

❷ *Clarithromycin:* Reduced clearance of ritonavir; ritonavir reduces clearance of clarithromycin; reduce clarithromycin dose for renal insufficiency

▲ *Clorazepate:* Increased plasma levels of clorazepate

▲ *Clozapine:* Increased plasma levels of clozapine

❸ *Despiramine:* Ritonavir increases AUC of desipramine by 145%

▲ *Diazepam:* Increased plasma levels of diazepam

❸ *Didanosine:* Separate dosing by 2.5 hr to avoid formulation incompatibility

❷ *Disulfiram:* Ritonavir (gel capsules and solution) contain ethanol; disulfiram-like reaction possible

▲ *Encainide:* Increased plasma levels of encainide

▲ *Ergot alkaloids:* Increased plasma levels of ergot alkaloids

❸ *Erythromycin:* Reduced clearance of ritonavir; ritonavir reduces clearance of erythromycin

▲ *Estazolam:* Increases plasma levels of estazolam

▲ *Flecainide:* Increased plasma levels of flecainide

▲ *Flurazepam:* Increased plasma levels of flurazepam

❸ *Indinavir:* Increased plasma level of indinavir; reduce dose to 400 mg bid when ritonavir dose is 400 mg bid

❸ *Ketoconazole:* Ritonavir reduces clearance of ketoconazole; reduce ketoconazole dose

▲ *Lovastatin:* Ritonavir reduces clearance of lovastatin

▲ *Meperidine:* Increased plasma levels of of normeperidine which has analgesic and CNS stimulant activity (seizures)

❸ *Methadone:* Ritonavir reduces methadone plasma concentration by 37%

❷ *Metronidazole:* Ritonavir (gel capsules and solution) contain ethanol; disulfiram-like reaction possible

▲ *Midazolam:* Increased plasma levels of midazolam and prolonged effect

❸ *Nelfinavir:* Increased plasma level of nelfinavir; reduce nelfinavir dose to 750 mg bid when ritonavir dose is 400 mg bid

❸ *Oral contraceptives:* Ritonavir may reduce efficacy

❸ *Phenytoin:* Increased clearance of ritonavir; reduced clearance of phenytoin

▲ *Pimozide:* Increased plasma levels of pimozide

▲ *Piroxicam:* Increased plasma levels of piroxicam

▲ *Propafenone:* Increased plasma levels of propafenone

▲ *Propoxyphene:* Increased plasma levels of propoxyphene

▲ *Quinidine:* Increased plasma levels of quinidine

---

* = non-FDA-approved use

❷ *Rifabutin:* Increased clearance of ritonavir; reduced clearance of rifabutin; reduce rifabutin dose to 150 mg qod

❸ *Rifampin:* Increased clearance of ritonavir

▲ *St. John's wort (hypericum perforatum):* Substantial decrease in plasma ritonavir concentrations with loss of virologic response

❸ *Saquinavir:* Decreased clearance of saquinavir; reduce dose of saquinavir (Fortovase or Invirase) to 400 bid with ritonavir 400 mg bid

❷ *Sildenafil:* Substantial increases in serum sildenafil concentrations

▲ *Simvastatin:* Ritonavir reduces clearance of simvastatin

▲ *Terfenadine:* Increased plasma levels of terfenadine

❸ *Theophylline:* Ritonavir reduces theophylline plasma concentration

▲ *Triazolam:* Increased plasma levels of triazolam and prolonged effect

❸ *Troleandomycin:* Reduced clearance of ritonavir; ritonavir reduces clearance of troleandomycin

❸ *Warfarin:* Decreased plasma warfarin concentrations

▲ *Zolpidem:* Increased plasma levels of zolpidem

SPECIAL CONSIDERATIONS

• As with other protease inhibitors, ritonavir will predominantly be used in combination regimens; the ability of ritonavir (alone or in combinations) to modify clinical endpoints (e.g., time to 1st AIDS-defining illness or death) will be important in determining the ultimate role of this agent in HIV; potential for drug interaction is troublesome; as with other protease inhibitors, resistance has been problematic after several mo of treatment

PATIENT/FAMILY EDUCATION

• Store capsules in the refrigerator until dispensed; refrigeration of capsules by patient not required if used within 30 days and stored below 77°F; store oral solution at room temperature, do not refrigerate, shake well; avoid exposure to excessive heat

• Take with food

MONITORING PARAMETERS

• Therapeutic: serum HIV-1 RNA, and CD4+ cell counts (every 2-4 wk)

• Toxicity: complete blood counts, routine blood chemistry, liver function tests, and serum lipid and lipoprotein profiles

---

rivastigmine

(riv-a-stig′meen)

Rx: Exelon

Chemical Class: Carbamate derivative

Therapeutic Class: Acetyl cholinesterase inhibitor

CLINICAL PHARMACOLOGY

Mechanism of Action: Increases the concentration of available acetylcholine via reversible inhibition of cholinesterase, thus improving the neuronal function of the basal forebrain, cerebral cortex, and hippocampus, all of which are involved in memory, attention learning, and other cognitive processes; no evidence that the drug alters the course of the underlying dementing process

Pharmacokinetics

PO: Peak concentration 1 hr; linear pharmacokinetics up to 3 mg bid; non-linear at higher doses; rapidly and completely absorbed (PO bioavailability 40%), administration with food delays T_{max} (90 min), lowers C_{max} (30%) and increases AUC

---

italic = common side effects　　　　**bold italic** = life-threatening reactions

(30%); widely distributed, including penetration of the blood brain barrier, 40% bound to plasma proteins; extensively metabolized by liver (not involving cytochrome P-450 systems), primarily to decarbamylated metabolite); excreted renally, 97% in urine, 0.4% in feces in 120 hr; t$_{1/2}$ 1.5 hr

INDICATIONS AND USES: Mild to moderate dementia of the Alzheimer's type, dementia with Lewy bodies*

DOSAGE

Adult

• 3-6 mg bid (higher doses tend to be more beneficial); initial dose 1.5 mg bid, with 3 mg/day increases q2wk, if tolerated (i.e., revert back to last tolerated dose in the event of nausea, vomiting, abdominal pain, loss of appetite); note: if treatment interrupted for more than several days, treatment should be reinitiated with the lowest daily dose and retitrated as above

• Both renal and hepatic dysfunction increase rivastigmine blood levels significantly; however, because dosage titrated to tolerance individually, dosage alteration is not necessary

§ AVAILABLE FORMS/COST OF THERAPY

• Cap—Oral: 1.5, 3, 4.5, 6 mg, 60's (all): **$139.73**
• Liq—Oral: 2 mg/ml, 120 ml dispenser bottle: **$257.25**

CONTRAINDICATIONS: Hypersensitivity

PRECAUTIONS: Peptic ulcers/gastrointestinal bleeding, anesthesia (see succinylcholine, Drug Interactions), cardiovascular conditions, conditions predisposing to urinary obstruction, history of seizures, asthma, obstructive pulmonary disease

PREGNANCY AND LACTATION: Pregnancy category B; excretion into human breast milk unknown

SIDE EFFECTS/ADVERSE REACTIONS

CNS: Ataxia, confusion, dizziness, abnormal gait, headache, paranoid reactions, paresthesia, seizures, syncope

CV: Atrial fibrillation, bradycardia, cardiac failure, edema, hypotension, palpitation, postural hypotension, vagotonic effects

EENT: Cataract, epistaxis, tinnitus

GI: Abdominal pain, *anorexia (17%)*, fecal incontinence, gastritis, *nausea (47%), vomiting (14%), weight loss (26%)*

HEME: Anemia

MS: Arthritis, leg cramps, myalgia, tremor

RESP: Allergy

SKIN: Rash (maculopapular, eczema, bullous, exfoliative, psoriaform, erythematous), sweating

METAB: Dehydration, hypokalemia

MISC: Asthenia, fatigue, fever, hot flushes, influenza-like symptom, malaise

INTERACTIONS

Drugs

3 *Anticholinergic drugs:* Interference with anticholinergic activity

3 *Cholinomimetics (cholinergics and other cholinesterase inhibitors i.e., bethanechol and succinylcholine):* Potential synergistic effects

3 *Clozapine:* Antagonistic effect on cholinesterase inhibitor activity

3 *Inhaled anesthetics:* Decreased neuromuscular blocking effects

3 *Local anesthetics:* Increased risk of local anesthetic toxicity (pseudocholinesterase competition)

3 *Neuromuscular blockers, nondepolarizing:* Antagonistic effects, reversal of neuromuscular blockade

---

* = non-FDA-approved use

SPECIAL CONSIDERATIONS
PATIENT/FAMILY EDUCATION
• Patient and caregiver should be advised of high incidence of gastrointestinal effects and directions for resource and resolution

MONITORING PARAMETERS
• Cognitive function (e.g., ADAS, Mini-Mental Status Exam (MMSE)), activities of daily living, global functioning, blood chemistry, complete blood counts, heart rate, blood pressure

---

rizatriptan
(rize-a-trip'tan)
Rx: Maxalt; Maxalt MLT
Chemical Class: Serotonin derivative
Therapeutic Class: Antimigraine agent

CLINICAL PHARMACOLOGY
Mechanism of Action: Selectively activates vascular 5-HT$_1$-receptors in cranial arteries causing vasoconstriction and inhibition of proinflammatory neuropeptide release, actions correlating with the relief of migraine in humans

Pharmacokinetics
PO: 45% bioavailability, peak 1-1.5 hr

MLT: (orally disintegrating tablet): Peak 1.6-2.5 hr 14% bound to plasma proteins; metabolism mainly via oxidative deamination by MAO-A; 82% excreted in urine (14% unchanged), 12% in feces; t$_{1/2}$ 2-3 hr

INDICATIONS AND USES: Acute migraine headache with or without aura

DOSAGE
Adult
• PO 5-10 mg at first sign of headache; may repeat after 2 hr if partial response or headache returns (max 30 mg/24 hr)

💲 AVAILABLE FORMS/COST OF THERAPY
• Tab—Oral: 5 mg, 10 mg, 6's: **$96.99**
• Tab, Orally Disintigrating—Oral: 5 mg, 10 mg, 6's: **$96.98**

CONTRAINDICATIONS: Ischemic heart disease; hemiplegic or basilar migraine; Prinzmetal's angina; uncontrolled hypertension; within 24 hr of ergotamine-containing products or other 5-HT$_1$-receptor agonist; concurrent use of MAO inhibitor therapy (or within 2 wk of discontinuing an MAO inhibitor)

PRECAUTIONS: Atypical headache; dialysis patients or hepatic impairment; elderly; children; phenylketonuric patients (MLT formulation contains phenylalanine)

PREGNANCY AND LACTATION: Pregnancy category C; use caution in nursing mothers

SIDE EFFECTS/ADVERSE REACTIONS
CNS: Paresthesia, dizziness, fatigue, drowsiness, vertigo, tremors, cognitive function disorders, sleep disorders, equilibrium disorders

CV: Palpitations, increased blood pressure, tachyarrhythmias, abnormal ECG, syncope

EENT: Photophobia, blurred vision, tinnitus

GI: Nausea, hyposalivation, vomiting, dyspeptic symptoms, diarrhea, constipation

GU: Bladder inflammation, polyuria, diuresis

HEME: Increased white cells

METAB: Thirst, polydipsia, dehydration, fluid retention

R

---

italic = common side effects   **bold italic** = life-threatening reactions

MS: Muscle pain, arthralgia, articular rheumatism, muscle cramps/spasms, joint/muscle stiffness, tightness, rigidity

RESP: Bronchitis, cough, pneumonia

SKIN: Sweating, rash, pruritus, urticaria

MISC: Pain/pressure sensations in neck/throat/jaw; chills, fever

INTERACTIONS
Drugs

⚠ *Ergotamine-containing drugs:* Increased vasoconstriction

⚠ *MAO inhibitors:* Potential for decreased metabolism of rizatriptan

3 *Propranolol:* Propranolol has been shown to increase the plasma concentrations of rizatriptan by 70%; patients receiving propranolol should use 5 mg tablets (max 15 mg/24 hr)

2 *Sibutramine:* Increased risk of serotonin syndrome

SPECIAL CONSIDERATIONS
• Safety of treating, on average, more than 4 headaches in a 30-day period has not been established

• MLT does not provide faster absorption or onset of effect because almost the entire dose is swallowed with saliva and absorbed in the GI tract

PATIENT/FAMILY EDUCATION
• Use only to treat migraine headache, not for prevention

• MLT, administration with liquid is not necessary; orally disintegrating tablet is packaged in a blister within an outer aluminum pouch, do not remove the blister from the outer pouch until just prior to dosing; blister pack should then be peeled open with dry hands and the orally disintegrating tablet placed on the tongue, where it will dissolve and be swallowed with the saliva

---

rofecoxib
(ro-fe-coks'ib)
Rx: Vioxx
Chemical Class: Cyclooxygenase-2 (COX-2) inhibitor
Therapeutic Class: Nonsteroidal antiinflammatory drug (COX-2 specific inhibitor)

CLINICAL PHARMACOLOGY
Mechanism of Action: Inhibition of prostaglandin synthesis, via inhibition of cyclooxygenase-2 (COX-2) provides nonsteroidal antiinflammatory, analgesic, and antipyretic; at therapeutic concentrations, does not inhibit the cyclooxygenase-1 (COX-1) isoenzyme

Pharmacokinetics

PO: C_{max} 3286 ng/ml
Well absorbed (PO), food effect only on T_{max} (1.2 hr delay), bioavailability 93%; tablets and oral suspension bioequivalent; 87% plasma protein bound; Vd 91 L; metabolized primarily by hepatic reduction by cytosolic enzymes with a minor contribution from cytochrome P450 (CYP3A), major metabolites inactive, <1% recovered unchanged; 72% excreted in urine as metabolites; $t_{1/2}$ 17 hr; crosses placenta and blood-brain barrier in animals

INDICATIONS AND USES: Osteoarthritis, rheumatoid arthritis*, acute pain, primary dysmenorrhea

DOSAGE
Adult and Child >16 yr
• *Osteoarthritis:* 12.5 mg qd; max 25 mg qd
• *Acute pain, primary dysmenorrhea:* 50 mg qd for up to 5 days (with or without food)

---

* = non-FDA-approved use

$ AVAILABLE FORMS/COST OF THERAPY

• Liq—Oral: 12.5 mg/5 ml, 150 ml: **$122.61**; 25 mg/5 ml, 150 ml: **$122.61**
• Tab—Oral: 12.5 mg, 30's: **$275.19**; 25 mg, 30's: **$262.33**; 50 mg, 30's: **$383.13**

CONTRAINDICATIONS: Hypersensitivity, patients who have experienced asthma, urticaria or allergic-type reactions with aspirin or other NSAIDs (aspirin triad)

PRECAUTIONS: History of GI ulceration, concomitant treatment with oral corticosteroids, anticoagulants, smokers, alcoholism, older age, or poor general health status - increased risk for GI ulceration, bleeding or perforation; severe renal dysfunction; pregnancy (3rd trimester) - premature closure of patent ductus arteriosus; diminished utility of signs of fever and inflammation in detecting infectious complications; moderate to severe hepatic dysfunction; impaired renal function, heart failure, elderly, concomitant diuretics and ACE inhibitors; hypertension

PREGNANCY AND LACTATION: Pregnancy category C; (teratogenic and nonteratogenic effects in animals); decreases the diameter of the patent ductus arteriosus in animals; no adequate and controlled trials in humans; excreted into breast milk of animals

SIDE EFFECTS/ADVERSE REACTIONS

CNS: Asthenia, dizziness, fatigue, headache
CV: Fluid retention, edema
EENT: Upper respiratory infection, sinusitis
GI: Diarrhea, dyspepsia, epigastric discomfort, heart burn, nausea
GU: Papillary necrosis, renal failure, urinary tract infection
HEME: Anemia
MS: Back pain

INTERACTIONS

Drugs

3 *Angiotensin-converting enzyme inhibitors:* Diminished antihypertensive effects
3 *Aspirin:* Increased risk of GI ulceration; negation of cardioprotective effects of aspirin
3 *Diuretics (loop, thiazides):* Reduced naturetic effect
3 *Lithium:* Elevation of plasma lithium levels, potential lithium toxicity
3 *Rifampin:* 50% reduction of rofecoxib plasma concentrations
3 *Warfarin:* Slight increases (10%) in PT/INRs expected; monitor appropriately

Labs

• *Transaminases:* Elevations of ALT or AST (approximately 3 or more times the upper limit of normal)

SPECIAL CONSIDERATIONS

• May be safer than conventional nonsteroidal antiinflammatory agents, particularly with respect to gastrointestinal tolerability, and offer comparable efficacy; other complications may arise, including cardiovascular complications from selective inhibition of the COX isoenzyme

PATIENT/FAMILY EDUCATION

• Alertness for the signs and symptoms of adverse effects (e.g., GI ulceration and bleeding, renal dysfunction, hepatitis)

MONITORING PARAMETERS

• Decreased pain and stiffness of affected joints; decreased pain, cramps; baseline hemogram and fecal occult blood and routine monitoring every 6-12 months; serum electrolytes, BUN, serum creatinine, weight gain, edema, decreased urine output every 6-12 months;

R

AST, ALT, nausea, vomiting, right upper abdominal pain, anorexia, jaundice

---

ropinirole
(ro-pin′i-role)
Rx: ReQuip
Chemical Class: Propylaminobenzothiazole (non-ergoline)
Therapeutic Class: Antiparkinson agent, dopaminergic

CLINICAL PHARMACOLOGY
Mechanism of Action: Selective dopamine-2 (D2) receptor agonist
Pharmacokinetics
PO: Peak 1-2 hr; $t_{1/2}$ 3-4 hr
INDICATIONS AND USES: Parkinson's disease
DOSAGE
Adult
• *Parkinson's disease:* Slow initiation titration necessary; titration kit available from company; dose titration schedule: Week 1, 0.25 mg tid; week 2, 0.5 mg tid; week 3, 0.75 mg tid; week 4, 1 mg tid; then increase by 1.5 mg/day weekly to a total of 24 mg/day if necessary
§ AVAILABLE FORMS/COST OF THERAPY
• Tab—Oral: 0.25, 0.5, 1, 2, 100's: **$115.26**; 3, 4, 5 mg, 100's: **$215.73**
PRECAUTIONS: Cardiovascular disease, breast feeding, pregnancy
PREGNANCY AND LACTATION: Pregnancy category D; inhibits lactation
SIDE EFFECTS/ADVERSE REACTIONS
CNS: Drowsiness, euphoria, somnolence
CV: Bradycardia, postural hypotension, supraventricular ectopy (rare)
GI: Nausea

INTERACTIONS
Drugs
3 *Ciprofloxacin, enoxacin, pefloxacin:* Addition increases ropinirole concentrations
3 *Dopamine antagonists:* Diminished anti-Parkinson's effect
3 *Estrogens:* Reduced ropinirole clearance, may need to decrease ripinirole if estrogen stopped
SPECIAL CONSIDERATIONS
• Domperidone 20 mg 1 hr prior to ropinirole prevents drug-induced postural effects
• Discontinue slowly over 1 wk

---

rosiglitazone
(roz-ih-gli′ta-zone)
Rx: Avandia
Chemical Class: Thiazolidinedione
Therapeutic Class: Oral hypoglycemic; insulin resistance reducer

---

CLINICAL PHARMACOLOGY
Mechanism of Action: Potent and selective agonist for peroxisome proliferator-activated receptor-gamma (PPARγ) which regulate the control of glucose production, transport, and utilization as well as fatty acid metabolism; improves glycemic control and reduces circulating insulin levels via improving sensitivity to insulin in muscle and adipose tissue and inhibiting hepatic glyconeogenesis
Pharmacokinetics
PO: Peak 1 hr; well absorbed (PO), absolute bioavailability 99%; concomitant food reduces C_{max} 25% and delays T_{max} 1.75 hr - insignificant; 99.8% bound to plasma proteins; extensively metabolized by liver (CYP2C8, CYP2C9) with no

unchanged drug or significantly active metabolites available for urinary excretion

INDICATIONS AND USES: Monotherapy (adjunct to diet and exercise) or added to sulfonylurea or metformin in the treatment of diabetes mellitus, type 2; polycystic ovaries syndrome (PCOS)*

DOSAGE

Adult and Child >16 yr

• PO 4-8 mg qd or divided bid

Renal Impairment

• No dosage changes required

Elderly

• No dosage adjustment required

$ AVAILABLE FORMS/COST OF THERAPY

• Tab, Film-Coated—Oral: 2 mg, 60's: **$108.75**; 4 mg, 100's: **$266.76**; 8 mg, 100's: **$493.59**

CONTRAINDICATIONS: Hypersensitivity

PRECAUTIONS: Cardiac failure (NYHA Class 3, 4), edema; hypoglycemia (in combination with other hypoglycemic agents); weight gain, anemia, premenopausal anovulatory women

PREGNANCY AND LACTATION: Pregnancy category C; no adequate and well controlled studies in pregnant women available; abnormally high glucose levels during pregnancy associated with higher incidence of congenital anomolaies, morbidity, and mortality, insulin monotherapy preferred agent; drug detected in lactating rats; no information in humans

SIDE EFFECTS/ADVERSE REACTIONS

CNS: Headache

CV: Edema (5%), CHF

EENT: Upper respiratory infection, sinusitis

GI: Diarrhea, elevated AST, ALT (>3 × normal), hepatotoxicity (rare - <0.1%)

GU: Ovulation in premenopausal anovulatory women

HEME: Anemia (1 g/dL drop in hemoglobin) during 1st 4-8 weeks of therapy (increased plasma volume)

METAB: Hyperglycemia, hypoglycemia, lipid changes, weight gain (1.2-3.5 kg over 26 weeks in clinical trials)

MS: Back pain

MISC: Injury, fatigue

INTERACTIONS

Drugs

3 *Fenugreek, ginseng, glucomannan:* Additive blood glucose lowering; increased risk of hypoglycemia

Labs

• Elevations of AST, ALT, bilirubin, LDH, LDL-cholesterol (15%); HDL-cholesterol (15%); decreases in hematocrit, hemoglobin, alkaline phosphatase

SPECIAL CONSIDERATIONS

• *Expected hypoglycemic effects:* Decreases in serum glucose: 50-75 mg/dL; decreases in HbA1c 1.2-1.5%

PATIENT/FAMILY EDUCATION

• Caloric restriction, weight loss, and exercise essential adjuvant therapy

• Blood draws for LFT monitoring along with routine diabetes mellitus labs; review symptoms of hepatitis (unexplained nausea, vomiting, abdominal pain, fatigue, anorexia or dark urine)

• Notify clinician of rapid increases in weight or edema or symptoms of heart failure (shortness of breath)

• OK to take with food

• Review hypoglycemia risks and symptoms when added to other hypoglycemic agents

MONITORING PARAMETERS

• "Poly" diabetes mellitus symptoms, periodic serum glucose and HbA1c measurements; LFT (AST,

R

---

italic = common side effects   ***bold italic*** = life-threatening reactions

ALT) prior to initiation of therapy and periodically thereafter; hemoglobin/hematocrit

---

salicylic acid
(sal-i-sill'ik)

OTC: Compound W, DuoFilm, DuoPlant, Freezone, Gets-it, Gordofilm, Keralyt, Mediplast, Mosco, Occlusal-HP, Off-Ezy, Sal-Acid, Salactic Film, Sal-Plant, Trans-Ver-Sal, Wart Away, Wart Fix, Wart Remover Combinations

  Rx: with sodium thiosulfate (Versiclear)

Chemical Class: Salicylate derivative

Therapeutic Class: Keratolytic

CLINICAL PHARMACOLOGY

Mechanism of Action: Produces desquamation of hyperkeratotic epithelium; dissolves intracellular cement substance

Pharmacokinetics

TOP: Peak 5 hr when occlusive dressing used; 50%-80% bound to plasma proteins; metabolized and excreted in urine

INDICATIONS AND USES: Removal of excessive keratin in hyperkeratotic skin disorders, including common and plantar warts, psoriasis, calluses, corns

DOSAGE

Adult and Child

• Gel: TOP apply thin layer to affected area(s) qd-bid

• Plaster: TOP cut to size that covers corn or callus, apply and leave in place for 48 hr; do not exceed 5 applications over 2 wk period

• Liq: TOP apply thin layer directly to wart qd as directed for 1 wk or until wart is removed

S   AVAILABLE FORMS/COST OF THERAPY

• Film—Top: 15%, 10's: **$10.04**; 17%, 18's: **$7.19**

• Gel—Top: 6%, 30 g: **$15.56**; 17%, 7.5, 15 g: **$5.50-$7.19**

• Liq—Top: 12%, 9 ml: **$2.87**; 17%, 10, 15 ml: **$1.25-$8.50**

• Plaster, Adhesive—Top: 40%, 14's: **$12.00**

CONTRAINDICATIONS: Prolonged use; diabetes; impaired circulation; use on moles, birthmarks, or warts with hair growing from them; genital or facial warts; warts on mucous membranes; irritated skin; infected skin

PRECAUTIONS: Children

PREGNANCY AND LACTATION: Pregnancy category C

SIDE EFFECTS/ADVERSE REACTIONS

SKIN: Burning, local irritation

MISC: Salicylism (tinnitus, hearing loss, dizziness, confusion, headache, hyperventilation)

SPECIAL CONSIDERATIONS
PATIENT/FAMILY EDUCATION

• For external use only; avoid contact with face, eyes, genitals, mucous membranes, and normal skin surrounding warts

• May cause reddening or scaling of skin

• Soaking area in warm water for 5 min prior to application may enhance effect (remove any loose tissue with brush, washcloth, or emery board and dry thoroughly prior to application)

---

* = non-FDA-approved use

salmeterol

(sal-me'te-rol)

Rx: Serevent, Serevent Diskus

Combinations

Rx: with fluticasone (Advair Diskus)

Chemical Class: Sympathomimetic amine; β_2-adrenergic agonist

Therapeutic Class: Antiasthmatic, bronchodilator

CLINICAL PHARMACOLOGY

Mechanism of Action: Causes long-lasting bronchodilation by β_2-stimulation, resulting in relaxation of bronchial smooth muscle; inhibits mast cell degranulation; stimulates cilia to remove secretions; approximately 50 times more selective for β_{-2}-adrenergic receptors than albuterol

Pharmacokinetics

INH: Onset within 20 min, peak effect 2 hr, duration 12 hr; low systemic absorption; 94%-98% bound to plasma proteins; metabolized in liver, eliminated in feces; $t_{1/2}$ 3-4 hr

INDICATIONS AND USES: Maintenance of bronchodilation and prevention of symptoms of asthma, including nocturnal asthma; prevention of exercise-induced bronchospasm; maintenance treatment of bronchospasm associated with chronic bronchitis and emphysema (COPD)

DOSAGE

Adult and Child >12 yr

• *Asthma, COPD:* MDI 2 puffs q12h

• *Exercise-induced asthma:* MDI 2 puffs 30-60 min before exercise; do not repeat earlier than 12 hr following initial dose

💲 AVAILABLE FORMS/COST OF THERAPY

• MDI—INH: 21 µg/puffs, 6.5 g (60 puffs): **$49.84**; 21 µg/puffs, 13 g (120 puffs): **$77.08**

• Powder, Disk—INH: 50 µg/INH, 28's: **$42.00**; 50 µg/INH, 60's: **$72.58**

CONTRAINDICATIONS: Significantly worsening or acutely deteriorating asthma, acute symptoms

PRECAUTIONS: Cardiovascular disorders, coronary insufficiency, cardiac dysrhythmias, hypertension, convulsive disorders, thyrotoxicosis, children <12 yr, psychosis, diabetes, history of stroke

PREGNANCY AND LACTATION: Pregnancy category C

SIDE EFFECTS/ADVERSE REACTIONS

CNS: Anxiety, dizziness, headache, insomnia, nervousness, stimulation, tremors

CV: ***Cardiac arrest, dysrhythmias,*** hypertension, lengthened QT segment, palpitations, tachycardia

EENT: Throat irritation

GI: Bad taste, GI distress, nausea, vomiting

METAB: Hyperglycemia, hypokalemia

MS: Muscle cramps in extremities

RESP: Cough, dyspnea, ***paradoxical bronchospasm***

INTERACTIONS

Drugs

❷ *β-blockers:* Decreased action of salmeterol, cardioselective β-blockers preferable if concurrent use necessary

❸ *Furosemide:* Potential for additive hypokalemia

SPECIAL CONSIDERATIONS

PATIENT/FAMILY EDUCATION

• Proper inhalation technique is vital

• Excessive use may lead to adverse effects

• Notify clinician if no response to usual doses, or if palpitations, rapid heartbeat, chest pain, muscle tremors, dizziness, headache occur
• **Do not use to treat acute symptoms or on an as-needed basis**

---

salsalate

(sal´sa-late)

Rx: Amigesic, Argesic-SA, Disalcid, Marthritic, Mono-Gesic, Salflex, Salsitab
Chemical Class: Salicylate derivative
Therapeutic Class: Nonnarcotic analgesic; NSAID

CLINICAL PHARMACOLOGY
Mechanism of Action: Inhibits prostaglandin synthesis; analgesic, anti-inflammatory, antipyretic actions
Pharmacokinetics
PO: Onset of anti-inflammatory action 3-4 days; 75%-90% bound to plasma proteins; hydrolyzed in liver to salicylic acid (active); excreted in urine; $t_{1/2}$ 7-8 hr
INDICATIONS AND USES: Mild to moderate pain, rheumatoid arthritis, osteoarthritis, related rheumatic disorders
DOSAGE
Adult
• PO 3 g/day divided bid-tid
🟥 **AVAILABLE FORMS/COST OF THERAPY**
• Cap, Gel—Oral: 500 mg, 100's: **$65.58**
• Tab, Coated—Oral: 500 mg, 100's: **$7.37-$62.88**; 750 mg, 100's: **$13.50-$83.94**
CONTRAINDICATIONS: Hypersensitivity to NSAIDs, hemophilia, bleeding ulcers, hemorrhagic states

PRECAUTIONS: Children or teenagers with chickenpox or influenza (association with Reye's syndrome), impaired hepatic or renal function, history of peptic ulcer disease, diabetes mellitus, gout, anemia, diabetes
PREGNANCY AND LACTATION: Pregnancy category C; excreted into breast milk; use caution in nursing mothers due to potential adverse effects in nursing infant
SIDE EFFECTS/ADVERSE REACTIONS
CNS: Confusion, dizziness, drowsiness, headache
EENT: Dimness of vision, reversible hearing loss, tinnitus
GI: Acute reversible hepatotoxicity, anorexia, diarrhea, *dyspepsia,* epigastric discomfort, **GI bleeding,** heartburn, *nausea*
HEME: Decreased plasma iron concentration, **leukopenia,** shortened erythrocyte survival time, **thrombocytopenia**
RESP: Hyperpnea, wheezing
SKIN: Angioedema, bruising, hives, rash, urticaria
MISC: Fever, thirst
INTERACTIONS
Labs
• *False increase:* Serum bicarbonate, CSF, protein, serum theophylline
• *False decrease:* Urine cocaine, urine estrogen, serum glucose, urine 17-hydroxycorticosteroids, urine opiates
• *False positive:* Urine ferric chloride test
SPECIAL CONSIDERATIONS
• Consider for patients with GI intolerance to aspirin or patients in whom interference with normal platelet function by aspirin or other NSAIDs is undesirable

---

* = non-FDA-approved use

MONITORING PARAMETERS
• AST, ALT, bilirubin, creatinine, CBC, hematocrit if patient is on long-term therapy

---

saquinavir

(sa-kwin′a-veer)
Rx: Fortovase, Invirase
Chemical Class: HIV protease inhibitor
Therapeutic Class: HIV infection

CLINICAL PHARMACOLOGY
Mechanism of Action: Inihibits HIV protease preventing cleavage of the viral polyproteins, resulting in the formation of immature noninfectious viral particles
Pharmacokinetics
PO: Absolute bioavailability 4%, increased by high-fat meal; 98% bound to plasma proteins; metabolized by hepatic cytochrome P450 enzymes, excreted in feces (88%) and urine (1%); mean residence time 7 hr
NOTE: Fortovase delivers more drug for prolonged periods compared to Invirase
INDICATIONS AND USES: Advanced HIV infection in combination with nucleoside analogues
DOSAGE
Adult
• Invirase PO 400 mg bid with ritonavir; Invirase otherwise not recommended
• Fortovase PO 1200 mg (6 × 200 mg caps) tid
• Adjust dose when used with delavirdine, efavirenz, nelfinavir, ritonavir
• For latest treatment guidelines, see www.hivatis.org

⑤ AVAILABLE FORMS/COST OF THERAPY
• Fortovase Cap—Oral: 200 mg, 180's: **$250.34**
• Invirase Cap—Oral: 200 mg, 270's: **$622.07-$673.91**
CONTRAINDICATIONS: Concurrent use of rifampin
PRECAUTIONS: Children <16 yr, hepatic insufficiency; concurrent use of ritabutin
PREGNANCY AND LACTATION: Pregnancy category B
SIDE EFFECTS/ADVERSE REACTIONS
CNS: Asthenia, dizziness, extremity numbness, headache, paresthesia, peripheral neuropathy
GI: **Abdominal discomfort,** abdominal pain, appetite disturbance, buccal mucosa ulceration, *diarrhea,* dyspepsia, mucosa damage, *nausea*
MS: Musculoskeletal pain, myalgia
SKIN: Pruritis, rash
INTERACTIONS
Drugs
⚠ *Astemizole:* Increased plasma levels of astemizole
❸ *Barbiturates:* Increased clearance of saquinavir; reduced clearance of barbiturates
❷ *Carbamazepine:* Increased clearance of saquinavir, reduced clearance of carbamazepine
⚠ *Cisapride:* Increased plasma levels of cisapride
❸ *Clarithromycin:* Reduced clearance of saquinavir; saquinavir reduces clearance of clarithromycin
❸ *Delavirdine:* Decreased clearance of saquinavir; reduce dose of Fortovase (saquinavir soft gel capsule) to 800 mg tid
❸ *Dexamethasone:* Reduced saquinavir level
⚠ *Efavirenz:* Reduced saquinavir level
⚠ *Ergot alkaloids:* Increased plasma levels of ergot alkaloids

S

---

italic = common side effects   ***bold italic*** = life-threatening reactions

3 *Erythromycin:* Reduced clearance of saquinavir; saquinavir reduces clearance of erythromycin

3 *Grapefruit juice:* Increased saquinavir level

▲ *Indinavir:* Decreased clearance of saquinavir

▲ *Lovastatin:* Saquinavir reduces clearance of lovastatin

▲ *Midazolam:* Increased plasma levels of midazolam and prolonged effect

3 *Nelfinavir:* Decreased clearance of saquinavir; reduce dose of Fortovase (saquinavir soft gel capsule) to 800 mg tid

3 *Oral contraceptives:* Saquinavir may reduce efficacy

3 *Phenytoin:* Increased clearance of saquinavir; reduced clearance of phenytoin

▲ *Rifabutin:* Increased clearance of saquinavir

▲ *Rifampin:* Increased clearance of saquinavir

3 *Ritonavir:* Decreased clearance of saquinavir; decrease saquinavir dose to 400 mg bid, or less, depending on ritonavir dose

▲ *Simvastatin:* Saquinavir reduces clearance of simvastatin

▲ *Terfenadine:* Increased plasma levels of terfenadine

▲ *Triazolam:* Increased plasma levels of triazolam and prolonged effect

SPECIAL CONSIDERATIONS

• Invirase and fortovase not considered bioequivalent; no food effect on Invirase when taken with ritonavir; take Fortovase with large meal

---

scopolamine

(skoe-pol'a-meen)

Rx: *Transdermal:*
Transderm-Scop
Ophth: Isopto Hyoscine
Oral: Scopace
Chemical Class: Belladonna alkaloid
Therapeutic Class: Mydriatic; cycloplegic; antiemetic; antivertigo agent; anticholinergic

CLINICAL PHARMACOLOGY
Mechanism of Action: Cholinergic receptor blocker decreases production of GI secretions and stomach acid; central muscarinic receptor blocker decreases involuntary movements; inhibition of vestibular input to the CNS, inhibits vomiting reflex; direct inhibitory effect on vomiting center in brain stem; ophth blocks cholinergic response of iris sphincter and accommodation of ciliary body to cholinergic stimulation resulting in dilation, paralysis of accommodation

Pharmacokinetics
SC/IM: Onset 30 min, duration 4 hr
IV: Peak 10-15 min, duration 4 hr
TRANSDERMAL: Onset 3 hr, duration, up to 72 hr
OPHTH: Peak 20-30 min, duration 3-7 days
Excreted in urine, bile, feces (unchanged), $t_{1/2}$ 8 hr

INDICATIONS AND USES: Systemic: Reduction of secretions before surgery; calm delirium; transdermal: motion sickness, vertigo; nausea and vomiting*; ophth: uveitis, iritis, cycloplegia, mydriasis

DOSAGE
Geriatric and pediatric patients more sensitive to anticholinergic effects

---

Adult

• *Preoperatively:* SC/IM/IV 0.32-0.65 mg; dilute IV with sterile water; transderm 1.5 mg

• OPHTH instill 1-2 gtt before refraction or 1-2 gtt qd-tid for iritis or uveitis

• *Motion Sickness:* Place 1 patch behind ear 4-5 hr before travel; replace q72h prn

• *Nausea associated with analgesia and opiate anesthesia:* Transderm 1.5 mg q72h

Child

• OPHTH: instill 1 gtt bid × 2 days before refraction

• *Preoperatively:* SC 0.006 mg/kg or 0.2 mg/m^2

💲 AVAILABLE FORMS/COST OF THERAPY

• Film, Cont Rel—Transdermal: 0.5 mg/24 hr, 4 discs: **$18.21**

• Inj, Sol—IM, IV, SC: 0.4 mg/ml, 1 ml: **$1.44-$1.98**; 1 mg/ml, 1 ml: **$1.20-$1.76**

• Sol—Ophth: 0.25%, 5, 15 ml: **$15.56**/5 ml

• Tab—Oral: 0.4 mg, 100's: **$34.95**

CONTRAINDICATIONS: Narrow-angle glaucoma, increased intraocular pressure, adhesions between iris and lens, unstable cardiovascular status (tachycardia, myocardial ischemia), myasthenia gravis, GI or GU obstruction

PRECAUTIONS: Children, elderly blondes, prostatic hypertrophy, Down's syndrome, debilitated COPD, asthma, CHF, hypertension, dysrhythmia, hiatal hernia

PREGNANCY AND LACTATION: Pregnancy category C; no reports of adverse effects reported; compatible with breast feeding

SIDE EFFECTS/ADVERSE REACTIONS

CNS: Anxiety, confusion, delirium, delusions, depression, dizziness, *drowsiness,* excitement, flushing,

hallucinations, headache, incoherence, irritability, restlessness, sedation, weakness

CV: Palpitations, paradoxical bradycardia, postural hypotension, tachycardia

EENT: Blurred vision, difficulty swallowing, dilated pupils, nasal congestion, photophobia

GI: Abdominal distress, *constipation, dryness of mouth,* nausea, paralytic ileus, vomiting

GU: Hesitancy, retention

METAB: Decreased sweating, fever

SKIN: Urticaria

MISC: Nasal congestion, suppression of lactation

INTERACTIONS

Drugs

🖪 *Antihistamines, phenothiazines, tricyclics:* Additive anticholinergic effect

SPECIAL CONSIDERATIONS
PATIENT/FAMILY EDUCATION

• Avoid abrupt discontinuation (taper off over 1 wk)

• Wash hands thoroughly after handling transdermal patches before contacting eyes

---

secobarbital

(see-koe-bar'bi-tal)

Rx: Seconal

Combinations

  Rx: with amobarbital (Tuinal)

Chemical Class: Barbituric acid derivative

Therapeutic Class: Sedative/hypnotic; anesthesia adjunct; anticonvulsant

DEA Class: Controlled Substance Schedule II

CLINICAL PHARMACOLOGY

Mechanism of Action: CNS depressant: Depresses the sensory cortex, decreases motor activity, alters cerebellar function, produces drowsiness, sedation, and hypnosis; little analgesic action at subanesthetic doses (may increase reaction to painful stimuli); anticonvulsant activity in anesthetic doses; dose-dependent respiratory depression (hypnotic doses produce respiratory depression similar to physiologic sleep)

Pharmacokinetics

PO: Onset 10-15 min, duration 3-4 hr

IM: Onset 10-15 min, duration 3-4 hr

Metabolized by liver; excreted by kidneys (metabolites); $t_{1/2}$ 15-40 hr

INDICATIONS AND USES: Sedative, hypnotic; preanesthetic medication; status epilepticus,* acute tetanus convulsions*; acute psychotic agitation*

DOSAGE

Adult

• *Insomnia:* PO 100-200 mg hs

• *Sedation/preoperatively:* PO 200-300 mg 1-2 hr preoperatively

Child

• *Sedation/preoperatively:* PO 50-100 mg 1-2 hr preoperatively

$ AVAILABLE FORMS/COST OF THERAPY

• Cap, Gel—Oral: 100 mg, 100's: **$22.64**

CONTRAINDICATIONS: Respiratory depression, severe liver impairment, porphyria

PRECAUTIONS: Anemia, hepatic disease, renal disease, hypertension, elderly, acute or chronic pain (paradoxical reaction to pain possible)

PREGNANCY AND LACTATION: Pregnancy category D; small amounts excreted in breast milk, drowsiness in infant reported; compatible with breast feeding

SIDE EFFECTS/ADVERSE REACTIONS

CNS: Ataxia, CNS depression, dependency, dizziness, *drowsiness, hangover, lethargy,* lightheadedness, mental depression, nightmares, paradoxical stimulation in the elderly and children, slurred speech

CV: Bradycardia, hypotension

GI: Constipation, diarrhea, nausea, vomiting

HEME: **Agranulocytosis, megaloblastic anemia** (long-term treatment), **thrombocytopenia**

RESP: **Apnea, bronchospasm,** hypoventilation, **laryngospasm**

SKIN: Abscesses at inj site, angioedema, pain, *rash,* **Stevens-Johnson syndrome,** thrombophlebitis, urticaria

MISC: Withdrawal symptoms, minor (anxiety, muscle twitching, tremor, weakness, dizziness, distortion in visual perception, nausea, vomiting, insomnia, orthostatic hypotension), major (**seizures,** delirium)

INTERACTIONS

Drugs

▣ *Acetaminophen:* Enhanced hepatotoxic potential of acetaminophen overdoses

▣ *Antidepressants:* Reduced serum concentration of cyclic antidepressants

▣ *β-adrenergic blockers:* Reduced serum concentrations of β-blockers which are extensively metabolized

▣ *Calcium channel blockers:* Reduced serum concentrations of verapamil and dihydropyridines

▣ *Chloramphenicol:* Increased barbiturate concentrations; reduced serum chloramphenicol concentrations

▣ *Corticosteroids:* Reduced serum concentrations of corticosteroids; may impair therapeutic effect

* = non-FDA-approved use

3 *Cyclosporine:* Reduced serum concentration of cyclosporine

3 *Digitoxin:* Reduced serum concentration of digitoxin

3 *Disopyramide:* Reduced serum concentration of disopyramide

3 *Doxycycline:* Reduced serum doxycycline concentrations

3 *Estrogen:* Reduced serum concentration of estrogen

3 *Ethanol:* Excessive CNS depression

3 *Griseofulvin:* Reduced griseofulvin absorption

3 *MAOIs:* Prolonged effect of barbiturates

3 *Methoxyflurane:* Enhanced nephrotoxic effect

3 *Narcotic analgesics:* Increased toxicity of meperidine; reduced effect of methadone; additive CNS depression

3 *Neuroleptics:* Reduced effect of either drug

2 *Oral anticoagulants:* Decreased hypoprothrombinemic response to oral anticoagulants

3 *Oral contraceptives:* Reduced efficacy of oral contraceptives

3 *Phenytoin:* Unpredictable effect on serum phenytoin levels

3 *Propafenone:* Reduced serum concentration of propafenone

3 *Quinidine:* Reduced quinidine plasma concentration

3 *Tacrolimus:* Reduced serum concentration of tacrolimus

3 *Theophylline:* Reduced serum theophylline concentrations

3 *Valproic acid:* Increased serum concentrations of secobarbital

2 *Warfarin:* See oral anticoagulants

Labs
• *Glucose:* Falsely low with Clinistix, Diastix
• *17-Ketosteroids:* Falsely increased in urine

• *Phenobarbital:* Falsely increased in serum

SPECIAL CONSIDERATIONS
• Compared to the benzodiazepine sedative hypnotics, secobarbital is more lethal in overdosage, has a higher tendency for abuse and addiction, and is more likely to cause drug interactions via induction of hepatic microsomal enzymes; few advantages if any in safety or efficacy over benzodiazepines

PATIENT/FAMILY EDUCATION
• Avoid driving and other dangerous activities
• Withdrawal insomnia may occur after short-term use; do not start using drug again, insomnia will improve in 1-3 nights
• May experience increased dreaming

---

selegiline
(seh-leg'ill-ene)
Rx: Atapryl, Carbex, Eldepryl, Selpak
Chemical Class: Phenethylamine derivative
Therapeutic Class: Anti-Parkinson's agent

CLINICAL PHARMACOLOGY
Mechanism of Action: Inhibition of monoamine oxidase, type B, which blocks the catabolism of dopamine, increasing the net amount of dopamine available; other less well understood mechanisms also lead to an increase in dopaminergic activity
Pharmacokinetics
Rapidly absorbed, peak ½-2 hr; rapidly metabolized (active metabolites: Ndesmethyldeprenyl, $t_{1/2}$ 2 hr; amphetamine, $t_{1/2}$ 17.7 hr, methamphetamine, $t_{1/2}$ 20 ½ hr); metabolites excreted in urine (45% in 48 hr)

---

italic = common side effects   ***bold italic*** = life-threatening reactions

INDICATIONS AND USES: Adjunct management of Parkinson's disease in patients being treated with levodopa/carbidopa who have had a poor response to therapy; early Parkinson's disease to delay progression*; atypical depression,* Alzheimer's disease*

DOSAGE

Adult

• *Parkinson's disease:* PO 10 mg/day in divided doses 5 mg at breakfast and lunch; after 2-3 days, begin to reduce the dose of concurrent levodopa/carbidopa 10%-30%

⑧ AVAILABLE FORMS/COST OF THERAPY

• Cap—Oral: 5 mg, 60's: **$138.10-$162.00**

• Tab, Uncoated—Oral: 5 mg, 60's: **$109.90-$141.37**

CONTRAINDICATIONS: Concurrent use with meperidine

PRECAUTIONS: Doses above 10 mg/day (doses in the 30-40 mg/day range are associated with nonselective monoamine oxidase inhibition)

PREGNANCY AND LACTATION: Pregnancy category C; excretion in breast milk unknown

SIDE EFFECTS/ADVERSE REACTIONS

CNS: Anxiety, apathy, back and leg pain, blepharospasm, chorea, confusion, delusions, dizziness, dystonic symptoms, grimacing, hallucinations, headache, increased apraxia, increased bradykinesia, increased tremors, involuntary movements, lethargy, migraine, mood changes, muscle cramps, nightmares, numbness, overstimulation, personality change, restlessness, sleep disturbances, tardive dyskinesia, tiredness, vertigo

CV: Angina pectoris, **dysrhythmia,** edema, hypertension, hypotension, orthostatic hypotension, palpitations, sinus bradycardia, syncope, tachycardia

EENT: Blurred vision, diplopia, dry mouth, tinnitus

GI: Abdominal pain, anorexia, constipation, diarrhea, dysphagia, heartburn, nausea, poor appetite, rectal bleeding, vomiting, weight loss

GU: Frequency, hesitation, nocturia, prostatic hypertrophy, retention, sexual dysfunction, slow urination

RESP: Asthma, shortness of breath

SKIN: Alopecia, facial hair, hematoma, increased sweating, photosensitivity, rash

INTERACTIONS

Drugs

❷ *Antidepressants, serotonin reuptake inhibitors (fluoxetine, fluvoxamine, paroxetine, sertraline):* Serious, sometimes fatal, reactions including hyperthermia, autonomic instability and mental status changes

❷ *Dexfenfluramine, fenfluramine:* Increased risk of serotonin syndrome

❷ *Dextroamphetamine:* Severe hypertension

❷ *Dextromethorphan:* Increased risk of serotonin syndrome

❸ *Guanadrel, guanethidine:* May inhibit the antihypertensive effects of antihypertensive agents

❸ *Insulin:* Excessive hypoglycemia may occur when MAOIs are administered to patients with diabetes

❸ *Levodopa:* May precipitate hypertensive crisis

⚠ *Methylphenidate:* Increased risk of hypertensive reactions

❸ *Moclobemide:* Increased pressor effects of tyramine; increased risk of adverse drug or food interactions

❷ *Narcotic analgesics (meperidine):* Stupor, muscular rigidity, severe agitation, elevated temperature, hallucinations, and death

3 *Narcotic analgesics (morphine):* Stupor, muscular rigidity, severe agitation, elevated temperature, hallucinations, and death

▲ *Reserpine:* Loss of antihypertensive effects

▲ *Sibutramine:* Increased risk of serotonin syndrome

3 *Succinylcholine:* Prolonged muscle relaxation caused by succinylcholine

▲ *Sympathomimetics (metaraminol, phenylpropanolamine, pseudoephedrine):* Additive pressor response to sympathomimetic

3 *Sympathomimetics (norepinephrine, phenylephrine):* Additive pressor response to sympathomimetic

▲ *Venlafaxine:* Increased risk of serotonin syndrome

Labs

• *False positive:* Urine ketones, urine glucose

• *False negative:* Urine glucose (glucose oxidase)

• *False increase:* Uric acid, urine protein

SPECIAL CONSIDERATIONS

• At low doses, irreversible type B MAOI; at higher doses is metabolized to amphetamine, inhibiting both A and B subtypes of MAO

• Several placebo-controlled studies have demonstrated a significant delay in the need to initiate levodopa therapy in patients who receive selegiline in the early phase of the disease

• May have significant benefit in slowing the onset of the debilitating consequences of Parkinson's disease

---

selenium sulfide

(see-leen'ee-um)
Rx: Exsel, Selsun
OTC: Selsun Blue
Chemical Class: Trace metal
Therapeutic Class: Antiseborrheic; antifungal

CLINICAL PHARMACOLOGY
Mechanism of Action: Antimitotic action reducing turnover of epidermal cells; additional local irritant, antibacterial, and antifungal activity
Pharmacokinetics
TOP: Absorption may be increased if applied to inflamed skin
INDICATIONS AND USES: Dandruff, seborrheic dermatitis, tinea versicolor
DOSAGE
Adult and Child
• *Seborrheic dermatitis/dandruff:* TOP wash hair with 1-2 tsp, leave on 2-3 min, rinse, repeat; 2 applications/wk for control or as needed for maintenance

• *Tinea versicolor:* TOP apply to affected area (perhaps with small amount of water), allow to remain on skin for 10 min, rinse thoroughly, repeat daily × 7 days; repeat as needed for maintenance

$ **AVAILABLE FORMS/COST OF THERAPY**
• Lotion—Top: 1%, 240 ml: **$3.31-$5.04**
• Shampoo—Top: 1% 210 ml (OTC): **$4.00-$5.76**
• Lotion/Shampoo—Top: 2.5% 120 ml: **$2.10-$20.83**
CONTRAINDICATIONS: Hypersensitivity to sulfur preparations
PRECAUTIONS: Infants, inflamed skin
PREGNANCY AND LACTATION: Pregnancy category C; excretion into breast milk unknown

---

italic = common side effects   ***bold italic*** = life-threatening reactions

SIDE EFFECTS/ADVERSE REACTIONS

SKIN: Alopecia, discoloration of hair (minimized with thorough rinsing), oiliness of hair and scalp, *skin irritation*

SPECIAL CONSIDERATIONS
PATIENT/FAMILY EDUCATION

• External use only; avoid contact with eyes
• May damage jewelry (remove before using)

---

senna
(sen´na)

OTC: Black Draught, Fletcher's Castoria, Gentlax, Senexon, Senna-Gen, Senokot, Senokotxtra
Combinations
  OTC: with docusate (Senokot-S); with cascara sagrada (Herbal Laxative); with psyllium (Perdiem)
Chemical Class: Anthraquinone derivatives
Therapeutic Class: Stimulant laxative

CLINICAL PHARMACOLOGY
Mechanism of Action: Stimulates peristalsis by action on intramural nerve plexi; alters water and electrolyte secretion
Pharmacokinetics
PO: Onset 6-8 hr
PR: Onset 0.5-1 hr
Minimal absorption; metabolized by liver; fecal and/or renal elimination

INDICATIONS AND USES: Constipation; bowel evacuation or preparation for surgery or examination

DOSAGE
Adult
• PO up to 1600 mg/day; tabs (187-600 mg), 1-8 tabs/day; granules (163-1600 mg/½ tsp), ¼-½ tsp/day; syr (218 mg/5 ml), 5-20 ml/day; liq (33.3 mg/ml), 10-15 ml/day
• PR up to 1600 mg/day; supp (652 mg), 1-2/day
Child >6 yr; >27 kg
• Do not use Black Draught (granules) for children
• PO up to 800 mg/day; tabs (187-600 mg), 1-4 tabs/day; syr (218 mg/5 ml), 10-30 ml/day; liq (33.3 mg/ml), 10-15 ml/day
Child 2-5 yr
• PO up to 300-400 mg/day; liq 5-10 ml/day
Child 1 mo-1 yr
• PO up to 300-400 mg/day; syr 1.25-5 ml/day

💲 **AVAILABLE FORMS/COST OF THERAPY**
• Liq—Oral: 33.3 mg/ml, 150 ml: **$5.27**
• Syr—Oral: 218 mg/5 ml, 240 ml: **$15.00**
• Tab—Oral: 187 mg, 100's: **$2.55-$20.02**; 217 mg, 100's: **$7.33**; 374 mg, 12's; 600 mg, 30's: **$1.31-$4.38**

CONTRAINDICATIONS: GI bleeding, obstruction, fecal impaction, abdominal pain, nausea or vomiting, symptoms of appendicitis, acute surgical abdomen

PRECAUTIONS: Fluid and electrolyte imbalance can occur with abuse; abuse, dependency; children

PREGNANCY AND LACTATION: Pregnancy category C; not excreted into breast milk; compatible with breast feeding

SIDE EFFECTS/ADVERSE REACTIONS

GI: Anorexia, cramps, diarrhea, *nausea, vomiting*

---

* = non-FDA-approved use

METAB: Alkalosis, enteropathy, hypocalcemia, hypokalemia, tetany

SPECIAL CONSIDERATIONS

• Proposed laxative of choice for narcotic-induced constipation

---

sertraline

(sir'trall-een)

Rx: Zoloft

Chemical Class: Substituted nanphthalenamine derivative
Therapeutic Class: Selective serotonin reuptake inhibitor (SSRI) antidepressant

---

CLINICAL PHARMACOLOGY

Mechanism of Action: Inhibitor of CNS neuronal uptake of serotonin (5-HT); no significant activity for histaminergic α- or β-adrenergic, muscarinic, or dopaminergic receptors

Pharmacokinetics

PO: Peak 4.5-8.4 hr, extensive 1st pass metabolism; plasma protein binding 99%; elimination $t_{1/2}$ 26-65 hr; excreted in urine and feces

INDICATIONS AND USES: Major depression; obsessive-compulsive disorder, panic disorder, posttraumatic stress disorder

DOSAGE

Adult and Child >12 yr

• *Depression and obsessive-compulsive disorder:* PO 50 mg qd; max 200 mg/day; do not change dose at intervals of <1 wk

• *Panic disorder and posttraumatic stress disorder:* 25 mg qd × 1 wk then increase to 50 mg qd; max 200 mg/day; do not change dose at intervals of <1 wk

Child (6-12 yr)

• *Obsessive-compulsive disorder:* PO 25 mg qd; max 200 mg qd; do not change dose at intervals of <1 wk

• Reduce dose for hepatic or renal dysfunction

$ **AVAILABLE FORMS/COST OF THERAPY**

• Liq, Concentrate—Oral: 20 mg/ml, 60 ml: **$59.74**

• Tab, Uncoated—Oral: 25 mg, 50's: **$126.04**; 50 mg, 100's: **$230.51**; 100 mg, 100's: **$198.50**

CONTRAINDICATIONS: Concomitant use with MAOIs, concomitant use of oral concentrate and disulfiram due to alcohol content of the concentrate

PRECAUTIONS: Weight loss, hepatic disease, seizure disorder, history of mania, suicide ideation

PREGNANCY AND LACTATION: Pregnancy category C; excretion into breast milk unknown, use caution in nursing mother

SIDE EFFECTS/ADVERSE REACTIONS

CNS: Agitation, ataxia, confusion, *dizziness, fatigue, headache, insomnia,* paresthesia, *somnolence, tremor,* twitching

CV: Chest pain, hypotension, palpitations

EENT: Vision abnormalities

GU: Male sexual dysfunction, micturition disorder

GI: Anorexia, constipation, *diarrhea, dry mouth,* dyspepsia, flatulence, *nausea,* vomiting

INTERACTIONS

Drugs

❸ *Cimetidine:* Increased plasma sertraline concentrations

❸ *Cyproheptadine:* Serotonin antagonist may partially reverse antidepressant and other effects

❷ *Dexfenfluramine:* Duplicate effects on inhibition of serotonin reuptake; inhibition of dexfenfluramine metabolism (CYP2D6) exaggerates effect; both mechanisms increase risk of serotonin syndrome

---

italic = common side effects   ***bold italic*** = life-threatening reactions

❷ *Fenfluramine:* Duplicate effects on inhibition of serotonin reuptake; inhibition of dexfenfluramine metabolism (CYP2D6) exaggerates effect; both mechanisms increase risk of serotonin syndrome

❸ *Lithium:* Neurotoxicity (tremor, confusion, ataxia, dizziness, dysarthria, and absence seizures) reported in patients receiving fluoxetine-lithium combination; mechanism unknown

⚠ *MAOI's (isocarboxazid, phenelzine, tranylcypromine):* Increased CNS serotonergic effects has been associated with severe or fatal reactions with this combination

❷ *Selegiline:* Sporadic cases of mania and hypertension

❸ *Sumatriptan:* Concomitant use of SSRI and sumatriptan may increase adverse effects

❸ *Tricyclic antidepressants (clomipramine, desipramine, doxepin, imipramine, nortriptyline, trazodone):* Marked increases in tricyclic antidepressant levels due to inhibition of metabolism (CYP2D6)

❷ *Tryptophan:* Additive serotonergic effects

❸ *Warfarin:* Increased hypoprothrombinemic response to warfarin

SPECIAL CONSIDERATIONS
• SSRI of choice based on intermediate length $t_{1/2}$, linear pharmacokinetics, absence of appreciable age effect on clearance, substantially less effect on P450 enzymes, reducing potential for drug interactions
• Oral concentrate contains 12% alcohol; dropper contains natural rubber, caution if latex allergy
• Splitting 100 mg tablets to yield 50 mg dose cuts costs

PATIENT/FAMILY EDUCATION
• Oral concentrate must be diluted in water, ginger ale, lemon/lime soda, lemonade, or orange juice only, no other liquids should be used; do not mix in advance
• Avoid alcohol

---

sevelamer
(seh-vel′a-mer)
Rx: Renagel
Therapeutic Class: Phosphate adsorbent

CLINICAL PHARMACOLOGY
Mechanism of Action: Binds phosphate in GI tract, increases elimination
Pharmacokinetics
PO: Not systematically absorbed in healthy volunteers

INDICATIONS AND USES: Reduction of serum phosphorus in patients with end-stage renal disease (ESRD)

DOSAGE
Adult
• PO (serum phosphorus >6 and <7.5 mg/dL) 2 caps tid with meals; (serum phosphorus ≥7.5 and <9 mg/dL) 3 caps tid with meals; (serum phosphorus ≥9 mg/dL) 4 caps tid with meals; adjust dose to lower serum phosphorus to ≤6 mg/dL, increase or decrease dose by 1 cap/meal prn; max 30 caps/day

💲 AVAILABLE FORMS/COST OF THERAPY
• Cap—Oral: 403 mg, 200's: **$127.51**

CONTRAINDICATIONS: Hypophosphatemia; bowel obstruction

PRECAUTIONS: Dysphagia, swallowing disorders, GI motility disorders, major GI tract surgery

---

PREGNANCY AND LACTATION:

Pregnancy category C; use caution in nursing mothers due to potential for reductions in serum levels of various vitamins

SIDE EFFECTS/ADVERSE REACTIONS

CNS: Headache

CV: Hypertension, hypotension, ***thrombosis***

GI: Diarrhea, dyspepsia, vomiting, nausea, flatulence, constipation

INTERACTIONS

Drugs

3 *Antiarrhythmics, anticonvulsants:* Potential for decreased bioavailability of these drugs when concomitantly administered with sevelamer, administer >1 hr before or 3 hr after sevelamer

SPECIAL CONSIDERATIONS

• Has not been studied in ESRD patients not on hemodialysis

• Compared to calcium acetate, may reduce the risk of developing hypercalcemia

PATIENT/FAMILY EDUCATION

• A daily multivitamin supplement may prevent reduction in serum levels of vitamins D, E, K, and folic acid

• Do not chew or take caps apart prior to administration

MONITORING PARAMETERS

• Serum phosphorus, calcium, bicarbonate, and chloride levels

sibutramine

(sih-byoo′tra-meen)

Rx: Meridia

Chemical Class: Cyclobutane-methamine derivative

Therapeutic Class: Anorexiant

DEA Class: Schedule IV

CLINICAL PHARMACOLOGY

Mechanism of Action: Inhibits reuptake of norepinephrine, serotonin, and dopamine in the CNS

Pharmacokinetics

PO: Peak 1.2 hr, 77% absorption, extensive first pass metabolism in the liver; 97% bound to plasma proteins; metabolized in the liver by cytochrome P450(3A$_4$) to active desmethyl metabolites; excreted in urine (77%) and feces; t$_{1/2}$ 1.1 hr (14 and 16 hr for two active metabolites)

INDICATIONS AND USES: Management of obesity (initial body mass index ≥30 kg/m^2, or ≥27 kg/m^2 in the presence of other risk factors like hypertension, diabetes and dyslipidemia) in conjunction with a reduced calorie diet

DOSAGE

Adult

• PO 10 mg qd; may increase to 15 mg qd after 4 wk if inadequate results; safety and efficacy beyond 1 yr of therapy has not been determined

$ **AVAILABLE FORMS/COST OF THERAPY**

• Cap—Oral: 5 mg, 100's: **$310.35**; 10 mg, 100's: **$298.70**; 15 mg, 100's: **$386.25**

CONTRAINDICATIONS: Patients receiving MAO inhibitors or other centrally acting appetite suppressants; anorexia nervosa

PRECAUTIONS: Hypertension, CAD, CHF, arrhythmia, stroke, narrow angle glaucoma, seizure disorders, gallstones, renal or hepatic dysfunction

PREGNANCY AND LACTATION: Pregnancy category C; excretion into breast milk unknown, not recommended in nursing mothers

SIDE EFFECTS/ADVERSE REACTIONS

CNS: Anxiety, depression, dizziness, emotional lability, *headache, insomnia,* nervousness, paresthesia, somnolence, stimulation

CV: Generalized edema, hypertension, migraine, palpitation, tachycardia, vasodilation

EENT: Ear disorder, ear pain, taste perversion

GI: Anorexia, constipation, dry mouth, dyspepsia, gastritis, increased appetite, nausea, rectal disorder, vomiting

GU: Dysmenorrhea, metorrhagia

MS: Arthralgia, back pain, joint disorder, myalgia, tenosynovitis

RESP: Cough increase, laryngitis, pharyngitis, rhinitis, sinusitis

SKIN: Acne, rash, sweating

MISC: Abdominal pain, asthenia, chest pain, flu syndrome, neck pain, thirst

INTERACTIONS

Drugs

❷ *MAO inhibitors:* Potential for the development of serotonin syndrome; at least 14 days should elapse between administration of MAO inhibitors and sibutramine

SPECIAL CONSIDERATIONS

• Primary pulmonary hypertension and cardiac valve disorders have been associated with other centrally acting weight loss agents that cause release of serotonin from nerve terminals; although sibutramine has not been associated with these effects in pre-marketing clinical studies, patients should be informed of the potential for these side effects and monitored closely for their occurrence

• Substantially increases blood pressure in some patients

• Maintenance of weight loss beyond 1 yr has not been studied

MONITORING PARAMETERS

• Regular blood pressure monitoring

---

sildenafil

(sill-den´-a-fill)

Rx: Viagra

Chemical Class: cGMPspecific phosphodiesterase inhibitor

Therapeutic Class: Anti-impotence agent

CLINICAL PHARMACOLOGY

Mechanism of Action: Increases cGMP in the corpus cavernosum, causing smooth muscle relaxation and inflow of blood, resulting in penile erection

Pharmacokinetics

PO: Peak 30-120 min. Rapidly absorbed, metabolized by liver (cytochrome P450 3A4) to active metabolite, excreted in feces (80%) and urine (13%); $T_{1/2}$ 4 hr, rate of absorption decreased by fatty meal

INDICATIONS AND USES: Erectile dysfunction

DOSAGE

Adult

• PO: 50 mg approx 1 hr before sexual activity. Dosage range 25-100 mg. Max recommended use once/day. Decrease dose in elderly (>65), hepatic dysfunction, renal insufficiency (CrCl <30 ml/min)

💲 AVAILABLE FORMS/COST OF THERAPY

• Tab, Coated—Oral: 25 mg, 100's: **$287.67**; 50 mg, 100's: **$958.91**; 100 mg, 100's: **$958.91**

CONTRAINDICATIONS: Concurrent nitrate use

PRECAUTIONS: Elderly, hepatic dysfunction, renal insufficiency, penile deformity, cardiac disease, conditions predisposing to priapism (sickle cell anemia, leukemia, multiple myeloma), bleeding disorders, active peptic ulcer disease, retinitis pigmentosa (some have disorders of retinal phosphodiesterases), concurrent use of cytochrome P450 inhibitors

PREGNANCY AND LACTATION: Pregnancy category B, use not recommended in women

SIDE EFFECTS/ADVERSE REACTIONS

CNS: Headache (16%), abnormal vision (11% at 100 mg dose, 3% at lower dose) including color tinge, photosensitivity, ataxia, hypertonia, neuropathy, paresthesia, tremor, vertigo, depression, insomnia, somnolence, abnormal dreams

CV: **Cardiac arrest, death,** angina, AV block, syncope, tachycardia, palpitations, hypotension, **myocardial ischemia**

EENT: Dizziness, mydriasis, tinnitus, eye pain, ear pain

GI: Dyspepsia (17% at 100 mg dose, 7% at lower dose), diarrhea, vomiting, gastritis, esophagitis, stomatitis, abnormal LFTs

GU: Nocturia, frequency, breast enlargement, incontinence, abnormal ejaculation, anorgasmia, no cases of priapism reported

HEME: **Anemia, leukopenia**

METAB: Hyperglycemia, hypoglycemia, hyperuricemia, hypernatremia

MS: Arthritis, synovitis, myalgia

RESP: Asthma, dyspnea, laryngitis, cough

SKIN: Flushing (10%), urticaria, pruritus, dermatitis

INTERACTIONS

Drugs

❸ *Cimetidine, erythromycin, itraconazole, ketoconazole:* Increased sildenafil levels

⚠ *Nitrates:* Cardiac arrest, death

❸ *Rifampin:* Decreased sildenafil levels

SPECIAL CONSIDERATIONS

• Tablets are priced the same regardless of dose, 100-mg tablets can be broken in half

---

silver nitrate

Rx: Silver nitrate
Chemical Class: Heavy metal
Therapeutic Class: Antibiotic; cauterizing agent

CLINICAL PHARMACOLOGY

Mechanism of Action: Germicidal action via liberated silver ions, which precipitate bacterial proteins; also antiseptic, astringent, local epithelial stimulant, and caustic

INDICATIONS AND USES: Prevention, treatment of gonorrheal ophthalmia neonatorum; treatment of indolent wounds, ulcers, and fissures; cauterize vesicular, bullous, or aphthous lesions and provide styptic action; neurovascular helomas (10% oint, 10% sol); impetigo vulgaris (10% sol); pruritis, plantar warts (25% sol); granulation tissue, papillomatous growths, granuloma pyogenicum (50% sol); wet dressing in burns and acute dermatitis (0.1-0.5% sol)*

DOSAGE

Adult

• TOP (as wet dressing or irrigant) apply a cotton applicator dipped in sol to affected area 2-3 times/wk for approximately 2-3 wk prn; apply oint in an apertured pad on affected lesion or area for approximately 5 days prn; touch applicators to the bases of vesicular, bullous, or aphthous lesions

Neonate

• *Gonorrheal ophthalmia neonatorum:* Instill 2 gtt of 1% sol into each eye; do *not* follow with irrigation

$ AVAILABLE FORMS/COST OF THERAPY

• Applicators—Top: 100's: **$5.02-$7.80**

• Oint-Top: 10%, 30 g: **$32.50**

• Sol—Ophth: 1%, 1 ml, 100's: **$147.60**

• Sol—Top: 0.5%, 960 ml: **$19.33**; 10%, 30 ml: **$21.25**; 25%, 30 ml: **$33.75**; 50%, 30 ml: **$48.75**

PRECAUTIONS: Antibiotic hypersensitivity; *not* effective for neonatal chlamydial conjunctivitis; caustic and irritating to skin

SIDE EFFECTS/ADVERSE REACTIONS

EENT: Discharge, edema, redness, swelling (chemical conjunctivitis)

METAB: Sodium and chloride depletion with chronic wet dressings

SKIN: Discoloration

SPECIAL CONSIDERATIONS

PATIENT/FAMILY EDUCATION

• Stains skin and utensils (removable with iodine tincture followed by sodium thiosulfate solution)

---

silver sulfadiazine

(sul-fa-dye′a-zeen)

Rx: Silvadene, SSD, SSD AF, Thermazene

Chemical Class: Sulfonamide derivative

Therapeutic Class: Topical antibiotic

CLINICAL PHARMACOLOGY

Mechanism of Action: Interferes with bacterial cell wall synthesis (bactericidal); broad antimicrobial activity including many gram-negative and gram-positive bacteria and yeast; *not* a carbonic anhydrase inhibitor, and may be useful in situations where such agents are contraindicated

Pharmacokinetics

TOP: Absorption varies depending on surface area covered and integrity of skin; appreciable serum concentrations obtainable with extensive use (8-12 µg/ml)

INDICATIONS AND USES: Adjunct for the prevention and treatment of wound sepsis in patients with 2nd and 3rd degree burns

DOSAGE

Adult and Child

• TOP apply to affected area qd-bid; burned area should be covered with cream at all times

$ AVAILABLE FORMS/COST OF THERAPY

• Cre—Top: 1%, 20, 25, 30, 50, 85, 400, 1000 g: **$18.96-$47.08**/400 g

CONTRAINDICATIONS: Child <2 mo

PRECAUTIONS: Impaired hepatic or renal function; G-6-PD deficiency

PREGNANCY AND LACTATION: Pregnancy category B; contraindicated in neonates (kernicterus)

SIDE EFFECTS/ADVERSE REACTIONS

GU: Crystalluria

*HEME: **Reversible leukopenia***

SKIN: Burning, brownish-gray skin discoloration, erythema, itching, pain, rash, skin necrosis, stinging, urticaria

INTERACTIONS

Drugs

3 *Proteolytic enzymes:* Silver may inactivate enzymes

SPECIAL CONSIDERATIONS

• Prior to application, burn wounds should be cleansed and debrided (following control of shock and pain)

• Use sterile glove and tongue blade to apply medication; thin layer (1.5 mm) to completely cover wound; dressing as required only

• Continue until no chance of infection

---

simethicone

(si-meth′i-kone)

OTC: Gas-X, Mylicon, Phazyme

Combinations

    OTC: with calcium carbonate (Titralac Plus); with aluminum hydroxide, magnesium hydroxide (Mylanta Gelisil, Maalox Extra Strength); with calcium carbonate, magnesium hydroxide (Tempo, Rolaids); with Magaldrate, (Riopan Plus); with charcoal (Charcoal Plus, Flatulex)

Therapeutic Class: Antiflatulent

CLINICAL PHARMACOLOGY

Mechanism of Action: Defoaming action, disperses and prevents formation of gas pockets in GI system

Pharmacokinetics

PO: Fecal elimination, unchanged

INDICATIONS AND USES: Relief of painful symptoms and pressure of excess gas in digestive tract; adjunct in conditions in which gas retention may be problematic (postoperatively, endoscopic examination, air swallowing, functional dyspepsia, peptic ulcer, spastic or irritable colon, diverticulosis); infant colic*

DOSAGE

Adult

• PO 40-125 mg qid pc, hs

Child 2-12 yr

• PO 40 mg qid

Child <2 yr

• PO 20 mg pc, hs (up to 240 mg/day)

$ **AVAILABLE FORMS/COST OF THERAPY**

• Cap—Oral: 125 mg, 50's: **$8.36-$9.78**; 166 mg, 60's: **$10.85**

• Liq—Oral: 40 mg/0.6 ml, 30 ml: **$1.65-$10.36**; 50 mg/5 ml, 300 ml: **$5.00**

• Tab, Chewable—Oral: 80 mg, 100's: **$1.50-$15.85**; 125 mg, 24's: **$3.32-$3.50**; 166 mg, 60's: **$10.85**

• Tab—Oral: 60 mg, 100's: **$13.18**; 95 mg, 100's: **$14.89**

PREGNANCY AND LACTATION: Pregnancy category C

SIDE EFFECTS/ADVERSE REACTIONS

GI: Belching, rectal flatus

SPECIAL CONSIDERATIONS

• Commonly prescribed, little evidence for any beneficial effect

---

italic = common side effects   ***bold italic*** = life-threatening reactions

simvastatin

(sim´va-sta-tin)

Rx: Zocor
Chemical Class: Substituted hexahydronaphthalene
Therapeutic Class: Antilipemic (HMG-CoA reductase inhibitor); "statin"

CLINICAL PHARMACOLOGY

Mechanism of Action: Competitively inhibits 3-hydroxy-3-methylglutaryl-coenzyme A (HMG-CoA) reductase, an early rate-limiting step in cholesterol biosynthesis; increases HDL cholesterol mildly [8%-12%], dramatically decreases total and LDL cholesterol [23%-36%, 14%-47%, respectively], moderate lowering effect on triglycerides [11%-24%]

Pharmacokinetics

PO: Peak 1-2½ hr, 85% absorbed; extensive 1st-pass metabolism (CYP3A4, active metabolites); 95% protein bound; excreted primarily in bile, feces (60%)

INDICATIONS AND USES: Reduction of elevated total and LDL cholesterol in patients with primary hypercholesterolemia, mixed dyslipidemia (types IIa and IIb and homozygous familial hyperlipidemia); reduction of morbidity and mortality in patients with coronary heart disease and hypercholesterolemia (secondary prevention)

DOSAGE

Adult

• PO 5-10 mg qd in PM initially, usual range 5-40 mg/day qd in PM; max daily dose 80 mg; dosage adjustments may be made in 4-wk intervals

$ AVAILABLE FORMS/COST OF THERAPY

• Tab, Plain Coated—Oral: 5 mg, 90's: **$169.70**; 10 mg, 100's: **$237.50**; 20 mg, 90's: **$396.80**; 40 mg, 100's: **$413.25**; 80 mg, 90's: **$396.80**

CONTRAINDICATIONS: Active liver disease

PRECAUTIONS: Past liver disease, alcoholism, severe acute infections, trauma, hypotension, uncontrolled seizure disorders, severe metabolic disorders, electrolyte imbalances

PREGNANCY AND LACTATION: Pregnancy category X; breast milk excretion unknown; other drugs in this class are excreted in small amounts; manufacturer recommends against breast feeding

SIDE EFFECTS/ADVERSE REACTIONS

CNS: Dizziness, headache, insomnia, memory loss, peripheral neuropathy, tremor, vertigo

GI: Abdominal pain, constipation, diarrhea, dyspepsia, flatus, heartburn, liver dysfunction, nausea, *pancreatitis,* vomiting

GU: Erectile dysfunction, gynecomastia, loss of libido

HEME: **Eosinophilia, hemolytic anemia, leukopenia, thrombocytopenia**

MS: Muscle cramps, myalgia, myositis, *rhabdomyolysis*

SKIN: Alopecia, pruritus, rash, *Stevens-Johnson syndrome*

INTERACTIONS

Drugs

❷ *Azole antifungals (fluconazole, itraconazole, ketoconazole, miconazole):* Increased simvastatin levels via inhibition of metabolism with increased risk of rhabdomyolysis

❸ *Cholestyramine, colestipol:* Reduced bioavailability of simvastatin

3 *Cyclosporine:* Concomitant administration increases risk of severe myopathy or rhabdomyolysis

3 *Danazol:* Inhibition of metabolism (CYP3A4) thought to yield increased simvastatin levels with increased risk of rhabdomyolysis

2 *Fluoxetine:* Inhibits CYP3A4 hepatic metabolism with risk of rhabdomyolysis

2 *Gemfibrozil:* Small increased risk of myopathy with combination, especially at high doses of statin

3 *Isradipine:* Isradipine probably decreases simvastatin (like lovastatin) plasma concentrations minimally

3 *Macrolide antibiotics (clarithromycin, erythromycin, troleandomycin):* Increased simvastatin levels via inhibition of metabolism with increased risk of rhabdomyolysis

3 *Nefazadone:* Inhibit CYP3A4 hepatic metabolism (like lovastatin) with risk of rhabdomyolysis

3 *Niacin:* Concomitant administration increases risk of severe myopathy or rhabdomyolysis

3 *Warfarin:* Addition of simvastatin may increase hypoprothrombinemic response to warfarin via inhibition of metabolism (CYP2C9)

SPECIAL CONSIDERATIONS

• Superior to fibrates, cholestyramine, and probucol in lowering total and LDL cholesterol levels

• Statin selection based on lipid-lowering prowess, cost, and availability

PATIENT/FAMILY EDUCATION

• Report symptoms of myalgia, muscle tenderness, or weakness

• Take daily doses in the evening for increased effect

MONITORING PARAMETERS

• Cholesterol (max therapeutic response 4-6 wk)

• LFT's (AST, ALT) at baseline and at 12 wk of therapy; if no change, no further monitoring necessary (discontinue if elevations persist at >3 × upper limit of normal)

• CPK in patients complaining of diffuse myalgia, muscle tenderness, or weakness

---

sirolimus
(sir-oh-leem'-us)
Rx: Rapamune
Chemical Class: Macrolide derivative
Therapeutic Class: Immunosuppressant

CLINICAL PHARMACOLOGY

Mechanism of Action: Inhibits the mammalian Target Of Rapamycin (mTOR) a key regulatory kinase that suppresses cytokine-driven T-cell proliferation through inhibition of the cell cycle

Pharmacokinetics

PO: Peak 1-3 hr, low bioavailability (15%), extensively metabolized by cytochrome P450 in the liver (CYP3A4), metabolites have <10% activity of parent compound, $T_{1/2}$ 60 hr

INDICATIONS AND USES: Prevention of organ rejection in renal transplantation (in combination with corticosteroids and cyclosporine)

DOSAGE

Adult and Child ≥13 yr

• PO 2 mg qd; loading dose of 3 × the maintenance dose as soon as possible after transplantation is recommended; follow trough levels to adjust dose

• *Dosage adjustments:* Patiens ≥13 yr and <40 kg PO 1 mg/m²/day, loading dose 3 mg/m²; Hepatic impairment: Reduce maintenance dose by ⅓, no change in loading dose; Renal impairment: no dosage adjustment needed

AVAILABLE FORMS/COST OF THERAPY
• Liq—Oral: 1 mg/ml, 1, 2, 4, 15, 50 ml: **$431.25**/50 ml
• Tab—Oral: 1 mg, 100 ml: **$718.75**
PRECAUTIONS: History of lymphoma or other malignancies, infection, hyperlipidemia (especially hypertryglyceridemia), diabetes, coronary artery disease, myelosuppression, hepatic insufficiency, pregnancy, liver transplant (increased risk of hepatic artery thrombosis, use not recommended in liver transplant)
PREGNANCY AND LACTATION: Pregnancy category C; excretion into breast milk unknown, use caution in nursing mothers
SIDE EFFECTS/ADVERSE REACTIONS
CNS: Headache
CV: Peripheral edema
GI: Anorexia, weight loss, diarrhea, elevated transaminases
GU: Minimal nephrotoxicity in initial studies
HEME: **Thrombocytopenia** (dose related), **leukopenia** (nondose related, WBC <4800/mm^3 in 20%)
METAB: Hypertriglyceridemia, hyperlipidemia, hyperglycemia
MS: Arthralgia
INTERACTIONS
Drugs
3 *Azole antifungals, bromocriptine, calcium channel blockers, cimetidine, danazol, ethinyl estradiol, GI prokinetic agents, macrolide antibiotics, protease inhibitors:* Decreased metabolism or increased bioavailability of sirolimus
3 *Carbamazepine, phenobarbital, phenytoin, rifabutin, rifapentine:* Decreased sirolimus concentrations possible

3 *Cyclosporine:* Increased sirolimus concentrations when given concurrently. Sirolimus should be taken 4 hr after cyclosporine
3 *Diltiazem:* Increased sirolimus concentrations
A *Grapefruit juice:* Increased sirolimus concentrations, grapefruit juice should not be administered with sirolimus
A *Ketoconazole:* Significant increase in rate and extent of absorption of sirolimus, concurrent administration not recommended
A *Live vaccines:* Avoid use of live vaccines, vaccinations may be less effective
2 *Rifampin:* Sirolimus clearance significantly increased, decreased sirolimus concentrations; consider alternative therapeutic agents to rifampin
3 *St. John's wort (hypericum perforatum):* Potential for decreased plasma tacrolimus concentrations
SPECIAL CONSIDERATIONS
• Tablets and solution are not bioequivalent (tab has 27% > bioavailability), however 2 mg tabs clinically equivalent to 2 mg oral sol; not known if higher doses of oral sol are clinically equivalent to higher doses of tabs
• Allows cyclosporine dose reduction
• Experience limited with use as rescue therapy
• Black patients had higher rejection rates (56% vs 13%) than non-blacks given same regimen; no significant differences in trough sirolimus concentrations at equal doses between blacks and non-blacks
• IV formulation is under development
PATIENT/FAMILY EDUCATION
• Take medication the same each day with regard to timing of meals and other medications

* = non-FDA-approved use

• Limit UV/sunlight exposure, wear protective clothing and use sunreen due to increased risk of skin cancer

• Due to potential risks to fetus, effective contraception should be used before, during and 12 wks after sirolimus therapy in women of childbearing potential

MONITORING PARAMETERS

• Whole-blood sirolimus levels (drawn 1 hr prior to next dose), 5-7 days after initiation or dose change. Maintain levels at 10-15 ng/ml for first month, then consider increasing to 15-20 ng/ml, especially in patients receiving little cyclosporine

• CBC, platelets, lipids

---

sodium bicarbonate

Combinations

OTC: with alginic acid, (AlOH, Mg Trisilicate Gastrocote); with sodium citrate (Citrocarbonate)

Chemical Class: Monosodium salt of carbonic acid

Therapeutic Class: Systemic/urinary alkalinizing agent; antacid; electrolyte supplement

---

CLINICAL PHARMACOLOGY

Mechanism of Action: Orally neutralizes gastric acid, which forms water, $NaCl$, CO_2; increases plasma bicarbonate, buffers H^+ ion concentration, raises pH, reverses acidosis

Pharmacokinetics

Excreted in urine and by lungs (CO_2)

INDICATIONS AND USES: Metabolic acidosis (e.g., renal disease, cardiac arrest, circulatory insufficiency); systemic and urinary alkalinization (renal calculi, treatment of drug intoxications); antacid; electrolyte replacement (diarrhea); sickle cell anemia treatment*

DOSAGE

Adult

• *Acidosis:* IV INF 100-350 mEq over 4-8 hr depending on CO_2 and pH

• *Cardiac arrest:* IV bolus 1 mEq/kg, then 0.5 mEq/kg q10min prn while arrest continues (based on ABGs)

• *Alkalinization of urine:* PO 325 mg-2 g qid

• *Antacid:* PO 300 mg-2 g chewed, taken with H_2O qd-qid

Child 6-12 yr

• *Acidosis:* IV INF 2-5 mEq/kg over 4-8 hr depending on CO_2 and pH

• *Cardiac arrest:* IV bolus 1 mEq/kg, then 0.5 mEq/kg q10 min prn while arrest continues (based on ABGs)

• *Alkalinization of urine:* PO 12-120 mg/kg/day

• *Antacid:* 520 mg; may repeat in 30 min

Infant

• *Acidosis:* IV INF not to exceed 8 mEq/kg/day based on ABGs (4.2% sol)

$ AVAILABLE FORMS/COST OF THERAPY

• Inj, Sol—IV: 4.2%, 10 ml: **$3.14-$13.75**; 5%, 500 ml: **$14.06-$39.25**; 7.5%, 50 ml: **$4.46-$18.96**; 8.4%, 10 ml: **$2.89-$17.20**

• Tab, Coated—Oral: 325 mg, 1000's: **$11.55**; 650 mg, 100's: **$0.65-$7.93**

CONTRAINDICATIONS: Continued losses from vomiting or GI suction; diuretic-induced hypochloremic alkalosis

PRECAUTIONS: CHF, cirrhosis, hypertension, hypocalcemia, toxemia, renal disease

PREGNANCY AND LACTATION: Pregnancy category C

---

italic = common side effects   ***bold italic*** = life-threatening reactions

SIDE EFFECTS/ADVERSE REACTIONS

CNS: Confusion, headache, *hyperreflexia,* irritability, **seizures** caused by alkalosis, stimulation, tetany, tremors, *twitching,* weakness

CV: **Cardiac arrest,** edema, irregular pulse, water retention, weight gain

GI: Acid rebound, *belching,* cramps, *distension,* flatulence, increased thirst, **paralytic ileus**

GU: Calculi

METAB: Alkalosis, hypercalcemia or milk-alkali syndrome, hypokalemia

RESP: **Apnea,** cyanosis, shallow, slow respirations

INTERACTIONS

Drugs

3 *Amphetamines:* Sodium bicarbonate inhibits the elimination and increases the effects of amphetamines

3 *Beta blockers:* Reduced absorption

3 *Cefpodoxime:* Reduced absorption

3 *Cefuroxime:* Reduced serum levels with reduced antibiotic efficacy

3 *Ephedrine:* Large doses of sodium bicarbonate increase the serum concentrations of ephedrine

3 *Flecainide:* Increased urine pH will increase flecainide serum concentration

3 *Glipizide:* Enhanced rate of glipizide absorption

3 *Glyburide:* Enhanced rate of glyburide absorption

3 *Iron:* Reduced iron absorption

3 *Ketoconazole:* Decreased ketoconazole absorption

3 *Lithium:* Sodium bicarbonate may lower lithium plasma concentrations

3 *Methenamine compound:* Sodium bicarbonate-induced urinary pH changes interfere with antibacterial activity of methenamine compounds

3 *Mexiletine:* Increased urine pH increases mexiletine concentrations

3 *Pseudoephedrine:* Sodium bicarbonate-induced urinary pH changes may markedly inhibit the elimination of pseudoephedrine

3 *Quinidine:* Sodium bicarbonate-induced urinary pH changes may increase quinidine concentrations

3 *Quinolones:* Reduced absorption

3 *Salicylates:* Sodium bicarbonate-induced urinary pH changes can decrease serum salicylate concentrations

3 *Tetracyclines:* Reduced absorption

Labs

• *Protein:* Falsely elevates urine protein

SPECIAL CONSIDERATIONS
PATIENT/FAMILY EDUCATION

• Milk-alkali syndrome (may result from excessive antacid use): confusion, headache, nausea, vomiting, anorexia, urinary stones, hypercalcemia

• To avoid drug interactions due to reduced absorption, separate intake by 2 hr

MONITORING PARAMETERS

• Electrolytes, blood pH, PO_2, HCO_3, during treatment

• ABGs frequently during emergencies

---

* = non-FDA-approved use

sodium chloride

OTC: *Nasal:* Afrin Saline Mist, Ayr, Breathe Free, Dristan Saline, HuMist, NāSal, Ocean, Pretz, SalineX, SeaMist
Ophth: Adsorbonac, AK-NaCl, Muro-128, Muroptic-5
Chemical Class: Sodium salt
Therapeutic Class: Electrolyte supplement; irrigant; moisturizing agent

CLINICAL PHARMACOLOGY

Mechanism of Action: Major electrolytes necessary for the maintenance of plasma tonicity; moisturizes dry mucous membranes; reduces corneal edema by osmosis of water through the semipermeable corneal epithelium

INDICATIONS AND USES: Electrolyte replacement, flushing IV catheters, extracellular fluid replacement, abortifacient; prevention of muscle cramps and heat prostration; GU irrigation; nasal mucous moisturization; diluent for IV, IM, or SC injections; corneal edema (ophth)

DOSAGE

Adult

• *Electrolyte replacement:* IV sodium deficiency (mEq/kg) = [% dehydration (L/kg)/100 × 70 (mEq/L)] + [0.6(L/kg) × (140 − serum sodium)(mEq/L)]

• *Severe hyponatremia:* IV mEq sodium = [desired sodium (mEq/L) − [actual sodium (mEq/L) × 0.6 × wt (kg)]; for acute correction, use 125 mEq as the desired serum sodium; acutely correct serum sodium in 5 mEq/L dose increments; more gradual correction in increments of 10 mEq/L/day is indicated in the asymptomatic patient

• *Chloride maintenance electrolyte requirement in parenteral nutrition:* IV 2-4 mEq/kg/24 hr or 25-40 mEq/1000 kcal/24 hr; max 100-150 mEq/24 hr

• *Sodium maintenance electrolyte requirement in parenteral nutrition:* IV 3-4 mEq/kg/24 hr or 25-40 mEq/1000 kcal/24 hr; max 100-150 mEq/24 hr

• *Heat cramps:* PO 0.5-1 g with full glass of water (up to 4.8 g/day)

• *GU irrigant:* 1-3 L/day

• *Nasal:* prn

• *Corneal edema:* Instill 1-2 gtt q3-4h or ointment hs

• *Abortifacient:* 20% (250 ml) transabdominal intra-amniotic instillation

Child

• *Electrolyte replacement:* IV sodium deficiency (mEq/kg) = [% dehydration (L/kg)/100 × 70 (mEq/L)] + [0.6(L/kg) × (140 − serum sodium)(mEq/L)]

• *Nasal:* prn

• *Corneal edema:* Instill 1-2 gtt q3-4h or ointment hs

Newborn

• *Electrolyte requirement:* Premature, 2-8 mEq/kg/24 hr; term, 0-48 hr 0-2 mEq/kg/24 hr; >48 hr 1-4 mEq/kg/24 hr

🅂 AVAILABLE FORMS/COST OF THERAPY

• Oint—Ophth: 5%, 3.5 g: **$10.22-$14.40**

• Sol, Bacteriostatic Diluent: 0.9%, 30 ml: **$0.56-$3.74**

• Sol, Electrolyte—IV: 0.45%, 1000 ml: **$1.38-$2.30**; 0.9%, 1000 ml: **$1.27-$1.56**; 3%, 500 ml: **$1.62**; 5%, 500 ml: **$11.88**; 14.6%, 20 ml (for dilution): **$0.98-$2.26**; 23.4%, 30 ml (for dilution): **$0.62-$1.51**

• Sol, Isotonic—INH: 0.45%, 3 ml × 100: **$10.00-$17.00**; 0.9%, 3 ml × 100: **$10.00-$22.00**

---

italic = common side effects   ***bold italic*** = life-threatening reactions

• Sol-Genitourinary Irrigant: 0.45%, 2000 ml (hypotonic): **$6.65-$12.74**; 0.9% (isotonic), 2000 ml: **$6.65-$12.74**

• Sol—Nasal: 0.4%; 15 ml: **$3.87**; 0.9%; 30 ml: **$2.38**

• Sol—Ophth: 2%, 15 ml: **$13.68-$17.58**; 5%, 15 ml: **$10.22-$21.25**

• Tab, Electrolyte—Oral: 1 g, 100's: **$3.25-$6.15**

CONTRAINDICATIONS: Hypernatremia, bacteriostatic solutions in newborns

PRECAUTIONS: Uncompensated cardiovascular, cirrhotic, or nephrotic disease; circulatory insufficiency; hypoproteinemia; hypervolemia; urinary tract obstruction; CHF; patients with concurrent edema and sodium retention, those receiving corticosteroids, and those retaining salt

PREGNANCY AND LACTATION: Pregnancy category C

SIDE EFFECTS/ADVERSE REACTIONS

CNS: Coma, irritability, obtundation, restlessness, *seizures,* weakness

*CV: **CHF,*** hypervolemia

EENT: Stinging

GI: Abdominal cramps, diarrhea, nausea, vomiting

METAB: Sodium chloride excess or deficit

*RESP: **Pulmonary edema***

MISC: Rapid infusion may cause local pain at inj site

INTERACTIONS

Drugs

3 *Lithium:* High sodium intake may reduce serum lithium concentrations, while restriction of sodium tends to increase serum lithium

SPECIAL CONSIDERATIONS

• One g of sodium chloride provides 17.1 mEq sodium and 17.1 mEq chloride

---

sodium citrate and citric acid sodium citrate and potassium citrate

Rx: *Sodium citrate and citric acid:* Bicitra, Oracit
Sodium citrate and potassium citrate: Citrolith, Polycitra, Polycitra-K, Polycitra-LC
Therapeutic Class: Oral alkalinizing agents

CLINICAL PHARMACOLOGY

Mechanism of Action: Sodium citrate is absorbed and metabolized to sodium bicarbonate, thus acting as a systemic alkalinizer; the effects of these salts are essentially those of chlorides before absorption and those of bicarbonates subsequently

Pharmacokinetics

PO: <5% of citrate is excreted unchanged

INDICATIONS AND USES: Alkalinizing agent; useful where long-term maintenance of an alkaline urine is desirable; alleviation of chronic metabolic acidosis (i.e., chronic renal insufficiency or the syndrome of renal tubular acidosis); buffers and neutralizes gastric acid

DOSAGE

Adult

• *Systemic alkalinization:* Sodium citrate and citric acid, PO 10-30 ml diluted pc, hs; sodium citrate and potassium citrate, PO 15-30 ml diluted pc, hs

• *Neutralizing buffer:* PO 15 ml diluted taken as a single dose

Child

• *Systemic alkalinization:* Sodium citrate and citric acid, PO 5-15 ml diluted pc, hs; sodium citrate and potassium citrate, PO 5-15 ml diluted pc, hs

---

* = non-FDA-approved use

$ AVAILABLE FORMS/COST OF THERAPY

Sodium Citrate/Citric Acid
• Sol—Oral: 480 ml: **$7.80**
Sodium Citrate/Potassium Citrate
• Liq/Syr—Oral: 480 ml: **$13.94-$16.95**
• Tab—Oral: 50 mg-950 mg, 100's: **$10.70**

CONTRAINDICATIONS: Sodium-restricted diets; severe renal impairment

PRECAUTIONS: Low urinary output; patients with cardiac failure, hypertension, impaired renal function, peripheral and pulmonary edema, and toxemia of pregnancy

SPECIAL CONSIDERATIONS
PATIENT/FAMILY EDUCATION
• Sugar free
• Dilute adequately with water and, preferably, take each dose after meals to avoid saline laxative effect

MONITORING PARAMETERS
• Serum electrolytes, particularly serum bicarb level
NOTE: Sodium citrate and potassium citrate known as Sholl's Solution, sodium citrate and citric acid as modified Sholl's

---

sodium polystyrene sulfonate

(pol-ee-stye'reen)
Rx: Kayexalate, Kionex
Chemical Class: Cation exchange resin
Therapeutic Class: Antihyperkalemic

CLINICAL PHARMACOLOGY
Mechanism of Action: Removes potassium by exchanging sodium for potassium in body; occurs primarily in large intestine

Pharmacokinetics
PO/PR: Not absorbed from the GI tract

INDICATIONS AND USES: Hyperkalemia (in conjunction with other measures)

DOSAGE
Administer in approx 25% sorbitol susp or concurrently treat with 70% oral sorbitol syrup 10-20 ml q2h to produce 1 or 2 watery stools/day
Adult
• PO 15 g qd-qid
• PR 30-50 g/100 ml of sorbitol warmed to body temp q6h
Child
• PO/PR 1g/kg q6h

$ AVAILABLE FORMS/COST OF THERAPY

• Powder—Oral: 454 g: **$81.25-$225.01**
• Susp—Oral: 15 g/60 ml, 60 ml: **$5.85-$8.65**
• Susp—Rect: 50 mg/200 ml, 200 ml: **$29.00**

CONTRAINDICATIONS: Hypokalemia

PRECAUTIONS: Renal failure, CHF, severe edema, severe hypertension

PREGNANCY AND LACTATION: Pregnancy category C; excretion in breast milk not expected

SIDE EFFECTS/ADVERSE REACTIONS
CV: CHF
METAB: Alkalosis
GI: Anorexia, constipation, diarrhea (sorbitol), fecal impaction, gastric irritation, nausea, vomiting
METAB: Hypocalcemia, hypokalemia, hypomagnesemia, sodium retention

INTERACTIONS
Drugs
3 *Antacids:* Combined use of magnesium- or calcium-containing antacids with resin may result in systemic alkalosis

---

italic = common side effects   ***bold italic*** = life-threatening reactions

SPECIAL CONSIDERATIONS
• Exchange efficacy of resin is approx 33%; 1 g of resin (4.1 mEq of sodium) exchanges approximately 1 mEq of potassium
• Rectal route is less effective than oral administration

PATIENT/FAMILY EDUCATION
• Don't mix with orange juice

MONITORING PARAMETERS
• Serum K, Ca, Mg, Na, acid-base balance, bowel function, possibly ECG

---

somatropin/somatrem (growth hormone)
(soe-ma-troe´pin)
Rx: *Somatropin:* Genotropin, Norditropin, Nutropin, Nutropin AQ, Humatrope, Saizen, Serostim
Somatrem: Protropin
Chemical Class: Recombinant DNA product; somatropin is identical to human growth hormone, somatrem contains an additional amino acid
Therapeutic Class: Growth hormone; anticachexic

CLINICAL PHARMACOLOGY
Mechanism of Action: Stimulates skeletal growth in growth hormone deficiency, reduces fat stores, induces insulin resistance

Pharmacokinetics
SC: Peak 7.5 hr; localizes to highly perfused organs; metabolized by kidney, liver

INDICATIONS AND USES: Pituitary growth hormone deficiency; growth failure associated with chronic renal insufficiency (somatropin only); AIDS wasting or cachexia (Serostim); Turner's syndrome in girls (Neutropin only)

DOSAGE
Adult
• *AIDs wasting or cachexia:* SC >55 kg 6 mg qhs, 45-55 kg 5 mg qhs, 35-45 kg 4 mg qhs, <35 kg 0.1 mg/kg qhs
Child
• *Somatropin*
• *Growth hormone inadequacy:* SC weekly dose of up to 0.3 mg/kg via daily injections (Nutropin); SC/IM up to 0.06 mg/kg 3 times/wk (Humatrope)
• *Chronic renal insufficiency:* SC weekly dose of up to 0.35 mg/kg via daily injections (Nutropin); therapy may be continued up to time of transplantation
• *Somatrem:* SC/IM up to 0.1 (0.26 IU) mg/kg 3 times/wk

⑤ AVAILABLE FORMS/COST OF THERAPY
Somatropin
• Inj, Dry-Sol—IM, SC: 1.5 mg: **$68.90**; 4 mg: **$168.00**; 5 mg: **$210.01**; 5.8 mg: **$229.69**; 6 mg: **$252.00**; 10 mg: **$441.00**; 12 mg: **$575.50**; 24 mg: **$1,151.01**
Somatrem
• Inj, Lyphl-Sol—IM, SC: 5 mg/vial: **$420.00**; 10 mg/vial: **$882.00**

CONTRAINDICATIONS: Hypersensitivity to benzyl alcohol, closed epiphyses, evidence of tumor activity and/or active neoplasia; sensitivity to m-cresol or glycerin (Humatrope)

PRECAUTIONS: Diabetes mellitus, hypothyroidism

PREGNANCY AND LACTATION: Pregnancy category C; excretion into breast milk unknown

SIDE EFFECTS/ADVERSE REACTIONS
CNS: Headache, *intracranial hypertension*
HEME: **Leukemia** (uncertain relationship)

METAB: Glycosuria, hypercalciuria, hypothyroidism, ketosis, mild hyperglycemia

SKIN: Inflammation at inj site, pain, rash, urticaria

MISC: Antibodies to growth hormone

SPECIAL CONSIDERATIONS
MONITORING PARAMETERS
• Individualize doses for growth hormone inadequacy
• Check for hypothyroidism, malnutrition, antibodies or opportunistic infections (AIDs patients) if no response to initial dose
• TSH
• Evaluate if child limps
• Follow with fundoscopy (papilledema)

---

sorbitol
(sor'bi-tole)
Rx: Sorbitol
Chemical Class: Polyalcoholic sugar
Therapeutic Class: Osmotic laxative; osmotic diuretic

CLINICAL PHARMACOLOGY
Mechanism of Action: Hyperosmolar; acts as diuretic, laxative
Pharmacokinetics
PO/PR: Absorption poor, onset of action 15-60 min; when used as urologic irrigant, variable systemic absorption occurs; metabolized to CO_2 and dextrose by liver or excreted by kidneys

INDICATIONS AND USES: Irrigant sol during transurethral prostatic surgery; laxative*; facilitates passage of sodium polystyrene sulfonate through intestinal tract*

DOSAGE
Adult
• *Laxative:* PO 30-150 ml (70% sol)

• *Rectal enema:* 120 ml (25%-30% sol)
• *Adjunct to polystyrene sulfonate:* 15 ml (70% sol) until diarrhea, or 20-100 ml as oral vehicle for the resin
• *Irrigant:* Top 3.3% sol
Child 2-11 yr
• *Laxative:* PO 2 ml/kg (70% sol)
• *Rectal enema:* 30-60 ml (25%-30% sol)
🅂 AVAILABLE FORMS/COST OF THERAPY
• Sol—Irrigation: 3.3%, 4000 ml: **$28.26**
• Sol—Oral: 70%, 480 ml: **$2.93-$17.50**

CONTRAINDICATIONS: Anuria
PRECAUTIONS: Significant cardiopulmonary, renal dysfunction; diabetes mellitus, hyponatremia, hypovolemia
SIDE EFFECTS/ADVERSE REACTIONS
CNS: **Seizures,** vertigo
CV: Angina, **CHF,** hypotension
EENT: Blurred vision, rhinitis, thirst
GI: Colonic necrosis, diarrhea, nausea, vomiting
GU: Acidosis, diuresis, edema, fluid retention, urinary retention
METAB: Acidosis, hyperglycemia, hypernatremia, hyponatremia
MISC: Chills, urticaria

---

sotalol
(soe'ta-lole)
Rx: Betapace
Chemical Class: Nonselective β-adrenergic blocker
Therapeutic Class: Antidysrhythmic

CLINICAL PHARMACOLOGY
Mechanism of Action: PO Competitive β-adrenergic antagonist; produces negative inotropic and chronotropic responses; slows AV

---

italic = common side effects   **bold italic** = life-threatening reactions

nodal conduction; decreases heart rate; decreases myocardial oxygen consumption; antiarrhythmic effects (class II); reduction in platelet aggregation and blood viscosity; suppression of renin release; inhibition of central sympathetic outflow; decreases presynaptic receptor neurotransmitter release; no intrinsic sympathomimetic or membrane stabilizing activity; low lipid solubility

Pharmacokinetics

PO: Onset 1-2 hr, peak effect 3-4 hr; $t_{1/2}$ 12 hr; excreted unchanged by kidney; low lipid solubility; not protein bound; absorption decreased 20%-30% by meals

INDICATIONS AND USES: Ventricular arrhythmias (tachycardia, fibrillation), angina pectoris,* hypertension,* postmyocardial infarction,* supraventricular arrhythmias,* congestive heart failure

DOSAGE

Adult and Child >16 yr

• *Arrhythmias (supraventricular and ventricular):* IV 0.2-1.5 mg/kg over 5 min; PO 80 mg bid (ac); increased q2-3 days in 40-80 mg increments to a total daily dose between 160-320 mg

NOTE: Gradually withdraw previous antiarrhythmic therapy prior to starting oral sotalol (2-3 half-lives); not a significant problem with lidocaine

• Renal failure adjustment: CrCl > 60 ml/min administer q12h; CrCl 30-60 ml/min administer q24h; CrCl 10-30 ml/min administer q36-48h; individualize dose for CrCl <10 ml/min; increase dose after 5-6 doses prn

💲 AVAILABLE FORMS/COST OF THERAPY

• Tab, Coated—Oral: 80 mg, 100's: **$51.25-$295.88**; 120 mg, 100's: **$68.38-$394.69**; 160 mg, 100's: **$85.49-$493.50**; 240 mg, 100's: **$111.13-$641.44**

CONTRAINDICATIONS: Bronchial asthma, cardiogenic shock, overt cardiac failure, 2nd and 3rd degree AV block, severe sinus bradycardia

PRECAUTIONS: Anesthesia/surgery (myocardial depression), avoid abrupt withdrawal, bronchospastic airways, congestive heart failure, diabetes mellitus, hyperthyroidism/thyrotoxicosis, concurrent clonidine (discontinue atenolol several days prior to withdrawal of clonidine), peripheral vascular disease, renal disease

PREGNANCY AND LACTATION: Pregnancy category B; similar drug, atenolol, frequently used in the third trimester for treatment of hypertension (many studies of efficacy and safety of atenolol in pregnancy-induced hypertension); long-term use has been associated with intrauterine growth retardation; concentrated in breast milk (levels 3-5 times those of plasma); symptoms of β-blockade possible in infant, but considered compatible with breast feeding

SIDE EFFECTS/ADVERSE REACTIONS

CNS: Anxiety, confusion, depression, *dizziness,* drowsiness, *fatigue,* hallucinations, insomnia, nightmares, weakness

CV: Bradycardia, chest pain, ***CHF,*** hypotension, Raynaud's phenomena, ***ventricular dysrhythmias including torsade de points***

GI: Constipation, diarrhea, nausea, stomach discomfort, vomiting

GU: Sexual dysfunction

HEME: ***Agranulocytosis***

---

* = non-FDA-approved use

RESP: ***Bronchospasm,*** cough, dyspnea

INTERACTIONS
Drugs

▣ *Adenosine:* Bradycardia aggravated

▣ *Alpha-1 adrenergic blockers:* Potential enhanced first dose response (marked initial drop in blood pressure), particularly on standing (especially prazocin)

▣ *Amiodarone:* Combination yielded bradycardia and hypotension in case reports

▣ *Antacids:* Reduced sotalol absorption

▣ *Calcium channel blockers:* See dihydropyridine calcium channel blockers and verapamil

▣ *Cimetidine:* Renal clearance reduced; AUC increased with cimetidine coadministration

▣ *Cisapride:* Dual prolongation of QT interval; increased risk of ventricular tachyarrhythmias

▣ *Clonidine, guanabenz, guanfacine:* Exacerbation of rebound hypertension upon discontinuation of clonidine

▣ *Cocaine:* Cocaine-induced vasoconstriction potentiated; reduced coronary blood flow

▣ *Contrast media:* Increased risk of anaphylaxis

▣ *Digitalis:* Enhances bradycardia

▣ *Dihydropyridine calcium channel blockers:* Additive pharmacodynamic effects

▣ *Dipyridamole:* Bradycardia aggravated

▣ *Epinephrine, isoproterenol, phenylephrine:* Potentiates pressor response; resultant hypertension and bradycardia

▣ *Flecainide:* Additive negative inotropic effects; case report of bradycardia, AV block, and cardiac arrest following switch from flecainide to sotalol

▣ *Fluoxetine:* Increased β-blockade activity

▣ *Fluroquinolones:* Reduced clearance of sotalol

▣ *Hypoglycemic agents:* Masked hypoglycemia, hyperglycemia

▣ *Insulin:* Altered response to hypoglycemia; increased blood glucose concentrations; impaired peripheral circulation

▣ *Lidocaine:* Increased serum lidocaine concentrations possible

▣ *Neostigmine:* Bradycardia aggravated

▣ *Neuroleptics:* Both drugs inhibit each other's metabolism; additive hypotension

▣ *NSAIDs:* Reduced hemodynamic effects of sotalol

▣ *Physostigmine:* Bradycardia aggravated

▣ *Prazosin:* First-dose response to prazosin may be enhanced by β-blockade

▣ *Tacrine:* Bradycardia aggravated

❷ *Terbutaline:* Antagonized bronchodilating effects of terbutaline

❷ *Theophylline:* Antagonistic pharmacodynamic effects

▣ *Verapamil:* Enhanced effects of both drugs; particularly AV nodal conduction slowing; reduced sotalol clearance

Labs

• *Metanephrines total:* Falsely increases urine levels (may be double)

SPECIAL CONSIDERATIONS
PATIENT/FAMILY EDUCATION

• Do not discontinue abruptly; may require taper; rapid withdrawal may produce rebound hypertension or angina

MONITORING PARAMETERS

• Angina: Reduction in nitroglycerin usage; frequency, severity, onset, and duration of angina pain; heart rate

---

italic = common side effects   ***bold italic*** = life-threatening reactions

- Arrhythmias: Heart rate and rhythm; monitor QT intervals (discontinue or reduce dose if QT >550 msec)
- Congestive heart failure: Functional status, cough, dyspnea on exertion, paroxysmal nocturnal dyspnea, exercise tolerance, and ventricular function
- Hypertension: Blood pressure
- Toxicity: Blood glucose, bronchospasm, hypotension, bradycardia, depression, confusion, hallucination, sexual dysfunction
- Because of prodysrhythmic risk, begin and increase drug in setting with cardiac rhythm monitoring

---

sparfloxacin

(spar-floks′a-sin)

Rx: Zagam
Chemical Class: Fluoroquinolone derivative
Therapeutic Class: Antibiotic

CLINICAL PHARMACOLOGY

Mechanism of Action: Interferes with the enzyme DNA gyrase needed for the synthesis of bacterial DNA; bactericidal

Pharmacokinetics

PO: Peak 3-6 hr; 45% bound to plasma proteins, penetrates well into body fluids and tissues; metabolized in liver (primarily by glucuronidation), excreted in feces (50%) and urine (50%); $t_{1/2}$ 20 hr

INDICATIONS AND USES: Community-acquired pneumonia, acute bacterial exacerbations of chronic bronchitis caused by susceptible organisms

Antibacterial spectrum usually includes:

- Gram-positive organisms: *Staphylococcus aureus, Streptococcus pneumoniae* (penicillin-susceptible strains)
- Gram-negative organisms: *Enterobacter cloacae, Haemophilus influenzae, H. parainfluenzae, Klebsiella pneumoniae, Moraxella catarrhalis*
- Other organisms: *Chlamydia pneumoniae, Mycoplasma pneumoniae*

DOSAGE

Adult

- PO 400 mg × 1, then 200 mg qd for 9 days; for CrCl <50 ml/min, 400 mg × 1, then 200 mg q48h for 9 days

$ AVAILABLE FORMS/COST OF THERAPY

- Tab—Oral: 200 mg, 11's: **$73.58**

CONTRAINDICATIONS: History of photosensitivity reactions, known prolonged QT_c interval, children <18 yr

PRECAUTIONS: Seizure disorder, dehydration, renal impairment, hepatic impairment

PREGNANCY AND LACTATION: Pregnancy category C; excretion into breast milk unknown; due to the potential for arthropathy and osteochondrosis, use extreme caution in nursing mothers

SIDE EFFECTS/ADVERSE REACTIONS

CNS: Anxiety, depression, dizziness, fatigue, headache, insomnia, seizures, somnolence
CV: QT_c interval prolongation
EENT: Dizziness, visual disturbances
GI: Abdominal pain, anorexia, diarrhea, dry mouth, flatulence, heartburn, increased AST, ALT; *nausea,* pseudomembranous colitis, vomiting
GU: Vaginal moniliasis
SKIN: Photosensitivity, pruritus, rash

---

* = non-FDA-approved use

INTERACTIONS
Drugs

3 *Aluminum:* Reduced absorption of sparfloxacin; do not take within 4 hr of dose

3 *Antacids:* Reduced absorption of sparfloxacin; do not take within 4 hr of dose

3 *Antipyrine:* Inhibits metabolism of antipyrine; increased plasma antipyrine level

3 *Calcium:* Reduced absorption of sparfloxacin; do not take within 4 hr of dose

3 *Diazepam:* Inhibits metabolism of diazepam; increased plasma diazepam level

3 *Didanosine:* Markedly reduced absorption of sparfloxacin; take sparfloxacin 2 hr before didanosine

3 *Foscarnet:* Coadministration increases seizure risk

3 *Iron:* Reduced absorption of sparfloxacin; do not take within 4 hr of dose

3 *Magnesium:* Reduced absorption of sparfloxacin; do not take within 4 hr of dose

3 *Metoprolol:* Inhibits metabolism of metoprolol; increased plasma metoprolol level

3 *Phenytoin:* Inhibits metabolism of phenytoin; increased plasma phenytoin level

3 *Propranolol:* Inhibits metabolism of propranolol; increased plasma propranolol level

3 *Ropinirole:* Inhibits metabolism of ropinirole; increased plasma ropinirole level

3 *Sodium bicarbonate:* Reduced absorption of sparfloxacin; do not take within 4 hr of dose

3 *Sucralfate:* Reduced absorption of sparfloxacin; do not take within 4 hr of dose

3 *Warfarin:* Inhibits metabolism of warfarin; increases hypoprothrombinemic response to warfarin

3 *Zinc:* Reduced absorption of sparfloxacin; do not take within 4 hr of dose

SPECIAL CONSIDERATIONS
PATIENT/FAMILY EDUCATION

• Avoid direct or indirect sunlight during treatment and for 5 days after completion of therapy; drink fluids liberally

---

spectinomycin
(spek-ti-noe-mye′sin)
Rx: Trobicin
Chemical Class: Aminoglycoside derivative
Therapeutic Class: Antibiotic

CLINICAL PHARMACOLOGY
Mechanism of Action: Inhibits bacterial synthesis by binding to 30S subunit on ribosomes; bacteriostatic
Pharmacokinetics
IM: Peak 1-2 hr, duration 8 hr, $t_{1/2}$ 1-3 hr (10-30 hr if CrCl <20 ml/min); excreted in urine (unchanged); poor distribution into saliva

INDICATIONS AND USES: Gonorrhea (except pharyngeal infection) in patients who cannot take ceftriaxone
DOSAGE
Adult
• IM 2-4 g as single dose; 2 g q12h for disseminated infection
Child <45 kg
• IM 30-40 mg/kg as single dose
$ AVAILABLE FORMS/COST OF THERAPY
• Inj, Dry-Susp—IM: 400 mg/ml, 2 g: **$28.21**
CONTRAINDICATIONS: Infants (diluent contains benzyl alcohol)
PRECAUTIONS: Children
PREGNANCY AND LACTATION: Pregnancy category B; excretion into breast milk unknown

---

SIDE EFFECTS/ADVERSE REACTIONS

CNS: Anxiety, chills, dizziness, fever, headache, insomnia

GI: Nausea, vomiting

GU: Decreased urine output

HEME: Anemia

SKIN: Fever, *pain at inj site,* pruritus, rash, urticaria

SPECIAL CONSIDERATIONS

• Follow with doxycycline 100 mg bid for 7 days (erythromycin if pregnant or allergic)

• Ineffective against syphilis and may mask symptoms

• Give in gluteal muscle; dose >2 g must be divided in 2 gluteal injections

---

spironolactone

(speer-on-oh-lak′tone)

Rx: Aldactone

Combinations

  Rx: with hydrochlorothiazide (Aldactazide, Spirozide)

Chemical Class: Aldosterone antagonist

Therapeutic Class: Potassium-sparing diuretic, antihypertensive

---

CLINICAL PHARMACOLOGY

Mechanism of Action: Competitive aldosterone inhibitor; interferes with sodium reabsorption in the distal tubule, thus decreasing potassium secretion; weak diuretic and antihypertensive effects when used alone unless primary or secondary hyperaldosteronism present (more potent); other actions: interferes with testosterone synthesis and conversion of testosterone to estradiol

Pharmacokinetics

PO: Peak serum concentration: 1-3 hr; peak effect, 48-72 hr; >90% bound to plasma proteins; metabolized in liver, excreted in feces (50%) urine (40%); crosses placenta; $t_{1/2}$ 1.4 hr

INDICATIONS AND USES: Edema, hypertension, CHF, diuretic-induced hypokalemia, primary hyperaldosteronism, nephrotic syndrome, cirrhosis of the liver with ascites, polycystic ovary disease,* premenstrual syndrome,* female hirsutism*

DOSAGE

Adult

• *Edema or hypertension:* PO 25-200 mg/day in single or divided doses

• *Hypokalemia:* PO 25-100 mg/day in single or divided doses *CHF:* PO 25 mg/day

• *CHF:* PO 25 mg/day

• *Primary hyperaldosteronism diagnosis:* PO 400 mg/day for 4 days (short test) or 4 wk (long test), then 100-400 mg/day maintenance

• *Polycystic ovary disease or hirsutism:* PO 100-200 mg/day

Child

• *Diuretic or antihypertensive or ascites:* PO 1-3 mg/kg/day in single or divided doses

$ **AVAILABLE FORMS/COST OF THERAPY**

• Tab, Plain Coated—Oral: 25 mg, 100's: **$6.25-$55.75**; 50 mg, 100's: **$81.59-$97.91**; 100 mg, 100's: **$142.28-$164.16**

CONTRAINDICATIONS: Anuria, severe renal disease, hyperkalemia, antikaliuretic therapy (including angiotensin-converting enzyme inhibitors, angiotensin receptor blockers, and potassium supplements)

PRECAUTIONS: Dehydration, diabetes, hepatic disease, hyponatremia, renal insufficiency, potassium supplements, menstrual abnormalities, gynecomastia, acidosis, elderly

---

* = non-FDA-approved use

PREGNANCY AND LACTATION:
Pregnancy category D; feminization occurs in male rat fetuses; active metabolite excreted in breast milk; compatible with breast feeding but alternate options preferred; therapy for existing hypertension can be continued throughout pregnancy with minimal risk; initiating for simple edema not recommended; few unequivocal indications for diuretic therapy in pregnancy except for pulmonary edema or congestive heart failure

SIDE EFFECTS/ADVERSE REACTIONS

CNS: Ataxia, confusion, drowsiness, headache, lethargy

CV: Bradycardia, ***CHF,*** hypotension

GI: Anorexia, ***bleeding,*** constipation, cramps, *diarrhea,* gastritis, nausea, *vomiting*

GU: Amenorrhea, deepening voice, gynecomastia, hirsutism, impotence, irregular menses, post-menopausal bleeding

METAB: Hyperchloremic metabolic acidosis, hyperkalemia, hyponatremia

SKIN: Pruritus, rash, urticaria

MISC: Breast cancer

INTERACTIONS

Drugs

🟥 *Ammonium chloride:* Combination may produce systemic acidosis

🟥 *Angiotensin-converting enzyme inhibitors:* Concurrent mechanisms to decrease potassium excretion; increased risk of hyperkalemia

🟥 *Angiotensin II receptor antagonists:* Concurrent mechanisms to decrease potassium excretion; increased risk of hyperkalemia

🟥 *Digitalis glycosides:* False or true increase in digoxin concentrations

🟥 *Disopyramide:* Increased potassium concentrations may enhance disopyramide effects on myocardial conduction

🔺 *Mitotane:* Spironolactone antagonizes the activity of mitotane

❷ *Potassium:* Increased risk of hyperkalemia

🟥 *Salicylates:* Decreased diuretic (not antihypertensive effect) due to decreased tubular secretion of active metabolite

Labs

• *Corticosteroids:* Marked false increase in plasma corticosteroids

• *Cortisol:* Falsely increased fluorometric methods of measurement

• *Digoxin:* False increases in digoxin concentrations

• *17-Hydroxycorticosteroids:* False increases in urine measurements

• *17-Ketogenic steroids:* Falsely increases urine concentrations

SPECIAL CONSIDERATIONS
MONITORING PARAMETERS

• When used for diagnosis of primary hyperaldosteronism, positive results are: (long test) correction of hyperkalemia and hypertension; (short test) serum potassium increases during administration, but falls upon discontinuation

• Blood pressure, edema, urine output, ECG (if hyperkalemia exists), urine electrolytes, BUN, creatinine, gynecomastia, impotence

S

---

stanozolol

(stan-oh′zoe-lole)

Rx: Winstrol
Chemical Class: Halogenated testosterone derivative
Therapeutic Class: Androgen; antiangioedema agent
DEA Class: Schedule III

CLINICAL PHARMACOLOGY

Mechanism of Action: Promotes body tissue-building processes and reverses catabolic processes when administered with adequate calories and protein; increases erythropoietin; increases C1 esterase inhibitor (deficient in hereditary angioedema) and resulting C2 and C4 concentrations; androgenic

INDICATIONS AND USES: Prophylaxis to decrease the frequency and severity of attacks of hereditary angioedema; possibly effective for aplastic anemia*

DOSAGE

Adult

• *Angioedema:* PO 2 mg tid, then decrease q1-3 mo to 2 mg qd or qod
• *Aplastic anemia:* PO 2 mg tid

Child

• *Angioedema:* PO up to 2 mg qd (6-12 yr); PO 1 mg qd (<6 yr)
• *Aplastic anemia:* PO up to 2 mg tid (6-12 yr); PO 1 mg bid (<6 yr)

💲 AVAILABLE FORMS/COST OF THERAPY

• Tab, Uncoated—Oral: 2 mg, 100's: **$90.07**

CONTRAINDICATIONS: Severe renal disease, severe cardiac disease, severe hepatic disease, genital bleeding (abnormal), prostate cancer, male breast cancer, female breast cancer with hypercalcemia; nephrosis; enhancement of physical appearance or athletic performance

PRECAUTIONS: Diabetes mellitus, CV disease, or risk factors for atherosclerosis, hepatic disease, seizure disorder, headache, children

PREGNANCY AND LACTATION: Pregnancy category X (masculinization); excretion into breast milk unknown; use extreme caution in nursing mothers

SIDE EFFECTS/ADVERSE REACTIONS

CNS: Anxiety, carpal tunnel syndrome, dizziness, fatigue, flushing, headache, insomnia, lability, paresthesias, sweating, tremors

CV: Increased blood pressure, edema

EENT: Conjunctival edema, deepening of voice in women, nasal congestion

GI: Cholestatic jaundice, diarrhea, ***hepatocellular necrosis, hepatic tumors, peliosis hepatis,*** nausea, vomiting, weight gain

GU: Clitoral hypertrophy, decreased breast size, decreased libido, epididymitis, gynecomastia, hematuria, impotence, menstrual irregularities, oligospermia, phallic enlargement in prepubertal males, priapism, testicular atrophy, vaginitis

METAB: Abnormal glucose tolerance, decreased HDL, electrolyte imbalance

MS: Cramps, spasms, premature epiphyseal closure (children)

SKIN: Acneiform lesions; acne vulgaris, alopecia, flushing, hirsutism and male pattern baldness in women, oily hair, skin; rash; sweating

INTERACTIONS

Drugs

❷ *Oral anticoagulants:* Enhanced hypoprothrombinemic response
❸ *Antidiabetic agents:* Enhanced hypoglycemic response
❷ *Cyclosporine:* Increased cyclosporine concentrations

---

* = non-FDA-approved use

3 *HMG-CoA reductase inhibitors (lovastatin, pravastatin):* Myositis risk increased

SPECIAL CONSIDERATIONS

• Anabolic steroids have potential for abuse, especially in the athlete

MONITORING PARAMETERS

• LFTs, lipids

• Growth rate in children (X-rays for bone age q6 mo)

---

stavudine (d4T)

(stav´yoo-deen)
Rx: Zerit
Chemical Class: Nucleoside analog
Therapeutic Class: Antiretroviral

CLINICAL PHARMACOLOGY

Mechanism of Action: Phosphorylated intracellularly to stavudine triphosphate, which inhibits HIV reverse transcriptase by competing with deoxythymidine triphosphate and inhibits viral DNA synthesis by causing DNA chain termination

Pharmacokinetics

PO: Peak 1 hr, bioavailability 85% (not affected by food); plasma $t_{1/2}$ 1½ hr, intracellular $t_{1/2}$ 3½ hr; not protein bound; only slightly metabolized; renal clearance by filtration and tubular secretion; urinary excretion of unchanged drug over 24 hr after oral dose 40%

INDICATIONS AND USES: Adults with advanced HIV infection who have received zidovudine therapy

DOSAGE

Adult

• *PO:* 40 mg q12h if weight ≥60 kg, 30 mg q12h if weight <60 kg; reduce dose by ½ if resuming therapy after resolution of side effect (neuropathy, transaminitis); adjust dose for renal insufficiency: CrCl 26-50 ml/min, 20 mg q12h if weight ≥60 kg, 15 mg q12h if weight <60 kg; CrCl 10-25 ml/min, 20 mg q24h if weight ≥60 kg, 15 mg q24h if weight <60 kg

• For latest treatment guidelines see www.hivatis.org

$ **AVAILABLE FORMS/COST OF THERAPY**

• Cap, Gel—Oral: 15 mg, 60's: **$221.98**; 20 mg, 60's: **$230.73**; 30 mg, 60's: **$240.80**; 40 mg, 60's: **$271.16**

• Sol—Oral: 1 mg/ml, 200 ml: **$61.26**

PRECAUTIONS: Peripheral neuropathy, pancreatitis, renal insufficiency, folate or vitamin B_{12} deficiency

PREGNANCY AND LACTATION: Pregnancy category C; excreted in breast milk

SIDE EFFECTS/ADVERSE REACTIONS

CNS: Dementia, headache, insomnia, *peripheral neuropathy* (15%-21%)

GI: Abdominal pain, diarrhea, *increased transaminases,* nausea, ***pancreatitis***

HEME: **Neutropenia**

MS: Myalgia

SKIN: Rash

MISC: Asthenia, fever

SPECIAL CONSIDERATIONS
PATIENT/FAMILY EDUCATION

• Report neuropathic symptoms (numbness, tingling, or pain in the feet or hands)

MONITORING PARAMETERS

• CBC, SGOT, SGPT

---

italic = common side effects   ***bold italic*** = life-threatening reactions

streptokinase

(strep-toe-kye′nase)

Rx: Kabikinase, Streptase
Chemical Class: Purified β-hemolytic streptococcus filtrate
Therapeutic Class: Thrombolytic

CLINICAL PHARMACOLOGY

Mechanism of Action: Promotes thrombolysis by promoting conversion of plasminogen to plasmin

Pharmacokinetics

IV/INTRACORONARY: Onset immediate; $t_{1/2}$ of streptokinase activator complex 23 min; mechanism of elimination unknown; no metabolites identified

INDICATIONS AND USES: Acute evolving transmural myocardial infarction; pulmonary embolism; deep venous thrombosis; arterial thrombosis or embolism; arteriovenous cannulae occlusion not responsive to heparin flush

DOSAGE

Adult

• *Acute evolving transmural MI:* IV INF 1,500,000 IU diluted to a volume of 45 ml; administer over 1 hr; intracoronary (IC) dilute 250,000 IU vial to total volume of 125 ml, give 20,000 IU (10 ml) by bolus followed by 2000 IU/min for 60 min for total dose 140,000 IU

• *Thrombosis or embolism:* IV INF 250,000 IU over ½ hr; then 100,000 IU/hr for 72 hr for deep vein thrombosis or 100,000 IU/hr for 24 hr for pulmonary embolism or 100,000 IU/hr for 24-72 hr for arterial thrombosis or embolism

• *Arteriovenous cannula occlusion:* IV INF 250,000 IU/2 ml sol into each occluded limb of cannula slowly; clamp for 2 hr; aspirate contents; flush with saline sol and reconnect cannula

💲 AVAILABLE FORMS/COST OF THERAPY

• Inj, Lyphl-Sol—Intracoronary; IV: 250,000 U/vial: **$127.83-$138.90**; 750,000 U/vial: **$306.58-$362.15**; 1,500,000 U/vial: **$561.16-$681.70**

CONTRAINDICATIONS: Active internal bleeding; recent (within 2 mo) CVA; intracranial or intraspinal surgery; intracranial neoplasm; severe uncontrolled hypertension

PRECAUTIONS: Recent (within 10 days) surgery, obstetrical delivery, organ biopsy, trauma including CPR; high likelihood of left heart thrombus (e.g., mitral stenosis with atrial fibrillation); subacute bacterial endocarditis; hemostatic defects; age ≥75 yr; diabetic hemorrhagic retinopathy; septic thrombophlebitis or infected occluded AV cannula at seriously infected site; recent streptococcal infection; repeat administration (between 5 days and 12 mo of prior streptokinase)

PREGNANCY AND LACTATION: Pregnancy category C; no data available for breast feeding

SIDE EFFECTS/ADVERSE REACTIONS

CNS: Fever, headache

CV: Hypotension, ***reperfusion dysrhythmias***

EENT: Periorbital edema

GI: Nausea, vomiting

HEME: Anemia, ***bleeding (GI, GU, intracranial, retroperitoneal,*** *surface)*

RESP: Altered respirations, ***bronchospasm, non-cardiogenic pulmonary edema,*** shortness of breath

SKIN: Flushing, itching, phlebitis at IV INF site, rash, urticaria

MISC: Chills, sweating

INTERACTIONS
Drugs
3 *Heparin, oral anticoagulants, drugs that alter platelet function (i.e., aspirin, dipyridamole, abciximab, eptifibitide, tirofiben):* May increase the risk of bleeding
Labs
• *Fibrinogen:* False increase with certain methods
• *Lactate dehydrogenase isoenzymes:* False positive

---

streptomycin
(strep-toe-mye´sin)
Rx: Streptomycin
Chemical Class: Aminoglycoside
Therapeutic Class: Antibiotic; antituberculosis agent

CLINICAL PHARMACOLOGY
Mechanism of Action: Interferes with protein synthesis in bacterial cell by binding to ribosomal subunit, causing inaccurate peptide sequence to form in protein chain, causing bacterial death
Pharmacokinetics
IM: Onset rapid, peak 1-2 hr, plasma $t_{1/2}$ 2-2½ hr; not metabolized, excreted unchanged in urine; crosses placenta
INDICATIONS AND USES: In combination with other drugs (INH, rifampin, pyrazinamide) in the treatment of tuberculosis; also indicated when 1 or more of the above drugs contraindicated; part of multidrug treatment for *Mycobacterium avium* complex*; secondary choice for nontubercular infections caused by sensitive strains of gram-negative organisms: *Hemophilus influenzae* (with another agent); *H. ducreyi* (chancroid); *Klebsiella pneumoniae* pneumonia (with another agent);

Yersinia pestis (plague); *Brucella* sp.; *Francisella tularensis* (tularemia); UTIs caused by *E. coli, Proteus* sp., *Klebsiella pneumonia* gram-positive organisms: *Streptococcus viridans* endocarditis (in combination with penicillin); *Enterococcus faecalis* (UTI and endocarditis); gram-negative bacillary bacteremia (with another agent); granuloma inguinale
DOSAGE
Adult
• *Tuberculosis:* IM 15 mg/kg/day (max 1 g qd); should ultimately be discontinued or reduced to 1 g 2-3 × /wk; given in combination with other antitubercular drugs
• *Streptococcal endocarditis:* IM 1 g q12h for 1 wk with penicillin, then 500 mg bid for 1 wk; if >60 yr, give 500 mg bid for entire 2 wk
• *Enterococcal endocarditis:* IM 1 g q12h for 2 wk, then 500 mg q12h for 4 wk with penicillin
• *Tularemia:* IM 1-2 g qd in divided doses for 7-14 days or until afebrile for 5-7 days
• *Plague:* IM 2-4 g qd in divided doses until afebrile for 3 days
• *Moderate to severe infections:* IM 1-2 g qd in divided doses q6-12h, max 4 g qd
Child
• *Tuberculosis:* IM 20-40 mg/kg/day in divided doses q6-12h given with other antitubercular drugs, max 1 g/day
$ **AVAILABLE FORMS/COST OF THERAPY**
• Inj, Sol—IM: 1 g: **$5.87**
CONTRAINDICATIONS: Severe renal disease
PRECAUTIONS: Neonates (renal immaturity) and especially those born to mothers on magnesium sulfate therapy (respiratory arrest), mild renal disease, hearing deficits, elderly

---

italic = common side effects   ***bold italic*** = life-threatening reactions

PREGNANCY AND LACTATION:
Pregnancy category D; small amounts excreted into breast milk; compatible with breast feeding (oral absorption poor)

SIDE EFFECTS/ADVERSE REACTIONS

CNS: Confusion, depression, muscle twitching, neurotoxicity, numbness, *seizures,* tremors

CV: Hypotension, myocarditis, palpitations

EENT: Deafness, ototoxicity (especially vestibular toxicity), visual disturbances

GI: Anorexia, nausea, vomiting

GU: Azotemia, hematuria, *nephrotoxicity,* oliguria, *renal damage, renal failure*

HEME: Agranulocytosis, eosinophilia, leukopenia, thrombocytopenia

SKIN: Alopecia, burning, dermatitis, rash, urticaria

INTERACTIONS

Drugs

3 *Amphotericin B, cephalosporins, cyclosporine, NSAIDs:* Additive nephrotoxicity

3 *Carboplatin:* Additive ototoxicity

2 *Ethacrynic Acid:* Additive ototoxicity

3 *Methoxyflurane:* Additive nephrotoxicity

2 *Neuromuscular blocking agents:* Respiratory depression

3 *Oral anticoagulants:* Enhanced hypoprothrombinemic response

3 *Penicillins, extended-spectrum:* Inactivation of aminoglycoside

Labs

• *Protein:* Falsely increases CSF-protein

• *Sugar:* Falsely increased urine levels via copper reduction methods

• *Urea Nitrogen:* Decreases serum levels

SPECIAL CONSIDERATIONS

• Not usually used for long term therapy secondary to nephrotoxicity and ototoxicity

MONITORING PARAMETERS

• Serum drug levels; therapeutic peak levels 20-30 µg/ml, toxic peak levels (1 hr after IM administration) >50 µg/ml

• Keep patient well hydrated

---

succimer
(sux′sim-mer)
Rx: Chemet
Chemical Class: Dimercaprol derivative
Therapeutic Class: Lead antidote

CLINICAL PHARMACOLOGY

Mechanism of Action: Forms water-soluble chelates with heavy metals that are excreted renally

Pharmacokinetics

PO: Rapidly but incompletely absorbed, peak 1-2 hr; metabolized to mixed succimer-cysteine disulfides; excreted in urine (mostly as metabolite) and feces; $t_{1/2}$ 2 days

INDICATIONS AND USES: Treatment of lead poisoning in children with blood levels >45 µg/dl; not for prophylaxis; may be of benefit in mercury* and arsenic* poisoning

DOSAGE

Adult and Child

• PO 10 mg/kg q8h for 5 days, then 10 mg/kg q12h for 14 days; may repeat if indicated by blood lead level; allow 2 wk between courses

$ **AVAILABLE FORMS/COST OF THERAPY**

• Cap, Gel—Oral: 100 mg, 100's: **$450.83**

PRECAUTIONS: Reduced renal function, history of liver disease, children <1 yr

---

* = non-FDA-approved use

PREGNANCY AND LACTATION:
Pregnancy category C; excretion in breast milk unknown; discourage mothers from breast feeding during therapy

SIDE EFFECTS/ADVERSE REACTIONS

CNS: Dizziness, drowsiness, headache, paresthesias

GI: Anorexia, diarrhea, metallic taste, nausea, vomiting

GU: Proteinuria, voiding difficulty

RESP: Cough

SKIN: Mucocutaneous eruptions, pruritus, rash

MISC: Chills, fever, flu-like symptoms

INTERACTIONS

Drugs

❷ *Other chelators (e.g., EDTA):* Coadministration not recommended

SPECIAL CONSIDERATIONS

PATIENT/FAMILY EDUCATION

• In children unable to swallow capsule, separate capsule and sprinkle beads on food or on spoon followed by fruit drink

MONITORING PARAMETERS

• Serum transaminases at start of therapy then qwk during therapy

• After therapy, monitor for rebound (because of redistribution of lead from bound stores to soft tissues, blood) qwk until stable

---

sucralfate

(soo-kral'fate)

Rx: Carafate

Chemical Class: Aluminum complex of sulfated sucrose

Therapeutic Class: Gastrointestinal antiulcer agent

CLINICAL PHARMACOLOGY

Mechanism of Action: Forms a complex that adheres to ulcer site, protects against acid, pepsin, bile salts

Pharmacokinetics

PO: Minimally absorbed, duration up to 5 hr; excreted in feces (90%)

INDICATIONS AND USES: Treatment and maintenance of duodenal ulcer; gastric ulcers*; reflux esophagitis*; NSAID-induced GI symptoms*; prevention of stress ulcers*;oral and esophageal radiation-induced ulcers (suspension)*

DOSAGE

Adult

• *Active ulcer:* PO 1 g qid 1 hr ac, hs for 4-8 wk

• *Maintenance:* PO 1 g bid

Ⓢ AVAILABLE FORMS/COST OF THERAPY

• Susp—Oral: 1 g/10 ml, 420 ml: **$40.82**

• Tab, Uncoated—Oral: 1 g, 100's: **$68.20-$97.91**

PRECAUTIONS: Renal failure, dialysis (small amounts aluminum absorbed with sucralfate)

PREGNANCY AND LACTATION: Pregnancy category B; little systemic absorption, so minimal, if any, excretion into milk expected

SIDE EFFECTS/ADVERSE REACTIONS

CNS: Dizziness, drowsiness, headache, vertigo

EENT: **Laryngospasm**

GI: Constipation, diarrhea, *dry mouth,* gastric pain, indigestion, nausea, vomiting

SKIN: Pruritus, rash, urticaria

INTERACTIONS

Drugs

🛚 *Ketoconazole:* Reduces plasma levels of antifungal

🛚 *Phenytoin:* Modest reduction in GI absorption of phenytoin

🛚 *Quinolones:* Reduced antibiotic levels

🛚 *Warfarin:* Isolated cases of reduced hypoprothrombinemic response to warfarin

SPECIAL CONSIDERATIONS

PATIENT/FAMILY EDUCATION

• Take antacids prn for pain relief, but not within ½ hr before or after sucralfate

---

sulfacetamide

(sul-fa-see′ta-mide)

Rx: AK-Sulf, Bleph-10, Klaron, Ocu-Sul, Ocusulf-10, Sebizon, Sodium Sulamyd, Sulf-10, Sulfac

Combinations

Rx: with prednisolone (Blephamide, Dioptimyd, Metamyd, Vasocidin, Isopto Cetapred); with sulfer (Sulfacet-R); with sulfabenzamide (Sulfathiazole, Sulfa-Gyn, Sulnac, Trysul); with phenylepherine (Vasosulf); with fluorometholone (FML-S)

Chemical Class: Sulfonamide derivative

Therapeutic Class: Antibiotic

CLINICAL PHARMACOLOGY

Mechanism of Action: Inhibits bacterial synthesis of dihydrofolic acid, which bacteria require for growth, through competitive inhibition of the enzyme dihydropteroate synthetase; bacteriostatic

Pharmacokinetics

OPHTH: Some systemic absorption; excreted mostly unchanged in urine; $t_{1/2}$ 7-13 hr

INDICATIONS AND USES: Conjunctivitis, corneal ulcer, superficial ocular infections, trachoma (adjunct to systemic sulfonamide therapy); seborrheic dermatitis, seborrhea sicca (dandruff); secondary bacterial infections of skin, acne vulgaris

DOSAGE

Adult and Child >2 mo (>12 yr for TOP lotion)

• *Conjunctivitis/corneal ulcer:* OPHTH instill 1 gtt in lower conjunctival sac(s) q1-3h according to severity of infection; apply ¼ in ribbon of ointment to lower conjunctival sac(s) 1-4 times/day and hs

• *Trachoma:* Ophth instill 2 gtt of 30% sol q2h (in conjunction with systemic sulfonamide therapy)

• *Seborrheic dermatitis and dandruff:* TOP apply lotion hs and allow to remain overnight; may use bid for severe cases with crusting, heavy scaling, and inflammation

• *Acne:* Top apply 1-3 times/day

🛚 **AVAILABLE FORMS/COST OF THERAPY**

• Lotion—Top: 10%, 60 ml: **$52.21**; 85 g: **$23.72**

• Oint—Ophth: 10%, 3.5 g: **$1.65-$23.09**

• Sol—Ophth: 10%, 1, 2, 2.5, 5, 15 ml: **$1.80-$31.79**/15 ml; 15%, 2, 5, 15 ml: **$2.10-$19.25**/15 ml; 30%, 15 ml: **$2.40-$25.01**

CONTRAINDICATIONS: Infants <2 mo; epithelial herpes simplex keratitis, vaccinia, varicella, and many other viral diseases of the cornea and conjunctiva; mycobacterial infection or fungal diseases of the ocular structures

PRECAUTIONS: Severe dry eye, children

PREGNANCY AND LACTATION: Pregnancy category B (category D if used near term); compatible with breast feeding in healthy, full-term infants

SIDE EFFECTS/ADVERSE REACTIONS

CNS: Fever, headache

EENT: Blurred vision (especially with ointment), browache, burning, conjunctival edema, itching, local irritation, reactive hyperemia, transient epithelial keratitis, transient stinging

*METAB: **Bone marrow depression***

*SKIN: **Exfoliative dermatitis,*** photosensitivity, rash, ***Stevens-Johnson syndrome, toxic epidermal necrolysis***

INTERACTIONS

Drugs

❷ *Silver preparations:* Incompatible with sulfacetamide

SPECIAL CONSIDERATIONS

PATIENT/FAMILY EDUCATION

• May cause sensitivity to bright light

• Do not touch tip of container to any surface

---

sulfamethoxazole

(sul-fa-meth-ox´a-zole)

Rx: Gantanol

Combinations

Rx: with trimethoprim, (Bactrim, Septra, Sulfaprim); see co-trimoxazol monograph

Chemical Class: Sulfonamide derivative

Therapeutic Class: Antibiotic

CLINICAL PHARMACOLOGY

Mechanism of Action: Inhibits bacterial synthesis of folic acid through competitive inhibition of the enzyme dihydropteroate synthetase; bacteriostatic

Pharmacokinetics

PO: Peak 3-4 hr; widely distributed into most body tissues; 50%-70% bound to plasma proteins; metabolized in liver by acetylation (inactive metabolite contributes to nephrotoxicity), excreted mainly in urine (20% unchanged, 70% acetylated metabolite); $t_{1/2}$ 7-12 hr (prolonged in renal failure)

INDICATIONS AND USES: Chancroid, trachoma, inclusion conjunctivitis, nocardiosis, UTI, toxoplasmosis (adjunctive therapy with pyrimethamine), malaria (adjunctive therapy of chloroquine-resistant strains of *Plasmodium falciparum),* meningococcal meningitis prophylaxis (when sulfonamide-sensitive group A strains prevail), acute otitis media due to *Hemophilus influenzae* (when used concomitantly with penicillin or erythromycin), pneumonia due to *pneumocystis carinii*

Antibacterial spectrum usually includes:

• Gram-positive organisms: Some strains of staphylococci, streptococci, *Bacillus anthracis, Clostrid-*

S

---

ium tetani, C. perfringens, many strains of *Nocardia asteroides* and *N. brasiliensis*

• Gram-negative organisms: *Enterobacter, Escherichia coli, Klebsiella, Proteus mirabilis, P. vulgaris, Salmonella, Shigella*

• Miscellaneous organisms: *Pneumocystis carinii, Toxoplasma gondii, Plasmodium*

DOSAGE

Adult

• PO, mild to moderate infections, 2 g initially, then 1 g bid; or when combined with trimethoprim, 800 mg bid; severe infections, 2 g initially, then 1 g tid; dose modification for renal insufficiency: CrCl >30 ml/min: use normal dose; CrCl 15-30 ml/min: use one half of normal dose; CrCl <15 ml/min: use not recommended

Child >2 mo

• PO 50-60 mg/kg initially, then 25-30 mg/kg bid; do not exceed 75 mg/kg/day

S AVAILABLE FORMS/COST OF THERAPY

• Tab, Uncoated—Oral: 500 mg, 100's: **$53.12**

• Tab, Uncoated—Oral: 400 mg SMX/80 mg TMP, 100's: **$7.88-$102.49**; 800 mg SMX/160 mg TMP, 100's: **$9.09-$161.48**

CONTRAINDICATIONS: Infants <2 mo (except as adjunctive therapy with pyrimethamine for congenital toxoplasmosis), porphyria, megaloblastic anemia due to folate deficiency, pregnant women at term

PRECAUTIONS: Group A β-hemolytic streptococcal infections (do not use for treatment), renal or hepatic function impairment, allergy or asthma, G-6-PD deficiency

PREGNANCY AND LACTATION: Pregnancy category C (if used near term; may cause jaundice, hemolytic anemia, and kernicterus in newborns); excreted into breast milk in low concentrations; compatible with breast feeding in healthy, full-term infants

SIDE EFFECTS/ADVERSE REACTIONS

CNS: Apathy, ataxia, drowsiness, hallucinations, headache, insomnia, mental depression, peripheral neuropathy, *seizures,* transient lesions of posterior spinal column, transverse myelitis

CV: Allergic myocarditis

EENT: Conjunctival and scleral infection, hearing loss, tinnitus, vertigo

GI: Abdominal pains, anorexia, diarrhea, glossitis, hepatitis, *hepatocellular necrosis, nausea, pancreatitis, pseudomembranous colitis,* stomatitis, *vomiting*

GU: Crystalluria, elevated creatinine, hematuria, *nephrotic syndrome,* proteinuria, *toxic nephrosis with oliguria and anuria*

HEME: Agranulocytosis, aplastic anemia, hemolytic anemia, leukopenia, megaloblastic anemia, methemoglobinemia, purpura, *thrombocytopenia*

MS: Arthralgia

RESP: Pulmonary infiltrates, transient pulmonary changes

SKIN: Erythema multiforme, *exfoliative dermatitis,* photosensitivity, *Stevens-Johnson syndrome*

INTERACTIONS

Drugs

❷ *Para-aminobenzoic acid-(PABA):* PABA may interfere with the antibacterial activity of sulfamethoxazole

❸ *Phenytoin:* Sulfamethoxazole increases phenytoin concentrations, requiring dosage adjustment

3 *Warfarin:* Trimethoprim-sulfamethoxazole, sulfamethoxazole increase the hypoprothrombinemic response to warfarin via inhibition of metabolism

Labs

• α-*Amino-Nitrogen:* Increased in plasma

• *Clindamycin:* False positive

• *Colistin:* False positive

• *Creatinine-kinase:* Falsely decreases serum levels

• *Creatinine:* Falsely increases serum creatinine levels

SPECIAL CONSIDERATIONS
PATIENT/FAMILY EDUCATION

• Avoid prolonged exposure to sunlight

• Administer with full glass of water

MONITORING PARAMETERS

• CBC, renal function tests, urinalysis

---

sulfasalazine

(sul-fa-sal′a-zeen)

Rx: Azaline, Azaline-EC, Azulfidine, Azulfidine EN-Tabs

Chemical Class: Sulfonamide derivative; salicylate derivative

Therapeutic Class: Gastrointestinal antiinflammatory; disease-modifying arthritis drug (DMARD)

CLINICAL PHARMACOLOGY

Mechanism of Action: Metabolized in gut to sulfapyridine and 5-aminosalicylic acid (mesalamine); therapeutic action may be result of antibacterial action of sulfapyridine or antiinflammatory action of 5-aminosalicylic acid on the colon; 5-aminosalicylic acid is the active moiety in inflammatory bowel disease; in rheumatoid arthritis, intact sulfasalazine and sulfapyridine both have beneficial effects: sulfasalazine is thought to interact with the mucosa-associated lymphoid tissue in the gut whereas sulfapyridine primarily targets the synovium

Pharmacokinetics

PO: Unchanged drug 10%-15% absorbed, sulfapyridine rapidly absorbed, little 5-aminosalicylic acid absorbed; peak 1.5-6 hr; sulfapyridine distributed to most body tissues and metabolized via acetylation in liver, excreted in urine (unchanged 15%, sulfapyridine and metabolites 60%, 5-aminosalicylic acid and metabolites 20%-33%), unabsorbed 5-aminosalicylic acid excreted in feces; $t_{1/2}$ 8.4-10.4 hr

INDICATIONS AND USES: Ankylosing spondylitis,* atrophic balance,* collagenous colitis,* Crohn's disease,* dermatitis herpetiformis,* hypertrophic scars,* inflammatory bowel disease,* polyarticular-course juvenile rheumatoid arthritis, proctosigmoiditis—radiation induced,* psoriasis,* psoriatic arthritis,* pyoderma gangrenosum,* reactive arthritis,* Reiter's syndrome,* rheumatoid arthritis, scleroderma,* ulcerative colitis, urticaria*

DOSAGE

Adult

• *Ulcerative colitis:* PO 1 g tid-qid; do not exceed 6 g/day; maintenance 2 g/day divided q6h

• *Rheumatoid arthritis:* 500 mg qd initially, increase by 500 mg weekly to 1 g bid; may increase to 1.5 g bid if inadequate response after 12 wk

Child >6 yr

• *Ulcerative colitis:* PO 40-60 mg/kg/day in 3-6 divided doses; maintenance 30 mg/kg/day in 4 divided doses; max dose 2 g/day

• *Juvenile rheumatoid arthritis:* 30-50 mg/kg/day in 2 divided doses; begin with ¼ to ⅓ of planned main-

S

---

tenance dose and increase weekly to maintenance dose at 1 month; max dose 2 g/day

💲 AVAILABLE FORMS/COST OF THERAPY

• Tab, Uncoated—Oral: 500 mg, 100's: **$12.75-$33.38**
• Tab, Enteric Coated—Oral: 500 mg, 100's: **$39.99**

CONTRAINDICATIONS: Infants <2 yr, porphyria, intestinal or urinary tract obstructions

PRECAUTIONS: Renal or hepatic function impairment, allergy or asthma, G-6-PD deficiency, blood dyscrasias, slow acetylator phenotypes

PREGNANCY AND LACTATION: Pregnancy category B; excreted into breast milk; should be given to nursing mothers with caution because significant adverse effects (bloody diarrhea) may occur in some nursing infants

SIDE EFFECTS/ADVERSE REACTIONS

CNS: Ataxia, cauda equina syndrome, drowsiness, fever, *Guillain-Barré syndrome,* hallucinations, *headache,* insomnia, mental depression, peripheral neuropathy, *seizures,* transient lesions of the posterior spinal column, transverse myelitis, vertigo

CV: Allergic myocarditis, pericarditis with or without tamponade, vasculitis

EENT: Conjunctival and scleral infection, hearing loss, periorbital edema, tinnitus

GI: Abdominal pains, *anorexia,* bloody diarrhea, diarrhea, *gastric distress, hepatic necrosis,* hepatitis, impaired folic acid absorption, *nausea,* neutropenic enterocolitis, *pancreatitis,* stomatitis, *vomiting*

GU: Crystalluria, hematuria, *hemolytic-uremic syndrome,* nephritis, nephrotic syndrome, proteinuria, *reversible oligospermia, toxic nephrosis with oliguria and anuria*

HEME: Agranulocytosis, aplastic anemia, congenital neutropenia, Heinz body anemia, hemolytic anemia, hypoprothrombinemia, leukopenia, megaloblastic anemia, *methemoglobinemia, myelodysplastic syndrome,* purpura, *thrombocytopenia*

MS: Arthralgias, *rhabdomyolysis*

RESP: Cyanosis, fibrosing alveolitis, pleuritis, pneumonitis with or without eosinophilia

SKIN: Alopecia, *epidermal necrolysis (Lyell's syndrome) with corneal damage,* erythema multiforme, *exfoliative dermatitis,* parapsoriasis varioliformis acuta (Mucha-Habermann syndrome), photosensitization, pruritus, skin rash, *Stevens-Johnson syndrome,* urticaria

MISC: Anaphylaxis, polyarteritis nodosa, serum sickness syndrome

INTERACTIONS

Drugs

🔳 *Digoxin:* Sulfasalazine reduces digoxin serum concentrations

🔳 *Folic acid:* Reduced absorption of folic acid

🔳 *Methenamine:* Combination of sulfadiazine and methenamine can result in crystalluria

🔳 *Phenytoin:* Some sulfonamides (sulfaphenazole, sulmethoxazole) increase phenytoin concentrations, requiring dosage adjustment

🔳 *Tolbutamide:* Several sulfonamides (sulfamethizole, sulfaphenazole, sulfisoxasole) can increase plasma sulfonylurea levels and enhance their hypoglycemic effects

🔳 *Warfarin:* Several sulfonamides (trimethoprim-sulfamethoxazole, sulfamethoxazole, sulfamethizole, sulfaphenazole) increase the hypoprothrombinemic response to warfarin via inhibition of metabolism

Labs

• *Bilirubin, conjugated:* Falsely increased in serum

• *Bilirubin, unconjugated:* Falsely decreased in serum

• *Creatinine:* Falsely increased in serum

• *Potassium:* Falsely decreased in serum

• *False positive:* Urinary glucose tests (Benedict's method)

SPECIAL CONSIDERATIONS

PATIENT/FAMILY EDUCATION

• Adequate hydration and urinary output are essential to prevent crystalluria and stone formation

• Avoid prolonged exposure to sunlight

MONITORING PARAMETERS

• Inflammatory bowel disease: Decrease in rectal bleeding or diarrhea in conjunction with mucosal healing

• Rheumatoid arthritis: Tender, swollen joints, visual analogue scale for pain; acute phase reactants (ESR, C-reactive protein), duration of early morning stiffness, preservation of function

• Baseline CBC with differential and liver function tests then every second week during the first 3 months of therapy, monthly during the second 3 months of therapy, then every 3 months thereafter; urinalysis and renal function tests periodically

---

sulfathiazole/ sulfacetamide/ sulfabenzamide (triple sulfa)

(sul-fa-thye′a-zole/sul-fa-see′ta-mide/sul-fa-ben′za-mide)

Rx: Gyne-Sulf, Sultrin Triple Sulfa, Triple Sulfa, Trysul, V.V.S.

Chemical Class: Sulfonamide derivatives

Therapeutic Class: Antibiotic

CLINICAL PHARMACOLOGY

Mechanism of Action: Inhibits bacterial synthesis of folic acid through competitive antagonism of para-aminobenzoic acid (PABA); bacteriostatic

INDICATIONS AND USES: Bacterial vaginosis

DOSAGE

Adult

• VAG (cream) insert 1 applicatorful bid for 4-6 days, treatment can then be reduced 25%-50%, repeat prn; (tablet) insert 1 tablet bid for 10 days, may repeat course prn

🛇 AVAILABLE FORMS/COST OF THERAPY

• Cre—Vag: 3.7% sulfabenzamide/ 2.86% sulfacetamide/3.42% sulfathiazole, 78, 82.5 g: **$6.54-$37.93**/78 g

• Tab—Vag: 3.7% sulfabenzamide/ 2.86% sulfacetamide/3.42% sulfathiazole, 100's: **$2.69**

CONTRAINDICATIONS: Kidney disease, pregnancy at term

PRECAUTIONS: Children

PREGNANCY AND LACTATION: Pregnancy category B (category D if used near term; may cause jaundice, hemolytic anemia, and kernicterus in newborns); excreted into breast

---

milk in low concentrations; compatible with breast feeding in healthy, full-term infants

SIDE EFFECTS/ADVERSE REACTIONS

GU: Local irritation

HEME: **Agranulocytosis**

SKIN: **Stevens-Johnson syndrome** (rare)

MISC: Allergic reactions

SPECIAL CONSIDERATIONS

PATIENT/FAMILY EDUCATION

• Insert high into vagina

• Do not engage in vaginal intercourse during treatment

---

sulfinpyrazone
(sul-fin-pyr´a-zone)
Rx: Anturane
Chemical Class: Pyrazolidine derivative
Therapeutic Class: Antigout agent; uricosuric; antithrombotic agent

---

CLINICAL PHARMACOLOGY

Mechanism of Action: Uricosuric: Inhibits tubular reabsorption of uric acid; *Antithrombotic:* Prostaglandin synthetase inhibitor; lacks anti-inflammatory and analgesic properties

Pharmacokinetics

PO: Well absorbed; max plasma concentration, 1.6 hr; hepatic metabolism, 2 active metabolites, 98%-99% bound to plasma proteins; 50% excreted in urine unchanged; $t_{1/2}$ 2.2-3 hr

INDICATIONS AND USES: Chronic and intermittent gouty arthritis, prevention of recurrent MI (further study indicated),* prevention of systemic embolism in rheumatic mitral stenosis,* preservation of life of hemodialysis shunts

* = non-FDA-approved use

DOSAGE

Adult

• PO 200-400 mg/day in 2 divided doses initially, increase to 400-800 mg/day in 2 divided doses; use lowest dose that will control blood uric acid level

$ **AVAILABLE FORMS/COST OF THERAPY**

• Cap, Gel—Oral: 200 mg, 100's: **$18.90-$76.27**

• Tab, Uncoated—Oral: 100 mg, 100's: **$12.53-$68.86**

CONTRAINDICATIONS: Active peptic ulcer, symptoms of GI inflammation or ulceration, hypersensitivity to phenylbutazone or other pyrazoles, blood dyscrasias

PRECAUTIONS: Renal function impairment, healed peptic ulcer, dehydration, acute gout attack

PREGNANCY AND LACTATION: Pregnancy category C

SIDE EFFECTS/ADVERSE REACTIONS

GI: Aggravation or reactivation of peptic ulcer, *upper GI disturbances*

HEME: **Agranulocytosis, aplastic anemia, anemia, leukopenia, thrombocytopenia**

GU: Interstitial nephritis, *renal failure*

RESP: Bronchospasm (patients with aspirin-induced asthma)

SKIN: Rash

INTERACTIONS

Drugs

3 *Acetaminophen:* Increased metabolism of acetaminophen by about 20%; increased risk of acetaminophen toxicity

3 *Beta-blockers:* Reduced hypotensive effects of β-blockers

• *Heparinoids:* Risk of augmented bleeding and epidural or spinal hematomas is increased when used concurrently with another agent that affects hemostasis

❷ *Methotrexate:* Increased methotrexate levels with subsequent increased effect and potential toxicity

❷ *Oral anticoagulants:* Inhibit warfarin metabolism and possibly other oral anticoagulants, increasing prothrombin time response; concomitant antiplatelet effects further complicate combined therapy

❸ *Salicylates:* Inhibited uricosuric effect of each other

Labs

• *Cyclosporine:* Falsely decreased serum levels

SPECIAL CONSIDERATIONS

PATIENT/FAMILY EDUCATION

• Take with food, milk, or antacids to decrease stomach upset

• Avoid aspirin and other salicylate-containing products

• Drink plenty of fluids

MONITORING PARAMETERS

• Serum uric acid concentrations, renal function, CBC

---

sulfisoxazole

(sul-fi-sox′a-zole)

Rx: Gantrisin

Combinations

   Rx: with erythromycin (Pediazole, Sulfimycin)

Chemical Class: Sulfonamide derivative

Therapeutic Class: Antibiotic

CLINICAL PHARMACOLOGY

Mechanism of Action: Inhibits bacterial synthesis of folic acid (pteroylglutamic acid) from aminobenzoic acid through competitive inhibition of the enzyme dihydropteroate synthetase; bacteriostatic

Pharmacokinetics

PO: Peak 1-4 hr; 85% bound to plasma proteins; parent drug and acetylated metabolites excreted in urine; $t_{1/2}$ 4.6-7.8 hr

INDICATIONS AND USES: Chancroid, trachoma, inclusion conjunctivitis, nocardiosis, UTI, toxoplasmosis (adjunctive therapy with pyrimethamine), malaria (adjunctive therapy of chloroquine-resistant strains of *Plasmodium falciparum),* meningococcal meningitis prophylaxis (when sulfonamide-sensitive group A strains prevail), meningococcal meningitis, acute otitis media due to *Hemophilus influenzae* (when used concomitantly with penicillin or erythromycin), *H. influenzae* meningitis (adjunctive therapy with parenteral streptomycin), recurrent otitis media*

Antibacterial spectrum usually includes:

• Gram-positive organisms: some strains of staphylococci, streptococci, *Bacillus anthracis, Clostridium tetani, C. perfringens,* many strains of *Nocardia asteroides* and *N. brasiliensis*

• Gram-negative organisms: *Enterobacter, Escherichia coli, Klebsiella, Proteus mirabilis, P. vulgaris, Salmonella, Shigella*

• Miscellaneous organisms: *Toxoplasma gondii, Plasmodium*

DOSAGE

Adult

• PO 4-8 g/day in 4-6 divided doses

Child >2 mo

• PO 75 mg/kg initially, then 120-150 mg/kg/day in 4-6 divided doses; max 6 g/day

⑤ AVAILABLE FORMS/COST OF THERAPY

• Sol—Ophth 4%: 15 ml: **$9.44-$15.76**

• Susp—Oral: 500 mg/5 ml, 480 ml: **$42.22**

• Tab, Uncoated—Oral: 500 mg, 100's: **$3.35-$23.40**

CONTRAINDICATIONS: Infants <2 mo, porphyria, megaloblastic anemia due to folate deficiency, pregnant women at term

PRECAUTIONS: Group A β-hemolytic streptococcal infections (do not use for treatment), renal or hepatic function impairment, allergy or asthma, G-6-PD deficiency

PREGNANCY AND LACTATION: Pregnancy category C (if used near term; may cause jaundice, hemolytic anemia, and kernicterus in newborns); excreted into breast milk in low concentrations; compatible with breast feeding in healthy, full-term infants

SIDE EFFECTS/ADVERSE REACTIONS

CNS: Apathy, ataxia, drowsiness, hallucinations, headache, insomnia, mental depression, peripheral neuropathy, *seizures,* transient lesions of posterior spinal column, transverse myelitis

CV: Allergic myocarditis

EENT: Conjunctival and scleral infection, hearing loss, tinnitus, vertigo

GI: Abdominal pains, anorexia, diarrhea, glossitis, hepatitis, *hepatocellular necrosis, nausea, pancreatitis, pseudomembranous colitis,* stomatitis, *vomiting*

GU: Crystalluria, elevated creatinine, hematuria, nephrotic syndrome, proteinuria, *toxic nephrosis with oliguria and anuria*

HEME: Agranulocytosis, aplastic anemia, hemolytic anemia, leukopenia, megaloblastic anemia, methemoglobinemia, purpura, *thrombocytopenia*

MS: Arthralgia

RESP: Pulmonary infiltrates, transient pulmonary changes

SKIN: Erythema multiforme, *exfoliative dermatitis,* photosensitivity, *Stevens-Johnson syndrome*

INTERACTIONS

Drugs

❷ *Para-aminobenzoic acid-(PABA):* PABA may interfere with the antibacterial activity of sulfamethoxazole

3 *Phenytoin:* Sulfamethoxazole increases phenytoin concentrations, requiring dosage adjustment

3 *Tolbutamide:* Sulfisoxazole can increase plasma sulfonylurea levels and enhance their hypoglycemic effects

3 *Warfarin:* Trimethoprim-sulfamethoxazole, sulfamethoxazole increase the hypoprothrombinemic response to warfarin via inhibition of metabolism

Labs

• *Folate:* Falsely decreased serum levels

• *Protein:* Falsely increased in CSF

• *Urobilinogen:* Decreased falsely in feces

SPECIAL CONSIDERATIONS

PATIENT/FAMILY EDUCATION

• Avoid prolonged exposure to sunlight

• Administer with glass of water

MONITORING PARAMETERS

• CBC, renal function tests, urinalysis

---

* = non-FDA-approved use

---

sulindac
(sul-in'dak)
Rx: Clinoril
Chemical Class: Acetic acid derivative
Therapeutic Class: NSAID with analgesic and antipyretic activity

---

CLINICAL PHARMACOLOGY
Mechanism of Action: Reversible cyclooxygenase (i.e., prostaglandin synthetase) inhibitor; non-selectively decreases the formation of both prostaglandins and thromboxane A2; variable effects on lipoxygenase synthesis and subsequent leukotriene production; antiinflammatory, antipyretic, and analgesic activity; inhibits platelet aggregation
Pharmacokinetics
PO: Onset of antirheumatic action within 7 days, peak 1-2 wk, peak serum levels 2-4 hr; sulindac is inactive until metabolized to active sulfide metabolite, excreted in urine primarily in biologically inactive forms (may possibly affect renal function to lesser extent than other NSAIDs), 25% excreted in feces; t₁/₂ 7.8 hr (sulfide metabolite 16.4 hr)
INDICATIONS AND USES: Osteoarthritis, rheumatoid arthritis, ankylosing spondylitis, prevention of cognitive decline,* prevention of colon cancer,* colon polyposis,* acute gouty arthritis, pain—mild to moderate, tendonitis/bursitis, painful shoulder, amnioreduction,* cough—angiotensin-converting enzyme inhibitor,* diabetic neuropathy,* antihypertensive/diuretic requiring patient—less negating effects,* pain—cancer,* preterm labor,* soft tissue injuries,* SLE

DOSAGE
Adult
• PO 150-200 mg bid with food; max 400 mg/day
Child
• PO dose not established although 4 mg/kg/day divided bid has been used

$ AVAILABLE FORMS/COST OF THERAPY
• Tab, Uncoated—Oral: 150 mg, 100's: **$37.73-$122.54**; 200 mg, 100's: **$87.90-$150.59**

CONTRAINDICATIONS: Bronchospasm, nasal polyps, angioedema precipitated by aspirin or other NSAIDs
PRECAUTIONS: History of GI ulceration, bleeding, or perforation; renal dysfunction, hypertension or cardiac conditions aggravated by fluid retention and edema, history of liver dysfunction, history of coagulation
PREGNANCY AND LACTATION: Pregnancy category B (category D if used in 3rd trimester); could cause constriction of the ductus arteriosus *in utero,* persistent pulmonary hypertension of the newborn, or prolonged labor
SIDE EFFECTS/ADVERSE REACTIONS
CNS: Dizziness, headache, lightheadedness
CV: Chest pain, *CHF,* dysrhythmias, edema, hypertension, hypotension, palpitation, tachycardia
EENT: Dry eyes, hearing disturbances, photophobia, tinnitus, visual disturbances
GI: Abdominal cramps, constipation, diarrhea, *dyspepsia,* flatulence, *gastric or duodenal ulcer with bleeding or perforation,* hepatitis, *pancreatitis,* vomiting
GU: Acute renal failure

---

italic = common side effects   **bold italic** = life-threatening reactions

HEME: **Agranulocytosis,** eosinophilia, **leukopenia, neutropenia, pancytopenia, thrombocytopenia**
METAB: Hyperglycemia, hyperkalemia, hypoglycemia, hyponatremia
RESP: Bronchospasm, dyspnea, pulmonary infiltrates
SKIN: Photosensitivity, rash, urticaria

INTERACTIONS
Drugs

■ *Aminoglycosides:* Reduced clearance with elevated aminoglycoside levels and potential for toxicity (especially indomethacin in premature infants; other NSAIDs probably)

■ *Anticoagulants:* Excessive hypoprothrombinemia, decreased platelet aggregation with increased risk of GI bleeding

■ *Antihypertensives (α-blockers, angiotensin-converting enzyme inhibitors, angiotensin II receptor blockers, β-blockers, diuretics):* Inhibition of antihypertensive and other favorable hemodynamic effects

■ *Corticosteroids:* Increased risk of GI ulceration

■ *Cyclosporine:* Increased nephrotoxicity risk

■ *Lithium:* Decreased clearance of lithium (mediated via prostaglandins) resulting in elevated serum lithium levels and risk of toxicity

■ *Methotrexate:* Decreased renal secretion of methotrexate resulting in elevated methotrexate levels and risk of toxicity

■ *Phenylpropanolamine:* Possible acute hypertensive reaction

■ *Potassium-sparing diuretics:* Additive hyperkalemia potential

■ *Triamterene:* Acute renal failure reported with addition of indomethacin; caution with other NSAIDs

SPECIAL CONSIDERATIONS
• No significant advantage over other NSAIDs; cost should govern use

PATIENT/FAMILY EDUCATION
• Avoid aspirin and alcoholic beverages
• Take with food, milk, or antacids to decrease GI upset
• Antirheumatic action may not be apparent for several weeks

MONITORING PARAMETERS
• Initial hemogram and fecal occult blood test within 3 mo of starting regular chronic therapy; repeat every 6-12 mo (more frequently in high-risk patients >65 years, peptic ulcer disease, concurrent steroids or anticoagulants); electrolytes, creatinine, and BUN within 3 mo of starting regular chronic therapy; repeat every 6-12 mo

---

sumatriptan
(soo-ma-trip′tan)
Rx: Imitrex
Chemical Class: Serotonin derivative
Therapeutic Class: Antimigraine agent

CLINICAL PHARMACOLOGY
Mechanism of Action: Selectively activates vascular 5-HT$_1$-receptors in cranial arteries causing vasoconstriction, and inhibiting proinflammatory neuropeptide release, actions correlating with the relief of migraine in humans

Pharmacokinetics
PO: Poor bioavailability (15%); onset 1-1½ hr, peak 2-2½ hr
SC: Onset within 1 hr, peak 12 min Metabolized by microsomal monoamine oxidase (MAO), excreted in urine (60%) and feces (40%); t$_{1/2}$ 2½ hr

---

INDICATIONS AND USES: Acute migraine headache with or without aura; cluster headache

DOSAGE

Adult

• SC 6 mg at 1st sign of headache or after completion of aura; may repeat if partial relief after 1 hr; max 12 mg/24 hr

• PO 25-100 mg at 1st sign of headache; may repeat q2h prn up to 300 mg/24 hr max; no evidence that doses larger than 25 mg provide substantially greater relief

• PO following SC, single tablets (25-50 mg) may be repeated at 2 hr intervals up to 200 mg/24 hr max

• Nasal 5-20 mg at 1st sign of headache or after completion of aura; may repeat if partial relief after 2 hr, max 40 mg/24 hr

§ AVAILABLE FORMS/COST OF THERAPY

• Inj, Sol—SC: 6 mg/0.5 ml, 2's: **$39.04-$103.62**

• Spray, Sol—Nasal: 5 mg/spray, 6's: **$143.38**; 20 mg/spray, 6's: **$143.38**

• Tab, Uncoated—Oral: 25 mg, 9's: **$96.66-$165.44**; 50 mg, 9's: **$122.17-$154.56**; 100 mg, 9's: **$154.56**

CONTRAINDICATIONS: Hemiplegic or basilar migraine, IV inj (potential for coronary vasospasm), ischemic heart disease, Prinzmetal's angina, uncontrolled hypertension, within 24 hr of ergotamine-containing products

PRECAUTIONS: Atypical headache, renal or hepatic function impairment, elderly, children

PREGNANCY AND LACTATION: Pregnancy category C; excreted in breast milk in animals, no data in humans

SIDE EFFECTS/ADVERSE REACTIONS

CNS: Anxiety, *dizziness,* drowsiness, fatigue, headache

CV: Chest discomfort, **dysrhythmia,** hypertension, hypotension, **myocardial ischemia**

EENT: Sinus discomfort, throat discomfort, vertigo, vision alterations

GI: Diarrhea, discomfort of mouth and tongue, reflux

MS: Jaw discomfort, muscle cramps, myalgias, neck pain and stiffness, weakness

SKIN: Flushing, *inj site reaction,* sweating

MISC: Atypical sensations, (tingling, warm or hot sensation, burning sensation, feeling of heaviness, pressure sensation, feeling of tightness, numbness; feeling strange, tight feeling in head; cold sensation)

INTERACTIONS

Drugs

3 *Ergot-containing drugs:* Potential for prolonged vasospastic reactions and additive vasoconstriction, theoretical precaution

2 *Sibutramine:* Increased risk of serotonin syndrome

SPECIAL CONSIDERATIONS

• First inj should be administered under medical supervision

PATIENT/FAMILY EDUCATION

• Use only to treat migraine headache; not for prevention

T

---

tacrine

(tack'rin)

Rx: Cognex

Chemical Class: Monoamine acridine derivative

Therapeutic Class: Antidementia agent

CLINICAL PHARMACOLOGY

Mechanism of Action: Centrally acting cholinesterase inhibitor; presumably elevates acetylcholine concentrations; a deficiency of acetylcholine may account for some clinical manifestations of mild to moderate dementia

Pharmacokinetics

PO: Rapidly absorbed; peak serum concentrations 1-2 hr; 55% bound to plasma proteins; metabolized by cytochrome P450 system in liver; elimination $t_{1/2}$ 2-4 hr

INDICATIONS AND USES: Treatment of mild to moderate dementia of the Alzheimer's type

DOSAGE

Adult

• PO 10 mg qid for 4 wk, then 20 mg qid for 4 wk; increase at 4-wk intervals, if patient tolerating drug well, to dose of 120-160 mg/day in divided doses qid

$ AVAILABLE FORMS/COST OF THERAPY

• Cap, Gel—Oral: 10, 20, 30, 40 mg, 120's: **$147.01**

CONTRAINDICATIONS: Patients treated with this drug who developed jaundice (total bilirubin >3 mg/dl)

PRECAUTIONS: Sick sinus syndrome, history of ulcers, GI bleeding, hepatic disease, bladder obstruction, asthma

PREGNANCY AND LACTATION: Pregnancy category C; excretion into breast milk unknown

SIDE EFFECTS/ADVERSE REACTIONS

CNS: Abnormal thinking, agitation, anxiety, ataxia, chills, confusion, depression, dizziness, fever, hallucinations, hostility, insomnia, somnolence, tremor

CV: Bradycardia, hypertension, hypotension

GI: Anorexia, diarrhea, dyspepsia, flatulence, **hepatotoxicity,** nausea, transaminase elevation, vomiting

GU: Frequency, incontinence, UTI

MS: Myalgia

SKIN: Flushing, rash

RESP: Asthma, cough, pharyngitis, rhinitis

INTERACTIONS

Drugs

🔳 *Anticholinergics:* Inhibits anticholinergic effect, centrally acting anticholinergics may inhibit effect of tacrine

🔳 *Beta-blockers:* Additive bradycardia

🔳 *Cholinergics:* Increased cholinergic effects

🔳 *Cimetidine:* Increased tacrine levels

🔳 *Levodopa:* Decreased levodopa effect

🔳 *Quinolones:* Inhibition of tacrine metabolism

🔳 *Serotonin reuptake inhibitors:* Increased tacrine concentrations

🔳 *Smoking:* Markedly reduces tacrine levels

🔳 *Theophylline:* Increased theophylline concentrations

SPECIAL CONSIDERATIONS

• Transaminase elevation is the most common reason for withdrawal of drug (8%); monitor ALT q wk for 1st 18 wk, then decrease to q 3 mo; when dose is increased, monitor q wk for 6 wk

• If elevations occur, modify dose as follows: ALT ≤3 times upper limit normal (ULN) continue current dose; ALT >3 to ≤5 times ULN reduce dose by 40 mg qd and resume dose titration when within normal limits; ALT >5 times ULN stop treatment; rechallenge may be tried if ALT is <10 times ULN

• Do not rechallenge if clinical jaundice develops

• Improvement in symptoms of dementia statistically, but perhaps not clinically significant; discontinue therapy if improvement not evident to family members and clinician

---

tacrolimus

(tak-roe-leem'us)
Rx: Prograf
Chemical Class: Macrolide derivative
Therapeutic Class: Immunosuppressant

CLINICAL PHARMACOLOGY

Mechanism of Action: Inhibits T-lymphocyte activation; suppresses humoral immunity and cell-mediated reactions such as allograft rejection

Pharmacokinetics
PO: Peak 1.5-3.5 hr, absolute bioavailability 14.4-17.4%, food reduces absorption and bioavailability; 75-99% bound to plasma proteins, crosses the placenta; extensively metabolized by liver, CYP3A; $t_{1/2}$ 11.7 hr

INDICATIONS AND USES: Prophylaxis of organ rejection in allogeneic liver and kidney transplants (in conjunction with adrenal corticosteroids); kidney, bone marrow, cardiac, pancreas, pancreatic island cell and small bowel transplantation*; autoimmune disease*; severe recalcitrant psoriasis*; moderate to severe atopic dermatitis

DOSAGE
Adult

• IV 0.03-0.05 mg/kg/day continuous IV infusion; initiate no sooner than 6 hr post transplant; convert to oral therapy as soon as possible, wait 8-12 hr after stopping IV infusion; adult patients should start at doses at low end of range; titrate dose based on clinical assessments of rejection and tolerability

• *Liver transplant:* PO 0.10-0.15 mg/kg/day in divided doses q12h

• *Kidney transplant:* PO 0.2 mg/kg/day in divided doses q12h

• *Atopic dermatitis:* TOP apply thin layer of 0.03% or 0.1% ointment to affected areas bid; do not use occlusive dressings; continue for 1 wk after clearing of signs and symptoms

• *Renal or hepatic impairment:* Initiate doses at low end of range; further reductions in dose may be required

Child

• *Liver transplant:* IV 0.03-0.05 mg/kg/day continuous IV infusion; PO 0.15-0.20 mg/kg/day; pediatric patients require higher doses than adults

• *Atopic dermatitis:* TOP child ->2 yr apply thin layer of 0.03% ointment to affected areas bid; do not use occlusive dressings; continue for 1 wk after clearing of signs and symptoms

🅂 AVAILABLE FORMS/COST OF THERAPY

• Cap —Oral: 0.5 mg, 60's: **$116.87**; 1 mg, 100's: **$325.18**; 5 mg, 100's: **$1,625.84**

• Inj, Sol—IV: 5 mg/ml: **$119.10**

• Oint—Top: 0.03%, 30, 60 g: **$59.95**/30 g; 0.1%, 30, 60 g: **$64.09**/30 g

CONTRAINDICATIONS: Hypersensitivity to HCO-60 polyoxyl 60 hydrogenated castor oil (used in ve-

---

italic = common side effects   ***bold italic*** = life-threatening reactions

hicle for injection), concomitant use with cyclosporine (see Interactions, Drugs)

PRECAUTIONS: Impaired renal and hepatic function, hypertension, myocardial hypertrophy, Netherton's syndrome (increased systemic absorption of ointment), topical use in chicken pox, shingles, herpes simplex, eczema herpeticum

PREGNANCY AND LACTATION: Pregnancy category C; excreted in breast milk, avoid nursing

SIDE EFFECTS/ADVERSE REACTIONS

CNS: **Coma,** delirium, *neurotoxicity (tremor, headache, changes in motor function, mental status and sensory function),* paresthesia, **seizures**
CV: *Hypertension, peripheral edema*
GI: *Abdominal pain, anorexia, constipation, diarrhea, elevated liver function tests, nausea, vomiting*
GU: **Nephrotoxicity**
HEME: Anemia, leukocytosis, **thrombocytopenia**
METAB: Hyperglycemia, hyperkalemia (10-44%), hyperuricemia, hypokalemia, hypomagnesemia
MS: Back pain
RESP: Atelectasis, dyspnea, pleural effusion
SKIN: Pruritus, rash
MISC: **Anaphylaxis** (with injection), *asthenia, fever,* **lymphoma,** *pain*

INTERACTIONS
Drugs
❸ *Azole antifungals, bromocriptine, calcium channel blockers, cimetidine, danazol, ethinyl estradiol, GI prokinetic agents, macrolide antibiotics, nefazodone, omeprazole, protease inhibitors:* Decreased metabolism or increased bioavailability of tacrolimus
❸ *Carbamazepine, phenobarbital, phenytoin, rifamycins:* Decreased tacrolimus blood levels

⚠ *Cyclosporine:* Additive/synergistic nephrotoxicity, do not coadminister, discontinue tacrolimus or cyclosporine for 24 hr before starting the other
⚠ *Live vaccines:* Avoid use of live vaccines, vaccinations may be less effective
❷ *Nephrotoxic agents (aminoglycosides, amphotericin B, cisplatin, ganciclovir):* Potential for additive/synergistic nephrotoxicity
❷ *Potassium-sparing diuretics:* Increased risk of hyperkalemia
❸ *St. John's wort (hypericum perforatum):* Potential for decreased plasma tacrolimus concentrations

SPECIAL CONSIDERATIONS
• Black patients may need higher doses in kidney transplant

MONITORING PARAMETERS
• Regularly assess serum creatinine, potassium, and fasting glucose
• Whole blood tacrolimus concentrations as measured by ELISA may be helpful in assessing rejection and toxicity, median trough concentrations measured after the second week of therapy ranged from 9.8 to 19.4 mg/ml

---

tamoxifen
(ta-mox'i-fen)
Rx: Nolvadex
Chemical Class: Triphenylethylene derivative
Therapeutic Class: Antineoplastic

CLINICAL PHARMACOLOGY
Mechanism of Action: Competes with estrogen for receptor sites; nonsteroidal antiestrogen
Pharmacokinetics
PO: Extensively metabolized; peak 4-7 hr, $t_{1/2}$ 14 days (active metabolite); excreted primarily in feces

INDICATIONS AND USES: Adjuvant therapy of axillary node-negative breast cancer and of node positive cancer in post-menopausal women following mastectomy, axillary dissection, and breast irradiation; treatment of metastatic breast cancer in both women and men; most beneficial in estrogen receptor-positive tumors; reduction in incidence of breast cancer in high-risk women (defined as ≥35 yr with a 5-yr predicted risk of breast cancer ≥1.67% as calculated by the Gail Model); also used in mastalgia,* gynecomastia*

DOSAGE
Adult
• PO 10-20 mg bid
• *Gynecomastia/mastalgia:* PO 10 mg qd
§ AVAILABLE FORMS/COST OF THERAPY
• Tab, Uncoated—Oral: 10 mg, 60's: **$109.57-$123.45**
• Tab—Oral: 20 mg, 90's: **$328.71-$370.35**
PRECAUTIONS: Leukopenia, thrombocytopenia, cataracts, liver disease, hypercalcemia, undiagnosed abnormal vaginal bleeding
PREGNANCY AND LACTATION: Pregnancy category D; excretion into breast milk unknown
SIDE EFFECTS/ADVERSE REACTIONS
CNS: Depression, *headache, hot flashes, (33%) lightheadedness*
CV: Chest pain
EENT: Blurred vision (high doses), corneal opacity, ocular lesions, retinopathy
GI: Abnormal liver function tests, altered taste, anorexia, ***hepatic necrosis,*** *nausea, vomiting*
GU: ***Endometrial cancer,*** *menstrual changes (irregularity, oligomenorrhea, amenorrhea),* pruritus vulvae, vaginal bleeding

HEME: ***Deep vein thrombosis, leukopenia, thrombocytopenia***
METAB: Hypercalcemia
RESP: ***Pulmonary embolism***
SKIN: Alopecia, rash
INTERACTIONS
Drugs
❷ *Aminoglutethimide:* Reduces tamoxifen concentrations
SPECIAL CONSIDERATIONS
• Treatment duration >5 yr may provide no further benefit and increase risk of endometrial cancer for some women; reevaluate the need for continued therapy
• The Gail Model Risk Assessment Tool is available to health care professionals by calling (800) 456-3669 (ext. 3838)
• Premenopausal women should use nonhormonal contraception during treatment
MONITORING PARAMETERS
• Endometrial biopsy indicated for abnormal vaginal bleeding

---

tamsulosin
(tam-sool'o-sin)
Rx: Flomax
Chemical Class: Quinazoline
Therapeutic Class: α₁-adrenergic blocker: symptomatic benign prostatic hypertrophy

CLINICAL PHARMACOLOGY
Mechanism of Action: Selective and preferential postsynaptic alpha₁-adrenergic receptor blockade in lower urinary tract and prostate; results in smooth muscle relaxation in bladder neck and prostate without affecting bladder contractility; minimal effect on cardiovascular system (i.e., minimal hypotensive response)
Pharmacokinetics
PO: Peak 4-5 hr (6-7 hr with food)

---

italic = common side effects   ***bold italic*** = life-threatening reactions

Absorption >90% fasting; food reduces peak concentrations by 40-70% and AUC by 30%; extensive hepatic metabolism; excreted in urine as inactive metabolites; $t_{1/2}$ 9-13 hr

INDICATIONS AND USES: BPH, symptomatic relief of signs and symptoms

DOSAGE

Adult

• *BPH:* 0.4-0.8 mg qd (administered approx. 30 min following the same meal each day)

$ AVAILABLE FORMS/COST OF THERAPY

• Cap—Oral: 0.4 mg 100's: **$170.14**

PRECAUTIONS: Like all alpha blockers, potential for "first-dose" phenomenon: marked hypotension with first couple of doses; elderly patients and those receiving calcium channel antagonists, diuretics, and β-blockers, have increased risks; anticipate the same effect if therapy is interrupted for several days

PREGNANCY AND LACTATION: Pregnancy category B; not indicated for use in women

SIDE EFFECTS/ADVERSE REACTIONS

CNS: Asthenia, dizziness, insomnia, somnolence, syncope, vertigo

CV: Orthostatic hypotension

GI: Bitter taste, elevations in ALT, AST; nausea, stomach discomfort

GU: Abnormal ejaculation, decreased libido

MS: Back pain

RESP: Cough, rhinorrhea

INTERACTIONS

Drugs

3 *β-blockers:* Enhanced "first-dose" phenomenon

SPECIAL CONSIDERATIONS

PATIENT/FAMILY EDUCATION

• Consider administration of first dose at bedtime; caution following first 12 hr after initiation or reinitiation of therapy for "first dose phenomenon"

---

tazarotene

(ta-zar'o-teen)

Rx: Tazorac

Chemical Class: Vitamin A derivative (retinoid prodrug)

Therapeutic Class: Antiacne, antipsoriatic agent

CLINICAL PHARMACOLOGY

Mechanism of Action: Prodrug, tazarotene rapidly converted to active metabolite, tazarotenic acid, following topical application; modulates differentiation and proliferation of epithelial tissue and exerts some antiinflammatory and immunological activity

Pharmacokinetics

TOP: Minimal (<1%) absorption of tazarotene and active metabolite (tazarotenic acid); retained in skin for prolonged periods (up to 3 months); eventually metabolized in liver with predominantly biliary excretion; active metabolite $t_{1/2}$ 18 hr

INDICATIONS AND USES: Acne (facial, mild to moderate); psoriasis (stable, plaque, ≤20% of body surface area)

DOSAGE

Adult and Child >16 yr

• *Acne:* TOP apply 0.05%-0.1% gel qd (evening)

• *Psoriasis:* TOP apply to plaques only qd (evening)

---

* = non-FDA-approved use

• Cre—Top: 0.05%, 15, 30, 60 g: **$70.10**/30 g; 0.1%, 15, 30, 60 g: **$74.48**/30 g
• Gel—Top: 0.05%, 30, 100 g: **$70.10**/30 g; 0.1%, 30, 100 g: **$74.48**/30 g

PRECAUTIONS: Eczema, concurrent use with other photosensitizers (thiazides, tetracyclines, fluoroquinolones, phenothiazines, sulfonamides)

PREGNANCY AND LACTATION: Pregnancy category X (some evidence to suggest potential increased safety margin vs. other retinoids based on minimal absorption and short half life); excreted into breast milk of rats; no human data

SIDE EFFECTS/ADVERSE REACTIONS

SKIN: Burning, desquamation, dry skin, erythema, fissuring, irritation, localized edema, *pruritus,* skin discoloration, skin pain, *stinging*

SPECIAL CONSIDERATIONS

• Attractive alternative to oral retinoid therapy in psoriasis (e.g., etretinate), primarily due to less toxicity. Structural changes to the basic retinoid structure (e.g., conformational rigidity) are claimed to enhance therapeutic efficacy and reduce the local toxicity associated with topical tretinoin (retinoic acid). However, place in therapy should await direct comparisons vs. standard regimens in terms of efficacy, toxicity, and cost

telmisartan
(tel-meh-sar′-tan)
Rx: Micardis
Chemical Class: Angiotensin II receptor antagonist
Therapeutic Class: Antihypertensive

CLINICAL PHARMACOLOGY
Mechanism of Action: Antihypertensive (inhibition of vasoconstrictor and aldosterone secretion), smooth muscle hypoproliferative, and cardioprotective effects are attributable to selective blockade of angiotensin II receptors found throughout the cardiovascular and renal systems; effects independent of angiotensin II synthesis
Pharmacokinetics
PO: Peak 0.5-1 hr; bioavailability, 42%, dose dependent, minimal food effect; 99.5+% plasma protein bound (albumin and α_1-acid glycoprotein); <3% metabolized by liver, 97% excreted unchanged in urine; $t_{1/2}$ 24 hr

INDICATIONS AND USES: Hypertension, myocardial ischemia,* congestive heart failure (left ventricular dysfunction),* chronic renal failure,* diabetic nephropathy*

DOSAGE
Adult and Child >16 yr
• *Hypertension:* 20 to 80 mg PO qd

• Tab—Oral: 20 mg, 40 mg, 28's: **$40.98**; 80 mg, 28's: **$43.81**

PRECAUTIONS: Angioedema (associated with aspirin and/or penicillin allergy), aortic or mitral valve stenosis, biliary cirrhosis or biliary obstruction, breast feeding period, coronary artery disease, elderly patients, hepatic dysfunction (adjust dose), hypertrophic cardiomyopa-

T

thy, hypotension (sodium- or volume-depleted patients), pregnancy, renal artery stenosis, solitary kidney, or congestive heart failure

PREGNANCY AND LACTATION: Pregnancy category C, first trimester—category D, second and third trimesters; drugs acting directly on the renin-angiotensin-aldosterone system are documented to cause fetal harm (hypotension, oligohydramnios, neonatal anemia, hyperkalemia, neonatal skull hypoplasia, anuria, and renal failure); neonatal limb contractures, craniofacial deformities, and hypoplastic lung development

SIDE EFFECTS/ADVERSE REACTIONS

CNS: Headache, dizziness, insomnia, somnolence, migraine, vertigo, paresthesia, involuntary muscle contractions, and hypoesthesia (0.3%-1%)

CV: Hypertension, chest pain, peripheral edema, palpitation, dependent edema, angina pectoris, tachycardia, leg edema, abnormal electrocardiogram, anxiety, depression, and nervousness (0.3%-1%)

EENT: Conjunctivitis

GI: Diarrhea (3%), dyspepsia, abdominal pain, nausea, flatulence, constipation, gastritis, vomiting, dry mouth, hemorrhoids, gastroenteritis, enteritis, gastroesophageal reflux, and toothache

GU: Impotence, urinary tract infection, increased frequency of urination, and cystitis (0.3%-1%)

MS: Back pain (3%), myalgia, arthritis, arthralgia, and leg cramps (0.3%-1%)

RESP: Angioedema (1 case in premarketing trials), upper respiratory tract infection (7%), sinusitis (7%), cough (1.6%), pharyngitis (1%), influenza-like symptoms, asthma, bronchitis, rhinitis, dyspnea, and epistaxis (0.3%-1%)

SKIN: Increased sweating, dermatitis, rash, eczema, and pruritus (0.3%-1%)

MISC: Angioedema

INTERACTIONS

Drugs

3 *Digoxin:* 49% increase in digoxin peak, 20% increase in trough digoxin concentrations

SPECIAL CONSIDERATIONS

• Potentially as or more effective than angiotensin-converting enzyme inhibitors, without cough; no evidence for reduction in morbidity and mortality as first-line agents in hypertension, yet; whether they provide the same cardiac and renal protection also still tentative; like ACE inhibitors, less effective in black patients

PATIENT/FAMILY EDUCATION

• Call your clinician immediately if note following side effects: wheezing; lip, throat, or face swelling; hives or rash

MONITORING PARAMETERS

• Baseline electrolytes, urinalysis, blood urea nitrogen and creatinine with recheck at 2-4 wk after initiation (sooner in volume-depleted patients); monitor sitting blood pressure; watch for symptomatic hypotension, particularly in volume-depleted patients

temazepam

(te-maz´e-pam)

Rx: Restoril

Chemical Class: Benzodiazepine

Therapeutic Class: Hypnotic

DEA Class: Schedule IV

CLINICAL PHARMACOLOGY

Mechanism of Action: CNS depressant via facilitation of inhibitory GABA at benzodiazepine receptor sites (BZ_1—associated with sleep; BZ_2—associated with memory, motor, sensory, and cognitive function); effects include muscle relaxation (spinal cord), anticonvulsant activity (brain stem), ataxia (cerebellum), emotional behavior (limbic and cortical areas), and anxiolytic effects (separate from general CNS depression); decreases sleep latency, the number of awakenings, and the time spent in stage 0 (awake) sleep; stage 2 (unequivocal sleep) is increased; in sum, sleep time increased

Pharmacokinetics

Onset 30-45 min, peak 2-4 hr, duration 6-8 hr; $t_{1/2}$ 9.5-10.4 hr; metabolized by liver to inactive metabolites; excreted by kidneys; crosses placenta, excreted in breast milk

INDICATIONS AND USES: Insomnia

DOSAGE

Adult

• PO 15-30 mg hs; 7.5 mg hs may be sufficient for elderly or debilitated patients

🔳 AVAILABLE FORMS/COST OF THERAPY

• Cap, Gel—Oral: 7.5 mg, 100's: **$46.67-$92.10**; 15 mg, 100's: **$7.50-$100.11**; 30 mg, 100's: **$8.25-$170.75**

PRECAUTIONS: Anemia, hepatic disease, renal disease, suicidal individuals, drug abuse, elderly, depression, psychosis, children <18 yr, acute narrow-angle glaucoma, seizure disorders, lung disease

PREGNANCY AND LACTATION: Pregnancy category X; may cause sedation and poor feeding in nursing infant

SIDE EFFECTS/ADVERSE REACTIONS

CNS: Anxiety, confusion, *daytime sedation,* dizziness, *drowsiness,* headache, irritability, *lethargy,* lightheadedness, rebound insomnia

CV: Chest pain, hypotension, tachycardia

GI: Abdominal pain, anorexia, constipation, diarrhea, heartburn, nausea, vomiting

HEME: **Granulocytopenia** (rare), **leukopenia**

RESP: **Respiratory depression,** sleep apnea

INTERACTIONS

Drugs

3 *Cimetidine, disulfiram:* Increased benzodiazepine levels

3 *Clozapine:* Possible increased risk of cardiorespiratory collapse

3 *Ethanol:* Adverse psychomotor effects

3 *Rifampin:* Reduced benzodiazepine levels

SPECIAL CONSIDERATIONS

• Good benzodiazepine choice for elderly and patients with liver disease (phase II metabolism and lack of active metabolites)

PATIENT/FAMILY EDUCATION

• Withdrawal symptoms may occur if administered chronically and discontinued abruptly; symptoms include dysphoria, abdominal and muscle cramps, vomiting, sweating, tremor, and seizure

T

---

italic = common side effects   ***bold italic*** = life-threatening reactions

• May cause impairment the day following administration, exercise caution with hazardous tasks and driving

---

tenofovir
(ten-oh'foh-veer)
Rx: Viread
Chemical Class: Nucleotide analog
Therapeutic Class: Antiviral

CLINICAL PHARMACOLOGY
Mechanism of Action: Tenofovir is phosphorylated to tenofovir diphosphate which competitively inhibits HIV reverse transcriptase and also leads to DNA chain termination
Pharmacokinetics
PO: Administered as a prodrug hydrolyzed to tenofovir; bioavailability 25% (increased by high fat meal); peak 1-1½ hr; 1% protein binding; not metabolized by liver; excreted in urine (40% unchanged after 24 hr; 80% unchanged after 72 hr) and stool
INDICATIONS AND USES: HIV-1 infection, in combination with other antiretroviral agents
DOSAGE
Adult
• PO 300 mg qd with a meal
$ **AVAILABLE FORMS/COST OF THERAPY**
• Tab, Coated—Oral: 300 mg, 100's: **$408.00**
PRECAUTIONS: Children, lactic acidosis, hepatic disease, hepatic steatosis, renal disease (do not administer if CrCl <60 ml/min)
PREGNANCY AND LACTATION: Pregnancy category B; breast milk excretion unknown; the CDC recommends that HIV-infected mothers not breast-feed their infants to avoid risking postnatal transmission of HIV
SIDE EFFECTS/ADVERSE REACTIONS
CNS: Asthenia, *headache*
GI: Abdominal pain, abnormal transaminase levels (4%), *diarrhea* (9%), flatulence, *hepatic steatosis*, *nausea* (11%), *vomiting*
GU: Increase in BUN, creatinine
METAB: **Lactic acidosis**
INTERACTIONS
Drugs
3 *Didanosine (buffered formulation):* Tenofovir decreases didanosine AUC by 44% (When co-administered with didanosine, tenofovir should be administered 2 hours before or 1 hour after administration of didanosine)
3 *Lopinavir/ritonavir:* Increases tenofovir AUC by 34%; tenofovir decreases AUC of lopinavir/ritonavir by 24% (when co-administered with lopinavir/ritonavir, tenofovir should be administered 2 hours before or 1 hour after administration of lopinavir/ritonavir)
SPECIAL CONSIDERATIONS
• For latest treatment guidelines see www.hivatis.org
PATIENT/FAMILY EDUCATION
• When co-administered with didanosine or lopinavir/ritonavir, take tenofovir 2 hours before or 1 hour after taking them
MONITORING PARAMETERS
• CBC with platelet count, renal function, liver enzymes

---

terazosin

(ter-a'zoe-sin)

Rx: Hytrin
Chemical Class: Quinazoline derivative
Therapeutic Class: α_1-adrenergic blocker; antihypertensive; symptomatic benign prostatic hypertrophy

CLINICAL PHARMACOLOGY

Mechanism of Action: Selectively blocks postsynaptic α_1-adrenergic receptors; dilates both arterioles and veins, reducing peripheral vascular resistance and blood pressure; no reflex tachycardia or changes in renin release; blockade of α_1-adrenoceptors in bladder neck and prostate relaxes smooth muscle, improving urine flow rates in benign prostatic hypertrophy

Pharmacokinetics

PO: Completely absorbed, peak 1 hr; 90%-94% bound to plasma proteins; $t_{1/2}$ 12 hr; excreted in urine (40%) and feces (60%), 70% as metabolites

INDICATIONS AND USES: Hypertension; benign prostatic hypertrophy (BPH), Raynaud's vasospasm,*

DOSAGE

Adult

• *BPH:* PO 1 mg hs, increase to 2 mg, 5 mg, 10 mg/day (usual dose); not to exceed 20 mg/day; treatment at dose of 10 mg qd for 4-6 wk necessary to determine response

• *Hypertension:* PO 1 mg hs, increase to desired response; usual dose 1-5 mg qd, max 20 mg/day; measure BP at end of dosing interval to determine if bid dose needed

$ AVAILABLE FORMS/COST OF THERAPY

• Cap, Gel—Oral: 1, 2, 5, 10 mg, 100's: **$117.40-$203.90**

PRECAUTIONS: Patients needing to perform hazardous tasks where syncope or dizziness could be dangerous

PREGNANCY AND LACTATION: Pregnancy category C; excretion into breast milk unknown

SIDE EFFECTS/ADVERSE REACTIONS

CNS: Depression, *dizziness, drowsiness,* fatigue, *headache,* paresthesia, syncope (especially 1st days of therapy), vertigo, weakness

CV: Edema, hypotension, palpitations, *postural hypotension*

EENT: Blurred vision, dry mouth, epistaxis, *nasal congestion,* red sclera, *sinusitis,* tinnitus

GI: Nausea

GU: Impotence, incontinence, urinary frequency

RESP: Dyspnea

MISC: Weight gain

INTERACTIONS

Drugs

🔢 *Angiotensin converting enzyme inhibitors (enalapril):* Potential for exaggerated first dose hypotensive episode when alpha blockers added

🔢 *Nonsteroidal antiinflammatory drugs (ibuprofen, indomethacin):* NSAIDs may inhibit antihypertensive effects

🔢 *β-adrenergic blockers:* Potential for exaggerated first dose hypotensive episode when alpha blockers added

Labs

• False positive urinary metabolites of norepinephrine and VMA

• No effect on prostate specific antigen (PSA)

SPECIAL CONSIDERATIONS

• The doxazosin arm of the ALLHAT study was stopped early; the doxazosin group had a 25% greater risk of combined cardiovascular disease events which was primarily accounted for by a doubled risk of

T

CHF vs the chlorthalidone group; doxazosin was also found to be less effective at controlling systolic BP an average of 3 mm Hg; may want to consider primary antihypertensives in addition to alpha blockers for BPH symptoms

• Use as a single antihypertensive agent limited by tendency to cause sodium and water retention and increased plasma volume

PATIENT/FAMILY EDUCATION

• Alert patients to the possibility of syncopal and orthostatic symptoms, especially with the 1st dose ("1st dose syncope"); initial dose should be administered at bedtime in the smallest possible dose

---

terbinafine

(ter-been′a-feen)
Rx: Lamisil (tab)
OTC: Lamisil (cream)
Chemical Class: Synthetic allylamine derivative
Therapeutic Class: Antifungal

CLINICAL PHARMACOLOGY
Mechanism of Action: Inhibits fungal sterol biosynthesis, causing accumulation of squalene within the fungal cell and cell death

Pharmacokinetics
TOP: Variable systemic absorption
PO: Peak 2 hr
>99% bound to plasma proteins; distributed to sebum and skin; terminal t½ 200-400 hr; extensively metabolized; eliminated via urine

INDICATIONS AND USES: Tinea cruris, tinea corporis, tinea pedis; onychomycosis due to dermatophytes; cutaneous candidiasis*; tinea versicolor; active against *Epidermophyton floccosum, Trichophyton mentagrophytes, Trichophyton rubrum*

DOSAGE
Adult
• *Tinea pedis:* Top apply bid for 1-4 wk, until symptoms resolved
• *Tinea cruris, tinea corporis:* Top apply qd-bid for 1-4 wk
• *Onychomycosis:* PO 250 mg qd for 6 wk (fingernail) or 12 wk (toenail)

$ AVAILABLE FORMS/COST OF THERAPY
• Cre—Top: 1%, 15, 30 g: **$53.23**/30 g
• Sol—Top: 1%, 30 ml: **$62.21**
• Tab—Oral: 250 mg, 30's: **$271.37**

CONTRAINDICATIONS: Pre-existing renal or hepatic disease (oral therapy)

PRECAUTIONS: Children <12 (safety and efficacy not established)

PREGNANCY AND LACTATION: Pregnancy category B; it is recommended that treatment of onychomycosis be delayed until after pregnancy; small amounts of terbinafine are excreted into breast milk when administered orally, not recommended in nursing mothers; avoid application to the breast when breast feeding

SIDE EFFECTS/ADVERSE REACTIONS
CNS: Headache
EENT: Visual disturbance
GI: Abdominal pain, diarrhea, dyspepsia, elevated transaminases, flatulence, nausea, taste disturbance
SKIN: Burning, dryness, irritation, itching

SPECIAL CONSIDERATIONS
PATIENT/FAMILY EDUCATION
• Optimal clinical effect in onychomycosis may not be apparent for several mo following completion of therapy

---

* = non-FDA-approved use

terbutaline

(ter-byoo´te-leen)

Rx: Brethaire, Brethine, Bricanyl

Chemical Class: Sympathomimetic amine; β_2-adrenergic agonist

Therapeutic Class: Antiasthmatic, bronchodilator; tocolytic

CLINICAL PHARMACOLOGY

Mechanism of Action: Causes bronchodilation by β_2-stimulation, resulting in relaxation of bronchial smooth muscle; inhibits mast cell degranulation; stimulates cilia to remove secretions; relaxes uterine smooth muscle

Pharmacokinetics

PO: Onset ½ hr, peak 1-2 hr, duration 4-8 hr

SC: Onset 5-15 min, peak ½-1 hr, duration 1½-4 hr

INH: Onset 5-30 min, peak 1-2 hr, duration 3-6 hr

Metabolized in gut wall and liver; excreted in urine; $t_{1/2}$ 3-4 hr

INDICATIONS AND USES: Bronchial asthma; reversible bronchospasm associated with bronchitis and emphysema; premature labor*

DOSAGE

Adult

• *Bronchospasm:* MDI 2 puffs separated by 1 min q4-6h; PO 2.5-5 mg q8h to max 15 mg qd; SC 0.25 mg, may repeat once in 15-30 min

• *Premature labor:* SC 0.25 mg qh; IV INF 0.01 mg/min, titrate upward to max of 0.08 mg/min; maintain at minimum effective dose for 4 hr; PO 5 mg q4h for 48 hr, then 5 mg q6h as maintenance for above doses

Child

• MDI 1-2 puffs q 4-6h; PO 0.05 mg/kg/dose q8h, increased gradually to 0.15 mg/kg/dose to max daily dose 5 mg (<12 yr); SC 0.005-0.01 mg/kg/dose to max 0.4 mg/kg/dose q 15-20 min for 2 doses

Ⓢ AVAILABLE FORMS/COST OF THERAPY

• Inj, Sol—SC: 1 mg/ml, 1 ml: **$3.17-$5.87**

• MDI-INH: 0.2 mg/inh, 7.5 ml: **$23.26-$26.27**

• Tab, Uncoated—Oral: 2.5 mg, 100's: **$33.48-$48.15**; 5 mg, 100's: **$48.06-$69.27**

PRECAUTIONS: Ischemic heart disease, cardiac dysrhythmias, hyperthyroidism, diabetes mellitus, prostatic hypertrophy, hypertension

PREGNANCY AND LACTATION: Pregnancy category B; compatible with breast feeding

SIDE EFFECTS/ADVERSE REACTIONS

CNS: Anxiety, dizziness, headache, insomnia, *nervousness, shakiness, tremor*

CV: Angina, ***cardiac arrest, dysrhythmias,*** hypertension, *palpitations, tachycardia*

GI: Elevated liver enzymes, *nausea, vomiting*

INTERACTIONS

Drugs

❷ *Beta-blockers:* Decreased action of terbutaline, cardioselective beta-blockers preferable if concurrent use necessary; metoprolol inhibits terbutaline metabolism

❸ *Furosemide:* Potential for additive hypokalemia

T

---

italic = common side effects　　　***bold italic*** = life-threatening reactions

terconazole

(ter-kon´a-zole)
Rx: Terazol 3, Terazol 7
Chemical Class: Triazole derivative
Therapeutic Class: Antifungal

CLINICAL PHARMACOLOGY
Mechanism of Action: Uncertain; may disrupt fungal cell membrane permeability
Pharmacokinetics
Systemic absorption 5%-16%
INDICATIONS AND USES: Local treatment of vulvovaginal candidiasis
DOSAGE
Adult
• VAG (cre) 5 g (1 applicator) qhs for 3 (0.8%) or 7 (0.4%) days
• VAG (supp) 1 qhs for 3 days
$ AVAILABLE FORMS/COST OF THERAPY
• Cre—Vag: 0.4%, 45 g: **$26.22-$36.39**; 0.8%, 20 g: **$32.23-$36.39**
• Supp—Vag: 80 mg, 3's: **$26.22-$36.39**
PREGNANCY AND LACTATION: Pregnancy category C, systemic absorption occurs; excretion into breast milk unknown
SIDE EFFECTS/ADVERSE REACTIONS
CNS: Headache
GI: Abdominal pain
GU: Genital pain, *itching,* vulvovaginal burning
SKIN: Photosensitivity reactions with repeated application under artificial UV light
SPECIAL CONSIDERATIONS
• No significant advantage over less expensive OTC products

testosterone

(tess-toss´ter-one)
Rx: *Testosterone aqueous:*
Testamone-100, Testro AQ
Testosterone cypionate:
Depo-Testosterone, Depotest, T-Cypionate, Virilon IM
Testosterone enanthate:
Delatestryl, Everone, Testro-L.A.
Testosterone propionate:
Generics only
Transdermal: Androderm, Testoderm, AndroGel
Pellet: Testopel
Chemical Class: Testosterone
Therapeutic Class: Androgen; antineoplastic
DEA Class: Schedule III

CLINICAL PHARMACOLOGY
Mechanism of Action: Promotes weight gain via retention of nitrogen, potassium, and phosphorous, increased protein anabolism and decreased catabolism; endogenous androgens essential for normal growth and development of male sex organs and maintenance of secondary sex characteristics
Pharmacokinetics
Testosterone: IM $t_{1/2}$ 10-100 min; transdermal peak 2-4 hr, returns to baseline 2 hr after removal (Testoderm)
Testosterone cypionate: IM $t_{1/2}$ 8 days; 98% protein bound; metabolized in liver; excreted in urine, breast milk; crosses placenta
INDICATIONS AND USES: Male primary and secondary hypogonadism (aqueous, transdermal, cypionate, enanthate, propionate); delayed puberty in males (enanthate, propionate); advanced metastatic breast cancer in women (enanthate,

propionate), postpartum breast pain and engorgement (propionate); male contraceptive (enanthate)*

DOSAGE

Adult and Child

• *Hypogonadism:* IM 25-50 mg 2-3 times/wk (aqueous); 40-50 mg/m^2 monthly to initiate pubertal growth, increasing to 100 mg/m^2 monthly during terminal growth phase, maintenance dose 50-400 mg q2-4wk (propionate); 50-400 mg q2-4wk (enanthate, cypionate); transdermal 4-6 mg/day system applied to clean, dry, shaved scrotal skin, wear for 22-24 hr/day (Testoderm); 5 mg/day (2 × 2.5 mg/day systems) applied nightly to clean, dry area of upper back, arms, abdomen or thighs; adjust dose, based on patient response and serum testosterone levels, by increasing to 3 systems or decreasing to 1 system/day (Androderm)

• *Delayed puberty:* IM 40-50 mg/m^2 monthly for 6 months (propionate); 50-200 mg q2-4wk for a limited duration (enanthate, cypionate)

• Postpartum breast engorgement: IM 25-50 mg for 3-4 days starting at the time of delivery (propionate)

• *Breast cancer:* IM 50-100 mg 3 times/wk (propionate) or 200-400 mg q2-4wk (cypionate or enanthate)

💲 AVAILABLE FORMS/COST OF THERAPY

Testosterone

• Film, Cont Rel—Percutaneous: 2.5 mg/24 hr, 60's: **$110.08-$148.47**; 4 mg/24 hr, 6 mg/24 hr, 30's: **$111.81**; 5 mg/24 hr, 30's: **$110.08-$148.47**

• Pellet—SC: 75 mg/pellet: **$15.00**

Testosterone Aqueous

• Inj, Susp—IM: 50 mg/ml, 10 ml: **$3.95-$12.00**; 100 mg/ml, 10 ml: **$6.50-$45.00**

Testosterone Cypionate

• Inj, Sol—IM: 100 mg/ml, 10 ml: **$13.27-$49.53**; 200 mg/ml, 10 ml: **$18.46-$85.98**

Testosterone Enanthate

• Inj, Sol—IM: 200 mg/ml, 10 ml: **$9.15-$42.10**

Testosterone Propionate

• Inj, Sol—IM: 100 mg/ml, 10 ml: **$5.85-$18.38**

CONTRAINDICATIONS: Severe renal disease, severe cardiac disease, severe hepatic disease, genital bleeding (abnormal), male breast cancer, prostate cancer

PRECAUTIONS: Diabetes mellitus, cardiovascular disease, risk factors for atherosclerosis, hepatic disease, seizure disorder, renal disease

PREGNANCY AND LACTATION: Pregnancy category X; excretion into breast milk unknown, use extreme caution in nursing mothers

SIDE EFFECTS/ADVERSE REACTIONS

CNS: Aggressive behavior, anxiety, depression, dizziness, emotional lability, fatigue, flushing, headache, insomnia, paresthesias, sweating, tremors

CV: **CHF,** edema, increased blood pressure

EENT: Conjunctival edema, deepening of voice, nasal congestion

GI: Cholestatic jaundice, constipation, *hepatocellular neoplasm,* nausea, vomiting, weight gain, *peliosis hepatis*

GU: Amenorrhea, clitoral hypertrophy, decreased breast size, gynecomastia, increased or decreased libido, priapism, testicular atrophy, vaginitis, virilization in females, oligospermia, menstrual irregularities

HEME: Polycythemia, suppression of clotting factors

T

---

italic = common side effects   ***bold italic*** = life-threatening reactions

METAB: Hypercalcemia (in breast cancer), hypercholesterolemia, hyperglycemia, increased potassium, premature epiphyseal closure (children)

SKIN: Acneiform lesions, acne vulgaris, alopecia, flushing, hirsutism, oily hair and skin, rash, sweating

MISC: Carpal tunnel syndrome

INTERACTIONS

Drugs

3 *Cyclosporine:* Increased cyclosporine concentrations

2 *Oral anticoagulants:* Increased hypoprothrombinemic response

SPECIAL CONSIDERATIONS

MONITORING PARAMETERS

• LFTs, lipids, Hct

• Growth rate in children (X-rays for bone age q6 mo)

---

tetracaine

(tet´ra-cane)

Rx: Opticaine, Pontocaine, Tetcaine HCl Ophthalmic

OTC: Pontocaine

Chemical Class: Benzoic acid derivative

Therapeutic Class: Local anesthetic

CLINICAL PHARMACOLOGY

Mechanism of Action: Decreases neuronal membrane permeability to sodium ions, blocking nerve impulses

Pharmacokinetics

INJ: Onset of action rapid, duration 2-3 hr

OPHTH: Onset of action 15 sec, duration 10-20 min

TOP: Peak 3-8 min, duration 3060 min

Hydrolyzed by plasma esterases; excreted by kidney

INDICATIONS AND USES: TOP: pruritus, sunburn, toothache, sore throat, cold sores, oral pain, rectal pain and irritation; control of gagging prior to performing bronchoscopy, bronchography, and esophagoscopy; OPHTHAL: cataract extraction, tonometry, gonioscopy, removal of foreign objects, corneal suture removal, glaucoma surgery; INJ: spinal anesthesia

DOSAGE

Adult and Child

• TOP apply to affected area

• OPHTH instill 1-2 gtt before procedure

• INJ 0.2%-0.3% sol for spinal anesthesia; for prolonged anesthesia (2-3 hr) 1% sol

$ **AVAILABLE FORMS/COST OF THERAPY**

• Cre—Top: 1%, 30 g: **$9.95**

• Inj, Sol—IV: 0.2%, 2 ml: **$5.47**; 0.3%, 5 ml: **$6.99**; 1%, 2 ml: **$5.62**

• Oint—Ophth: 0.5%, 3.5 g: **$11.79-$16.21**

• Oint—Top: 0.5%, 30 g: **$9.32**

• Sol—Ophth: 0.5%, 15 ml: **$2.31-$27.02**

• Sol—Top: 2%, 30 ml: **$13.66-$27.00**

CONTRAINDICATIONS: Hypersensitivity to ester anesthetics; infants less than 1 yr; application to large areas

PRECAUTIONS: Child <6 yr, sepsis, denuded skin

PREGNANCY AND LACTATION: Pregnancy category C; excretion into breast milk unknown

SIDE EFFECTS/ADVERSE REACTIONS

SKIN: Burning, irritation, rash, sensitization, stinging, tenderness

INTERACTIONS

Drugs

3 *Propranolol:* Enhanced sympathomimetic side effects resulting in hypertensive reactions; acute discontinuation of beta-blockers prior to local anesthesia may increase side effects of tetracaine

Labs
• *Interference:* CSF protein

SPECIAL CONSIDERATIONS
• Also used as a component of "Magic Numbing Solution" or TAC Sol (epinephrine 1:2,000, tetracaine 0.5%, cocaine 11.8%) and LET Sol (lidocaine 4%, epinephrine 0.1%, tetracaine 0.5%), which are used as topical anesthesia for repair of minor lacerations, especially in pediatric patients

---

tetracycline
(tet-ra-sye′kleen)
Rx: *Systemic:* Ala-Tet, Brodspec, Emtet-500, Panmycin, Sumycin, Tetra 500, Tetracap, Tetracon, Wesmycin
Topical: Topicycline
Peridontal fiber: Actisite
Chemical Class: Tetracycline
Therapeutic Class: Antibiotic

CLINICAL PHARMACOLOGY
Mechanism of Action: Inhibition of microbial protein synthesis; bacteriostatic

Pharmacokinetics
PO: Peak 2-3 hr, duration 6 hr; excreted in urine (60% unchanged); crosses placenta, excreted in breast milk; 20%-60% protein bound; $t_{1/2}$ 6-10 hr

INDICATIONS AND USES: *Systemic:* Infections caused by Rickettsiae (Rocky Mountain spotted fever, typhus fever, Q fever, rickettsial pox and tick fever), *Mycoplasma pneumoniae,* agents of psittacosis and ornithosis, agents of lymphogranuloma venerium and granuloma inguinale, relapsing fever *(Borrelia recurrentis)*

Antimicrobial spectrum usually includes:
• Gram-positive organisms: streptococcus sp. (up to 44% of *S. pyogenes* and 74% of *S. faecalis* are resistant), *Diplococcus pneumoniae, Staph. aureus* (skin and soft tissue infections)
• Gram-negative organisms: *Hemophilus ducreyi* (chancroid), *Pasturella pestis, P. tularensis, Bartonella bacilliformis, Bacteroides* spp.; *Vibrio colera* and *V. fetus, Brucella* spp. (in combination with streptomycin); *Chlamydia trachomatis:* susceptibility should be demonstrated for *E. coli, Enterobacter aerogenes, Shigella* spp., *H. influenzae* (respiratory infections), *Klebsiella* spp. (respiratory and urinary infections)
• Anaerobic organisms: *Propionibacterium acnes* (acne)
• Alternative to penicillin for *Neisseria gonorrhoeae, Treponema pallidum,* and *T. pertenue* (syphilis and yaws); *Listeria monocytogenes, Clostridium* spp.; *Bacillus anthracis, Fugobacterium fusiforme* (Vincent's infection); *Actinomyces* spp.
Topical: Acne vulgaris

DOSAGE
Adult
• PO 250-500 mg q6h
• *Gonorrhea:* PO 1.5 g, then 500 mg qid for a total of 9 g
• *Chlamydia:* PO 500 mg qid for 7 days
• *Syphilis:* (Benzathine penicillin is the drug of choice for syphilis) PO 2-3 g in divided doses for 10-15 days; if syphilis duration >1 yr, must treat 30 days
• *Brucellosis:* PO 500 mg qid for 3 wk with 1 g streptomycin IM bid for 1 wk, and qd the 2nd wk

---

• *Acne:* PO 250 mg qid; maintenance 125-500 mg qd; TOP apply sol bid to affected area

Child >8 yr

• PO 25-50 mg/kg/d in divided doses q6h

💲 **AVAILABLE FORMS/COST OF THERAPY**

• Cap, Gel—Oral: 100 mg, 1000's: **$31.20**; 250 mg, 100's: **$0.54-$18.96**; 500 mg, 100's: **$0.67-$14.09**
• Fiber—Peridontal: 12.7 mg, 10's: **$262.80**
• Sol—Top: 2.2 mg/ml, 70 ml: **$59.83**
• Susp—Oral: 125 mg/5 ml, 480 ml: **$6.00-$13.98**
• Tab, Coated—Oral: 250 mg, 100's: **$7.25**; 500 mg, 100's: **$14.11**

CONTRAINDICATIONS: Children <8 yr (systemic)

PRECAUTIONS: Renal disease, hepatic disease

PREGNANCY AND LACTATION: Pregnancy category D (systemic), category B (topical); systemic tetracycline excreted into breast milk in low concentrations; theoretically, dental staining could occur, but serum levels in infants undetectable, so considered compatible with breast feeding

SIDE EFFECTS/ADVERSE REACTIONS

CNS: Fever, headache, paresthesia, ***pseudotumor cerebri***

CV: Pericarditis

EENT: Dysphagia, esophagitis, oral candidiasis, oral ulcers

GI: Abdominal cramps, abdominal pain, anorexia, decreased calcification of deciduous teeth (children <8 yr), *diarrhea,* enterocolitis, epigastric burning, flatulence, glossitis, ***hepatotoxicity,*** nausea, stomatitis, *vomiting*

GU: Increased BUN, renal failure (associated with use of outdated products)

HEME: Eosinophilia, ***hemolytic anemia, neutropenia, thrombocytopenia***

SKIN: Angioedema, ***exfoliative dermatitis,*** increased pigmentation, photosensitivity, pruritus, *rash,* stinging (top), *urticaria*

INTERACTIONS

Drugs

3 *Antacids:* Reduced tetracycline concentrations

2 *Bismuth subsalicylate:* Reduced tetracycline concentrations

3 *Calcium:* Reduced tetracycline concentrations

3 *Cholestyramine colestipol:* Reduced tetracycline concentrations

3 *Digoxin:* Decreased digoxin concentrations due to reduced GI flora

3 *Food:* Reduced tetracycline concentrations

3 *Iron:* Reduced tetracycline concentrations

3 *Magnesium:* Reduced tetracycline concentrations

2 *Methoxyflurane:* Increased renal toxicity

3 *Oral contraceptives:* Possible decreased contraceptive effect

3 *Penicillin:* Impaired efficacy of penicillin

3 *Sodium bicarbonate:* Reduced tetracycline concentrations

3 *Zinc:* Reduced tetracycline concentrations

Labs

• *False negative:* Urine glucose with Clinistix or TesTape
• *False increase:* Serum glucose
• *False decrease:* Serum acetaminophen concentration, serum folate
• *Interference:* Plasma catecholamines, urinary porphyrins, CSF protein

SPECIAL CONSIDERATIONS
PATIENT/FAMILY EDUCATION
• Avoid milk products, antacids, or separate by 2 hr; take with a full glass of water
• Use in children ≤8 yr causes permanent discoloration of teeth, enamel hypoplasia, and retardation of skeletal development; risk greatest for children <4 yr and receiving high doses
• Side effects noted for systemic administration not observed with topical formulations

---

tetrahydrozoline
(tet-ra-hi-droz′o-leen)
Rx: *Nasal:* Tyzine, Tyzine Pediatric
OTC: *Ophthalmic:* Collyrium Fresh Eye Drops, Eyesine, Murine Plus Eye Drops, Optigene 3 Eye Drops, Visine Eye Drops
Chemical Class: Sympathomimetic amine
Therapeutic Class: Decongestant

CLINICAL PHARMACOLOGY
Mechanism of Action: Local α-adrenergic-mediated vasoconstriction dilated conjunctival and nasal mucosal blood vessels
Pharmacokinetics
TOP: Duration 2-3 hr
INDICATIONS AND USES: NASAL: Decongestion of nasal and nasopharyngeal mucosa; OPHTHAL: ocular congestion, irritation, itching, redness
DOSAGE
Adult
• NASAL, instill 2-4 gtt/sprays 0.1% sol in each nostril q4-8h
• OPHTH, instill 1-2 gtt in affected eye up to qid

Child (2-6 yr)
• NASAL, instill 2-3 gtt 0.05% sol in each nostril q4-6h

💲 AVAILABLE FORMS/COST OF THERAPY
• Aer, Spray—Nasal: 0.1%, 15 ml: **$9.53**
• Sol—Nasal: 0.05%, 15 ml: **$14.93**; 0.1%, 30 ml: **$17.24**
• Sol—Ophth: 0.05%, 30 ml: **$2.88-$5.96**

CONTRAINDICATIONS: Narrow-angle glaucoma
PRECAUTIONS: Severe hypertension, diabetes, hyperthyroidism, elderly, severe arteriosclerosis, cardiac disease, infants, diabetes, asthma, CAD
PREGNANCY AND LACTATION: Pregnancy category C; excretion into breast milk unknown
SIDE EFFECTS/ADVERSE REACTIONS
CNS: Dizziness, headache, weakness
CV: **CV collapse, dysrhythmias,** hypertension, palpitation, reflex bradycardia, tachycardia
EENT: Blurred vision, conjunctival allergy, lacrimation, stinging
SPECIAL CONSIDERATIONS
• Manage rebound congestion by stopping tetrahydrozoline: one nostril at a time, substitute systemic decongestant, substitute inhaled steroid
PATIENT/FAMILY EDUCATION
• Do not use for >3-5 days or rebound congestion may occur

T

---

thalidomide
(thal-e-doe-mide)
Rx: Thalomid
Chemical Class: Glutamic acid
derivative
Therapeutic Class: Leprostatic

CLINICAL PHARMACOLOGY
Mechanism of Action: Reduces inflammation by cytokine modulation. Reduces levels of tumor necrosis factor-alpha in patients with erythema nodosum leprosum
Pharmacokinetics
PO: Slowly absorbed from GI tract, peak 3-6 hr; highly protein bound; major metabolic pathway is nonenzymatic hydrolysis in plasma to multiple metabolites; minimal amount metabolized by liver; metabolites excreted in urine (1% unchanged after 24 hr); $t_{1/2}$ 5-7 hr
INDICATIONS AND USES: Erythema nodosum leprosum, discoid lupus erythematosus,* graft vs. host disease,* oral aphthous ulcers in immunocompromised patients*
DOSAGE
Adult
• *Aphthous ulceration:* PO 100-200 mg qd until response, then 50-100 mg qd
• *Discoid lupus erythematosus:* PO 400 mg qd until response, then 50-100 mg qd
• *Erythema nodosum leprosum:* PO 100-400 mg qd until response, then 25-100 mg qd
• *Graft vs. host disease:* PO 800-1600 mg qd until response, then taper by 25% every 2 wk
⑤   AVAILABLE FORMS/COST OF THERAPY
• Cap—Oral: 50 mg, 14's: **$105.00-$145.76**

CONTRAINDICATIONS: Women of child-bearing potential unless: 1. An effective form of contraception has been used for at least 1 mo before therapy, during therapy, and for 1 mo following   discontinuation   of therapy, and 2. Pregnancy has been definitely excluded through a negative pregnancy test within 2 wk prior to thalidomide therapy. Men must use barrier contraception if sexually active with women of child-bearing potential
PRECAUTIONS: Bradycardia, photosensitization
PREGNANCY AND LACTATION: Pregnancy category X; breast milk excretion unknown
SIDE EFFECTS/ADVERSE REACTIONS
CNS: Anxiety, *dizziness, headache (12%), neuropathy,* paresthesia, *somnolence (38%),* tremor, *vertigo*
CV: Edema
EENT: Dry mouth
GI: Anorexia, constipation, *elevated transaminase levels (10%),* nausea
GU: Impotence
HEME: Anemia, **leukopenia (20%)**
METAB: Hypothyroidism
SKIN: Pruritus, rash (25%)
INTERACTIONS
Drugs
③ *Barbiturates:* Additive sedative effects
③ *Chlorpromazine:* Additive sedative effects
③ *Ethanol:* Additive sedative effects
③ *Reserpine:* Additive sedative effects
SPECIAL CONSIDERATIONS
PATIENT/FAMILY EDUCATION
• Teratogenic in human whether taken by male or female
• Sedation common; usually taken at bedtime

---

* = non-FDA-approved use

MONITORING PARAMETERS
• Pregnancy test (weekly during first mo of use, then monthly)
• ALT, AST
• CBC

---

theophylline

(thee-off'i-lin)
Rx: *Immediate release tabs:*
Quibron-T, Slo-Phylline, Theolair
Liquids: Asmalix, Elixophyllin, Slo-Phyllin, Theolair, Truxophylline
Sustained release caps
Aerolate Slo-Bid Gyrocaps, Theo-24
Sustained release tabs:
Quibron-T/SR, Respbid, Theochron, Theo-Dur, Theolair-SR, Theo-X, Uni-Dur, Theo-Time, T-Phyl, Uniphyl
Combinations
  Rx: with guaifenesin (Elixophyllin-GG, Quibron, Slo-Phyllin-GG); with potassium iodide (Elixophylline KI)
Chemical Class: Xanthine derivative
Therapeutic Class: Antiasthmatic, bronchodilator; COPD agent

CLINICAL PHARMACOLOGY
Mechanism of Action: Directly relaxes bronchial and pulmonary blood vessel smooth muscle; stimulates CNS; induces diuresis; increases gastric acid secretion, lowers lower esophageal sphincter pressure; is a central respiratory stimulant; exact mechanism unproven but may involve antagonism of pulmonary adenosine receptors

Pharmacokinetics
PO: Well absorbed from GI tract, absorption altered by food; peak 2 hr (immediate release), 4-6 hr (Sus Action); crosses placenta, excreted into breast milk; metabolized in liver; excreted (15% unchanged) in urine; $t_{1/2}$ 3-15 hr in non-smokers, 4-5 hr in smokers, 1-9 hr in children, 20-30 hr in premature neonates (who may accumulate the caffeine metabolite)
INDICATIONS AND USES: Bronchial asthma; reversible bronchospasm of chronic bronchitis and emphysema; apnea and bradycardia of prematurity*
DOSAGE
(Based on ideal body weight) When converting to sustained release products, total daily dose remains the same but is divided q8h-q24h depending on product and dose (doses >1200 mg/day should be divided q8h, doses <1200 mg/day can be given q12h)
Adult
• *Acute symptoms:* PO 5 mg/kg load, maintenance 3 mg/kg q8h (non-smokers), 3 mg/kg q6h (smokers), 2 mg/kg q8h (older patients), 1-2 mg/kg q12h (CHF); IV 5 mg/kg load over 20 min, maintenance 0.2 mg/kg/hr (CHF, elderly), 0.43 mg/kg/hr (non-smokers), 0.7 mg/kg/hr (young adult smokers), measure serum level for patients currently receiving theophylline, approx 0.5 mg/kg theophylline increases serum level 1 µg/ml
• *Slow titration:* PO initial dose 16 mg/kg/24h or 400 mg/24 hr, whichever is less, doses divided q6-8h
• *PO dosage adjustment after serum theophylline measurement:*
• Serum level 5-10 µg/ml, increase dose by 25%, recheck level in 3 days
• Serum level 10-20 µg/ml, maintain dosage if tolerated, recheck level q6-12mo

T

• Serum level 20-25 µg/ml, decrease dose by 10%, recheck level in 3 days
• Serum level 25-30 µg/ml, skip next dose, decrease dose by 25%, recheck level in 3 days
• Serum level >30 µg/ml, skip next 2 doses, decrease dose by 50%, recheck level in 3 days

Child
• 9-16 yr: PO 5 mg/kg load, maintenance 3 mg/kg q6h; IV 5 mg/kg load over 20 min, maintenance 0.7 mg/kg/h
• 1-9 yr: PO 5 mg/kg load, maintenance 4 mg/kg q6h; IV 5 mg/kg load over 20 min, maintenance 0.8 mg/kg/hr
• Infants: PO [(0.2 × age in weeks) + 5] × kg = 24 hr dose in mg; divide into q8h dosing (6 wk-6 mo), q6h dosing (6-12 mo); IV 5 mg/kg load over 20 min, maintenance dose in mg/kg/hr [(.0008 × age in weeks) + 0.21]
• Premature infants: IV 1 mg/kg q12h (≤24 days postnatal), 1.5 mg/kg q12h (>24 days postnatal)

💲 **AVAILABLE FORMS/COST OF THERAPY**
• Cap—Oral: 100 mg, 100's: **$39.02-$49.45**; 200 mg, 100's: **$51.93-$65.72**; 300 mg, 100's: **$20.82**
• Cap, Gel, Sus Action—Oral: 50 mg, 100's: **$17.33-$25.68**; 65 mg, 100's: **$17.00**; 75 mg, 100's: **$19.75-$28.34**; 100 mg, 100's: **$19.61-$32.80**; 125 mg, 100's: **$24.77-$41.10**; 130 mg, 100's: **$16.00-$18.25**; 200 mg, 100's: **$29.48-$48.93**; 250 mg, 100's: **$45.07**; 260 mg, 100's: **$20.00-$23.40**; 300 mg, 100's: **$35.10-$58.28**; 400 mg, 100's: **$112.11**; 100 mg/24 hr, 100's: **$43.55**; 200 mg/24 hr, 100's: **$64.91**; 600 mg/24 hr, 100's: **$65.14**
• Elixir—Oral: 80 mg/15 ml, 480 ml: **$3.84-$91.40**

• Inj, Sol—IV: 0.4 mg/ml, 1000 ml: **$11.45**; 0.8 mg/ml, 1000 ml: **$15.16**; 1.6 mg/ml, 500 ml: **$16.21**; 2 mg/ml, 100 ml: **$9.48**; 3.2 mg/ml, 250 ml: **$10.95**; 4 mg/ml, 100 ml: **$9.77**
• Sol—Oral: 80 mg/15 ml, 480 ml: **$2.50-$28.86**
• Syr—Oral: 80 mg/15 ml, 480 ml: **$14.78-$27.58**
• Tab, Coated, Sus Action—Oral: 100 mg, 100's: **$7.40-$22.75**; 200 mg, 100's: **$7.58-$58.22**; 250 mg, 100's: **$34.24-$52.20**; 300 mg, 100's: **$10.23-$68.13**; 400 mg, 100's: **$101.83-$110.34**; 450 mg, 100's: **$27.75-$57.55**; 500 mg, 100's: **$49.54-$77.94**; 600 mg, 100's: **$129.89-$147.13**
• Tab, Uncoated—Oral: 100 mg, 100's: **$8.50-$24.00**; 125 mg, 100's: **$53.19**; 200 mg, 100's: **$31.88**; 250 mg, 100's: **$82.56**; 300 mg, 100's: **$46.75-$60.48**

CONTRAINDICATIONS: Tachydysrhythmias; as sole treatment of status asthmaticus; active peptic ulcer disease; seizure disorders

PRECAUTIONS: Elderly, CHF, cor pulmonale, hepatic disease, diabetes mellitus, hyperthyroidism, hypertension, active alcoholism, children, neonates

PREGNANCY AND LACTATION: Pregnancy category C; no reports of malformations; compatible with breast feeding with precaution that rapidly absorbed preparations may cause irritability in the infant

SIDE EFFECTS/ADVERSE REACTIONS
CNS: Anxiety, *dizziness,* headache, insomnia, lightheadedness, muscle twitching, restlessness, *seizures*
CV: Dysrhythmias, fluid retention with tachycardia, hypotension, palpitations, pounding heartbeat, sinus tachycardia

---

* = non-FDA-approved use

GI: Anorexia, bitter taste, diarrhea, dyspepsia, gastroesophageal reflux, *nausea, vomiting*
GU: Urinary frequency
RESP: Increased rate
SKIN: Flushing, urticaria

INTERACTIONS
Drugs

3 *Adenosine:* Inhibited hemodynamic effects of adenosine

3 *Allopurinol, amiodarone, cimetidine, ciprofloxacin, disulfiram, erythromycin, interferon alfa, isoniazid, methimazole, metoprolol, norfloxacin, pefloxacin, pentoxyfylline, propafenone, propylthiouracil, radioactive iodine, tacrine, thiabendazole, ticlopidine, verapamil:* Increased theophylline concentrations

3 *Aminoglutethamide, barbiturates, carbamazepine, moricizine, phenytoin, rifampin, ritonavir, thyroid hormone:* Reduced theophylline levels; decreased serum phenytoin concentrations

3 *Beta-blockers:* Reduced bronchodilating response to theophylline

2 *Enoxacin, fluvoxamine, mexiletine, propranolol, troleandomycin:* Markedly increased theophylline concentrations

3 *Imipenem:* Some patients on theophylline have developed seizures following the addition of imipenem

3 *Lithium:* Reduced lithium concentrations

3 *Smoking:* Increased theophylline dosing requirements

Labs

• *False increase:* Serum barbiturate concentrations, urinary uric acid
• *False decrease:* Serum bilirubin
• *Interference:* Plasma somatostatin

SPECIAL CONSIDERATIONS
PATIENT/FAMILY EDUCATION
• Contents of beaded capsules may be sprinkled over food for children
MONITORING PARAMETERS
• Blood levels; therapeutic level is 10-20 µg/ml (6-14 µg/ml for apnea, bradycardia of prematurity); toxicity may occur with small increase above 20 µg/ml and occasionally at levels below this; obtain serum levels 1-2 hr after administration for immediate release products and 5-9 hr after the AM dose for sustained release formulations
• Recent evidence indicates that blood levels of 8-12 µg/ml may provide adequate therapeutic effect with a lower risk of adverse events
• Signs of toxicity include nausea, vomiting, anxiety, insomnia, seizures, ventricular dysrhythmias

---

thiabendazole
(thye-a-ben′da-zole)
Rx: Mintezol
Chemical Class: Benzimadazole derivative
Therapeutic Class: Anthelmintic

CLINICAL PHARMACOLOGY
Mechanism of Action: May inhibit the helminth-specific enzyme, fumarate reductase
Pharmacokinetics
PO: Peak 1-2 hr, metabolized completely to 5-hydroxy form, excreted in urine as glucuronide or sulfate conjugates, most within 24 hr
INDICATIONS AND USES: Vermicidal and/or vermifugal against *Enterobius vermicularis* (pinworm), *Ascaria lumbricoides* (roundworm), *Strongyloides stercoralis* (threadworm), *Trichuris trichiura* (whipworm), trichinosis, *Ancylos-*

---

italic = common side effects   ***bold italic*** = life-threatening reactions

toma duodenale (hookworm), *Necator americanus, Ancylostoma braziliense* (dog and cat hookworm)

DOSAGE

Adult and Child

• PO 22 mg/kg/dose given bid for 2-7 days, not to exceed 3 g/day (strongyloidiasis 2 days; cutaneous larva migrans 2 days; visceral larva migrans 7 days; trichinosis 2-4 successive days per response; roundworms, including ascariasis, uncinariasis, and trichuriasis 2 days)

$ **AVAILABLE FORMS/COST OF THERAPY**

• Susp—Oral: 500 mg/5 ml, 120 ml: **$26.32**

• Tab, Chewable—Oral: 500 mg, 36's: **$45.35**

PRECAUTIONS: Severe malnutrition, hepatic disease, renal disease, anemia, severe dehydration, child <14 kg

PREGNANCY AND LACTATION: Pregnancy category C

SIDE EFFECTS/ADVERSE REACTIONS

CNS: Behavioral changes, dizziness, drowsiness, fever, flushing, headache, *seizures*

CV: Bradycardia, hypotension

EENT: Blurred vision, tinnitus, xanthopsia

GI: Anorexia, diarrhea, epigastric distress, increased AST, jaundice, liver damage, *nausea, vomiting*

GU: Abnormal smell of urine, enuresis, hematuria, *nephrotoxicity*

SKIN: Erythema, pruritus, rash, *Stevens-Johnson syndrome*

INTERACTIONS

Drugs

3 *Carbamazepine:* Decreased thiabendazole concentrations, therapeutic failure possible

3 *Theophylline:* May inhibit metabolism of xanthines, potentially elevating serum concentrations

SPECIAL CONSIDERATIONS

PATIENT/FAMILY EDUCATION

• Take after meals; chew before swallowing

• Proper hygiene after bowel movement, including handwashing technique; change bed linen

---

thiamine (vitamin B$_1$)

(thy′a-min)

Rx: Thiamine

OTC: Thiamilate

Chemical Class: B complex vitamin

Therapeutic Class: Vitamin

CLINICAL PHARMACOLOGY

Mechanism of Action: Acts as coenzyme, as an oxidation-reduction agent, or possibly as a mitochondrial agent in pyruvate metabolism

Pharmacokinetics

PO/IM: Rapid and complete absorption; widely distributed (highest concentrations in liver, brain, kidney, and heart); rapidly metabolized; excess excreted in urine; body depletion of vitamin B$_1$ can occur after approx 3 wk of total absence of thiamine in the diet

INDICATIONS AND USES: Vitamin B$_1$ deficiency syndromes including polyneuritis, beriberi, pellagra, Wernicke-Korsakoff syndrome; metabolic disorders (maple syrup urine disease, subacute necrotizing encephalitis); parenteral thiamine is recommended for alcoholic patients with altered sensorium admitted to the hospital and in all patients presenting with coma or hypothermia of unknown etiology; essential component of total parenteral nutrition therapy

---

* = non-FDA-approved use

DOSAGE
Adult
• *Beriberi:* IM/IV 10-500 mg tid × 2 wk, then 5-10 mg PO qd × 1 mo
• *Beriberi with cardiac failure:* IV 100-500 mg
• *Metabolic disorders:* PO 10-20 mg qd
• *Anemia or pellagra:* PO 100 mg qd
• *Wernicke's encephalopathy:* IV 100 mg, then 50-100 mg qd until patient is consuming a regular, well-balanced diet

Child
• *Beriberi:* IM 10-50 mg qd × 46 wk
• *Anemia or pellagra:* PO 10-50 mg qd
• *Beriberi with cardiac failure:* IV 100-500 mg

§ AVAILABLE FORMS/COST OF THERAPY
• Inj, Sol—IM, IV: 100 mg/ml, 1 ml: **$1.00-$2.11**
• Tab—Oral: 50 mg, 100's: **$1.33-$2.30**; 100 mg, 100's: **$1.88-$4.50**; 500 mg, 100's: **$7.35**

PREGNANCY AND LACTATION: Pregnancy category A; excreted into breast milk; U.S. recommended daily allowance for thiamine during lactation is 1.5-1.6 mg; supplement women with inadequate intake; compatible with breast feeding

SIDE EFFECTS/ADVERSE REACTIONS

CNS: Restlessness, weakness
CV: **Collapse,** hypotension, **pulmonary edema**
EENT: Tightness of throat
GI: Diarrhea, hemorrhage, *nausea*
SKIN: Angioneurotic edema, cyanosis, pruritus, sweating, urticaria, warmth

SPECIAL CONSIDERATIONS
• Worsening of Wernicke's encephalopathy is possible following glucose administration, administer thiamine before or along with dextrose-containing fluids

• Single vitamin B₁ deficiency is rare—suspect multiple vitamin deficiencies

---

thiethylperazine
(thye-eth-il-per′azeen)
Rx: Torecan
Chemical Class: Piperazine phenothiazine derivative
Therapeutic Class: Antiemetic

CLINICAL PHARMACOLOGY
Mechanism of Action: Acts centrally by blocking chemoreceptor trigger zone and blocking vomiting center

Pharmacokinetics
PO: Onset 45-60 min, duration 4 hr; metabolized by liver; excreted by kidneys; crosses placenta

INDICATIONS AND USES: Nausea and vomiting

DOSAGE
Adult
• PO/IM 10 mg qd-tid

§ AVAILABLE FORMS/COST OF THERAPY
• Inj, Sol—IV: 5 mg/ml, 2 ml: **$4.84**
• Tab, Uncoated—Oral: 10 mg, 100's: **$55.99**

CONTRAINDICATIONS: Coma
PRECAUTIONS: Children <2 yr, elderly, sulfite sensitivity, bone marrow depression, seizure disorder

PREGNANCY AND LACTATION: Pregnancy category C; excretion into breast milk unknown, use caution in nursing mothers

SIDE EFFECTS/ADVERSE REACTIONS

CNS: Depression, drowsiness, *euphoria,* extrapyramidal symptoms, restlessness, **seizures**
CV: **Circulatory failure,** ECG changes, postural hypotension, tachycardia

T

GI: Anorexia, constipation, cramps, diarrhea, dry mouth, metallic taste, weight loss

GU: Dark urine, urinary retention

RESP: **Respiratory depression**

INTERACTIONS

Drugs

❸ *Anticholinergics, antiparkinson drugs, antidepressants:* Increased anticholinergic action

❸ *Barbiturates:* Induction, decreased effect of thiethylperazine

❸ *Beta-blockers:* Augmented pharmacologic action of both drugs

❸ *Bromocriptine:* Neuroleptic drugs inhibit bromocriptine's ability to lower prolactin concentration

❸ *Epinephrine:* Reversed pressor response to epinephrine

❸ *Levodopa:* Inhibited antiparkinsonian effect of levodopa

❸ *Lithium:* Lowered serum concentration of both drugs in combination

❸ *Narcotic analgesics:* Hypotension with meperidine, caution with other narcotic analgesics

❸ *Orphenadrine:* Lower thiethylperazine concentration and excessive anticholinergic effects

SPECIAL CONSIDERATIONS

• Effective antiemetic agent for the treatment of postoperative nausea and vomiting, nausea and vomiting secondary to mildly emetic chemotherapeutic agents, and vomiting secondary to radiation therapy and toxins

• No comparisons with prochlorperazine

• More extrapyramidal reactions than chlorpromazine and promazine; thiethylperazine would be less desirable than these agents in patients where the occurrence of a dystonic reaction would be hazardous (i.e., head and neck surgery patients, patients with severe pulmonary disease, patients with a history of dyskinetic reactions)

PATIENT/FAMILY EDUCATION

• Avoid hazardous activities, activities requiring alertness

MONITORING PARAMETERS

• Respiratory status initially

---

thioridazine

(thye-or-rid′a-zeen)

Rx: Mellaril

Chemical Class: Piperidine phenothiazine derivative

Therapeutic Class: Antipsychotic

CLINICAL PHARMACOLOGY

Mechanism of Action: Dopamine receptor antagonist, with higher affinity for D_2 over D_1-receptors, and variable selectivity among the cortical dopamine tracts; also activity on nondopaminergic sites, i.e., cholinergic, α-adrenergic and histaminic receptors (explaining side effects); high rates of sedation, anticholinergic effects, and orthostatic hypotension; minimal risk of extrapyramidal reaction

Pharmacokinetics

PO: Onset erratic, peak 2-4 hr; metabolized by liver; excreted in urine; crosses placenta; $t_{1/2}$ 26-36 hr

INDICATIONS AND USES: Psychotic disorders; behavioral problems in children (combativeness, explosive hyperexcitable behavior); alcohol withdrawal as adjunct; short-term treatment of anxiety, major depressive disorders, organic brain syndrome

DOSAGE

Adult

NOTE: 100 mg equivalent to chlorpromazine 100 mg

---

* = non-FDA-approved use

• *Psychosis:* PO 25-100 mg tid, max dose 800 mg/day; dose is gradually increased to desired response, then reduced to maintenance

• *Depression, behavioral problems, organic brain syndrome:* PO 25 mg tid, range from 10 mg bid-qid to 50 mg tid-qid

Child 2-12 yr

• PO 0.5-3 mg/kg/day in divided doses

$ AVAILABLE FORMS/COST OF THERAPY

• Conc—Oral: 30 mg/ml, 120 ml: **$14.50-$220.34**; 100 mg/ml, 120 ml: **$25.00-$43.20**

• Susp—Oral: 25 mg/5 ml, 480 ml: **$68.47**; 100 mg/5 ml, 480 ml: **$140.47**

• Tab, Coated—Oral: 10 mg, 100's: **$5.25-$44.88**; 15 mg, 100's: **$7.75-$50.79**; 25 mg, 100's: **$7.50-$63.14**; 50 mg, 100's: **$9.88-$76.65**; 100 mg, 100's: **$14.50-$90.00**; 150 mg, 100's: **$30.00-$96.64**; 200 mg, 100's: **$34.50-$115.47**

CONTRAINDICATIONS: Coma, severe CNS depression, child <2 yr, brain damage, severe hypertension or hypotension

PRECAUTIONS: Seizure disorders, hypertension, hepatic disease, cardiac disease, COPD

PREGNANCY AND LACTATION: Pregnancy category C

SIDE EFFECTS/ADVERSE REACTIONS

CNS: Confusion, extrapyramidal symptoms (rare) including pseudo-parkinsonism, akathisia, dystonia, tardive dyskinesia, *headache, seizures*

CV: **Cardiac arrest,** ECG changes, orthostatic hypotension, tachycardia

EENT: Blurred vision, dry eyes, glaucoma, pigmentary retinopathy

GI: Anorexia, constipation, diarrhea, *dry mouth;* increased ALT, AST, jaundice, *nausea, vomiting,* weight gain

GU: Amenorrhea, enuresis, galactorrhea, gynecomastia, impotence, urinary frequency, urinary retention

HEME: **Agranulocytosis,** anemia, **leukocytosis, leukopenia**

RESP: Dyspnea, **laryngospasm, respiratory depression**

SKIN: Dermatitis, photosensitivity, rash

INTERACTIONS

Drugs

3 *Anticholinergics, antiparkinson drugs, antidepressants:* Increased anticholinergic action

3 *Barbiturates:* Induction, decreased effect of thioridazine

3 *Beta-blockers:* Augmented pharmacologic action of both drugs

3 *Bromocriptine:* Neuroleptic drugs inhibit bromocriptine's ability to lower prolactin concentration; reverse not common

3 *Epinephrine:* Reversed pressor response

3 *Levodopa:* Inhibited antiparkinsonian effect

3 *Lithium:* Lowered serum concentration of both drugs in combination

3 *Narcotic analgesics:* Hypotension with meperidine, caution with other narcotic analgesics

3 *Orphenadrine:* Lower thioridazine concentration and excessive anticholinergic effects

3 *Phenylpropanolamine:* Patient on thioridazine died after single dose of phenylpropanolamine; a causal relationship was not established

Labs

• *False positive:* Pregnancy tests, serum tricyclic antidepressants screen

T

---

italic = common side effects   ***bold italic*** = life-threatening reactions

SPECIAL CONSIDERATIONS

- Phenothiazine with weak potency, low incidence of EPS, but high incidence of sedation, anticholinergic effects, and cardiovascular effects

PATIENT/FAMILY EDUCATION

- Arise slowly from reclining position
- Avoid abrupt withdrawal
- Use a sunscreen during sun exposure
- Caution with activities requiring complete mental alertness (e.g., driving), may cause sedation
- Provide full information on risks of tardive dyskinesia

---

thiothixene

(thye-oh-thix'een)

Rx: Navane
Chemical Class: Thioxanthene derivative
Therapeutic Class: Antipsychotic

CLINICAL PHARMACOLOGY

Mechanism of Action: Dopamine receptor antagonist, with higher affinity for D_2- over D_1-receptors, and variable selectivity among the cortical dopamine tracts; also activity on nondopaminergic sites, i.e., cholinergic, α-adrenergic and histaminic receptors (explaining side effects); minimal sedation and anticholinergic effects; moderate orthostatic hypotension; high risk of extrapyramidal reactions

Pharmacokinetics
PO: Onset slow, peak 2-8 hr, duration up to 12 hr
IM: Onset 15-30 min, peak 1-6 hr, duration up to 12 hr
Metabolized by liver, excreted in urine; crosses placenta; $t_{1/2}$ 34 hr

INDICATIONS AND USES: Psychotic disorders; acute agitation*

DOSAGE

NOTE: 4 mg equivalent to chlorpromazine 100 mg

Adult
- PO 2-5 mg bid-qid depending on severity of condition; dose gradually increased to 15-30 mg/day if needed; max 60 mg/day
- IM 4 mg bid-qid; max dose 30 mg/day; administer PO dose as soon as possible

💲 AVAILABLE FORMS/COST OF THERAPY

- Cap, Gel—Oral: 1 mg, 100's: **$15.77-$45.44**; 2 mg, 100's: **$11.33-$63.10**; 5 mg, 100's: **$15.57-$98.69**; 10 mg, 100's: **$47.15-$132.08**; 20 mg, 100's: **$190.88**
- Conc—Oral: 5 mg/ml, 120 ml: **$31.25-$91.88**
- Inj, Powder—IM: 10 mg/vial: **$35.35**

CONTRAINDICATIONS: Blood dyscrasias, child <12 yr, circulatory collapse, CNS depression, coma

PRECAUTIONS: Lactation, seizure disorders, hypertension, hepatic disease, cardiovascular disease, glaucoma, COPD

PREGNANCY AND LACTATION: Pregnancy category C

SIDE EFFECTS/ADVERSE REACTIONS

CNS: Akathisia, drowsiness, dystonia, *extrapyramidal symptoms* including pseudoparkinsonism, *headache, seizures,* tardive dyskinesia
CV: **Cardiac arrest,** ECG changes, hypertension, orthostatic hypotension, tachycardia
EENT: Blurred vision, glaucoma, mydriasis
GI: Anorexia, constipation, diarrhea, dry mouth; increased ALT, AST, jaundice, weight gain
GU: Amenorrhea, enuresis, galactorrhea, gynecomastia, impotence, urinary frequency, urinary retention

---

* = non-FDA-approved use

HEME: **Agranulocytosis,** anemia, **leukocytosis, leukopenia**
RESP: Dyspnea, **laryngospasm, respiratory depression**
SKIN: Dermatitis, photosensitivity, rash
MISC: **Neuroleptic malignant syndrome**

INTERACTIONS
Drugs
3 *Anticholinergics, antiparkinson drugs, antidepressants:* Increased anticholinergic action
3 *Barbiturates:* Induction, decreased effect of thiothixene
3 *Beta-blockers:* Augmented pharmacologic action of both drugs
3 *Bromocriptine:* Thiothixene inhibits bromocriptine's ability to lower prolactin concentration, reverse not common
3 *Epinephrine:* Reversed pressor response
3 *Guanethidine:* Inhibited antihypertensive response to guanethidine
3 *Levodopa:* Inhibited antiparkinsonian effect
3 *Lithium:* Lowered serum concentration of both drugs in combination
3 *Narcotic analgesics:* Hypotension with meperidine, caution with other narcotic analgesics
3 *Orphenadrine:* Lower thiothixene concentration and excessive anticholinergic effects

SPECIAL CONSIDERATIONS
• High-potency antipsychotic with a relatively high incidence of EPS, but a low incidence of sedation, anticholinergic effects, and cardiovascular effects

PATIENT/FAMILY EDUCATION
• Informed consent regarding risks of tardive dyskinesia; orthostatic hypotension

thyroid
(thye'roid)
Rx: Armour Thyroid, Nature-Throid, Westhroid
Chemical Class: Thyroid hormone in natural state
Therapeutic Class: Thyroid hormone

CLINICAL PHARMACOLOGY
Mechanism of Action: Increases metabolic rate, increases cardiac output, O_2 consumption, body temperature, blood volume, growth, development at cellular level, metabolism of carbohydrates, lipids, and proteins; exerts profound influence on every organ system, especially CNS
Pharmacokinetics
PO: Peak 12-48 hr, partially absorbed (48%-79%, T_3 >T_4); 99% bound to plasma proteins; deiodinated in liver, kidney; enterohepatically circulated; neither T_3 or T_4 cross placenta; $t_{1/2}$ 6-7 days
INDICATIONS AND USES: Replacement or supplemental therapy (hypothyroidism, cretinism, myxedema); pituitary TSH suppression in the treatment or prevention of various types of euthyroid goiters, including thyroid nodules, subacute or chronic lymphocytic thyroiditis (Hashimoto's), multinodal goiter, and in the management of thyroid cancer; diagnostic agent in suppression tests to differentiate suspected mild hyperthyroidism or thyroid gland autonomy
DOSAGE
Adult
• *Hypothyroidism:* PO 30 mg qd, increased by 15-30 mg q30d until desired response; maintenance dose 65-120 mg qd

---

italic = common side effects · **bold italic** = life-threatening reactions

• *Myxedema:* After stabilization with IV levothyroxine or liothyronine and concurrent correction of electrolyte disturbances and administration of corticosteroids, switch to PO thyroid; initial PO 15 mg qd, double dose q2wk, maintenance 65-120 mg/day

• *Thyroid cancer, thyroid suppression therapy:* PO TSH should be suppressed to low or undetectable levels; therefore, larger doses of thyroid hormone than those used for replacement therapy are required.

• *Geriatric:* PO 7.5-15 mg qd, double dose q4-6wk until desired response, maintenance dose

Child

• *Cretinism, juvenile hypothyroidism:* [age, mg/day (mg/kg/day))]: 0-6 mo, 15-30 mg (4.8-6 mg); 6-12 mo, 30-45 mg (3.6-4.8 mg); 1-5 yr, 45-60 mg (3-3.6 mg); 6-12 yr, 60-90 mg (2.4-3 mg); >12 yr, >90 mg (1.21.8 mg)

$ AVAILABLE FORMS/COST OF THERAPY

• Tab, Uncoated—Oral: 15 mg, 100's: **$11.41-$15.75**; 30 mg, 100's: **$4.62-$21.01**; 60 mg, 100's: **$0.79-$24.34**; 65 mg: **$1.85-$8.98**; 90 mg: **$20.90-$23.51**; 120 mg, 100's: **$0.98-$42.01**; 130 mg: **$3.06-$16.56**; 180 mg, 100's: **$5.25-$43.79**; 240 mg, 100's: **$65.49**; 300 mg, 90's: **$81.19**

CONTRAINDICATIONS: Adrenal insufficiency (uncorrected), thyrotoxicosis, MI

PRECAUTIONS: Cardiovascular disease, diabetes mellitus or insipidus, elderly

PREGNANCY AND LACTATION: Pregnancy category A; little or no transplacental passage at physiologic serum concentrations; excreted into breast milk in low concentrations (inadequate to protect a hypothyroid infant; too low to interfere with neonatal thyroid screening programs)

SIDE EFFECTS/ADVERSE REACTIONS

CNS: Headache, *insomnia, tremors*

CV: Angina, **cardiac arrest, dysrhythmias,** hypertension, *palpitations, tachycardia*

GI: Cramps, diarrhea, increased or decreased appetite, nausea

METAB: Bone demineralization (osteoporosis)

MISC: Fever, heat intolerance, menstrual irregularities, sweating, weight loss

INTERACTIONS

Drugs

3 *Carbamazepine, phenytoin, rifampin:* Increases elimination of thyroid hormones; may increase dosage requirements

3 *Bile acid sequestrants:* Reduced serum thyroid hormone concentrations

3 *Oral anticoagulants:* Thyroid hormones increase catabolism of vitamin K–dependent clotting factors; an increase or decrease in clinical thyroid status will increase or decrease the hypoprothrombinemic response to oral anticoagulants

3 *Theophylline:* Reduced serum theophylline concentrations with initiation of thyroid therapy

SPECIAL CONSIDERATIONS

• Although used traditionally, natural hormones less clinically desirable due to varying potencies, inconsistent clinical effects, and more adverse stimulatory effects; synthetic derivatives (i.e., levothyroxine) preferred

MONITORING PARAMETERS

• TSH yearly

---

* = non-FDA-approved use

tiagabine

(ti-ah-ga'bean)
Rx: Gabitril
Chemical Class: Nipecotic acid derivative
Therapeutic Class: Anticonvulsant

CLINICAL PHARMACOLOGY

Mechanism of Action: Gamma-aminobutyric acid (GABA) uptake inhibitor; inhibits uptake into neurons and glia with anticonvulsant, anxiolytic and analgesic effects

Pharmacokinetics

PO: Peak serum levels 0.5-1 hr with no accumulation with chronic dosing

Well absorbed (oral bioavailability, 95%; food reduces Cmax 40%, but not AUC); 95% plasma protein bound; metabolized by liver (CYP3A); undergoes enterohepatic recirculation; $t_{1/2}$ 7-9 hr

INDICATIONS AND USES: Adjunctive therapy in the treatment of refractive partial seizures (simple, complex, secondarily generalized)

DOSAGE

Adult

• PO 4 mg qd for first wk; then increase 4-8 mg/day, weekly up to maximum of 56 mg/day prn desired effect/tolerance

(NOTE: no changes for patients with renal impairment or elderly patients; hepatic impairment may require reduced initial and maintenance doses)

Child >12 yr; <18 yr

• PO 4 mg qd for first wk; 4 mg bid second week; then increase 4-8 mg/day, weekly up to maximum of 32 mg/day prn desired effect/tolerance

$ AVAILABLE FORMS/COST OF THERAPY

• Tab, Coated—Oral: 4 mg, 100's: **$130.00**; 12 mg, 100's: **$172.50**; 16 mg, 100's: **$230.00**; 20 mg, 100's: **$218.75**

PRECAUTIONS: Liver disease (dosage reductions may be necessary); concurrent neurologic disorders (Alzheimer's dementia, organic brain disease, stroke) given potential for exacerbation; withdrawal seizures with abrupt withdrawal

PREGNANCY AND LACTATION: Pregnancy category C

SIDE EFFECTS/ADVERSE REACTIONS

CNS: Confusion, dizziness, emotional lability, headache, *impaired concentration, speech or language,* memory impairment, *nervousness, sedation, somnolence*
EENT: Binds to eye and other melanin containing tissue
GI: Abdominal pain
SKIN: Rash
MISC: Generalized weakness

INTERACTIONS

Drugs

3 *Anticonvulsants (hepatic enzyme inducers—i.e., barbiturates, carbamazepine, phenytoin, primidone):* Decreased tiagabine levels and effect

3 *Rifampin:* Decreased tiagabine levels and effect via hepatic enzyme induction

3 *Valproate:* Increased tiagabine free blood levels

SPECIAL CONSIDERATIONS

• Patients should exercise caution with initiation and dosage titration when driving, operating hazardous machinery, or other activities requiring mental concentration; patients should be advised to take the medi-

T

cation with food, to delay peak effects to avoid many CNS adverse effects

ticarcillin
ticarcillin/clavulanic
acid

(tye-kar-sill'in)
Rx: *Ticarcillin:* Ticar
Ticarcillin/clavulanic acid:
Timentin
Chemical Class: Penicillin derivative; β-lactamase inhibitor
Therapeutic Class: Antibiotic

CLINICAL PHARMACOLOGY
Mechanism of Action: Inhibits bacterial wall synthesis; bactericidal; clavulanate protects ticarcillin from degradation by β-lactamase enzymes

Pharmacokinetics
IM: Peak ½-1 hr, duration 4-6 hr
IV: Peak 30-45 min, duration 4 hr
t₁/₂ 70 min; protein binding 45%; small amount metabolized in liver, excreted in urine (glomerular filtration and tubular secretion); addition of clavulanic acid doesn't affect pharmacokinetics of ticarcillin

INDICATIONS AND USES: Infections of the respiratory tract, skin and soft tissue, bones and joints, urinary tract, and bacterial septicemia; intra-abdominal and gynecological infections caused by susceptible organisms
Antibacterial spectrum usually includes:
• Gram-positive organisms: *Staphylococcus aureus, Streptococcus faecalis, Streptococcus pneumoniae*
• Gram-negative organisms: *Neisseria gonorrhoeae, Escherichia coli, Proteus mirabilis, Salmonella,*

Morganella morganii, Providencia rettgeri, Enterobacter, Pseudomonas aeruginosa, Serratia
• Anaerobes: *Bacteroides* spp. including *Bacteroides fragilis; Fusobacterium* spp.; *Veillonella* spp.; *Clostridium; Eubacterium* spp.; *Peptococcus* spp.; *Peptostreptococcus* spp. **Ticarcillin/clavulanic acid:** Addition of clavulanic acid expands spectrum to include bacteria caused by β-lactamase-producing strains of above organisms and also includes:
• Gram-positive organisms: *Staphylococcus epidermidis*
• Gram-negative organisms: *Klebsiella* spp., *Hemophilus influenzae, Citrobacter* spp., *Serratia marcescens*
• Anaerobes: *Bacteroides melaninogenicus*

DOSAGE
Adult
• Ticarcillin: IV/IM 12-24 g/day in divided doses q3-6h; infuse over ½-2 hr (usual dose 3 g q4h or 4 g q6h); dosage adjustments for decreased clearance: for CrCl (ml/min): >60, 3 g q4h; 30-60, 2 g q4h; 10-30, 2 g q8h; <10, 2 g q12h; <10 with hepatic dysfunction, 2 g q24h; peritoneal dialysis, 3 g q12h; hemodialysis, 2 g q12h supplemented with 3 g after each dialysis
• Ticarcillin/clavulanic acid: IV 3.1 g (contains 3 g ticarcillin, 100 mg clavulanic acid) q4-6h; for patients weighing ≤60 kg 200 mg-300 mg/kg/day (based on ticarcillin content) given in divided doses q4-6h
Child
• IV/IM 50-300 mg/kg/day in divided doses q4-8h
Neonates
• IV INF 75-100 mg/kg/8-12 hr

AVAILABLE FORMS/COST OF THERAPY

• Inj, Dry-Sol—IM, IV: 3 g/vial: **$11.40**

Ticarcillin/Clavulanic Acid

• Inj, Dry-Sol—IV: 0.1 g/3 g: **$15.70**

PRECAUTIONS: Hypersensitivity to cephalosporins, renal and hepatic dysfunction

PREGNANCY AND LACTATION: Pregnancy category B; excreted into breast milk in low concentrations; compatible with breast feeding

SIDE EFFECTS/ADVERSE REACTIONS

CNS: Anxiety, coma, depression, hallucinations, lethargy, *seizures,* twitching

GI: Abdominal pain, *diarrhea,* glossitis, increased AST, ALT; *nausea,* **pseudomembranous colitis,** *vomiting*

GU: Glomerulonephritis, hematuria, *moniliasis,* oliguria, proteinuria, *vaginitis*

HEME: **Bone marrow depression,** increased bleeding

METAB: Hypokalemia

SKIN: Pruritus, rash, urticaria

MISC: Drug fever, local reactions (phlebitis)

INTERACTIONS

Drugs

3 *Aminoglycosides:* Inactivation of aminoglycosides *in vitro* and *in vivo,* reducing the aminoglycoside effect

Labs

• *False increase:* Urine glucose

SPECIAL CONSIDERATIONS

• Synergistic with aminoglycosides
• Sodium content, 5.2 mEq/g ticarcillin
• For reliable activity against *Pseudomonas,* must be dosed q4h

ticlopidine

(tye-klo´pa-deen)
Rx: Ticlid
Chemical Class: Thienpyridine derivative
Therapeutic Class: Antiplatelet agent

CLINICAL PHARMACOLOGY

Mechanism of Action: Selectively and irreversibly inhibits ADP-induced platelet aggregation by inhibiting the binding of ADP to its receptors on platelets, thereby affecting ADP-dependent activation of the glycoprotein IIb/IIIa complex, the major site of platelet-fibrinogen binding

Pharmacokinetics

PO: Peak 2 hr, rapidly absorbed (decreased 20% by meals); 98% bound to plasma proteins; extensively hepatically metabolized, excreted in urine (60%) and feces (23%); nonlinear pharmacokinetics (clearance decreases on repeated dosing); $t_{1/2}$ after a single 250 mg dose, 12.6 hr; with repeat dosing at 250 mg bid, $t_{1/2}$ rises to 4-5 days (steady state levels after approximately 14-21 days)

INDICATIONS AND USES: Reducing the risk of thrombotic stroke in aspirin intolerant patients or aspirin failures; prevention of thrombosis following intracoronary stent placement*; intermittent claudication*; chronic arterial occlusion*; sickle cell disease*

DOSAGE

Adult

• PO 250 mg bid with food

AVAILABLE FORMS/COST OF THERAPY

• Tab, Uncoated—Oral: 250 mg, 100's: **$186.00**

CONTRAINDICATIONS: Current blood dyscrasia (neutropenia, thrombocytopenia); history of TTP; hemostatic disorder or active pathological bleeding (such as bleeding peptic ulcer or intracranial bleeding); patients with severe liver impairment

PRECAUTIONS: Past liver disease, renal disease, elderly, children, increased bleeding risk (trauma, surgery, or pathological conditions, dental procedures)

PREGNANCY AND LACTATION: Pregnancy category B; use caution in nursing mothers

SIDE EFFECTS/ADVERSE REACTIONS

GI: (40% have GI effects): Cholestatic jaundice, *diarrhea, GI discomfort,* hepatitis; increased cholesterol, LDL, VLDL; *nausea, vomiting*

HEME: **Agranulocytosis,** bleeding (epistaxis, hematuria, conjunctival hemorrhage, GI bleeding), **neutropenia, thrombocytopenia**

SKIN: Pruritus, *rash*

INTERACTIONS

Drugs

🔳 *Cyclosporine:* Potential for reduction in blood cyclosporine concentrations

🔳 *Phenytoin:* Inhibition of hepatic metabolism (CYP2C9) of phenytoin; potential for development of phenytoin toxicity, reduction in phenytoin dose may be necessary

🔳 *Theophylline:* Increased theophylline level via inhibition of metabolism, increased risk of toxicity

SPECIAL CONSIDERATIONS

• Due to the risk of life-threatening neutropenia or agranulocytosis and cost, ticlopidine should be reserved for patients intolerant to aspirin or who fail aspirin

MONITORING PARAMETERS

• CBC q2wk for 1st 3 mo of therapy, then periodically thereafter

---

tiludronate
(ti-loo′dro-nate)
Rx: Skelid
Chemical Class: Synthetic analog of pyrophosphate
Therapeutic Class: Bisphosphonate

CLINICAL PHARMACOLOGY

Mechanism of Action: Binds to hydroxyapatite at sites of bone resorption, inhibiting normal and abnormal bone resorption ("crystal poison"); minimal secondary reduction in bone formation (resorption coupled to formation); suppresses the pagetic disease process

Pharmacokinetics

PO: Poorly absorbed, 3% bioavailability (reduced 90% by food), high affinity for bone, 90% protein bound, renal excretion, elimination $t_{1/2}$ 40-150 hr

INDICATIONS AND USES: Paget's disease, postmenopausal osteoporosis,* hyperparathyroidism,* bone pain in prostatic carcinoma and metastatic breast cancer,* hypercalcemia of malignancy*

DOSAGE

Adult

• *Paget's disease:* PO 400 mg qd for 3-6 months

• *Osteoporosis:* PO 100 mg qd for 6 months

💲 AVAILABLE FORMS/COST OF THERAPY

• Tab—Oral: 200 mg, 56's: **$420.89**

CONTRAINDICATIONS: Renal failure (CrCl <30 ml/min), due to lack of clinical experience

PRECAUTIONS: Esophageal, gastric disease, GERD

---

* = non-FDA-approved use

PREGNANCY AND LACTATION:
Pregnancy category C; dose-related
scoliosis; avoid exposure in children

**SIDE EFFECTS/ADVERSE REAC-
TIONS**

CV: Chest pain, peripheral edema

GI: Diarrhea, dysphagia, esophageal
ulcer, esophagitis, flatulence, gastric ulcer, nausea, vomiting

SKIN: Rash

INTERACTIONS

Drugs

❷ *Food:* Reduces bioavailability
90%

❷ *Antacids/calcium:* Reduces bioavailability 60-80%

❸ *Aspirin:* Decreases bioavailability of tiludronate by 50%

❸ *Indomethacin:* Bioavailability of
NSAID increased 2-4 fold

SPECIAL CONSIDERATIONS

• Studies needed to assess place in
therapy with other bisphosphonates

• Inhibition of bone loss in osteoporosis may persist up to 2 yr after 6 mo of treatment and discontinuation of drug

PATIENT/FAMILY EDUCATION

• Take with 6-8 oz plain water; do
not take within 2 hr of food or other
medications

timolol

(tim′oh-lole)

Rx: *Oral:* Blockadren,
Ophthalmic: Betimol,
Timoptic, Timoptic-XE
Combinations

   Rx: Ophthalmic with dorzol
amide (Cosopt)

Chemical Class: Nonselective,
β-adrenergic blocker

Therapeutic Class: Antihypertensive; antianginal; antiglaucoma agent

CLINICAL PHARMACOLOGY

Mechanism of Action: PO: Competitive β-adrenergic antagonist;
produces negative inotropic and
chronotropic responses; slows AV
nodal conduction; decreases heart
rate; decreases myocardial oxygen
consumption; antiarrhythmic effects (class II); reduction in platelet
aggregation and blood viscosity;
suppression of renin release; inhibition of central sympathetic outflow;
decreases presynaptic receptor neurotransmitter release; no intrinsic
sympathomimetic or membrane stabilizing activity; low to moderate
lipid solubility; OPHTH: reduces
intraocular pressure via reduction in
production of aqueous humor

Pharmacokinetics

OPHTH: Onset 0.5-20 min, peak 1-2
hr, duration 24 hr

PO: Peak 2 hr (0.5-3 hr); rapidly and
completely absorbed; excreted
30%-45% unchanged, 60%-65%
metabolized by liver; $t_{1/2}$ 4 hr

INDICATIONS AND USES: Aphakic
glaucoma, glaucoma, migraine
headache, hypertension, post-myocardial infarction, supraventricular
arrhythmias (atrial fibrillation, atrial
flutter, paroxysmal supraventricular
tachycardia), aggressive behavior,*

---

italic = common side effects   ***bold italic*** = life-threatening reactions

angina pectoris,* anxiety,* cataract extraction prophylaxis,* congestive heart failure,* hyperthyroidism,* neuroleptic-induced akathisia,* retinal detachment,* tremor*

DOSAGE

Adult

• OPHTH 1 gtt 0.25% sol in affected eye(s) bid, then 1 gtt qd for maintenance, may increase to 1 gtt 0.5% sol bid if needed

• *Hypertension:* PO 10 mg bid initially, usually maintenance 20-40 mg/day divided bid, not to exceed 60 mg/day

• *Post-MI prophylaxis:* PO 10 mg bid

• *Migraine:* 10 mg bid, up to 30 mg/day divided bid

• *Angina pectoris:* PO 10-60 mg daily (usually bid)

• *Arrythmias:* PO 20-30 mg daily (usually bid) for supraventricular arrythmias

§ AVAILABLE FORMS/COST OF THERAPY

• Gel—Ophth: 0.25%, 2, 5 ml: **$25.97-$29.03**/5 ml; 0.5%, 2.5, 5 ml: **$30.90-$35.72**/5 ml

• Sol—Ophth: 0.25%, 2.5, 5, 10, 15 ml: **$9.25-$38.29**/10 ml; 0.5%, 2.5, 5, 10, 15 ml: **$27.98-$45.58**/10 ml

• Tab, Uncoated—Oral: 5 mg, 100's: **$22.15-$53.45**; 10 mg, 100's: **$31.80-$66.11**; 20 mg, 100's: **$64.79-$108.26**

CONTRAINDICATIONS: Bronchial asthma, cardiogenic shock, overt cardiac failure, second and third degree AV block, severe sinus bradycardia

PRECAUTIONS: Anesthesia/surgery (myocardial depression), abrupt withdrawal, bronchospastic airways, congestive heart failure, diabetes mellitus, hyperthyroidism/thyrotoxicosis, concurrent clonidine (discontinue timolol several days prior to withdrawal of clonidine), peripheral vascular disease, renal disease

PREGNANCY AND LACTATION: Pregnancy category C; similar drug, atenolol, frequently used in the third trimester for treatment of hypertension (many studies of efficacy and safety of atenolol in pregnancy induced hypertension; long term use has been associated with intrauterine growth retardation; mean milk: plasma ratio, 0.80 in one study; quantity of drug ingested by breast feeding infant unlikely to be therapeutically significant

SIDE EFFECTS/ADVERSE REACTIONS

CNS: Anxiety, confusion, depression, *dizziness,* fatigue, hallucinations, headache, insomnia, weakness

CV: Bradycardia, claudication, *CHF, dysrhythmias,* edema, *heart block, hypotension, syncope*

EENT: Conjunctivitis, *double vision,* dry burning eyes, eye irritation, keratitis, sore throat, *visual changes*

GI: Abdominal pain, anorexia, diarrhea, dyspepsia, *ischemic colitis, mesenteric arterial thrombosis, nausea*

GU: Frequency, impotence

HEME: Agranulocytosis, purpura, thrombocytopenia

METAB: Hyperglycemia, mask hypoglycemia

MS: Joint pain

RESP: Bronchospasm, cough, dyspnea, rales

SKIN: Alopecia, fever, pruritus, rash, urticaria

INTERACTIONS

Drugs

§ *α-1 adrenergic blockers:* Potential enhanced first dose response (marked initial drop in blood pressure, particularly on standing (especially prazocin)

---

3 *Amiodarone:* Combined therapy may lead to bradycardia, cardiac arrest, or ventricular dysrhythmia

3 *Antidiabetics:* β-blockers increase blood glucose and impair peripheral circulation; altered response to hypoglycemia by prolonging the recovery of normoglycemia, causing hypertension, and blocking tachycardia

3 *Clonidine:* Hypertension occurring upon withdrawal of clonidine may be exacerbated by timolol

3 *Digoxin:* Additive prolongation of atrioventricular (AV) conduction time

3 *Dihydropyridine calcium channel blockers:* Additive hypotension (kinetic and dynamic)

3 *Diltiazem:* Potentiates β-adrenergic effects; hypotendion, left ventricular failure, and AV conduction disturbances problemmatic in elderly, patients with left ventricular dysfunction, aortic stenosis, or with large doses of either drug

3 *Disopyramide:* Additive negative inotropic cardiac effects

3 *Epinephrine:* Enhanced pressor response (hypertension and bradycardia)

3 *Hypoglycemic agents:* Masked hypoglycemia, hyperglycemia

3 *Isoproterenol:* Reduced isoproterenol efficacy in asthma

3 *Methyldopa:* Potential for development of hypertension in the presence of increased catecholamines

3 *Nonsteroidal anti-inflammatory drugs:* Reduced antihypertensive effects of timolol

3 *Phenylephrine:* Potential for hypertensive episodes when administered together

3 *Prazosin:* First-dose response to prazosin may be enhanced by β-blockade

3 *Quinidine:* Increased timolol concentrations

3 *Tacrine:* Additive bradycardia

3 *Theophylline:* Antagonistic pharmacodynamic effects

3 *Verapamil:* Potentiates β-adrenergic effects; hypotendion, left ventricular failure, and AV conduction disturbances problemmatic in elderly, patients with left ventricular dysfunction, aortic stenosis, or with large doses of either drug

SPECIAL CONSIDERATIONS

• Currently available β-blockers appear to be equally effective; cardioselective or combined α- and β-adrenergic blockade are less likely to cause undesirable effects and may be preferred

PATIENT/FAMILY EDUCATION

• Do not discontinue abruptly; may require taper; rapid withdrawal may produce rebound hypertension or angina

MONITORING PARAMETERS

• Angina: reduction in nitroglycerin usage; frequency, severity, onset, and duration of angina pain; heart rate

• Arrhythmias: heart rate

• Congestive heart failure: functional status, cough, dyspnea on exertion, paroxysmal nocturnal dyspnea, exercise tolerance, and ventricular function

• Hypertension: Blood pressure

• Migraine headache: reduction in the frequency, severity, and duration of attacks

• Post myocardial infaction: left ventricular function, lower resting heart rate

• Toxicity: blood glucose, bronchospasm, hypotension, bradycardia, depression, confusion, hallucination, sexual dysfunction

---

italic = common side effects   ***bold italic*** = life-threatening reactions

tinzaparin
(tin-za-pair'in)
Rx: Innohep
Chemical Class: Depolymerized heparin derivative (low-
molecular-weight heparin)
Therapeutic Class: Anticoagulant

CLINICAL PHARMACOLOGY
Mechanism of Action: Enhances
the inhibition of Factor Xa and
thrombin by binding to and accelerating antithrombin activity; preferentially inhibits Factor Xa; aPTT not
affected
Pharmacokinetics
SC: Onset 2-3 hr, peak 4-5 hr; well
absorbed (SC bioavailability 87%);
partially metabolized by desulph-
ation and depolymerization; elimination is primarily renal; t$_{1/2}$ 3-4 hr
INDICATIONS AND USES: Treatment of acute symptomatic deep
vein thrombosis (DVT) with or
without pulmonary embolism (PE)
in conjunction with warfarin
therapy
DOSAGE
Adult
• SC: 175 anti-Xa IU/kg qd; initiate
warfarin therapy concurrently and
continue tinzaparin for a minimum
of 5 days and until therapeutic oral
anticoagulant effect has been
achieved (INR 2-3)
**§ AVAILABLE FORMS/COST
OF THERAPY**
• Inj, Sol—SC: 20,000 anti-Xa
IU/ml, 2 ml: **$161.28**
CONTRAINDICATIONS: Active
major bleeding; history of heparin-
induced thrombocytopenia (HIT);
hypersensitivity to sulfites, benzyl
alcohol or pork products; IM administration

PRECAUTIONS: Bacterial endocarditis; bleeding disorders; active ulcerative and angiodysplastic
GI disease; hemorrhagic stroke; recent brain, spinal or ophthalmological surgery; renal function impairment; children; neuraxial anesthesia; uncontrolled hypertension; diabetic retinopathy
PREGNANCY AND LACTATION:
Pregnancy category B; low-molecular-weight heparins have been used
to prevent and treat thromboembolic
disease during pregnancy in lieu of
warfarin which is a known teratogen; excretion into breast milk unknown but thought to be minimal
based on pharmacokinetic parameters, use caution in nursing
mothers
**SIDE EFFECTS/ADVERSE REAC-
TIONS**
CNS: Dizziness
CV: Hypotension, hypertension,
tachycardia
GI: Increased ALT, AST
GU: Priapism
HEME: **Hemorrhage, thrombocytopenia,** anemia
SKIN: Local irritation, pain, hematoma and ecchymosis at injection
site; rash
MISC: Insomnia, confusion
INTERACTIONS
Drugs
3 *Antiplatelet agents (aspirin,
ticlopidine, clopidogrel, dipyridamole, NSAIDs), thrombolytics:*
Increased risk of hemorrhage
3 *Oral anticoagulants:* Additive
anticoagulant effects
Labs
• *Increase:* AST, ALT
SPECIAL CONSIDERATIONS
• Cannot be used interchangeably
with unfractionated heparin or other
low-molecular-weight heparin
products

* = non-FDA-approved use

PATIENT/FAMILY EDUCATION
• Administer by deep SC inj into abdominal wall; alternate inj sites
• Do not rub inj site after completion of the inj
• Report any unusual bruising or bleeding to clinician
MONITORING PARAMETERS
• Periodic CBC with platelets
• Monitoring aPTT is not required
• Consider anti-Factor Xa monitoring in patients with impaired renal function, during pregnancy, and in very small or obese patients

---

tioconazole
(tyo-con′a-zole)
OTC: Vagistat-1
Chemical Class: Imidazole derivative
Therapeutic Class: Antifungal

CLINICAL PHARMACOLOGY
Mechanism of Action: Alteration of the fungal cell membrane, which allows leakage of essential intracellular components; fungicidal against *Candida*
Pharmacokinetics
VAG: Negligible systemic absorption
INDICATIONS AND USES: Local treatment of vulvovaginal candidiasis
DOSAGE
Adult
• VAG 1 applicatorful hs × 1
$ **AVAILABLE FORMS/COST OF THERAPY**
• Oint—Vag: 6.5%, 4.6 g single dose: **$14.38-$24.19**
PRECAUTIONS: Discontinue if irritation or sensitization occurs; chronic or recurrent candidiasis may be a symptom of unrecognized diabetes or a compromised immune system

PREGNANCY AND LACTATION: Pregnancy category C; excretion into breast milk unknown
SIDE EFFECTS/ADVERSE REACTIONS
GU: Burning, desquamation, discharge, dryness of vaginal secretions, dysuria, irritation, itching, nocturia, vaginal pain, vulvar edema
SPECIAL CONSIDERATIONS
• Similar in efficacy to miconazole, econazole, and clotrimazole for the topical management of fungal skin infections; choice determined by cost and availability; additional efficacy vs. trichomoniasis with longer course of therapy

---

tiopronin
(tye-o-pro′nen)
Rx: Thiola
Chemical Class: Thiol derivative
Therapeutic Class: Anti-kidney stone agent

CLINICAL PHARMACOLOGY
Mechanism of Action: Undergoes thiol-disulfide exchange with cysteine to form a mixed, water-soluble disulfide of tiopronin-cysteine; the amount of sparingly soluble cysteine is reduced
Pharmacokinetics
PO: 48% appears in urine in 4 hr; 78% by 72 hr; reduction of urinary cysteine of 250-500 mg on 1-2 g/day may be expected; rapid onset and offset of action
INDICATIONS AND USES: Prevention of kidney stone formation in patients with severe homozygous cystinuria with urinary cysteine greater than 500 mg/day, who are resistant to conservative treatment

---

italic = common side effects   ***bold italic*** = life-threatening reactions

DOSAGE

Adult

• PO 800-1000 mg/day, given in divided doses tid at least 1 hr before or 2 hr after meals

Child

• PO 15 mg/kg/day, given in divided doses tid at least 1 hr before or 2 hr after meals

$ AVAILABLE FORMS/COST OF THERAPY

• Tab, Uncoated—Oral: 100 mg, 100's: **$71.25**

CONTRAINDICATIONS: History of agranulocytosis, thrombocytopenia, aplastic anemia on this medication

PRECAUTIONS: Goodpasture's syndrome, children <9 yr

PREGNANCY AND LACTATION: Pregnancy category C; excreted in breast milk and may cause adverse effects in nursing infant, mothers taking tiopronin should avoid nursing

SIDE EFFECTS/ADVERSE REACTIONS

METAB: Vitamin B_6 deficiency

SKIN: Erythema, lupus-like syndrome (fever, arthralgia, lymphadenopathy), maculopapular, pruritus, wrinkling skin

MISC: Blunting of taste, *drug fever*

SPECIAL CONSIDERATIONS

• May be associated with fever and less severe adverse reactions than d-penicillamine

---

tirofiban

(tye-roe-fye'ban)

Rx: Aggrastat

Chemical Class: Glycoprotein (GP) IIb/IIIa inhibitor

Therapeutic Class: Antiplatelet agent

CLINICAL PHARMACOLOGY

Mechanism of Action: Reversibly prevents fibrinogen, von Willebrand's factor, and other adhesion ligands from binding to platelet GP IIb/IIIa receptors, thereby inhibiting platelet aggregation

Pharmacokinetics

65% bound in human plasma; 65% cleared by renal excretion (significantly decreased in patients with creatinine clearance <30 ml/min, including patients requiring hemodialysis); $t_{1/2}$ 2 hr

INDICATIONS AND USES: Acute coronary syndromes in combination with heparin, including patients who are to be managed medically and those undergoing percutaneous transluminal coronary angioplasty (PCTA), or atherectomy

DOSAGE

Adult

• *Acute coronary syndrome:* IV initial 0.4 µg/kg/min × 30 min, maintenance 0.1 µg/kg/min; administer in combination with heparin for 48-108 hr according to schedule below; INF should be continued through angiography and for 12-24 hr after angioplasty or artherectomy

• Injection must first be diluted to same strength as injection premixed (50 µg/ml)

• *Renal impairment (CrCl <30 ml/min):* IV half the usual rate of infusion; initial 0.2 µg/kg/min × 30 min, maintenance 0.05 µg/kg/min

---

$ AVAILABLE FORMS/COST OF THERAPY

• Inj, Sol—IV: 250 µg/ml, 25 ml (vial): **$243.24**; 50 µg/ml, 500 ml (premixed): **$840.00**

CONTRAINDICATIONS: Active internal bleeding or history of bleeding diathesis within previous 30 days; history of stroke within 30 days; history of hemorrhagic stroke; major surgical procedure or severe physical trauma within previous month; systolic blood pressure >180 mm Hg or diastolic blood pressure >110 mm Hg; history of intracranial hemorrhage, intracranial neoplasm, arteriovenous malformation or aneurysm; history, symptoms or findings of aortic dissection, acute pericarditis

PRECAUTIONS: Platelet count <150,000/mm^3; hemorrhagic retinopathy; IM injections, urinary catheters, nasotracheal intubation, nasogastric tubes; elderly; severe renal insufficiency (creatinine clearance <30 ml/min)

PREGNANCY AND LACTATION: Pregnancy category B; excretion into breast milk unknown, use caution in nursing mothers

SIDE EFFECTS/ADVERSE REACTIONS

*HEME: **Bleeding*** (major bleeding 1.4% to 2.2%, minor bleeding 10.5% to 12%)

INTERACTIONS

Drugs

3 *Antithrombotics (aspirin, heparin, warfarin, ticlopidine, clopidogrel):* Increased risk of bleeding

SPECIAL CONSIDERATIONS

• When bleeding cannot be controlled with pressure discontinue INF

• Most major bleeding occurs at arterial access site for cardiac catheterization; prior to pulling femoral artery sheath, discontinue heparin for 3-4 hr and document activated clotting time (ACT) <180 sec or aPTT <45 sec; achieve sheath hemostasis ≥4 hr before discharge

• In clinical studies, patients received ASA unless it was contraindicated

• Tirofiban, eptifibitide, and abciximab can all decrease the incidence of cardiac events associated with acute coronary syndromes; direct comparisons are needed to establish which, if any, is superior; for angioplasty, until more data become available, abciximab appears to be the drug of choice

MONITORING PARAMETERS

• Platelet count, hemoglobin, hematocrit, PT/aPTT (baseline, within 6 hr following bolus dose, then daily thereafter)

---

tizanidine

(tye-zan′i-deen)

Rx: Zanaflex

Chemical Class: Imidazoline derivative

Therapeutic Class: Skeletal muscle relaxant

CLINICAL PHARMACOLOGY

Mechanism of Action: Centrally acting agonist at α_2-adrenergic receptor sites; presumably reduces spasticity by increasing presynaptic inhibition of motor neurons

Pharmacokinetics

PO: Peak 1.5 hr, bioavailability 40% due to extensive first-pass metabolism; 30% bound to plasma proteins; metabolized by liver to inactive metabolites, excreted in urine (60%) and feces (20%); half-life 2.5 hr

---

INDICATIONS AND USES: Acute and intermittent management of increased muscle tone associated with spasticity (e.g., with multiple sclerosis and spinal cord injuries)

DOSAGE

Adult

• PO 4-8 mg q4-6h prn; not to exceed 36 mg/day prn

$ **AVAILABLE FORMS/COST OF THERAPY**

• Tab—Oral: 2 mg, 4 mg, 150's: **$203.66**

PRECAUTIONS: Renal impairment, hypotension, impaired hepatic function, children

PREGNANCY AND LACTATION: Pregnancy category C; lipid soluble, may pass into breast milk

SIDE EFFECTS/ADVERSE REACTIONS

CNS: Asthenia, *dizziness,* dyskinesia, nervousness, *somnolence,* speech disorder

CV: Hypotension, orthostatic hypotension

EENT: Blurred vision, pharyngitis, rhinitis

GI: Abnormal liver function tests, constipation, *dry mouth,* vomiting

GU: Urinary frequency

MS: Increased spasm or muscle tone

INTERACTIONS

Drugs

❷ *Clonidine, guanabenz, guanadrel, guanethidine, guanfacine:* Potential for hypotension, avoid concurrent use

❸ *Oral contraceptives:* Decreased clearance of tizanidine

SPECIAL CONSIDERATIONS

PATIENT/FAMILY EDUCATION

• Arise slowly from a reclining position

---

tobramycin

(toe-bra-mye′sin)

Rx: *Systemic:* Nebcin

Ophthalmic: AKTob, Tobralcon, Tobrex, Tomycine, Tobrasol

Combinations

  Rx: Ophthalmic: with dexamethasone (Tobradex)

Chemical Class: Aminoglycoside

Therapeutic Class: Antibiotic

CLINICAL PHARMACOLOGY

Mechanism of Action: Interferes with protein synthesis in bacterial cell by binding to ribosomal subunit, causing inaccurate peptide sequence to form in protein chain; bactericidal

Pharmacokinetics

IM: Onset rapid, peak 30-90 min

IV: Onset immediate, peak 1 hr

Not metabolized, excreted unchanged in urine (clearance proportional to creatinine clearance); crosses placental barrier; $t_{1/2}$ 2-3 hr

INDICATIONS AND USES: Severe infections of CNS, respiratory, GI, urinary tract, bone, skin, soft tissues, intra-abdominal infections, septicemia caused by susceptible organisms

OPHTH: External infections of the eye and its adnexa caused by susceptible bacteria

Antibacterial spectrum usually includes:

• Gram-positive aerobes: *S. aureus* (Low order of activity against most gram-positive organisms, including *Str. pyogenes, Str. pneumoniae,* and enterococci)

• Gram-negative aerobes: *Citrobacter* spp., *Enterobacter* spp., *Escherichia coli; Klebsiella* spp., *Morganella morganii, Pseudomonas*

---

aeruginosa, Proteus mirabilis, P. vulgaris, Providencia spp., *Serratia* spp.

DOSAGE

Base dosage calculations on lean body weight

Adult

• IM/IV 3 mg/kg/day in divided doses q8h; may give up to 5 mg/kg/day in divided doses q6-8h; adjust dose according to serum peak and trough concentrations; careful monitoring of serum concentrations and dose adjustment required in renal function impairment

Child

• IM/IV 6-7.5 mg/kg/day in 3-4 equal divided doses

Neonates <1 wk

• IM up to 4 mg/kg/day in divided doses q12h; IV up to 4 mg/kg/day in divided doses q12h

• OPHTH: Oint ¼ in ribbon to conjunctiva q8-12h; SOL: 1 gtt q4h

$ AVAILABLE FORMS/COST OF THERAPY

• Inj, Dry-Sol—IV: 80 mg/vial: **$3.82-$22.50**

• Oint—Ophth: 0.3%, 3.5 g: **$25.60-$41.87**

• Sol—Ophth: 0.3%, 5 ml: **$4.44-$38.25**

CONTRAINDICATIONS: Severe renal disease, hypersensitivity to sulfites (contains sodium bisulfite)

PRECAUTIONS: Neonates, mild renal disease, myasthenia gravis, hearing deficits, Parkinson's disease, extensive burns (altered pharmacokinetics)

PREGNANCY AND LACTATION: Pregnancy category D (ophth category B); excreted into breast milk; given poor oral absorption, toxicity minimal; limited to modification of bowel flora and interference with interpretation of culture results if fever workup required

SIDE EFFECTS/ADVERSE REACTIONS

CNS: Confusion, depression, dizziness, muscle twitching, neurotoxicity, numbness, *seizures,* tremors, vertigo

CV: Hypertension, hypotension, palpitation

EENT: Deafness, ototoxicity, tinnitus

OPHTH: blurred vision, burning, stinging of eyes, visual disturbances

GI: Anorexia, hepatomegaly, hepatic necrosis, increased ALT, AST, bilirubin; nausea, splenomegaly, vomiting

GU: Azotemia, hematuria, *nephrotoxicity,* oliguria, renal damage, *renal failure*

HEME: **Agranulocytosis,** anemia, eosinophilia, *leukopenia, thrombocytopenia*

SKIN: Alopecia, burning, dermatitis, *rash,* urticaria

INTERACTIONS

Drugs

3 *Amphotericin B:* Synergistic nephrotoxicity

2 *Atracurium:* Tobramycin potentiates respiratory depression by atracurium

3 *Carbenicillin:* Potential for inactivation of tobramycin in patients with renal failure

3 *Carboplatin:* Additive nephrotoxicity or ototoxicity

3 *Cephalosporins:* Increased potential for nephrotoxicity in patients with preexisting renal disease

3 *Cisplatin:* Additive nephrotoxicity or ototoxicity

3 *Cyclosporine:* Additive nephrotoxicity

2 *Ethacrynic acid:* Additive ototoxicity

3 *Indomethacin:* Reduced renal clearance of tobramycin in premature infants

---

italic = common side effects   ***bold italic*** = life-threatening reactions

3 *Methoxyflurane:* Additve nephrotoxicity

2 *Neuromuscular blocking agents:* Tobramycin potentiates respiratory depression by neuromuscular blocking agents

3 *NSAIDs:* May reduce renal clearance of tobramycin

3 *Penicillins (extended spectrum):* Potential for inactivation of tobramycin in patients with renal failure

3 *Piperacillin:* Potential for inactivation of tobramycin in patients with renal failure

2 *Succinylcholine:* Tobramycin potentiates respiratory depression by succinylcholine

3 *Ticarcillin:* Potential for inactivation of tobramycin in patients with renal failure

3 *Vancomycin:* Additive nephrotoxicity or ototoxicity

2 *Vecuronium:* Tobramycin potentiates respiratory depression by vecuronium

SPECIAL CONSIDERATIONS
• Gentamicin is 1st-line aminoglycoside of choice; differences in toxicity between gentamicin and tobramycin not likely to be clinically important in most patients with normal renal function given short courses of treatment; consider tobramycin in patients who are more likely to develop toxicity (prolonged and/or recurrent aminoglycoside therapy, those with renal failure) and in patients infected with *Pseudomonas aeruginosa* because of increased antibacterial activity
• Has been administered via nebulizer to treat resistant pneumonia in patients with cystic fibrosis
MONITORING PARAMETERS
• Serum Ca, Mg, Na; serum concentrations, peak (30 min following IV INF or 1 hr after IM inj) and trough (just prior to next dose); prolonged concentrations above 12 µg/ml or

trough levels above 2 µg/ml may indicate tissue accumulation; such accumulation, advanced age, and cumulative dosage may contribute to ototoxicity and nephrotoxicity; perform serum concentration assays after 2 or 3 doses, so that the dosage can be adjusted if necessary, and at 3- to 4-day intervals during therapy; in the event of changing renal function, more frequent serum concentrations should be obtained and the dosage or dosage interval adjusted according to more detailed guidelines

---

tocainide

(toe-kay´nide)
Rx: Tonocard
Chemical Class: Lidocaine derivative
Therapeutic Class: Antidysrhythmic (Class IB)

CLINICAL PHARMACOLOGY
Mechanism of Action: Decreases sodium and potassium conductance, resulting in decreased excitability of myocardial cells; no clinically significant changes in sinus nodal function, effective refractory periods or intracardiac conduction times; failure to respond to lidocaine predicts failiure to tocainide
Pharmacokinetics
PO: Peak ½-2 hr; oral bioavailability 100%; metabolized by liver (negligible 1st-pass metabolism), excreted in urine; $t_{1/2}$ 10-17 hr
INDICATIONS AND USES: Life-threatening ventricular dysrhythmias (i.e., sustained ventricular tachycardia)

DOSAGE

Adult

• PO initial 400 mg q8h; usual maintenance dose 1200 to 1800 mg/day divided tid

$ AVAILABLE FORMS/COST OF THERAPY

• Tab, Plain Coated—Oral: 400 mg, 100's: **$83.48**; 600 mg, 100's: **$106.40**

CONTRAINDICATIONS: Hypersensitivity to amides, severe heart block (2nd or 3rd degree)

PRECAUTIONS: Children, renal disease, liver disease, CHF, respiratory depression, myasthenia gravis, blood dyscrasias

PREGNANCY AND LACTATION: Pregnancy category C

SIDE EFFECTS/ADVERSE REACTIONS

CNS: Confusion, dizziness, headache, involuntary movement, irritability, paresthesias, psychosis, restlessness, *seizures,* tremors

CV: Angina, bradycardia, *cardiovascular collapse,* chest pain, *CHF, heart block,* hypotension, *prodysrhythmic effect,* PVCs, tachycardia

EENT: Blurred vision, hearing loss, tinnitus

GI: Anorexia, diarrhea, hepatitis, nausea, vomiting

HEME: Agranulocytosis, blood dyscrasias, hypoplastic anemia, leukopenia, thrombocytopenia

MS: Lupus-like illness, positive ANA

RESP: Dyspnea, *pulmonary fibrosis, respiratory depression*

SKIN: Edema, rash, swelling, urticaria

INTERACTIONS

Drugs

3 *Antacids:* Antacids which increase urinary pH may increase tocainide serum concentrations

3 *Rifampin:* Reduction of serum tocainide concentrations

SPECIAL CONSIDERATIONS

• Can be considered oral lidocaine; antidysrhythmic drugs have not been shown to improve survival in patients with ventricular dysrhythmias; class I antidysrhythmic drugs (e.g., tocainide) have increased the risk of death when used in patients with non-life-threatening dysrhythmias

• Initiate therapy in facilities capable of providing continuous ECG monitoring and managing life-threatening dysrhythmias

MONITORING PARAMETERS

• Blood concentrations (therapeutic concentrations 4-10 µg/ml)

---

tolazamide

(tole-az'a-mide)

Rx: Tolinase

Chemical Class: Sulfonylurea (1st generation)

Therapeutic Class: Oral hypoglycemic

CLINICAL PHARMACOLOGY

Mechanism of Action: Decreases blood sugar via stimulation of insulin secretion and increased tissue responsiveness to insulin; initial hypoglycemic effects due to stimulation of pancreatic islets (dependent upon functioning β-cells); extrapancreatic effect predominantly due to inhibition of hepatic glucose production, but may also facilitate improved insulin-insulin receptor binding

Pharmacokinetics

PO: Onset 4-6 hr, peak 4-8 hr, duration 12-24 hr, completely absorbed by GI route; metabolized in liver, excreted in urine (active metabolites); highly protein bound; $t_{1/2}$ 7 hr

T

---

italic = common side effects   ***bold italic*** = life-threatening reactions

INDICATIONS AND USES: Type II (non-insulin-dependent) diabetes mellitus; adjunct to insulin in selected patients*

DOSAGE

Adult

• PO 100 mg/day for fasting blood sugar <200 mg/dl or 250 mg/day for fasting blood sugar >200 mg/dl; dose should be titrated to patient response; divide doses >500 mg/day bid; max dose 1 g/day

$ AVAILABLE FORMS/COST OF THERAPY

• Tab, Uncoated—Oral: 100 mg, 100's: **$10.40-$43.29**; 250 mg, 100's: **$13.12-$96.08**; 500 mg, 100's: **$28.88-$162.83**

CONTRAINDICATIONS: Juvenile or brittle diabetes

PRECAUTIONS: Elderly, cardiac disease, thyroid disease, severe hypoglycemic reactions, renal disease, hepatic disease

PREGNANCY AND LACTATION: Pregnancy category C; inappropriate for use during pregnancy due to inadequacy for blood glucose control, potential for prolonged neonatal hypoglycemia, and risk for congenital abnormalities; insulin is the drug of choice for control of blood sugars during pregnancy; breast milk excretion data is not available—again, the potential for neonatal hypoglycemia dictates caution in nursing mothers

SIDE EFFECTS/ADVERSE REACTIONS

CNS: Dizziness, fatigue, headache, lethargy, weakness

EENT: Tinnitus, vertigo

GI: Constipation, diarrhea, gas, heartburn, ***hepatotoxicity,*** jaundice, *nausea, vomiting*

*HEME: **Agranulocytosis, aplastic anemia, hemolytic anemia, leukopenia, pancytopenia, thrombocytopenia***

METAB: Hypoglycemia

SKIN: Allergic reactions, eczema, erythema, photosensitivity, pruritus, rash, urticaria

INTERACTIONS

Drugs

3 *Anabolic steroids, chloramphenicol, clofibrate, cyclic antidepressants, MAOIs, sulfonamides:* Enhanced hypoglycemic effects

3 *β-blockers:* Alter response to hypoglycemia, increase blood glucose concentrations

3 *Clonidine:* Diminished symptoms of hypoglycemia

3 *Ethanol:* Altered glycemic control, usually hypoglycemia

3 *Oral anticoagulants:* Dicoumarol, not warfarin, enhances hypoglycemic response

3 *Oral contraceptives:* Impaired glucose tolerance

3 *Rifampin:* Reduced serum levels, reduced hypoglycemic activity

SPECIAL CONSIDERATIONS

• Similar clinical effect as 2nd generations (e.g., glyburide, glipizide); usually less expensive

PATIENT/FAMILY EDUCATION

• Home blood glucose monitoring

• Multiple drug interactions, including alcohol and salicylates

• Symptoms of hypoglycemia: tingling lips/tongue, nausea, confusion, fatigue, sweating, hunger, visual changes (spots)

MONITORING PARAMETERS

• Self-monitored blood glucoses; glycosolated hemoglobin q 3-6 mo

---

* = non-FDA-approved use

tolazoline

(toe-laz′a-leen)

Rx: Priscoline

Chemical Class: Imidoline derivative

Therapeutic Class: Direct peripheral vasodilator

CLINICAL PHARMACOLOGY

Mechanism of Action: Peripheral vasodilation occurs by direct relaxation of vascular smooth muscle; moderate α-adrenergic blocking properties; decreases peripheral resistance and increases venous capacity; other actions: sympathomimetic (cardiac stimulation), parasympathomimetic (GI tract stimulation), histamine-like (gastric secretion and peripheral vasodilation)

Pharmacokinetics

IM/SC: Peak 30-60 min, duration 3-4 hr; excreted in urine; $t_{1/2}$ 3-10 hr

INDICATIONS AND USES: Persistent pulmonary hypertension of newborn; hypoxic pulmonary hypertension,* arterial trauma,* clonidine overdose,* cor pulmonale,* lumbar puncture headache,* peripheral vascular disease,* spasmodic torticollis*

DOSAGE

Newborn

• IV 1-2 mg/kg via scalp vein followed by IV INF 1-2 mg/kg/hr

§ AVAILABLE FORMS/COST OF THERAPY

• Inj, Repository—IV: 25 mg/ml, 4 ml: **$68.80**

PRECAUTIONS: Active peptic ulcer, mitral stenosis

PREGNANCY AND LACTATION: Pregnancy category C

SIDE EFFECTS/ADVERSE REACTIONS

CV: ***Cardiovascular collapse, dysrhythmias,*** edema, hypertension, *orthostatic hypotension,* tachycardia

GI: Diarrhea, ***GI hemorrhage,*** hepatitis, nausea, peptic ulcer, vomiting

GU: Hematuria, oliguria

HEME: ***Leukopenia, thrombocytopenia***

RESP: ***Pulmonary hemorrhage***

SKIN: Chills, *flushing,* increased pilomotor activity, rash, sweating, tingling

INTERACTIONS

Drugs

③ *Epinephrine, norepinephrine, phenylephrine:* Decrease blood pressure response; rebound hypertension

SPECIAL CONSIDERATIONS
MONITORING PARAMETERS

• Vital signs, oxygenation, acid-base status, fluid, and electrolytes

---

tolbutamide

(tole-byoo′ta-mide)

Rx: Orinase

Chemical Class: Sulfonylurea (1st generation)

Therapeutic Class: Oral hypoglycemic

CLINICAL PHARMACOLOGY

Mechanism of Action: Decreases blood sugar via stimulation of insulin secretion and increased tissue responsiveness to insulin; initial hypoglycemic effects due to stimulation of pancreatic islets (dependent upon functioning β-cells); extrapancreatic effect predominantly due to inhibition of hepatic glucose production, but may also facilitate improved insulin-insulin receptor binding

---

italic = common side effects   ***bold italic*** = life-threatening reactions

Pharmacokinetics

PO: Onset 30-60 min, peak 3-5 hr, duration 6-12 hr, completely absorbed by GI route, metabolized in liver, excreted in urine (active metabolites); 90%-95% plasma protein bound; $t_{1/2}$ 4-5 hr

INDICATIONS AND USES: PO diabetes mellitus type 2; IV diagnostic test (Fajan's test) for pancreatic islet cell adenoma

DOSAGE

Adult

• PO 1-2 g/day in divided doses, titrated to patient response, max 3 g/day

• *Diagnostic test:* IV 1 g at constant rate over 2-3 min

$ **AVAILABLE FORMS/COST OF THERAPY**

• Inj, Lyphl-Sol—IV: 1 g/vial, 20 ml: **$88.02**

• Tab, Uncoated—Oral: 500 mg, 100's: **$3.65-$37.56**

CONTRAINDICATIONS: Diabetes mellitus, type 1; ketoacidosis

PRECAUTIONS: Elderly, cardiac disease, thyroid disease, severe hypoglycemic reactions, renal disease, hepatic disease

PREGNANCY AND LACTATION: Pregnancy category C; inappropriate for use during pregnancy due to inadequacy for blood glucose control, potential for prolonged neonatal hypoglycemia, and risk of congenital abnormalities; insulin is the drug of choice for control of blood sugars during pregnancy; milk-to-plasma ratio of 0.25 reported; the potential for neonatal hypoglycemia dictates caution in nursing mothers

SIDE EFFECTS/ADVERSE REACTIONS

CNS: Dizziness, *headache,* paresthesia, *weakness*

EENT: Tinnitus, vertigo

GI: Cholestatic jaundice, diarrhea, *fullness, heartburn,* **hepatotoxicity,** increased AST, ALT, alk phosphatase, *nausea,* taste alteration

HEME: **Agranulocytosis, aplastic anemia, leukopenia, thrombocytopenia**

METAB: **Hypoglycemia**

MS: Joint pains

SKIN: Allergic reactions, eczema, erythema, photosensitivity, pruritus, rash, urticaria

INTERACTIONS

Drugs

3 *Anabolic steroids, aspirin, chloramphenicol, MAOIs, sulfonamides:* Enhanced hypoglycemic effects

3 *β-blockers:* Alter response to hypoglycemia

A *Ethanol:* Altered glycemic control, usually hypoglycemia; "Antabuse"-like reaction

3 *Fluconazole, halofenate, itraconazole, ketoconazole, miconazole:* Increased serum concentrations of tolbutamide and other sulfonylureas

3 *Oral anticoagulants:* Dicoumarol, not warfarin, enhances hypoglycemic response to tolbutamide

2 *Phenylbutazone:* Increased hypoglycemic action

3 *Rifabutin, rifampin:* Reduced serum levels, reduced hypoglycemic activity

Labs

• *False increase:* Serum AST, CSF protein

• *Interference:* Urinary albumin

SPECIAL CONSIDERATIONS

• Possible differences exist for tolbutamide (short duration of action, hepatic clearance), potential preferred choice in older patients with poor general physical status and renal impairment

PATIENT/FAMILY EDUCATION
• Multiple drug interactions, including alcohol and salicylates
• Symptoms of hypoglycemia: tingling lips/tongue, nausea, confusion, fatigue, sweating, hunger, visual changes (spots)

MONITORING PARAMETERS
• Self-monitored blood glucoses; glycosolated hemoglobin q 3-6 mo

---

tolcapone
(toll´ka-pone)
Rx: Tasmar
Chemical Class: Catechol-O-methyl-tranferase (COMT) inhibitor
Therapeutic Class: Anti-Parkinson's agent

CLINICAL PHARMACOLOGY
Mechanism of Action: Alters the plasma pharmacokinetics of levodopa; when given in combination with levodopa/carbidopa, plasma levels of levodopa are more sustained and result in more constant dopaminergic stimulation in the brain, leading to greater effects on the signs and symptoms of Parkinson's disease; may allow decrease in levodopa dose requirements
Pharmacokinetics
PO: Peak 2 hr; bioavailability 65% (decreased by food); >99.9% bound to plasma proteins (mainly albumin); almost completely metabolized prior to excretion; 60% excreted in urine, 40% in feces; $t_{1/2}$ 2-3 hr

INDICATIONS AND USES: As an adjunct to levodopa/carbidopa for the treatment of signs and symptoms of idiopathic Parkinson's disease

DOSAGE
Adult
• PO 100 mg tid, with or without food always as an adjunct to levodopa/carbidopa therapy (immediate or sustained release); in clinical trials the first dose of tolcapone was administered with the first levodopa/carbidopa dose of the day, and subsequent doses were given 6-12 hr later; doses of 200 mg should be used only if anticipated clinical benefit is justified (elevations in ALT may occur more frequently with 200 mg doses)
• Reduction of daily levodopa dose may be necessary, especially if levodopa dose >600 mg/day or in patients with severe dyskinesia before beginning treatment

§ AVAILABLE FORMS/COST OF THERAPY
• Tab, Film Coated—Oral: 100 mg, 90's: **$227.71**; 200 mg, 90's: **$244.41**

CONTRAINDICATIONS: Clinical evidence of liver disease or ALT or AST values greater than twice upper limit of normal; retreatment in patients who develop evidence of hepatocellular injury during tolcapone therapy; history of nontraumatic rhabdomyolysis or hyperpyrexia and confusion possibly related to medication

PRECAUTIONS: Severe dystonia or dyskinesia; renal function impairment

PREGNANCY AND LACTATION: Pregnancy category C; use caution in nursing mothers

SIDE EFFECTS/ADVERSE REACTIONS
CNS: Dyskinesia, sleep disorder, dystonia, excessive dreaming, somnolence, confusion, dizziness, headache, hallucination
CV: Orthostatic complaints, chest pain, hypotension, chest discomfort

EENT: Sinus congestion

GI: **Hepatotoxicity,** *diarrhea, nausea,* anorexia, vomiting, constipation, dry mouth, abdominal pain, dyspepsia, flatulence

GU: Urine discoloration, micturition disorder

MS: Muscle cramps, stiffness, arthritis, neck pain

RESP: Dyspnea

SKIN: Increased sweating

MISC: Fatigue

INTERACTIONS

Drugs

❷ *Nonselective MAO inhibitors (phenelzine, tranycypromine):* Inhibition of the majority of the pathways responsible for normal catecholamine metabolism

❸ *Warfarin:* Possible increased hypoprothrombinemic effect of warfarin

SPECIAL CONSIDERATIONS

• Because of the risk of liver failure, use only in patients who are experiencing symptom fluctuations and are not responding to, or are not candidates for, other adjunctive therapies

• Withdraw drug from patients who fail to show substantial clinical benefit within 3 wk of initiation

• Consider having patients sign informed consent alerting them to potential risks and benefits of this drug

PATIENT/FAMILY EDUCATION

• Monitor for signs of liver disease (clay-colored stools, jaundice, dark urine, right upper quadrant tenderness, pruritus, fatigue, appetite loss, lethargy)

MONITORING PARAMETERS

• ALT/AST at baseline then q2 wk for first yr of therapy, q4 wk for next 6 mo, then q8 wk thereafter; repeat this cycle if dose increased to 200 mg tid; **discontinue tolcapone if ALT or AST exceeds upper limit of** normal or if clinical signs and symptoms suggest onset of hepatic failure

---

tolmetin

(tole′met-in)

Rx: Tolectin

Chemical Class: Acetic acid derivative

Therapeutic Class: NSAID with analgesic and antipyretic activity

---

CLINICAL PHARMACOLOGY

Mechanism of Action: Reversible cyclooxygenase (i.e., prostaglandin synthetase) inhibitor; nonselectively decreases the formation of both prostaglandins and thromboxane A2; variable effects on lipoxygenase synthesis and subsequent leukotriene production; antiinflammatory, antipyretic, and analgesic activity; inhibits platelet aggregation

Pharmacokinetics

PO: Peak 2 hr; metabolized in liver, excreted in urine (metabolites); 99% protein binding; $t_{1/2}$ 3-3½ hr

INDICATIONS AND USES: Osteoarthritis, rheumatoid arthritis, ankylosing spondylitis,* prevention of cognitive decline,* prevention of colon cancer,* dysmenorrhea,* acute gout,* pain*

DOSAGE

Adult

• PO 400 mg tid-qid, not to exceed 2 g/day

Child >2 yr

• PO 15-30 mg/kg/day in 3 or 4 divided doses

$ **AVAILABLE FORMS/COST OF THERAPY**

• Cap, Gel—Oral: 400 mg, 100's: **$68.95-$148.95**

---

* = non-FDA-approved use

• Tab—Oral: 200 mg, 100's: **$49.75-$72.53**; 600 mg, 100's: **$85.92-$180.74**

CONTRAINDICATIONS: Bronchospasm, nasal polyps, angioedema precipitated by aspirin or other NSAIDs

PRECAUTIONS: History of GI ulceration, bleeding, or perforation; renal dysfunction, hypertension or cardiac conditions aggravated by fluid retention and edema, history of liver dysfunction, history of coagulopathy

PREGNANCY AND LACTATION: Pregnancy category B (category D near term); small amounts excreted into breast milk, compatible with breast feeding

SIDE EFFECTS/ADVERSE REACTIONS

CNS: Anxiety, confusion, depression, dizziness, drowsiness, fatigue, insomnia, tremors

CV: **Dysrhythmias,** hypertension, palpitations, peripheral edema, tachycardia

EENT: Blurred vision, hearing loss, tinnitus

GI: Anorexia, **bleeding,** cholestatic hepatitis, constipation, cramps, diarrhea, dry mouth, flatulence, jaundice, nausea, peptic ulcer, perforation, ulceration, vomiting

GU: Azotemia, dysuria, hematuria, **nephrotoxicity,** oliguria, pseudoproteinuria

HEME: **Blood dyscrasias**

SKIN: Pruritus, purpura, rash, sweating

INTERACTIONS

Drugs

3 *Aminoglycosides:* Reduced clearance with elevated aminoglycoside levels and potential for toxicity (especially indomethacin in premature infants; other NSAIDs probably)

3 *Anticoagulants:* Excessive hypoprothrombinemia, decreased platelet aggregation with increased risk of GI bleeding

3 *Antihypertensives (α-blockers, angiotensin-converting enzyme inhibitors, angiotensin II receptor blockers, β-blockers, diuretics):* Inhibition of antihypertensive and other favorable hemodynamic effects

3 *Corticosteroids:* Increased risk of GI ulceration

3 *Cyclosporine:* Increased nephrotoxicity risk

3 *Lithium:* Decreased clearance of lithium (mediated via prostaglandins) resulting in elevated serum lithium levels and risk of toxicity

3 *Methotrexate:* Decreased renal secretion of methotrexate resulting in elevated methotrexate levels and risk of toxicity

3 *Phenylpropanolamine:* Possible acute hypertensive reaction

3 *Potassium-sparing diuretics:* Additive hyperkalemia potential

3 *Triamterene:* Acute renal failure reported with addition of indomethacin; caution with other NSAIDs

Labs

• *False positive:* Proteinuria (use dye-impregnated reagent strips), urinary drugs of abuse screen

SPECIAL CONSIDERATIONS

MONITORING PARAMETERS

• Initial hemogram and fecal occult blood test within 3 mo of starting regular chronic therapy; repeat every 6-12 mo (more frequently in high-risk patients [>65 years, peptic ulcer disease, concurrent steroids or anticoagulants]); electrolytes, creatinine, and BUN within 3 mo of starting regular chronic therapy; repeat every 6-12 mo

---

italic = common side effects **bold italic** = life-threatening reactions

tolnaftate
(tole-naf'tate)
OTC: Aftate, NP-27, Tinactin, Ting
Chemical Class: Carbamothioic acid derivative
Therapeutic Class: Antifungal

CLINICAL PHARMACOLOGY
Mechanism of Action: Fungicidal
INDICATIONS AND USES: Topical fungal infections (tinea pedis, tinea manuum, tinea cruris, tinea corporis, tinea capitis, tinea versicolor) due to susceptible strains of the following dermatophytes: *Trichophyton rubrum, T. mentagrophytes, T. tonsurans, Microsporum canis, M. audouini Epidermophyton floccosum, Melassezia furfur*
DOSAGE
Adult and Child
• TOP apply to affected area bid for 2-6 wk
§ **AVAILABLE FORMS/COST OF THERAPY**
• Cre—Top: 1%, 15, 30 g: **$1.56-$8.44**/15 g
• Oint—Top: 1%, 30, 100 g: **$1.90**/30 g
• Powder—Top: 1%, 45, 90 g: **$1.92-$5.99**/45 g
• Powder, Aer—Top: 1%, 100, 105, 150 g: **$3.95**/105 g
• Sol—Top: 1%, 10, 15, 30, 60, 120 ml: **$1.60-$4.79**/10 ml
• Spray—Top: 1%, 105, 120 ml: **$2.00-$4.10**/105 ml
PREGNANCY AND LACTATION: Pregnancy category C
SIDE EFFECTS/ADVERSE REACTIONS
SKIN: Rash, stinging, urticaria
SPECIAL CONSIDERATIONS
• Non-prescription topical antifungal agent not effective in the treatment of deeper fungal infections of the skin, nor is it reliable in the treatment of fungal infections involving the scalp or nail beds; *Candida* is resistant; useful for patients desiring self-medication of mild tinea infections; patients must be advised of limitations
• Powders generally used as adjunctive therapy, but may be acceptable as primary therapy in very mild cases

tolteridine
(toll-ter'eh-deen)
Rx: Detrol, Detrol LA
Chemical Class: Substituted amine
Therapeutic Class: Genitourinary muscle relaxant

CLINICAL PHARMACOLOGY
Mechanism of Action: Blocks urinary bladder muscle contraction by competitive muscarinic receptor antagonism
Pharmacokinetics
PO: Well absorbed, peak 1-2 hr; bioavailability increased by 53% with food; 96% protein bound; 98% metabolized by liver (CYP2D6 and CYP3A4 to active metabolite 5-hydroxymethyl tolteridine); 77% excreted in urine, 17% in stool; $t_{1/2}$ 2-4 hr
INDICATIONS AND USES: Overactive bladder with symptoms of urinary frequency, urgency, or urge incontinence
DOSAGE
Adult
• PO 2 mg bid; Sus Action PO 4 mg qd
• Reduce dose by half if significantly reduced hepatic or renal function or concomitant CYP3A4 inhibitors

💲 AVAILABLE FORMS/COST OF THERAPY

• Tab—Oral: 1 mg, 60's: **$88.70**; 2 mg, 60's: **$91.04**

• Tab, Sus Action—Oral: 2 mg, 90's: **$245.25**; 4 mg, 90's: **$251.70**

CONTRAINDICATIONS: Urinary retention, gastric retention, uncontrolled narrow-angle glaucoma

PRECAUTIONS: Bladder outflow obstruction, controlled narrow-angle glaucoma, liver disease, renal disease

PREGNANCY AND LACTATION: Pregnancy category C; probably excreted in breast milk. Not recommended during lactation

SIDE EFFECTS/ADVERSE REACTIONS

CNS: Anxiety, *headache (11%)*, paresthesia, somnolence, *vertigo*

CV: Hypertension

EENT: Blurred vision, dry eyes, *dry mouth (40%)*

GI: Abdominal pain, constipation, dyspepsia

RESP: Bronchitis, cough

SKIN: Dry skin

INTERACTIONS

Drugs

3 *Clarithromycin:* Increased blood tolteridine concentration

3 *Cyclosporine:* Increased blood tolteridine concentration

3 *Erythromycin:* Increased blood tolteridine concentration

3 *Itraconazole:* Increased blood tolteridine concentration

3 *Ketoconazole:* Increased blood tolteridine concentration

3 *Vinblastine:* Increased blood tolteridine concentration

SPECIAL CONSIDERATIONS
PATIENT/FAMILY EDUCATION

• Dry mouth occurs in 40% of treated patients at a dose of 2 mg bid; incidence is dose-dependent

topiramate

(toe-peer´a-mate)

Rx: Topamax

Chemical Class: Sulfamate-substituted monosaccharide derivative

Therapeutic Class: Anticonvulsant

CLINICAL PHARMACOLOGY

Mechanism of Action: Blocks voltage-dependent sodium and calcium channels and spread of seizure activity; does not affect reuptake or binding of neurotransmitters; weak carbonic anhydrase inhibitor

Pharmacokinetics

PO: Well absorbed; 75% bioavailable; peak 2-4 hr; excreted unchanged in urine; $t_{1/2}$ 20 hr

INDICATIONS AND USES: Adjunctive therapy for partial onset seizure treatment in adults

DOSAGE

Adult

• PO initiate at 50 mg/day and titrate upward, usual dose 200 mg bid, range 100-400 mg bid; maximum 1600 mg/day

💲 AVAILABLE FORMS/COST OF THERAPY

• Tab—Oral: 15 mg, 60's: **$81.94**; 25 mg, 60's: **$79.28-$105.00**; 100 mg, 60's: **$203.11**; 200 mg, 60's: **$237.79**

PREGNANCY AND LACTATION: Pregnancy category C

SIDE EFFECTS/ADVERSE REACTIONS

CNS: Ataxia, cognitive dysfunction (83% in 1 study), dizziness, nystagmus, paresthesia, sedation, visual disturbances

GI: Constipation, decreased appetite, diarrhea, dyspepsia, nausea, weight loss

---

italic = common side effects   ***bold italic*** = life-threatening reactions

GU: Breast pain, dysmenorrhea, kidney stones
HEME: Leukopenia
INTERACTIONS
Drugs
3 *Phenytoin, carbamazepine, valproic acid:* Lowers topiramate concentrations
3 *Ethinyl estradiol:* Increased clearance of estrogen
SPECIAL CONSIDERATIONS
PATIENT/FAMILY EDUCATION
• Drink plenty of fluids to prevent kidney stone formation

---

torsemide
(tor'se-mide)
Rx: Demadex
Chemical Class: Pyridine-sulfonamide derivative
Therapeutic Class: Loop diuretic

CLINICAL PHARMACOLOGY
Mechanism of Action: Inhibits the $Na^+/K^+/Cl^-$ carrier system in the thick ascending portion of the loop of Henle where it increases urinary excretion of Na, Cl, and water, but does not significantly alter glomerular filtration rate, renal plasma flow, or acid-base balance
Pharmacokinetics
IV: Onset 10 min, peak 1 hr
PO: Onset 1 hr, peak 1-2 hr
Bioavailability 80%; minimal 1st-pass metabolism; volume of distribution 12-15 L (doubled in CHF, renal failure); cleared via hepatic metabolism (80%) and renal excretion (20%); $t_{1/2}$ 3½ hr
INDICATIONS AND USES: Edema (CHF, hepatic cirrhosis and chronic renal failure); hypertension

DOSAGE
Adult
NOTE: Because of high bioavailability, IV and PO doses are interchangeable
• *CHF, chronic renal failure:* PO/IV 10-20 mg qd, titrate upward to response (usually doubling) to max 200 mg/day
• *Cirrhosis:* PO/IV 5-10 mg qd (usually with aldosterone antagonist or potassium-sparing diuretic), titrate upward to response (usually by doubling) to max 40 mg/day
• *Hypertension:* 5-10 mg qd
§ AVAILABLE FORMS/COST OF THERAPY
• Inj, Sol—IV: 10 mg/ml, 2 ml: **$3.99**
• Tab, Uncoated—Oral: 5 mg, 100's: **$50.26**; 10 mg, 100's: **$55.70**; 20 mg, 100's: **$65.06**; 100 mg, 100's: **$241.20**
CONTRAINDICATIONS: Anuria, hepatic coma
PRECAUTIONS: Fluid and electrolyte imbalance (including sodium, chloride, potassium, magnesium, calcium), renal disease, hepatic disease (may precipitate hepatic encephalopathy), gout, COPD, lupus erythematosus, diabetes mellitus, hyperparathyroidism, vomiting, diarrhea, elevated cholesterol/triglycerides
PREGNANCY AND LACTATION: Pregnancy category B; cardiovascular disorders such as pulmonary edema, severe hypertension, or CHF are probably the only valid indications for loop diuretics during pregnancy
SIDE EFFECTS/ADVERSE REACTIONS
CNS: Asthenia, dizziness, *headache (7%)*, insomnia, nervousness
CV: Atrial fibrillation, chest pain, ***ventricular tachycardia***

---

* = non-FDA-approved use

GI: Constipation, diarrhea, dyspepsia, edema

METAB: Hypocalcemia, hypokalemia, hypomagnesemia, increases in BUN, creatinine, uric acid, glucose, total cholesterol

MS: Arthralgia, myalgia

RESP: Cough, rhinitis

SKIN: Rash

INTERACTIONS

Drugs

❷ *Aminoglycosides (gentamicin, kanamycin, neomycin, streptomycin):* Additive ototoxicity (ethacrynic acid > furosemide, torsemide, bumetanide)

❸ *Angiotensin converting enzyme inhibitors:* Initiation of ACEI with intensive diuretic therapy may result in precipitous fall in blood pressure; ACEIs may induce renal insufficiency in the presence of diuretic-induced sodium depletion

❸ *Barbiturates (phenobarbital):* Reduced diuretic response

❸ *Bile acid-binding resins (cholestyramine, colestipol):* Resins markedly reduce the bioavailability and diuretic response of furosemide

❸ *Carbenoxolone:* Severe hypokalemia from coadministration

❸ *Cephalosporins (cephaloridine, cephalothin):* Enhanced nephrotoxicity with coadministration

❷ *Cisplatin:* Additive ototoxicity (ethacrynic acid > furosemide, torsemide, bumetanide)

❸ *Clofibrate:* Enhanced effects of both drugs, especially in hypoalbuminemic patients

❸ *Corticosteroids:* Concomitant loop diuretic and corticosteroid therapy can result in excessive potassium loss

❸ *Digitalis glycosides (digoxin, digitoxin):* Diuretic-induced hypokalemia may increase risk of digitalis toxicity

❸ *Nonsteroidal antiinflammatory drugs (flurbiprofen, ibuprofen, indomethacin, naproxen, piroxicam, aspirin, sulindac):* Reduced diuretic and antihypertensive effects

❸ *Phenytoin:* Reduced diuretic response

❸ *Serotonin-reuptake inhibitors (fluoxetine, paroxetine, sertraline):* Case reports of sudden death; enhanced hyponatremia proposed; causal relationships not established

❸ *Terbutaline:* Additive hypokalemia

❸ *Tubocurarine:* Prolonged neuromuscular blockade

SPECIAL CONSIDERATIONS

• Offers potential advantages over other loop diuretics, including a longer duration of action and fewer adverse electrolyte and metabolic effects; available data not extensive or convincing enough at present to recommend replacement of standard loop diuretic (furosemide); considered alternative in refractory patients

MONITORING PARAMETERS

• Urine volume, creatinine clearance, BUN, electrolytes, reduction in edema, increased diuresis, decrease in body weight, reduction in blood pressure, glucose, uric acid, serum calcium (tetany), tinnitus, vertigo, hearing loss (especially in those at risk for ototoxicity—IV doses >120 mg; concomitant ototoxic drugs; renal disease)

T

---

tramadol

(traah´ma-doll)

Rx: Ultram

Chemical Class: Substituted-cyclohexanol derivative

Therapeutic Class: Centrally acting synthetic analgesic

CLINICAL PHARMACOLOGY

Mechanism of Action: Complementary binding to μ-opiate receptors and inhibition of reuptake of norepinephrine and serotonin

Pharmacokinetics

PO: Onset of analgesia/plasma concentrations 1 hr, peak plasma concentrations 2-3 hr, rapid/complete absorption; volume of distribution 2.6-2.9 L/kg; 20% protein binding; extensively metabolized, mostly inactive metabolites, 60% excreted in urine; $t_{1/2}$ 6-7 hr

INDICATIONS AND USES: Moderate to moderately severe pain management

DOSAGE

Adult

• PO 50-100 mg q4-6h, not to exceed 400 mg/day; not necessary to reduce dose for elderly (<300 mg/day suggested)

• *Renal impairment:* CrCl <30 ml/min, extend dosing interval q12h

• *Hepatic impairment:* (cirrhosis) 50 mg q12h

🟦 AVAILABLE FORMS/COST OF THERAPY

• Tab, Uncoated—Oral: 50 mg, 100's: **$85.00-$135.10**

CONTRAINDICATIONS: Acute intoxication with alcohol, hypnotics, centrally acting analgesics, opioids or psychotropic drugs

PRECAUTIONS: Respiratory depression, increased intracranial pressure or head trauma, acute abdominal conditions, drug abuse and dependence, seizure disorder

PREGNANCY AND LACTATION: Pregnancy category C; small amounts excreted into breast milk

SIDE EFFECTS/ADVERSE REACTIONS

CNS: Anxiety, asthenia, CNS stimulation, confusion, coordination disturbance, dizziness, euphoria, headache, nervousness, *seizures,* sleep disorder, somnolence, vertigo

CV: Vasodilation

EENT: Visual disturbance

GI: Abdominal pain, anorexia, constipation, diarrhea, dry mouth, dyspepsia, flatulence, nausea, vomiting

GU: Menopausal symptoms, urinary retention and frequency

SKIN: Pruritus, rash

INTERACTIONS

Drugs

🟦 *Carbamazepine:* CNS depression; increased tramadol metabolism, may require significantly increased tramadol dosing for equianalgesic effects

🟦 *Ethanol, opioids, anesthetic agents, phenothiazines, tranquilizers, sedative-hypnotics:* CNS depression

🟦 *MAOIs:* Potential exaggerated norepinephrine and serotonin effects, as tramadol inhibits reuptake

🟦 *SSRIs:* Increased risk of seizures

SPECIAL CONSIDERATIONS

• Expensive, nonnarcotic, "narcotic"-tricyclic antidepressant combination analgesic; potential use in chronic pain; demonstrated efficacy in a variety of pain syndromes; minimal cardiovascular and respiratory side effects

• Does not completely bind to opioid receptors; caution in addicted patients

- Has more potential for abuse than previously thought
- Tolerance and withdrawal symptoms milder than with opiates
- Not chemically related to opiates

---

trandolapril

(tran-doe'la-pril)
Rx: Mavik
Combinations
  Rx: with verapamil (Tarka)
Chemical Class: Nonsulfhydryl angiotensin-converting enzyme (ACE) inhibitor
Therapeutic Class: Antihypertensive

CLINICAL PHARMACOLOGY
Mechanism of Action: Antihypertensive, hypoproliferative, and cardioprotective effects attributable to competitive inhibition of angiotensin-converting enzyme (ACE) yielding decreased plasma concentrations of angiotensin II, plasma aldosterone concentrations, systemic vascular resistance, blood pressure, preload, and afterload, not accompanied by changes in heart rate, pressor sensitivity to exogenous norepinephrine, or baroreceptor sensitivity

Pharmacokinetics
PO: Prodrug—peak 1 hr (4-10 hr trandolaprilat), metabolized by liver to active metabolite (trandolaprilat); 80% protein bound to plasma proteins; eliminated in urine (30%) and feces (66%); $t_{1/2}$ of trandolaprilat 10 hr

INDICATIONS AND USES: Hypertension, CHF (left ventricular dysfunction),* MI (left ventricular salvage),* erythrocytosis,* nephropathy,* retinopathy*

DOSAGE
Adult and Child >16 yr
- *Hypertension:* PO initial dose: 0.5 mg qd (for renal or hepatic impairment or patients receiving diuretics), 1 mg qd (non-African American), 2 mg (African American patient); maintenance dose: titrate to 4 mg qd - 4 mg bid at 2 wk intervals
- *Dosage in renal failure:* CrCl 30-60 ml/min, initial dose 0.5 mg qd; maximal dose 2 mg qd; patients with CrCl <30 ml/min not recommended (resultant serum concentrations double)

$ **AVAILABLE FORMS/COST OF THERAPY**
- Tab—Oral: 1 mg, 2 mg, 4 mg, 100's: **$88.01**

PRECAUTIONS: History of anaphylaxis, renal insufficiency (<30 ml/min), hypotension (CHF, elderly, volume depletion—diuretics, dialysis, cirrhosis), aortic stenosis, hyperkalemia (potassium supplements, potassium-sparing diuretics, renal disease, diabetes), neutropenia (autoimmune diseases, collagen vascular, febrile illness, immunosuppressant drug therapy), proteinuria, renal artery stenosis, surgery/anesthesia (excessive hypotension, correctable with fluids)

PREGNANCY AND LACTATION: Pregnancy category C (1st trimester), category D (2nd and 3rd trimesters); ACE inhibitors can cause fetal and neonatal morbidity and death when administered to pregnant women; when pregnancy is detected, discontinue ACE inhibitors as soon as possible

SIDE EFFECTS/ADVERSE REACTIONS
CNS: Anxiety, *dizziness, fatigue, headache,* insomnia, paresthesia
CV: Angina, hypotension, palpitations, postural hypotension, syncope (especially with 1st dose)

---

italic = common side effects   ***bold italic*** = life-threatening reactions

GI: Abdominal pain, constipation, melena, nausea, vomiting

GU: Decreased libido, impotence, increased BUN, creatinine; urinary tract infection

HEME: **Agranulocytosis, neutropenia**

METAB: Hyperkalemia, hyponatremia

MS: Arthralgia, arthritis, myalgia

RESP: Asthma, bronchitis, *cough,* dyspnea, sinusitis

SKIN: Angioedema, flushing, rash, sweating

INTERACTIONS

Drugs

❸ *Azathioprine:* Increased myelosuppression

❸ *Lithium:* Increased risk of serious lithium toxicity

❸ *Loop diuretics:* Initiation of ACE inhibitor therapy in the presence of intensive diuretic therapy results in a precipitous fall in blood pressure in some patients; ACE inhibitors may induce renal insufficiency in the presence of diuretic-induced sodium depletion

❸ *NSAIDs:* Inhibition of the antihypertensive response to ACE inhibitors

❸ *Potassium-sparing diuretics:* Increased risk for hyperkalemia

❸ *Trimethoprim:* Additive risk of hyperkalemia, especially in patient predisposed to renal insufficiency

Labs

• ACE inhibition can account for approximately 0.5mEq/L rise in serum potassium

SPECIAL CONSIDERATIONS

PATIENT/FAMILY EDUCATION

• Caution with salt substitutes containing potassium chloride

• Rise slowly to sitting/standing position to minimize orthostatic hypotension

• Dizziness, fainting, lightheadedness may occur during 1st few days of therapy

• May cause altered taste perception or cough; persistent dry cough usually does not subside unless medication is stopped; notify clinician if these symptoms persist

MONITORING PARAMETERS

• BUN, creatinine, potassium within 2 wk after initiation of therapy (increased levels may indicate acute renal failure)

---

tranylcypromine

(tran-ill-sip′roe-meen)

Rx: Parnate

Chemical Class: Substituted cyclopropylamine; nonhydrazine derivative

Therapeutic Class: Monoamine oxidase inhibitor (MAOI) antidepressant

---

CLINICAL PHARMACOLOGY

Mechanism of Action: MAOI resulting in increased endogenous concentrations of serotonin, norepinephrine, epinephrine, and dopamine in the CNS; chronic administration results in down regulation (desensitization) of α_2- or β-adrenergic and serotonin receptors, which may correlate with antidepressant activity

Pharmacokinetics

PO: Onset 10 days, well absorbed; metabolized by liver, excreted by kidneys (within 24 hr); monoamine oxidase activity is recovered in 3-5 days (possibly up to 10 days) after withdrawal

INDICATIONS AND USES: Atypical depression; bulimia*; panic disorder with agoraphobia*

---

* = non-FDA-approved use

DOSAGE

Adult

• PO 10 mg bid; may increase to 30 mg/day after 2 wk; max 60 mg/day

$ AVAILABLE FORMS/COST OF THERAPY

• Tab, Plain Coated—Oral: 10 mg, 100's: **$65.65**

CONTRAINDICATIONS: Hypertension, CHF, severe hepatic disease, pheochromocytoma, severe renal disease, severe cardiac disease, cerebrovascular defects

PRECAUTIONS: Suicidal patients, convulsive disorders, severe depression, schizophrenia, hyperactivity, diabetes mellitus

PREGNANCY AND LACTATION: Pregnancy category C

SIDE EFFECTS/ADVERSE REACTIONS

CNS: Anxiety, confusion, *dizziness, drowsiness,* fatigue, headache, hyperreflexia, insomnia, mania, stimulation, tremors, weakness, weight gain

CV: **Dysrhythmias,** *hypertension,* **hypertensive crisis,** *orthostatic hypotension*

EENT: Blurred vision

GI: Anorexia, constipation, diarrhea, dry mouth, nausea, vomiting, weight gain

GU: Change in libido, urinary frequency

HEME: Anemia

METAB: Syndrome of inappropriate antidiuretic hormone release-like syndrome

SKIN: Flushing, increased perspiration, rash

INTERACTIONS

Drugs

⚠ *Amphetamines, ephedrine, metaraminol, phenylephrine, phenylpropanolamine, pseudoephedrine, tyramine-containing foods:* Severe hypertensive reactions

❸ *Antidiabetics:* Prolonged hypoglycemia

❸ *Barbiturates:* Prolonged effect of barbiturates

⚠ *Clomipramine, fluoxetine, fluvoxamine, paroxetine, sertraline:* Severe or fatal reactions, serotonin related

⚠ *Ethanol:* Hypertensive response with alcoholic beverages containing tyramine

❸ *Guanethidine:* Inhibited antihypertensive response to guanethidine

❸ *Levodopa:* Hypertensive response; carbidopa minimizes the reaction

❷ *Lithium:* Hyperpyrexia with phenelzine

⚠ *Meperidine:* Serotonin accumulation—agitation, blood pressure elevations, hyperpyrexia, **seizures**

❸ *Norepinephrine:* Increased pressor response to norepinephrine

❸ *Reserpine:* Severe hypertensive reactions

⚠ *Sumatriptan:* Increased sumatriptan concentrations, possible toxicity

SPECIAL CONSIDERATIONS

• Irreversible nonselective MAOI effective for typical and atypical depression; equal efficacy to other MAOIs with quicker onset of action, and an amphetamine-like activity with a higher potential for abuse; no anticholinergic or cardiac effects

PATIENT/FAMILY EDUCATION

• Therapeutic effects may take 1-4 wk

• Avoid alcohol ingestion, CNS depressants, OTC medications (cold, weight loss, hay fever, cough syrup)

• Prodromal signs of hypertensive crisis are increased headache, palpitations; discontinue drug immediately

• Do not discontinue medication abruptly after long-term use

T

---

italic = common side effects   ***bold italic*** = life-threatening reactions

• Avoid high-tyramine foods (aged cheese, sour cream, beer, wine, pickled products, liver, raisins, bananas, figs, avocados, meat tenderizers, chocolate, yogurt)

---

trazodone
(tray´zoe-done)
Rx: Desyrel
Chemical Class: Triazolopyridine derivative
Therapeutic Class: Antidepressant

CLINICAL PHARMACOLOGY
Mechanism of Action: Selective inhibition (high) of presynaptic serotonin uptake, prolonging neuronal activity; slight anticholinergic, moderate orthostatic, and very high sedation side effects; cardiac conduction effects less pronounced than those seen with tricyclic antidepressants

Pharmacokinetics
PO: Peak 1-2 hr, onset of therapeutic effect 2-4 wk; 85%-95% bound to plasma proteins; extensively metabolized in liver, excreted mainly in urine with some fecal elimination; $t_{1/2}$ 4-7½ hr

INDICATIONS AND USES: Depression, aggressive behavior,* panic disorder,* agoraphobia with panic attacks,* insomnia*

DOSAGE
Adult
• PO 150 mg/day divided tid initially, increase by 50 mg/day q3-4d; adjust dose to lowest effective level; max 400 mg/day (outpatients), 600 mg/day (inpatients)
Child 6-18 yr
• PO 1.5-2 mg/kg/day in divided doses initially, increase gradually q3-4d as needed; max 6 mg/kg/day divided tid

* = non-FDA-approved use

---

⑤ AVAILABLE FORMS/COST OF THERAPY
• Tab, Plain Coated—Oral: 50 mg, 100's: **$7.25-$225.41**; 100 mg, 100's: **$15.44-$393.90**; 150 mg, 100's: **$70.35-$339.34**; 300 mg, 100's: **$426.52-$603.98**

PRECAUTIONS: Pre-existing cardiac disease, initial recovery phase of MI, children <18 yr, suicidal ideation, electroconvulsive therapy
PREGNANCY AND LACTATION: Pregnancy category C; excreted into human breast milk; effects on nursing infant unknown, but of possible concern

SIDE EFFECTS/ADVERSE REACTIONS
CNS: Agitation, akathisia, anger, confusion, decreased concentration, delusions, disorientation, *dizziness, drowsiness,* excitement, extrapyramidal symptoms, fatigue, hallucinations, headache, hostility, hypomania, impaired memory, impaired speech, incoordination, insomnia, lightheadedness, mania, nervousness, nightmares or vivid dreams, numbness, paresthesia, psychosis, *seizures,* stupor, tardive dyskinesia, tremors, weakness
CV: Atrial fibrillation, bradycardia, *cardiac arrest,* chest pain, conduction block, *dysrhythmias,* edema, hypertension, hypotension, *MI,* orthostatic hypotension, palpitations, syncope, tachycardia, vasodilation, ventricular ectopic activity
EENT: Blurred vision, diplopia, nasal and sinus congestion, red eyes, tinnitus, vertigo
GI: Abdominal or gastric disorder, bad taste in mouth, constipation, *diarrhea,* dry mouth, flatulence, hyperbilirubinemia, hypersalivation, inappropriate antidiuretic hormone syndrome, intrahepatic cholestasis, jaundice, liver enzyme alterations, nausea, vomiting

GU: Breast enlargement and engorgement, decreased or increased libido, delayed urine flow, early menses, hematuria, increased urinary frequency, impotence, lactation, missed periods, priapism, retrograde ejaculation, urinary incontinence or retention

MS: Aches and pains, ataxia, muscle twitches

RESP: Apnea, shortness of breath

SKIN: Alopecia, clamminess, pruritis, rash, sweating, urticaria

MISC: Decreased appetite, malaise, weight gain or loss

INTERACTIONS

Drugs

3 *Clonidine:* Inhibited antihypertensive response to clonidine

3 *Ethanol:* Additive impairment of motor skills; abstinent alcoholics may eliminate cyclic antidepressants more rapidly than non-alcoholics

3 *Fluoxetine:* Increased plasma trazodone concentrations

A *MAOIs:* Potential for fatal serotonin syndrome

3 *Neuroleptics:* Additive hypotension

SPECIAL CONSIDERATIONS

• Very sedating antidepressant with minimal anticholinergic effects; good choice for elderly patients in whom sedating properties would be desirable

PATIENT/FAMILY EDUCATION

• Take with food

• Use caution driving or performing other tasks requiring alertness

tretinoin

(tret'i-noyn)

Rx: Topical: Avita, Retin-A, Renova

Oral: Vesanoid

(Tretinoin/Retinoic Acid)

Chemical Class: Vitamin A derivative

Therapeutic Class: Antiacne agent

CLINICAL PHARMACOLOGY

Mechanism of Action: Decreases cohesiveness of follicular epithelial cells with decreased microcomedone formation; stimulates mitotic activity and increases turnover of follicular epithelial cells causing extrusion of comedones

INDICATIONS AND USES: Topical treatment of acne vulgaris; lamellar ichthyosis,* mollusca contagiosa,* verrucae plantaris,* verrucae planae juveniles,* ichthyosis vulgaris,* bullous congenital icthyosiform and pityriasis rubra pilaris,* improvement of photoaged skin (especially wrinkling and liver spots)*; PO induction of remission in patients with acute promyelocytic leukemia (APL)

DOSAGE

Adult and Child >12 yr

• TOP apply qd before retiring; begin therapy with 0.025% cream or 0.01% gel and increase concentration as tolerated; if stinging or irritation develops, decrease frequency of application

• PO 45 mg/m^2/day divided bid until complete remission documented; discontinue 30 days after achievement of complete remission or after 90 days of treatment, whichever comes first; follow with standard consolidation and/or maintenance chemotherapy

T

💲 AVAILABLE FORMS/COST OF THERAPY

• Cap—Oral: 10 mg, 100's: **$1,576.20**

• Cre—Top: 0.025%, 20, 45 g: **$28.48-$57.94**/20 g; 0.05%, 20, 45, 60 g: **$30.20-$43.91**/20 g; 0.10%, 20, 45 g: **$38.17-$51.13**/20 g

• Gel—Top: 0.01%, 15, 45 g: **$25.73**/15 g; 0.02%, 40 g: **$65.74**; 0.025%, 15. 20, 45 g: **$25.35-$32.60**/15 g; 0.1%, 20, 45 g: **$36.76**/20 g

• Liq—Top: 0.05%, 28 ml: **$41.58-$63.61**

PRECAUTIONS: Eczematous skin, sunburned skin (do not use until skin is fully recovered)

PREGNANCY AND LACTATION: Pregnancy category B; teratogenic risk when used topically is thought to be close to zero; minimal absorption occurring after topical application probably precludes detection of clinically significant amounts in breast milk

SIDE EFFECTS/ADVERSE REACTIONS

CNS: Dizziness, fever, headache

CV: **CHF, dysrhythmia,** *hypertension*

EENT: Visual disturbance

GI: Constipation, diarrhea, dyspepsia, mucositis, nausea, vomiting

MS: Bone pain

SKIN: Alopecia, blistering, crusting, edema, *erythema, excessive dryness, increased sweating, initial acne flare-up, irritation,* photosensitivity, *pruritis, rash,* temporary hyperpigmentation or hypopigmentation

INTERACTIONS

Drugs

🖪 *Sulfur, resorcinol, benzoyl peroxide, salicylic acid:* Concomitant topical acne products may cause significant skin irritation

SPECIAL CONSIDERATIONS

• Oral therapy should be prescribed only by those knowledgeable in the treatment of APL

PATIENT/FAMILY EDUCATION

• Keep away from eyes, mouth, angles of nose, and mucous membranes

• Avoid exposure to ultraviolet light

• Acne may worsen transiently

• Normal use of cosmetics is permissible

---

triamcinolone

(trye-am-sin'oh-lone)

Rx: *Oral:* Aristocort, Aristopak

Injectable: Acetocot, Amcort, Aristocort, Aristocort Forte, Aristospan, Cinonide-40, Clinalog, TAC-3, Kenalog, Kenaject-40, Triam-A, Triam Forte, Triamcot, Tristoject

Inhalation: Azmacort

Nasal: Nasacort, Nasacort AQ

Topical: Aristocort, Cinalog, Cinolar, Kenalog, Kenalog in Orabase, Triacet, Triamcot

Chemical Class: Synthetic glucocorticoid

Therapeutic Class: Inhaled corticosteroid; systemic corticosteroid; topical corticosteroid, low potency (0.025%), intermediate potency (0.1%), high potency (0.5%)

CLINICAL PHARMACOLOGY

Mechanism of Action: Controls the rate of protein synthesis, depresses the migration of polymorphonuclear leukocytes and fibroblasts, reverses capillary permeability, and causes lysosomal stabilization at the cellular level to prevent or control inflammation

---

* = non-FDA-approved use

Pharmacokinetics

TOP: Absorbed through the skin (increased by inflammation and occlusive dressings)

IM: Peak within 8-10 hr

Metabolized in liver, excreted in urine and bile; biologic $t_{1/2}$ 18-36 hr

INDICATIONS AND USES: *Nasal:* Seasonal or perennial rhinitis, nasal polyps

Inhaled: Prophylaxis of asthma

Systemic: Anti-inflammatory or immunosuppressant agent in the treatment of diseases of hematologic, allergic, inflammatory, neoplastic, and autoimmune origin

Topical: Psoriasis, eczema, contact dermatitis, pruritus, oral inflammatory and ulcerative traumatic lesions (dental paste)

Intraarticular: Synovitis, osteoarthritis

Intradermal: Keloids, alopecia areata, inflammatory skin lesions

DOSAGE

Adult

• PO 4-60 mg/day

• IM (diacetate) 40 mg per wk; (acetonide) 2.5-60 mg/day

• Intra-articular/intrasynovial/intralesional/sublesional (acetonide) 2.5-5 mg (small joints), 5-15 mg (large joints), 1 mg/inj site using only 3 mg/ml or 10 mg/ml strength (intradermal); (diacetate) 5-40 mg, do not use more than 12.5 mg/inj site, usual dose is 25 mg/lesion (intralesional or sublesional); (hexacetonide) 2-20 mg (intra-articular); 10-20 mg (large joints); 2-6 mg (small joints); up to 0.5 mg/in² of affected area (intralesional or sublesional)

• TOP apply to affected area bid-tid

• INH 2 inhalations tid-qid up to 16 INH/day

• NASAL 2 sprays in each nostril qd-bid

Child

• IM (acetonide or hexacetonide) 0.03-0.2 mg/kg at 1-7 day intervals

• INH 1-2 inhalation tid-qid up to 12 INH/day

• NASAL (6-11 yr) 2 sprays in each nostril qd (Nasacort AQ)

• Intra-articular/intrasynovial/intralesional/sublesional (acetonide) 2.5-15 mg, repeated prn

• TOP apply bid-tid

💲 AVAILABLE FORMS/COST OF THERAPY

Triamcinolone

• Syr—Oral: 4 mg/5 ml, 120 ml: **$33.25**

• Tab, Uncoated—Oral: 1 mg, 50's: **$17.00**; 2 mg, 100's: **$75.00**; 4 mg, 100's: **$5.50-$147.84**; 8 mg, 50's: **$107.57**

Triamcinolone Acetate

• Aer—INH: 100 μg/inh, 100 sprays: **$55.40-$68.58**

• Aer—Nasal: 55 μg/inh, 10 g: **$43.64-$53.05**; 55 μg/inh, 16.5 g (AQ): **$38.71**

• Aer, Spray—Top: 0.147 mg/g, 63 g: **$32.98**

• Cre—Top: 0.025%, 15, 30, 60, 80, 454 g: **$2.55-$12.75**/80 g; 0.1%, 15, 30, 60, 80, 240, 454, 480 g: **$3.80-$46.52**/80 g; 0.5%, 15, 20, 100, 240 g: **$2.96-$36.62**/15 g

• Inj, Susp—Intra-articular, IM: 40 mg/ml, 5 ml: **$4.95-$38.52**

• Inj, Susp—Intra-articular, Intradermal: 10 mg/ml, 5 ml: **$8.02**

• Inj, Susp—Intradermal: 3 mg/ml, 5 ml: **$10.43**

• Lotion—Top: 0.025%, 60 ml: **$7.50-$44.22**; 0.1%, 60 ml: **$8.28-$49.65**

• Oint—Top: 0.025%, 15, 30, 80, 454 g: **$2.80-$6.25**/80 g; 0.1%, 15, 30, 60, 80, 240, 454 g: **$2.80-$13.35**/60 g; 0.5%, 15 g: **$3.35-$24.00**/15 g

• Paste—Dental: 0.1%, 5 g: **$4.44-$17.70**

T

Triamcinolone Diacetate
• Inj, Susp—Intra-articular, IM: 40 mg/ml, 5 ml: **$8.98-$27.13**
• Inj, Sol—IV: 25 mg/ml, 5 ml: **$23.30**

Triamcinolone Hexacetonide
• Inj, Sol—IV: 5 mg/ml, 5 ml: **$13.71**; 20 mg/ml, 5 ml: **$2.11-$18.40**

CONTRAINDICATIONS: Systemic fungal infections, bacterial infection of nose (nasal); primary treatment of status asthmaticus (inhalation)

PRECAUTIONS: Psychosis, diabetes mellitus, glaucoma, osteoporosis, seizure disorders, ulcerative colitis (intestinal perforation), CHF, hypertension, myesthenia gravis (if used with anticholinesterase agents), renal disease, esophagitis, peptic ulcer, latent tuberculosis or amebiasis (reactivation of disease). Topical: use on face, groin, or axilla, ocular herpes simplex

PREGNANCY AND LACTATION: Pregnancy category C; excreted in breast milk and could interfere with infant's growth and endogenous corticosteroid production

SIDE EFFECTS/ADVERSE REACTIONS

CNS: Depression, headache, *mood changes, seizures,* vertigo (systemic)

CV: CHF, hypertension, tachycardia

EENT: Blurred vision, *Candida* infection of oral cavity, cataract; dysphonia, hoarseness, increased intraocular pressure, *sore throat* (inhalation); dryness, epistaxis, nasal irritation and stinging, rebound congestion, sneezing (nasal)

GI: Abdominal distension, diarrhea, **GI hemorrhage,** increased appetite, *nausea, pancreatitis*

METAB: Cushingoid state, decreased glucose tolerance, growth suppression in children, HPA suppression

MS: Aseptic necrosis of femoral and humeral heads, fractures, muscle mass loss, osteoporosis, weakness

SKIN: Acne, allergic contact dermatitis, atrophy, bruising, burning, dryness, ecchymosis, folliculitis, hypertrichosis, hypopigmentation, irritation, itching, miliaria, perioral dermatitis, petechiae, poor wound healing, secondary infection (topical), striae; suppression of skin test reactions; thin, fragile skin

MISC: Systemic absorption of topical corticosteroids has produced reversible HPA axis suppression (more likely with occlusive dressings, prolonged administration, application to large surface areas, liver failure, and in children)

INTERACTIONS

Drugs

3 *Aminoglutethamide:* Increased clearance of steroid; doubling of dose may be necessary

3 *Antidiabetics:* Increased blood glucose

3 *Barbiturates, carbamazepine:* Reduced serum concentrations of corticosteroids

3 *Cholestyramine, colestipol:* Possible reduced absorption of corticosteroids

3 *Cyclosporine:* Possible increased concentration of both drugs, seizures

3 *Erythromycin, troleandomycin, clarithromycin, ketoconazole:* Possible enhanced steroid effect

3 *Estrogens, oral contraceptives:* Enhanced effects of corticosteroids

3 *Isoniazid:* Reduced plasma concentrations of isoniazid

3 *IUDs:* Inhibition of inflammation may decrease contraceptive effect

3 *NSAIDs:* Increased risk of GI ulceration

3 *Rifampin:* Reduced therapeutic effect of corticosteroids

---

* = non-FDA-approved use

3 *Salicylates:* Increased elimination of salicylates

Labs

• *False increase:* Urinary amino acids

SPECIAL CONSIDERATIONS
PATIENT/FAMILY EDUCATION

• May cause GI upset, take with meals or snacks (systemic)

• Do not give live virus vaccines to patients on prolonged systemic therapy

• Take PO as single daily dose in AM

• Signs of adrenal insufficiency include fatigue, anorexia, nausea, vomiting, diarrhea, weight loss, weakness, dizziness, and low blood sugar

• Avoid abrupt withdrawal of therapy following high-dose or long-term therapy

• Increased dose of rapidly acting corticosteroids may be necessary in patients subjected to unusual stress

• To be used on a regular basis, not for acute symptoms (nasal and inhalation)

• Use bronchodilators before oral inhaler (for patients using both)

• Rinse mouth to prevent oral candidiasis

• Nasal sol may cause drying and irritation of nasal mucosa, clear nasal passages prior to use

MONITORING PARAMETERS

• Serum K and glucose

• Growth of children on prolonged therapy

---

triamterene

(try-am'ter-een)
Rx: Dyrenium
Combinations
  Rx: with hydrochlorothiazide (Dyazide, Maxzide)
Chemical Class: Pteridine derivative
Therapeutic Class: Potassium-sparing diuretic, antihypertensive

---

CLINICAL PHARMACOLOGY

Mechanism of Action: Inhibits reabsorption of sodium ions in exchange for potassium and hydrogen ions directly in the distal renal tubule (not aldosterone inhibitor); weak diuretic and antihypertensive effects when used alone

Pharmacokinetics

PO: Onset 2-4 hr, peak 3 hr, duration 7-9 hr; primarily metabolized to sulfate conjugate of hydroxytriamterene (active), 21% excreted in urine unchanged; $t_{1/2}$ 1½-2 hr

INDICATIONS AND USES: Edema (CHF, cirrhosis of the liver, nephrotic syndrome, steroid-induced, idiopathic, and secondary hyperaldosteronism); may be used alone or with other diuretics either for its added diuretic effect or its potassium-conserving potential

DOSAGE

Adult

• PO 100 mg bid pc; do not exceed 300 mg/day; when combined with other diuretics or antihypertensives, decrease total daily dosage initially and adjust to patient's needs

Child

• PO 2-4 mg/kg/day in 1-2 divided doses; max 6 mg/kg/day or 300 mg/day

---

• Cap, Gel—Oral: 50 mg, 100's: **$90.75**; 100 mg, 100's: **$98.46**

CONTRAINDICATIONS: Anuria, severe renal disease, hyperkalemia, antikaliuretic therapy (including angiotensin-converting enzyme inhibitors, angiotensin II receptor blockers, and potassium supplements)

PRECAUTIONS: Diabetes, renal function impairment, hepatic function impairment, children, electrolyte imbalance, renal stones, predisposition to gouty arthritis

PREGNANCY AND LACTATION: Pregnancy category B; therapy for preexisting hypertension can be continued throughout pregnancy with minimal risk; initiating for simple edema not recommended; few unequivocal indications for diuretic therapy in pregnancy except for pulmonary edema or congestive heart failure; may decrease placental perfusion; excreted in cow's milk, no human data

SIDE EFFECTS/ADVERSE REACTIONS

CNS: Dizziness, headache
GI: Diarrhea, dry mouth, jaundice, liver enzyme abnormalities, *nausea,* vomiting
GU: Elevated BUN and creatinine, has been found in renal stones, *interstitial nephritis*
HEME: Megaloblastic anemia, *thrombocytopenia*
METAB: Electrolyte imbalance, hyperkalemia, hypokalemia
SKIN: Photosensitivity, rash
MISC: Fatigue, weakness

INTERACTIONS
Drugs
🔁 *ACE inhibitors:* Hyperkalemia in predisposed patients
🔁 *Amantadine:* Increased toxicity of amantadine

🔁 *Angiotensin II receptor antagonists:* Concurrent mechanisms to decrease potassium excretion; increased risk of hyperkalemia
🔁 *Cimetidine:* Increased triamterene bioavailability and decreased renal clearance
🔁 *NSAIDs:* Acute renal failure with indomethacin and possibly other NSAIDs
❷ *Potassium preparation:* Concurrent use increases the risk of hyperkalemia
Labs
• *False increase:* Serum digoxin concentrations
• *Interference:* Urinary catecholamines

SPECIAL CONSIDERATIONS
PATIENT/FAMILY EDUCATION
• Take with meals
• Avoid prolonged exposure to sunlight
• Take single daily doses in AM
MONITORING PARAMETERS
• Blood pressure, edema, urine output, urine electrolytes, BUN, creatinine, ECG (if hyperkalemic), gynecomastia, impotence

---

triazolam
(trye-ay´zoe-lam)
Rx: Halcion
Chemical Class: Benzodiazepine
Therapeutic Class: Hypnotic
DEA Class: Schedule IV

CLINICAL PHARMACOLOGY
Mechanism of Action: CNS depressants via facilitation of inhibitory GABA at benzodiazepine receptor sites (BZ_1—associated with sleep; BZ_2—associated with memory, motor, sensory, and cognitive function); effects include muscle relaxation (spinal cord), anticonvulsant

activity (brain stem), ataxia (cerebellum), emotional behavior (limbic and cortical areas), and anxiolytic effects (separate from general CNS depression); decreases sleep latency, the number of awakenings, and the time spent in stage 0 (awake) sleep; stage 2 (unequivocal sleep) is increased; in sum, sleep time increased

Pharmacokinetics

PO: Onset 15-30 min, peak 42 min, duration 6-7 hr; 89% bound to plasma proteins; extensively metabolized in liver, excreted in urine as unchanged drug and metabolites; $t_{1/2}$ 1.7-5 hr

INDICATIONS AND USES: Short-term treatment of insomnia (generally 7-10 days); use for more than 2-3 wk requires complete reevaluation of the patient

DOSAGE

Adult

• PO 0.125-0.5 mg hs

Elderly or debilitated patients

• PO 0.125-0.25 mg hs; initiate with 0.125 mg until individual response is determined

$ **AVAILABLE FORMS/COST OF THERAPY**

• Tab, Plain Coated—Oral: 0.125 mg, 100's: **$58.14-$64.87**; 0.25 mg, 100's: **$64.73-$95.10**

CONTRAINDICATIONS: Narrow-angle glaucoma, psychosis, children <18 yr

PRECAUTIONS: Elderly, debilitated, hepatic disease, renal disease, history of drug abuse, abrupt withdrawal, respiratory depression, prolonged use

PREGNANCY AND LACTATION: Pregnancy category X (according to manufacturer); no congenital anomalies have been attributed to use during human pregnancies; other benzodiazepines have been suspected of producing fetal malformations after 1st-trimester exposure

SIDE EFFECTS/ADVERSE REACTIONS

CNS: Abnormal thinking, agitation, anterograde amnesia, anxiety, apathy, *asthenia,* ataxia, decreased reflexes, early morning insomnia, emotional lability, hangover, hostility, *hypokinesia,* neuritis, **seizures,** sleep disorder, *somnolence,* stupor

CV: **Dysrhythmia,** syncope

EENT: Ear pain; epistaxis, eye irritation, pain, pharyngitis, photophobia, rhinitis, sinusitis, swelling

GI: Abdominal pain, decreased or increased appetite, dyspepsia, enterocolitis, flatulence, gastritis, increased AST, ALT, melena, mouth ulceration

GU: Decreased libido, frequent urination, hematuria, menstrual cramps, nocturia, oliguria, penile discharge, urinary hesitancy and urgency, urinary incontinence, vaginal discharge and itching

HEME: **Agranulocytosis**

MS: Back pain, lower extremity pain

RESP: Asthma, cough, dyspnea, hyperventilation

SKIN: Acne, dry skin, photosensitivity, urticaria

INTERACTIONS

Drugs

3 *Carbamazepine, phenytoin:* Reduced effect of triazolam

3 *Cimetidine, clarithromycin, disulfiram, erythromycin, fluvoxamine, grapefruit juice, isoniazid, troleandomycin:* Increased plasma triazolam concentrations

2 *Ethanol:* Enhanced adverse psychomotor effects of benzodiazepines

2 *Fluconazole, itraconazole, ketoconazole:* Increased plasma triazolam concentrations

---

italic = common side effects **bold italic** = life-threatening reactions

SPECIAL CONSIDERATIONS
• **Prescriptions should be written for short-term use (7-10 days); drug should not be prescribed in quantities exceeding a 1 mo supply**
PATIENT/FAMILY EDUCATION
• Avoid alcohol and other CNS depressants
• Do not discontinue abruptly after prolonged therapy
• May cause drowsiness or dizziness, use caution while driving or performing other tasks requiring alertness
• May be habit forming

---

trientine
(trye-en′teen)
Rx: Syprine
Chemical Class: Thiol derivative
Therapeutic Class: Copper antidote

CLINICAL PHARMACOLOGY
Mechanism of Action: Chelating agent that binds copper and facilitates its excretion from the body (cupriuresis)
INDICATIONS AND USES: Treatment of Wilson's disease in patients intolerant of penicillamine
DOSAGE
Adult
• PO 750-1250 mg/day divided bid-qid; may increase to max of 2 g/day
Child ≤12 yr
• PO 500-750 mg/day divided bid-qid; may increase to max of 1.5 g/day
$ AVAILABLE FORMS/COST OF THERAPY
• Cap, Gel—Oral: 250 mg, 100's: **$112.84**

CONTRAINDICATIONS: Cystinuria, rheumatoid arthritis, biliary cirrhosis
PRECAUTIONS: Iron deficiency anemia, children
PREGNANCY AND LACTATION: Pregnancy category C
SIDE EFFECTS/ADVERSE REACTIONS
GI: Epigastric pain, heartburn
HEME: Iron deficiency anemia
MS: Cramps, muscle pain
SKIN: Tenderness, thickening and fissuring of skin
MISC: Malaise, systemic lupus erythematosus
SPECIAL CONSIDERATIONS
PATIENT/FAMILY EDUCATION
• Take on empty stomach
MONITORING PARAMETERS
• Free serum copper (goal is <10 μg/dl); increase daily dose only when clinical response is not adequate or concentration of free serum copper is persistently above 20 μg/dl (determine optimal long-term maintenance dosage at 6-12 mo intervals)
• 24 hr urinary copper analysis at 6-12 mo intervals (adequately treated patients will have 0.5-1 mg copper/24 hr collection of urine)

---

trifluoperazine
(trye-floo-oh-per′a-zeen)
Rx: Stelazine
Chemical Class: Piperazine phenothiazine derivative
Therapeutic Class: Antipsychotic

CLINICAL PHARMACOLOGY
Mechanism of Action: Dopamine receptor antagonist, with higher affinity for D_2 over D_1 receptors, and variable selectivity among the cortical dopamine tracts; also activity on

nondopaminergic sites, i.e., cholinergic, α_1-adrenergic and histaminic receptors (explaining side effects); high rates of extrapyramidal reactions; minimal sedation, anticholinergic effects and rates of orthostatic hypotension

Pharmacokinetics

PO: Peak 1½-4½ hr, duration ≥12 hr; ≥90% bound to plasma proteins; extensive liver metabolism, excreted in urine and bile; $t_{1/2}$ >24 hr with chronic use (7-18 hr after single dose)

INDICATIONS AND USES: Psychotic disorders, short-term treatment of non-psychotic anxiety (not drug of choice for most patients)

DOSAGE

NOTE: 5 mg equivalent to chlorpromazine 100 mg

Adult

• *Psychotic disorders:* PO 2-5 mg bid, most patients show optimum response with 15-20 mg/day, some may require ≥40 mg/day; IM (for prompt control of symptoms) 1-2 mg q4-6h prn, doses >6 mg/24 hr are rarely necessary

• *Non-psychotic anxiety:* PO 1-2 mg bid, do not administer >6 mg/day or for >12 wk

Child

• PO 1 mg qd-bid initially, usually not necessary to exceed 15 mg/day: IM 1 mg qd-bid (little experience in children)

💲 AVAILABLE FORMS/COST OF THERAPY

• Conc—Oral: 10 mg/ml, 60 ml: **$143.36**

• Inj, Sol—IM: 2 mg/ml, 10 ml: **$65.81**

• Tab, Plain Coated—Oral: 1 mg, 100's: **$20.28-$80.91**; 2 mg, 100's: **$40.30-$119.33**; 5 mg, 100's: **$40.48-$150.20**; 10 mg, 100's: **$60.00-$213.56**

CONTRAINDICATIONS: Severe toxic CNS depression, coma, subcortical brain damage, bone marrow depression

PRECAUTIONS: Elderly, children <12 yr, prolonged use, severe cardiovascular disorders, epilepsy, hepatic or renal disease, glaucoma, prostatic hypertrophy, severe asthma, emphysema, hypocalcemia (increased susceptibility to dystonic reactions)

PREGNANCY AND LACTATION: Pregnancy category C; has been used as an antiemetic during normal labor without producing any observable effect on newborn; bulk of evidence indicates safety for mother and fetus

SIDE EFFECTS/ADVERSE REACTIONS

CNS: Agitation, anxiety, confusion, depression, *drowsiness,* euphoria, exacerbation of psychotic symptoms including hallucinations, catatonic-like behavioral states, *extrapyramidal symptoms (pseudoparkinsonism, akathisia, dystonia), headache,* insomnia, lethargy, **neuroleptic malignant syndrome,** restlessness, **seizures,** tardive dyskinesia

CV: ECG changes, hypertension, hypotension, tachycardia

EENT: Blurred vision, cataracts, dry eyes, glaucoma, pigmentation of retina or cornea, retinopathy, vertigo

GI: Anorexia, *constipation,* diarrhea, *dry mouth,* dyspepsia, hypersalivation, *nausea,* vomiting

GU: Gynecomastia, impotence, increased libido, menstrual irregularities, priapism, urinary retention

HEME: **Agranulocytosis,** anemia, **aplastic anemia, hemolytic anemia,** leukocytosis, minimal decreases in red blood cell counts, transient leukopenia

---

italic = common side effects　　　**bold italic** = life-threatening reactions

METAB: Breast engorgement, hyperglycemia, hypoglycemia, hyponatremia, lactation, mastalgia

RESP: **Bronchospasm,** increased depth of respiration, *laryngospasm*

SKIN: Diaphoresis, loss of hair, maculopapular and acneiform skin reactions, photosensitivity

MISC: Heat or cold intolerance

INTERACTIONS

Drugs

❸ *Anticholinergics:* Inhibited therapeutic response to antipsychotic; enhanced anticholinergic side effects

❸ *Antidepressants:* Increased serum concentrations of some cyclic antidepressants

❸ *Barbiturates:* Reduced effect of antipsychotic

❸ *Bromocriptine, lithium:* Reduced effects of both drugs

❸ *Guanethidine:* Inhibited antihypertensive response to guanethidine

❷ *Levodopa:* Inhibited effect of levodopa on Parkinson's disease

❸ *Narcotic analgesics:* Excessive CNS depression, hypotension, respiratory depression

❸ *Orphenadrine:* Reduced serum neuroleptic concentrations; excessive anticholinergic effects

Labs

• *False increase:* Urinary protein

SPECIAL CONSIDERATIONS

PATIENT/FAMILY EDUCATION

• Arise slowly from reclining position

• Do not discontinue abruptly

• Use a sunscreen during sun exposure; take special precautions to stay cool in hot weather

MONITORING PARAMETERS

• Observe closely for signs of tardive dyskinesia

• Periodic CBC with platelets during prolonged therapy

---

triflupromazine
(trye-floo-proe´ma-zeen)

Rx: Vesprin

Chemical Class: Aliphatic phenothiazine derivative

Therapeutic Class: Antipsychotic; antiemetic

CLINICAL PHARMACOLOGY

Mechanism of Action: Dopamine receptor antagonist, with higher affinity for D_2- over D_1-receptors, and variable selectivity among the cortical dopamine tracts; also activity on nondopaminergic sites, i.e., cholinergic, α_1-adrenergic and histaminic receptors (explaining side effects); high rates of sedation and anticholinergic effects; moderate risk of extrapyramidal reactions and orthostatic hypotension

Pharmacokinetics

IM: Onset 15-30 min, peak 1 hr, duration 4-6 hr; metabolized by liver, excreted in urine and feces

INDICATIONS AND USES: Psychotic disorders, control of severe nausea and vomiting

DOSAGE

NOTE: 25 mg equivalent to chlorpromazine 100 mg

Adult

• *Psychotic disorders:* IM 60 mg, up to max of 150 mg/day

• *Nausea and vomiting:* IV 1 mg up to a max total 3 mg/day; IM 5-15 mg as a single dose, may repeat q4h up to max of 60 mg/day

Elderly or debilitated patients

• *Nausea and vomiting:* IM 2.5 mg up to a max of 15 mg/day

Child >2 yr

• IM 0.2-0.25 mg/kg, up to max total dose of 10 mg/day

---

* = non-FDA-approved use

🔳 AVAILABLE FORMS/COST OF THERAPY

• Inj, Sol—IM, IV: 10 mg/ml, 10 ml: **$57.53**; 20 mg/ml, 1 ml: **$13.00**

CONTRAINDICATIONS: Severe toxic CNS depression, coma, subcortical brain damage, bone marrow depression, narrow-angle glaucoma

PRECAUTIONS: Elderly, prolonged use, severe cardiovascular disorders, epilepsy, hepatic or renal disease, glaucoma, prostatic hypertrophy, severe asthma, emphysema, hypocalcemia (increased susceptibility to dystonic reactions)

PREGNANCY AND LACTATION: Pregnancy category C; bulk of evidence indicates phenothiazines are safe for mother and fetus

SIDE EFFECTS/ADVERSE REACTIONS

CNS: Agitation, anxiety, confusion, depression, *drowsiness,* euphoria, exacerbation of psychotic symptoms including hallucinations, catatonic-like behavioral states, *extrapyramidal symptoms (pseudoparkinsonism, akathisia, dystonia), headache,* insomnia, lethargy, **neuroleptic malignant syndrome,** restlessness, **seizures,** tardive dyskinesia

CV: ECG changes, hypertension, hypotension, tachycardia

EENT: Blurred vision, cataracts, dry eyes, glaucoma, pigmentation of retina or cornea, retinopathy, vertigo

GI: Anorexia, constipation, diarrhea, *dry mouth,* dyspepsia, hypersalivation, *nausea,* vomiting

GU: Gynecomastia, impotence, increased libido, menstrual irregularities, priapism, urinary retention

HEME: **Agranulocytosis,** anemia, **aplastic anemia, hemolytic anemia,** leukocytosis, minimal decreases in red blood cell counts, transient leukopenia

METAB: Breast engorgement, hyperglycemia, hypoglycemia, hyponatremia, lactation, mastalgia

RESP: **Bronchospasm,** increased depth of respiration, **laryngospasm**

SKIN: Diaphoresis, loss of hair, maculopapular and acneiform skin reactions, photosensitivity

MISC: Heat or cold intolerance

INTERACTIONS

Drugs

🔳 *Anticholinergics:* Inhibited therapeutic response to antipsychotic; enhanced anticholinergic side effects

🔳 *Barbiturates:* Reduced effect of antipsychotic

🔳 *Bromocriptine, lithium:* Reduced effects of both drugs

🔳 *Guanethidine:* Inhibited antihypertensive response to guanethidine

❷ *Levodopa:* Inhibited effect of levodopa on Parkinson's disease

🔳 *Narcotic analgesics:* Excessive CNS depression, hypotension, respiratory depression

🔳 *Orphenadrine:* Reduced serum neuroleptic concentrations; excessive anticholinergic effects

SPECIAL CONSIDERATIONS

PATIENT/FAMILY EDUCATION

• Arise slowly from reclining position

---

italic = common side effects   **bold italic** = life-threatening reactions

trifluridine

(trye-flure´i-deen)
Rx: Viroptic
Chemical Class: Nucleoside
analog
Therapeutic Class: Ophthalmic
antiviral

CLINICAL PHARMACOLOGY
Mechanism of Action: Interferes
with DNA synthesis in cultured
mammalian cells; antiviral mechanism of action not completely
known
Pharmacokinetics
Penetrates the intact cornea; systemic absorption following therapeutic dosing appears to be negligible
INDICATIONS AND USES: Primary
keratoconjunctivitis and recurrent
epithelial keratitis; epithelial keratitis; epithelial keratitis resistant to
topical vidarabine; antiviral spectrum usually includes herpes simplex virus 1 and 2 and vaccinia virus;
some strains of adenovirus are also
inhibited in vitro
DOSAGE
Adult
• OPHTH instill 1 gtt onto cornea of
affected eye(s) q2h while awake until ulcer has completely reepithelial-
ized, max 9 gtt/day; after reepithe-
lialization, 1 gtt q4h while awake for
an additional 7 days, minimum 5
gtt/day; do not exceed 21 days due to
potential for ocular toxicity
$ **AVAILABLE FORMS/COST**
OF THERAPY
• Sol—Ophth: 1%, 7.5 ml: **$51.97-
$99.01**
PRECAUTIONS: Prolonged use
(>21 days); not effective for bacterial, fungal, or chlamydial infections
of the cornea or trophic lesions

PREGNANCY AND LACTATION:
Pregnancy category C
**SIDE EFFECTS/ADVERSE REAC-
TIONS**
EENT: Burning, epithelial keratopa-
thy, hyperemia, hypersensitivity reaction, increased intraocular pressure, irritation, keratitis sicca,
palpebral edema, stinging, stromal
edema, superficial punctate kerat-
opathy
SPECIAL CONSIDERATIONS
PATIENT/FAMILY EDUCATION
• Notify clinician if no improvement
after 7 days

trihexyphenidyl

(trye-hex-ee-fen´i-dill)
Rx: Artane
Chemical Class: Synthetic ter-
tiary amine
Therapeutic Class: Anticholin-
ergic, anti-Parkinson's agent

CLINICAL PHARMACOLOGY
Mechanism of Action: Blocks striatal cholinergic receptors, which
helps balance cholinergic and
dopaminergic activity
Pharmacokinetics
PO: Onset within 1 hr, peak effects
last 2-3 hr, duration 6-12 hr; excreted in urine
INDICATIONS AND USES: Adjunctive treatment of all forms of Parkinson's syndrome; drug-induced extrapyramidal symptoms
DOSAGE
Adult
• *Parkinsonism:* PO 1-2 mg on 1st
day, increase by 2 mg q3-5d to 6-10
mg/day divided tid-qid; postencephalitic patients may require
12-15 mg/day; when used with
levodopa, 3-6 mg/day in divided
doses is usually adequate

• *Drug-induced extrapyramidal symptoms:* PO 1 mg initially, progressively increase subsequent doses if reaction not controlled in a few hr; maintenance 5-15 mg/day in divided doses

$ AVAILABLE FORMS/COST OF THERAPY

• Elixir—Oral: 2 mg/5 ml, 480 ml: **$20.00-$42.84**
• Tab, Uncoated—Oral: 2 mg, 100's: **$9.09-$21.30**; 5 mg, 100's: **$10.00-$42.38**

CONTRAINDICATIONS: Narrow-angle glaucoma, myasthenia gravis, GI or GU obstruction, peptic ulcer, megacolon, prostatic hypertrophy

PRECAUTIONS: Elderly, tachycardia, liver or kidney disease, drug abuse history, dysrhythmias, hypotension, hypertension, psychosis, children, tardive dyskinesia

PREGNANCY AND LACTATION: Pregnancy category C; nursing infants may be particularly sensitive to anticholinergic effects

SIDE EFFECTS/ADVERSE REACTIONS

CNS: Anxiety, confusion, delusions, depression, dizziness, hallucinations, headache, incoherence, irritability, memory loss, restlessness, *sedation*

CV: Flushing, hypotension, mild bradycardia, palpitations, postural hypotension, tachycardia

EENT: Angle-closure glaucoma, blurred vision, difficulty swallowing, dilated pupils, dry eyes, increased intraocular tension, mydriasis, photophobia

GI: Abdominal distress, *constipation, dry mouth,* epigastric distress, nausea, ***paralytic ileus,*** vomiting

GU: Dysuria, erectile dysfunction, hesitancy, retention

MS: Cramping, muscular weakness

SKIN: Dermatoses, rash, urticaria

MISC: Decreased sweating, heat stroke, hyperthermia, numbness of fingers

INTERACTIONS

Drugs

3 *Amantadine:* Potentiates the side effects of amantadine

3 *Anticholinergics:* Increased anticholinergic side effects

3 *Neuroleptics:* Inhibition of therapeutic response to neuroleptics; excessive anticholinergic effects

3 *Tacrine:* Reduced therapeutic effects of both drugs

Labs

• *False increase:* Serum T_3 and T_4

SPECIAL CONSIDERATIONS

PATIENT/FAMILY EDUCATION

• Do not discontinue abruptly
• Use caution in hot weather; drug may increase susceptibility to heat stroke

---

trimethadione
(trye-meth-a-dye'one)
Rx: Tridione
Chemical Class: Oxazolidinedione derivative
Therapeutic Class: Anticonvulsant

CLINICAL PHARMACOLOGY

Mechanism of Action: Decreases seizures in cortex, basal ganglia; decreases synaptic stimulation to low-frequency impulses

Pharmacokinetics

PO: Peak 30-120 min; demethylated in liver to active metabolite (dimethadione), excreted by kidneys; $t_{1/2}$ 16-24 hr (dimethadione 6-13 days)

INDICATIONS AND USES: Refractory absence (petit mal) seizures

DOSAGE
Adult
• PO 300-600 mg tid-qid; give 900 mg/day initially, increase by 300 mg at weekly intervals until therapeutic results are seen or toxicity appears
Child
• PO 300-900 mg/day divided tid-qid

$ AVAILABLE FORMS/COST OF THERAPY
• Cap, Gel—Oral: 300 mg, 100's: **$44.19**
• Tab, Chewable—Oral: 150 mg, 100's: **$40.50**

PRECAUTIONS: Hepatic disease, renal disease, abrupt discontinuation, diseases of retina or optic nerve, intermittent porphyria, myasthenia gravis

PREGNANCY AND LACTATION: Pregnancy category D; has demonstrated both clinical and experimental fetal risk greater than other anticonvulsants; avoid use in pregnancy

SIDE EFFECTS/ADVERSE REACTIONS
CNS: Dizziness, *drowsiness,* fatigue, headache, insomnia, irritability, paresthesia
CV: Hypertension, hypotension
EENT: Diplopia, epistaxis, photophobia, retinal hemorrhage
GI: Abdominal pain, abnormal liver function tests, bleeding gums, *nausea, vomiting*
GU: Albuminuria, nephrosis, vaginal bleeding
HEME: **Agranulocytosis, aplastic anemia,** eosinophilia, **hemolytic anemia,** increased prothrombin time, **leukopenia, neutropenia, thrombocytopenia**
SKIN: Alopecia, erythema, *exfoliative dermatitis,* petechiae, rash
MISC: Lupus erythematosus

SPECIAL CONSIDERATIONS
PATIENT/FAMILY EDUCATION
• Take with food if GI upset occurs

• Avoid prolonged exposure to sunlight

MONITORING PARAMETERS
• CBC at baseline and qmo thereafter; satisfactory control usually occurs when serum dimethadione levels are ≥700 µg/ml

---

trimethobenzamide
(trye-meth-oh-ben′za-mide)
Rx: Benzacot, Stemetic, Tigan
Chemical Class: Ethanolamine derivative
Therapeutic Class: Antiemetic

CLINICAL PHARMACOLOGY
Mechanism of Action: Exact mechanism unknown; appears to directly affect the medullary chemoreceptor trigger zone (CTZ) by inhibiting stimuli at the CTZ
Pharmacokinetics
PO: Onset 10-40 min, duration 3-4 hr
IM: Onset 15-35 min, duration 2-3 hr
Exact metabolic fate unclear, 30%-50% excreted unchanged in urine

INDICATIONS AND USES: Nausea and vomiting

DOSAGE
Adult
• PO 250 mg tid-qid; PR/IM 200 mg tid-qid
Child
• PO (13.6-45 kg) 100-200 mg tid-qid; PR (<13.6 kg) 100 mg tid-qid; (13.6-45 kg) 100-200 mg tid-qid

$ AVAILABLE FORMS/COST OF THERAPY
• Cap, Gel—Oral: 100 mg, 100's: **$42.68-$64.44**; 250 mg, 100's: **$27.00-$77.70**; 300 mg, 100's: **$106.25**
• Inj, Sol—IM: 100 mg/ml, 20 ml: **$8.68-$48.88**

---

* = non-FDA-approved use

• Supp—Rect: 100 mg, 10's: **$4.31-$24.78**; 200 mg, 10's: **$4.85-$29.40**

CONTRAINDICATIONS: Hypersensitivity to benzocaine or similar anesthetics; parenteral use in children; suppositories in premature infants or neonates

PRECAUTIONS: Acute febrile illness, encephalitis, Reye's syndrome, gastroenteritis, dehydration, electrolyte imbalance

PREGNANCY AND LACTATION: Pregnancy category C; has been used to treat nausea and vomiting during pregnancy

SIDE EFFECTS/ADVERSE REACTIONS

CNS: **Coma,** depression, disorientation, dizziness, *drowsiness,* dystonic reactions, headache, Parkinson-like symptoms, **seizures**

CV: Hypotenstion (IM)

EENT: Blurred vision

GI: Diarrhea, jaundice

HEME: **Blood dyscrasias**

MS: Muscle cramps

SKIN: Allergic-type skin reactions, burning and stinging at inj site (IM)

INTERACTIONS

Drugs

3 *Alcohol:* Increased adverse reactions

Labs

• *False positive:* Urinary amphetamine

SPECIAL CONSIDERATIONS

• Less effective than phenothiazines

trimethoprim

(trye-meth´oh-prim)

Rx: Proloprim, Trimpex

Combinations

> **Rx:** with sulfamethoxazole (see co-trimoxazole monograph); with polymyxin B sulfate (Polytrim Ophthalmic)

Chemical Class: Synthetic folate-antagonist

Therapeutic Class: Antibiotic

CLINICAL PHARMACOLOGY

Mechanism of Action: Selectively interferes with bacterial biosynthesis of nucleic acids and proteins by blocking production of tetrahydrofolic acid from dihydrofolic acid via binding to and reversibly inhibiting the required enzyme, dihydrofolate reductase; binding much stronger for bacterial enzyme than for corresponding mammalian enzyme

Pharmacokinetics

PO: Peak 1-4 hr; widely distributed into body tissues and fluids; 42%-46% bound to plasma proteins; metabolized in liver to oxide and hydroxylated metabolites, excreted in urine (80% unchanged); $t_{1/2}$ 8-11 hr (prolonged in renal failure)

INDICATIONS AND USES: Acute uncomplicated UTI, prophylaxis of chronic and recurrent UTI,* *Pneumocystis carinii* pneumonia (in conjunction with dapsone or sulfamethoxazole),* travelers' diarrhea,* otitis media, and chronic bronchitis and shigella (with sulfamethoxazole)

Antibacterial spectrum usually includes:

• Gram-positive organisms: *Streptococcus pneumoniae,* group A β-hemolytic streptococci, coagulase-negative staphylococci

---

italic = common side effects   ***bold italic*** = life-threatening reactions

• Gram-negative organisms: *Acinetobacter, Citrobacter, Enterobacter, Escherichia coli, Klebsiella pneumoniae, Proteus mirabilis, Salmonella, Shigella, Haemophilus influenzae*

DOSAGE
Adult
• PO 100 mg q12h or 200 mg q24h, each for 10 days
• Dosing in renal failure (CrCl 15-30 ml/min): PO 50 mg q12h. Combination with sulfamethoxazole: see co-trimoxazole

🛡 AVAILABLE FORMS/COST OF THERAPY
• Sol—Oral: 50 mg/ml, 473 ml: **$59.13**
• Tab, Uncoated—Oral: 100 mg, 100's: **$18.74-$111.24**; 200 mg, 100's: **$32.00-$222.31**

CONTRAINDICATIONS: Megaloblastic anemia due to folate deficiency, infants <2 mo, CrCl <15 ml/min

PRECAUTIONS: Renal or hepatic impairment, children <12 yr, folate deficiency (folates may be administered concurrently without interfering with antibacterial action)

PREGNANCY AND LACTATION: Pregnancy category C; because trimethoprim is a folate antagonist, caution should be used during the 1st trimester; excreted into breast milk in low concentrations; compatible with breast feeding

SIDE EFFECTS/ADVERSE REACTIONS
CNS: Fever
GI: Elevation of serum transaminases and bilirubin, epigastric distress, glossitis, **hepatic necrosis, nausea, vomiting**
GU: Increased BUN and serum creatinine
HEME: **Leukopenia, megaloblastic anemia, methemoglobinemia, neutropenia, thrombocytopenia**

SKIN: Pruritus, rash, **Stevens-Johnson syndrome, toxic epidermal necrolysis**

INTERACTIONS
Drugs
3 *Dapsone:* Increased serum concentrations of both drugs
3 *Phenytoin:* Increased serum phenytoin concentrations, potential for toxicity
3 *Procainamide:* Increased serum concentrations of procainamide and N-acetylprocainamide

SPECIAL CONSIDERATIONS
• Good alternative to co-trimoxazole in patients taking warfarin

---

trimipramine
(trye-mip′ra-meen)
Rx: Surmontil
Chemical Class: Dibenzazepine derivative: tertiary amine
Therapeutic Class: Tricyclic antidepressant

CLINICAL PHARMACOLOGY
Mechanism of Action: Inhibits the reuptake of norepinephrine and serotonin (slightly) at the presynaptic neuron prolonging neuronal activity; inhibition of histamine and acetylcholine activity; mild peripheral vasodilator effects and possible quinidine-like action on cardiac conduction; moderate anticholinergic and orthostatic hypotensive effects; high sedative activity

Pharmacokinetics
PO: Peak within 6 hr; 95% protein bound; metabolized in liver to desmethyltrimipramine, excreted in urine; $t_{1/2}$ 20-26 hr

INDICATIONS AND USES: Depression, chronic urticaria and angioedema,* nocturnal pruritus in atopic dermatitis*

---

* = non-FDA-approved use

DOSAGE

Adult

• PO 75-100 mg/day in divided doses initially, increase to 150-200 mg/day, max 300 mg/day

Adolescent and Elderly

• PO 50 mg/day initially, increase to 100 mg/day

§ AVAILABLE FORMS/COST OF THERAPY

• Cap, Gel—Oral: 25 mg, 100's: **$85.58**; 50 mg, 100's: **$140.01**; 100 mg, 100's: **$203.54**

CONTRAINDICATIONS: Acute recovery phase of MI, concurrent use of MAOIs

PRECAUTIONS: Suicidal patients, seizure disorders, prostatic hypertrophy, psychiatric disease, severe depression, increased intraocular pressure, narrow-angle glaucoma, urinary retention, cardiac disease, hepatic disease, renal disease, hyperthyroidism, electroshock therapy, elective surgery, elderly, abrupt discontinuation

PREGNANCY AND LACTATION: Pregnancy category C; excreted into breast milk; effect on nursing infant unknown, but may be of concern

SIDE EFFECTS/ADVERSE REACTIONS

CNS: Anxiety, confusion (especially in elderly), *dizziness, drowsiness,* fatigue, headache, increased psychiatric symptoms, insomnia, memory impairment, nightmares, stimulation, tremors, weakness

CV: **Dysrhythmias,** ECG changes, hypertension, *orthostatic hypotension,* palpitations, tachycardia

EENT: Blurred vision, mydriasis, nasal congestion, ophthalmoplegia, tinnitus

GI: Constipation, cramps, diarrhea, *dry mouth,* epigastric distress, hepatitis, increased appetite, jaundice, nausea, **paralytic ileus,** stomatitis, vomiting

GU: Urinary retention

HEME: **Agranulocytosis,** eosinophilia, **leukopenia, thrombocytopenia**

SKIN: Photosensitivity, pruritus, rash, sweating, urticaria

INTERACTIONS

Drugs

3 *Anticholinergics, propantheline:* Excessive anticholinergic effects

3 *Barbiturates, carbamazepine:* Reduced serum concentrations of cyclic antidepressants

3 *Cimetidine:* Increases trimipramine level

2 *Clonidine:* Reduced antihypertensive response to clonidine; enhanced hypertensive response with abrupt clonidine withdrawal

2 *Epinephrine, norepinephrine:* Markedly enhanced pressor response to IV epinephrine

3 *Ethanol:* Additive impairment of motor skills; abstinent alcoholics may eliminate cyclic antidepressants more rapidly than non-alcoholics

3 *Fluoxetine:* Marked increases in cyclic antidepressant plasma concentrations

2 *Guanadrel, guanethidine:* Inhibited antihypertensive response to guanethidine

⚠ *MAOIs:* Excessive sympathetic response; mania or hyperpyrexia possible

2 *Moclobemide:* Potential association with fatal or non-fatal serotonin syndrome

3 *Phenylephrine:* Markedly enhanced pressor response to IV epinephrine

3 *Propoxyphene:* Enhanced effect of cyclic antidepressants

3 *Quinidine:* Increased cyclic antidepressant serum concentrations

T

---

italic = common side effects   **bold italic** = life-threatening reactions

SPECIAL CONSIDERATIONS
PATIENT/FAMILY EDUCATION
• Therapeutic effects may take 2-3 wk
• Avoid rising quickly from sitting to standing, especially elderly
• Do not discontinue abruptly after long-term use
MONITORING PARAMETERS
• CBC, ECG

---

trioxsalen
(trye-ox′a-len)
Rx: Trisoralen
Chemical Class: Psoralen derivative
Therapeutic Class: Pigmenting agent

CLINICAL PHARMACOLOGY
Mechanism of Action: Exact mechanism unknown; may involve increased tyrosinase activity in melanin-producing cells, which enhances melanin production; successful pigmentation requires the presence of functioning melanocytes
Pharmacokinetics
PO: Onset 1-2 hr, maximal effects 2-4 hr, duration 7-8 hr; 80% appears in urine within 8 hr as hydroxylated or glucuronide derivatives
INDICATIONS AND USES: Repigmentation in the treatment of vitiligo, in conjunction with UVA—treatment known as PUVA (psoralen plus ultraviolet light A); increasing tolerance to sunlight and enhancing pigmentation (in conjunction with controlled exposure to UVA light or sunlight)
DOSAGE
Adult and Child >12 yr
• *Idiopathic vitiligo:* PO 5-10 mg qd 2-4 hr before measured periods of sunlight or UVA exposure

• *Other uses:* PO 10 mg qd 2 hr before measured periods of sunlight or UVA exposure; do not exceed 14 days of therapy or 140 mg total dose
💲 AVAILABLE FORMS/COST OF THERAPY
• Tab, Uncoated—Oral: 5 mg, 100's: **$238.31**
CONTRAINDICATIONS: Diseases associated with photosensitivity, melanoma, invasive squamous cell carcinoma, aphakia, children <12 yr
PRECAUTIONS: Cardiac disease, hepatic disease, contains tartrazine (FD&C #5), photosensitizing agents
PREGNANCY AND LACTATION: Pregnancy category C; excretion into breast milk unknown, use caution in nursing mothers
SIDE EFFECTS/ADVERSE REACTIONS
CNS: Depression, dizziness, headache, insomnia, malaise, nervousness
CV: Edema, hypotension
EENT: Cataract formation
GI: Nausea
MS: Leg cramps
SKIN: Basal cell epitheliomas, cutaneous tenderness, *erythema,* extension of psoriasis, folliculitis, hypopigmentation, *pruritus,* severe burns, urticaria, vesiculation and bullae formation
INTERACTIONS
Drugs
3 *Anthralin, coal tar, griseofulvin, phenothiazines, nalidixic acid, halogenated salicylanilides, sulfonamides, tetracyclines, thiazides:* Increased photosensitivity to these agents
SPECIAL CONSIDERATIONS
PATIENT/FAMILY EDUCATION
• Do not sunbathe during 24 hr prior to ingestion and UVA exposure

---

• Wear UVA-absorbing sunglasses for 24 hr following treatment to prevent cataract

• Avoid sun exposure for at least 8 hr after ingestion

• Avoid furocoumarin-containing foods (e.g., limes, figs, parsley, parsnips, mustard, carrots, celery)

• Repigmentation may begin after 2-3 wk but full effect may require 6-9 mo

---

tripelennamine

(tri-pel-enn´a-meen)
Rx: PBZ, PBZ-SR
Chemical Class: Ethylenediamine derivative
Therapeutic Class: Antihistamine

CLINICAL PHARMACOLOGY

Mechanism of Action: Decreases allergic response by blocking histamine at H_1-receptors

Pharmacokinetics

PO: Onset within 30 min, duration 4-6 hr (Sus Action 8 hr); metabolized in liver, excreted in urine

INDICATIONS AND USES: Perennial and seasonal allergic rhinitis; vasomotor rhinitis; allergic conjunctivitis due to inhalants, allergens and food; allergic skin manifestations of urticaria and angioedema; dermographism; adjunctive anaphylactic therapy

DOSAGE

Adult

• PO 25-50 mg q4-6h, max 600 mg/day; PO Sus Action 100 mg bid, may also be given q8h in difficult cases

Child

• PO 5 mg/kg/day or 150 mg/m²/day in 4-6 divided doses, max 300 mg/day

AVAILABLE FORMS/COST OF THERAPY

• Tab, Uncoated—Oral: 25 mg, 100's: **$17.91**; 50 mg, 100's: **$3.54-$27.20**

• Tab, Coated, Sus Action—Oral: 100 mg, 100's: **$44.71**

CONTRAINDICATIONS: Narrow-angle glaucoma, bladder neck obstruction

PRECAUTIONS: Liver disease, elderly, increased intraocular pressure, hyperthyroidism, cardiovascular disease, hypertension, urinary retention, renal disease, stenosed peptic ulcers

PREGNANCY AND LACTATION: Pregnancy category B; manufacturer considers the drug contraindicated in nursing mothers, possibly due to increased sensitivity of newborn or premature infants to antihistamines; anecdotal evidence indicates safety in pregnancy

SIDE EFFECTS/ADVERSE REACTIONS

CNS: Anxiety, confusion, *dizziness, drowsiness,* euphoria, fatigue, poor coordination

CV: Hypotension, palpitations, tachycardia

EENT: Blurred vision, dilated pupils, dry nose, throat, nasal stuffiness, tinnitus

GI: Anorexia, *constipation,* diarrhea, *dry mouth,* nausea, vomiting

GU: Dysuria, frequency, impotence, retention

HEME: ***Agranulocytosis, hemolytic anemia, thrombocytopenia***

RESP: Increased thick secretions, wheezing

SKIN: Photosensitivity

---

triprolidine

(trye-proe´li-deen)
Combinations
Rx: with pseudoephedrine,
codeine (Triprolidine-C):
OTC: with pseudoephedrine
(Actifed)
Chemical Class: Alkylamine
derivative
Therapeutic Class: Antihistamine

CLINICAL PHARMACOLOGY
Mechanism of Action: Decreases
allergic response by blocking histamine at H_1-receptors
Pharmacokinetics
PO: Onset 20-60 min, duration 8-12
hr; metabolized in liver, excreted in
urine
INDICATIONS AND USES: Perennial and seasonal allergic rhinitis
and other allergic symptoms including urticaria
DOSAGE
Adult
• PO 2.5 mg q4-6h
Child 6-12 yr
• PO 1.25 mg q4-6h
💲 AVAILABLE FORMS/COST
OF THERAPY
• Syr—Oral: 1.25 mg/5 ml (with 30
mg pseudoephedrine), 120 ml:
$1.20-$6.34; 1.25 mg/5 ml (with 30
mg pseudoephedrine and 10 mg codeine), 480 ml: **$9.17-$50.26**
• Tab, Uncoated—Oral: 2.5 mg
(with 60 mg pseudoephedrine),
100's: **$1.92-$14.32**
CONTRAINDICATIONS: Narrow-angle glaucoma, bladder neck obstruction
PRECAUTIONS: Liver disease, elderly, increased intraocular pressure,
hyperthyroidism, cardiovascular
disease, hypertension, urinary retention, newborn or premature infants, renal disease, GI outlet obstruction
PREGNANCY AND LACTATION:
Pregnancy category C (but no teratogenicity documented); excreted
into breast milk; compatible with
breast feeding
SIDE EFFECTS/ADVERSE REACTIONS
CNS: Anxiety, confusion, *dizziness,
drowsiness,* euphoria, fatigue, poor
coordination
CV: Hypotension, palpitations,
tachycardia
EENT: Blurred vision, dilated pupils,
dry nose, throat, nasal stuffiness; tinnitus
GI: Anorexia, *constipation,* diarrhea, *dry mouth,* nausea, vomiting
GU: Dysuria, frequency, impotence,
retention
HEME: **Agranulocytosis, hemolytic
anemia, thrombocytopenia**
RESP: Increased thick secretions,
wheezing
SKIN: Photosensitivity
INTERACTIONS
Labs
• *False increase:* Urinary amino acids

tromethamine

(troe-meth´a-meen)
Rx: Tham
Chemical Class: Organic amine
buffer
Therapeutic Class: Alkalinizing agent

CLINICAL PHARMACOLOGY
Mechanism of Action: Acts as a
proton acceptor preventing or correcting acidosis by actively binding
hydrogen ions (H^+); binds cations
of fixed or metabolic acids, and hydrogen ions of carbonic acid, thus

increasing bicarbonate anion (HCO_3^-); also acts as an osmotic diuretic, increasing urine flow, urinary pH, and excretion of fixed acids, carbon dioxide, and electrolytes

Pharmacokinetics

IV: Rapidly eliminated by kidney (75% or more appears in the urine after 8 hr), urinary excretion continues over a period of 3 days

INDICATIONS AND USES: Metabolic acidosis associated with cardiac bypass surgery and cardiac arrest; correction of acidity of acid citrate dextrose (ACD) blood in cardiac bypass surgery

DOSAGE

Dosage may be estimated from the buffer base deficit of extracellular fluid (mEq/L) using the following formula as a general guide: ml of 0.3 M tromethamine solution = body weight (kg) × base deficit (mEq/L) × 1.1

Adult

• *Acidosis during cardiac bypass surgery:* IV INF total single dose of 500 ml (150 mEq or 18 g) is adequate for most adults; larger single doses (up to 1000 ml) may be required in severe cases; do not exceed individual doses of 500 mg/kg given over at least 1 hr

• *Acidity of ACD-priming blood:* Use from 0.5-2.5 g (15-77 ml) added to each 500 ml of ACD blood; 62 ml added to 500 ml of ACD blood is usually adequate

• *Acidosis associated with cardiac arrest:* IV 3.6-10.8 g (111-333 ml) into large peripheral vein; if chest is open, inject 2-6 g (62-185 ml) directly into ventricular cavity

$ **AVAILABLE FORMS/COST OF THERAPY**

• Inj, Sol—IV: 3.6 g/100 ml (0.3 M), 500 ml: **$177.61**

CONTRAINDICATIONS: Anuria, uremia

PRECAUTIONS: Respiratory depression, perivascular infiltration, neonates, renal function impairment, children

PREGNANCY AND LACTATION: Pregnancy category C

SIDE EFFECTS/ADVERSE REACTIONS

GI: ***Hemorrhagic hepatic necrosis***

METAB: Hypovolemia, transient depression of blood glucose

RESP: ***Respiratory depression***

SKIN: Local reactions (febrile response, infection, venous thrombosis or phlebitis)

INTERACTIONS

Labs

• *False decrease:* Plasma ammonia, serum ionized calcium

SPECIAL CONSIDERATIONS

• Avoid overdosage and alkalosis

MONITORING PARAMETERS

• Pretreatment and subsequent blood gas values

• Urine output

• ECG

• Serum glucose and electrolytes before, during, and after administration

• Experience limited to short-term use; may administer for >1 day in life-threatening situation

T

---

italic = common side effects   ***bold italic*** = life-threatening reactions

trovafloxacin/ alatrofloxacin

(troh-vah-floks´-uh-sin)

Rx: Trovan
Combinations
  Rx: with azithromycin (Trovan/Zithromax compliance pak)
  Chemical Class: Fluoroquinolone derivative
  Therapeutic Class: Antibiotic

CLINICAL PHARMACOLOGY

Mechanism of Action: Inhibts DNA gyrase and topoisomerase 4, which are needed for the synthesis of bacterial DNA. Alatrofloxacin is the L-alanyl prodrug of trovafloxacin

Pharmacokinetics

IV: (alatrofloxacin): Rapidly converted to trovafloxacin, peak plasma level 1 hr, $t_{1/2}$ 9-11 hr

PO: (trovafloxacin): Bioavailability 88%, not affected by food; peak plasma level 1-2 hr; widely distributed (concentrated in lung, bile, and urine), 76% protein bound; 51% metabolized by conjugation in the liver (CYP450 independent), excreted unchanged in stool (43%), urine (6%), and as metabolites in urine; $t_{1/2}$ 9-12 hr

INDICATIONS AND USES: Serious life- or limb-threatening infections of the following types: Acute bacterial exacerbations of chronic bronchitis; acute sinusitis; cellulitis; diabetic foot infections; gonorrhea (urethral in males); endocervical and rectal in females); gynecologic and pelvic infections; intraabdominal infections; nongonococcal urethritis (female) and cervicitis; pelvic inflammatory disease; pneumonia, community or hospital acquired; bacterial prostatis; urinary tract infection (cystitis) caused by susceptible organisms. **Based on FDA advisory June 9, 1999 (see precautions), patients should receive their initial therapy in an inpatient health care facility.**

Antibacterial spectrum usually includes:

• Gram-positive organisms: *Enterococcus faecalis* (many strains are only moderately susceptible), *Staphylococcus aureus* (methicillin-susceptible strains), *S. epidermidis* (methicillin-susceptible strains), *Streptococcus pneumoniae, S. pyogenes, Viridans*-group *streptococci*

• Gram-negative organisms: *Citrobacter freundii, Enterobacter aerogenes, Escherichia coli, Gardnerella vaginalis, H. influenzae, H. parainfluenza, Klebsiella pneumoniae, Moraxella catarrhalis, Morganella morganii, N. gonorrhoeae, Proteus mirabilis, P. vulgaris, Pseudomonas aeruginosa*

• Other: *Chlamydia pneumoniae, Chlamydia trachomatis, Legionella pneumophila, Mycoplasma hominis, Mycoplasma pneumoniae;* Anaerobes: *Bacteroides fragilis, Bacteroides distasonis, Clostridium perfringens, Peptostreptococcus species*

DOSAGE

Adult

• *Acute bacterial exacerbations of chronic bronchitis:* PO 100 mg qd × 7-10 days

• *Acute sinusitis:* PO 200 mg qd × 10 days

• *Cellulitis (uncomplicated):* PO 100 mg qd × 7-10 days

• *Cellulitis (complicated) including diabetic foot infections:* PO 200 mg qd × 10-14 days

• *Gonorrhea (urethral in males):* PO 100 mg (single dose)

---

* = non-FDA-approved use

• *Gonorrhea (endocervical and rectal in females):* PO 200 mg qd × 5 days

• *Gynecologic and pelvic infections:* IV 300 mg, then PO 200 mg qd × 7-14 days

• *Intraabdominal infections:* IV 300 mg, then PO 200 mg qd × 7-14 days

• *Nongonococcal urethritis (female) and cervicitis:* PO 200 mg qd × 5 days

• *Pelvic inflammatory disease:* PO 200 mg qd × 14 days

• *Pneumonia, community acquired:* PO 200 mg qd × 7-14 days

• *Pneumonia, hospital acquired:* IV 300 mg, then PO 200 mg qd × 10-14 days

• *Chronic bacterial prostatitis:* PO 200 mg qd × 28 days

• *Cystitis:* PO 100 mg qd × 3 days

• *Prophylaxis of infection associated with elective colorectal surgery or hysterectomy:* IV 200 mg or PO 200 mg

• Dose change for renal disease: none

• Dose change for hepatic disease (mild-moderate cirrhosis): for 300 mg IV, substitute 200 mg IV; for 200 mg IV or PO, substitute 100 mg IV or PO; for 100 mg PO, no change

💲 AVAILABLE FORMS/COST OF THERAPY

• Inj, Sol—IV (alatrofloxacin): 200 mg/40 ml, 1's: **$37.93**

• Tab—Oral (trovafloxacin): 100 mg, 30's: **$183.20**; 200 mg, 30's: **$228.86**

PRECAUTIONS: Pregnancy, lactation, age <18 yr, chronic liver disease (e.g., cirrhosis), **reported to cause unpredictable life-threatening hepatotoxicity, which is more common with therapy longer than 14 days (see http://www.fda.gov/cder/news/trovan/trovan-advisory.htm for more information)**

PREGNANCY AND LACTATION: Pregnancy category C; excreted in breast milk

SIDE EFFECTS/ADVERSE REACTIONS

CNS: Anxiety, dizziness (11%), headache, light-headedness

GI: Abdominal pain, diarrhea, *elevated transaminases (9% with 28-day course),* **hepatic failure (1 per 25,000 patients receiving trovafloxacin),** *nausea (8%),* vomiting

GU: Vaginitis

HEME: Prolonged INR (even if not taking warfarin)

MS: Arthralgia, tendinitis

SKIN: Photosensitivity, rash

INTERACTIONS
Drugs

3 *Aluminum:* Reduced absorption of trovafloxacin; do not take within 4 hr of dose

3 *Antacids:* Reduced absorption of trovafloxacin; do not take within 4 hr of dose

3 *Antipyrine:* Inhibits metabolism of antipyrine; increased plasma antipyrine level

3 *Calcium:* Reduced absorption of trovafloxacin; do not take within 4 hr of dose

3 *Diazepam:* Inhibits metabolism of diazepam; increased plasma diazepam level

3 *Didanosine:* Markedly reduced absorption of trovafloxacin; take trovafloxacin 2 hr before didanosine

3 *Foscarnet:* Coadministration increases seizure risk

3 *Iron:* Reduced absorption of trovafloxacin; do not take within 4 hr of dose

3 *Magnesium:* Reduced absorption of trovafloxacin; do not take within 4 hr of dose

3 *Metoprolol:* Inhibits metabolism of metoprolol; increased plasma metoprolol level

---

italic = common side effects   ***bold italic*** = life-threatening reactions

3 *Morphine:* Reduced absorption of trovafloxacin; do not take within 2 hr of dose

3 *Pentoxifylline:* Inhibits metabolism of pentoxifylline; increased plasma pentoxifylline level

3 *Phenytoin:* Inhibits metabolism of phenytoin; increased plasma phenytoin level

3 *Propranolol:* Inhibits metabolism of propranolol; increased plasma propranolol level

3 *Ropinirole:* Inhibits metabolism of ropinirole; increased plasma ropinirole level

3 *Sodium bicarbonate:* Reduced absorption of trovafloxacin; do not take within 4 hr of dose

3 *Sucralfate:* Reduced absorption of trovafloxacin; do not take within 4 hr of dose

3 *Warfarin:* Inhibits metabolism of warfarin; increases hypoprothrombinemic response to warfarin

3 *Zinc:* Reduced absorption of trovafloxacin; do not take within 4 hr of dose

SPECIAL CONSIDERATIONS
PATIENT/FAMILY EDUCATION
• Do not take antacids (aluminum, calcium, or magnesium-containing) or iron within 2 hr of taking trovafloxacin. Take at bedtime or with food to minimize dizziness associated with trovafloxacin. Avoid excessive sunlight during treatment
MONITORING PARAMETERS
• Transaminases if given for more than 7 days

---

undecylenic acid
(un-de-sye-len´ik)
OTC: Caldesene, Cruex, Desenex, Fungoid Topical Solution, Protectol
Chemical Class: Hendecenoic acid derivative
Therapeutic Class: Antifungal

CLINICAL PHARMACOLOGY
Mechanism of Action: Interferes with fungal cell membrane permeability; fungistatic
Pharmacokinetics
Improvement may be seen within 1 wk
INDICATIONS AND USES: Tinea cruris, tinea pedis, tinea corporis, diaper rash
DOSAGE
Adult and Child
• TOP apply to affected areas bid for 2-4 wk
§ AVAILABLE FORMS/COST OF THERAPY
• Cre—Top: 20%, 15 g: **$5.28**
• Oint—Top: 25%, 15, 30, 454 g: **$1.80-$7.40**/30 g
• Powder—Top: 25%, 45, 60, 90, 165 g: **$5.36**/90 g
• Spray—Top: 1%, 113 g: **$5.00-$5.50**; 19%, 54, 90, 105, 165 g: **$4.64**/105 g; 25%, 45 g: **$3.85**
• Tincture—Top: 25%, 30 ml: **$9.75**
PRECAUTIONS: Impaired circulation; diabetes mellitus; broken, pustular skin; puncture wounds; children <2 yr
PREGNANCY AND LACTATION: Problems not documented in breast feeding
SIDE EFFECTS/ADVERSE REACTIONS
SKIN: Skin irritation
SPECIAL CONSIDERATIONS
• Newer topical antifungals more effective

• Powders are generally used as adjunctive therapy, but may be useful for primary therapy in very mild cases

---

urea
(yoor-ee´a)
Rx: *Parenteral:* Ureaphil
Topical: Gordon's Urea 40%;
OTC: *Topical:* Aqua Care,
Carmol, Gormel, Lanaphilic
Ultramide, Nutraplus,
Ureacin
Chemical Class: Carbonic acid
diamide salt
Therapeutic Class: Osmotic
agent; antiglaucoma agent

CLINICAL PHARMACOLOGY
Mechanism of Action: Systemic; elevates plasma osmolality, increasing flow of water from tissues into blood, including the brain and the eye; Topical: promotes hydration; removes excess keratin
Pharmacokinetics
IV: Onset of action 10 min, peak effect 1-2 hr, duration of action 3-10 hr (diuresis and decreased CSF pressure), 5-6 hr (reduced intraocular pressure); excreted in urine; crosses placenta; excreted in breast milk
INDICATIONS AND USES: Parenteral: cerebral edema, glaucoma; has been used for induction of abortion by intra-amniotic injection; topical: emollient, hydration, and removal of hyperkeratotic skin
DOSAGE
Adult and Child >2 yr
• IV 0.5-1.5 g/kg as 30% sol in 5% or 10% dextrose over ½-2 hr at rate not exceeding 4 ml/min, max 2 g/kg/day
• TOP apply bid-qid
Child <2 yr
• IV 0.1-1.5 g/kg as sol as described and administered for adults

💲 AVAILABLE FORMS/COST OF THERAPY
• Cre—Top: 10%, 75, 90, 454 g: **$6.42**/75 g; 20%, 75, 90, 120, 454, 480 g: **$7.59**/90 g; 22%, 30 g: **$13.12**; 30%, 60 g: **$6.50**; 40%, 30, 90, 120 g: **$24.08-$31.25**/30 g
• Inj, Dry-Sol—IV: 40 g/150 ml: **$84.43**
• Lotion—Top: 10%, 90, 180, 240, 480 ml: **$2.95-$12.00**/240 ml; 15%, 120 g: **$5.90**; 25%, 105, 240 ml: **$10.54**/240 ml
• Oint—Top: 10%, 180. 454 g: **$3.85**/180 g; 20%, 454 g: **$7.50**/480 g
• Paste—Top: 50%, 60 g: **$14.79**
CONTRAINDICATIONS: Severe renal disease, active intracranial bleeding (except during craniotomy), severe dehydration, liver failure
PRECAUTIONS: Hepatic disease, renal disease, electrolyte imbalances, cardiac disease, CHF, hypovolemia
PREGNANCY AND LACTATION: Pregnancy category C; no data on breast feeding available
SIDE EFFECTS/ADVERSE REACTIONS
For systemic use:
CNS: Disorientation, dizziness, fever, *headache,* syncope
CV: Postural hypotension, tachycardia, venous thrombosis
GI: Nausea, vomiting
HEME: **Hemolysis, intraocular bleeding**
METAB: Dehydration, hypokalemia, hyponatremia
SKIN: Extravasation, phlebitis
SPECIAL CONSIDERATIONS
• Do not infuse into lower extremity veins
• Monitor for extravasation, tissue necrosis may occur

U

---

italic = common side effects   ***bold italic*** = life-threatening reactions

urokinase

(yoor-oh-kine´ase)
Rx: Abbokinase, Abbokinase
Open-Cath (not for systemic
administration)
Chemical Class: Renal enzyme
Therapeutic Class: Throm-
bolytic

CLINICAL PHARMACOLOGY
Mechanism of Action: Promotes
thrombolysis by directly converting
plasminogen to plasmin
Pharmacokinetics
Onset of fibrinolysis is rapid, duration ≥4 hr; cleared by liver, small
amount excreted in urine and bile;
unknown if crosses placenta or if excreted in breast milk; $t_{1/2}$ 10-20 min
INDICATIONS AND USES: Massive
pulmonary embolism (PE); arteriovenous cannula occlusion; acute
myocardial infarction; thrombotic
stroke*; arterial thrombosis,* arterial embolism*
DOSAGE
Adult and Child
• *Pulmonary embolism and arterial
or venous thrombosis:* IV 4400
IU/kg over 10 min followed by 4400
IU/kg/hr for 12 hr; after thrombin
time has decreased to less than twice
normal control value (approx 3-4
hr), begin heparin (no loading dose)
• *Venous catheter occlusion:* Instill
into catheter a volume of urokinase
(5000 IU/ml) equal to the internal
volume of catheter over 1-2 min; aspirate from catheter 1-4 hr later,
flush catheter with saline, may repeat with 10,000 U/ml sol if not
cleared
• *Acute   myocardial   infarction
(adult):* Intracoronary (following
IV heparin bolus of 2500 to 10,000
units) 6000 IU/min for up to 2 hr (average dose 500,000 IU); repeat angiography q15min until artery maximally opened; continuing heparin
therapy recommended

**§   AVAILABLE FORMS/COST
OF THERAPY**
• Inj, Lyphl-Sol—IV: 5000 U/ml, 1
ml: **$56.61** (not for systemic admin-
istration); 9000 U/vial: **$98.72** (not
for   systemic   administration);
250,000 U/vial: **$466.17**

CONTRAINDICATIONS: (Systemic therapy only, no contraindications to use for declotting catheter);
active bleeding, intraspinal surgery,
CNS neoplasms; ulcerative colitis,
enteritis; coagulation defects, rheumatic valvular disease; cerebral embolism,   thrombosis,   hemorrhage
within 2 mo; intra-arterial diagnostic procedure, surgery, or trauma
within 10 days; severe hypertension
PRECAUTIONS: Moderate hypertension, recent lumbar puncture, patients receiving IM medications, renal disease, hepatic disease, childbirth within 10 days, diabetic retinopathy, age >75 yr
PREGNANCY AND LACTATION:
Pregnancy   category   B;   no   data
available on breast feeding
**SIDE EFFECTS/ADVERSE REAC-
TIONS**
*CV: **MI,*** tachycardia, transient hypertension or hypotension
GI: Nausea, vomiting
*HEME: **Internal bleeding (GI, GU,
vaginal, IM, retroperitoneal or in-
tracranial sites),*** surface bleeding
METAB: Acidosis
*RESP: **Bronchospasm,*** dyspnea, hy-
poxemia
SKIN: Rash
MISC: Chills, fever

---

* = non-FDA-approved use

INTERACTIONS
Drugs
3 *Heparin, oral anticoagulants, drugs that alter platelet function (i.e., aspirin, dipyridamole, abciximab, eptifibitide, tirofiban):* May increase the risk of bleeding

---

ursodiol
(your-soo'dee-ol)
Rx: Actigall, Urso
Chemical Class: Ursodeoxycholic acid
Therapeutic Class: Cholelitholytic

CLINICAL PHARMACOLOGY
Mechanism of Action: Decreases cholesterol content of bile and gallstones by reducing hepatic cholesterol secretion and reabsorption of cholesterol by the intestine
Pharmacokinetics
PO: 90% absorption from small bowel; 1st-pass hepatic clearance; conjugates secreted into bile; peak concentration 1-3 hr, $t_{1/2}$ 100 hr

INDICATIONS AND USES: Dissolution of radiolucent, non-calcified gallbladder stones (<20 mm in diameter) for which surgery is not indicated; chronic cholestatic liver disease*

DOSAGE
Adult
• PO 8-10 mg/kg/day in 2-3 divided doses; perform gallbladder ultrasound q6mo to determine if stones have dissolved; if so, continue therapy, repeat ultrasound within 1-3 mo; maintenance therapy 250 mg qhs for 6-12 mo; safety beyond 24 mo not established
Child
• *Cholestatic liver disease:* PO 10-18 mg/kg/day

$ AVAILABLE FORMS/COST OF THERAPY
• Cap, Gel—Oral: 300 mg, 100's: **$242.95-$327.98**
• Tab—Oral: 250 mg, 100's: **$194.64-$210.21**

CONTRAINDICATIONS: Calcified cholesterol stones, radiopaque stones, stones >20 mm in diameter, bile pigment stones, patients with compelling reasons for cholecystectomy (cholangitis, biliary obstruction)

PRECAUTIONS: Children, chronic liver disease, non-visualizing gallbladder

PREGNANCY AND LACTATION: Pregnancy category B; excretion into breast milk unknown

SIDE EFFECTS/ADVERSE REACTIONS
CNS: Anxiety, depression, fatigue, headache, insomnia
EENT: Metallic taste, rhinitis
GI: Abdominal pain, constipation, diarrhea, dyspepsia, flatulence, nausea, stomatitis, vomiting
MS: Arthralgia, back pain, myalgia
RESP: Cough
SKIN: Alopecia, dry skin, pruritus, rash, sweating, urticaria

SPECIAL CONSIDERATIONS
• Complete dissolution may not occur; likelihood of success is low if partial stone dissolution not seen by 12 mo
• Stones recur within 5 yr in 50% of patients

PATIENT/FAMILY EDUCATION
• Administer with food to facilitate dissolution in the intestine

V

---

valacyclovir

(val-a-sye′kloe-ver)

Rx: Valtrex
Chemical Class: Acyclovir
derivative
Therapeutic Class: Antiviral

CLINICAL PHARMACOLOGY
Mechanism of Action: Converted to acyclovir triphosphate, causing decreased viral DNA synthesis
Pharmacokinetics
PO: Rapidly absorbed from GI tract and converted to acylovir by 1st-pass intestinal or hepatic metabolism; bioavailability 55% not altered by food; plasma protein binding 14%-18%; excreted in urine (89%) and feces; $t_{1/2}$ of acyclovir 2.5-3.3 hr (14 hr in end-stage renal disease)
INDICATIONS AND USES: Herpes zoster in immunocompetent adults; initial episode and episodic treatment of recurrent genital herpes in immunocompetent adults; suppression of recurrent episodes of genital herpes in immunocompetent adults
DOSAGE
Herpes zoster: PO 1 g tid for 7 days within 72 hr of onset of rash; for CrCl 30-49 ml/min 1 g q12h, CrCl 10-29 ml/min 1 g q24h, CrCl <10 ml/min 500 mg q24h
Initial episode genital herpes: PO 1 g bid for 10 days; for CrCl 10-29 ml/min 1 g qd, CrCl <10 ml/min 500 mg qd
Recurrent genital herpes: PO 500 mg bid for 5 days; for CrCl <30 ml/min, 500 mg qd
Chronic suppression of genital herpes: PO 500-1000 mg qd (if <9 attacks per year, start with 500 mg); for CrCl <30 ml/min, 500 mg q48h

$ **AVAILABLE FORMS/COST OF THERAPY**
• Cap—Oral: 500 mg, 42's: **$142.09-$186.56**
• Tab—Oral: 1 g, 21's: **$72.83-$135.31**
PRECAUTIONS: Renal insufficiency, hepatic insufficiency, elderly, children
PREGNANCY AND LACTATION: Pregnancy category B; acyclovir excreted into breast milk, safety not established but should be compatible with breast feeding
SIDE EFFECTS/ADVERSE REACTIONS
CNS: Dizziness, headache
GI: Abdominal pain, anorexia, constipation, diarrhea, nausea, vomiting
GU: Renal dysfunction
*HEME: **Anemia, thrombocytopenia***
SPECIAL CONSIDERATIONS
• Acyclovir 400 mg PO bid less expensive for chronic suppression of genital herpes

valdecoxib

(val-de-cocks′ib)

Rx: Bextra
Chemical Class: Cyclooxygenase-2 (COX-2) inhibitor
Therapeutic Class: Nonsteroidal antiinflammatory drug (COX-2 specific inhibitor)

CLINICAL PHARMACOLOGY
Mechanism of Action: Inhibition of prostaglandin synthesis, via inhibition of cyclooxygenase-2 (COX-2) provides nonsteroidal antiinflammatory, analgesic, and antipyretic actions; at therapeutic concentrations, does not inhibit cyclooxygenase-1 (COX-1) isoenzyme

Pharmacokinetics

PO: Peak 3 hr Well absorbed, 80% bioavailability without food/antacid effect (PO); extensively metabolized by liver (active major metabolite, no contribution to clinical effects), renal excretion (only 5% unchanged); $t_{1/2}$ 8-11 hr; crosses placenta in rats (human information unavailable)

INDICATIONS AND USES: Osteoarthritis, rheumatoid arthritis, dysmenorrhea, postoperative pain*

DOSAGE

Adult and Child >16 yr

• *Osteoarthritis, rheumatoid arthritis:* PO 10 mg qd

• *Dysmenorrhea:* PO 20-40 mg qd or 20 mg bid

• *Pain:* PO 20-40 mg qd

Renal and Hepatic Dysfunction

• No change in dose in renal failure; significant increases (130%) in valdecoxib levels seen in moderate liver dysfunction; don't exceed 10 mg qd with close monitoring for edema; avoid in patients with severe liver dysfunction

💲 AVAILABLE FORMS/COST OF THERAPY

• Tab, film-coated, capsule shaped—Oral: 10, 20 mg 100's: **$291.50**

CONTRAINDICATIONS: Hypersensitivity; patients who have experienced asthma, urticaria or allergic-type reactions with aspirin or other NSAIDs (aspirin triad); acute peptic ulcer disease or GI bleeding; severe hepatic or renal disease

PRECAUTIONS: History of GI ulceration, concomitant treatment with oral corticosteroids, anticoagulants, smokers, alcoholism, older age, stress, or poor general health status (increased risk for GI ulceration, bleeding, or perforation); mild or moderate renal and liver dysfunction; concurrent diseases increasing risk for renal dysfunction (i.e., diabetes, preexisting edema, hypovolemia, sepsis); pregnancy (1st and 3rd trimesters); CHF, elderly, concurrent diuretics and ACE inhibitors, hypertension

PREGNANCY AND LACTATION: Pregnancy category C; excreted into breast milk of animals

SIDE EFFECTS/ADVERSE REACTIONS

CNS: Dizziness, headache

CV: Hypertension, edema

EENT: Sinusitis

GI: Nausea, dyspepsia, abdominal pain, abdominal fullness, diarrhea, flatulence, ***ulceration***

GU: Serum creatinine, BUN increases

HEME: Anemia

MS: Back pain, myalgia

RESP: Upper respiratory tract infection

SKIN: Rash

INTERACTIONS

Drugs

3 *Angiotensin-converting enzyme inhibitors:* Diminished antihypertensive effects

3 *Aspirin:* Increased risk of GI ulceration; negation of cardioprotective effects of aspirin

3 *Diuretics (loop, thiazides):* Reduced naturetic effect

3 *Lithium:* Elevation of plasma lithium levels, potential lithium toxicity

SPECIAL CONSIDERATIONS

• May be safer that conventional nonsteroidal antiinflammatory agents, particularly with respect to gastrointestinal tolerability, and offer comparable efficacy. Other complications may arise, including cardiovascular complications from selective inhibition of the COX-2 isozyme (see rofecoxib)

V

PATIENT/FAMILY EDUCATION
• Alert for symptoms of adverse effects (e.g., GI ulceration and bleeding, renal dysfunction)
MONITORING PARAMETERS
• Improvement in clinical symptoms (pain, stiffness, mobility, swollen/tender joints); blood pressure in patients with cardiovascular disease, upper gastrointestinal tests are suggested in patients with persistent dyspepsia, nausea, cramps, hematemesis

---

valganciclovir
(val-gan-sye′kloh-veer)
Rx: Valcyte
Chemical Class: Synthetic nucleoside analog
Therapeutic Class: Antiviral

CLINICAL PHARMACOLOGY
Mechanism of Action: Valganciclovir is an L-valyl ester (prodrug) of ganciclovir, converted to ganciclovir by intestinal and hepatic esterases; ganciclovir preferentially phosphorylated in virus-infected cells to ganciclovir-triphosphate, which inhibits viral DNA synthesis by: (1) competitive inhibition of viral DNA polymerases and (2) direct incorporation into viral DNA, causing termination of viral DNA elongation
Pharmacokinetics
PO: Bioavailability 60%; rapidly and completely metabolized to ganciclovir; peak ganciclovir level 1-3 hr; protein binding 1-2%; crosses blood-brain barrier; ganciclovir excreted unchanged by kidney; elimination half life 3-6 hr (prolonged in renal insufficiency); AUC for 900 mg valganciclovir PO same as ganciclovir 5 mg/kg IV and double that of ganciclovir 1000 mg tid PO

INDICATIONS AND USES: Treatment of cytomegalovirus (CMV) retinitis in AIDS patients
DOSAGE
Adult
• Treatment of CMV retinitis: PO 900 mg bid with meals for 21 days; follow with maintenance treatment, PO 900 mg qd with meals
• Renal function impairment (dosage for CrCl in ml/min):
CrCl ≥60 PO 900 mg bid (induction) and 900 mg qd (maintenance);
CrCl 40-59 PO 450 mg bid (induction) and 450 mg qd (maintenance);
CrCl 25-39 PO 450 mg qd (induction) and 450 mg every 2 days (maintenance);
• CrCl 10-24 PO 450 mg every 2 days (induction) and 450 mg twice weekly (maintenance)
AVAILABLE FORMS/COST OF THERAPY
• Tab—Oral: 450   mg,   60's: **$1,798.50**
PRECAUTIONS: Renal insufficiency (CrCl <10 ml/min or dialysis patient), do not administer valganciclovir if the absolute neutrophil count is less than 500 cells/μl, the platelet count is less than 25,000/μl, or the hemoglobin is less than 8 g/dL
PREGNANCY AND LACTATION: Pregnancy category C (teratogenic in animals); breast milk excretion unknown but breast feeding not recommended if taking valganciclovir; do not resume nursing for at least 72 hr after last dose of valganciclovir
SIDE EFFECTS/ADVERSE REACTIONS
CNS: Agitation, confusion, convulsion, *headache* (22%), *insomnia* (16%), *paresthesia* (8%), *peripheral neuropathy,* psychosis
EENT: Retinal detachment
GI: Abdominal pain (15%), *diarrhea* (41%), *nausea* (30%), *vomiting* (21%)

---

* = non-FDA-approved use

GU: Increase in BUN, creatinine

HEME: **Agranulocytosis, thrombo-cytopenia** (6%), **neutropenia** (27%), **anemia** (26%)

MISC: Pyrexia (31%)

INTERACTIONS

Drugs

3 *Didanosine:* Didanosine may increase valganciclovir level; increased hematological toxicity possible

❷ *Mycophenolate:* Mycophenolate may increase valganciclovir level; valganciclovir may increase mycophenolate level; increased hematological toxicity possible

❷ *Probenecid:* Probenecid reduces ganciclovir clearance; increased hematological toxicity possible

A *Zidovudine:* Additive hematological toxicity

SPECIAL CONSIDERATIONS
PATIENT/FAMILY EDUCATION

• Take with food
• Do not take during pregnancy or lactation
• Men should use a condom during sex while using this medicine for at least 3 months after treatment ends because valganciclovir interferes with normal sperm formation

MONITORING PARAMETERS

• CBC, platelet count, creatinine

---

valproate/divalproex
(val-proe´ate)
Rx: *Valproate Sodium:*
Depacon
Valproic acid: Depakene
Divalproex: Depakote,
Depakote Sprinkle
Chemical Class: Carboxylic
acid derivative
Therapeutic Class: Anticonvulsant

CLINICAL PHARMACOLOGY
Mechanism of Action: Increases levels of gamma-aminobutyric acid (GABA), inhibitory neurotransmitter in brain; divalproex dissociates to the valproate ion in the GI tract

Pharmacokinetics
PO: Onset 15-30 min, peak 1-5 hr (slower absorption with sprinkles and food), $t_{1/2}$ 6-16 hr (shorter with younger age and serum levels lower in polytherapy; 40-60 hr in newborns)

RECT: Onset slow, duration 4-6 hr, $t_{1/2}$ 6-16 hr

Metabolized by liver, excreted by kidneys and in feces; crosses placenta; excreted into breast milk

INDICATIONS AND USES: Simple, complex (petit mal) absence, mixed, tonic-clonic (grand mal) seizures, mania in bipolar disorders in adults (divalproex sodium), prophylaxis of adult migraine (divalproex sodium)

DOSAGE
Adult
• *Epilepsy:*
• PO for monotherapy 5-15 mg/kg/day divided in 1-3 doses, may increase by 5-10 mg/kg/day qwk; for polytherapy, initial dose 10-30 mg/kg/day, if dose exceeds 250 mg qd, divide into 2 or more

---

doses, max 60 mg/kg/day; IV same as PO; administer as 60 min infusion at a rate not exceeding 20 mg/min

• *Mania:* (Divalproex sodium)

• PO 750 mg/day in divided doses; increase until desired effect or plasma concentration at trough of 50-125 µg/ml; max 60 mg/kg/day

• *Migraine:*

• PO 250 mg bid; dose may be increased up to 1000 mg/d if necessary

Child

• PO same as adult; children receiving polytherapy may require doses up to 100 mg/kg/day in 3-4 divided doses

• RECT dilute syr 1:1 with water; give loading dose 17-20 mg/kg once as retention enema; maintenance 10-15 mg/kg/day q8h

$ AVAILABLE FORMS/COST OF THERAPY

Valproic Acid

• Cap, Elastic—Oral: 250 mg, 100's: **$22.00-$188.51**

• Syr—Oral: 250 mg/5 ml, 480 ml: **$29.00-$192.70**

Divalproex Sodium

• Cap, Enteric Coated (Sprinkle)—Oral: 125 mg, 100's: **$50.43**

• Tab, Enteric Coated—Oral: 125 mg, 100's: **$50.15**; 250 mg, 100's: **$98.48**; 500 mg, 100's: **$181.63**

Valproate Sodium

• Inj—IV: 100 mg/ml, 5 ml: **$12.18**

CONTRAINDICATIONS: Hepatic disease

PRECAUTIONS: Renal disease, Addison's disease, blood dyscrasias; children <2 yr, patients with organic brain disease, and patients on multiple anticonvulsants (polytherapy) at increased risk of hepatotoxicity

PREGNANCY AND LACTATION: Pregnancy category D; teratogenic; increased risk of neural tube defects (1%-2% when used between day 17-30 after fertilization); compatible with breast feeding

SIDE EFFECTS/ADVERSE REACTIONS

CNS: Ataxia, behavioral changes, **coma,** depression, diplopia, dizziness, *drowsiness,* **encephalopathy,** hallucinations, headache, incoordination, nystagmus, paresthesia, *sedation,* tremors

GI: Anorexia, *constipation,* cramps, *diarrhea, heartburn,* **hepatic failure,** *nausea,* **pancreatitis,** stomatitis, *vomiting*

GU: Amenorrhea, breast enlargement, enuresis, galactorrhea, irregular menses

HEME: **Anemia, hypofibrinogenemia, leukopenia,** lymphocytosis, **thrombocytopenia**

METAB: Abnormal thyroid function tests, carnitine deficiency, hyperammonemia, hyperglycemia, hyponatremia, syndrome of inappropriate antidiuretic hormone release

SKIN: Alopecia, **erythema multiforme,** pruritis, *rash,* **Stevens-Johnson syndrome**

INTERACTIONS

Drugs

▪ *Carbamazepine, phenytoin:* Increase, decrease, or no effect on carbamazepine and phenytoin concentrations

▪ *Cholestyramine, colestipol:* Reduced absorption of valproic acid

▪ *Clarithromycin, erythromycin, troleandomycin:* Increased valproic acid concentrations

▪ *Clonazepam:* Absence seizure reported with concurrent use

▪ *Clozapine:* Reduced serum clozapine concentrations

▪ *Felbamate:* Increased valproic acid concentrations

3 *Isoniazid:* Increased valproic acid concentrations

3 *Lamotrigine:* Increased plasma lamotrigine concentrations; decreased valproic acid concentrations

3 *Nimodipine:* Increased nimodipine area under the plasma concentration-time curve

3 *Phenobarbital, primidone:* Increased phenobarbital levels

3 *Salicylates:* Increased valproate levels

3 *Zidovudine:* Increased zidovudine levels

Labs

• *False increase:* Serum free fatty acids

• *False positive:* Urinary ketones

SPECIAL CONSIDERATIONS

PATIENT/FAMILY EDUCATION

• Administer with food to decrease GI side effects

• Do not administer with carbonated beverages or milk

MONITORING PARAMETERS

• Therapeutic levels (draw just before next dose) 50-100 µg/ml

• ALT, AST, coagulation studies, and platelet count prior to and during therapy, especially 1st 6 mo

• Minor elevations in ALT, AST are frequent and dose related

valsartan
(val-sar'tan)
Rx: Diovan
Combinations
  Rx: with hydrochlorothiazide (Diovan HCT)
Chemical Class: Angiotensin II receptor antagonist
Therapeutic Class: Antihypertensive

CLINICAL PHARMACOLOGY

Mechanism of Action: Antihypertensive (inhibition of vasoconstriction and aldosterone secretion), smooth muscle hypoproliferative, and cardioprotective effects are attributable to selective blockade of angiotensin II (AT1) receptors found throughout the cardiovascular and renal systems; effects independent of angiotensin II synthesis

Pharmacokinetics

PO: Peak 2-4 hr, duration 24 hr; steady state maximal reduction in blood pressure 2-4 wk; bioavailability approx 25%; food decreases exposure significantly; elimination as unchanged drug in feces (83%) and urine (13%); $t_{1/2}$ 6 hr

INDICATIONS AND USES: Hypertension; CHF,* myocardial infarction,* diabetic nephropathy*

DOSAGE

Adult

• *Hypertension:* PO 80-320 mg qd

$ **AVAILABLE FORMS/COST OF THERAPY**

• Cap—Oral: 80 mg, 100's: **$139.75**; 160 mg, 100's: **$151.70**; 320 mg, 100's: **$193.75**

• Tab—Oral (with hydrochlorothiazide): 12.5 mg-80 mg, 100's: **$153.19**; 12.5 mg-160 mg, 100's: **$164.96**

V

PRECAUTIONS: Angioedema (associated with aspirin and/or penicillin allergy), aortic or mitral valve stenosis, biliary cirrhosis or biliary obstruction, breast feeding period, coronary artery disease, elderly patients, hepatic dysfunction (adjust dose), hypertrophic cardiomyopathy, hypotension (sodium- or volume-depleted patients), pregnancy, renal artery stenosis, solitary kidney, or congestive heart failure

PREGNANCY AND LACTATION: Pregnancy category C, first trimester—category D, second and third trimesters; drugs acting directly on the renin-angiotensin-aldosterone system are documented to cause fetal harm (hypotension, oligohydramnios, neonatal anemia, hyperkalemia, neonatal skull hypoplasia, anuria, and renal failure); neonatal limb contractures, craniofacial deformities, and hypoplastic lung development

SIDE EFFECTS/ADVERSE REACTIONS

CNS: Dizziness, headaches
CV: Palpitations
GI: Abdominal pain, constipation, diarrhea, dyspepsia, flatulence, liver function test abnormalities
GU: Impotence
METAB: Hyperkalemia
MS: Back pain, muscle cramps, myalgia
RESP: Cough, dyspnea, pharyngitis, rhinitis, sinusitis
SKIN: Pruritus and rash
MISC: Anemia, fatigue, angioedema

SPECIAL CONSIDERATIONS

• Potentially as or more effective than angiotensin-converting enzyme inhibitors, without cough; no evidence for reduction in morbidity and mortality as first-line agents in hypertension, yet; whether they provide the same cardiac and renal protection also still tentative; like ACE inhibitors, less effective in black patients

PATIENT/FAMILY EDUCATION

• Call your clinician immediately if note following side effects: wheezing; lip, throat, or face swelling; hives or rash

MONITORING PARAMETERS

• Baseline electrolytes, urinalysis, BUN and creatinine with recheck at 2-4 wk after initiation (sooner in volume-depleted patients); monitor sitting blood pressure; watch for symptomatic hypotension, particularly in volume-depleted patients

---

vancomycin

(van-koe-mye'sin)
Rx: Lyphocin, Vancocin, Vancoled
Chemical Class: Tricyclic glycopeptide derivative
Therapeutic Class: Antibiotic

CLINICAL PHARMACOLOGY

Mechanism of Action: Inhibits bacterial cell wall synthesis, cell membrane permeability, and RNA synthesis; bactericidal against Gram-positive organisms, except bacteriostatic against enterococci

Pharmacokinetics

PO: Absorption poor
IV: 15 mg/kg over 60 min yields mean plasma concentration of 63, 23, and 8 µg/ml immediately, 2 hr, and 8 hr after INF; penetrates inflamed meninges, and into inflamed pleural, pericardial, ascitic, and synovial fluids, urine, peritoneal dialysis fluid, atrial appendage tissue, and bile; 55% protein bound; $t_{1/2}$ 4-8 hr; excreted in urine (active form); linearly associated with creatinine

clearance; therapeutic serum concentrations, peak 25-40 µg/ml, trough <5-10 µg/ml

INDICATIONS AND USES: Serious or severe Gram-positive infections not treatable with other antimicrobials, including penicillins and cephalosporins, caused by susceptible organisms (e.g., endocarditis, osteomyelitis, pneumonia, and pseudomembranous colitis)

Antibacterial spectrum usually includes:

• Gram-positive organisms: Staphylococci, streptococci, *enterococcus*
• Anaerobes: *C. difficile*

DOSAGE

NOTE: Administer IV doses over 60 min; prevents "red-neck syndrome"

Adult

• *Serious staphylococcal infections:* IV 500 mg q6h or 1 g q12h
• *Pseudomembranous, staphylococcal enterocolitis:* PO 500 mg to 2 g/day in 3-4 divided doses for 7-10 days
• *Dosage adjustment for renal impairment:* After initial loading dose of 750 mg to 1 g, CrCl 50-80 ml/min 1 g q1-3d, CrCl 10-50 ml/min 1 g q3-7d, CrCl <10 1 g q7-14d; guided by serum vancomycin concentrations

Child

• *Serious staphylococcal infections:* IV 40 mg/kg/day divided q6h

Neonates

• *Serious staphylococcal infections:* IV 15 mg/kg initially followed by 10 mg/kg q8-12h
• *Pseudomembranous, staphylococcal enterocolitis:* PO 40 mg/kg/day divided q6h, not to exceed 2 g/day

$ AVAILABLE FORMS/COST OF THERAPY

• Cap, Gel—Oral: 125 mg, 20's: **$134.00**; 250 mg, 20's: **$268.01**

• Inj, Conc-Sol—IV: 500 mg/vial: **$7.80-$13.76**; 1 g/vial: **$1.56-$24.54**
• Powder, Reconst—Oral: 250 mg/5 ml, 10, 20 ml: **$37.08**; 500 mg/6 ml, 120 ml: **$340.58**

CONTRAINDICATIONS: Decreased hearing

PRECAUTIONS: Renal disease, elderly, neonates

PREGNANCY AND LACTATION: Pregnancy category C (oral), B (IV); excreted into breast milk, milk level 4 hr after steady state dose, 12.7 µg/ml (similar to mother's trough level); poorly absorbed orally, systemic absorption not expected; problems limited to modification of bowel flora, allergic sensitization, and interference with interpretation of culture results during fever workup

SIDE EFFECTS/ADVERSE REACTIONS

CV: **Cardiac arrest, vascular collapse**

EENT: Ototoxicity, permanent deafness, tinnitus

HEME: Eosinophilia, **leukopenia, neutropenia**

GI: Nausea

GU: **Nephrotoxicity**

RESP: Dyspnea, wheezing

SKIN: Chills, fever, necrosis with extravasation (red man's syndrome or "red-neck syndrome"), pruritus, rash, thrombophlebitis at inj site, urticaria

INTERACTIONS

Drugs

3 *Aminoglycosides:* Enhanced nephrotoxicity

3 *Indomethacin:* Increased vancomycin in neonates, possible vancomycin toxicity

3 *Methotrexate:* Reduced methotrexate concentrations with oral vancomycin

Labs
• *False increase:* CSF protein
SPECIAL CONSIDERATIONS
MONITORING PARAMETERS
• Audiograms, BUN, creatinine, serum vancomycin concentrations

---

vasopressin

(vay-soe-press'in)
Rx: Pitressin
Chemical Class: Arginine vasopressin
Therapeutic Class: Antidiuretic; hemostatic

CLINICAL PHARMACOLOGY
Mechanism of Action: A posterior pituitary hormone product; has ADH activity (promotes renal tubular reabsorption of water) and vasopressor activity (vascular smooth muscle contraction)
Pharmacokinetics
IM/SC: Antidiuretic activity duration 2-8 hr
Metabolized or destroyed in liver, kidneys; excreted in urine; $t_{1/2}$ 15 min
INDICATIONS AND USES: Neurogenic diabetes insipidus, treatment of abdominal distension postoperatively, prior to abdominal x-rays to dispel interfering gas shadows, bleeding esophageal varices*
DOSAGE
Adult
• *Diabetes insipidus:* IM/SC 5-10 U bid-tid as needed
• *Abdominal distension:* IM 5 U, increasing to 10 U after 3-4 hr if needed
• *Abdominal x-rays:* IM/SC 10 U given 2 hr and then ½ hr prior to x-rays
• *Esophageal varices:* IV or selective intra-arterial: 0.2 U/min initially, increased to 0.4 U/min if bleeding continues (max 0.9 U/min)

Child
• *Diabetes insipidus:* IM/SC 2.5-10 U bid-qid as needed
$ **AVAILABLE FORMS/COST OF THERAPY**
• Inj, Sol—IM, SC: 20 U/ml, 2 ml: **$8.06-$9.07**
CONTRAINDICATIONS: Chronic nephritis
PRECAUTIONS: Vascular disease (especially CAD), epilepsy, migraine, asthma, CHF
PREGNANCY AND LACTATION: Pregnancy category C; breast feeding reported without complications
SIDE EFFECTS/ADVERSE REACTIONS
CNS: Drowsiness, flushing, headache, lethargy, tremor, vertigo
CV: Angina, *cardiac arrest,* circumoral pallor, decreased cardiac output, *dysrhythmias,* gangrene, hypertension, *MI,* peripheral vasoconstriction
GI: Cramps, flatus, heartburn, nausea, vomiting
GU: Uterine cramping, vulvar pain
METAB: Hyponatremia
RESP: Bronchial constriction
SKIN: Sweating, urticaria, vasoconstriction or necrosis with extravasation
SPECIAL CONSIDERATIONS
• For diabetes insipidus, vasopressin sol for injection may be administered intranasally on cotton pledgets, by nasal spray or by dropper; dose must be individualized
PATIENT/FAMILY EDUCATION
• Common adverse effects (skin blanching, abdominal cramps, and nausea) may be reduced by taking 1-2 glasses of water with the dose of vasopressin; self-limited in minutes
MONITORING PARAMETERS
• ECG, fluid and electrolyte status
• Extravasation may cause tissue necrosis

---

* = non-FDA-approved use

venlafaxine

(ven-la-fax´een)

Rx: Effexor, Effexor XR
Chemical Class: Phenethyl-amine derivative
Therapeutic Class: Antidepressant

CLINICAL PHARMACOLOGY

Mechanism of Action: Potentiation of neurotransmitter activity in the CNS by strong inhibition of neuronal serotonin and norepinephrine reuptake and weak inhibition of dopamine reuptake; no anticholinergic, sedation, or orthostatic hypotensive activity

Pharmacokinetics

PO: Peak level 1-2 hr, steady state level of drug and active metabolites achieved in 3 days; absorption 92% (no change with food); protein binding 27%; metabolized by cytochrome p450 system in liver, unchanged drug and metabolites excreted in urine; elimination $t_{1/2}$ 3-7 hr for drug, 9-13 hr for active metabolites; clearance of drug and active metabolites reduced by 50% in cirrhotics, reduced by 25% if CrCl 10-70 ml/min, and reduced by 60% in dialysis patients

INDICATIONS AND USES: Depression, obsessive-compulsive disorder,* generalized anxiety disorder

DOSAGE

Adult

• PO starting dose 75 mg/day, given bid or tid (qd for Sus Action); increase daily dose by 75 mg up to 225 mg/day, given bid or tid (qd for Sus Action) (375 mg/day for severe depression) at intervals of no less than 4 days

• Reduce total daily dose 25% in patients with mild to moderate renal impairment, by 50% in patients with severe renal impairment; dialysis patients should receive dose after dialysis; reduce total daily dose by 50% in patients with moderate hepatic impairment

• When discontinuing drug, taper over 2 wk

💲 AVAILABLE FORMS/COST OF THERAPY

• Cap, Sus Action—Oral: 37.5 mg, 100's: **$233.56**; 75 mg, 100's: **$253.01**; 150 mg, 100's: **$285.00**
• Tab, Uncoated—Oral: 25 mg, 100's: **$137.88**; 37.5 mg, 100's: **$142.00**; 50 mg, 100's: **$146.23**; 75 mg, 100's: **$155.05**; 100 mg, 100's: **$164.33**

CONTRAINDICATIONS: Concurrent use of MAOIs (at least 14 days should elapse between discontinuation of an MAOI and initiation of venlafaxine; at least 7 days should be allowed after stopping venlafaxine before starting an MAOI), age <18 yr

PRECAUTIONS: Hypertension, anxiety, seizures, aggravation of bipolar disorder (0.5%)

PREGNANCY AND LACTATION: Pregnancy category C; excretion into breast milk unknown

SIDE EFFECTS/ADVERSE REACTIONS

*CNS: Anxiety, dizziness, insomnia, nervousness, **seizures (0.3%)**, somnolence, tremor*

CV: Hypertension (dose dependent; frequency 3%-13%), *vasodilation*

EENT: Blurred vision, dry mouth, dysgeusia, mydriasis, tinnitus

GI: Anorexia, dyspepsia, nausea, vomiting

GU: Abnormal ejaculation or orgasm; impotence, urinary retention

RESP: Yawning

SKIN: Sweating

MISC: Asthenia

SPECIAL CONSIDERATIONS

• Do not stop abruptly

V

verapamil

(ver-ap′a-mill)
Rx: Calan, Calan SR, Covera HS, Isoptin, Isoptin SR, Verelan
Combinations
   Rx: with trandolapril (Tarka)
Chemical Class: Phenylalkylamine
Therapeutic Class: Calcium channel blocker, antihypertensive; antianginal; antidysrhythmic (Class IV)

CLINICAL PHARMACOLOGY
Mechanism of Action: Inhibits calcium ion influx across cell membrane during cardiac depolarization; produces relaxation of coronary vascular smooth muscle; dilates coronary arteries; slows SA/AV node conduction; dilates peripheral arteries; hemodynamics: decreases myocardial contractility and peripheral vascular resistance; can decrease or increase cardiac output
Pharmacokinetics
IV: Onset 3 min, peak 3-5 min, duration 10-20 min
PO: Onset variable (30 min for non-sustained-release preparations), peak serum concentration 1-2.2 hr, duration 17-24 hr, 90% absorption; extensive 1st-pass metabolism; bioavailability 20%-35%; 83%-90% protein bound; metabolized by liver to norverapamil (20% activity of verapamil), excreted in urine (96% as metabolites); $t_{1/2}$ (biphasic) 4 min, 3-7 hr (terminal)
INDICATIONS AND USES: Chronic stable angina pectoris, vasospastic angina, unstable angina, dysrhythmias (atrial flutter, atrial fibrillation, paroxysmal supraventricular tachycardia [PSVT]), hypertension, pro-

phylaxis of migraine headaches,* cardiomyopathy (diastolic dysfunction)
DOSAGE
Adult
• *Angina:* PO initial 80-120 mg tid; titrate to 480 mg/day based on response (adjust dose weekly)
• *Dysrhythmias (atrial fibrillation/digitalized):* PO 240-320 mg/day in tid or qid dosage
• *Dysrhythmias (supraventricular tachycardia):* IV bolus initial 5-10 mg over 2 min; repeat dose 10 mg, 30 min after 1st if ineffective
• *Hypertension:* PO 80 mg bid initially, increase as need to 480 mg/d divided bid; Sus Action 180-240 mg qd initially, increase as need up to 360 mg/day
Child 0-1 yr
• *Dysrhythmias (PSVT):* IV bolus 0.1-0.2 mg/kg over >2 min with ECG monitoring; repeat if necessary in 30 min
Child 1-15 yr
• *Dysrhythmias (PSVT):* IV bolus 0.1-0.3 mg/kg over >2 min; repeat in 30 min; not to exceed 10 mg in a single dose
$ AVAILABLE FORMS/COST OF THERAPY
• Cap, Sus Action: 100 mg, 100's: **$135.00**; 120 mg, 100's: **$129.05-$185.08**; 180 mg, 100's: **$135.16-$193.81**; 200 mg, 100's: **$173.88**; 240 mg, 100's: **$152.54-$218.74**; 300 mg, 100's: **$252.79**; 360 mg, 100's: **$209.94-$301.08**
• Inj, Sol—IV: 2.5 mg/ml, 2 ml: **$1.65-$12.25**
• Tab, Coated, Sus Action—Oral: 120 mg, 100's: **$86.79-$135.55**; 180 mg, 100's: **$22.93-$171.79**; 240 mg, 100's: **$27.74-$196.54**
• Tab, Plain Coated—Oral: 40 mg, 100's: **$26.15-$49.85**; 80 mg, 100's: **$9.36-$71.70**; 120 mg, 100's: **$12.30-$106.50**

* = non-FDA-approved use

CONTRAINDICATIONS: Sick sinus syndrome, 2nd or 3rd degree heart block, hypotension less than 90 mm Hg systolic, cardiogenic shock, severe CHF

PRECAUTIONS: CHF, hypotension, hepatic injury, children, renal disease, concomitant IV β-blocker therapy, cirrhosis, Duchenne's muscular dystrophy

PREGNANCY AND LACTATION: Pregnancy category C; excreted in breast milk (approx 25% of maternal serum); compatible with breast feeding

SIDE EFFECTS/ADVERSE REACTIONS

CNS: Asthenia, dizziness, headache, lightheadedness

CV: **AV block,** bradycardia, **CHF,** edema, hypotension, palpitations

GI: Constipation, nausea

GU: Nocturia, polyuria

SKIN: Rash

INTERACTIONS

Drugs

3 *Amiodarone:* Cardiotoxicity with bradycardia and decreased cardiac output

3 *Barbiturates:* Reduced plasma concentrations of verapamil

3 *Benzodiazepines:* Marked increase in midazolam concentrations, increased sedation likely to result

3 *Beta-blockers:* β-blocker serum concentrations increased *(atenolol, metoprolol, propranolol);* increased risk of bradycardia, hypotension, AV conduction, and myocardial contractility

2 *Carbamazepine:* Increased carbamazepine toxicity when verapamil added to chronic anticonvulsant regimens; reduced metabolism

3 *Cimetidine:* Increased verapamil concentrations and effect by cimetidine

3 *Cyclosporine, tacrolimus:* Increased concentrations of these drugs, nephrotoxicity possible

3 *Dantrolene:* Hyperkalemia and myocardial depression may occur; consider a dihydropyridine calcium blocker

3 *Diclofenac:* Reduced verapamil concentrations

3 *Digitalis glycosides:* Increased digoxin concentrations by approximately 70%

3 *Doxazosin, prazosin, terazosin:* Enhanced hypotensive effects

3 *Doxorubicin:* Increased doxorubicin concentrations

3 *Encainide:* Increased encainide concentrations

3 *Ethanol:* Increased ethanol concentrations, prolonged and increased levels of intoxication

3 *Fentanyl:* Severe hypotension or increased fluid volume requirements

3 *Histamine H_2-antagonists:* Increased blood levels of verapamil with cimetidine

3 *Hydantoins:* Serum verapamil levels may fall if used concurrently

3 *Imipramine:* Increased imipramine concentrations

3 *Lithium:* Potential for neurotoxicity

3 *Neuromuscular blocking agents:* Prolonged neuromuscular blockade

3 *Quinidine:* Quinidine toxicity via inhibition of metabolism

3 *Rifampin, rifabutin:* Induced metabolism; reduced verapamil concentrations

3 *Sulfinpyrazone:* Increased clearance of verapamil

3 *Theophylline:* Verapamil inhibits metabolism, increases theophylline levels

3 *Vitamin D:* Therapeutic efficacy of verapamil may be reduced

V

---

italic = common side effects   ***bold italic*** = life-threatening reactions

SPECIAL CONSIDERATIONS

• Dihydropyridine calcium channel blockers preferred over verapamil and diltiazem in patients with sinus bradycardia, conduction disturbances, and for combination with a β-blocker

• Differentiate PSVT from narrow complex ventricular tachycardia prior to IV administration; failure to do so has resulted in fatalities

---

vidarabine

(vye-dare'a-been)

Rx: Vira-A

Chemical Class: Nucleoside analog

Therapeutic Class: Antiviral

CLINICAL PHARMACOLOGY

Mechanism of Action: Inhibits bacterial and viral replication by preventing DNA synthesis

Pharmacokinetics

OPHTH: Minimal systemic absorption

INDICATIONS AND USES: Acute keratoconjunctivitis and recurrent epithelial keratitis; superficial keratitis caused by susceptible organisms

Antiviral spectrum usually includes herpes simplex virus 1 and 2, varicella zoster, and vaccinia viruses, except for rhabdovirus and oncornavirus; minimal activity against other RNA or DNA viruses

DOSAGE

Adult and Child

• OPHTH: ½ inch ribbon to lower lid 5 times daily (q3h); after re-epithelialization, treat for 7 more days at bid

💲 AVAILABLE FORMS/COST OF THERAPY

• Oint—Ophth: 3%, 3.5 g: **$24.81**

PREGNANCY AND LACTATION: Pregnancy category C

SIDE EFFECTS/ADVERSE REACTIONS

EENT: Burning, pain, photophobia, stinging, temporary visual haze

INTERACTIONS

Drugs

🔢 *Allopurinol:* Increased vidarabine toxicity

SPECIAL CONSIDERATIONS

• Trifluridine is more effective; vidarabine is not the drug of choice in any viral infection; however, it may be a useful alternative in patients who cannot tolerate or have failed other antiviral therapy

---

vitamin A

Rx: Aquasol A

Chemical Class: Fat soluble vitamin

Therapeutic Class: Vitamin

CLINICAL PHARMACOLOGY

Mechanism of Action: Involved in bone and tooth development, visual dark adaptation, skin disease, mucosa tissue repair, assists in production of adrenal steroids, cholesterol, RNA

Pharmacokinetics

PO/IM: Stored in liver, kidneys, fat; transported in plasma as retinol, bound to retinol-binding protein, excreted (metabolites) in bile bound to glucuronide and small amount in urine

INDICATIONS AND USES: Vitamin A deficiency

DOSAGE

Adult and Child >8 yr

• PO 100,000-500,000 IU qd × 3 days, then 50,000 qd × 2 wk; dose based on severity of deficiency; maintenance 10,000-20,000 IU qd for 2 mo

---

* = non-FDA-approved use

Child 1-8 yr
• IM 5,000-15,000 IU qd × 10 days; then maintenance as follows:
Child 4-8 yr
• IM 15,000 IU qd × 2 mo
Child <4 yr
• IM 10,000 IU qd × 2 mo
Infants <1 yr
• IM 5,000-15,000 IU × 10 days

$ AVAILABLE FORMS/COST OF THERAPY
• Cap, Elastic—Oral: 25,000 U, 100's: **$3.50-$50.08**; 50,000 U, 100's: **$5.50-$87.10**
• Inj, Sol—IM: 50,000 U/ml, 2 ml: **$22.17-$27.67**

CONTRAINDICATIONS: Malabsorption syndrome (PO)

PRECAUTIONS: Impaired renal function

PREGNANCY AND LACTATION: Pregnancy category A; safety of exceeding 5000/6000 IU PO/IV recommended daily allowance (RDA) not established; naturally present in breast milk, deficiency rare, RDA during lactation is 6000 IU; danger of higher doses unknown

SIDE EFFECTS/ADVERSE REACTIONS
CNS: Headache, increased intracranial pressure, intracranial hypertension, lethargy, malaise
EENT: Exophthalmos, gingivitis, inflammation of tongue and lips, papilledema
GI: Abdominal pain, anorexia, jaundice, nausea, vomiting
METAB: Hypercalcemia, hypomenorrhea
MS: Arthralgia, hard areas on bone, retarded growth
SKIN: Alopecia, drying of skin, increased pigmentation, night sweats, pruritus

INTERACTIONS
Drugs
3 *Acitretin, etretinate:* Large doses of vitamin A should be avoided with these retinoids
SPECIAL CONSIDERATIONS
PATIENT/FAMILY EDUCATION
• Administer with food for better PO absorption
• Foods high in vitamin A: yellow and dark green vegetables, yellow and orange fruits, A-fortified foods, liver, egg yolks

---

vitamin D (cholecalciferol, vitamin D₃; ergocalciferol, vitamin D₂)

(cole′ee-cal-sif′er-ol; er′go-cal-sif′erol)
Rx: Calciferol, Drisdol
OTC: Calciferol, Drisdol
Chemical Class: Fat soluble vitamin
Therapeutic Class: Vitamin

CLINICAL PHARMACOLOGY
Mechanism of Action: Participates in regulation of calcium, phosphate, bone development, parathyroid activity, neuromuscular functioning; synthesis in two steps: hydroxylation in the liver (to 25-hydroxy vitamin D) and in the kidneys (to 1,25-dihydroxy vitamin D); parathyroid hormone is responsible for regulation of metabolism in the kidneys
Pharmacokinetics
PO/INJ: Lag of 10 to 24 hr between the administration of vitamin D and the initiation of its action in the body due to the necessity of synthesis of active metabolites; max hypercalcemic effects at 4 wk, duration 2 mo, readily absorbed from small intestine (bile is essential for adequate

V

absorption), $t_{1/2}$ 7-12 hr; stored in liver; excreted in bile (metabolites) and urine

INDICATIONS AND USES: Dietary supplement, vitamin D deficiency, refractory rickets, renal osteodystrophy, hypoparathyroidism, hypophosphatemia, hypocalcemic tetany, osteoporosis

DOSAGE

NOTE: The range between therapeutic and toxic doses is narrow; calcium intake should be adequate; cholecalciferol 1 mg provides 40,000 U vitamin D activity; ergocalciferol 1.25 mg provides 50,000 IU of vitamin D activity

Adult

• Dietary supplementation (including prevention of osteoporosis): PO 400-800 IU qd

• *Vitamin D deficiency:* PO/IM 12,000 IU qd, then increase to 500,000 IU qd

• *Vitamin D-resistant rickets:* PO/IM 12,000 to 500,000 IU qd

• *Hypoparathyroidism:* PO/IM 25,000 to 200,000 IU qd concomitantly with calcium lactate 4 g, administered 6 times/day

• Refractory rickets: PO/IM 12,000-500,000 IU qd (with phosphate supplements)

• Familial hypophosphatemia: PO/IM 10,000-80,000 IU qd (with 1-2 g/day elemental phosphorous)

Child

• Dietary supplementation: PO 400 IU qd

• *Vitamin D deficiency:* PO/IM 1500-5000 IU qd × 2-4 wk, may repeat after 2 wk or 600,000 IU as single dose

• *Hypoparathyroidism:* PO/IM 50,000-200,000 IU qd (with calcium supplements)

• Refractory rickets: PO/IM 400,000-800,000 IU qd (with phosphate supplements)

§ AVAILABLE FORMS/COST OF THERAPY

• Cap, Elastic—Oral: 50,000 U D_2, 100's: **$3.57-$36.00**

• Inj—IM: 500,000 IU/ml, D_2, 1 ml amp: **$32.45**

• Liq—Oral: 8000 U/ml D_2, 60 ml (OTC): **$18.72-$88.86**

• Tab—Oral: 400 IU D_3, 100's: **$3.33**

CONTRAINDICATIONS: Hypercalcemia, renal dysfunction, hyperphosphatemia, abnormal sensitivity to the toxic effects of vitamin D and hypervitaminosis D

PRECAUTIONS: Cardiovascular disease, renal calculi, elderly

PREGNANCY AND LACTATION: Pregnancy category A (400 IU/d); category D (doses above recommended daily allowance) associated with supravalvular aortic stenosis, elfin facies, and mental retardation; caution should be exercised when ergocalciferol is administered to nursing women; vitamin D and metabolites appear in breast milk; compatible with breast feeding, but infant should be monitored for hypercalcemia if doses exceed recommended daily allowance

SIDE EFFECTS/ADVERSE REACTIONS

CNS: Drowsiness, fatigue, headache, psychosis, *seizures,* weakness, anorexia

CV: **Dysrhythmias,** hypertension, vascular calcification

GI: Constipation, cramps, diarrhea, dry mouth, metallic taste, nausea, vomiting, *pancreatitis,* elevated ALT/AST

GU: Albuminuria, decreased libido, hematuria, nocturia, polyuria, reversible azotemia

METAB: Hypercholesterolemia, mild acidosis

MS: Bone pain, muscle pain, weakness

* = non-FDA-approved use

SKIN: Photophobia, pruritus
MISC: Weight loss

INTERACTIONS

Labs

• *Interference:* Serum cholesterol

SPECIAL CONSIDERATIONS

• IM therapy should be reserved for patients with GI, liver, or biliary disease associated with vitamin D malabsorption

• Ensure adequate calcium intake; maintain serum calcium levels between 9-10 mg/dL

MONITORING PARAMETERS

• Serum calcium and phosphorus levels (vitamin D levels also helpful, although less frequently)

• Height and weight in children

• X-ray bones monthly until condition is corrected and stabilized

• Periodically determine magnesium and alk phosphatase

• Serum calcium times phosphorous should not exceed 70 mg/dL to avoid ectopic calcification

---

vitamin E

OTC: Aquasol E, E-400, Gordon's Vite E

Chemical Class: Fat soluble vitamin

Therapeutic Class: Vitamin

CLINICAL PHARMACOLOGY

Mechanism of Action: Involved in digestion and metabolism of polyunsaturated fats, decreases platelet aggregation, decreases blood clot formation, promotes normal growth and development of muscle tissue, prostaglandin synthesis

Pharmacokinetics

PO: Metabolized in liver, excreted in bile

INDICATIONS AND USES: Vitamin E deficiency, impaired fat absorption,* hemolytic anemia in premature neonates,* prevention of retrolental fibroplasia,* sickle cell anemia,* supplement in malabsorption syndrome*; reduction of the risk of second MI in patients with CAD*

DOSAGE

Adult

• *Vitamin E deficiency:* PO/IM 6075 IU qd, not to exceed 300 IU/day

• *Secondary prevention of MI:* PO 400-800 IU/d

Child

• *Vitamin E deficiency:* PO/IM 1 IU/kg/day

$ AVAILABLE FORMS/COST OF THERAPY

• Cap, Gel—Oral: 100 IU, 100's: **$2.70-$88.74**; 200 IU, 100's: **$2.20-$6.53**; 400 IU, 100's: **$2.90-$12.50**; 600 IU, 100's: **$9.15**; 1000 IU, 100's: **$5.99-$27.30**

• Sol, Drops—Oral: 50 IU/0.3 ml, 12 ml: **$24.68**

PREGNANCY AND LACTATION: Pregnancy category A (C if used above recommended daily allowance doses); recommended daily allowance in pregnancy is 15 IU; excreted into breast milk, 5 times richer in vitamin E than cow's milk; U.S. recommended daily allowance of vitamin E during lactation is 16 IU

SIDE EFFECTS/ADVERSE REACTIONS

CNS: Fatigue, headache

EENT: Blurred vision

GI: Cramps, diarrhea, nausea

GU: Gonadal dysfunction

METAB: Altered metabolism of thyroid, pituitary, and adrenal hormones

MS: Weakness

SKIN: Contact dermatitis, sterile abscess

---

italic = common side effects   ***bold italic*** = life-threatening reactions

INTERACTIONS
Drugs

☒ *Iron:* Impaired hematological response to iron in children with iron-deficiency anemia

☒ *Oral anticoagulants:* Vitamin E increases hypoprothrombinemic response to oral anticoagulants, especially in doses >400 IU/day

SPECIAL CONSIDERATIONS

• Recommended daily allowance adult male 15 IU, adult female 12 IU

---

warfarin
(war´far-in)

Rx: Coumadin, Warfilone
Chemical Class: Coumarin derivative
Therapeutic Class: Oral anticoagulant

CLINICAL PHARMACOLOGY

Mechanism of Action: Interferes with hepatic synthesis of vitamin K dependent clotting factors, causing depression in the activity of factors II, VII, IX, X and proteins C and S in a dose-dependent manner; has no direct effect on established thrombus, but prevents further extension of formed clot

Pharmacokinetics

PO: Rapidly and completely absorbed, peak activity 1½-3 days, duration 2-5 days; 97%-99% bound to plasma proteins; metabolized by hepatic microsomal enzymes; excreted in urine and feces (inactive metabolites); $t_{1/2}$ 36 hr

INDICATIONS AND USES: Prophylaxis and treatment of: venous thrombosis; pulmonary embolism; atrial fibrillation with embolism; thromboembolic complications associated with cardiac valve replacement; and death, recurrent MI, and systemic embolism after MI; recurrent transient ischemic attack,* hypercoagulable states*

DOSAGE
Adult

• PO initiate with 5 mg qd for 2-4 days; adjust dosage according to INR determinations; make dose adjustments in 5-20% increments based on weekly dose of warfarin; usual maintenance dose 2-10 mg qd based on INR determinations

Child

• PO 0.1 mg/kg/day with a range of 0.05-0.34 mg/kg/day; adjust dosage according to INR determinations; consistent anticoagulation may be difficult to maintain in children <5 yr

🄢 **AVAILABLE FORMS/COST OF THERAPY**

• Sol, Inj—IV: 5 mg: **$22.58**
• Tab, Uncoated—Oral: 1 mg, 100's: **$53.35-$65.40**; 2 mg, 100's: **$55.67-$68.24**; 2.5 mg, 100's: **$57.45-$70.43**; 3 mg, 100's: **$60.55-$70.69**; 4 mg, 100's: **$57.83-$70.88**; 5 mg, 100's: **$58.21-$71.32**; 6 mg, 100's: **$86.69-$101.21**; 7.5 mg, 100's: **$85.43-$104.71**; 10 mg, 100's: **$88.61-$108.61**

CONTRAINDICATIONS: Active bleeding, hemorrhagic blood dyscrasias; hemorrhagic tendencies, history of bleeding diathesis, recent cerebral hemorrhage; active ulceration of the GI tract; ulcerative colitis; open traumatic or surgical wounds; recent or contemplated brain, eye, spinal cord surgery, or prostatectomy; regional or lumbar block anesthesia; bacterial endocarditis; pericarditis; visceral carcinoma; severe or malignant hypertension; eclampsia or pre-eclampsia; threatened abortion; emacia-

---

* = non-FDA-approved use

tion; pregnancy; history of warfarin-induced skin necrosis; uncooperative patient

PRECAUTIONS: Trauma, infection, renal insufficiency, hypertension, vasculitis, indwelling catheters, severe diabetes, active tuberculosis, postpartum, protein C deficiency, hepatic insufficiency, elderly, children, hyperthyroidism, hypothyroidism, CHF, polyarteritis, diverticulitis, antibiotic therapy, malnutrition

PREGNANCY AND LACTATION: Pregnancy category X; use in 1st trimester carries significant risk to the fetus; exposure in the 6th-9th wk of gestation may produce a pattern of defects termed the fetal warfarin syndrome with an incidence up to 25% in some series; compatible with breast feeding for normal, full-term infants

SIDE EFFECTS/ADVERSE REACTIONS

GI: Anorexia, cholestatic jaundice, ***hepatotoxicity,*** mouth ulcers, nausea, paralytic ileus, sore mouth, vomiting

GU: Albuminuria, anuria, red-orange urine, ***renal tubular necrosis***

HEME: ***Hemorrhage, leukopenia***

SKIN: Alopecia, dermatitis, ***exfoliative dermatitis, necrosis or gangrene of skin and other tissues,*** urticaria

MISC: Systemic cholesterol microembolization ("purple toe" syndrome)

INTERACTIONS

Drugs

3 *Acetaminophen:* Repeated doses of acetaminophen may increase the hypoprothrombinemic response to warfarin

3 *Allopurinol, amiodarone, ciprofloxacin, clarithromycin, erythromycin, fluconazole, fluorouracil, fluvastatin, fluvoxamine, glucagon, isoniazid, itraconazole, ketoconazole, lovastatin, miconazole, nalidixic acid, neomycin (oral), norfloxacin, ofloxacin, propafenone, propoxyphene, quinidine, sertraline, sulfonamides, sulfonylureas, thyroid hormones, triclofos, troleandomycin, vitamin E, zafirlukast:* Enhanced hypoprothrombinemic response to warfarin

3 *Aminoglutethimide, carbamazepine, cyclophosphamide, ethchlorvynol, griseofulvin, mercaptopurine, methimazole, mitotane, nafcillin, propylthiouracil, vitamin K:* Reduced hypoprothrombinemic response to warfarin

2 *Aspirin:* Increased risk of bleeding complications

2 *Azathioprine, chloramphenicol, cimetidine, clofibrate, co-trimoxazole, danazole, dextrothyroxine, disulfiram, gemfibrozil, metronidazole, sulfinpyrazone, testosterone derivatives:* Enhanced hypoprothrombinemic response to warfarin

2 *Barbiturates, glutethimide, rifampin:* Reduced hypoprothrombinemic response to warfarin

3 *Bile acid-binding resins:* Variable effect on hypoprothrombinemic effect of warfarin

2 *Cephalosporins:* Enhanced hypoprothrombinemic response to warfarin with moxalactam, cefoperazone, cefamandole, cefotetan, and cefmetazole

3 *Chloral hydrate:* Transient increase in hypoprothrombinemic response to warfarin

3 *Ethanol:* Enhanced hypoprothrombinemic response to warfarin with acute ethanol intoxication

3 *Heparin:* Prolonged activated partial thromboplastin time in patients receiving heparin; prolonged prothrombin times in patients receiving warfarin

w

---

italic = common side effects   ***bold italic*** = life-threatening reactions

3 *Mesalamine:* Warfarin effect inhibited in one case report

2 *NSAIDs:* Increased risk of bleeding in anticoagulated patients

2 *Oral contraceptives:* Increase or decrease in anticoagulant response; increased risk of thromboembolic disorders

3 *Phenytoin:* Transient increase in hypoprothrombinemic response to warfarin with initiation of phenytoin therapy, followed within 1-2 wk by inhibition of hypoprothrombinemic response to warfarin

3 *Salicylates:* Increased risk of bleeding in anticoagulated patients; enhanced hypoprothrombinemic response to warfarin with large salicylate doses

Labs
• *Interference:* May cause orange-red discoloration of urine, which may interfere with some lab tests

SPECIAL CONSIDERATIONS
• Avoid use of initial doses >5 mg
• INR during 1st 5 days of therapy does not correlate with degree of anticoagulation
• Anticoagulant effect of warfarin may be reversed by administration of vitamin K or fresh frozen plasma; should only use in situations where INR is severely elevated >10, or when patient is actively bleeding

PATIENT/FAMILY EDUCATION
• Strict adherence to prescribed dosage schedule is necessary
• Avoid alcohol, salicylates, and drastic changes in dietary habits
• Do not change from one brand to another without consulting clinician

MONITORING PARAMETERS
• Dosage of anticoagulants must be individualized and adjusted according to INR determinations; it is recommended that INR determinations be performed prior to initiation of therapy, at 24-hr intervals while maintenance dosage is being established, then once or twice weekly for the following 3-4 wk, then at 1-4 wk intervals for the duration of treatment
• Maintain INR at 2-3 (2.5-3.5 for mechanical valves, recurrent systemic thromboembolism)

---

xylometazoline
(zye-loe-met-az'oh-leen)
OTC: Otrivin
Chemical Class: Imidazoline derivative
Therapeutic Class: Decongestant

CLINICAL PHARMACOLOGY
Mechanism of Action: Local α-adrenergic-mediated vasoconstriction on dilated nasal mucosal blood vessels
Pharmacokinetics
NASAL: Onset 5-10 min, duration 5-6 hr, occasionally enough drug is absorbed to produce systemic effects
INDICATIONS AND USES: Relief of nasal congestion associated with acute or chronic rhinitis, common cold, sinusitis, and hay fever or other allergies

DOSAGE
Adult
• INSTILL 2-3 gtt or sprays of 0.1% sol into each nostril q8-10h; do not exceed 3 administrations in 24 hr; should not be used for longer than 3-5 days
Child 2-12 yr
• INSTILL 2-3 gtt of 0.05% sol into each nostril q8-10h; do not exceed 3 administrations in 24 hr; should not be used for longer than 3-5 days

§ AVAILABLE FORMS/COST OF THERAPY
• Sol, Drops—Nasal: 0.05%, 25 ml: **$5.38-$6.44**; 0.1%, 25 ml: **$6.24-$7.48**

• Sol, Spray—Nasal: 0.1%, 20 ml: **$4.88-$5.86**

CONTRAINDICATIONS: Angle-closure glaucoma

PRECAUTIONS: Children <2 yr, hyperthyroidism, heart disease, hypertension, diabetes mellitus

PREGNANCY AND LACTATION: Pregnancy category C

SIDE EFFECTS/ADVERSE REACTIONS

CNS: Dizziness, headache, nervousness, weakness

CV: Cardiac irregularities, hypertension

EENT: Anosmia; dryness, rebound congestion and hyperemia, sneezing, stinging, transient burning, ulceration of nasal mucosa

GI: Nausea

SKIN: Sweating

SPECIAL CONSIDERATIONS

• Manage rebound congestion by stopping xylometazoline: one nostril at a time, substitute systemic decongestant, substitute inhaled steroid

PATIENT/FAMILY EDUCATION

• Do not use for >3-5 days or rebound congestion may occur

---

yohimbine

(yoe-him'been)

Rx: Actibine, Aphrodyne, Dayto-Himbin, Testomar, Yocon, Yohimar, Yohimex, Yoman

Chemical Class: Indolalkylamine derivative

Therapeutic Class: Anti-impotence agent

CLINICAL PHARMACOLOGY

Mechanism of Action: Blocks presynaptic α_2-adrenergic receptors; increases parasympathetic (cholinergic) and decreases sympathetic (adrenergic) activity in peripheral autonomic nervous system; may increase penile blood inflow, decrease penile blood outflow, or both

Pharmacokinetics

No data available

INDICATIONS AND USES: No FDA sanctioned indications; impotence of vascular or diabetic origins (data are sparse),* sexual dysfunction caused by selective serotonin reuptake inhibitors,* orthostatic hypotension*

DOSAGE

Adult

• *Impotence:* PO 5.4 mg tid

• *Orthostatic hypotension:* PO 12.5 mg/day in divided doses

$ AVAILABLE FORMS/COST OF THERAPY

• Tab, Uncoated—Oral: 5.4 mg, 100's: **$7.00-$64.39**

CONTRAINDICATIONS: Renal disease, children

PRECAUTIONS: History of gastric or duodenal ulcer; generally not for use in females

PREGNANCY AND LACTATION: Do not use during pregnancy

SIDE EFFECTS/ADVERSE REACTIONS

CNS: Central excitation, dizziness, headache, increased motor activity, irritability, nervousness, tremor

CV: Increased or decreased blood pressure, increased heart rate

GI: Nausea, vomiting

GU: Antidiuresis

SKIN: Skin flushing, sweating

---

italic = common side effects   ***bold italic*** = life-threatening reactions

zafirlukast

(za-feer'loo-kast)
Rx: Accolate
Chemical Class: Tolylsulfonyl benzamide derivative
Therapeutic Class: Antiasthmatic; leukotriene receptor antagonist

CLINICAL PHARMACOLOGY
Mechanism of Action: Competitive and reversible antagonist of the leukotriene D_4 receptor; leukotriene D_4 increases airway reactivity and vascular permeability and causes bronchoconstriction
Pharmacokinetics
PO: Onset 1 hr, peak 2-4 hr, duration 12-14 hr; metabolized in liver by cytochrome 3A4 and 2C9, elimination $t_{1/2}$ 2 hr

INDICATIONS AND USES: Asthma (maintenance treatment), exercise-induced asthma*

DOSAGE
Adult and Children ≥12 yr
• *Asthma:* PO 20 mg bid on an empty stomach
• *Exercise-induced asthma:* PO 20 mg, taken 2 hr before exercise

$ **AVAILABLE FORMS/COST OF THERAPY**
• Tab—Oral: 10, 20 mg, 60's: **$73.81**

PRECAUTIONS: Liver disease, severe asthma
PREGNANCY AND LACTATION: Pregnancy category C; breast milk excretion unknown

SIDE EFFECTS/ADVERSE REACTIONS
CNS: Headache (18%), somnolence, weakness
EENT: Pharyngitis (20%), rhinitis (9%)
GI: Dry mouth, elevated transaminase levels, gastritis

RESP: Cough, exacerbation of asthma

INTERACTIONS
Drugs
3 *Astemizole, terfenadine:* Zafirlukast inhibits drug metabolism with potential for cardiac dysrhythmias
3 *Warfarin:* Zafirlukast increases hypoprothrombinemic effect

SPECIAL CONSIDERATIONS
PATIENT/FAMILY EDUCATION
• Take regularly, even during symptom-free periods
MONITORING PARAMETERS
• ALT, AST, CBC

zalcitabine (ddc)

(zal-site'a-been)
Rx: Hivid
Chemical Class: Nucleoside analog
Therapeutic Class: Antiretroviral

CLINICAL PHARMACOLOGY
Mechanism of Action: Converted to active metabolite, dideoxycytidine 5'-triphosphate (ddCTP), by cellular enzymes; ddCTP serves as an alternative substrate to deoxycytidine triphosphate (dCTP) for HIV reverse transcriptase and inhibits the *in vitro* replication of HIV-1 by inhibition of viral DNA synthesis; incorporation into growing DNA chain leads to premature chain termination; ddCTP serves as a competitive inhibitor of the natural substrate, dCTP, for the active site of DNA polymerase, further inhibiting viral and cellular DNA synthesis

* = non-FDA-approved use

Pharmacokinetics

PO: Peak serum level 0.8 hr; bioavailability 80% (reduced by food); <4% bound to plasma proteins; phosphorylated intracellularly to ddCTP; excreted in urine; $t_{1/2}$ 1-3 hr

INDICATIONS AND USES: Combination therapy with zidovudine in advanced HIV infection (CD4 cell count ≤300/mm^3 with significant clinical or immunologic deterioration); monotherapy for advanced HIV in patients who are either intolerant to zidovudine or have disease progression while receiving zidovudine

DOSAGE

Adult and Children >12 yr, >30 kg
• PO 0.75 mg with 200 mg zidovudine q8h; for monotherapy 0.75 mg q8h; interrupt therapy with zalcitabine if signs or symptoms of peripheral neuropathy appear, reinstitute at 0.375 mg q8h if all findings related to peripheral neuropathy improve to mild symptoms
• *Renal function impairment:* PO (CrCl 10-40 ml/min) 0.75 mg q12h; (CrCl <10 ml/min) 0.75 mg q24h
• For latest treatment guidelines, see www.hivatis.org

$ **AVAILABLE FORMS/COST OF THERAPY**
• Tab, Uncoated—Oral: 0.375 mg, 100's: **$204.98**; 0.75 mg, 100's: **$229.92**

PRECAUTIONS: Low CD4 cell counts (<50/mm^3), existing peripheral neuropathy, history of pancreatitis, ethanol abuse, cardiomyopathy, CHF, renal or hepatic function impairment, children <13 yr

PREGNANCY AND LACTATION: Pregnancy category C

SIDE EFFECTS/ADVERSE REACTIONS

CNS: Dizziness, fever, headache, *peripheral neuropathy (28%)*
EENT: Pharyngitis

GI: Abdominal pain, anorexia, constipation, diarrhea, dry mouth, dyspepsia, dysphagia, esophageal ulcers, exacerbation of hepatic dysfunction, glossitis, nausea, *oral ulcers,* **pancreatitis,** vomiting
MS: Arthralgia, myalgia
SKIN: Night sweats, pruritus, rash
MISC: Fatigue, weight decrease

SPECIAL CONSIDERATIONS
• Consult the most recent guidelines for HIV antiviral therapy prior to prescribing

MONITORING PARAMETERS
• Periodic CBC, serum chemistry tests, transaminase levels
• Serum amylase and triglyceride concentrations in patients with history of elevated amylase, pancreatitis, ethanol abuse, or receiving parenteral nutrition

---

zaleplon
(zal′e-plon)
Rx: Sonata
Chemical Class: Pyrazolopyrimidine derivative
Therapeutic Class: Sedative/hypnotic
DEA Class: Schedule IV

CLINICAL PHARMACOLOGY
Mechanism of Action: Interacts with a specific sub-unit of the GABA-BZ complex responsible for sedative effects; other effects modulated by the GABA-BZ receptor include anxiolytic, muscle relaxant, and anticonvulsive effects

Pharmacokinetics

PO: Peak 1 hr Rapid and nearly complete absorption (PO), absolute bioavailability 30% (significant first pass metabolism); Vd 1.4 L/kg, 60% bound to plasma proteins; extensively metabolized by liver

(CYP3A4 and aldehyde oxidase) to 5-oxo-zapelon; (inactive); 70% excreted in urine over 48 hr; $t_{1/2}$ 1 hr

INDICATIONS AND USES: Short term treatment of insomnia

DOSAGE

Adult

• 10 mg hs (at least 4 hr before becoming active again); max 20 mg hs

• 5 mg hs for mild-moderate hepatic impairment, low body weight, elderly, or concomitant metabolism inhibitors

• No dosage adjustments for mild-moderate renal dysfunction

$ AVAILABLE FORMS/COST OF THERAPY

• Cap—Oral: 5 mg, 100's: **$191.41**; 10 mg, 100's: **$235.44**

PRECAUTIONS: Hepatic impairment, compromised respiratory function, debilitated, depression

PREGNANCY AND LACTATION: Pregnancy category C; small amount excreted in breast milk, with highest excreted amount during a feeding 1 hr after zaleplon administration

SIDE EFFECTS/ADVERSE REACTIONS

CNS: Anxiety, depression, depersonalization, difficulty concentrating, drowsiness, amnesia, paresthesia, migraine, nervousness

EENT: Abnormal vision, conjunctivitis, hyperacusis, parosmia

GI: Abdominal pain, anorexia, constipation, dry mouth, dyspepsia

MS: Arthralgia, arthritis, back pain, chest pain, myalgia

RESP: Bronchitis

SKIN: Pruritus, rash

MISC: Fever

INTERACTIONS

Drugs

❷ *Alcohol:* Additive CNS depression

❸ *Carbamazepine:* CYP3A4 inducer; may reduce efficacy of zaleplon by lowering AUC, C_{max}

❷ *Cimetidine:* Inhibits both CYP3A4 and aldehyde oxidase; concomitant administration increases zaleplon AUC and C_{max} 85%

❸ *Diphenhydramine:* Weak inhibitor of aldehyde oxidase; might reduce hepatic clearance of zaleplon; additive CNS depressant effects

❸ *Imipramine:* Additive effects on decreased alertness and psychomotor performance

❸ *Phenytoin:* CYP3A4 inducer; may reduce efficacy of zaleplon by lowering AUC, C_{max}

❸ *Phenobarbital:* CYP3A4 inducer; may reduce efficacy of zaleplon by lowering AUC, C_{max}

❸ *Rifampin:* Inducer of CYP3A4; reduced AUC, C_{max} of zaleplon 80% - may compromise efficacy

❸ *Thioridazine:* Additive effects on decreased alertness and psychomotor performance

Labs

• *Liver function tests:* Transaminases (ALT, AST), bilirubin increased

• *Cholesterol:* Increased

• *Uric acid:* Increased

• *Glucose:* Increased or decreased

SPECIAL CONSIDERATIONS

• Because of the short $t_{1/2}$, agent best for problems with sleep latency, rather than duration of sleep or number of awakenings (e.g., shift workers)

• Abuse potential similar to benzodiazepines

• Advantage over triazolam, given big cost difference, difficult to justify, if used correctly

---

* = non-FDA-approved use

PATIENT/FAMILY EDUCATION

• *Timing of administration:* Immediately before bedtime or after the patient has gone to bed and has experienced difficulty falling asleep
• Do not take with alcohol or OTC cimetidine

MONITORING PARAMETERS

• Sleep latency, number of awakenings, daytime function (hangover effect), dizziness, confusion

---

zanamivir

(za-na'mi-veer)
Rx: Relenza
Chemical Class: Carboxylic acid ethyl ester
Therapeutic Class: Antiviral

CLINICAL PHARMACOLOGY

Mechanism of Action: Inhibits influenza virus neuraminidase; may alter virus particle aggregation and release

Pharmacokinetics

INH: Of inhaled dose, 4-17% systemically absorbed; peak plasma level 1-2 hr; less than 10% protein bound; excreted in urine (100% unchanged after 24 hr); $t_{1/2}$ 2.5-5 hr; crosses placenta

INDICATIONS AND USES: Uncomplicated influenza A and B infection in adults and children 7 years and older who have been symptomatic for no more than 2 days, prevention of influenza in family members of influenza patients* (see Special Considerations)

DOSAGE

Adult and Child >7 yr

• *Treatment of influenza:* INH (oral) 10 mg q12h for 5 days
• *Prevention of influenza in family contacts:* INH (oral) 10 mg qd for 10 days

💲 AVAILABLE FORMS/COST OF THERAPY

• INH: Supplied in a circular pack (a ROTADISK) containing 4 blisters (5 mg of zanamivir powder each); 5 ROTADISKS packaged in a white tube: **$52.23** for course of therapy

PRECAUTIONS: Asthma, chronic obstructive pulmonary disease

PREGNANCY AND LACTATION: Pregnancy category C; breast milk excretion unknown

SIDE EFFECTS/ADVERSE REACTIONS

CNS: Dizziness, headache
EENT: ENT infections, nasal signs and symptoms, sinusitis
GI: Diarrhea, nausea, vomiting
RESP: Bronchitis, cough
SKIN: Facial edema

SPECIAL CONSIDERATIONS

• Off-label use to prevent influenza in family members of influenza patients (N Engl J Med 2000 Nov 2;343(18):1282-9): Attack rate reduced from 19% to 4%

PATIENT/FAMILY EDUCATION

• Expected benefit of zanamivir is one day of shortening of overall symptoms
• Patients with less severe symptoms get less benefit from therapy
• Influenza vaccine remains the best way to prevent influenza and use of zanamivir should not affect the evaluation of individuals for annual influenza vaccination
• Patients scheduled to use an inhaled bronchodilator at the same time as zanamivir should use their bronchodilator before taking zanamivir
• Two doses should be taken on the first day of treatment whenever possible provided there is at least 2 hours between doses

---

italic = common side effects   ***bold italic*** = life-threatening reactions

zidovudine

(zyde-o'vue-deen)

Rx: Retrovir

Combinations

Rx: with lamivudine (Combivir)

Chemical Class: Nucleoside analog

Therapeutic Class: Antiretroviral

CLINICAL PHARMACOLOGY

Mechanism of Action: Converted by cellular thymidine kinase to zidovudine monophosphate, which is further converted to diphosphate by cellular thymidylate kinase and to triphosphate derivative by other cellular enzymes; triphosphate interferes with the HIV reverse transcriptase thus inhibiting viral replication

Pharmacokinetics

PO: Peak 30-90 min; 25%-38% bound to plasma proteins; metabolized in liver to inactive metabolites, 63%-95% excreted in urine as metabolites and unchanged drug; terminal $t_{1/2}$ 60 min

INDICATIONS AND USES: Treatment of HIV infection when antiretroviral therapy is indicated (should not be used as monotherapy); prevention of maternal-fetal HIV transmission

DOSAGE

Adult

• PO 600 mg/d in divided doses in combination with other antiretroviral agents; IV 1 mg/kg/dose infused over 1 hr q4h while awake (5 mg/kg/day)

• *End-stage renal disease CrCl <15 ml/min:* PO 100 mg q6-8h; IV 1 mg/kg q6-8h

• *Hepatic impairment:* Dose reduction may be necessary

• *Maternal-fetal HIV transmission:* Maternal dose (>14 wk of pregnancy) PO 100 mg 5 times/day until start of labor; during labor and delivery, IV zidovudine should be administered at 2 mg/kg (total body weight) over 1 hr followed by continuous IV INF of 1 mg/kg/hr (total body weight) until clamping of the umbilical cord; infant dose PO 2 mg/kg q6h starting within 12 hr after birth and continuing through 6 wk of age; IV 1.5 mg/kg, infused over 30 min q6h

• For latest treatment guidelines see www.hivatis.org

Child 3 mo-12 yr

• PO 180 mg/m² taken q6h, max 200 mg q6h; IV INF 0.5-1.8 mg/kg/hr; IV 100 mg/m²/dose q6h

• For latest treatment guidelines see www.hivatis.org

§ AVAILABLE FORMS/COST OF THERAPY

• Cap, Gel—Oral: 100 mg, 100's: **$148.25-$205.15**

• Inj, Conc, w/Buffer—IV: 10 mg/ml, 20 ml: **$17.23-$22.19**

• Syr—Oral: 50 mg/5 ml, 240 ml: **$42.47-$49.24**

• Tab—Oral: 300 mg, 60's: **$318.52-$369.27**

PRECAUTIONS: Bone marrow compromise (granulocyte count <1000 cells/mm³ or Hgb <9.5 g/dl); hepatomegaly, hepatitis, or other known risk factor for liver disease; severely impaired renal or hepatic function; children

PREGNANCY AND LACTATION: Pregnancy category C; indicated for pregnant women >14 wk gestation for prevention of maternal-fetus HIV transmission; excreted in breast milk; breast feeding by HIV+ mothers not recommended

---

* = non-FDA-approved use

SIDE EFFECTS/ADVERSE REACTIONS

CNS: Anxiety, chills, confusion, depression, dizziness, emotional lability, fever, *headache, insomnia,* loss of mental acuity, paresthesia, *somnolence,* tremor, twitching

EENT: Hearing loss, photophobia, vertigo

GI: Anorexia, cholestatic hepatitis, constipation, cramps, *diarrhea, dyspepsia,* dysphagia, flatulence, mouth ulcer, *nausea,* taste change, vomiting

GU: Dysuria, polyuria, urinary frequency or hesitancy

*HEME: **Anemia, granulocytopenia, leukopenia, thrombocytopenia***

MS: Arthralgia, muscle spasm, *myalgia*

RESP: Dyspnea

SKIN: Acne, diaphoresis, pigmentation of nails (blue), pruritus, *rash,* urticaria

MISC: Malaise

INTERACTIONS

Drugs

▲ *Doxorubicin:* Antagonism of therapeutic effect; concomitant use should be avoided

❸ *Fluconazole:* Increased plasma concentrations of zidovudine

▲ *Ganciclovir:* Increased hematologic toxicity

▲ *Interferon-alpha:* Increased hematologic toxicity

❸ *Probenecid:* Increased plasma concentration of zidovudine

▲ *Ribavirin:* Antagonism of therapeutic effect; concomitant use should be avoided

❸ *Rifampin:* Reduced plasma concentrations of zidovudine

▲ *Stavudine:* Antagonism of therapeutic effect; concomitant use should be avoided

❸ *Valproic acid:* Increased plasma concentrations of zidovudine

SPECIAL CONSIDERATIONS

• Consult the most recent guidelines for HIV antiviral therapy prior to prescribing

PATIENT/FAMILY EDUCATION

• Close monitoring of blood counts is extremely important; does not reduce risk of transmitting HIV to others through sexual contact or blood contamination

MONITORING PARAMETERS

• CBC with differential and platelets q2wk initially for 2 mo, then q4-8 wk

---

zileuton

(zi-loo'ton)

Rx: Zyflo
Chemical Class: Urea derivative
Therapeutic Class: Antiasthmatic; lipoxygenase inhibitor

CLINICAL PHARMACOLOGY

Mechanism of Action: Specific inhibitor of 5-lipoxygenase, the 1st enzymatic step in conversion of arachidonic acid to leukotrienes

Pharmacokinetics

PO: Onset 30 min, peak 1-3 hr, duration of effect 5-8 hr, oral absorption rapid; extensive 1st-pass metabolism primarily by glucuronidation with renal excretion of inactive metabolites; elimination $t_{1/2}$ 2-3 hr

INDICATIONS AND USES: Asthma (maintenance treatment); aspirin-induced wheezing,* allergic rhinitis,* ulcerative colitis*

DOSAGE

Adult and child ≥12 yr

• *Asthma:* PO 600 mg qid

💲 AVAILABLE FORMS/COST OF THERAPY

• Tab—Oral: 600 mg, 120's: **$103.19**

italic = common side effects   ***bold italic*** = life-threatening reactions

CONTRAINDICATIONS: Active liver disease, unexplained transaminase elevation

PRECAUTIONS: Renal insufficiency, hepatic insufficiency

PREGNANCY AND LACTATION: Pregnancy category C; breast milk excretion unknown

SIDE EFFECTS/ADVERSE REACTIONS

CNS: Dizziness, fatigue, *headache,* insomnia, paresthesia

GI: Abdominal pain, *dyspepsia (8%),* elevated transaminase levels, nausea

SKIN: Rash, urticaria

SPECIAL CONSIDERATIONS

PATIENT/FAMILY EDUCATION

• Must be taken regularly, even during symptom free periods

• Not a bronchodilator, do not use to treat acute episodes of asthma

MONITORING PARAMETERS

• CBC, renal function, and transaminase levels periodically during 1st year of prolonged therapy

---

zinc sulfate/zinc acetate

Rx: Injection: Zinca-Pak
Oral: Galzin, Zincate
OTC: Oral: Orazinc 110, Orazinc 220, Verazinc, Zinc Sulfate 15, Zinc 15, Zinc 220; Ophthalmic: Eye-Sed
Chemical Class: Zinc salt
Therapeutic Class: Ophthalmic astringent; trace element; chelating agent

---

CLINICAL PHARMACOLOGY

Mechanism of Action: Vasoconstriction occurs by action on conjunctiva; needed for adequate healing, bone and joint development; in patients with Wilson's disease induces the production of metallothronein in the enterocyte, a protein that binds copper thereby preventing its transfer into the blood, the bound copper is then lost in the stool following desquamation of the intestinal cells

Pharmacokinetics

PO: Poorly absorbed, excreted mainly through the intestine

INDICATIONS AND USES: Dietary supplement, treatment or prevention of zinc deficiency; temporary relief of minor eye irritation (ophthalmic); chelation therapy maintenance in Wilson's disease (zinc acetate)

DOSAGE

ZINC SULFATE

Adult

• PO 110-220 mg (15-50 mg zinc) qd, recommended daily allowance 66 mg (15 mg zinc) qd; IV 2.5-4 mg/day in metabolically stable adults (add 2 mg/day for acute catabolic states)

• *Minor eye irritation:* Instill 1 gtt bid-tid

Child

• PO 0.3 mg/kg/day

• *Minor eye irritation:* Instill 1 gtt bid-tid

ZINC ACETATE

Adult

• PO 50 mg tid; 25 mg tid may be appropriate in children >10 or pregnant women

$ AVAILABLE FORMS/COST OF THERAPY

Zinc Acetate

• Cap—Oral: 25 mg, 250's: **$154.00**; 50 mg, 250's: **$258.00**

Zinc Sulfate

• Cap, Gel—Oral: 220 mg, (50 mg zinc), 100's: **$3.38-$26.51**

• Inj, Sol—IV: 1 mg/ml, 10 ml: **$1.89-$2.50**; 5 mg/ml, 5 ml: **$2.40-$5.00**

• Sol—Ophth: 0.25%, 15 ml: **$3.24**

• Tab—Oral: 66 mg (15 mg zinc), 100's: **$1.45**; 110 mg (25 mg zinc), 100's **$4.08**

PRECAUTIONS: Narrow-angle glaucoma (ophthalmic), excessive doses

PREGNANCY AND LACTATION: Pregnancy category A (in doses not exceeding recommended daily allowance); for zinc acetate, zinc has appeared in breast milk and zinc-induced copper deficiency may occur, nursing not recommended

SIDE EFFECTS/ADVERSE REACTIONS

EENT: Burning (ophthalmic), eye irritation

GI: Nausea, vomiting

INTERACTIONS

Drugs

3 *Ciprofloxacin, enoxacin, norfloxacin:* Reduced serum concentrations of these drugs

3 *Tetracycline:* Reduced serum tetracycline concentrations

SPECIAL CONSIDERATIONS

• Acetate not recommended for initial therapy of symptomatic Wilson's disease (should be treated initially with chelating agents)

PATIENT/FAMILY EDUCATION

• Take acetate on an empty stomach

MONITORING PARAMETERS

• 24 hr urine copper, LFTs (acetate)

---

ziprasidone

(zye-pray'za-done)

Rx: Geodon

Chemical Class: Benzisothiazole derivative

Therapeutic Class: Atypical antipsychotic (neuroleptic)

CLINICAL PHARMACOLOGY

Mechanism of Action: Efficacy in schizophrenia mediated through combination of dopamine type 2 (D_2) and serotonin type 2 ($5HT_2$) receptor antagonism; additionally, high *in vitro* affinity for dopamine D_3, serotonin $5HT_{2A}$, $5HT_{2C}$, $5HT_{1A}$, $5HT_{1D}$, and α_1-adrenergic receptors and moderate affinity for histamine H_1 receptor; these actions account for potential side effects (i.e., sedation and orthostatic hypotension)

Pharmacokinetics

PO: T_{max} 6-8 hr

Well absorbed (PO); bioavailability with food, 60% (doubles with food); 99% plasma protein bound, but minimal displacement drug interactions; extensively hepatically metabolized (4 major metabolites - reduction via aldehyde oxidase; CYP3A4, CYP1A2), excreted in urine - 20%; in feces - 66% (<1% excreted unchanged); $t_{1/2}$ 7 hr

INDICATIONS AND USES: Schizophrenia, schizoaffective disorder

DOSAGE

Adult

• *Initial dose:* 20 mg bid with food; adjust subsequently based on clinical status (steady state achieved within 1-3 days) generally following several weeks of observation; max dose, 100 mg bid

• Dosage adjustments not required on the basis of age, gender, race, renal, or hepatic function

AVAILABLE FORMS/COST OF THERAPY

• Capsule—Oral: 20 mg, 40 mg, 60 mg, 80 mg, 60's (all): **$243.75**

CONTRAINDICATIONS: QT prolongation, hypersensitivity

PRECAUTIONS: *QT prolongation:* Certain circumstances increase the risk of torsades de pointes and/or sudden death in association with the use of drugs that prolong the QTc interval: bradycardia, hypokalemia or hypomagnesemia, concomitant use of other drugs that prolong QTc in-

---

italic = common side effects   ***bold italic*** = life-threatening reactions

terval (see Drug Interactions), presence of congenital prolongation of the QT interval

PREGNANCY AND LACTATION:
Pregnancy category C; animal, not human studies demonstrated developmental toxicity, including possible teratogenic effects at doses similar to human therapeutic doses; breast milk excretion - unknown

SIDE EFFECTS/ADVERSE REACTIONS

CNS: Agitation, confusion, extrapyramidal syndrome (5%), hostility, paresthesia, somnolence (14%), tremor

*CV: **ECG changes (QTc prolongation)**,* increased heart rate, orthostatic hypotension

EENT: Vertigo

GI: Abdominal pain, vomiting

METAB: Fever, weight gain (10%), hypothermia

MS: Flank pain

RESP: Dyspnea, flu syndrome, respiratory disorder (8%)

SKIN: Photosensitivity reaction

MISC: Face edema

INTERACTIONS

Drugs

3 *Ketoconazole:* Added ketoconazole (inhibits CYP3A4) results in increased AUC and C_{max} (35-40%); other inhibitors predicted to produce similar effects: cisapride, clarithromycin, erythromycin, fluconazole, itraconazole (all azole antifungals), quinine

3 *Carbamazepine:* Added carbamazepine decreased AUC 35%

SPECIAL CONSIDERATIONS

• Atypical agents with less risk of movement disorders best for: Patients resistant to standard antipsychotic agents; patients with therapy-limiting extrapyramidal symptoms, other adverse effects; comparisons with other atypical agents, shorter

half-life and bid dosing requirement potential disadvantage, but perhaps less weight gain

PATIENT/FAMILY EDUCATION

• Review presentation of cardiac (prolonged QT - torsades de pointes) and movement disorders; avoid electrolyte disturbance and drug interactions

MONITORING PARAMETERS

• Improvement of symptomatology (both positive and negative symptoms), complete blood counts, liver function tests, serum prolactin, routine chemistry (especially K^+, Mg^{++} during prolonged therapy); signs/symptoms of akathisia, abnormal movements, persistent constipation

---

zoledronic acid

(zole-eh-drone'ick)

Rx: Zometa

Chemical Class: Bisphosphonic acid

Therapeutic Class: Bisphosphonate

CLINICAL PHARMACOLOGY

Mechanism of Action: Antiresorptive mechanisms include inhibition of osteoclastic activity, induction of osteoclast apoptosis, and binding to bone which blocks resorption mineralized bone and cartilage; single doses associated with decreases in serum calcium and phosphorus and increases in urinary calcium and phosphorus excretion

Pharmacokinetics

IV: Initial response: 1 week; low plasma concentrations observed up to 28 days post dose; low plasma protein binding (22%); no biotransformation; <3% found in feces, eliminated primarily intact via kidney; $t_{1/2}$ 167 hr

INDICATIONS AND USES: Treatment of hypercalcemia of malignancy, Paget's disease of bone*, osteolytic bone metastases*

DOSAGE

Adult and Child >16 yr

• *Hypercalcemia of malignancy:* 4 mg single-dose IV infusion over no less than 15 minutes

• *Paget's disease of bone:* 400 µg single-dose IV infusion over no less than 15 minutes

$ AVAILABLE FORMS/COST OF THERAPY

• Inj, Sol—IV: 4 mg vial: **$892.06**

CONTRAINDICATIONS: Hypersensitivity

PRECAUTIONS: Renal insufficiency, dehydration

PREGNANCY AND LACTATION: Pregnancy category C (developmental and embryocidal effects noted in animals, no adequate and well controlled studies in pregnant women); information on excretion into human breast milk is not available

SIDE EFFECTS/ADVERSE REACTIONS

CNS: Agitation, anxiety, asthenia, confusion, insomnia, somnolence
CV: Chest pain, edema, hypotension
EENT: Conjunctivitis
GI: Abdominal pain, anorexia, constipation, diarrhea, dysphagia, nausea, vomiting
GU: Deterioration in renal function, **renal failure,** UTI
HEME: Anemia, **granulocytopenia, pancytopenia, thrombocytopenia**
METAB: Fever, flu like syndrome (fever, chills, bone pain, arthralgias, myalgias); hypomagnesemia, hypokalemia, hypophosphatemia
RESP: Coughing, dyspnea
SKIN: Rash, mucositis, pruritus
MISC: Local reactions at injection site (redness, swelling), moniliasis

INTERACTIONS

Drugs

3 *Aminoglycosides:* Additive nephrotoxicity
3 *Diuretics (loop):* Additive hypocalcemia

SPECIAL CONSIDERATIONS

• Reconstitute with 5 ml sterile water, then further diluted in 100 ml 0.9% sodium chloride or 5% dextrose; do not mix with calcium-containing infusion solutions (i.e., lactated Ringer's)

• Most potent bisphosphonate available

MONITORING PARAMETERS

• Serum creatinine, electrolytes, phosphate, magnesium, CBC

---

zolmitriptan

(zohl-mih-trip′tan)
Rx: Zomig, Papimeh
Chemical Class: Serotonin derivative
Therapeutic Class: Antimigraine agent

CLINICAL PHARMACOLOGY

Mechanism of Action: Selectively activates vascular 5-HT$_1$ receptors in cranial arteries causing vasoconstriction and inhibition of pro-inflammatory neuropeptide release, actions correlating with the relief of migraine in humans

Pharmacokinetics

PO: Well absorbed, peak 2 hr (2-3 hr for active metabolite), absolute bioavailability 40%; 25% bound to plasma proteins; converted to an active N-desmethyl metabolite with 2 to 6 times the potency of the parent compound; excreted in urine (65%) and feces (30%); t$_{1/2}$ 3 hr (mean of parent drug and active metabolite)

Z

INDICATIONS AND USES: Treatment of acute migraine with or without aura

DOSAGE

Adult

• PO 1.25-2.5 mg at first sign of headache; may repeat initial dose after 2 hr; max 10 mg/24 hr period; the safety of treating an average of more than 3 headaches in a 30 day period has not been established

⑤ AVAILABLE FORMS/COST OF THERAPY

• Tab, Film-Coated—Oral: 2.5 mg, 6's: **$88.19**; 5 mg, 3's: **$52.24**
• Tab, Disintigrating—Oral: 2.5 mg, 6's: **$91.86**; 5 mg, 3's: **$52.24**

CONTRAINDICATIONS: Ischemic heart disease, coronary artery vasospasm, significant underlying cardiovascular disease; uncontrolled hypertension; use within 24 hr of another 5-HT$_1$ agonist, or an ergotamine-containing or ergot-type medication (e.g. dihydroergotamine or methysergide); hemiplegic or basilar migraine; within 2 weeks MAO inhibitor therapy; symptomatic Wolff-Parkinson-White syndrome

PRECAUTIONS: Hypertension, hypercholesterolemia, smokers, obesity, diabetes, strong family history of early CAD, peripheral vascular disease, impaired hepatic function (initiate therapy with low dose)

PREGNANCY AND LACTATION: Pregnancy category C; excretion into breast milk unknown, use caution in nursing mothers

SIDE EFFECTS/ADVERSE REACTIONS

CNS: Agitation, anxiety, depression, dizziness, emotional lability, insomnia, somnolence, vertigo

CV: Bradycardia, chest pain, *dysrhythmia;* edema, extrasystoles, hypertension, palpitations; postural hypotension, pressure or heaviness; syncope, tightness

EENT: Dry eyes, ear pain, eye pain, tinnitus

GI: Dry mouth, dyspepsia, dysphagia, nausea

GU: Hematuria, polyuria, urinary frequency, urinary urgency

MS: Myalgia, myasthenia

RESP: **Bronchospasm,** hiccup, laryngitis, yawning

SKIN: Pruritus, rash, sweating, urticaria

MISC: Asthenia; hyperesthesia, neck, throat, jaw pain, paresthesia, pressure or tightness, warm or cold sensations

INTERACTIONS

Drugs

❸ *Cimetidine:* Increased zolmitriptan concentration

❸ *Ergot-containing drugs:* Potential for prolonged vasospastic reactions and additive vasoconstrictions, theoretical precaution

❷ *MAO inhibitors:* Increased zolmitriptan concentrations, increased potential for serotonin-related toxicity

❷ *Sibutramine:* Increased risk for serotonin syndrome

SPECIAL CONSIDERATIONS

• Alternative to sumatriptan for the treatment of migraine headache; has not been compared head-to-head with sumatriptan; choice should be based on cost and availability

• First dose should be administered in medical office in case cardiac symptoms occur; take great care to exclude the possibility of silent cardiovascular disease prior to prescribing

• Doses >2.5 mg were not associated with more headache relief, but were associated with increased side effects; if no relief is obtained after first dose, a second dose is unlikely to provide any benefit

---

zolpidem

(zole-pi'dem)

Rx: Ambien

Chemical Class: Imidazopyridine derivative
Therapeutic Class: Hypnotic
DEA Class: Schedule IV

CLINICAL PHARMACOLOGY
Mechanism of Action: Subunit modulation of the GABA receptor is responsible for pharmacologic effects: sedative, anticonvulsant, anxiolytic, and myorelaxant properties; selective binding to the BZ, or omega, receptor may explain the preservation of deep sleep (stages 3 and 4) and the relative absence of myorelaxant and anticonvulsant effects

Pharmacokinetics
PO: Peak 1.6 hr (delayed by food); 92% bound to plasma proteins; converted in liver to inactive metabolites, eliminated primarily by renal excretion; $t_{1/2}$ 2½ hr

INDICATIONS AND USES: Short-term treatment of insomnia

DOSAGE
Adult
• PO 5-10 mg immediately before hs; do not exceed 10 mg/day

$ AVAILABLE FORMS/COST OF THERAPY
• Tab, Uncoated—Oral: 5 mg, 100's: **$207.56**; 10 mg, 100's: **$255.30**

PRECAUTIONS: Psychiatric disorders, elderly and/or debilitated patients, depression, abrupt discontinuation, concomitant systemic illness, compromised respiratory function, hepatic impairment, history of drug abuse, children <18 yr

PREGNANCY AND LACTATION: Pregnancy category B; excreted into breast milk in small amounts

SIDE EFFECTS/ADVERSE REACTIONS

CNS: Amnesia, anxiety, confusion, daytime drowsiness, dizziness, *headache,* irritability, lethargy, lightheadedness, poor coordination
CV: Chest pain, palpitation
GI: Abdominal pain, constipation, diarrhea, heartburn, nausea, vomiting
HEME: **Granulocytopenia (rare), leukopenia**

SPECIAL CONSIDERATIONS
PATIENT/FAMILY EDUCATION
• Take immediately prior to retiring
• Avoid alcohol
• Use caution driving or performing other tasks requiring alertness

---

zonisamide

(zoh-nis'a-mide)

Rx: Zonegran
Chemical Class: Sulfonamide
Therapeutic Class: Anticonvulsant

CLINICAL PHARMACOLOGY
Mechanism of Action: Anticonvulsant activity via sodium channel blockade, reducing voltage-dependent, transient inward currents (T-type Ca^{++} currents), stabilizing neuronal membranes and suppressing neuronal hypersynchronization; no GABA activity; weak carbonic anhydrase inhibiting activity; facilitates both dopaminergic and serotonergic neurotransmission

---

Pharmacokinetics

PO: C_{max} 2-5 µg/ml after 200-400 mg dose); T_{max} 2-6 hr Food delays T_{max} to 4 hr, but not AUC; Vd 1.45 L/kg, 40% plasma protein bound; 65% metabolized - acetylation/reduction (CYP3A4) (N-acetyl zonisamide, major metabolite), excreted in primarily in urine - 65% by 10 days); $t_{1/2}$ 63 hr

INDICATIONS AND USES: Adjunctive therapy of partial seizures in adults with epilepsy; partial and generalized seizures*, tonic-clonic seizures*, absence seizures in patients unresponsive to other anticonvulsants*, myoclonic epilepsy*, Lennox-Gastaut syndrome*, infantile spasms*

DOSAGE

Adult and Child >16 yr

• *Partial seizures:* Initial dose: 100 mg qd; increase 100 mg/day increments every 2 weeks to 300-400 mg qd; little experience with doses greater than 600 mg qd

§ AVAILABLE FORMS/COST OF THERAPY

• Cap—Oral (white/red): 100 mg, 100's: **$189.60**

CONTRAINDICATIONS: Hypersensitivity to sulfonamides

PRECAUTIONS: Seizures upon abrupt withdrawal, kidney stones

PREGNANCY AND LACTATION: Pregnancy category C (teratogenic, embryolethal in animals; no adequate and well-controlled studies in pregnant women ; breast milk excretion in women unknown

SIDE EFFECTS/ADVERSE REACTIONS

CNS: Agitation, anxiety, ataxia (6%), confusion, depression, difficulty concentrating, somnolence, dizziness, headache, insomnia, irritability, memory problems, mental slowing, nystagmus, paresthesia

EENT: Taste perversion, diplopia, rhinitis

GI: Abdominal pain, anorexia, constipation, diarrhea, dry mouth, dyspepsia, flu syndrome, *fulminant hepatic necrosis,* nausea, vomiting, weight loss

HEME: **Agranulocytosis, aplastic anemia,** ecchymosis

METAB: **Oligohydrosis, hyperthermia,** weight loss

SKIN: Rash, **Stevens-Johnson syndrome, toxic epidermal necrolysis**

MISC: Fatigue (6%)

INTERACTIONS

Drugs

3 *Carbamazepine:* Increased clearance of zonisamide via CYP3A4 induction ($t_{1/2}$ decreased to 38 hr); no appreciable effect on carbamazepine kinetics

3 *Phenytoin:* Increased clearance of zonisamide via CYP3A4 induction ($t_{1/2}$ decreased to 27 hr); no appreciable effect on phenytoin kinetics

3 *Phenobarbital:* Increased clearance of zonisamide via CYP3A4 induction ($t_{1/2}$ decreased to 38 hr)

3 *Valproic acid:* Increased clearance of zonisamide via CYP3A4 induction ($t_{1/2}$ decreased to 46 hr); no appreciable effect on valproate kinetics

Labs

• *Liver function tests (ALT/AST/ LDH):* Increased

• *Glucose:* Decreased

• *Sodium:* Decreased

SPECIAL CONSIDERATIONS

• Due to long $t_{1/2}$, steady state achievable with stable dosing for 2 weeks

• Adjunctive therapy for wide variety of seizure disorders, especially those refractory to other drugs

* = non-FDA-approved use

PATIENT/FAMILY EDUCATION
• Low threshold for discussing signs and symptoms related to skin rash, liver problems, or blood problems with clinician
MONITORING PARAMETERS
• Frequency and severity of seizures, neurotoxicity, hypersensitivity reactions, serum creatinine, BUN

Appendix A

Comparative Tables

The following comparative drug tables were developed by the authors to assist providers in choosing medications of a given therapeutic class. These tables allow clinicians to compare drugs on the basis of important pharmacologic or clinical characteristics. Whenever possible, the information is based on definitive drug data and should help the reader obtain maximal therapeutic effect with minimal adverse effects. When applicable, accepted clinical practice guidelines have been incorporated into the tables.

Tables:

Acid Secretion Inhibitors

Drug Name	Trade Name	Usual Adult Starting Oral Dose	Nonprescription Strength	Generic Formulation Available	Drug Interaction Potential	Dose Adjustment in Renal Dysfunction
H2 Blockers						
Cimetidine	Tagamet, Tagamet HB	300 mg qid, 400 mg bid, or 800 mg hs	100 mg	Yes	++++	Yes (CrCl <30 ml/min)
Famotidine	Pepcid, Pepcid AC Pepcid RPD	20 mg bid or 40 mg hs	10 mg	Yes	+	Yes (CrCl <50 ml/min)
Nizatidine	Axid, Axid AR	150 mg bid or 300 mg hs	75 mg	No	+	Yes (CrCl <50 ml/min)
Ranitidine	Zantac, Zantac 75 Zantac EFFERdose Zantac GELdose	150 mg bid or 300 mg hs	75 mg	Yes	+	Yes (CrCl <50 ml/min)
Proton Pump Inhibitors						
Esomeprazole	Nexium	20 mg qd	NA	No	+++	No
Lansoprazole	Prevacid	15-30 mg qd	NA	No	+++	No
Omeprazole	Prilosec	20 mg qd	NA	No	+++	No
Pantoprazole	Protonix	40 mg qd	NA	No	++	No
Rabeprazole	Aciphex	20 mg qd	NA	No	++	No

Nonopioid Analgesics

Drug Name	Trade Name	Usual Adult Dose	Maximum Adult Dose	Chemical Class	Comments
Acetaminophen	Tylenol, Panadol, Tempra, Generics	325-650 mg q4-6h	4000 mg/day	Para-aminophenol	Hepatotoxic in large doses, with alcohol or cirrhosis–limit dose to 2 g/day
Salicylates					
Acetylsalicylic acid (aspirin)	Generics	325-975 mg q4h (3.6-5.4 g/day)	6000 mg/day	Salicylate	Antagonizes effect of probenecid; increases effect of sulfonylureas; reduces renal clearance of methotrexate
Choline magnesium trisalicylate	Trilisate (500, 750, 1000 mg—total mg of salicylate)	See choline or magnesium salicylate		Combined salicylates	
Choline salicylate	Arthropan	870 mg q3-4h	5.2 g/day	Salicylate	Fewer side effects than aspirin
Diflunisal	Dolobid, Generics	500 mg bid	1.5 g/day	Salicylate	Not metabolized to salicylate; increases acet-aminophen level by 50% when coadministered
Magnesium salicylate	Extra Strength Doan's, Magan, Mobidin, Generics	650 mg tid	3.6-4.8 g/day	Salicylate	Sodium-free salicylate derivative; fewer side effects than aspirin
Salsalate	Disalcid, Salfex, Generics	1 g tid, 750 mg qid	3 g/day	Salicylate	Antagonizes effect of probenecid; increases effect of sulfonylureas; reduces renal clearance of methotrexate
Sodium salicylate	Generics	325-650 mg q4h		Salicylate	Less effective than equal doses of aspirin
Sodium thiosalicylate	Rexolate	100 mg qd-bid	600 mg/day × 2 days (acute gout)	Salicylate	Intramuscular administration

Continued

Nonopioid Analgesics—cont'd

Drug Name	Trade Name	Usual Adult Dose	Maximum Adult Dose	Chemical Class	Comment
Short-acting NSAIDs					
Diclofenac	Cataflam, Voltaren, Voltaren SR, Generic	25-75 mg bid-tid	200 mg/day	Acetic acid	Formulation is delayed release; also available in qd dose form
Fenoprofen	Nalfon, Generics	300-600 mg tid/bid	3200 mg/day	Propionic acid	Highly protein bound (to albumin); greater renal toxicity
Ibuprofen	Advil, Medalol, Motrin, Rufen, Generics	300-800 mg tid/qid	3200 mg/day	Propionic acid	Also approved for primary dysmenorrhea; available in combination with hydrocodone (Vicoprofen)
Indomethacin	Indocin, Indocin SR, Generics	25-50 mg bid/tid	200 mg/day	Acetic acid	Available in suppository, suspension, and sustained-release forms
Ketoprofen	Orudis, Oruvail, Generics	25-50 mg q6-8h	75 mg/day	Propionic acid	High rate of dyspepsia (11%), available in sustained-release form
Ketorolac	Toradol, Generics	PO: 10 mg q4-6h IM/IV: 30-60 mg initially, then 15-30 mg q6h	40 mg/day 150 mg first day, then 120 mg/day	Acetic acid Acetic acid	Approved only for continuation of parenteral ketorolac, 5 days only 30 mg equal to 6-12 mg morphine sulfate; 10 times more expensive
Meclofenamate	Meclomen	50-100 mg tid/qid	400 mg/day	Anthranilic acid	High rate of diarrhea (10%-33%)
Mefenamic acid	Ponstel, Generic	250 mg q6h	1 g/day	Anthranilic acid	Primarily used for primary dysmenorrhea
Tolmetin	Tolectin, Tolectin DS, Generics	200-600 mg tid	1800 mg/day	Acetic acid	High rate of nausea (11%)

Intermediate-acting NSAIDs					
Etodolac	Lodine, Lodine XL, Generics	200 mg qid-500 mg bid	1200 mg/day	Acetic acid	Antacids reduce peak concentration by 20%
Flurbiprofen	Ansaid, Generics	50-100 mg bid-tid	300 mg/day	Phenylalkanoic acid	May cause CNS stimulation
Naproxen	Naprosyn, EC-Naprosyn, Naprelan, Generics	250-500 mg q8-12h	1.25 g/day	Propionic acid	Approved for acute gout; may increase effect of protein-bound drugs such as phenytoin, sulfonylureas, and warfarin; available in qd dose form
Naproxen Sodium	Anaprox, Generics	275-550 mg q8-12h	1.375 g/day	Propionic acid	Approved for acute gout; may increase effect of protein-bound drugs such as phenytoin, sulfonylureas, and warfarin
Sulindac	Clinoril, Generics	150-200 mg q12h	400 mg/day	Acetic acid	Approved for acute gout; less renal toxicity
Long-acting NSAIDs					
Meloxicam	Mobic	7.5-15 mg qd	15 mg/day	Oxicam	15 mg IM effective; COX-2 selectivity
Nabumetone	Relafen	500 mg-1g qd-bid	2 g/day	Nonacidic	High rate of diarrhea (14%); metabolized to active agent
Piroxicam	Feldene, Generics	10-20 mg qd	20 mg/day	Oxicam	High rate of dyspepsia (20%); may increase effect of protein-bound drugs such as phenytoin, sulfonylureas, and warfarin
Oxaprozin	Daypro	600-1200 mg qd	1800 mg/day	Proprionic acid	
COX-2 selective NSAIDs					
Celecoxib	Celebrex	100-200 mg bid	400 mg/day		Immediate duration
Rofecoxib	Vioxx	12.5-50 mg qd	50 mg/day		Long-acting duration
Valdecoxib	Bextra	10-20 mg qd	20 mg/day		Immediate duration

Opioid and Opioid-Like Analgesics

Drug Name	Trade Name	Usual Adult Dose (mg) and Routes	Parenteral Dose (mg) Equal to 10 mg Morphine Sulfate IM	Oral Dose (mg) Equal to Listed Parenteral Dose	Comment
Opioid-like agents					
Buprenorphine	Buprenex	0.3-0.6 q6h IM	0.3-0.6	0.4-0.8 (SL)	Mixed agonist-antagonist; schedule V controlled substance
Butorphanol	Stadol	1-4 q3-4h IM, Nasal 0.5-2 q3-4 IV	2-3	NA	Mixed agonist-antagonist; not a controlled substance
Nalbuphine	Nubain	10 q6h IM, IV, or SC	10-20	50-60	Mixed agonist-antagonist; not a controlled substance
Tramadol	Ultram	50-100 q4-6h PO	NA	NA	100 mg equianalgesic to 60 mg codeine; long term use may cause dependence and withdrawal syndromes; toxicity includes seizures
Opioids					
Fentanyl	Sublimaze, Duragesic (transdermal)	0.05-0.1 q1-2h IM or IV; 25-100 μg/h transdermal (base dose on total morphine dose); 0.2-0.4 as lozenge	0.1-0.2	NA	Primary use is IV or epidural for perioperative or patient-controlled analgesia; transdermal form available but costly
Oxymorphone	Numorphan	1-1.5 q4-6h IM; 5 q4-6h PR; 0.5 IV	1-1.5	10	Major use is perioperative
Hydromorphone	Dilaudid	2 q4-6h PO; 1-2 q4-6h IM; 3 q6-8h PR	1.5-2	6-7.5	High abuse potential

Levorphanol	Levo-Dromoran	2 q6-8h PO	2-3	4	Long acting
Methadone	Dolophine	5-10 q4-6h PO: 2.5-10 q3-4h IM, SC	7.5-10	15	Different $t_{1/2}$ for analgesia and prevention of opiate withdrawal
Morphine sulfate	Roxanol, MSIR, MS Contin, Oramorph, Kadian, Astramorph	5-20 q4h IM: 5-20 q6h PR; 10 q4h SL: 10-30 mg q4h PO	10	30-40	Oral bioavailability poor; sublingual form useful for breakthrough pain
Morphine, sustained release	MS Contin	15-60 q6-12h PO	NA	30	Not appropriate for prn use
Oxycodone	Percocet, Percodan, Tylox, Oxycontin, Roxicodone	5-10 q4-6h PO	NA	15-30	Often combined with aspirin (Percodan) or acetaminophen (Percocet, Tylox); available in long-acting form (Oxycontin)
Hydrocodone	Vicodin, Vicoprofen	5-10 q4-6h PO	NA	30	Only available combined with acetaminophen, aspirin, ibuprofen, or decongestants
Pentazocine	Talacen, TalwinNX	30-60 q3-4h IM: 50-100 q4h PO	60	180	Mixed narcotic agonist-antagonist
Meperidine	Demerol	50-150 q3-4h IM: 50-150 q4h PO	75-100	300	May be used IV; metabolite normeperidine may accumulate with prolonged use causing excitation or seizures
Codeine	Codeine	15-60 q4h PO	130	200	Schedule II unless combined with acetaminophen or aspirin; used as cough suppressant
Propoxyphene	Darvon	32-100 q4h PO		180-240	Less abuse potential than codeine at usual doses

Cephalosporin Antibiotics

Drug Name (Generation in Parentheses)	Trade Name	Usual Adult Dose (g)	Adjust Dose for Renal Insufficiency	Comment
Oral				
Cefadroxil (1)	Duricef	0.5-1.0 q12-24h	Y	
Cephalexin (1)	Keflex	0.25-0.5 q6h	Y	Cheapest in its therapeutic class
Cephradine (1)	Velosef	0.5 q6h	Y	
Cefaclor (2)	Ceclor	0.25-0.5 q8h	N	
Cefpodoxime proxetil (2)	Vantin	0.1-0.4 q12h	Y	
Cefprozil (2)	Cefzil	0.25-0.5 q12h	Y	
Cefuroxime axetil (2)	Ceftin	0.25-0.5 q12h	Y	
Loracarbef (2)	Lorabid	0.2-0.4 q12h	Y	Carbacephem derivative rather than true cephalosporin
Ceftibuten (3)	Cedax	0.4 q24h	Y	
Cefixime (3)	Suprax	0.4 q24h	Y	Single dose therapy (400 mg) for gonococcal genital and pharyngeal infections
Cefdinir (3)	Omnicef	0.6 qd or 0.3 q12h	Y	
Cefditoren (3)	Spectracef	0.2-0.4 q12h	Y	
Parenteral (IV/IM)				
Cefazolin (1)	Ancef, Kefzol	1-2 q6-8h	Y	
Cephalothin (1)	Keflin	1-2 q4-6h	Y	

Cephapirin (1)	Cefadyl	1 q4-6h	Y	
Cefamandole (2)	Mandol	0.5-1.0 q4-8h	Y	
Cefmetazole (2)	Zefazone	2 q6-12h	Y	
Cefonicid (2)	Monocid	1-2 q24h	Y	May be useful in outpatient therapy of endocarditis
Ceforanide (2)	Precef	0.5-1.0 q12h	Y	
Cefotetan (2)	Cefotan	1-2 q12h	Y	Covers GI anaerobes
Cefoxitin (2)	Mefoxin	1-2 q4-6h	Y	Covers GI anaerobes
Cefuroxime (2)	Zinacef	0.75-1.5 q8h	Y	Crosses blood-brain barrier
Cefepime (3)	Maxipime	0.5-2.0 q12h	Y	
Cefoperazone (3)	Cefobid	1-2 q8-12h	N	
Cefotaxime (3)	Claforan	1-2 q4-6h	Y	Crosses blood-brain barrier
Ceftazidine (3)	Fortaz	1-2 q6-8h	Y	
Ceftizoxime (3)	Cefizox	1-2 q6-8h	Y	Crosses blood-brain barrier
Ceftriaxone (3)	Rocephin	1-2 q12-24h	N	May be useful in outpatient therapy of endocarditis; single-dose (250 mg IM) therapy for gonococcal genital and pharyngeal infections; crosses blood-brain barrier

Macrolide Antibiotics

Drug Name	Trade Name	Usual Adult Dose (mg)	Comment
Azithromycin	Zithromax	500, followed by 250 q24h	Single dose therapy for chlamydial urethritis or cervicitis (1000 mg); antibacterial spectrum includes *Hemophilus influenzae;* indicated to prevent *Mycobacterium avium-intracellulare* infection (1200 mg qwk); available in parenteral form
Clarithromycin	Biaxin, Biaxin XL	250-500 q12h (Biaxin) or 500-1000 q24h (Biaxin XL)	Antibacterial spectrum includes *H. influenzae;* used to treat *Helicobacter pylori* and to prevent *Mycobacterium avium-intracellulare* infection; multiple drug interactions
Dirithromycin	Dynabac	500 q24h	Antibacterial spectrum same as erythromycin
Erythromycin	Erythromycin	250-500 q6-12h	Available as combination product with sulfisoxazole (extends spectrum to include Group A streptococci); coating does not decrease GI side effects; available in parenteral form; multiple drug interactions

Penicillin Antibiotics

Drug Name	Trade Name	Usual Adult Dose (g)	Comment
ORAL			
Penicillin V	Penicillin VK	0.25-0.5 q6h	
Broad Spectrum Penicillins			
Amoxicillin	Amoxicillin	0.25-0.5 q8-12h	May take with meals
Amoxicillin-Potassium Clavulanate	Augmentin	One tablet (0.25 or 0.5 amoxicillin/0.125 clavulanate) q8h, or one tablet (0.875 mg amoxicillin/0.125 clavulanate) q12h	Spectrum extended to include beta-lactamase producers such as *Hemophilus influenza, Moraxella catarrhalis, Staphylococcus aureus* (except MRSA), and *Escherichia coli*
Ampicillin	Ampicillin	0.5-1.0 q6h	Do not take with food
Bacampicillin	Spectrobid	0.4-0.8 q12h	Gives higher and more sustained serum levels of ampicillin
Penicillinase Resistant Penicillins			
Cloxacillin	Tegopen	0.25-0.5 q6h	Oral penicillin of choice for *S. aureus* (except MRSA)
Dicloxacillin	Dycill	0.25-0.5 q6h	Oral penicillin of choice for *S. aureus* (except MRSA)
PARENTERAL (IV)			
Penicillin G	Penicillin	1-3 million U q4-6h	Procaine and benzathine forms available for IM use
Broad Spectrum Penicillins			
Ampicillin	Ampicillin	1-2 q4-6h	
Ampicillin-Sulbactam	Unasyn	1-2/0.5-1.0 q6h	Spectrum extended to include beta-lactamase producers such as *H. influenza, M. catarrhalis, S. aureus* (except MRSA), and *E. coli*

Continued

Penicillin Antibiotics—cont'd

Drug Name	Trade Name	Usual Adult Dose (g)	Comment
Carbenicillin	Geopen, Geocillin	4-5 q4-6h	Carbenicillin indanyl sodium available for oral use
Ticarcillin	Ticar	2-3 q4-6h	
Ticarcillin-Potassium Clavulanate	Timentin	3.1 (3.0 ticarcillin, 0.1 potassium clavulanate) q4-6h	Spectrum extended to include beta-lactamase producers such as *S. aureus* (except MRSA), *E. coli*, *Klebsiella* spp., and *Bacteroides fragilis*
Mezlocillin	Mezlin	2-4 q4-8h	Spectrum includes enterococci, *Klebsiella*, *Enterobacter*, and *Serratia* spp.
Piperacillin	Pipracil	3-4 q4-6h	Spectrum includes enterococci, *Klebsiella*, *Enterobacter*, *Acinetobacter*, and *Serratia* spp.
Piperacillin-Tazobactam	Zosyn	3.375 (3.0 piperacillin, 0.375 tazobactam) q4-6h	Spectrum includes enterococci, *Klebsiella*, *Enterobacter*, *Acinetobacter*, and *Serratia* spp; extended to include beta-lactamase producers such as *S. aureus* (except MRSA) and *B. fragilis*
Penicillinase Resistant Penicillins			
Methicillin	Methicillin	1-2 q4-6h	Parenteral penicillin of choice for *S. aureus* (except MRSA)
Nafcillin	Nafcillin	0.5-2.0 q4-6h	Parenteral penicillin of choice for *S. aureus* (except MRSA)
Oxacillin	Oxacillin	0.5-2.0 q4-6h	Parenteral penicillin of choice for *S. aureus* (except MRSA)

NOTE: MRSA = Methicillin resistant *S. aureus*.

Quinolone Antibiotics

Drug Name	Trade Name	Usual Adult Dose (mg)	Comment
Cinoxacin	Cinobac	PO: 250 q6h or 500 q12h	Approved only to treat UTIs; *Enterococcus, Staphylococcus,* and *Pseudomonas* spp. are resistant
Ciprofloxacin	Cipro	PO: 500-750 q12h (250 q12h for UTIs) IV: 200-400 q12h	Available for ophthalmic use; useful in oral therapy of osteomyelitis; approved for *Campylobacter, Salmonella,* and *Shigella* infections; antibacterial spectrum includes *Mycobacterium avium-intracellulare*
Enoxacin	Penetrex	PO: 400 q12h	Approved only to treat UTIs
Gatifloxacin	Tequin	PO: 400 q24h IV: 400 q24h	Enhanced activity against gram-positive cocci and anaerobes including *Bacteroides fragilis*; no drug interaction with warfarin
Levofloxacin	Levaquin	PO: 250-750 q24h	Levo-form of ofloxacin; enhanced activity against gram-positive cocci and oral anaerobes
Lomefloxacin	Maxaquin	PO: 400 q24h	Not effective for *Pseudomonas aeruginosa* infections outside of the urinary tract
Moxifloxacin	Avelox	PO: 400 q24h IV: 400 q24h	Enhanced activity against gram-positive cocci and anaerobes including *Bacteroides fragilis*; no drug interaction with warfarin
Norfloxacin	Noroxin	PO: 400 q12h	Available for ophthalmic use; approved only to treat UTIs and conjunctivitis
Ofloxacin	Floxin	PO: 200-400 q12h IV: 200-400 q12h	Available for ophthalmic use
Trovafloxacin	Trovan	PO: 100-200 q24h	Restricted use; enhanced activity against gram-positive cocci and anaerobes including *Bacteroides fragilis*; no drug interaction with warfarin; rare reports of fatal hepatitis

Systemic Antifungal Antibiotics

Drug Name	Trade Name	Usual Adult Dose	Common Indications	Comment
Amphotericin B	Abelcet, AmBisome, Amphotec, Fungizone	IV: 0.4-0.6 mg/kg/d for 8-10 wk (nonlipid form only)	Histoplasmosis, blastomycosis, candidiasis, cryptococcosis, coccidioidomycosis, aspergillosis, mucormycosis	Used topically in bladder; causes multiple electrolyte abnormalities (hypokalemia, renal tubular acidosis, hypomagnesemia, azotemia); give 1 mg test dose prior to giving full dose; three lipid-complexed forms available with different doses but lower nephrotoxicity
Fluconazole	Diflucan	PO or IV: 100-400 qd	Blastomycosis, histoplasmosis, candidiasis, coccidioidomycosis	Increases serum rifabutin levels and toxicity; increases effect of cyclosporine, terfenadine, astemizole, warfarin, sulfonylureas, and others; single dose oral treatment for vaginal infection
Flucytosine	Ancobon	PO: 12.5-37.5 mg/kg q6h	Cryptococcosis, candidiasis, chromoblastomycosis	Usually used in combination with amphotericin B (allows lower dose); converted to 5-fluorouracil in fungal cell
Griseofulvin	Fulvicin, Gris-PEG	PO: 500 mg qd-bid (microcrystalline) PO: 330 mg qd-bid (ultra microcrystalline)	Dermatophytes	Cytochrome P450 inducer; absorption enhanced when taken with fatty foods
Itraconazole	Sporanox	PO: 100-200 mg qd-bid	Onychomycosis, blastomycosis, histoplasmosis, candidiasis, coccidioidomycosis, sporotrichosis, cryptococcosis, aspergillosis	Cytochrome P450 3A inhibitor—affects cyclosporine, terfenadine, astemizole, warfarin, sulfonylureas, and others; tablet and solution forms not interchangeable
Ketoconazole	Nizoral	PO: 200-400 mg qd-bid	Blastomycosis, histoplasmosis, candidiasis, coccidioidomycosis, dermatophytes	Cytochrome P450 3A inhibitor—affects cyclosporine, terfenadine, astemizole, warfarin, sulfonylureas, and others; requires acid pH for absorption; reduces testosterone synthesis; available in topical form
Terbinafine	Lamisil	PO: 250 mg qd	Onychomycosis	Hepatic clearance increased by rifampin, decreased by cimetidine
Voriconazole	Viread	IV: 6 mg/kg q12h × 2 doses, then 4 mg/kg PO: >40 kg: 400 mg q12h × 2 doses, then 200 mg q12h; <40 kg: 200 mg q12h × 2 doses, then 100 mg q12h	Aspergillosis, candidiasis (resistant)	Transient visual disturbances in 30% of patients

Selective Serotonin Reuptake Inhibitor (SSRI) Antidepressants

Drug Name	Brand Name	Usual Adult Dose (mg/d)	Drug and Active Metabolite (t½ [hr])	Serotonin Reuptake Inhibition	Anticholinergic Effect	Drowsiness	Degree of Cytochrome P450 System Inhibition	Comment
Citalopram	Celexa	20-40	33-37	4+	1+	0	0	Dose up to 80 mg/d occasionally needed
Fluoxetine	Prozac	20-60 (starting dose 10 in elderly)	24-72 (acute); 96-144 (chronic); (norfluoxetine: 96-384)	4+	0-1+	0	3+ (2D6)	Up to 60 mg/d for obsessive-compulsive disorder
Fluvoxamine	Luvox	50-300	15-26 (no active metabolite)	4+	0	0	2+	Indicated only for obsessive-compulsive disorder
Paroxetine	Paxil	20-60 (starting dose 10 in elderly)	21 (no active metabolite)	4+	2	1+	2+ (2D6)	May cause weight gain
Sertraline	Zoloft	75-200 (starting dose 12.5-25 in elderly)	26 (desmethylsertraline: 62-104)	4+	0-1+	0-1+	1+ (2D6)	Metabolite weakly active

Tricyclic and Tetracyclic Antidepressants

Drug Name	Brand Name	Usual Adult Dose (mg) for Acute Therapy (Maintenance Dose is ½–⅔ of this; lower doses recommended for elderly persons)	Relative Sedation	Relative Anticholinergic Effect	Relative Delay of Cardiac Conduction	Relative Postural Hypotension	Comment
Tricyclic							
Amitriptyline	Elavil	75–300	3+	4+	3+	4+	Used for chronic pain
Clomipramine	Anafranil	25–250	3+	3+	2+	4+	Primary use is for obsessive-compulsive disorder; may lower seizure threshold; may increase plasma concentration of protein bound drugs (e.g., digoxin, warfarin)
Desipramine	Norpramin	75–300	1+	2+	3+	2+	Used for chronic pain; metabolite of imipramine
Doxepin	Sinequan	75–300	4+	3+	1+	4+	Potent antihistamine
Imipramine	Tofranil	50–300	2+	3+	3+	3+	Used for chronic pain, panic disorder, and headache
Nortriptyline	Pamelor	50–150	1+	2+	2+	3+	Used for chronic pain, panic disorder, and headache; metabolite of amitriptyline

							Comments
Protriptyline	Vivactil	15-60	2+	4+	2+	2+	
Trimipramine	Surmontil	50-300	4+	3+	3+	4+	
Tetracyclic							
Amoxapine	Asendin	200-400	2+	1+	1+	3+	Metabolite has neuroleptic side effect
Maprotiline	Ludiomil	75-300	3+	1+	1+	3+	May lower seizure threshold
Heterocyclic							
Nefazodone	Serzone	200-600	+/-	1+	0+	2+	Divided doses on bid schedule; do not administer with astemizole, cisapride, lovastatin, or simvastatin; may increase plasma concentration of protein bound drugs (e.g., digoxin, warfarin); cytochrome 3A4 inhibitor
Trazodone	Desyrel	150-600	2+	0+	0+	4+	Risk of priapism in males and similar phenomenon in females; may increase plasma concentration of protein bound drugs (e.g., digoxin, warfarin); should be given in divided doses

Miscellaneous Antidepressants, Including Foods that Interact with MAOIs

Drug Name	Brand Name	Usual Adult Dose (mg/d)	Anticholinergic Effect	Drowsiness	Orthostatic Hypotension	Cardiac Dysrhythmias	Comment
Bupropion	Wellbutrin, Zyban	225-450	0	+/−	+/−	1+	Single dose should not exceed 150 mg; inhibits dopamine reuptake; given bid or tid; FDA-approved as an aid to smoking cessation
Mirtazapine	Remeron	15-45	2+	3+	0	0-1+	Do not use with MAOIs
Venlafaxine	Effexor, Effexor XR	75-375	0	0	0	4+	Inhibits serotonin and norepinephrine reuptake; given bid or tid or as long-acting form; associated with elevated blood pressure
Monoamine oxidase inhibitors (MAOIs)							Avoid foods rich in amines (see below) and selected medications while taking MAOI and for 14 days after last dose
Isocarboxazid	Marplan	10-30	1+	1+	2+	1+	May be given as single daily dose
Phenelzine	Nardil	15-90	1+	1+	2+	1+	Given in divided doses
Tranylcypromine	Parnate	30-60	1+	1+	1+	1+	Given in divided doses

Avoid the following foods if taking MAOIs (contain tyramine and other amines, often as a result of aging or fermenting): broad beans; red wines; yeast extracts; beer with yeast; chicken or beef liver; caviar, anchovies, and pickled herring; fermented sausages (bologna, pepperoni, salami, and summer sausage); and aged cheeses (Boursault, Brie, Camembert, cheddar, Emmenthaler, Gruyere, mozzarella, parmesan, romano, Roquefort, and Stilton).

Systemic Antihistamines

Drug Name	Trade Name	Usual Adult Dose	Sedative Effects	Comment
First-Generation Agents				
Azatidine	Optimine	1-2 mg q12h	++	
Azelastine	Astelin	0.5 mg q12h	+/−	Nasal spray
Brompheniramine	Dimetapp Allergy	4 mg q4-6h	+	Also available as injection and in combination with decongestants
Chlorpheniramine	Aller-Chlor, Chlo-Amine, Chlor-Trimeton	4 mg q4-6h	+	Also available as syrup, extended release tablets, and in combination with decongestants
Clemastine	Antihist-1, Tavist	1 mg q12h	++	Also available as syrup and in combination with decongestants
Cyproheptadine	Periactin	4 mg q8h	+	Also available as syrup
Dexchlorpheniramine	Polaramine	2 mg q4-6h	+	Active dextro-isomer of chlorpheniramine; also available as syrup and extended release tablets
Diphenhydramine	AllerMax, Banophen, Benadryl, Diphen AF, Diphenhist, Genahist	25-50 mg q6-8h	+++	Also available as syrup, liquid, solution, elixir, injection, and in combination with decongestants
Hydroxyzine	Atarax, Vistaril	25-100 mg q4-8h	+++	Also available as syrup; often used as antipruritic
Phenindamine	Nolahist	25 mg q4-6h	+/−	Less sedating OTC alternative
Tripelennamine	PBZ, PBZ-SR	25-50 mg q4-6h	++	Also available as extended release tablet; often recommended for pregnant patients

Continued

Systemic Antihistamines—cont'd

Drug Name	Trade Name	Usual Adult Dose	Sedative Effects	Comment
Second-Generation Agents				
Cetirizine	Zyrtec	5-10 mg qd	+/-	Also available as syrup
Desloratidine	Clarinex	5 mg qdh	+/-	Active metabolite of loratidine
Fexofenadine	Allegra	60 mg q12h	+/-	Active metabolite of terfenadine
Loratadine	Claritin	10 mg qd	+/-	Also available as syrup and rapidly disintegrating tablet
Miscellaneous Agents				
Doxepin	Sinequan	10-50 mg q8-24h	+++	Sedating tricyclic antidepressant; antipruritic
Promethazine	Phenergan	12.5 mg q6-8	++	Phenothiazine derivative; well tolerated by children; available as syrup, suppositories, and injection

Systemic Corticosteroids

Drug Name	Trade Name	Oral or Parenteral Dose for Equivalent Glucocorticoid Effect (mg)*	Relative Mineralocorticoid Effect	Biologic Half-life (hrs)†
Betamethasone	Celestone	0.75	0	36-54
Cortisone	Cortone	25	1	8-12
Dexamethasone††	Decadron, Dexone, Hexadrol	0.75	0	36-54
Hydrocortisone	Cortef, Solu-Cortef	20	1	8-12
Methylprednisolone	Medrol	4	0	18-36
Prednisolone	Delta-Cortef	5	0.5	18-36
Prednisone	Deltasone, Orasone	5	0.5	18-36
Triamcinolone	Aristocort, Atolone, Kenacort	4	0	18-36

*Not all preparations are suitable for IV injection.
†Because chemical half-life of all agents is 0.5-4.0 hrs, endogenous cortisol level can be measured 24 hrs after last corticosteroid dose (*JAMA* 1999; 282:671-676).
††Dexamethasone is only corticosteroid that does not cross-react with cortisol assay.

Inhaled Antiinflammatory Drugs

Drug Name	Trade Name	Dose per Inhalation	Usual Adult Dose	Maximum Adult Daily Dose (# of inhalations)
Respiratory Corticosteroids				
Beclomethasone	Vanceril	42 µg	84 µg tid-qid or 168 µg bid	840 µg (20)
	Vanceril Double Strength	84 µg	168 µg bid	840 µg (10)
	QVAR	40, 80 µg	40-80 µg bid	640 µg (8-16)
Budesonide	Pulmicort	200 µg	200-800 µg bid	1,600 µg (8)
Flunisolide	AeroBid, AeroBid-M	250 µg	500 µg bid	2,000 µg (8)
Fluticasone	Flovent	44, 110, 220 µg	88-220 µg bid	880 µg (4-20)
	Flovent Roatadisk (powder)	50, 100, 250 µg	100-250 µg bid	1,000 µg
Triamcinolone	Azmacort	100 µg	200 µg tid-qid or 400 µg bid	1,600 µg (16)
Intranasal Corticosteroids				
Beclomethasone	Beconase, Vancenase, Vancenase Pockethaler (metered dose inhaler); Beconase AQ (solution with metering pump)	42 µg	42 µg each nostril bid-qid	336 µg (8)
	Vancenase AQ 84 µg (solution with metering pump)	84 µg	84-168 µg each nostril qd	336 µg (4)
Budesonide	Rhinocort (metered dose inhaler); Rhinocort Aqua (solution with metering pump)	32 µg	64 µg each nostril bid	256 µg (8)

Flunisolide	Nasalide (metered dose inhaler); Nasarel (solution with metering pump)	25 μg	50 μg each nostril bid	400 μg (16)
Fluticosone	Flonase	50 μg	100 μg each nostril bid	200 μg (4)
Mometasone	Nasonex	50 μg	100 μg each nostril qd	200 μg (4)
Triamcinolone	Nasacort (metered dose inhaler); Nasacort AQ (solution with metering pump)	55 μg	110 μg each nostril qd	440 μg (8)
	Tri-Nasal	50 μg	100 μg each nostril qd	400 μg (8)
Noncorticosteroids				
Cromolyn (inhaled)	Intal	800 μg	1600 μg qid	6400 μg (8)
Cromolyn (intranasal)	Nasalcrom	5.2 mg	5.2 mg each nostril q3-6 hours	62.4 mg (12)
Nedocromil (inhaled)	Tilade	1.75 mg	3.5 mg bid-qid	14 mg (8)

Inhaled Bronchodilators

Drug Name	Trade Name	Dose per Inhalation with Metered Dose Inhaler	Usual Adult Dose
Albuterol	Proventil, Ventolin, Combivent (with ipratropium)	90 μg	1-2 inhalations q 4-6h
Bitolterol	Tornalate	2 mg/ml*	2.5 mg tid-qid via nebulizer
Epinephrine	Primatene Mist	220 μg	1-2 inhalations q 3-4 h (max 12 per day)
Formoterol	Foradil	12μg†	12 μg q12h
Ipratropium	Atrovent, Combivent (with albuterol)	18 μg	2 inhalations q 4-6 h (max 12 per day)
Levalbuterol	Xopenex	0.63-1.25 mg/3 ml*	0.63-1.25 mg tid via nebulizer
Metaproterenol	Alupent	650 μg	2-3 inhalations q 3-4 h (max 12 per day)
Pirbuterol	Maxair	200 μg	1-2 inhalations q 4-6 h (max 12 per day)
Salmeterol	Serevent Serevent Diskus	25 μg* 50 mg†	2 inhalations q 12h 50 μg q12h

*Solution for inhalation via nebulizer.
†Inhalation powder.

Noncontraceptive Estrogens

Drug Name	Trade Name	Available Strengths	Usual Adult Dose	Comment
Systemic				
Conjugated estrogens, oral	Premarin	0.3 mg, 0.625 mg, 0.9 mg, 1.25 mg, 2.5 mg	0.625-1.25 mg qd	Available in IV form; available in combination with medroxyprogesterone acetate (2.5/5 mg-Prempro; 5 mg Premphase); dose for bone loss prevention 0.625 mg qd
Esterified estrogens	Estratab, Menest	0.3 mg, 0.625 mg, 1.25 mg, 2.5 mg	0.625-1.25 mg qd	Contains 80% sodium estrone sulfate
Estradiol oral	Estrace	0.5 mg, 1 mg, 2 mg	0.5-2 mg qd	Dose for bone loss prevention 0.5 mg qd
Estradiol transdermal systems	Vivelle, Climara, Estraderm	0.0375 mg/24 hr 0.05 mg/24 hr 0.075 mg/24 hr 0.1 mg/24 hr	0.05-0.1 mg/24 hr	Estraderm and Vivelle applied twice weekly; Climara applied weekly; dose for bone loss prevention 0.05 mg qd
Estradiol valerate in oil	Delestrogen, Dioval, Estra-L, Gynogen LA	10 mg/ml; 20 mg/ml; 40 mg/ml	10-20 mg q 4 weeks	Oil suspension gives long action
Estrone	Aquest, Kestrone	2 mg/ml; 5 mg/ml	0.1-2 mg per week in single or divided doses	Aqueous solution of estrone

Continued

Noncontraceptive Estrogens—cont'd

Drug Name	Trade Name	Available Strengths	Usual Adult Dose	Comment
Estropipate	Ortho-Est, Ogen	0.75 mg, 1.5 mg, 3 mg	0.75-1.5 mg qd	0.75 mg estropipate equivalent to 0.625 mg conjugated estrogens; dose for bone loss prevention 0.75 mg qd
Ethinyl estradiol	Estinyl	0.02 mg, 0.05 mg, 0.5 mg	0.02-0.05 mg qd	
Topical				
Conjugated estrogens	Premarin	0.625 mg conjugated estrogens per g	0.5-2 g cream qd	
Dienestrol	Ortho Dienestrol	0.01% cream	1 applicatorful qd-bid	
Estradiol	Estrace	0.1 mg estradiol per g	2-4 g cream qd	
Estradiol	Estring	2 mg estradiol per ring	Insert vaginal ring and leave in place for 90 days	Low systemic estradiol exposure
Estropipate	Ogen	1.5 mg estropipate per g	2-4 g cream qd	

Oral Hypoglycemic Agents

Drug	Trade Name	Dosage Range	Cost	Comments
Sulfonylureas: **First Generation***				
Chlorpropamide	Diabinese	100-500 mg/day (max 750 mg/day)	$0.43-0.87/250 mg tablet	Active metabolite—caution in elderly; ↓ renal function; 24-72 hr duration of effect; disulfiram reactions, hyponatremia
Tolazamide	Tolinase	250-500 mg qd (max 500 mg bid)	$0.18-0.92/250 mg tablet	Active metabolite—caution in elderly; ↓ renal function; 12-24 hr duration of effect
Tolbutamide	Orinase	250-3000 mg/day (divide doses bid)	$0.23/500 mg tablet	Negligible metabolites; OK with ↓ renal function; 6-12 hr duration of effect
Sulfonylureas: **Second Generation**				
Glimepiride	Amaryl	1-4 mg qd (max 8 mg/day)	$0.83/4 mg tablet	Minimal added effect > 4 mg/day
Glipizide	Glucotrol, Glucotrol-XL, generics	2.5-20 mg qd (max 40 mg/day); divide doses > 10 mg bid	$0.15-0.76/10 mg tablet	Minimal added effect > 20 mg/day; inactive metabolite; 24 hr duration of effect
Glyburide, micronized	Glynase	0.75-12 mg qd (max 12 mg/day)	$0.72/3 mg tablet	Extended-release product of long-acting drug (?)
Glyburide	DiaBeta, Micronase, generic	1.25-10 mg qd (max 20 mg/day)	$0.23-0.83/5 mg tablet	Minimal added effect > 10 mg/day; active metabolite with duration longer than parent
Meglitinides†				
Nateglinide	Starlix	60-120 mg tid, ac	$0.86/60 mg tablet	

*Mechanism: stimulate pancreatic insulin secretion (i.e., secretagogues).
†Mechanism: quick acting secretagogues.

Continued

Oral Hypoglycemic Agents—cont'd

Drug	Trade name	Dosage range	Cost	Comments
Sulfonylureas: Second Generation—cont'd				
Bioguanides‡				
Repaglinide	Prandin	0.5-4 mg tid ac (max 16 mg/day)	$0.81/2 mg tablet	
Metformin	Glucophage, Glucophage XR, generics	1000 mg bid; (max 2550 mg/day)	$1.46/1000 mg tablet	Excreted unchanged in urine; avoid in low clearance states (e.g., decreased renal function, CHF) because predisposed to lactic acidosis; caution in pre-radiological studies requiring contrast material
Thiazolidinediones¶				
Pioglitazone	Actos	15-30 mg qd (max 45 mg/day)	$4.37/30 mg tablet	Caution: weight gain, CHF
Rosiglitazone	Avandia	4-8 mg qd (max 8 mg/day)	$4.25/8 mg tablet	Caution: weight gain, CHF
α-Glucosidase Inhibitors§				
Acarbose	Precose	50-100 mg tid ac (max 100 mg tid)	$0.54/50 mg tablet	GI adverse effects expectedly
Miglitol	Glyset	50-100 mg tid ac (max 100 mg tid)	$0.57/50 mg tablet	GI adverse effects expectedly

‡Mechanism: decrease hepatic glucose production and increase insulin sensitivity.
¶Activate peroxisome proliferative-activated receptors, "insulin sensitizer."
§Inhibit starch breakdown, attenuate postprandial hyperglycemia.

Insulins

Preparation	Onset (hr)	Peak Effect (hr)	Duration (hr)	Mixing Compatibility
Rapid-Acting Insulins				
Regular	0.5	2-4	6-8	All
Semilente	1-1.5	5-10	12-16	Lente
Lispro	0.25	0.5-1.5	3.4-4.5	Ultralente, NPH
Aspart	0.25	1-3	3-5	
Intermediate-Acting Insulins				
Lente	1-3	6-12	18-24	Regular, semilente
NPH	1-1.5	6-12	18-24	Regular
Long-Acting Insulins				
Glargine	1.1	5	24	None
PZI	4-8	14-24	3	Regular
Ultralente	4-8	10-30	>36	Regular, semilente
Premixed Insulins				
70/30	0.5	2-12	18-24	
50/50	0.5	2-12	16-24	

Lipid Lowering Agents

Drug	Brand Name	Usual Adult Dose	Lipid-Lowering Effect	Cost($) per Dose
Bile Acid Binding Resins				
Cholestyramine	LoCholest, Prevalite, Questran	8-16 mg/day; max 24 g/day divided bid-tid	LDL ↓ 15%-25% HDL ↑ 3%-5% TG no change or ↑	$0.29-0.54/4 g powder
Colestipol	Colestid	5-30 g qd or divided		$1.00/5 g powder
Colesevelam	Welchol	625 mg tablets; 3-6 tablets qd or 3 tablets bid		$0.77/625 mg tablet
Niacin	Immediate-release: various, generic Extended-release: Niaspan, Niacor, Slo-Niacin	1.5-6 g/day divided bid-tid (following gradual titration)	LDL ↓ 15%-25% HDL ↑ 15%-25% TG ↓ 20%-50%	IR: $0.04/500 mg tablet ER: $0.70/500 mg tablet
Fibric Acid Derivatives			LDL ↓ 0-20% HDL ↑ 10%-20% TG ↓ 20%-50%	
Clofibrate	Atromid-S	1-2 g daily in divided doses		$0.92/500 mg capsule
Fenofibrate	Tricor	54-160 mg qd		$1.64/134 mg capsule
Gemfibrozil	Lopid	600 mg bid		$0.48-1.48/600 mg tablet

HMG CoA Reductase Inhibitors			LDL ↓ 18%–55% HDL ↑ 5%–15% TG ↓ 7%–30%	
Atorvastatin	Lipitor	10-80 mg qd		$2.81/20 mg tablet
Fluvastatin	Lescol	20-80 mg qPM		$1.60/40 mg tablet
Lovastatin	Mevacor, generic	10-80 mg qPM		$3.94/40 mg tablet
Pravastatin	Pravachol	10-40 qPM		$3.56/40 mg tablet
Simvastatin	Zocor	5-80 qPM		$357/20 mg tablet

Topical Steroids

Potency Category	Drug Name	Trade Name	Type of Preparation
I (very high)	Augmented betamethasone dipropionate (0.05%)	Diprolene	Ointment, gel, lotion
	Clobetasol propionate (0.05%)	Temovate	Cream, ointment, scalp application, gel
		Embeline E	Cream
	Diflorasone diacetate (0.05%)	Psorcon	Ointment
	Halobetasol propionate (0.05%)	Ultravate	Cream, ointment
II (high)	Amcinonide (0.1%)	Cyclocort	Cream, ointment, lotion
	Augmented betamethasone dipropionate (0.05%)	Diprolene AF	Cream
	Betamethasone dipropionate (0.05%)	Alphatrex, Diprosone, Maxivate	Cream, ointment
		Teladar	Cream
	Betamethasone valerate (0.1%)	Betatrex, Valisone	Ointment
	Desoximetasone (0.25%)	Topicort	Gel (0.05%), cream, ointment
	Diflorasone diacetate (0.05%)	Florone, Maxifor	Ointment (emollient base), cream
		Florone E, Psorcon	Cream
		Synalar-HP	Cream
	Fluocinolone acetonide (0.2%)	Lidex, Lidex E	Cream, ointment, solution, gel
	Fluocinonide (0.05%)	Halog, Halog-E	Cream, ointment, solution
	Halcinonide (0.1%)	Aristocort, Flutex, Kenalog	Cream, ointment
	Triamcinolone acetonide (0.5%)	Aristocort A	Cream
III (intermediate)	Betamethasone dipropionate (0.05%)	Alphatrex, Diprosone, Maxivate	Lotion
	Betamethasone valerate (0.1%)	Betatrex, Beta-Val, Valisone	Cream, lotion
	Clocortolone pivalate (0.1%)	Cloderm	Cream
	Desoximetasone (0.05%)	Topicort	Cream
	Fluocinolone acetonide (0.025%)	Flurosyn, Synalar	Cream, ointment
	Flurandrenolide (0.025%, 0.05%)	Cordran, Cordran SP	Cream, ointment (0.025%)
		Cordran, Cordran SP	Cream, ointment, lotion (0.05%)
		Cordran	Tape (4 µg/cm^2)
	Fluticasone propionate (0.005%, 0.05%)	Cutivate	Cream (0.05%), ointment (0.005%)
	Hydrocortisone butyrate (0.1%)	Locoid	Cream, ointment, solution
	Hydrocortisone valerate (0.2%)	Westcort	Cream, ointment
	Mometasone furoate (0.1%)	Elocon	Cream, ointment, lotion

IV (low)	Triamcinolone acetonide (0.025%, 0.1%)	Aristocort, Aristocort A, Delta-Tritex, Flutex, Kenalog	Cream, ointment (0.1%)
		Kenalog-H, Kenonel, Triacet, Triderm	Cream (0.1%)
		Flutex, Kenalog	Cream, ointment (0.025%)
		Aristocort, Aristocort A	Cream (0.025%)
		Kenalog	Lotion (0.025%, 0.1%)
	Aclometasone dipropionate (0.05%)	Aclovate	Cream, ointment
	Desonide (0.05%)	DesOwen, Tridesilon	Cream, ointment
		DesOwen	Lotion
	Dexamethasone (0.01%, 0.04%)	Aeroseb-Dex	Aerosol (0.01%)
		Decaspray	Aerosol (0.04%)
	Dexamethasone sodium phosphate (0.1%)	Decadron Phosphate	Cream
	Fluocinolone acetonide (0.01%)	Flurosyn, Synalar	Cream
		Fluonid, Synalar	Solution
		FS Shampoo	Shampoo
		Derma-Smoothe/FS	Oil
	Hydrocortisone (0.25%, 0.5%, 1%, 2%, 2.5%)	Cetacort	Lotion (0.25%)
		Cortizone-5, and others	Cream, ointment (0.5%)
		Cetacort, S-T Cort	Lotion (0.5%)
		Hycort, Hytone, and others	Cream, ointment (1%)
		Acticort, Ala-Cort, and others	Lotion (1%)
		Scalpicin, T/Scalp	Liquid (1%)
		Extra Strength CortaGel	Gel (1%)
		Penecort, Texacort	Solution (1%)
		Maximum Strength Cortaid, Procort	Spray (1%)
		Maximum Strength Cortaid Faststick	Stick, roll-on (1%)
		Ala-Scalp	Lotion (2%)
		Hytone and others	Cream, ointment (2.5%)
		Hytone, LactiCare-HC	Lotion (2.5%)
		Cortaid with Aloe, Lanacort-5, and others	Cream, ointment (0.5%)
	Hydrocortisone acetate (0.5%, 1%)	Maximum Strength Cortaid and others	Cream, ointment (1%)

Topical Antifungal Agents

Drug Name	Trade Name	Usual Adult Dose	Spectrum/Comment
Vaginal Preparations for Candidiasis			
Butoconazole	Femstat	2% vaginal cream, 5 g qhs × 3d (6d if pregnant)	Pregnancy category C
Clotrimazole	FemCare, Gyne-Lotrimin, Mycelex	1% vaginal cream, 1 applicatorful qhs × 7d; 100 mg vaginal tablet qhs × 7d; 500 mg vaginal tablet × 1	Pregnancy category B
Miconazole	Monistat	1% vaginal cream, 1 applicatorful qhs × 7d; 100 mg vaginal tablet qhs × 7d; 200 mg vaginal tablet × 3	Pregnancy category C
Nystatin	Mycostatin	100,000 units vaginal tablet qd × 14d	Pregnancy category A
Terconazole	Terazol	0.8% vaginal cream 1 applicatorful (5g) or 80 mg vaginal suppositories qhs × 3d	Pregnancy category C
Tioconazole	Vagistat	6.5% vaginal ointment, 1 applicatorful qhs × 1	Pregnancy category C
Dermatologic Preparations			
Amphotericin	Fungizone	3% cream, lotion, ointment, suspension	Candida
Butenafine	Mentax	1% cream	Tinea
Ciclopirox	Loprox	1% cream, ointment	Tinea, Candida, Tinea versicolor

Clioquinol	Vioform	3% cream, ointment	Tinea
Clotrimazole	Lotrimin, Mycelex	1% cream, lotion, solution	OTC-Tinea; Rx-Tinea, Candida, Tinea versicolor
Econazole	Spectazole	1% cream	Tinea, Candida, Tinea versicolor
Haloprogin	Halotex	1% cream, solution	Tinea, Tinea versicolor
Iodoquinol	Vytone	1% cream	Tinea, Candida
Ketoconazole	Nizoral	2% cream, shampoo	Tinea, Candida, Tinea versicolor; scalp seborrheic dermatitis
Miconazole	Micatin, Monistat-Derm	2% cream, powder, spray	Tinea, Candida, Tinea versicolor
Naftifine	Naftin	1% cream, gel	Tinea, Candida
Nystatin	Mycostatin, Nilstat, Nystex	100,000 units per gram, cream, ointment, powder	Candida
Oxiconazole	Oxistat	1% cream, lotion	Tinea, Candida, Tinea versicolor
Selenium sulfide	Selsun Blue, Exsel	1%, 2.5% lotion, shampoo	Tinea versicolor; scalp seborrheic dermatitis
Sulconazole	Exelderm	1% cream, solution	Tinea, Candida, Tinea versicolor
Terbinafine	Lamisil	1% cream	Tinea, Candida, Tinea versicolor
Tolnaftate	Aftate, Tinactin, Desenex	1% cream, gel, powder, solution, spray liquid, spray powder	Tinea, Tinea versicolor
Undecylenic acid	Cruex, Desenex, Pedi-Pro, Caldesene, Protectol	8-20% cream, foam, ointment, powder, soap	Tinea

Nucleoside Reverse Transcriptase Inhibitors*

Drug Name	Trade Name	Usual Adult Dose (mg)	Dose Change in Renal Insufficiency	Drug Interactions	Comment
Abacavir	Ziagen	300 q12h	No	Amprenavir	Hypersensitivity in 2-5% of recipients; rechallenge may be fatal; available as oral solution
Didanosine (ddI)	Videx, Videx EC	125-200 q12h on empty stomach (pills) or 250-400 q24h	Reduce dose if CrCl < 60 ml/min	Dapsone, ganciclovir, itraconazole, methadone, quinolones	Enteric coated form preferred; available as a powder (not bioequivalent to pills)
Lamivudine (3TC)	Epivir, Combivir	150 q12h	Reduce dose if CrCl < 50 ml/min		Available as oral solution; available in combination with zidovudine
Stavudine (D4T)	Zerit	30-40 q12h	Reduce dose if CrCl < 50 ml/min	Additive neuropathic effect with dapsone, isoniazid, metronidazole, phenytoin, vincristine	Antagonism with zidovudine; available as oral solution
Tenofovir	Viread	300 q24h	Do not use if CrCl < 60 ml/min	Cidofovir, ganciclovir	Take with food
Zalcitabine (ddC)	Hivid	0.75 q8h	Reduce dose if CrCl < 60 ml/min	Antacids, amphotericin, foscarnet, aminoglycosides, probenecid, cimetidine, pentamidine	
Zidovudine (AZT)	Retrovir, Combivir	100-200 q8h or 300 q12h	Reduce dose if CrCl < 10 ml/min	Ganciclovir, interferon, probenecid, rifampin, valproic acid	Available as syrup, injection; available in combination with lamivudine; avoid with ribavirin

*See *www.hivatis.org* for most current information.

Non-Nucleoside Reverse Transcriptase Inhibitors*

Drug Name	Trade Name	Usual Adult Dose (mg)	Dose Change in Renal Insufficiency	Drug Interactions	Comment
Delavirdine	Rescriptor	400 tid	No	Antacids, astemizole, barbiturates, carbamazepine, cisapride, clarithromycin, dapsone, didanosine, ergotamines, H2 blockers, indinavir, midazolam, nelfinavir, nifedipine, phenytoin, proton pump inhibitors, quinidine, rifabutin, rifampin, saquinavir, terfenadine, triazolam, warfarin, zidovudine	Do not use as monotherapy due to resistance induction; separate dosing with didanosine or antacids by 1 hour; cytochrome P-4503A4 inhibitor; coadministration with astemizole, cisapride, ergotamines, H2 blockers, lovastatin, midazolam, proton pump inhibitors, rifabutin, rifampin, simvastatin, terfenadine, triazolam not recommended
Efavirenz	Sustiva	600 qd	No	Amprenavir, astemizole, barbiturates, carbamazepine, cisapride, clarithromycin, ergotamines, ethinyl estradiol, indinavir, lopinavir, lovastatin, midazolam, nelfinavir, nifedipine, phenytoin, rifabutin, rifampin, ritonavir, saquinavir, simvastatin, terfenadine, triazolam, warfarin	Do not use as monotherapy due to resistance induction; CNS side effects very frequent; cytochrome P-450 mixed inducer and inhibitor; coadministration with astemizole, cisapride, clarithromycin, ergotamines, midazolam, saquinavir, terfenadine, triazolam not recommended
Nevirapine	Viramune	200 qd for 14d, then 200 bid	No	Clarithromycin, erythromycin, ethinyl estradiol, indinavir, ketoconazole, lopinavir, methadone, nelfinavir, rifabutin, rifampin, ritonavir, saquinavir	Do not use as monotherapy due to resistance induction; cytochrome P-4503A4 inducer; coadministration with ketoconazole, rifampin not recommended; may affect methadone dose needed; available as elixir

*See www.hivatis.org for most current information.

Protease Inhibitors*

Drug Name	Trade Name	Usual Adult Dose (mg)	Dose Change in Renal Insufficiency	Selected Drug Interactions (see individual monographs for complete list)	Comment
Amprenavir	Agenerase	1200 q12h	No	Astemizole, cisapride, ergot alkaloids, lovastatin, midazolam, rifampin, simvastatin, terfenadine, triazolam	Capsules of amprenavir contain 109 IU of vitamin E; liquid contains 46 IU per mL
Indinavir	Crixivan	800 q8h	No	Astemizole, cisapride, ergot alkaloids, lovastatin, midazolam, rifampin, saquinavir, simvastatin, terfenadine, triazolam	Do not take with large meal; associated with nephrolithiasis
Lopinavir	Kaletra	400 q12h with ritonavir 100 q12h	No	Astemizole, cisapride, ergot alkaloids, flecainide, lovastatin, midazolam, pimozide, propafenone, rifampin, simvastatin, terfenadine, triazolam	Only available in combination with ritonavir; capsules contain 133.3 mg lopinavir plus 33.3 mg ritonavir
Nelfinavir	Viracept	750 tid	No	Astemizole, cisapride, ergot alkaloids, lovastatin, midazolam, rifampin, simvastatin, terfenadine, triazolam	Diarrhea most common side effect
Ritonavir	Norvir	600 q12h	No	Amiodarone, astemizole, bepredil, bupropion, cisapride, clorazepate, clozapine, diazepam, encainide, ergot alkaloids, estazolam, flecainide, flurazepam, lovastatin, meperidine, midazolam, pimozide, piroxicam, propafenone, propoxyphene, simvastatin, terfenadine, triazolam, zolpidem	Take with food; start with 300 mg q12h, increase over 14 days in 100 mg increments to 600 mg q12h
Saquinavir	Invirase (hard capsule), Fortovase (soft capsule)	Hard capsule: 400 q12h with ritonavir; soft capsule: 1200 q8h	No	Astemizole, cisapride, efavirenz, ergot alkaloids, indinavir, lovastatin, midazolam, rifabutin, rifampin, simvastatin, terfenadine, triazolam	Take with high fat meal to enhance bioavailability; available in more bioavailable gel capsule form (Fortovase)

*See *www.hivatis.org* for most current information.

Ophthalmic Agents: Glaucoma

Drug	Brand Name	Strength	Indications	Dose	Duration of Effect (hr)	Comments
Sympathomimetics*						
Apraclonidine	Iopidine	0.5%-1%	Ocular hypertension, post-operative; glaucoma, open angle	1 hr before laser surgery and on completion: bid/tid	7-12	
Brimonidine	Alphagan	0.2%	↑ IOP	tid	12	
Dipivefrin	Propine	0.1%	Glaucoma, open angle; ↑ IOP	q12h	12	
Epinepherine	Epifrin, Glaucon	0.5%-2%	Glaucoma, open angle	qd-bid	12	
Beta Blockers*						
Betaxolol	Betoptic, Betoptic S	0.25%-0.5%	↑ IOP: glaucoma, open angle	bid	12	β_1 selective; onset <30 min; max effect 2 hr
Carteolol	Ocupress	1%	↑ IOP: glaucoma, open angle	bid	12	β_1 and β_2; max effect 2 hr
Levobunolol	AK-beta, Betagan	0.25%-0.5%	↑ IOP: glaucoma, open angle	qd-bid	12-24	β_1 and β_2; onset < 60 min; max effect 2-6 hr
Metipranolol	Optipranolol	0.3%	↑ IOP: glaucoma, open angle	bid	12-24	β_1 and β_2; onset ≤ 30 min; max effect approx 2 hr

Sympathomimetics—mechanism of action: ↓ IOP via aqueous suppression (↓ production). There are added effects with miotic agents.
Beta blockers—mechanism of action: ↓ IOP via aqueous suppression (↓ production). Standard drug packaging colors: blue, yellow, or both. Use alone or in combination. Beta blockers are more effective than pilocarpine or epinephrine. There is no effect on pupil size or accommodation.

Continued

Ophthalmic Agents: Glaucoma—cont'd

Drug	Brand Name	Strength	Indications	Dose	Duration of Effect (hr)	Comments
Beta Blockers*—cont'd						
Timolol	Timoptic, Betimol, Timoptic-XE	0.25%-0.5%	↑ IOP; open angle glaucoma	bid; XE qd	12-24	β_1 and β_2; onset < 30 min; max effect 2 hr; XE preparation is "gel forming"
Levobetaxolol	Betaxon	0.5%	↑ IOP; open angle glaucoma	bid	12	β_1 selective; onset <30; max effect 2 hr
Miotics, Direct Acting*						
Acetylcholine	Miochol-E	1%	Miosis during surgery	prn rapid effect (sec)	10-20 min	
Carbachol	Carbastat, Miostat	0.75%-3%	Miosis during surgery	prn—single use	6-8	
Pilocarpine	Isopto Carpine, Pilagen, Ocusert Pilo	0.25%-10%; ocular therapeutic systems	↑ IOP; open angle glaucoma; acute angle closure glaucoma; mydriasis; preoperative and postoperative	Solution: tid-qid Gel: HS Ocusert: weekly	4-8	
Miotics, Cholinesterase Inhibitors*						
Demecarium	Humorsol	0.25%	Open angle glaucoma; accommodative esotropia	bid-biw	Miosis: 3-10 days; ↓ IOP: 7-28 days	Reversible cholinesterase binding, long acting
Echothiophate	Phospholine Iodide	0.06%-0.25%	↑ IOP; open angle glaucoma; accommodative esotropia	bid	Miosis: 1-4 weeks; ↓ IOP: 7-28 days	Irreversible cholinesterase binding
Physostigmine		0.25%	↑ IOP; open angle glaucoma	qd-tid	Miosis: 12-36; ↓ IOP: 12-36 hr	Reversible cholinesterase binding, short acting

Carbonic Anhydrase Inhibitors*					
Dorzolamide	Trusopt	2%	tid	↑ IOP (ocular hypertension; open angle glaucoma)	8
Brinzolamide	Azopt	1%	tid	↑ IOP (ocular hypertension; open angle glaucoma)	4 weeks
Prostaglandin Analogues*					
Bimatoprost	Lumigan	0.03%	hs	↑ IOP (ocular hypertension; open angle glaucoma)	24	Onset: 4 hr, peak: 8-12 hr; eye pigment changes (increasing brown pigmentation)
Latanoprost	Xalatan	0.005%	hs	↑ IOP (ocular hypertension; open angle glaucoma)	24	Onset: 3-4 hr, peak: 8-12 hr; eye pigment changes (increasing brown pigmentation)
Travoprost	Travatan	0.004%	hs	↑ IOP (ocular hypertension; open angle glaucoma)	24	Onset: 2 hrs; peak: 12 hrs eye pigment; changes (increasing brown pigmentation)
Unoprostone	Rescula	0.15%	bid	↑ IOP (ocular hypertension; open angle glaucoma)	10	Eye pigment changes (increasing brown pigmentation)

Miotics, direct acting—mechanism of action: ↓ IOP via aqueous suppression (↓ outflow). Standard drug packaging color: green. Formerly first step in glaucoma treatment but yielded to beta blockers. Dark pigmented irides may require higher doses. There is an effect on accommodation.

Miotics, cholinesterase inhibitors—mechanism of action: ↓ IOP via (indirectly) ↓ resistance to aqueous outflow. Standard drug package color: green. Contraindications include angle closure glaucoma and demecarium during pregnancy. Side effects and systemic toxicity are more common and of greater significance than those of direct-acting miotics.

Carbonic anhydrase inhibitors—mechanism of action: ↓ IOP via ↓ aqueous humor secretion.

Prostaglandin analogues—mechanism of action: ↓ IOP via selective prostenoid receptor agonism, enhancing uveoscleral outflow. Concomitant use with other topical agents to ↓ IOP is appropriate.

APPENDIX A

Ophthalmic Agents: Mydriatics

Drug	Brand Name	Preparations	Dose	Mydriasis		Cycloplegia	
				Peak (min)	Recovery (days)	Peak (min)	Recovery (days)
Atropine	Isopto atropine, Atropine Care, Atropisol	Ointment 1%, solution 0.5%, 1%, 2%	Uveitis: qid Refraction: 1 hr before exam	30-40	7-10	60-180	6-12
Homatropine	Isopto Homatropine	2%, 5%	Uveitis: qid Refraction: 1 hr before exam	40-60	1-3	30-60	1-3
Scopolamine	Isopto Hyoscine	0.25%	Uveitis: qid Refraction: 1 hr before exam	20-30	3-7	30-60	3-7
Cyclopentolate	AK-Pentolate, Cyclogyl, Pentolair	0.5%, 1%, 2%	Refraction: 5-10 min before exam; repeat in 5-10 min prn	30-60	1	25-75	0.25-1
Tropicamide	Mydriacyl, Opticyl	0.5%, 1%	Refraction: 5-15 min before exam; may repeat within 20-30 min	0.25	20-35	20-35	<0.25
Miotic*				Reversal (min): 30-120 (post phenylephrine or tropicamide)			
Dapiprazole	Rev-Eyes	0.5%	Post-procedure; repeat 5 min later				

*Miotic—mechanism of action: α = adrenergic blockade producing miosis, no activity or ciliary muscle contraction or IOP; indications: reversal of iatrogenically induced mydriasis via adrenergic or parasympatholytic agents.

Ophthalmic Agents: Inflammation

Drug	Brand Name	Strength	Indications	Dose	Comments
Nonsteroidal Antiinflammatory Agents*					
Diclofenac	Voltaren	0.1%	Postoperative inflammation—cataract extraction; corneal refractive surgery	qid 24 hr before, 2 weeks after; qid 1 hr before, 15 min after, then × 3 days or less	Standard package color: grey; unlabeled uses: cystoid macular edema, inflammation after cataract, glaucoma laser surgery, and uveitis syndromes
Flurbiprofen	Ocufen	0.03%	Intraoperative miosis	q30min × 4 starting 30 min preoperative	Contraindications: epithelial herpes, simplex keratitis, soft contact lenses
Ketorolac	Acular	0.5%	Seasonal allergic conjunctivitis; postoperative inflammation—cataract extraction	qid prn; qid × 2 weeks	
Suprofen	Profenal	1%	Intraoperative miosis	q1h × 3 preoperative	
Corticosteroids*					
Dexamethasone	AK-Dex, Decadron, Maxidex	0.05%–0.1%	Ocular inflammatory conditions	Solution: q1-2h to response, then qid; ointment: qid to response, then bid-qid	Warnings: prolonged use may result in glaucoma, optic nerve damage, defects in visual acuity and fields of vision, posterior subcapsular cataract formation, secondary ocular infections, and delay healing after cataract surgery

*Nonsteroidal antiinflammatory agents—mechanism of action: inhibition of cyclooxygenase enzyme essential for biosynthesis of prostaglandins (mediators of intraocular inflammation), no effect on IOP, inhibition of miosis independent of cholinergic mechanisms.

Corticosteroids—mechanism of action: antiinflammatory actions due to potentiation of epinephrine vasoconstriction, stabilization of lysosomal membranes, retardation of macrophage movement, prevention of kinin release, inhibition of lymphocyte and neutrophil function, inhibition of prostaglandin synthesis, and decrease in antibody production regardless of source (mechanical, chemical, or immunological).

Continued

Ophthalmic Agents: Inflammation—cont'd

Drug	Brand Name	Strength	Indications	Dose	Comments
Corticosteroids*— cont'd					
Fluorometholone	Fluor-Op, FML, Flarex	0.1%-0.25%	Ocular inflammatory conditions	bid-qid	Contraindications: acute epithelial herpes simplex keratitis, fungal diseases of eye, vaccinia and varicella and other viral disease of the cornea and conjunctiva, ocular tuberculosis
Loteprednol	Lotemax, Alrex	0.2%-0.5%	Ocular inflammatory conditions; postoperative inflammation	qid	
Medrysone	HMS	1%	Ocular inflammatory conditions	q2h x 24, then bid-qid	
Prednisolone	Pred Mild, Econopred, PredForte, AK-Pred, Inflamase	0.125%-1%	Ocular inflammatory conditions	q1-2h, then qid	
Rimexolone	Vexol	1%	Ocular inflammatory conditions; postoperative inflammation	qid	

Ophthalmic Agents: Allergy and Congestion

Drug	Brand Name	Strengths	Indications	Dose	Comments
Mast Cell Stabilizers*					
Cromolyn	Crolom, Opticvom	4%	Conjunctivitis: vernal kerato-conjunctivitis, vernal conjunctivitis, vernal keratitis	4-6 x per day	Symptomatic response evident within a few days but often longer; appropriate use requires regular, non-prn dosing
Ketotifen	Zaditor	0.025%	Allergic conjunctivitis	q8-23h	Selective, noncompetitive histamine antagonist and mast cell stabilizer
Lodoxamide	Alomide	0.1%	Conjunctivitis: vernal kerato-conjunctivitis, vernal conjunctivitis, vernal keratitis	qid	
Nedocromil	Alocril	2%	Allergic conjunctivitis	bid	
Pemirolast	Alamast	0.1%	Allergic conjunctivitis	qid	
Antihistamines*					
Azelastine	Optivar	0.05% mg/ml	Allergic conjunctivitis	bid	Symptomatic response evident rapidly, without rebound congestion; appropriate use includes both chronic and prn dosing

Continued

Mast cell stabilizers—mechanism of action: inhibition of type I immediate hypersensitivity reaction via mast cell stabilization.

Antihistamines—mechanism of action: selective histamine (H_1) antagonists.

Ophthalmic Agents: Allergy and Congestion—cont'd

Drug	Brand Name	Strengths	Indications	Dose	Comments
Antihistamines*— cont'd					
Emedastine	Emadine	0.05%	Allergic conjunctivitis	bid (6-8 hr interval)	
Levocabastine	Livostin	0.05%	Allergic conjunctivitis	qid	
Olopatadine	Pantanol	0.1%	Allergic conjunctivitis	bid (6-8 hr interval)	
Vasoconstrictors*					
Naphazoline	otc: 20/20 eye drops, Al-Ierest, Clear Eyes, Degest 2, Naphcon, Allergy Drops, VasoClear, Comfort Rx: AK-Con, Albalon, Nafazair, Naphcon Forte, Vasocon	0.012%, 0.02%, 0.03% 0.1%	Relief of eye redness due to minor irritation	q3-4h prn	Duration of action: 3-4 hr
Oxymetazoline	otc: OcuClerar, Visine LR	0.025%,	Relief of eye redness due to minor irritation	q6h prn	Duration of action: 4-6 hr
Phenylepherine	otc (0.12%): AK-Nefrin, Prefrin, Relief Rx: AK-Dilate, Mydfrin, Neo-Synephrine, Phenoptic	0.12%, 2.5%, 10%	otc: Relief of eye redness due to minor irritation Rx: Pupil dilation in uveitis (posterior synechiae), open angle glaucoma, refraction without cycloplegia before surgery, ophthalmoscopic examination, diagnostic procedures (funduscopy)	up to qid prn Mydriasis produced in 15-30 min and lasts 1-3 hr	Duration of action: 0.5-1.5 hr

Vasoconstrictors*—cont'd				
Tetrahydrozoline	otc: Collyrium Fresh, Eye drops, Eyesine, Geneye, Mallazine, Murine, Optigene, Tetrasine, Visine	0.05%	Relief of eye redness due to minor irritation	qid	Duration of action: 1-4 hr
Combination Decongestant/ Antihistamines				
Phenylephrine/ pheniramine	otc: Zincfrin			
Naphzoline/ pheniramine	otc: Clear Eyes ACR, Vaso-Clear A, Naphcon-A, Rx: Opcon-A			
Naphzoline/ pheniramine	Vasocon-A			
Tetrahydrozoline/ antazoline	otc: Visine Allergy, Geneye AC			

Vasoconstrictors—mechanism of action: sympathomimetic

α: Pupil dilation, increase in outflow of aqueous humor, vasoconstriction.

β: Relaxation of ciliary muscle, decrease in formation of aqueous humor.

Contraindications: Narrow angle or anatomically narrow (occludable) angle and no glaucoma; rebound congestion occurs with frequent or extended use.

Appendix B

Bibliography

1. Mosby's GenRx, 9th ed., St. Louis, Mosby, 1999.
2. Briggs GG, Freeman RK, Yaffe SJ. Drugs in pregnancy and lactation, 5th ed. Baltimore, Williams and Wilkins, 1998.
3. Shepard TH. Catalog of teratogenic agents, 8th ed. Baltimore, Johns Hopkins University Press, 1995.
4. Hansten PD, Horn JR. Drug interactions analysis and management. Vancouver, Washington, Applied Therapeutics Incorporated, 1999.
5. Drug facts and comparisons. St. Louis, Facts and Comparisons, Incorporated, 1999.
6. McEvoy, GK, American Hospital Formulary Service: Drug information, Bethesda, American Society of Hospital Pharmacists, 1999.
7. Doherty MC. Drug topics red book 1999. Montvale, NJ, Medical economics data production company, 1999.
8. Young DS. Effects of Drugs on Clinical Lab Tests, 4th ed. Washington D.C., 1995, American Association for Clinical Press.

Therapeutic Index

The therapeutic index is arranged by condition/disorder. *Italics* indicate category of drug.

goserelin, 467-468
megestrol, 611-612
methyltestosterone, 660-661
nandrolone, 711-712
pamidronate, 780-781
risedronate, 910-911
tamoxifen, 976-977
testosterone, 986-988
tiludronate, 1006-1007

Bronchitis
Oral cephalosporins
azithromycin, 84-85
cefixime, 165
cefpodoxime, 172-173
cephalexin, 183-184
clarithromycin, 218-221
grepafloxacin, 469-470
ofloxacin, 752-754
Other
amoxicillin/clavulanate, 51-53
co-trimoxazole, 251-253
doxycycline, 337-339
lomefloxacin, 583-584
trovafloxacin/alatrofloxacin,
1054-1056

Bronchospasm
albuterol, 17-18
atropine, 76-78
bitolterol, 111-112
dyphylline, 341-342
epinephrine, 357-359
formoterol, 438-440
isoetharine, 530-531
isoproterenol, 533-534
metaproterenol, 627-628
pirbuterol, 832-833
salmeterol, 923-924
terbutaline, 985
theophylline, 993-995

Brucellosis
co-trimoxazole, 251-253
doxycycline, 337-339
gentamicin, 455-457
minocycline, 681-683
streptomycin, 959-960
tetracycline, 989-991

Bulimia
desipramine, 275-277
fluoxetine, 420-422
lithium, 581-583
tranylcypromine, 1030-1032

Burns
mafenide, 595
nitrofurazone, 738
pramoxine, 846
silver sulfadiazine, 938-939

Bursitis
Adrenal corticosteroids
betamethasone, 101-103
corticotropin (ACTH), 248-249
cortisone, 249-251
prednisone, 853-854
*Nonsteroidal antiinflammatory
drugs*
aspirin, 69-72
choline salicylate, 209
ibuprofen, 503-504
naproxen, 712-714
sulindac, 971-972

Cachexia
cyproheptadine, 262
dronabinol, 339-340
megestrol, 611-612
somatropin/somatrem, 948-949

Candidiasis
amphotericin b, 55-57
butoconazole, 129
ciclopirox, 210
clotrimazole, 237-238
econazole, 342-343
fluconazole, 410-412
flucytosine, 412-413
itraconazole, 540-542
ketoconazole, 545-547
miconazole, 674-675
nystatin, 750
terbinafine, 984
terconazole, 986
tioconazole, 1011

Carcinoid
octreotide, 751-752

Cardiac decomposition
dobutamine, 325-326

Index

Entries can be identified as follows: generic name, Trade Name.

Entries can be identified as follows: generic name, Trade Name.

Entries can be identified as follows: generic name, Trade Name.

Entries can be identified as follows: generic name, Trade Name.

Entries can be identified as follows: generic name, Trade Name.

Entries can be identified as follows: generic name, Trade Name.

Entries can be identified as follows: generic name, Trade Name.

Entries can be identified as follows: generic name, Trade Name.

Entries can be identified as follows: generic name, Trade Name.

Entries can be identified as follows: generic name, Trade Name.

Entries can be identified as follows: generic name, Trade Name.

Entries can be identified as follows: generic name, Trade Name.

Entries can be identified as follows: generic name, Trade Name.

Entries can be identified as follows: generic name, Trade Name.

Entries can be identified as follows: generic name, Trade Name.

Entries can be identified as follows: generic name, Trade Name.

Entries can be identified as follows: generic name, Trade Name.

Entries can be identified as follows: generic name, Trade Name.

Entries can be identified as follows: generic name, Trade Name.

Entries can be identified as follows: generic name, Trade Name.

Entries can be identified as follows: generic name, Trade Name.

Entries can be identified as follows: generic name, Trade Name.

Entries can be identified as follows: generic name, Trade Name.

Entries can be identified as follows: generic name, Trade Name.

Entries can be identified as follows: generic name, Trade Name.

Entries can be identified as follows: generic name, Trade Name.

Entries can be identified as follows: generic name, Trade Name.

Entries can be identified as follows: generic name, Trade Name.

Entries can be identified as follows: generic name, Trade Name.

Entries can be identified as follows: generic name, Trade Name.

Entries can be identified as follows: generic name, Trade Name.

Entries can be identified as follows: generic name, Trade Name.

Entries can be identified as follows: generic name, Trade Name.

Entries can be identified as follows: generic name, Trade Name.

Entries can be identified as follows: generic name, Trade Name.

IDEAL BODY WEIGHT (IBW)

ADULTS (>18 YRS):
Male IBW (kg) = 50 + 2.3 for each inch over 60 inches
Female IBW (kg) = 45.5 + 2.3 for each inch over 60 inches

CHILDREN:
Age 1 to 18 yrs, height <60 inches: IBW (kg) = $[1.65 \times height^2 (cm)]/1000$

BODY MASS INDEX (BMI)

$$BMI = \frac{weight\ (kg)}{height^2\ (m)}$$

Normal range:
    Male: 21.9-22.4
    Female: 21.3-22.1

CREATININE CLEARANCE CALCULATION

ADULTS (AGE >18; SERUM CREAT <5 MG/DL AND NOT CHANGING RAPIDLY):

$$CrCl\ (ml/min) = \frac{(140 - age)\ (weight\ in\ kg)}{(serum\ creat\ [mg/dl])\ (72)}$$

NOTES: 1. Multiply by 0.85 for females
        2. Use the following value for weight:
           a. If actual weight <IBW, use actual weight
           b. If actual weight is 100%-130% of IBW, use IBW
           c. If actual weight >130% of IBW, easiest approximation is by using IBW + (actual weight − IBW)/3
        3. Accuracy reduced in muscle wasting diseases (e.g., neuromuscular disease) and amputees

CHILDREN:
CrCl (ml/min/1.73m^2) = $[0.48 \times height\ (cm)]/serum\ creat\ (mg/dl)$

Conversion Information

WEIGHTS AND MEASURES

PREFIXES FOR FRACTIONS
deci = 10^{-1}
centi = 10^{-2}
milli = 10^{-3}
micro = 10^{-6}
nano = 10^{-9}
pico = 10^{-12}

TEMPERATURE MEASURES
$°C = 5/9 \times (°F -32)$
$°F = 9/5 \times (°C) + 32$

PERCENTAGE EQUIVALENTS
0.1% solution contains: 1 mg per ml
1% solution contains: 10 mg per ml
10% solution contains: 100 mg per ml

MILLIEQUIVALENT CONVERSIONS
1 mEq Na = 23 mg Na = 58.5 mg NaCl
1 g Na = 2.54 g NaCl = 43 mEq Na
1 g NaCl = 0.39 g Na = 17 mEq Na

1 mEq K = 39 mg K = 74.5 mg KCl
1 g K = 1.91 g KCl = 26 mEq K
1 g KCl = 0.52 g K = 13 mEq K

1 mEq Ca = 20 mg Ca
1 g Ca = 50 mEq Ca

1 mEq Mg = 0.12 g $MgSO_4 \cdot 7H_2O$
1 g Mg = 10.2 g $MgSO_4 \cdot 7H_2O$ = 82 mEq Mg

10 mmol P_i = 0.31 g P_i = 0.95 g PO_4
1 g P_i = 3.06 g PO_4 = 32 mmol P_i